Contents

List of contributors

Jangu E. Banatvala
MA MD FRCP FRCPath FMed Sci
Emeritus Professor of Clinical Virology, Guy's King's and St Thomas School of Medicine and Dentistry, St Thomas' Hospital, London, UK

Christine Baylis
PhD
Professor of Physiology, West Virginia University, Charlottesville, West Virginia 22903, USA

Martin M. Black
MD FRCP FRCPath
Chairman, Consultant Dermatologist, Department of Dermatopathology, Guy's, Kings and St Thomas' School of Medicine, St John's Institute of Dermatology, St Thomas' Hospital, London, UK

John Davison
BSc MD MSc FRCOG
Consultant Obstetrician and Gynecologist, Department of Obstetrics & Gynaecology, Royal Victoria Infirmary, Queen Victoria Road, Newcastle Upon Tyne, UK

James O. Donaldson
MD
Professor of Neurology, University of Connecticut School of Medicine, Farmington, Conneticut 06030-1845, USA

Elizabeth A. Fagan
MSc MD FRCPath FRCP FACP
Professor of Internal Medicine and Pediatrics, Sections of Hepatology and Pediatric Gastroenterology and Nutrition, Rush Presbyterian St Luke's Medical Center, Chicago, Illinois 60612, USA.

Joanna Girling
MA MRCP MRCOG
Consultant Obstetrician and Gynaecologist, West Middlesex Hospital, Twickenham Road, Isleworth, Middlesex, UK

Frank D. Johnstone
MD FRCOG
Senior Lecturer and Consultant, Obstetrics and Gynaecology, New Royal Infirmatory of Edinburgh, Edinburgh, UK

Elizabeth A. Letsky
MBBS FRCPath
Consultant Perinatal Haematologist, Queen Charlotte's & Chelsea Hospital, London, UK

Peter Liddle
BSc BMBCH PhD MRCPsych
Professor of Psychiatry, University of Nottingham, Queen's Medical Centre, Nottingham, UK

Laurent Mandelbrot
Professor of Obstetrics and Gynaecology, Hopital Louis Mourier, 178 rue des Renouillers, 92701 Colombes Cedex, France

Michael Maresh
MD FRCOG
Consultant Obstetrician, St Mary's Hospital for Women and Children, Whitworth Park, Hathersage Road, Manchester, UK

Marie-Louise Newell
MB PhD
Professor of Paediatric Epidemiology, Centre for Paediatric Epidemiology and Biostatistics, Institute of Child Health, University College, London, UK

Margaret R Oates
MB ChB DPM FRCPsych
Senior Lecturer in Psychiatry, University of Nottingham, Queen's Medical Centre, Nottingham, UK

Christopher W.G. Redman
FRCP
Professor of Obstetric Medicine, Nuffield Department of Obstetrics and Gynnaecology, John Radcliffe Hospital, Oxford, UK

G.L. Ridgway
MD BSc FRCP FRCPath
Consultant Microbiologist, Department of Clinical Microbiology, University College London Hospitals, Grafton Way, London, UK

Michael de Swiet
MD FRCP
Emeritus Professor of Obstetric Medicine, Faculty of Medicine, Imperial College, Consultant Physician, Queen Charlotihe's and Chelsta Hospital, London, UK

Samantha Vaughan Jones
MD FRCP
Consultant Dermatologist, Ashford and St Peter's Hospital NHS Trust, Guildford Road, Chertsey, Surrey, UK

Barry N.J. Walters
FRACP
Physician in Obstetric Medicine, Department of Obstetrics and Gyneacology, King Edward Memorial Hospital for Women, Perth, Western Australia 6000

Preface to the Fourth Edition

In this 4th edition of *Medical Disorders in Obstetric Practice* all the chapters have been revised and many have been extensively rewritten. I am most grateful to Miss Joanna Girling who has taken over and rewritten the chapter on thyroid disease (Chapter 12); also to Dr Geoff Ridgway and to Professor Jangu Banatvala who have split the former chapter on infectious diseases and written new chapters on bacteriological and viral disease respectively, emphasising the importance of infectious disease in modern obstetrics. Samantha Vaughan Jones has rewritten the chapter on skin disease. Margaret Oates has joined forces with Peter Liddle regarding psychiatry in pregnancy. Similarly, Laurent Mandelbrot and Marie-Louise Newell have joined Frank Johnstone to up-date the rapidly developing subject of HIV infection in pregnancy.

I am gratified by the success of *Medical Disorders in Obstetric Practice* and hope that the 4th edition will be a useful knowledge base for those continuing to practice and train in obstetric medicine. Anyone working in clinical obstetrics will recognise the subspecialty of obstetric medicine and the need for physicians and obstetricians who have special knowledge of the medical problems of pregnancy. This need is finally being recognised by those who have not responsibility for certification. I hope that in the not too distant future, perhaps even within the lifetime of this book, the Royal Colleges of Obstetricians and Gynaecologists, and Physicians will jointly sanction a training and certification process for obstetric medicine.

Acknowledgment

First and foremost, it is pleasure to acknowledge all the authors of this edition of Medical Disorder in Obstetric Practice who have been so generous of their time and so willing to write. I would also like to thank all those who have commented on previous editions and made invaluable suggestions regarding improvements. My thanks to Dr Stephen Wright who kindly checked the section on malaria (Chapter 16) and to Dr Ian Chrystie who supplied some of the figures for, and checked, Chapter 17. Finally, I would like to thank the staff at Blackwell Publishing for their help and expertise in editing and production.

Michael de Swiet
2002

Preface to the First Edition

This book has been produced to replace *Medical Disorders in Obstetric Practice* which was written by my predecessor, as Consultant Physician at Queen Charlotte's Maternity Hospital, Cyril Barnes. In many ways Cyril Barnes established the subspecialty of obstetric medicine in Great Britain. Some would argue that obstetric medicine is not a subspecialty at all; that the already established subspecialities, such as cardiology and haematology, embrace a sufficient body of knowledge to deal adequately with all medical complications of pregnancy. I disagree. The physiology of the pregnant woman is so altered, and the constraint of the welfare of the fetus is so important, that subspecialists who can oversee the two widely different fields of obstetrics and medicine are needed.

Barnes' text was a model of clarity, and a tribute to his considerable clinical experience. I hope that with this book, we have been able to continue in the tradition of my predecessor. In particular, I hope that the obstetrician who may not always have optimal medical support, will find practical answers to his medical problems here. In addition, this is now a multi-author book, and we have tried to include the latest advances in a very rapidly progressing subject.

M. De Swiet
1995

1 Diseases of the respiratory system

Michael de Swiet

Disorders of the lung severe enough to cause respiratory failure are rare in pregnancy [1] since the major causes, chronic bronchitis and emphysema, are more common in men, or in women past their childbearing years. Nevertheless, respiratory failure may occur in bronchial asthma, in cystic fibrosis in overwhelming infection, occasionally in connective tissue disorders and in neuromuscular problems such as Guillain–Barré syndrome or Charcot–Marie–Tooth disease [2]. The Report on Confidential Enquiries into Maternal Deaths in the UK recorded just seven deaths from such causes in 2.2 million maternities between 1994 and 1996 [3]. Respiratory failure may also be the cause of death in postanaesthetic complications but this is now becoming extremely rare.

Before considering these and other respiratory diseases in pregnancy, we should first review the physiological changes in the respiratory system that occur during pregnancy. For more detailed reviews of physiology see references [4–7].

Physiological adaptation to pregnancy

Oxygen consumption, P_{ao_2}, CO_2 production, P-50

During pregnancy oxygen consumption rises by about 45 mL/min [8,9]. Because oxygen consumption at rest is approximately 300 mL/min [10,11] the increase is about 18%. About one-third of the increased oxygen consumption is necessary for the metabolism of the fetus and placenta. The remainder is supplied for the extra metabolism of the mother, in particular the extra work of increased secretion and reabsorption by the kidney [5].

The majority of authors find little change in P_{ao_2} during pregnancy. The normal value is about 13.6 kPa (103 mmHg) at the end of pregnancy [12].

Those authors such as Lucius et al. [13] that have found a P_{ao_2} reduced to 11.3 kPa (85 mmHg) in pregnancy have usually not specified the position of their patients. P_{ao_2} may fall by up to 1.7 kPa (13 mmHg) on changing from the sitting to the supine position [14] probably due to a combination of haemodynamic alterations (e.g. reduction in cardiac output, Chapter 5) and changes in functional residual capacity and closing volume. These changes cause mismatching of ventilation and perfusion and subsequent hypoxaemia. Therefore arterial blood gas measurements should always be made in pregnancy in the sitting position if they are to be used for diagnostic purposes such as in suspected pulmonary embolism (see Chapter 4).

Although residence at extreme altitude is associated with decreased maternal P_{ao_2} and intrauterine growth restriction, modern aircraft are pressurized to about 2500 m (8200 ft) and at these pressures Huch et al. [15] found no evidence of ill-effects on mother or fetus in 10 pregnancies studied during commercial flights.

The increase in oxygen consumption is associated with a corresponding increase in CO_2 output. Because respiratory quotient increases from 0.76 before pregnancy to 0.83 in late pregnancy, the increase in CO_2 production is proportionately greater than the increase in oxygen uptake [10,16]. This effect is likely to be due to an increase in the proportion of carbohydrate to fat metabolized during pregnancy.

P-50, an inverse measure of affinity of haemoglobin for oxygen, is progressively increased from 26 mmHg in the non-pregnant state to 30 mmHg at term [17]. This represents a decrease in affinity induced by pregnancy and would allow easier 'unloading' of oxygen from maternal blood to fetal blood in the placenta.

Tidal volume

The increase in oxygen consumption is associated with a marked increase in ventilation of up to 40% in pregnancy. This increase in ventilation is achieved efficiently by increasing tidal volume from 500 to 700 mL [19] rather than by any increase in respiratory rate [11] (Fig. 1.1). It occurs early in pregnancy [20]. Effective alveolar ventilation is further increased by a reduction of 20% in residual volume—the volume of air in the lungs which remains at the end of expiration and with which the incoming air is diluted [8] (Fig. 1.2).

Ventilatory equivalent, $Paco_2$ and pH

The increase in ventilation of 40% compared to the increase in oxygen consumption of 20% causes a considerable

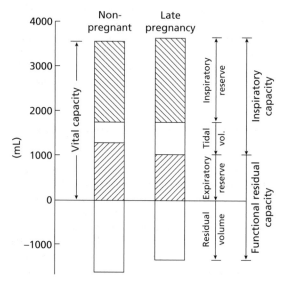

Fig 1.1 Subdivisions of lung volume and their alterations in pregnancy. (From [19].)

increase in ventilatory equivalent—the minute volume divided by oxygen consumption—which rises from 3.21/min/100 mL oxygen consumed to 4.01/min/100 mL oxygen consumed. Therefore, the $Paco_2$ falls in pregnancy from non-pregnant levels of 4.7–5.3 kPa (35–40 mmHg) to about 4 kPa (30 mmHg) [21]. Most authors (e.g. Milne [7]) find the $Paco_2$ falls early in pregnancy in parallel with the change in ventilation, but Lucius *et al.* [13] and Bouterline-Young and Bouterline-Young [22] found a progressive fall in $Paco_2$. The fall in $Paco_2$ is even greater at altitude where the mother is hyperventilating further in an attempt to maintain the Pao_2 as high as possible. Hellegers *et al.* [23] found a $Paco_2$ of 3.7 kPa (28 mmHg) at 4400 m, and Sobrevilla *et al.* [24] recorded a $Paco_2$ of 3.2 kPa (24 mmHg) at altitude.

The fall in $Paco_2$ is matched by an equivalent fall in plasma bicarbonate concentration and all the evidence suggests that arterial pH is not altered from normal non-pregnant levels of about 7.40.

The stimulus to hyperventilation

The increase in ventilation and associated fall in $Paco_2$ occurring in pregnancy is probably due to progesterone [25], which may act via a number of mechanisms. It lowers the threshold of the respiratory centre to CO_2 [26]. In addition, during pregnancy, the sensitivity of the respiratory centre increases [27] so that an increase in $Paco_2$ of 0.13 kPa (1 mmHg) increases ventilation by 5 L/min in pregnancy, compared to 1.5 L/min in the non-pregnant state [11,21,28]. It is also possible that progesterone acts as a primary stimulant to the respiratory centre independently of any change in CO_2 sensitivity or threshold [29]. Not only does progesterone stimulate ventilation, but it also increases the level of carbonic anhydrase B in the red cell [30,31]. An increase in carbonic anhydrase will facilitate CO_2 transfer, and also tend to decrease $Paco_2$ independently of any change in ventilation. The respiratory stimulant effect of progesterone has been used in the treatment of respiratory failure and emphysema with varying success [32–34]. A similar but smaller increase in ventilation is observed in the luteal phase of the menstrual cycle [35,36] and in patients taking some oral contraceptives [7].

Vital capacity

The vital capacity, the maximum volume of gas that can be expired after a maximum inspiration, probably does not change in pregnancy (Figs 1.1 & 1.2). Some have found that it increases [7,9], others have found that it decreases [21,37]; the majority have found no change [7,8,19]. Cugell *et al.* [19] found a transient fall in vital capacity in the puerper-

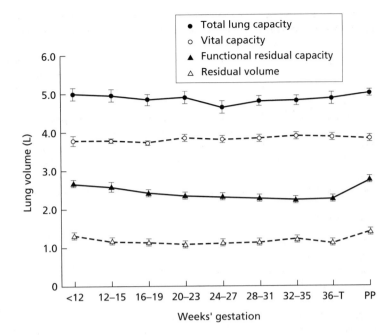

Total lung capacity

Fig 1.2 Serial values of static lung volume during normal pregnancy and after delivery. (Values are mean ± SEM.) (From [8].)

ium. As the authors themselves noted, it is likely that this was due to maternal discomfort from, for example, episiotomy sutures preventing full cooperation.

Anatomical changes

The findings of no change in vital capacity with a reduction in residual volume are in keeping with the observed changes in the configuration of the chest during pregnancy. The level of the diaphragm rises by about 4 cm early in pregnancy even before it is under pressure from the enlarging uterus. This would account for the decrease in residual volume because the lungs would be relatively compressed at forced expiration.

Airways resistance

The work performed in breathing may be partitioned into work done in overcoming the total airways resistance of the tracheobronchial tree—where the resistance of large airways (>2 mm in diameter) is much more important than small airways function [38]—and work done in expanding the lungs and chest wall, the compliance.

Measurements of forced expiratory volume in 1 s (FEV_1) and peak expiratory flow rate are indirect measurements that depend on both airways resistance and lung compliance. Neither measurement is affected by pregnancy [39], nor is airways conductance [20] nor lung compliance [40].

Bevan *et al.* [41] and Garrard *et al.* [42] found an increased closing volume in pregnancy with closure beginning during normal tidal volume in half their subjects. This would suggest that the calibre of small airways <2 mm in diameter decreases in pregnancy to the point where some airways close during respiration. However, others [43–45] have found no change in the point of airways closure during normal pregnancy, and Farebrother and McHardy [46] suggested that an increased closing volume was only a feature of complicated pregnancy. Certainly ventilation/perfusion imbalance occurs in severe pre-eclampsia [47]. More work is necessary in this field. If some airways do close during tidal breathing, this would lead to impairment of ventilation/perfusion ratio and a decreased efficiency of pulmonary gas exchange causing hypoxaemia.

Gas transfer (pulmonary diffusing capacity)

This factor is a measure of the ease with which carbon monoxide and therefore oxygen is transported across the pulmonary membrane. Some studies showed no change in transfer factor during pregnancy [48,49]. However, Milne *et al.* [50] showed a marked decrease in transfer factor early in pregnancy (Fig. 1.3). This could be related to the fall in haematocrit, but would be offset by the increase in cardiac output occurring early in pregnancy. A reduction in transfer factor would be one factor acting against the increase in ventilation to improve the efficiency of gas exchange in pregnancy.

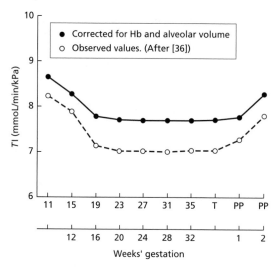

Fig 1.3 Change in pulmonary transfer factor during normal pregnancy and after delivery (PP).

In summary, the mother more than compensates for the increased oxygen consumption required by her and the fetus with a marked increase in tidal volume, leading to a considerable reduction in Pa_{CO_2}. This is driven by progesterone, and respiratory efficiency is augmented by the decrease in residual volume. These effects could be offset by an increase in closing volume and a decrease in transfer factor.

Exercise

The interactions between pregnancy and exercise are of particular relevance in view of current obsessions with physical fitness. However, the capacity for exercise in pregnancy has not been fully tested [51]. This is because weight-bearing exercise such as treadmill walking or step testing is heavily influenced by the change in weight associated with pregnancy. Sitting exercise (bicycle ergometry) should be less affected [52]. Also the capacity for maximum exercise depends on many other variables such as motivation, which may themselves be altered by pregnancy. One question of interest is whether in pregnancy exercise costs more or is performed less efficiently. Artal *et al.* [53] found on treadmill testing in late pregnancy, that women could not increase oxygen consumption to such an extent as in the non-pregnant state and that the ventilatory equivalent increased with higher grades of exercise, i.e. ventilation was less efficient at extreme exercise.

Nevertheless, short-term exercise does not appear to affect the normal fetus, at least as measured in terms of fetal cardiac function assessed by M-mode echocardiography [54]. Longer exercise lasting more than 20 min does increase fetal heart rate, although the mechanism is unknown [55]. Changes in uterine blood flow induced by maternal exercise may be compensated for by haemoconcentration (increasing oxygen carrying capacity) and increased oxygen extraction by the placenta [51]. In selected patients, participation in an exercise programme was associated with feeling good, improved American Paediatric Gross Assessment Record (APGAR) scores and a lower caesarean section rate [56]. The consensus view is that moderate exercise improves the pregnancy outcome in women with no contraindication such as hypertension [57].

Breathlessness in pregnancy

Breathlessness is a subjective symptom and the degree to which patients are aware of the profound changes in ventilation occurring in pregnancy as breathlessness varies enormously between patients and in the same patient in different pregnancies.

The degree of breathlessness felt by women in pregnancy has been documented by Thomson and Cohen [58], Cugell *et al.* [19] and Milne *et al.* [59]. Milne *et al.* found that about 50% of women were aware of breathlessness before 20 weeks' gestation. The maximum incidence of breathlessness at rest occurred between 28 and 31 weeks' gestation. However, the symptom of breathlessness cannot in general be correlated with any single parameter of respiratory function. Therefore, the reason for the maximum incidence of dyspnoea at 28–31 weeks' gestation remains unknown.

It is clearly important for the clinician to be aware that dyspnoea is a normal feature of pregnancy and does not necessarily represent cardiorespiratory disease. In the absence of any other symptoms of cardiorespiratory disease, normal findings on examination and a normal chest radiograph should be sufficient to exclude any serious pathology in the majority of women with breathlessness in pregnancy. Measurement of arterial blood gases and transfer factor should be reserved for those who are markedly breathless with particular relevance to pulmonary embolus and the possibility of diffuse infiltrative lung conditions, such as idiopathic pulmonary fibrosis.

One further test is to measure oxygen saturation transcutaneously and therefore non-invasively. The equipment to do this should now be widely available. The normal oxygen saturation is in excess of 95%. A fall in saturation on exercise, e.g. climbing stairs, indicates some form of cardiopulmonary disease and should be investigated further.

General comments on disorders of the respiratory system in pregnancy

Pregnancy stresses the respiratory system very little compared to its effect on the cardiovascular system. During pregnancy the minute ventilation increases by about 40% from 7.5 to 10.5 L/min and oxygen consumption increases by about 18% from about 250 to 300 mL/min. Yet, in exercise, minute ventilation can increase to 80 L/min [60], a 10-fold increase. Cardiac output also rises by approximately 40% from 4.5 to 6 L/min in pregnancy (see Chapter 5), but in contrast, the maximum cardiac output achieved in exercise is probably no greater than 12 L/min, a threefold increase. Thus, although cardiac output and minute ventilation both increase by an equal fraction in pregnancy, the increase in cardiac output represents a far greater proportion of the maximum that the woman can achieve, than does the increase in ventilation. Patients with respiratory disease are therefore less likely to deteriorate in pregnancy than those with cardiac disease because they have greater reserve.

Those chest diseases occurring frequently in pregnancy are described below. In addition, case reports suggest that fibrosing alveolitis may deteriorate in pregnancy [61] and that pulmonary fibrosis in association with systemic sclerosis is not affected [62].

Bronchial asthma

Asthma is a common condition affecting more than 3% of women in their childbearing years [63] and the prevalence may well be increasing [64]. For example in Halifax, Nova Scotia, the prevalence of asthma in pregnancy was 4.8% in 1991 and rose to 6.9% in 1993 [65].

More recently, Hernandez et al. [66] reported that 1% of 4529 pregnancies at Johns Hopkins Hospital were complicated by acute asthma: 0.15% had severe attacks requiring hospitalization. It is therefore the most common respiratory disorder complicating pregnancy. For other general reviews see [6,77].

The effect of pregnancy on asthma

Asthma is a very variable condition. Its severity depends on the patient's exposure to allergens and the presence of respiratory infection, both also dependent on the season of the year. In addition, the patient's emotional state is important. If sufficient patients are studied to allow for these influences, pregnancy has no consistent effect on asthma; an alternative viewpoint is that it is impossible to predict the effect of pregnancy on asthma [75].

For example, White et al. [78] found that pregnancy improved asthma, whereas Gordon et al. [79] found that pregnancy was associated with a deterioration in bronchial asthma. Turner et al. [71] reviewed 1054 cases reported in nine different publications: 48% showed no change in pregnancy, 29% improved and 23% deteriorated. Patients do not necessarily change in the same way during different pregnancies. Williams [80] found that 37% of 63 patients with asthma reacted differently in different pregnancies; this difference did not depend on the sex of the fetus [80]. In a prospective study, Juniper et al. [81] followed airways responsiveness and treatment requirement (amongst other variables) in 16 patients from before conception and showed that both improved in a significant majority during pregnancy. An intriguing study suggests that women pregnant with boys take less asthma medication than those carrying girls, possibly because of androgen production from the male fetus [82].

When we followed measurements of FEV_1, serially through pregnancy in 27 patients with asthma, we were unable to find any consistent changes during pregnancy, or between pregnancy and the non-pregnant state [39]; this is in keeping with studies in non-asthmatic patients reviewed above.

If pregnancy does not cause any net change in airways resistance either in normal subjects or in those with asthma, this is likely to be the sum of several factors acting in opposing directions. The bronchodilator influences are increased progesterone secretion [83], and increased free cortisol (see Chapter 13); the bronchoconstrictor influences are the reduced residual volume [84], reduced $Paco_2$ [85] and increased prostaglandin $F_{2\alpha}$ secretion [86]. Prostaglandin $F_{2\alpha}$ should therefore not be used in obstetric practice (therapeutic abortion, induction of labour) [86–90] unless there is a life-threatening emergency such as postpartum haemorrhage when it is injected directly into the uterus or occasionally intramuscularly. Prostaglandin E is used more widely and is the preferred prostaglandin for use in asthmatic patients, although there is some controversy as to whether it may be a bronchoconstrictor or a bronchodilator [91].

The most common cause for asthma to deteriorate in pregnancy is because the patient has reduced treatment either because of her own or her attendants' mistaken belief that such treatment will harm the fetus [92].

The effect of asthma on pregnancy

There has always been concern about a possible effect of asthma on the outcome of pregnancy. Large epidemiological studies do suggest increased risks of preterm delivery, low birthweight and congenital malformations with relative risks 1.3–2.2 compared to healthy controls [93–94]. However, these risks almost certainly relate to poor treatment, although the cause of the birth defects is not clear. There is also considerable variability between studies. For example Apter *et al.* [95] found no excess fetal morbidity in 21 adolescent patients with asthma even though these patients required aggressive treatment with multiple hospital admissions. By contrast it has been suggested that perinatal mortality is doubled in patients with asthma compared to controls, but this effect was largely confined to a black, presumably socially deprived, population [79]. In a study in Nova Scotia between 1991 and 1993 the only fetal problem shown in 871 women with asthma was a slight increase in hyperbilirubinaemia when compared to 13 709 non-asthmatics [65]. Other studies have shown no excess fetal risks when asthma specialists managed asthma in pregnancy and achieved good control of symptoms.

We found no statistically significant extra risk to the fetus if the mother suffered from asthma in pregnancy, although there was a tendency towards growth restriction, particularly amongst fetuses of mothers taking oral steroid therapy [39]. These patients were more severely affected by asthma, and may have been intermittently hypoxic. The relation between growth restriction and impaired respiratory function has been shown to be statistically significant in a group of 352 pregnant asthmatics [96]. Templeton [97] suggested that hypoxia was the cause of recurrent growth retardation that he noted in a patient with bronchiectasis. Alternatively, hyperventilation, which may be associated with acute attacks of asthma, often causes hypocapnia, and this also has been related to fetal hypoxia [98,99]. Animal data would suggest that maternal respiratory alkalosis also causes fetal hypoxia [100] and both respiratory alkalosis and hypocapnia may act via a reduction in maternal placental perfusion [98,101].

In summary, there is a slight increased risk to the fetus of the mother with asthma, but this effect is very small, and should not be exaggerated when counselling individual patients.

Management of asthma in pregnancy [102]

Pregnancy is a time when patients see their doctors frequently. This is a good opportunity to optimize the therapy of asthma, ideally in a combined medical or respiratory and obstetric clinic.

The diagnosis of bronchial asthma is made on the basis of the history of recurrent episodes of wheeze and breathlessness, often associated with trigger factors such as exposure to allergens (dust, pollen), infection and exacerbated by psychological factors. An arbitrary definition is a variation in peak expiratory flow rate or $FEV_1 > 20\%$, either spontaneously or as a result of treatment. Some patients may present with a history of cough only. Patients with attacks only at night or on exercise may have a primary cardiac cause rather than bronchial asthma, but these women usually have other signs of heart disease, or cardiomegaly on the chest radiograph. Inexpensive peak expiratory flow meters can be used at home to record peak flows throughout the day on diary cards. In patients with asthma these records show characteristic dips in peak flow at night or during the early morning.

Respiratory function may deteriorate before the patient is aware of it [103]. Home peak flow monitoring allows the patient to increase treatment (usually with inhaled or oral glucocorticoids) before her symptoms deteriorate.

In addition, pulmonary embolus may also rarely present as bronchospasm [104] and this should be remembered as a possibility in patients who have their first attack of severe 'asthma' in pregnancy [105] (see Chapter 4).

GENERAL MEASURES

Asthma is by definition a variable condition, which inevitably affects the patient's emotions. Also emotional upsets to which patients are particularly susceptible in pregnancy adversely affect asthma. It is therefore particularly important for obstetricians and physicians to foster a trusting relationship. In general all first-line drugs currently used for the treatment of asthma should be considered safe in pregnancy [106]. All authorities agree that the danger to the fetus from undertreated maternal asthma is far greater than any theoretical risk from the drugs themselves [92].

As in the non-pregnant state barbiturates and other sedative drugs should not be used because of the risk of respiratory depression; even diazepam is unsafe. Anxiety is much better treated by relief of symptoms with effective therapy. If the patient has any evidence of chest infection, as indicated by purulent sputum, this should be treated with an appropriate antibiotic (see below). However, eosinophilia may cause yellow sputum, which looks purulent. Chest infection is probably overdiagnosed as a cause of exacerbation of asthma, and such exacerbation should always be managed with an increase in bronchodilator therapy. In addition, it should be remembered that expectorants containing iodine should not be used in pregnancy, because the iodine may block thyroxine synthesis in the fetus making it hypothyroid or giving it a goitre [107,108]. Because iodine is preferentially excreted in breast milk [109], mothers who are breastfeeding should also not use iodine-containing expectorants or cough medicine.

Those clinicians who use desensitization in the treatment of asthma [110] or penicillin allergy [111] have not found any problems specific to pregnancy [110], although the risk of desensitization (i.e. anaphylaxis) remains.

Current recommendations for the treatment of asthma indicate a stepped care approach [112] and this should also be the policy in pregnancy. The stepped care scheme is outlined below. Comments on individual drugs and classes of drugs follow. Most treatment is now given by inhaler; it is very important to ensure that the patient uses the correct technique, particularly if the response to therapy seems suboptimal.

Step 1: occasional attacks of bronchospasm may be relieved by treatment with inhaled β-sympathomimetic drugs such as salbutamol 1–2 puffs (100–200 μg). If this is being used more than once per day:

Step 2: add a preventing drug, i.e. inhaled glucocorticoid, e.g. beclomethasone 100–400 μg twice daily. Alternatively add inhaled cromoglycate but this is increasingly less popular and in any case inhaled steroids should be used if the cromoglycate is not working.

Step 3: add high-dose inhaled steroid or long-acting inhaled β-sympathomimetic drug, i.e. inhaled short-acting β-sympathomimetic as required plus beclomethasone 800–2000 μg daily in divided doses. Alternatively, inhaled short acting μ-sympathomimetic plus beclomethasone 100–400 μg twice daily plus inhaled salmeterol 50 μg twice daily.

Step 4: inhaled high-dose steroid plus regular inhaled bronchodilator. The regular bronchodilator may be inhaled β-sympathomimetic or ipratropium, or theophylline tablets.

Step 5: add regular oral prednisolone to Step 4.

If there is any difficulty in controlling asthma the patient should be admitted to hospital, particularly in pregnancy. Status asthmaticus is difficult to define and has been renamed acute severe asthma, but deteriorating asthma that fails to respond promptly to regular medication is a life-threatening condition [38], which has been shown to be particularly dangerous in pregnancy [79]. It is likely that this is because the condition is managed initially by those with an obstetric orientation. It is notoriously easy to underestimate the severity of attacks of asthma [113]. Therefore all patients with acute severe asthma in pregnancy should be managed in cooperation with a physician interested in respiratory disease, preferably in an intensive care unit. Ominous signs include a heart rate >110/min, respiratory rate >25/min, pulsus paradoxus of >18–20 mmHg, and peak expiratory flow <200 L/min or less than 50% predicted [112]; also dyspnoea, accessory muscle use and wheeze [114]. Be very worried about patients who cannot complete sentences in one breath!

The patient should be monitored with regular measurements of peak flow rate and pulse oximetry to estimate oxygen saturation. Blood gas measurement can be reserved for those with saturation <92% or with life-threatening attacks. If this is done, there is no need for controlled oxygen therapy, and the patient can have oxygen, 40–60%, given via a facemask. Because of the maternal risk, the patient should be managed as if she were not pregnant, giving optimal therapy for the respiratory condition. This should be salbutamol 5 mg or terbutaline 10 mg given via an oxygen-driven nebulizer and prednisolone tablets 60 mg, hydrocortisone 200 mg i.v. or both. Life-threatening features require addition of nebulized ipratropium and/or intravenous aminophylline or salbutamol. In the future intravenous magnesium may be recommended as a bronchodilator. This should appeal to obstetricians, granted their experience with the use of magnesium for the treatment and prophylaxis of eclampsia (see Chapter 6)

A chest radiograph must always be taken to exclude pneumothorax. As outlined below, treatment with steroids, β-sympathomimetics or theophyllines is unlikely to affect the fetus. Indeed it has been shown that acute attacks of asthma if promptly treated do no affect fetal outcome [115]. The only drug that should not be used is tetracycline (see below), but fortunately there are other, better, broad-spectrum antibiotics available. Despite this, antibiotics should only be given if there is clear evidence of infection.

Ventilation is rarely necessary but should the patient require it, either because of exhaustion or rising $Paco_2$, it is clear that maternal $Paco_2$ should be maintained at as near physiological levels as possible; indeed, this is the usual purpose of ventilation. As noted previously, Wulf *et al.* [99] showed that as maternal Po_2 fell from 12.1 to 6.3 kPa (91–47 mmHg), fetal umbilical vein Po_2 fell from 4.3 to 3.6 kPa (32–27 mmHg). However, hypocapnia (Pco_2 2.3 kPa, 17 mmHg) and alkalosis (pH >7.6) should also be avoided, because these are associated with reduced fetal oxygenation, probably due to impaired placental transport [71,99]. If all therapy fails to improve the patient with acute severe asthma, termination of pregnancy may be life saving [116,117].

β-sympathomimetic drugs (isoprenaline, salbutamol, terbutaline, fenoterol)

An inhaled β-sympathomimetic is the first drug to use in treating patients who have occasional attacks of bronchospasm. It may be used prophylactically if the patient is particularly at risk, for example, from exercise-induced asthma. Although most of the β-sympathomimetics such as salbutamol, terbutaline and fenoterol that are used for the treatment of asthma are relatively selective, stimulating β_2 rather than β_1 receptors, the dosage given is still limited by cardiac side-effects of tachycardia and irregularities of heart rhythm. In addition, patients may notice tremor and a feeling of anxiety or apprehension. These effects are more marked with non-selective β-sympathomimetic drugs such as isoprenaline, which should not be used. There is little to choose between one selective β-sympathomimetic drug and another. My own preference is to use salbutamol, which has been widely studied in pregnant and non-pregnant patients, and to avoid fenoterol, which may be less selective and is possibly marketed at too high a dose [118].

There is considerable experience of the use of sympathomimetic agents in pregnancy, not only for the treatment of asthma, but also for preterm labour [119]. There is no evidence of teratogenicity and ephedrine in particular has been shown to be safe [120]. However, in the case of adrenaline (epinephrine) when given in the first 4 months of pregnancy there was a small non-specific increased risk of teratogenicity (minor eye and ear abnormalities) found by the Perinatal Collaborative Project [120]; but it is possible that the acute condition for which adrenaline was given, rather than the drug itself, was the cause of the malformations.

The most worrying side-effects in pregnancy are pulmonary oedema and metabolic acidosis [121]. High-dose intravenous therapy is much more likely to cause side-effects in patients receiving β-sympathomimetics for preterm labour, rather than in the treatment of asthma where intravenous sympathomimetic drugs have only been used in the treatment of acute severe asthma and where more patients receive inhaled β-sympathomimetics.

Because β-sympathomimetics are used in the treatment of preterm labour, their use for asthma might be expected to delay the onset or impede the progress of normal labour. The fact that this does not occur [39] is perhaps not surprising in view of doubts about their efficacy in preterm labour [122].

The newer, long-acting inhaled β₂ agonists such as salmeterol have proved to be effective and popular [123]. They can be used as an adjuvant to limit the amount of inhaled steroid [124] or to avoid the use of systemic steroids. Because very little inhaled salmeterol enters the maternal blood, it is unlikely that the fetus will be affected and there have not been any adverse reports in pregnancy.

Theophyllines

Aminophylline has been widely used and is safe in pregnancy [125]. However, theophylline has been replaced by inhaled β agonists and inhaled steroids for most patients. Therefore theophylline appears relatively late and only as an alternative in the stepped care plan of the British Thoracic Society Guidelines for Asthma Management [112]. The indications for theophylline use are likely to be failure of inhaled glucocorticoids or inability to use an inhaler. It is

available as a soluble preparation, a slow-release preparation or as rectal suppositories in varying dosages. The oral dose is up to 10 mg/kg/day. The slow-release preparation acts for up to 12 h and should therefore be used in preference to suppositories for the control of nocturnal and early morning asthma [126]. Theophylline is also available as an elixir, which is rapidly absorbed, giving therapeutic blood levels at 15 min [127]. Optimal treatment, particularly in acute severe asthma, is achieved by maintaining blood levels between 5 and 20 mg/mL [73,128]. The recommended infusion rate to achieve this in non-pregnant subjects is 0.7 mg/kg/h for the first 12 h after a 6 mg/kg bolus, followed by 0.5 mg/kg/h thereafter. Earlier reports [129] suggested that theophylline pharmacokinetics do not change during pregnancy and the above regimen could therefore be recommended for the pregnant state [130]. However, it may need to be modified according to the theophylline blood level particularly since a more recent study [131] suggests that clearance is increased in pregnancy (Fig. 1.4). In any case, blood levels should always be checked in acute severe asthma. Aminophylline may cause nausea and also causes tachydysrhythmias, especially when given intravenously. The bolus dose should therefore be given slowly. Because aminophylline is also a pulmonary vasodilator, the patient should be receiving oxygen during intravenous administration to avoid hypoxaemia.

Aminophylline is assumed to cross the placenta [73] and is excreted in breast milk in small quantities [132] but this has not been shown to cause any long-term harm to the fetus [133]. The safety of theophyllines in pregnancy is also suggested by a study in which aminophylline was given to women at risk of preterm delivery. Therapy was associated with decreases in the incidence

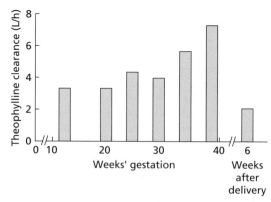

Fig 1.4 Theophylline clearance calculated from steady-state concentrations in a pregnant woman with asthma. Having been controlled before pregnancy on 250 mg every 12 h, by the end of pregnancy this patient had subtherapeutic concentrations despite receiving 1500 mg/day. (From [131].)

of neonatal respiratory distress syndrome and perinatal mortality. There were no adverse side-effects [134]. Stenius-Aarniala *et al.* [135] in a study of more than 500 women comparing those who had taken aminophylline in pregnancy with those who had not, found no adverse effects concerning the outcome of pregnancy, except a slight increase in jaundice in the treated group. However, there are reports [136,137] of three newborn infants who showed theophylline toxicity (jitteriness, tachycardia, opisthotonos) after the mother had been given theophylline or aminophylline in late pregnancy. There were no long-term sequelae in any of these infants.

Disodium cromoglycate

Disodium cromoglycate is inhaled from a Spinhaler or as a conventional aerosol but the aerosols only deliver a small dose. It is used as a prophylactic to prevent the occurrence of asthma attacks. It appears to be safe for the fetus [72,138]. Because the drug is taken by inhalation the quantity entering the blood (8%) is very small [138] and so little is transferred to the fetus. It occasionally causes bronchospasm at the time of inhalation and this can be avoided by using a combination preparation of disodium cromoglycate and isoprenaline.

Anticholinergic drugs, such as atropine or more recently ipratropium bromide given by aerosol, are also used in the prophylaxis of asthma [139]. Atropine has not been associated with any increased risk of teratogenesis [120], and fetal tachycardia is the only likely fetal side-effect.

Steroids

There is considerable debate concerning the use of steroids in pregnancy. Inhaled steroid therapy, e.g. beclomethasone, represents a considerable advance, because it permits the reduction or omission of oral therapy with prednisone. In one study only 4% of 257 women taking inhaled steroids at the beginning of pregnancy had an acute attack of asthma during pregnancy by comparison with 17% of women who were not taking steroids at the beginning of pregnancy [115]. Inhaled steroids given after an acute attack requiring hospital admission in pregnancy halve the subsequent remission rate [140].

Inhaled steroids act locally on the bronchi and are not absorbed except at high dosage, e.g. more than 1 mg/day (20 × 50 μg puffs) of Becotide [141]. Inhaled beclometasone has been used widely in pregnancy [125] and its safety is established [125] Preliminary data suggest that inhaled triamcinolone is similar in efficacy and safety to beclometasone in pregnancy [142]. The side-effects that occur with long-term use are monilial infections of the upper respiratory and gastrointestinal tracts, but these are not a specific risk of pregnancy and only a problem in 5% of users. If patients are changed from *chronic* oral to inhaled steroid therapy, the dosage of oral steroid therapy should be reduced very slowly—no more rapidly than 1 mg reduction of prednisone per day every 4 weeks, if the dosage of prednisone is <10 mg/day. More rapid reduction has been associated with Addisonian collapse, a flare-up of other atopic manifestations such as allergic rhinitis, or just lethargy and non-specific malaise.

If patients require oral corticosteroid therapy for asthma, this should not be withheld because they are pregnant. Corticosteroids are said to cause cleft palate [143] but this risk appears to be confined to the rabbit [144]. The controversy has recently been reopened by a case–controlled study suggesting an odds ratio of 6.55 (confidence interval 1.44–29.76) for oral clefts in patients taking corticosteroids [145]. However, as suggested by the wide confidence intervals, the numbers involved in this study were small: amongst 1184 patients with oral clefts five came from women taking corticosteroids in early pregnancy. In a similar number of matched controls only one mother took corticosteroids in early pregnancy. But of the five mothers taking corticosteroids, one was taking triamcinolone, a fluorinated corticosteroid very rarely used as oral therapy, and another was taking hydrocortisone in physiological replacement doses, i.e. a replacement of a natural hormone that is unlikely to be teratogenic. If these patients were to be omitted, the study, already suspect because of its small size, would not show statistically significant results. Furthermore Schatz *et al.* [146] did not find any excess of congenital malformations in 70 pregnancies complicated by asthma, treated with corticosteroids (average daily dose of prednisone, 8 mg) and this has been confirmed in other clinical studies [120,147,148] and reviewed by Turner *et al.* [71].

Steroid therapy will depress maternal adrenal activity. This can lead to a reduction in the adrenal and urinary secretion of oestriol if the dose is more than 30 mg of prednisone a day [149–151]. The effect, which is important if oestriol levels are used as an index of fetal well-being, may occur at dosages below 30 mg prednisone per day, but this has not been documented. In any case the urinary secretion of oestriol is now rarely used as an index of fetal well-being. However, note that serum oestriol measurements are a component of some schemes using biochemical markers to screen for Down's syndrome

There is always concern that the hypothalamo-pituitary–adrenal axis of the fetus may be suppressed by maternal steroid therapy [152]; this would make the infant liable to collapse in the neonatal period. In practice this does not occur with prednisone, perhaps because little of this drug crosses the placenta. The maternal–fetal concentration of prednisone is 10 : 1 [153], in comparison to hydrocortisone 6 : 1 and beclometasone 3 : 1 [154]. Also the fetoplacental unit is relatively lacking in the enzymes to convert prednisone to its active metabolite prednisolone [154], and placental 11, β-ol-dehydrogenase is very efficient, deactivating 87% of an injected dose of prednisone [155]. Nevertheless, perhaps 15% of maternal hydrocortisone does cross the placenta and could account for 30–50% of fetal cortisol levels [156]: as always corticosteroids should not be used unless there is a good reason. As indicated above, other glucocorticoids do cross the placenta and indeed have been given to the mother for treatment of the fetus, e.g. the use of beclometasone to 'mature' the preterm fetal lung and dexamethasone to suppress the fetal adrenal gland in congenital adrenal hyperplasia (see Chapter 13). Studies that have assessed the fetal benefits of beclometasone given to mature the fetal lung, i.e. given specifically to affect the fetus, are also encouraging in terms of long-term psychological [157] and physical [158] development in the child; however, there is a suggestion that such children are at increased risk of infection in later life.

Leukotriene antagonists

There is insufficient experience to recommend the use of leukotriene antagonists such as montelukast or zafirlukast in pregnancy.

THE MANAGEMENT OF LABOUR

It is unusual for labour to be complicated by attacks of asthma. Perhaps this is because of an even greater secretion of glucocorticoids from the adrenal cortex [159] and possibly also catecholamines from the adrenal medulla. Increased prostaglandin secretion during labour may also cause bronchodilatation. For attacks of asthma that do occur in labour, conventional treatment with inhaled β-sympathomimetics should be used first, with earlier recourse to parenteral steroid therapy if the patient does not improve rapidly.

Patients who have taken glucocorticoids equivalent to more than 5 mg prednisone daily (or very high dose of inhaled steroids, e.g. beclometasone 1.5 mg/day) within the preceding 3 months are at risk of Addisonian collapse during labour because of adrenal suppression. Nevertheless, Addisonian collapse in labour is very rare. Those taking high-dose steroids, i.e. prednisone 40 mg daily, should receive hydrocortisone 50 mg i.v. or i.m. 8 hourly for 72 h; this can be reduced to 25 mg 8 hourly for 48 h in those taking a low dose such as prednisone 5 mg daily.

Oral steroids can be substituted once the patient is eating with confidence.

Except for cases of severe postpartum haemorrhage, prostaglandin $F_{2\alpha}$ should not be used because of its bronchoconstrictor action (see above); also syntocinon should be used rather than ergometrine because of concern that the latter may cause bronchospasm in patients with asthma [160,161].

ANAESTHESIA AND ANALGESIA

Epidural anaesthesia is preferable to general anaesthesia [162] because of the risk of atelectasis and subsequent chest infection following the latter. If a general anaesthetic cannot be avoided, halothane should be considered because of its bronchodilating properties. Nebulized salbutamol can be given pre- and postoperatively. Opiates such as pethidine are best avoided because they cause bronchoconstriction and respiratory depression; but these remain relative rather than absolute contraindications and it would not be correct to deny a patient with asthma any effective analgesia at all, if epidural anaesthesia were not available.

BREASTFEEDING

Breastfeeding should be encouraged [163]. There is some evidence that women with asthma in particular should breastfeed because it may confer protection from food allergy in atopic individuals [163]. A recent study from Western Australia indicated that exclusive breastfeeding up to 4 months of age decreased the risks of asthma and other atopic manifestations by about 20% [164].

Turner *et al.* [71] have reviewed the secretion of drugs used in the treatment of asthma in breast milk. None of these drugs, including steroids, is likely to be secreted in sufficient quantities to harm the neonate, except tetracycline and iodides. In general, patients with asthma should therefore breastfeed their infants.

GENETIC COUNSELLING

The overall risk of any child having asthma is about 4%. If one parent has asthma, the risk that the child will have asthma increases to 8–16%, depending on whether the parent is also atopic. If both parents have asthma, and are also atopic, the risk may be as high as 30% [165]. However, evidence is increasing that maternal factors are particularly important for the development of atopic illness in the child [166] and current recommendations include the avoidance during pregnancy and lactation of potential allergens such as peanuts, which might cross the placenta or be secreted in breast milk. Alternatively maternal IgE may enter amniotic fluid and be swallowed thus transmitting allergy to the fetus [167,168]. Further work is necessary in this area [168].

In conclusion, asthma is a common condition affecting many women who are pregnant. It is not usually a problem in pregnancy, either to the mother or the fetus. The major difficulties lie in realizing that the majority of drugs used in the treatment of pregnancy do not harm the fetus, and in maintaining the treatment of a potentially life-threatening illness despite the mother's pregnancy.

Allergic rhinitis

The symptoms of allergic rhinitis are often worse in pregnancy. This is because the nasal mucosa shares in the generalized vasodilatation of pregnancy so the nasal passages become more congested. Treatment should be with intranasal preparations of beclometasone and cromoglycate [169]. Based on the experience of use of similar preparations in asthma (see above) there should be no concern about adverse affects of these drugs on the fetus. First-generation antihistamines such as chlopheniramine are also considered safe in pregnancy.

Churg–Strauss syndrome

Churg–Strauss syndrome is a rare allergic granulomatosis characterized by asthma, allergic rhinitis and systemic vasculitis. Although single-case reports suggest that Churg–Strauss syndrome improves in pregnancy [170], it may also become more obvious in pregnancy because of the inadvertent withdrawal of steroid therapy [171].

Tuberculosis

Pulmonary tuberculosis is now a rare complication of pregnancy in the general population of the UK, although some subgroups such as the Gujurati Indians and those with human immunodeficiency virus (HIV) infection (see Chapter 18) have an incidence that is up to 100 times greater than the national figure. At Queen Charlotte's Hospital, London, we see up to three cases every year, delivering approximately 4500 patients per year. For this reason we and others [172–176] do not routinely perform chest radiographs in pregnancy, despite contrary recommendations [176a]. In our population, routine chest radiographs are not worth the financial cost, or the very minimal extra risk to the fetus of irradiating the mother.

Even in a population with 16 times the national average incidence of tuberculosis, a screening programme in 1983 based on skin testing followed up by chest radiograph in positive cases did not detect any cases in pregnancy that were not detected by clinical criteria (fever, cough or weight loss) [176]. When this study was repeated in 1994 [177, 178], recent immigrant status was the only positive predictor for a positive skin test. Nevertheless, there should be no hesitation in performing chest radiographs if there is any clinical indication. Also there should be a very high index of suspicion for tuberculosis in pregnant or puerperal women with unexplained cough and sputum: tuberculosis can spread very extensively among such patients [178] and active tuberculosis is probably more likely to be asymptomatic in pregnancy [179].

Before antituberculous drugs were available, the results of pregnancy complicated by tuberculosis were poor for both mother and fetus [180]; there was a particular tendency for patients to deteriorate in the puerperium [181,182]. However, Selikoff and Dormann [183] reported that pregnancy did not affect the 15–30% of patients with untreated active tuberculosis, who deteriorated in the first 30 months after diagnosis. De March [184] was unable to find any deleterious effect of pregnancy in 100 patients with tuberculosis who had been pregnant, compared with 108 patients with pulmonary tuberculosis who had not been pregnant. These findings have been confirmed in a group of women with HIV infection who became pregnant [185], i.e. although HIV predisposes to tuberculosis, pregnancy does not make the situation any worse.

There is also no conclusive evidence that the outcome of pregnancy is adversely affected by tuberculosis [186–188] providing treatment is instituted in the first half of pregnancy. However, Bjerkedal et al. [188] did notice an increased risk of abortion to 20 in 1000 patients with tuberculosis compared to two in 1000 controls. But two in 1000 is a very low incidence of abortion for the controls, and these data should therefore be questioned. There is certainly no longer any justification for therapeutic abortion in maternal tuberculosis either for the sake of maternal health or because the fetus would otherwise be at such risk. Tuberculosis only very rarely affects the fetus by transplacental passage. A recent review cited only 29 cases in the English literature since 1980. But if the mother has open tuberculosis, the neonate is also at risk from infection after delivery.

The criteria for congenital tuberculosis are:
1 the disease must be bacteriologically proven;
2 there must be a primary complex in the fetal or neonatal liver;
3 disease must appear early in the first days of life;
4 extrauterine infection must be excluded [189].

Infection may occur via the fetus swallowing infected amniotic fluid, or be blood-borne via the umbilical vein. If the diagnosis is made early, for which a high index of clinical suspicion is necessary, the outlook for the neonate is good. The mother may have a tuberculous infection of any severity from subclinical to miliary [190]. Postnatal transfer of tuberculosis from mother to neonate is discussed below.

In pregnancy, pulmonary tuberculosis may present because of symptoms—cough, purulent sputum, haemoptysis, fever, weight loss, chest pain (tuberculous pleural effusion)—or as an incidental finding when a chest radiograph is taken for a different reason. The diagnosis is based on the chest radiograph appearance, sputum culture and examination of the pleural effusion, pleural biopsy, liver biopsy or by bone-marrow aspiration. Up to 10% of patients with early culture-positive tuberculosis will have normal chest radiographs [191]. A significant number will be smear negative, i.e. the organism will only be demonstrated in culture [192]. The Mantoux test will become positive within 4–12 weeks after the initial infection. It is disputed whether Mantoux status is affected by pregnancy itself [193-195].

The problem in managing a pregnant patient with tuberculosis is not her potential respiratory impairment, but the possible effects on the fetus of the chemotherapeutic drugs used. This subject has recently been extensively reviewed by Snider *et al.* [190,196]. Overall, their findings were very encouraging, because 94% of all pregnancies resulted in the delivery of apparently normal infants, and only 3% of the infants exposed *in utero* were classified as having birth defects [190]. Before starting chemotherapy for tuberculosis, the obstetrician and/or general physician should consult a chest physician; since the general decline of tuberculosis in the community, chest physicians are the only specialists with sufficient experience of the varying regimens that are used.

The drugs for which there is considerable information are ethambutol, isoniazid, streptomycin and rifampicin. In addition, it is believed that ethionamide is teratogenic [197].

Ethambutol has replaced *para*-aminosalicylic acid (PAS) as a 'front-line' antituberculous drug, because it is so much easier for the patient to take, although ethambutol has in term been replaced by pyrazinamide for non-pregnant and most pregnant patients. Although ethambutol may cause retrobulbar neuritis in adults in high doses [198], there is no evidence from abortion specimens [199] or the neonate [200] that the fetus is affected. Snider *et al.* [190] found only 14 infants or fetuses with abnormalities in 655 pregnancies treated with ethambutol and none had optic nerve abnormalities. The drug must therefore be considered safe in pregnancy.

The same is true of isoniazid. There have been 16 abnormal fetuses reported in a total of 1480 pregnancies [190]. This abnormality rate is lower than in the normal hospital population. Monnet *et al.* [201] noted that four of five abnormal fetuses in their series of 125 patients treated with isoniazid, had central nervous system (CNS) abnormalities. Because isoniazid is known to cause peripheral neuritis, this is the potential difficulty in the use of isoniazid in pregnancy, but it must be emphasized that the high incidence of CNS abnormalities was only seen in one group of patients, all of whom had also received ethionamide [201]. In addition, the Collaborative Drug Project [120] found a small (twice excess) non-specific increase of congenital abnormalities in patients taking isoniazid. Because of the possible higher requirement of pyridoxine in pregnancy, all patients taking isoniazid in pregnancy should also take pyridoxine 50 mg/day [202] to reduce the risk of peripheral neuritis [203], although note the possibility of neonatal seizures due to withdrawal of maternal pyridoxine therapy [204]. Hepatitis is a recognized complication of isoniazid therapy, which seems to be more common in pregnancy and the puerperium [205]. Patients receiving isoniazid in pregnancy should have their liver function checked at baseline and monthly. If isoniazid is to be introduced as preventative therapy this should be delayed until 3 months after delivery [206].

The greatest worries concern the use of streptomycin, rifampicin and pyrazinamide. Although at one time it was considered that streptomycin was relatively innocuous in pregnancy [207], this cannot be the current opinion. Conway and Birt [207] found no disabled children from 17 patients in whom the mother had been treated with streptomycin in pregnancy, but eight children had abnormal caloric tests and/or abnormal audiograms. Severe hearing loss was reported by Robinson and Cambon [208]. Snider *et al.* [190] found 34 cases of eighth nerve damage amongst the reports of 206 patients treated with streptomycin. This incidence of over 10% appears excessive. Furthermore, the risk of eighth nerve damage will persist after the period of organogenesis, throughout gestation.

Initial concern about the teratogenic potential of rifampicin [190] has not been confirmed and this preparation is now recommended for use in pregnancy [209]. There is one curious report of a nearly fivefold increase in the risk of deep vein thrombosis in patients treated with rifampicin for tuberculosis but this study was not performed in pregnant patients.

Pyrazinamide is used in antituberculous regimens because it rapidly renders the sputum negative for acid-fast bacilli and because 6 month rather than 9 month treatment periods are effective [210]. Although there are few data about the safety of pyrazinamide in early pregnancy it has been used quite extensively in pregnancy without adverse effects [206] and there should certainly be no concern about using the drug after organogenesis is complete. It is probably safe even earlier in pregnancy.

In summary, the patient presenting with tuberculosis in the first trimester of pregnancy should be treated with isoniazid, ethambutol and rifampicin in standard doses. After organogenesis is complete at 14 weeks' gestation it is safe to use pyrazinamide and some would use it earlier. It may be necessary to admit the patient to establish the diagnosis, in which case she should be in a single room rather than have strict barrier nursing. The patient should also be in a single room when she is admitted for labour. However, now that antituberculous therapy is so effective, the majority of treatment can be given as an outpatient. Nine months' treatment with isoniazid and rifampicin is considered sufficient for pulmonary tuberculosis or 6 months' treatment if the regimen has included pyrazinamide.

Extrapulmonary tuberculosis is very rare in pregnancy because one of its principal manifestations, genital tract tuberculosis, is associated with infertility. Extrapulmonary tuberculosis confined to the lymph nodes has no effect on pregnancy outcome, but tuberculosis at other sites is associated with higher rates of hospitalization, and with low-birthweight infants that have poorer APGAR scores [211]. Brooks and Stirrat [212] have reported a case of tuberculous peritonitis in pregnancy with a temporary Addisonian state, which responded excellently to conventional antituberculous therapy. There are isolated reports of colonic tuberculosis [213] and pericardial disease [214] in pregnancy. Figueroa and Arredondo [215] have described the pregnancies of 12 women with renal and other extrapulmonary tuberculosis. Tuberculous meningitis was a frequent terminal manifestation of women with tuberculosis in pregnancy [216,217] but is now very uncommon.

After birth, babies should only be isolated from their mothers if the mothers are still smear positive. Because modern antituberculous regimens render the sputum sterile within 2 weeks and markedly reduce the number of organisms with 24 h, this should not occur frequently. The neonate should be treated with prophylactic isoniazid for 3 months. After this period BCG vaccination is given in the UK although not in the USA [218]. It is not clear whether neonatal BCG vaccination adds any further protection to isoniazid prophylaxis. It is not without risks: skin ulceration, osteitis and occasionally disseminated disease, particularly if the mother has an immunodeficiency state such as acquired immune deficiency syndrome (AIDS). As isoniazid therapy does not affect the immunogenicity of BCG vaccine, there is no longer any rationale for the use of isoniazid-resistant BCG neonatal vaccination [218]. Mothers taking antituberculous therapy should be encouraged to breastfeed since the infant will receive a maximum of 20% of the normal infant dose by this route [219].

Sarcoidosis

Although sarcoid is most common in women aged 20–40 years, pulmonary sarcoid is rarely reported as a complication of pregnancy—perhaps 0.05% of all pregnancies are affected by the condition [220]. Also, there have been few cases reported where there was any marked symptomatic impairment in respiratory function [220–222]. Nevertheless, specialist referral centres have experience of large numbers of patients with sarcoid in pregnancy [223]. The consensus of opinion is that sarcoidosis either does not change in pregnancy [224] or if it changes, improves, perhaps due to the increase in free as well as total cortisol (see Chapter 13); however, there is a tendency for the condition to relapse in the puerperium [72]. Nevertheless, the relapse is unlikely to be serious and should not be a contraindication to pregnancy, except in the rare patient who is severely affected. Apart from pulmonary complications of sarcoid, patients may occasionally have life-threatening heart, renal and neurological disease. Other risk factors are parenchymal lesions on chest radiograph, increasing maternal age and requirement for drugs other than steroids [221].

The usual presentation is with symmetrical bilateral hilar lymphadenopathy and mediastinal lymphadenopathy found on chest radiograph either by chance or in a patient with pyrexia or erythema nodosum. The patient may also have cervical lymphadenopathy. The differential diagnoses include lymphoma such as Hodgkin's disease [225] and tuberculosis. In tuberculosis and Hodgkin's disease the hilar lymphadenopathy is usually not symmetrical and tuberculosis is usually associated with parenchymal lung lesions in the acute attack in women of this age. The Kveim test is positive in the majority of women with sarcoid presenting with bilateral lymphadenopathy. If there is any doubt the patient should have fibre-optic bronchoscopy with transbronchial aspiration. If this is negative, mediastinotomy, mediastinoscopy or liver biopsy may be necessary to prove or disprove the diagnosis.

More advanced sarcoid is associated with diffuse lung infiltration, when the patient is more likely to be breathless and will frequently have a reduced transfer factor. Those patients who are symptomatic can be given alternate-day steroid therapy (see above), particularly if there is evidence of deteriorating pulmonary function. Because hilar lymphadenopathy may be absent, the differential diagnosis of diffuse lung infiltration is wide, ranging from hypersensitivity to drugs to connective tissue diseases and organic dust diseases. Lymphangioleiomyomatosis is a very rare cause of diffuse pulmonary infiltration that can occur in pregnancy and one that is specific to women in their childbearing years [226] (see below). In the absence of any clinical clues, transbronchial, fibre-optic lung biopsy is usually the definitive investigation. The late manifestations of sarcoid include lung fibrosis and cor pulmonale due to hypoxaemia. Steroid therapy rarely helps at this stage.

No special management is necessary for the average case in pregnancy. Angiotensin-converting enzyme levels have been reported to fall [227] or to remain unchanged in normal pregnancy [228]. In addition they showed diurnal variation [227]. Also levels vary markedly in patients with sarcoid in pregnancy independent of apparent disease activity [228]. Thus, converting enzyme levels may no longer be of value in monitoring patients with sarcoid who become pregnant [228].

Systemic steroids should not be withheld (see above) if they are indicated for the pulmonary condition. However, there is no evidence that steroid therapy influences the natural course of the disease. Sarcoid is not transmitted to the fetus [181], although sarcoid granulomata have been reported in the placenta in one patient [229] but not in others [222]. Because patients often take extra vitamins in pregnancy, they should be particularly warned not to take extra vitamin D, to which they may be very sensitive [223] thus causing hypercalcaemia.

Erythema nodosum

This topic is included here because erythema nodosum frequently complicates sarcoid and tuberculosis. However, it may also complicate other infections (streptococcal, pertussis, measles, coccidiomycosis), drug therapy (particularly sulphonamides) and inflammatory bowel disease. In patients with coccidiomycosis and pregnancy, erythema nodosum is associated with a better outcome and fewer complications [230]. For a general review of erythema nodosum in pregnancy see Bartelsmeyer and Petrie [231]. In many patients, the precipitating cause, if there is one, is not found. The rash consists of tender, pretibial red or purple nodules. Occasionally the nodules are present on the arms. New lesions appear while old ones are resolving, and each lesion lasts a few days to a few weeks. The whole illness may last several months, and be accompanied by fever and arthralgia.

Erythema nodosum occurs not infrequently in pregnancy. We see about one case per 1000 maternities at Queen Charlotte's Maternity Hospital, London. If the patient has none of the clinical conditions outlined above, a normal chest radiograph and a blood count that is normal for pregnancy, she may be reassured that the condition is most unlikely to have any sequelae and that her pregnancy will not be affected.

Salvatore and Lynch [232] reported 21 cases occurring in pregnancy, or in patients taking oral contraceptives. Because they could find no cause for 10 of these, they believed that pregnancy or oestrogen therapy could be precipitating factors. This remains unproven, because erythema nodosum occurs most frequently in women during their childbearing years.

Wegener's granulomatosis

This is a rare form of systemic vasculitis in which necrotizing granulomatous lesions affect the upper respiratory tract (particularly the nose—causing perforation of the septum), lungs and kidneys. It presents with nasal symptoms, haemoptysis, general malaise or renal failure. Untreated, it is rapidly fatal but the condition is now being diagnosed more frequently in [233,234] or before [235] pregnancy as less-severe cases are recognized and treated with prednisone and cyclophosphamide. The latter drug, an alkylating agent, is potentially teratogenic; at least three case reports have documented various abnormalities following first trimester use [155,236,237]. Therefore, patients who conceived taking cyclophosphamide should be offered termination and patients who have Wegener's granulomatosis should wait until they are in remission so that cyclophosphamide can be stopped before pregnancy. Cyclophosphamide also cause ovarian failure.

Cyclophosphamide has been used in the latter half of pregnancy in Wegener's granulomatosis [234] and other conditions [217]; the only fetal abnormality noted was leucopenia [238] but this is of concern in view of the potential for alkylating agents to induce leukaemia [239]. The titre of antineutrophil cytoplasmic antibody (ANCA) may be a guide to the necessity for restarting cyclophosphamide therapy [240] but this has not been evaluated in pregnancy. Furthermore, there is insufficient experience to comment whether the course of Wegener's granulomatosis is affected by pregnancy. On balance most reports suggest that pregnancy is associated with exacerbation of the disease but this may just represent selective reporting [241,242].

In a single case of pulmonary eosinophilic granuloma [243], respiratory function was not affected by pregnancy.

Pulmonary lymphangioleiomyomatosis

This is a very rare condition but it has attracted much interest and is of particular relevance because it occurs in young women during their childbearing years [244–246]. Pulmonary lymphangioleiomyomatosis is characterized by proliferation of smooth muscle in pulmonary mediastinal and retroperitoneal lymphatics, in pulmonary vessels and in the smaller airways [244]. Patients present with breathlessness or with symptoms from pneumothorax or chylothorax.

Chest radiology may be normal initially or show interstitial thickening, pneumothorax or pleural effusion [245]. High-resolution computed tomography (CT) scanning may be necessary to show the typical small cystic changes. Lung function tests show air-flow obstruction and characteristically low gas transfer factor (although note that this is decreased in pregnancy, see above). The differential diagnosis of pulmonary infiltration includes eosinophilic granuloma, sarcoidosis and idiopathic pulmonary fibrosis. Diagnosis is usually confirmed by lung biopsy, which can be performed safely in pregnancy.

Early reports [244] suggested that most patients died within 10 years of diagnosis. More recent studies, possibly in patients diagnosed earlier in the course of disease, are most optimistic. Taylor *et al.* [246] found that 78% of patients were alive 8 years after diagnosis. The evidence that oestrogen [247] and pregnancy [248,249] cause the condition to deteriorate is anecdotal. Nevertheless, in the desire to give some form of active treatment for an otherwise fatal condition, patients have been offered oophorectomy with or without additional progesterone and tamoxifen therapies [246]. Lung transplantation has been performed for some patients [250].

Pre-pregnancy counselling and decisions about termination of pregnancy can only be based on a frank discussion of the uncertainty about the natural history of this fascinating condition.

Pneumonia and other respiratory tract infections

Upper respiratory tract

At least half of the infections of the upper respiratory tract are viral and due to adeno-, rhino- and parainfluenza viruses. In addition, acute bronchitis may be bacterial in origin due to organisms such as *Haemophilus influenzae*. Viral upper respiratory tract infections require no specific treatment. The condition is self-limiting and the patient improves with symptomatic therapy—analgesics and antipyretics (e.g. paracetamol) and bed rest. A high fluid intake is encouraged. If the patient has purulent sputum,

a sample should be sent for culture and appropriate antibiotic therapy should be started. For acute bronchitis this should be broad-spectrum therapy with ampicillin, amoxicillin or a cephalosporin. Erythromycin can be used in patients who are sensitive to penicillin. The safety of cotrimoxazole has not been established in pregnancy and tetracycline should definitely not be used because of the risks of abnormal bone formation and permanent discolouration of the child's teeth [251]. In addition, tetracycline therapy has been related to multiple congenital abnormalities [252], and parenteral tetracycline has caused pancreatitis and fatal liver failure in pregnancy [253]. Treatment for bronchitis should also include steam inhalation to liquefy secretions, but iodine-containing expectorants should not be used because of the adverse effects of iodine on the fetus (see Chapter 12). Bronchodilators to relieve bronchospasm may also be helpful (see above).

Pneumonia

This is associated with the clinical and radiological signs of lung consolidation. The patient presents with fever, cough, purulent sputum or chest pain. Patients frequently have a history of antecedent chest illness and the majority are smokers. No cause for the infection can be found in up to 52% of cases [254]. The majority are bacterial in origin, due to *Streptococcus pneumoniae* (the pneumococcus) but many other organisms may be involved, particularly in epidemics. Hospital-acquired infection may be with *Haemophilus influenzae*, haemolytic streptococcus, *Staphylococcus aureus* or *Klebsiella pneumoniae* in the very debilitated. However, the influenza virus is an important cause of pneumonia during epidemics and chlamydia and mycoplasma may also cause pneumonia, although many cases previously thought to be due to mycoplasma may have been caused by *Legionella pneumophilia*.

Immunocompromised patients such as those with AIDS or those treated with immunosuppressive drugs are at risk of developing pneumonia due to atypical organisms; for example, nocardiosis infection in a pregnant patient with sarcoid treated with high-dose steroids [255] or *Pneumocystis carinii* infection in a patient with AIDS [256] (see also Chapter 18 for a discussion of pneumonia in pregnant patients with AIDS).

In patients who present with pneumonia outside hospital, therapy in the first instance should be with high-dose oral amoxicillin 1 g 8 hourly on the assumption that the patient has a *Strep. pneumoniae* infection. At present such therapy should cover the increasing number of penicillin-resistant pneumococci but this policy should be kept under review. Patients with underlying chest disease are more likely to have *H. influenzae* infection and should be given coamoxiclav.

If the patient is sensitive to penicillin, she should receive erythromycin, 500 mg 6 hourly; this will also treat legionnaire's disease and mycoplasma infection. If the patient is thought to have a hospital-acquired infection or is severely ill she should be treated with high-dose cefuroxime and erythromycin pending the results of sputum, blood culture and sensitivities tests, when further antibiotics may be necessary. Ampicillin dosage should be doubled in pregnancy [131] because of the increased drug clearance [257] due to increased renal blood flow. Patients should also receive paracetamol as an antipyretic and may require tepid sponging and full nursing care in an intensive care situation if they are very sick. Patients who are sick should be managed with a microbiologist and/or an infectious disease expert. Ominous signs include a respiratory rate greater than 30/min, significant hypoxaemia (Po_2 <60 mmHg, 7.98 kPa on room air), acidosis (pH <7.3), disseminated intravascular coagulation, hypotension, elevated blood urea and evidence of multiple organ failure.

Pneumonia used to have a bad reputation in pregnancy with many patients aborting and a 20% maternal mortality rate [258]. Now that effective antibiotics are available, this is no longer so, except for patients with HIV infection or those who are debilitated by drug abuse [259].

Preterm labour remains a definite risk, presumably related to pyrexia [258] and/or prostaglandin release.

It is generally believed that viral pneumonia has a high mortality in pregnancy [260]; during influenza epidemics pneumonia may be responsible for half the cases of maternal mortality [261] and there have been isolated severe cases requiring ventilation associated with influenza and pneumonia [262,263] (see Chapter 17). However, such high maternal mortalities have not been reported recently, and the additional risk of influenza pneumonia due to pregnancy has probably been exaggerated [264].

In contrast, 10% of maternal varicella infections may be complicated by pneumonia, and Parayani and Arvin [265] reported a series in which two patients required ventilation and one died. Not unreasonably, therefore, Parayani and Arvin [265] suggested that pregnant women who have close exposure to varicella zoster virus and no antibody to varicella should receive zoster immunoglobulin (zig) [265]. The effectiveness of zig in preventing fetal complications is not known [266]. Because of the high risk of infection in pregnancy, those patients who develop varicella should be treated with acyclovir 800 mg, five times daily for 7 days. Such treatment is much more effective when given early in the course of the disease particularly within 24 h of the appearance of vesicles.

Varicella pneumonia or those who are very sick with varicella should be treated with parenteral acyclovir 10–30 mg/kg daily in three divided doses for 5 days [267–270] (see Chapter 17). Parenteral acyclovir should be used with caution particularly in the first trimester, although it has been given without problem to large numbers of children with varicella from the age of 2 years [271].

Fungal lung infections are very uncommon in the UK. Cantanazaro [272] has reviewed the pulmonary mycoses that occur in pregnancy in North America. Cryptococcosis, blastomycosis and sporotrichosis are rare. However, coccidioidomycosis is more common and appears to be particularly dangerous in pregnancy possibly due to the stimulating effect of oestrogen and progesterone on coccidioides [273]. In 50 cases of coccidioidomycosis from North America, 22 became disseminated in pregnancy with a maternal mortality of nearly 100% if untreated with amphotericin B [274].

There have been no reports of fetal toxicity from amphotericin B despite its use in the first trimester [272–275]. Flucytosine is also used in the treatment of fungal infections but such therapy is much more worrying since flucytosine is metabolized to the antimetabolite fluorouracil [272].

Cystic fibrosis

Cystic fibrosis is the most common important genetic disorder in Caucasians with a gene frequency of one in 20 [276]. Because heterozygotes are asymptomatic, homozygous patients who suffer from the condition are relatively common. The incidence is about one in 2500 live births [277]. Recently the mortality has improved markedly, so that many more women are surviving to become pregnant [18]. The median age of survival for patients attending cystic fibrosis clinics in the USA in 1990 was 27.6 years [278]. In 1997 it was estimated that there were 2400 people with cystic fibrosis over the age of 16 years in the UK of whom about 43% would have been female [279].

Because of the large number of cystic fibrosis mutations that have been identified (more than 150) only 80% of all heterozygotes can be identified [280]. Nevertheless, cystic fibrosis carrier screening is a practical proposition in general practice [281]. In addition, first-trimester prenatal diagnosis is possible on genetic material prepared from chorionic villi using linked DNA probes in at least two-thirds of couples presenting with one affected child; Super *et al.* [282] have described their experience with this technique in 96 families. The expected false-negative and false-positive rates of this procedure are 2% and 6%, respectively [283]. Biochemical analysis of amniotic fluid is not sufficiently accurate at present to detect or exclude the affected fetus. The patient should also be aware that her child will be heterozygous for cystic fibrosis, even if it is not homozygous. This, in turn, is likely to increase the future genetic load in the community. An alternative approach is *in vitro* fertilization following preimplantation diagnostic testing to exclude the condition [284]. This technique consumes considerable resources and is likely to be applicable only in individual cases.

The improvement in mortality from cystic fibrosis has come from improved prophylactic bronchial toilet and widespread use of antibiotics, rather than any single therapeutic advance although the possibility of heart and lung transplantation could make a big difference to prognosis [285]. In addition, pancreatic enzymes and vitamins are added to a high-protein and low-fat diet. Carbohydrates are given as sugar to increase calorie intake.

For reviews of cystic fibrosis in pregnancy see [286–290]. The condition has been diagnosed in patients for the first time during pregnancy [286]. Such cases diagnosed later in life seem to have a better prognosis than those where the diagnosis is made in early childhood.

Phelan [290] reported only three successful pregnancies in 66 women aged over 16 years, attending the Royal Children's Hospital, Melbourne. He comments that the low incidence of pregnancy was possibly due to fear of producing affected children, as well as possible infertility due to unfavourable cervical mucus and low lean body mass. (Most males with the condition are infertile due to atresia of the vas and epididymis [291].)

Cohen *et al.* [292] surveyed 119 centres in North America and reported the outcome in 129 patients delivered before 1975. Although 19% of patients had therapeutic abortions, the incidence of spontaneous abortion (5%) was not elevated. However, both the perinatal mortality (11%) and the maternal mortality (12% within 6 months of delivery) were considerably greater than that in the rest of the population. Although the maternal mortality is alarming, it was not greater than reported for patients with cystic fibrosis who were not pregnant [293,294]. Corkey *et al.* [295] reported the outcome of 11 pregnancies in seven patients. Only one pregnancy required termination and these authors suggested that this prognosis is better when pancreatic function is maintained.

It has been reported that patients with cystic fibrosis show a decrease in residual volume as do normal women in pregnancy, but that they are unable to maintain vital capacity. Although they increase oxygen uptake, they do not show the 'hyperventilation' associated with normal pregnancy [263].

The judgement of individual physicians is likely to be influenced by their most recent experience of relatively few cases, and this would account for a wide diversity of clinical opinions regarding the advisability of pregnancy in patients with cystic fibrosis. Several indices have been suggested as a guide to the success of pregnancy, based on history, the nutritional status, the presence or absence of emphysema, cor pulmonale and such abnormalities in respiratory function as vital capacity less than 50% predicted for height [288,296]. Although a vital capacity of less than 50% than that predicted has been recommended as an indication for termination, many patients with a vital capacity of less than this in cystic fibrosis and other conditions such as kyphoscoliosis have a normal pregnancy. Because patients die of uncontrollable recurrent chest infection and cor pulmonale (which is in turn related to hypoxaemia) it is suggested that these should be the parameters considered when counselling patients.

Echocardiographic measurement of right ventricular cavity size at end diastole is a good estimate of clinical outcome [297,298] and this dimension is likely to be related to pulmonary artery pressure. If there is any doubt about the presence of hypoxaemia, the arterial blood gases should be measured. From the data of di Saint'Agnese and Davis [291], it would appear that an arterial Po_2 of <60 mmHg, when the patient is free from infection and breathing air, is associated with a National Institutes of Health (NIH) score of <50. This is the score at which pulmonary hypertension is present [299]. Pulmonary hypertension has a particularly poor outcome in pregnancy (see Chapter 5). The pulmonary artery pressure can be estimated fairly reliably by echocardiography. If the pulmonary artery systolic pressure is <35 mmHg, the patient does not have cor pulmonale. A recent study in a non-pregnant population [278] confirms the poor outcome if the Po_2 is <55 mmHg (2 years mortality >50%). Similar life expectancy was indicated by FEV_1 < 30% predicted or Pco_2 >50 mmHg.

Physicians should also be aware that patients with cystic fibrosis may have liver disease [300] and diabetes mellitus. However, the reported incidence of cirrhosis varies between 0.5% [18] and 90% [301] and this has not yet been reported to be a problem in pregnancy.

Apart from a high level of medical and obstetric care, paying particular attention to nutrition, there are no special measures that should be taken in the antenatal period once antenatal diagnosis of the fetus has been discussed. Because of the ototoxic and renal side-effects of the aminoglycosides reviewed above, intravenous and intramuscular use of these antibiotics should be avoided if possible in pregnancy, and the penicillins should be given instead. Nebulized gentamicin represents a real advantage here. However, it is reassuring that there were no congenital abnormalities amongst the 129 cases reviewed by Cohen *et al.* [292] of whom 26 received amino-glycosides during pregnancy.

During labour, particular care should be taken concerning fluid and electrolyte balance. Patients with cystic fibrosis lose large quantities of sodium in sweat and may easily become hypovolaemic. However, they will also be very intolerant of over hydration, if there is any degree of cor pulmonale. Oxygen may be freely administered if the $Paco_2$ is not elevated. Because of the risk of postanaesthetic atelectasis, inhalation anaesthesia should be avoided and epidural or caudal anaesthesia substituted. Chest pain arising in labour should raise the suspicion of pneumothorax to which these patients are particularly predisposed. Forceps delivery should be performed if the second stage is at all prolonged.

Whitelaw and Butterfield [302] reported that the sodium content of breast milk from women with cystic fibrosis may be as high as 280 mmol/L, and suggested that this was a reason for these mothers not to breastfeed. However, Alpert and Cormier [303] have found normal electrolyte content in milk from mothers with cystic fibrosis and believe that the sodium content found by Whitelaw and Butterfield was abnormally high because the milk was expressed from a woman who was not lactating freely. Such expressed milk was demonstrated to have abnormally high electrolyte content even if the mothers did not have cystic fibrosis. It would seem sensible to check the sodium content of breast milk from women with cystic fibrosis who are lactating, but it is unlikely that this will be a contraindication to breastfeeding.

Chronic bronchitis, emphysema and bronchiectasis

Because these conditions are now rarely important in patients during childbearing years, there is little information on their outcome in pregnancy. Although there have been reports of intrauterine growth restriction in patients with bronchiectasis [12,304], this does not regularly occur [305]. If pregnancy does occur in patients with bronchiectasis, they can be severely debilitated [304] and will need to be treated as high-risk patients with regular supervision and attention to postural drainage and physiotherapy. Chest infection and airways obstruction should be managed as described earlier. As suggested by Lalli and Raju [306] a successful outcome to pregnancy may be limited by the presence of pulmonary hypertension and hypoxaemia (see above).

In a single case report, emphysema due to α_1-antitrypsin deficiency did not affect the successful outcome of pregnancy [307], although another case was affected by severe pre-eclampsia [308]. This condition is now amenable to prenatal diagnosis by chorionic villus biopsy [310] and DNA polymorphism.

Kyphoscoliosis

The reported incidence of kyphoscoliosis is 0.1–0.7% of pregnancies [311] but much depends on the definition in mild cases. Kopenhager [311] noted a marked increase in perinatal mortality to 102 in 1000, due to maternal hypoxia. In Mendelson's series [312] only one patient had a vital capacity of <1 L, and she was in heart failure during labour. However, we have successfully delivered two patients with kyphoscoliosis who had vital capacities of <1 L with no overt problems. Lao *et al.* [313] studied 10 pregnancies in eight patients in Hong Kong with severe kyphoscoliosis (average vital capacity approximately 1000 mL). There were no major maternal problems but four infants were delivered before 37 weeks and one died. In one case of kyphoscoliosis, very severe chronic maternal hypoxia (Pao_2 =5.9 kPa) has caused fetal brain damage [314]. Less severe kyphoscoliosis has a universally good outcome [315]. As in cystic fibrosis, the limiting factors are hypoxaemia, pulmonary hypertension and the presence of muscular weakness.

However, Sawicka *et al.* [316] on the basis of six cases with paralytic or early-onset kyphoscoliosis suggest that patients with this form of the disease may be particularly at risk during pregnancy because four of their cases with vital capacities 1360 mL or less required long-term negative-pressure ventilation in a tank-lung before and after delivery. Certainly those patients with idiopathic scoliosis who have a primary curve >25° may deteriorate in pregnancy [317]; lesser curves are not affected by pregnancy [317]. All these patients are more likely to require caesarean section, because of associated abnormalities of the bony pelvis and of abnormal presentations of the fetus [313]. Notwithstanding the spinal deformities, epidural anaesthetic is preferable to general anaesthesia.

Patients with achondroplasia and other chondrodystrophies may have similar though less severe respiratory and pelvic problems [318].

Adult respiratory distress syndrome

This is the end point of several different types of obstetric disaster including inhalation of gastric contents during anaesthesia (see below). In addition, it may occur with disseminated intravascular coagulation (DIC) in pre-eclampsia, eclampsia, abruptio placentae, dead fetus syndrome and amniotic fluid embolism (see Chapter 3). The syndrome is also associated with hypovolaemic shock from postpartum haemorrhage with or without sepsis

[319], with endotoxin shock [320] and with severe anaphylaxis. It is also found with metastatic cancer or, in pregnancy, with hydatidiform mole.

Adult respiratory distress syndrome in association with pyelonephritis in pregnancy seems to be a particular problem in the USA [322,323]. Particular risk factors for the development of adult respiratory distress syndrome in a patient with pyelonephritis include maternal heart rate >110/min, pyrexia >39.4°C in patients with gestational age >20 weeks and the use of tocolytic agents.

In a group of 14 obstetric cases with adult respiratory distress syndrome, 12 were caused by strictly obstetric factors such as pre-eclampsia or haemorrhage. The mortality was 43% [90].

Changes in maternal physiology such as increased interstitial lung water [324] or activation of various pathways of arachidonic acid metabolism may be the reason for the apparent frequency of pregnancy as an underlying cause of adult respiratory distress in women. Alternatively, it may be that other secondary causes, such as anaesthesia, shock from haemorrhage and DIC (see Chapter 3) are more likely to be present in women in the pregnant than the non-pregnant state.

The patients are severely ill and should be managed in an intensive care unit. The clinical picture is of a patient who develops acute severe hypoxaemia despite a high inspired oxygen concentration, and shows diffuse infiltrates on the chest radiograph—where signs may take 24 h to develop. It has been suggested that an acute fall in white cell count occurring after the initial insult may be of value in predicting those patients who will develop adult respiratory distress syndrome [325]. It is assumed that the primary problem is in the lung, where compliance and permeability are reduced due to extravasation of liquid, rather than in the heart. However, it may be necessary to prove that there is not a primary cardiac abnormality by demonstrating a normal (<14 mmHg) pulmonary artery wedge pressure, i.e. a normal left-ventricular end-diastolic pressure, using a flow-guided Swan–Ganz catheter [326]. Such a catheter (if left in place) can be of great assistance for management, because it can provide measurements of pulmonary artery pressure and cardiac output by green dye or thermodilution. Peripheral oedema, elevated jugular venous pressure and cardiomegaly are unusual and suggest cardiac, rather than pulmonary, pathology.

The therapeutic options available are correction of the underlying cause, artificial ventilation, membrane oxygenation and medication with diuretics, antibiotics, vasoactive drugs, inotropes and steroids.

Correction of the underlying cause is usually limited to reversal of DIC with fresh frozen plasma (followed by delivery of the dead fetus if present) and treatment of infection. Andersen *et al*. [319] suggest ventilation, preferably with an inspired oxygen concentration of <60%, maintaining an end-expiratory pressure of 5–35 cmH$_2$O to try to keep the arterial Po_2 >60 mmHg. The use of positive end-expiratory pressure (PEEP) may help by thinning the layer of water in the alveolus and increasing alveolar area to improve gas exchange.

Fluid balance is crucial. If the patients are hypovolaemic, cardiac output and perfusion will decrease; hence infusion of albumin or blood (increasing oxygen carrying capacity) can be helpful, although there is a risk of further protein loss into the alveoli (see Chapter 3 for a further discussion of which fluid may be best in this situation). If they are hypervolaemic, there will be increased extravasation of fluid and increased preload, decreasing oxygenation and cardiac output. Diuretic therapy or dialysis will then be necessary. The necessity for manipulating blood volume and its effect can be assessed by repeated measurement of pulmonary artery wedge pressure and cardiac output, using the Swan–Ganz catheter. Corticosteroids may reverse excess capillary permeability [327], but they may also increase susceptibility to infection [328] and one study suggests that they do not affect outcome [329].

Despite these measures, the mortality of adult respiratory distress syndrome is 50–60% [330]. Nevertheless, every effort should be made in treating these patients because those who survive recover well. It is hoped, although not proven, that early aggressive treatment will reduce mortality of this condition [319].

Pneumothorax and pneumomediastinum

Both these conditions occur infrequently in pregnancy, but probably more commonly than in the non-pregnant state. They most commonly occur in susceptible individuals due to the expulsive efforts of labour [331,332], but pneumomediastinum in particular may occur at other times, for example in association with bronchial asthma [333] or ruptured oesophagus following vomiting [334]. Pneumothorax may occur in association with other chest conditions, such as emphysema, pulmonary tuberculosis or cystic fibrosis. In pneumomediastinum, which is more common in pregnancy than pneumothorax, a false passage is created between the airways and the mediastinal tissues. The condition usually, although not invariably, follows a strenuous labour. Air tracks through the mediastinum to the neck or pericardium (pneumopericardium) [336], and there may be widespread subcutaneous emphysema over the thorax or even the whole body. This produces a quite characteristic crackling sound and sensation on palpation, which does not occur in any other condition.

In addition, there may be a crunching noise (Hamman's sign [337]) synchronous with the heartbeat at the left sternal edge.

In pneumothorax there is a false passage between the airways and the pleural cavity. Pneumothorax accompanies about one-third of the cases of pneumomediastinum that occur in pregnancy but may also occur independently [338]. In both conditions, the patient complains of the sudden onset of chest pain and breathlessness, and the diagnosis is confirmed by chest radiography. In tension pneumothorax the patient will become cyanosed and hypotensive due to the reduction in the venous return. A similar variant of pneumomediastinum 'malignant mediastinum' [339] also occurs but is much more rare.

Pneumomediastinum normally clears spontaneously and the treatment is therefore usually conservative, with oxygen and analgesics. Malignant mediastinum requires urgent relief either by multiple incisions over the subcutaneous tissue where air is trapped [339] or by splitting the sternum. Pneumothorax should be drained via an underwater seal if the lung is more than 25% collapsed. Tension pneumothorax requires immediate relief by a large-bore needle inserted through the chest wall overlying the pneumothorax. If pneumothorax or pneumomediastinum has occurred in pregnancy, elective forceps delivery should be performed to minimize the chance of recurrence, caused by raised intrapulmonary pressure due to maternal straining.

Pleural effusion

Pleural effusion may arise in pregnancy secondary to conditions such as tuberculosis, pneumonia, pulmonary infarction and cardiac failure, which also cause effusions in the non-pregnant state. Small pleural effusions are said to be a common finding in the first 24 h postpartum [340]. Spring and Winston [341] found pleural effusions in a surprisingly high proportion (45–65% of normal women) postpartum. This was not confirmed by Udeshi et al. [342] who used a sensitive ultrasound technique. They only found pleural effusions after delivery in women who had pre-eclampsia, an association that has been noted previously by Suonio et al. [343]. Perhaps the increased lung water of pregnancy [324] and/or the profound changes that must occur in the maternal circulation after delivery are the causes.

Lung cancer

This is an uncommon cancer in pregnancy (the most common are breast, cervix and haematopoietic); the incidence is likely to increase because of increased smoking amongst women. About 10 cases have been reported. Metastasis may occur in the pericardium and the placenta. There are insufficient data to state whether the natural history of lung cancer is affected by pregnancy.

Anaesthetic considerations

Two recent Confidential Maternal Mortality reports, which examined all maternal deaths occurring in the UK in the years 1985–90, indicates that there were three deaths due to inhalation of stomach contents, out of a total of 590 cases [344,345]. This represents a significant improvement over the previous series in which there were eight deaths from inhalation in England and Wales out of a total of 176 cases [346]. The management of adult respiratory distress syndrome has been discussed above. Further treatment of inhalation includes bronchoscopy for the patient who becomes acutely cyanotic following regurgitation of large particles of food that have obstructed major airways. It is also important to realize that pulmonary aspiration may occur without frank vomiting and regurgitation. The differential diagnosis of amniotic fluid embolism and aspiration is considered in Chapters 3 and 4.

Much of modern obstetric medical practice involves prevention of the complication of gastric aspiration. The increasing use of regional anaesthesia (epidural or spinal block) is one way of reducing the problem. It is also common practice to starve women during labour, but the stomach will continue to secrete fluid, even though in reduced quantities; also gastric emptying from meals taken before the onset of labour is much reduced. On the assumption that it is the acid component of gastric content that is harmful, patients in labour are often given up to 30 mL of antacid (magnesium trisilicate mixture) every 2 h to maintain a pH >3.2 [347]. However, the Confidential Maternal Mortality series indicates that the number of deaths from aspiration during 1973–75, when antacid administration was widespread, was no less than the number occurring in 1970–72, before antacids were generally used [348]. Furthermore, Bond et al. [349] have described pulmonary aspiration syndrome after inhalation of stomach contents of pH 6.4, in a patient who had been given regular antacid therapy with magnesium and aluminium hydroxide. The one maternal death due to aspiration of stomach contents in the 1985–86 confidential enquiry [344] was in a woman who received adequate prophylaxis with ranitidine and sodium citrate. All this would suggest that the hydrogen ion concentration is not the only determinant of the pulmonary aspiration syndrome; either the antacid itself or other constituents of the gastric fluid must contribute. Although 0.3 mol/L sodium citrate solution may be a safer antacid [350], it is not so effective in reducing acidity [321]; both medicines increase the volume in the stomach, which may be crucial. Alternative approaches are to use an H_2 antagonist such as cimetidine [351–353], which decreases acid secretion, or metoclopramide therapy, which increases gastric emptying [354]. Large-scale comparative studies are necessary to determine which is the most effective.

Pending the results of such studies, a reasonable guide to prophylaxis is as follows [355].

1 Normal labour: starve patient; the place of additional antacid therapy is unclear.

2 High risk when general anaesthesia may be necessary: give oral antacid and H_2-receptor antagonist.

3 Elective caesarean section under general anaesthesia: oral H_2-receptor antagonist at least 90 min preoperatively. Antacid 15 mL preoperatively.

4 Emergency caesarean section under general anaesthetic: antacid preoperatively if none has been given recently. Metoclopramide 10 mg i.v. to promote gastric emptying. Ranitidine 50 mg i.v. preoperatively to prevent any further acid formation. The best preventative measure would be to use epidural rather than general anaesthesia whenever possible.

Furthermore, in the patient who has respiratory impairment, general anaesthesia should be avoided because of the risk of intrapartum hypoxia, due to deteriorating ventilation perfusion imbalance, and the greater risk of postoperative atelectasis. In addition pain is a potent stimulant to hyperventilation, which can increase oxygen consumption in labour as much as 100% [356]. Therefore, the efficacy of regional anaesthesia as an analgesic decreases oxygen consumption [357].

Because of the generalized muscular effort, labour is obviously a time when the patient with severe respiratory impairment is at risk of developing respiratory failure. But in addition, expulsive efforts specifically fatigue the diaphragm [358], exacerbating this risk. Epidural block can eliminate the desire to push, allowing forceps delivery at full dilation.

There are additional reasons for the use of epidural anaesthesia in any patient whose respiratory status is compromised. One caveat is that when used for caesarean section, even regional block is associated with reductions in FEV_1 of 19%, forced vital capacity of 17% and peak flow rate of 35% [359]. Similar data have been reported by Harrop-Griffiths et al. [360]. Regional block is the best way to manage these patients but it does have some adverse effects.

References

1 Gaensler EA, Paton WE et al. Pulmonary functions in pregnancy: III. Serial observations in patients with pulmonary insufficiency. Am Rev Tuberc 1953; 67: 779–97.

2 Bryne DL, Chappatte OA et al. Pregnancy complicated by Charcot–Marie–Tooth disease, requiring intermittent ventilation. Br J Obstet Gynaecol 1992; 9979–80.

3 Department of Health. Why Mothers Die: Report on Confidential Enquiries into Maternal Deaths in the United Kingdom 1994–96. 1998.

4 de Swiet M. The respiratory system. In: Chamberlain G, Broughton Pipkin F eds. Clinical Physiology in Obstetrics, 3rd edn. Blackwell Science, Oxford, 1998; 111–128.

5 de Swiet M. Maternal pulmonary disorders. In: Creasy RK, Resnik R, eds. Maternal Fetal Medicine: Principles and Practice, 3rd edn. W.B. Saunders, Philadelphia, 1993.

6 Fishburne JI. Physiology and disease of the respiratory system in pregnancy. A review. J Reprod Med 1979; 22: 177–89.

7 Milne JA. The respiratory response to pregnancy. Postgrad Med J 1979; 55: 318–24.

8 Alaily AB, Carrol KB. Pulmonary ventilation in pregnancy. Br J Obstet Gynaecol 1978; 85: 518–24.

9 Gazioglu K, Kaltreider NL et al. Pulmonary function during pregnancy in normal women and in patients with cardiopulmonary disease. Thorax 1970; 25: 445–50.

10 Knuttgen HG, Emerson K. Physiological response to pregnancy at rest and during exercise. J Appl Physiol 1974; 36: 549.

11 Pernoll ML, Metcalfe J et al. Ventilation during rest and exercise in pregnancy and postpartum. Resp Physiol 1975; 25: 295.

12 Templeton A, Kelman GR. Maternal blood gases (PAo_2, Pao_2) physiological shunt and V_D/V_T in normal pregnancy. Br J Anaesth 1976; 48: 1001–4.

13 Lucius H, Gahlenbeck H et al. Respiratory functions, buffer system and electrolyte concentrations of blood during human pregnancy. Resp Physiol 1970; 9: 311.

14 Ang CK, Tan TH et al. Postural influence on maternal capillary oxygen and carbon dioxide tension. Br Med J 1969; 4: 201.

15 Huch R, Baumann H et al. Physiologic changes in pregnant women and their fetuses during jet travel. Am J Obstet Gynecol 1986; 154: 996–1000.

16 Emerson K, Saxena BN et al. Caloric cost of normal pregnancy. Obstet Gynaecol 1972; 49: 786–94.

17 Kambam JR, Handte RE et al. Effect of pregnancy on oxygen dissociation. Anesthesiology 1983; 59: A395.

18 Crozier MD. Cystic fibrosis—a not-so-fatal disease. Pediatric Clin North Am 1974; 21: 935–7.

19 Cugell DW, Frank NR et al. Pulmonary function in pregnancy. I. Serial observations in normal women. Am Rev Tuberc 1953; 67: 568–97.

20 Milne JA, Mills RJ et al. Large airways function during normal pregnancy. Br J Obstet Gynaecol 1977; 84: 448–51.

21 Eng M, Butler J et al. Respiratory function in pregnant obese women. Am J Obstet Gynecol 1975; 123: 241.

22 Bouterline-Young H, Bouterline-Young E. Alveolar carbon dioxide levels in pregnant parturient and lactating subjects. J Obstet Gynaecol Br Empire 1956; 63: 509.

23 Hellegers A, Metcalfe J et al. The alveolar Pco_2 in pregnant and non-pregnant women at altitude. J Clin Invest 1959; 38: 1010.

24 Sobrevilla LA, Cassinelli MT et al. Human fetal and maternal oxygen tension, and acid-base status during delivery at high altitude. Am J Obstet Gynecol 1971; 111: 1111.

25 Doring GK, Loeschche HH. Atmung und Savre—Basengleichgewicht in der Schwangershaft Pflüger Archiv für die gesamte. Physiologie Des Menschen Terre 1947; 249: 437.

26 Wilbrand U, Porath CH et al. Der einfluss der Ovarialsteroide auf die Funktion des Aternzentrums. Arch Gynakologie 1952; 191: 507.

27 Lunell NO, Wager J *et al*. Metabolic effects of oral salbutamol in late pregnancy. *Eur J Clin Pharmacol* 1978; 14: 95–9.

28 Prowse CM, Gaensler EA. Respiratory and acid–base changes during pregnancy. *Anesthesiology* 1965; 26: 381.

29 Skatrud JB, Dempsey JA, Kaiser DG. Ventilatory response to the medroxy-progesterone acetate in normal subjects: time course and mechanism. *J Appl Physiol* 1978; 44: 939–44.

30 Paciorek J, Spencer N. An association between plasma progesterone and erythrocyte carbonic anhydrase 1 concentration in women. *Clin Sci* 1980; 58: 161–4.

31 Schenker JG, Ben-Joseph Y *et al*. Erythrocyte carbonic anhydrase B levels during pregnancy and use of oral contraceptives. *Obstet Gynecol* 1972; 39: 237–40.

32 Cullen JH, Brum VO *et al*. The respiratory effects of progesterone in severe pulmonary emphysema. *Am J Med* 1959; 27: 551–7.

33 Lyons HA, Huang CT. Therapeutic use of progesterone in alveolar hypoventilation associated with obesity. *Am J Med* 1968; 44: 881–8.

34 Sutton FD Jr, Zwillich CW *et al*. Progesterone for outpatient treatment of Pickwickian syndrome. *Ann Intern Med* 1975; 83: 476–9.

35 England SJ, Fahri LE. Fluctuations in alveolar CO_2 and in base excess during the menstrual cycle. *Resp Physiol* 1976; 26: 157.

36 Milne JA, Pack AI *et al*. Gas exchange and acid-base status during ovulatory cycles and those regulated by oral contraceptives. *J Endocrinol* 1977; 75: 17–P.

37 Rubin A, Russo N, Coucher D. The effect of pregnancy upon pulmonary function in normal women. *Am J Obstet Gynecol* 1956; 72: 2963.

38 Maklem PT, Mead J. Resistance of central and peripheral airways measured by a retrograde catheter. *J Appl Physiol* 1967; 22: 395.

39 Sims CD, Chamberlain GVP *et al*. Lung function tests in bronchial asthma during and after pregnancy. *Br J Obstet Gynaecol* 1976; 88: 434–7.

40 Gee JBL, Packer BS *et al*. Pulmonary mechanics during pregnancy. *J Clin Invest* 1967; 46: 945–52.

41 Bevan DR, Holdcroft A *et al*. Closing volume and pregnancy. *Br Med J* 1974; i: 13–15.

42 Garrard CG, Littler WAW *et al*. Closing volume during normal pregnancy. *Thorax* 1978; 33: 484.

43 Baldwin GR, Moorthi S *et al*. New lung functions and pregnancy. *Am J Obstet Gynecol* 1977; 127: 235.

44 Craig DR, Toole MA. Airway closure in pregnancy. *Can Anaesth Soc J* 1975; 22: 665.

45 Russell IF, Chambers WA. Closing volume in normal pregnancy. *Br J Anaesth* 1981; 53: 1043–7.

46 Farebrother MJ, McHardy GJR. Closing volume and pregnancy. *Br Med J* 1974; 1: 454.

47 Templeton A, Kelman GR. Arterial blood gases in pre-eclampsia. *Br J Obstet Gynaecol* 1977; 84: 290–3.

48 Bedell GN, Adams RS. Pulmonary diffusing capacity during rest and exercise. A study of normal persons and persons with atrial septal defect, pregnancy and pulmonary disease. *J Clin Invest* 1962; 41: 1908.

49 Krumholz RA, Echt CR *et al*. Pulmonary diffusing capacity, capillary blood volume, lung volumes and mechanics of ventilation in early and late pregnancy. *J Lab Clin Med* 1964; 63: 648.

50 Milne JA, Pack AI *et al*. Maternal gas exchange and acid-base status during normal pregnancy. *Scott Med J* 1977; 22: 108.

51 Lotgering FK, Gilbert RD *et al*. The interactions of exercise and pregnancy: a review. *Am J Obstet Gynecol* 1984; 149: 560–8.

52 Edwards MJ, Metcalfe J *et al*. Accelerated respiratory response to moderate exercise in late pregnancy. *Resp Physiol* 1981; 45: 229–41.

53 Artal R, Wiswell R *et al*. Pulmonary responses to exercise in pregnancy. *Am J Obstet Gynecol* 1986; 154: 378–83.

54 Sorensen KE, Borlum K. Fetal heart function in response to short-term maternal exercise. *Br J Obstet Gynaecol* 1986; 93: 310–3.

55 Clapp JF. Fetal heart rate response to running in mid pregnancy and late pregnancy. *Am J Obstet Gynecol* 1985; 153: 251–2.

56 Hall DC, Kaufmann DA. Effects of aerobic and strength conditioning on pregnancy outcomes. *Am J Obstet Gynecol* 1987; 157: 1199–203.

57 Huch R, Erkkola R. Pregnancy and exercise and pregnancy. A short review. *Br J Obstet Gynaecol* 1990; 97: 208–14.

58 Thornson KJ, Cohen ME. Studies on the circulation in pregnancy. II. Vital capacity observations in normal pregnant women. *Surg Gynecol Obstet* 1938; 66: 591.

59 Milne JA, Howie AD *et al*. Dyspnoea during normal pregnancy. *Br J Obstet Gynaecol* 1978; 84: 448.

60 Comroe JJ, Forster RE *et al*. *The Lung: Clinical Physiology and Pulmonary Function Tests*. Year Book Medical Publishers, Chicago, 1962.

61 Prichard MG, Musk AW. Adverse effect of pregnancy on familial fibrosing alveolitis. *Thorax* 1984; 39: 319–20.

62 Ballou SP, Morley JJ *et al*. Pregnancy and systemic sclerosis. *Arthritis Rheumatol* 1984; 27: 295–8.

63 Littlejohns P, Ebrahim S *et al*. Prevalence and diagnosis of chronic respiratory symptoms in adults. *Br Med J* 1989; 298: 1556–60.

64 Burney PG, Chinn S *et al*. Has the prevalence of asthma increased in children? Evidence from national study of health and growth 1973–86. *Br Med J* 1990; 300: 1306–10.

65 Alexander S, Dodds L *et al*. Perinatal outcomes in women with asthma during pregnancy. *Obstet Gynecol* 1998; 92 (3): 435–40.

66 Hernandez E, Angel CS *et al*. Asthma in pregnancy: current concepts. *Obstet Gynecol* 1980; 55: 739–43.

67 Greenberger PA, Patterson R. Betamethasone dipropionate for severe asthma in pregnancy. *Ann Intern Med* 1983; 98: 478–80.

68 Greenberger PA. Pregnancy and asthma. *Chest* 1985; 87: 855–75.

69 Spector SL. The treatment of the asthmatic mother during pregnancy and lactation. *Ann Allergy* 1983; 51: 173–8.

70 Stablein JF, Lockey RF. Managing asthma during pregnancy. *Comp Ther* 1984; 10: 45–52.

71 Turner ES, Creenberger PA *et al*. Management of the pregnant asthmatic patient. *Ann Intern Med* 1980; 6: 905–18.

72 Weinberger SE, Weiss ST *et al*. Pregnancy and the lung. *Am Rev Resp Med* 1980; 121: 559–81.

73 Weinstein AM, Dubin BD *et al*. Asthma and pregnancy. *J Am Med Assoc* 1980; 241: 1161–4.

74 Schatz M. Asthma and pregnancy. *Lancet* 1999; 353 (9160): 1202–4.

75 Schatz M. Interrelationships between asthma and pregnancy: a literature review. *J Allergy Clin Immunol* 1999; 103: S330–6.

76 Terr AI. Asthma and reproductive medicine. *Obstet Gynecol Surv* 1998; 53 (11): 699–707.

77 Moore-Gillon J. Asthma in pregnancy. *Br J Obstet Gynaecol* 1994; 101 (8): 658–60.

78 White RJ, Coutts II *et al*. A prospective study of asthma during pregnancy and the puerperium. *Obstet Gynecol Survey* 1989; 83: 240–1.

79 Gordon M, Niswander KR *et al.* Fetal morbidity following potentially anoxigenic obstetric conditions. VII. Bronchial asthma. *Am J Obstet Gynecol* 1970; 106: 421–9.

80 Williams DA. Asthma and pregnancy. *Acta Allergologica* 1957; 22: 311–23.

81 Juniper EF, Daniel EE *et al.* Improvement in airway responsiveness and asthma severity during pregnancy. *Am Rev Respir Dis* 1989; 140: 924–31.

82 Beecroft N, Cochrane GM *et al.* Effect of sex of fetus on asthma during pregnancy: blind prospective study. *Br Med J* 1998; 317: 856–7.

83 Beynon HL, Garbett ND *et al.* Severe premenstrual exacerbations of asthma: effect of intramuscular progesterone. *Lancet* 1988; ii: 370–2

84 Briscoe WA, Dubois AB. The relationship between airway resistance, airway conductance and lung volume in subjects of different age and body size. *J Clin Invest* 1958; 37: 1279.

85 Newhouse MT, Becklaile MR *et al.* Effect of alterations in endtidal CO_2 on flow resistance. *J Appl Physiol* 1964; 19: 745.

86 Hyman AL, Spannha KEEW *et al.* Prostaglandins and the lung: State of the art. *Am Rev Respir Dis* 1978; 177: 111–36.

87 Fishburne JI, Brenner WE *et al.* Bronchospasm complicating intravenous prostaglandin F2 for therapeutic abortion. *Obstet Gynecol* 1972; 39: 892–6.

88 Fishburne J, Brenner WE *et al.* Cardiovascular and respiratory responses to intravenous infusion of prostaglandin F2 in the pregnant woman. *Am J Obstet Gynecol* 1972; 114: 765–72.

89 Kreisman H, Van De Wiel N *et al.* Respiratory function during prostaglandin-induced labour. *Am Rev Respir Dis* 1975; 111: 564–6.

90 Smith JL, Thomas F *et al.* Adult respiratory distress syndrome during pregnancy and immediately postpartum. *Western J Med* 1990; 153: 508–10.

91 Smith AP. The effects of intravenous infusion of graded doses of prostaglandins F2 and E2 on lung resistance in patients undergoing termination of pregnancy. *Clin Sci* 1973; 44: 17–25.

92 Clark SL. Asthma in pregnancy. National Asthma Education Program Working Group on Asthma and Pregnancy. National Institutes of Health, National Heart, Lung and Blood Institute. *Obstet Gynecol* 1993; 82 (6): 1036–40.

93 Demissie K, Breckenridge MB *et al.* Infant and maternal outcomes in the pregnancies of asthmatic women. *Am J Respir Crit Care Med* 1998; 158 (4): 1091–5.

94 Kramer MS, Coates AL *et al.* Maternal asthma and idiopathic preterm labor. *Am J Epidemiol* 1995; 142 (10): 1078–88.

95 Apter AJ, Greenberger PA *et al.* Outcomes of pregnancy in adolescents with severe asthma. *Arch Intern Med* 1989; 149: 2571–5.

96 Schatz M, Zeiger RS *et al.* Intrauterine growth is related to gestational pulmonary function in pregnant asthmatic women. Kaiser Permanente Asthma and Pregnancy Group. *Chest* 1990; 98: 389–92.

97 Templeton A. Intrauterine growth retardation associated with hypoxia due to bronchiectasis. *Br J Obstet Gynaecol* 1977; 84: 389–90.

98 Moya F, Morishima HO *et al.* Influence of maternal hyperventilation on the new born infant. *Am J Obstet Gynecol* 1975; 91: 76–84.

99 Wulf KH, Kunzel S, Lehman V. Clinical aspects of placental gas exchange. In: Longo LD, Bartels H, eds. *Respiratory Gas Exchange and Blood Flow in the Placenta.* US Department of Health, Education and Welfare, Bethesda, Maryland, 1972.

100 Motoyama EK, Rivard G, Acheson F, Cook CD. The effect of changes in maternal pH and P_{CO_2} of fetal lambs. *Anesthesiology* 1967; 28: 891–903.

101 Motoyama EK, Rivard G *et al.* Adverse effect of maternal hyperventilation of the fetus. *Lancet* 1966; i: 286–8.

102 Fan Chung K, Barnes PJ. Prescribing in pregnancy. Treatment of asthma. *Br Med J* 1987; 294: 103–5.

103 Kendrick AH, Higgs CMB *et al.* Accuracy of perception of severity of asthma: patients treated in general practice. *Br Med J* 1999; 307: 422–4.

104 Windebank WJ, Boyd G *et al.* Pulmonary thromboembolism presenting as asthma. *Br Med J* 1973; i: 90.

105 Gurewich V, Sasahara AA *et al.* Pulmonary Embolic Disease. Grune & Stratton, New York, 1965.

106 Schatz M, Zeiger RS *et al.* The safety of asthma and allergy medications during pregnancy. *J Allergy Clin Immunol* 1997; 100 (3): 301–6.

107 Carswell F, Kerr MM *et al.* Congenital goitre and hypothyroidism produced by maternal ingestion of iodides. *Lancet* 1970; i: 1241.

108 Galina MP, Avnet NL *et al.* Iodides during pregnancy: Apparent cause of fetal death. *N Engl J Med* 1962; 267: 1124.

109 Varheer H. Drug excretion in breast milk. *Postgrad Med* 1974; 56: 97–104.

110 Metzger WJ, Turner E *et al.* The safety of immunotherapy during pregnancy. *J Allergy Clin Immunol* 1978; 61: 268–72.

111 Wendel GD, Stark BJ *et al.* Penicillin allergy and desensitization in serious infection during pregnancy. *N Engl J Med* 1985; 312: 1229–32.

112 British Thoracic Society *et al.* The British Guidelines on Asthma Management 1995 Review and Position Statement. *Thorax* 1997; 52 (Suppl. 1): S1–S21.

113 MacDonald JB, MacDonald ET *et al.* Asthma deaths in Cardiff 1963–74: 53 deaths in hospital. *Br Med J* 1976; 2: 721–3.

114 Fischl MA, Pitchenick A *et al.* An index predicting relapse and need for hospitalization in patients with acute bronchial asthma. *N Engl J Med* 1981; 305: 783–9.

115 Stenius Aarniala BS, Hedman J *et al.* Acute asthma during pregnancy. *Thorax* 1996; 51 (4): 411–14.

116 Gelber M, Sidi Y *et al.* Uncontrollable life-threatening status asthmaticus—an indicator for termination of pregnancy by caesarean section. *Respiration* 1984; 46: 320–2.

117 Shanies HM, Venkataraman MT *et al.* Reversal of intractable acute severe asthma by first-trimester termination of pregnancy. *J Asthma* 1997; 34 (2): 169–72.

118 Wong CS, Pavord ID *et al.* Bronchodilator, cardiovascular, and hypokalaernic effects of fenoterol, salbutamol, and terbutaline in asthma. *Lancet* 1990; 336: 1396–7.

119 Lewis PJ, de Swiet M *et al.* How obstetricians in the United Kingdom manage preterm labour. *Br J Obstet Gynaecol* 1980; 87: 574–7.

120 Heinonen OP, Slone D *et al. Birth Defects and Drugs in Pregnancy.* Publishing Sciences Group, Boston, Massachusetts, 1977.

121 de Swiet M, Fidler J. Heart disease in pregnancy: some controversies. *J R Coll Phys* 1981; 15: 183–6.

122 Hemminki E, Starfield B. Prevention and treatment of premature labour by drugs: review of clinical trials. *Br J Obstet Gynaecol* 1978; 85: 411–17.

123 Pearlman DS, Chervinsky P *et al.* A comparison of salmeterol with albuterol in the treatment of mild to moderate asthma. *N Engl J Med* 1992; 327: 1420–5.

124 Greening A, Ind PW *et al.* Added salmeterol versus higher-dose corticosteroid in asthma patients with symptoms on existing inhaled corticosteroid. *Lancet* 1994; 344: 219–24.

125 Greenberger P, Patterson R. Safety of therapy for allergic symptoms during pregnancy. *Ann Intern Med* 1978; 89: 234–7.

126 Alkader AA, Cole RB. Effect of aminophylline on FEV, in patients with nocturnal asthma. *Thorax* 1978; 88: 536–7.

127 Fixley M, Shen DD *et al.* Theophylline bioavailability. A comparison of the oral absorption of a theophylline elixir and two combination theophylline tablets to intravenous aminophylline. *Am Rev Respir Dis* 1977; 115: 955–62.

128 Abramowicz M. Drugs for asthma. *Med Lett Drugs Ther* 1978; 20: 69.

129 Sutton PL, Koup JR *et al.* The pharmacokinetics of theophylline in pregnancy. *J Allergy Clin Immunol* 1978; 61: 174.

130 Marx CM, Fraser DG. Treatment of asthma in pregnancy. *Obstet Gynecol* 1981; 57: 766–7.

131 Rubin PC. Prescribing in pregnancy. General principles. *Br Med J* 1986; 293: 1415–7.

132 Yurchak AM, Jusko WJ. Theophylline secretion in breast milk. *Pediatrics* 1976; 75: 518–20.

133 Nelson MM, Forfar JO. Associations between drugs administered during pregnancy and congenital abnormalities of the fetus. *Br Med J* 1971; i: 523–7.

134 Hadjigeogiou E, Kitsiou S *et al.* Antepartum aminophylline treatment for prevention of respiratory distress syndrome in premature infants. *Am J Obstet Gynecol* 1979; 135: 257–60.

135 Stenius-Aarniala B, Riikonen S *et al.* Slow-release theophylline in pregnant asthmatics. *Chest* 1996; 107 (3): 642–7 [Published erratum appears in *Chest* 109 (6): 1668.].

136 Arwood LL, Dasta JF *et al.* Placental transfer of theophylline: two case reports. *Pediatrics* 1979; 63: 844–6.

137 Yeh TF, Pildes RS. Transplacental arninophylline toxicity in a neonate. *Lancet* 1977; i: 910.

138 Dykes MHM. Evaluation of an anti-asthmatic agent cromolyn sodium (Aarare, Intal). *J Am Med Assoc* 1974; 227: 1061–2.

139 Van Arsdel PPJ, Paul GH. Drug therapy in the management of asthma. *Ann Intern Med* 1977; 87: 68–74.

140 Wendel PJ, Ramin SM *et al.* Asthma treatment in pregnancy: a randomized controlled study. *Am J Obstet Gynecol* 1996; 175 (1): 150–4.

141 Harris DM. Some properties of beclomethasone dipropionate and related steriods in man. *Postgrad Med J* 1975; 51 (Suppl. 4): 20–5.

142 Dombrowski MP, Brown CL *et al.* Preliminary experience with triamcinolone acetonide during pregnancy. *J Matern Fetal Med* 1996; 5 (6): 310–13.

143 Francis HH, Smellie J. General disease in pregnancy. *Br Med J* 1964; 1: 887–90.

144 Fainstalt T. Cortisone-induced congenital cleft palate in rabbits. *Endocrinology* 1954; 55: 502.

145 Rodriguez-Pinilla E, Martinez-Frias ML. Corticosteroids during pregnancy and oral clefts. A case-control study. *Teratology* 1998; 58: 2–5.

146 Schatz M, Patterson R *et al.* Corticosteroid therapy for the pregnant asthmatic patient. *J Am Med Assoc* 1975; 233: 804–7.

147 Bongionvanni AM, McPadden AJ. Steroids during pregnancy and possible fetal consequences. *Fertil Steril* 1960; 11: 181–6.

148 Synder RD, Synder DL. Corticosteroids for asthma during pregnancy. *Ann Allergy* 1978; 41: 340–1.

149 Driscoll AM. Urinary oestriol excretion in pregnant patients given large doses of prednisone. *Br Med J* 1969; 1: 556–7.

150 Morrison J, Kilpatrick N. Low urinary oestriol excretion in pregnancy associated with oral prednisone therapy. *J Obstet Gynaecol Br Commonwealth* 1969; 76: 719–20.

151 Wallace SJ, Michie EA. A follow-up study of infants born to mothers with low oestriol excretion during pregnancy. *Lancet* 1966; ii: 560–3.

152 Warrell DW, Taylor R. Outcome for the fetus of mother receiving prednisolone during pregnancy. *Lancet* 1968; i: 117–8.

153 Beitins R, Baynard F *et al.* The transplacental passage of prednisone and prednisolone in pregnancy near term. *J Pediatr* 1972; 81: 936–45.

154 Ballard PL, Granberg P *et al.* Glucocorticoid levels in maternal and cord serum after prenatal beclomethasone therapy to prevent respiratory distress syndrome. *J Clin Invest* 1975; 56: 1548–58.

155 Greenberg LM, Tanaka KR. Congenital anomalies probably induced by cyclophosphamide. *J Am Med Assoc* 1964; 188: 423–6.

156 Gitau R, Cameron A, *et al.* Fetal exposure to maternal cortisol *Lancet* 1998; 352: 707–8

157 Schmand B, Neuval J *et al.* Psychological development of children who were treated antenatally with corticosteroids to prevent respiratory distress syndrome: a 10–12 year follow-up. *Pediatrics* 1990; 86: 58–64.

158 Smolders de Haas H, Neuvel J. Physical development and medical history of children who were treated antenatally with corticosteroids to prevent respiratory distress syndrome: a 10–12 year follow-up. *Pediatrics* 1990; 86: 65–70 .

159 Jolivet A, Blanchier H *et al.* Blood cortisol variations during late pregnancy and labour. *Am J Obstet Gynecol* 1974; 119: 775–83.

160 Sellers WFS, Long DR. Bronchospasm following ergometrine. *Anaesthesia* 1979; 34: 909.

161 Selwyn Crawford J. Bronchospasm following ergometrine. *Anaesthesia* 1980; 35: 397–8.

162 Marx GF. Obstetric anesthesia in the presence of medical complications. *Clin Obstet Gynecol* 1974; 17: 165–81.

163 Jellife DB, Jellife EFP. 'Breast is Best': modern meanings. *N Engl J Med* 1977; 297: 912–15.

164 Oddy WH, Holt PG *et al.* Association between breast feeding and asthma in 6 year old children: findings of a prospective birth cohort study. *Br Med J* 1999; 319: 815–19.

165 Sibbald B. *A family study approach to the genetic basis of asthma.* University of London, PhD Thesis, 1981.

166 Martinez FD. Maternal risk factors in asthma. *Ciba Found Symposium* 1997; 206: 233–9.

167 Jones CA, Warner JA, Warner JO. Fetal swallowing of IgE. *Lancet* 1998; 351: 1859.

168 Ewan PW. Prevention of peanut allergy. *Lancet* 1998; 352: 4–5.

169 Mazzotta P, Loebstein R, Koren G. Treating allergic rhinitis in pregnancy. Safety considerations. *Drug Saf* 1999; 20 (4): 361–75.

170 Zielonka TM, Dabrowski A, Droszcz W. Efficacite de la betamethazone-retard dans le syndrome de Churg et Strauss. A propos d'un cas. [Efficacy of slow-release betamethasone in Churg–Strauss syndrome. Apropos of a case]. *Rev Pneumol Clin* 1994; 50 (2): 77–9.

171 Priori R, Tomassini M *et al.* Churg–Strauss syndrome during pregnancy after steroid withdrawal. *Lancet* 1998; 352: 1599–60.

172 Bonebrake CR, Noller KL *et al.* Routine chest roentography in pregnancy. *J Am Med Assoc* 1978; 240: 2747–8.

173 Glass DD, Ginburgh FW, Boucot KK. Screening procedures for pulmonary disease in prenatal patients. *Am Rev Respir Dis* 1960; 82: 689.

174 Mattox JH. The value of a routine prenatal chest X-ray. *Obstet Gynaecol* 1973; 41: 243–5.

175 Stanton SL. Routine radiology of the chest in antenatal care. *J Obstet Gynaecol Br Comonw* 1968; 75: 1161–4.

176 Plauche WC, Buechner HA, Diket AL. Tuberculosis prenatal screening and therapy during pregnancy. *J Louisiana State Assoc* 1983; 135: 13–15.

176a Sulavik SB. Pulmonary disease. In: Burrow GN & Ferris TF (eds) *Medical Complications during Pregancy*. WB Saunders, Philadelphia, 1975, p. 549.

177 Nolan TE, Espinosa TL *et al.* Tuberculosis skin testing in pregnancy: trends in apopulation. *J Perinatol* 1997; 17: 199–201.

178 Takamutsu I, Kameda M *et al.* Tuberculosis outbreak among inpatients. *Kekkaku* 1999; 74: 397–494.

179 Carter EJ, Mates S. Tuberculosis during pregnancy. The Rhode island experience; 1987 to 1991. *Chest* 1994. 106: 1466–70.

180 Cohen JD, Patton EA, Badger TL. The tuberculous mother. *Am Rev Tuberc* 1952; 65: 1–23.

181 Barnes CG. *Medical Disorders in Obstetric Practice*. Blackwell Scientific Publications, Oxford, 1974.

182 Hedvall E. Pregnancy and tuberculosis. *Acta Med Scand* 1953; 286 (Suppl. 147): 1–101.

183 Selikoff IJ, Dormann HL. Management of tuberculosis. In: *Medical, Surgical and Gynecologic Complications in Pregnancy*, 2nd edn. Williams & Wilkins, Baltimore, 1965.

184 de March P. Tuberculosis and pregnancy. Five to ten year review of 215 patients in their fertile age. *Chest* 1975 (68): 800–4.

185 Espinal MA, Reingold AL *et al.* Effect of pregnancy on the risk of developing active tuberculosis *J Infect Dis* 1996; 173: 488–91.

186 Schaefer G, Zervoudakis TA, Fuchs FF, David S. Pregnancy and pulmonary tuberculosis. *Obstet Gynecol* 1975; 46: 706–15.

187 Figueroa-Damian R, Arrendondo-Garcia JL. Neonatal outcome of children born to women with tuberculosis *Arch Med Res* 2001; 32: 66–69.

188 Bjerkedal T, Bahna SL, Lehmann EH. Cause and outcome of women with pulmonary tuberculosis. *Scand J Respir Dis* 1975; 56: 245–50.

189 Beitzki NK. Uber die angioborne tuberkulase infektion. *Ergeb Tuberk Fortschr* 1935; 7: 1–30.

190 Snider DE, Layde PM, Johnson NW, Lyle HA. Treatment of tuberculosis during pregnancy. *Am Rev Respir Dis* 1980; 122: 65–78.

191 Marciniuk DD, McNab BD *et al.* Detection of pulmonary tuberculosis in patients with a normal chest radiograph. *Chest* 1999; 115: 445–52

192 Doveren RF Block R. Tuberculosis and pregnancy—a provincial study. *Neth J Med* 1998; 52: 100–6.

193 Finn R, St Hill CA *et al.* Immunological responses in pregnancy and survival of fetal homograft. *Br Med J* 1972; 3: 150–2.

194 Present PA, Comstock GW. Tubercular sensitivity in pregnancy. *Am Rev Respir Dis* 1975; 122: 413–16.

195 Sepulveda RL Gonzalez B *et al.* The influence of BCG immunization on tuberculin reactivity in healthy Chilean women in the third trimester of pregnancy. *Tuber Lung Dis* 1995; 76: 28–34.

196 Snider DE. Pregnancy and tuberculosis. *Chest* 1984; 86: 10S–13S.

197 Potworoska M, Sianozeka E, Szufladowicz R. Ethionamide treatment in pregnancy. *Polish Med J* 1966; 5: 1152–8.

198 Citron K. Ethambutol: a review with special reference to ocular toxicity. *Tubercle* 1969; 50: (Suppl.) 32–6.

199 Lewitt T, Neibel L, Terracina S, Karman S. Ethambutol in pregnancy. Observations on embryogenesis. *Chest* 1974; 66: 25–6.

200 Brobowitz ID. Ethambutol in pregnancy. *Chest* 1974; 66: 20–4.

201 Monnet P, Kalb JC, De Pujol M. L'influence nocive de l'isoniazide sur le produit de conception. *Lyon Med* 1967; 218: 431–55.

202 Atkins NA. Maternal plasma concentrations of pyridoxal phosphate during pregnancy: adequacy of vitamin B6 supplementation during isoniazid therapy. *Am Rev Respir Med* 1982; 126: 714–16.

203 Brummer DL. Letter to the editor. *Am Rev Respir Dis* 1972; 106: 785.

204 South M Neonatal seizures after use of pyidoxine in pregnancy *Lancet* 1999; 353: 1940–1.

205 Franks AL Binkin NJ *et al.* Isoniazid hepatitis among pregnant and postpartum Hispanic patients. *Public Health Reports* 1989; 104: 151–5.

206 Davidson PT Le HQ. Drug treatment of tuberculosis. *Drugs* 1992; 43: 651–73.

207 Conway N, Birt BD. Streptomycin in pregnancy: effect on the foetal ear. *Br Med J* 1965; 2: 260–3.

208 Robinson GC, Cambon KG. Hearing loss in infants of tuberculous mothers treated with streptomycin during pregnancy. *N Engl J Med* 1964; 271: 949–51.

209 Brost BC Newman RB. The maternal and fetal effects of tuberculosis therapy. *Obstet Gynecol Clin North Am* 1997; 24: 659–73.

210 Cole RB. Modern management of pulmonary tuberculosis. *Prescr J* 1985; 25: 110–18.

211 Jana N, Vasishta K *et al.* Obstetrical outcomes among women with extrapulmonary tuberculosis. *N Engl J Med* 199; 341: 645–9.

212 Brooks JM, Stirrat GM. Tuberculous peritonitis in pregnancy. Case report. *Br J Obstet Gynaecol* 1986; 93: 1009–10.

213 Joshi MA, Balsarkar D *et al.* Massive rectal bleeding due to jejunal and colonic tuberculosis *Trop Gastroenterol* 1998; 19: 168–70.

214 Bowley DG Lloyd J *et al.* Tuberculous pericarditis presenting as pericardial tamponade. *J R Army Med Corps* 1998; 144: 31–3.

215 Figueroa-Damian R, Arrendondo-Garcia JL. Pregnancy and tuberculosis: influence of treatment on perinatal outcome *Am J Perinatol* 1998; 15: 303–6

216 Gordon-Nesbitt DC, Rajan G. Congenital TB successfully treated. *Br Med J* 1973; i: 233–4.

217 Mucklow ES. Tuberculous meningitis in labour. *J Obstet Gynecol* 1987; 8: 145.

218 Editorial. Perinatal prophylaxis of tuberculosis. *Lancet* 1990; 336: 1479–80.

219 Snider DE. Should women taking antituberculous drugs breast feed? *Arch Intern Med* 1984; 144: 589–90.

220 Grossman IIJH, Littler MD. Severe sarcoidosis in pregnancy. *Obstet Gynecol* 1976; 50 (Suppl.): 81S–84S.

221 Haynes de Reg R. Sarcoidosis and pregnancy. *Obstet Gynecol* 1987; 70: 369–72.

222 Reisfeld DR, Yahia C, Laurenz GA. Pregnancy and cardiorespiratory failure in Boeck's sarcoid. *Surg Gynecol Obstet* 1969; 109: 412–16.

223 James DG. Sarcoidosis. *Disease-a-Month* 1970; 1: 43.

224 Agha FP, Vade A, Amendola MA, Cooper RF. Effects of pregnancy on sarcoidosis. *Surg Gynecol Obstet* 1982; 155: 817–22.

225 Case BW, Benaroya S. Dyspnoea in a pregnant young woman. *Can Med Assoc J* 1980; 122: 890–6.

226 McCarty KS, Mossler JA, McLelland R, Seiker HO. Pulmonary lymphangiomyomatosis responsive to progesterone. *N Engl J Med* 1980; 303: 1461–5.

227 Cugini P, Letizia C *et al.* Circadian variation in serum angiotensin converting enzyme activity in normal and hypertensive pregnancy. *J Obstet Gynecol* 1989; 10: 124.

228 Erskine KJ, Taylor KS, Agnew RAL. Serial estimation of serum angiotensin converting enzyme activity during and after pregnancy in a woman with sarcoidosis. *Br Med J* 1985; 290: 269–70.

229 Keleman JT, Mandl L. Sarcoidose in der placenta. *Zent.t Alleg Pathologie Pathological* 1969; 112: 18.

230 Arsura EL, Kilgore WB *et al.* Erythema nodosum in pregnant patients with coccidioidomycosis *Clin Infect Dis* 1998; 27: 1201–3.

231 Bartelsmeyer JA, Petrie RH. Erythema nodosum, estrogens and pregnancy. *Clin Obstet Gynecol* 1990; 33: 777–81.

232 Salvatore MA, Lynch PJ. Erythema nodosum, estrogens and pregnancy. *Arch Dermatol* 1980; 116: 557–8.

233 Murty GE, Davison JM, Cameron DS. Wegener's granulomatosis complicating pregnancy. *Br J Obstet Gynaecol* 1990; 10: 399–400.

234 Talbot SF, Main DM, Levinson AI. Wegener's granulomatosis: first report of a case with onset during pregnancy. *Arthritis Rheumatol* 1984; 27: 109–11.

235 Cooper K, Stafford J, Turner Warwick M. Wegener's granuloma complicating pregnancy. *Br J Obstet Gynaecol* 1970; 77: 1028–30.

236 Coates A. Cyclophosphamide in pregnancy. *Aust NZ J Obstet Gynaecol* 1970; 10: 33–4.

237 Toledo TM, Harper RC, Moser RH. Fetal effects during cyclophosphamide and radiation therapy. *Ann Intern Med* 1971; 74: 87–91.

238 Wheeler GE. Cyclophosphamide associated leukaemia in Wegener's granulomatosis. *Ann Intern Med* 1981; 94: 161–2.

239 Casciato J. Leukaemia following cytotoxic therapy. *Medicine* 1979; 58: 32–47.

240 Cohen Tervaert JW, Huitema MG *et al.* Prevention of relapses in Wegener's granulomatosis by treatment based on antineutrophil cytoplasmic antibody titre. *Lancet* 1990; 336: 709–11.

241 Kumar A, Mohan A *et al.* Relapse of Wegener's granulomatosis in the first trimester of pregnancy: a case report. *Br J Rheumatol* 1998; 37: 331–3.

242 Pauzner R Mayan H *et al.* Exacerbation of Wegener's granulomatosis during pregnancy: report of a case with tracheal stenosis and literature review. *J Rheumatol* 1994; 21: 1153–6.

243 Lavin JP, Miodovaik M. Pulmonary eosinophilic granuloma complicating pregnancy. *Obstet Gynecol* 1981; 58: 516–19.

244 Corrin B, Liebow AA, Friedman PJ. Pulmonary lymphangiomyomatosis. A review. *Am J Pathol* 1975; 79: 348–67.

245 Silverstein EF, Ellis K, Wolff M, Jaretzki A. Pulmonary lymphangiomyomatosis. *Am Roentgenol Rad Ther Nucl Med* 1974; 120: 832–50.

246 Taylor RJ, Rym J, Colby TV, Raffin TA. Lymphangiomyomatosis—clinical course in 32 patients. *N Engl J Med* 1990; 323: 1254–60.

247 Shen A, Iseman MD, Waldron JA, King TE. Exacerbation of pulmonary lymphangioleiomyomatosis by exogenous estrogens. *Chest* 1987; 91: 782–5.

248 Hughes E, Hodder RV. Pulmonary lymphangiomyomatosis complicating pregnancy. A case report. *J Reprod Med* 1987; 32: 553–7.

249 Murata A, Takeda Y *et al.* A case of pulmonary lymphangiomyomatosis induced by pregnancy. *Nippon Kyobu Shikkan Gakkai Zasshi* 1989; 27: 1106–11.

250 Raffin TA, Taylor JR, Ryu J, Colby TV. Treatment of lymphangiomyomatosis. *N Engl J Med* 1991; 325: 64.

251 Elder HA, Santamarine BAG, Smith S, Kass EH. The natural history of asymptomatic bacteriuria during pregnancy: The effect of tetracycline on the clinical course and outcome of pregnancy. *Am J Obstet Gynecol* 1971; 111: 441–62.

252 Corcoran K, Castles JM. Tetracycline for acne vulgaris and possible teratogenesis. *Br Med J* 1977; 2: 807–8.

253 Kunelis CT, Peters JL, Edmondson HA. Fatty liver of pregnancy and its relationship to tetracycline therapy. *Am J Med* 1965; 38: 359–77.

254 White RJ, Harrison KJ, Clarke SKR. Causes of pneumonia presenting to a district general hospital. *Thorax* 1981; 36: 566–70.

255 Opsahl MS, O'Brien WF. Systemic nocardiosis in pregnancy. *J Reprod Med* 1983; 28: 621–3.

256 Jensen LP, O'Sullivan MJ *et al.* Acquired immunodeficiency (AIDS) in pregnancy. *Am J Obstet Gynecol* 1984; 148: 1145–6.

257 Philipson A. Pharmacokinetics of ampicillin during pregnancy. *J Infect Dis* 1977; 136: 3070–6.

258 Oxorn H. The changing aspects of pneumonia complicating pregnancy. *Obstet Gynecol* 1955; 70: 1057.

259 Berkowitz K, LaSala A. Risk factors associated with the increasing prevalence of pneumonia during pregnancy. *Am J Obstet Gynecol* 1990; 163: 981–5.

260 Greenberg M, Jacobziner H, Paketer J, Weisel BAG. Maternal mortality in the epidemic of Asian influenza New York City 1957. *Am J Obstet Gynecol* 1958; 76: 897–902.

261 Freeman DW, Barno A. Death with Asian influenza associated with pregnancy. *Am J Obstet Gynecol* 1959; 78: 1172–5.

262 Griffith ER. Viral pneumonia in pregnancy: report of a case complicated by disseminated intravascular coagulation and acute renal failure. *Am J Obstet Gynecol* 1974; 120: 201–2.

263 Novy MJ, Tyler JM *et al.* Cystic fibrosis and pregnancy. *Obstet Gynecol* 1967; 30: 530–6.

264 Editorial. Pregnant patients and swine flu vaccine. *Contemp Obstet Gynecology* 1976; 8: 74–5.

265 Parayani SG, Arvin AM. Intrauterine infection with varicella zoster after maternal varicella. *N Engl J Med* 1986; 314: 1542–6.

266 Gilbert GL. Chickenpox during pregnancy. *Br Med J* 1993; 306: 1079–80.

267 Boyd K, Walker E. Use of acyclovir to treat chickenpox in pregnancy. *Br Med J* 1988; 296: 393–4.

268 Cox SM, Cunningham FG, Luby J. Management of varicella pneumonia complicating pregnancy. *Am J Perinatol* 1990; 7: 300–1.

269 Glaser JB, Loftus J *et al.* Varicella zoster infection in pregnancy. *N Engl J Med* 1986; 315: 1416.

270 Haake DA, Zakowski PC, Haake DL, Bryson YJ. Early treatment with acyclovir for varicella pneumonia in otherwise healthy adults: retrospective controlled study and review. *Rev Infect Dis* 1990; 12: 788–98.

271 Dunkle LM, Arvin AM *et al.* A controlled trial of acyclovir for chickenpox in normal children. *N Engl J Med* 1991; 325: 1539–44.

272 Cantanazaro A. Pulmonary mycosis in pregnant women. *Chest* 1984; 68: 145–85.

273 Drutz DK, Muppert M, Sun SH, McCuire WL. Human sex hormones stimulate the growth and maturation of *Coccidioides immitis*. *Infect Immun* 1981; 32: 897–907.

274 Smale LE, Waechter KG. Dissemination of coccidiodomycosis. *Am J Obstet Gynecol* 1976; 107: 356–61.

275 Ismail MA, Lerner SA. Disseminated blastomycosis in a pregnant women. *Am Rev Respir Dis* 1982; 128: 350–3.

276 Editorial. Cystic fibrosis in adults. *Br Med J* 1979; 2: 626.

277 The British Paediatric Working Party of Cystic Fibrosis. Cystic fibrosis in the United Kingdom 1977–85: an improving picture. *Br Med J* 1988; 297: 1599–602.

278 Kerem E, Reisman J et al. Prediction of mortality in patients with cystic fibrosis. *N Engl J Med* 1992; 326: 1187–91.

279 Dodge JA, Morrison S et al. (the UK Cystic Fibrosis Survey Management Committee). Incidence, population and survival of cystic fibrosis in the United Kingdom 1968–1995. *Arch Dis Child* 1997; 77: 493–6.

280 Wald NJ. Couple screening for cystic fibrosis. *Lancet* 1991; 338: 1318–9.

281 Harris H, Scotcher D et al. Cystic fibrosis carrier testing in early pregnancy by general practitioners. *Br Med J* 1993; 306: 1580–3.

282 Super M, Ivinson A et al. Clinic experience of prenatal diagnosis of cystic fibrosis by use of linked DNA probes. *Lancet* 1987; ii: 782–4.

283 Farrall M, Law H et al. First-trimester prenatal diagnosis of cystic fibrosis with linked DNA probes. *Lancet* 1986; i: 1402–5.

284 Handyside AH, Lesko JG et al. Birth of a normal girl after *in vitro* fertilization and preimplantation diagnosis testing for cystic fibrosis. *N Engl J Med* 1992; 327: 905–9.

285 Scott J, Higenbottam T et al. Heart-lung transplantation for cystic fibrosis. *Lancet* 1988; ii: 192–4.

286 Johnson SR, Varner MW, Yates SJ, Hanson R. Diagnosis of maternal cystic fibrosis during pregnancy. *Obstet Gynecol* 1983; 61 (Suppl.): 2S–7S.

287 Matson JA, Capen CV. Pregnancy in the cystic fibrosis patient. *J Reprod Med* 1982; 27: 373–5.

288 Palmer J, Dillon-Baker C et al. Pregnancy in patients with cystic fibrosis. *Ann Intern Med* 1983; 99: 596–600.

289 Shaw LMA. Cystic fibrosis and reproductive function. *J Obstet Gynecology* 1985; 6: 1–5.

290 Phelan D. Cystic fibrosis and pregnancy. *Med J Aust* 1981; 1: 58.

291 di Saint'Agnese PA, Davis PB. Cystic fibrosis in adults. *Am J Med* 1979; 66: 121–32.

292 Cohen LF, di Saint'Agnese PA, Freidlander J. Cystic fibrosis and pregnancy. A national survey. *Lancet* 1980; ii: 842–4.

293 Cystic Fibrosis Foundation. *1974 Report on Survival of Patients with Cystic Fibrosis*. Cystic Fibrosis Foundation, Rockville, Maryland, 1976.

294 Warwick WJ, Progue RE, Gerber HM, Nesbitt CJ. Survival patterns in cystic fibrosis. *J Chron Dis* 1975; 28: 609–22.

295 Corkey CWB, Newth CJL, Corey M, Levison H. Pregnancy in cystic fibrosis: a better prognosis in patients with pancreatic function? *Am J Obstet Gynecol* 1981; 140: 737–42.

296 Taussig LM, Kattwinkel J, Freidwald WT, di Saint'Agnese PA. A new prognostic score and clinical evaluation system for cystic fibrosis. *J Pediatr* 1973; 82: 380–90.

297 Rosenthal A, Tucker CR et al. Echocardiographic assessment of cor pulmonale in cystic fibrosis. *Pediatr Clin North Am* 1976; 23: 327–44.

298 Ryssing E. Assessment of cor pulmonale in cystic fibrosis by echocardiography. *Acta Paediatr Scand* 1977; 66: 753–6.

299 Siassi B, Moss AJ, Dooley RR. Clinical recognition of cor pulmonale in cystic fibrosis. *J Pediatr* 1971; 78: 794.

300 Psacharopoulos HT, Howard ER et al. Hepatic complications of cystic fibrosis. *Lancet* 1981; ii: 78–80.

301 Isenberg JN, L'Heureuse DR. Clinical observation on the biliary system in cystic fibrosis. *Am J Gastroenterol* 1976; 65: 134–9.

302 Whitelaw A, Butterfield A. High breast milk sodium in cystic fibrosis. *Lancet* 1977; ii: 1288.

303 Alpert SE, Cormier AD. Normal electrolyte and protein content in milk from mothers with cystic fibrosis: an explanation for the initial report of elevated milk sodium concentration. *J Pediatr* 1983; 102: 77–80.

304 Thaler I, Bronstein M, Rubin AE. The course and outcome of pregnancy associated with bronchiectasis. Case report. *Br J Obstet Gynaecol* 1986; 93: 1006–8.

305 Howie AD, Milne JA. Pregnancy in patients with bronchiectasis. *Br J Obstet Gynaecol* 1978; 85: 197–200.

306 Lalli CM, Raju L. Pregnancy and chronic obstructive pulmonary disease. *Chest* 1981; 80: 759–61.

307 Giesler CF, Buchler JH, Depp R. Alpha-antitrypsin deficiency, severe obstructive lung disease and pregnancy. *Obstet Gynecol* 1977; 49: 31–4.

308 Kennedy SH. A case of pre-eclampsia in a woman with homozygous Pizz-alpha-$_1$-antitrypsin deficiency. *Br J Obstet Gynecol* 1987; 94: 1103–4.

309 Gustavii B, Edvall H et al. Acyclovir in prophylaxis and treatment of perinatal varicella. *Lancet* 1987; i: 161.

310 Editorial. Alpha$_1$–antitrypsin deficiency and prenatal diagnosis. *Lancet* 1987; i: 421–2.

311 Kopenhager T. A review of 50 pregnant patients with kyphoscoliosis. *Br J Obstet Gynaecol* 1977; 84: 585.

312 Mendelson CL. Pregnancy and kyphoscoliotic heart disease. *Am J Obstet Gynecol* 1958; 56: 457.

313 Lao TT, Yeung S, Leung BFH. Kyphoscoliosis and pregnancy. *J Obstet Gynaecol* 1986; 7: 11–15.

314 Barrett JFR, Dear PRF, Lilford RJ. Brain damage as a result of chronic intra-uterine hypoxia in a baby born of a severely kyphoscoliotic mother. *J Obstet Gynaecol* 1991; 11: 260–1.

315 Siegler D, Zorab PA. Pregnancy in thoracic scoliosis. *Br J Disord Chest* 1981; 75: 367–700.

316 Sawicka EH, Spencer GT, Branthwaite MA. Management of respiratory failure complicating pregnancy in severe kyphoscoliosis: a new use for an old technique? *Br J Dis Chest* 1986; 80: 191–6.

317 Berman AT, Cohen DL, Schwentker EP. The effects of pregnancy on idiopathic scoliosis. *Spine* 1982; 7: 76–7.

318 Allanson JE, Hall JG. Obstetric and gynecologic problems in women with chondrodystrophies. *Obstet Gynecol* 1986; 67: 74–80.

319 Andersen HF, Lynch JP, Johnson TRB. Adult respiratory distress syndrome in obstetrics and gynecology. *Obstet Gynecol* 1980; 55: 291–5.

320 Cunningham FG, Leveno KJ, Hawkins GDV, Whally PJ. Respiratory insufficiency associated with pyelonephritis during pregnancy. *Obstet Gynecol* 1984; 63: 121–5.

321 O'Sullivan GM, Bullingham RES. The assessment of gastric acidity and antacid effect in pregnant women by a non-invasive radiotelemetry technique. *Br J Obstet Gynaecol* 1984; 91: 973–8.

322 Ridgway LF, Martin RW *et al*. Acute gestational pyelonephritis: the impact of colloid osmotic pressure, plasma fibronectin, and arterial oxygen saturation. *Am J Perinatol* 1991; 8: 222–6.

323 Towers CV, Kaminskas CM *et al*. Pulmonary injury associated with antepartum pyelonephritis: can patients at risk be identified? *Am J Obstet Gynecol* 1991; 164: 974–8.

324 MacLennan FM. Maternal mortality from Mendelson's syndrome: an explanation. *Lancet* 1986; i: 587–9.

325 Thornmasen HY, Russell JA, Boyko WJ, Hogg JC. Transient leucopenia associated with adult respiratory distress syndrome. *Lancet* 1984; i: 809–12.

326 Keefer JR, Strauss RG, Givetta JM, Burke T. Noncardiogenic pulmonary edema and invasive cardiovascular monitoring. *Obstet Gynecol* 1981; 58: 46–51.

327 Wilson JW. Treatment or prevention of pulmonary cellular damage with pharmacological doses of corticosteroids. *Surg Gynecol Obstet* 1972; 134: 675.

328 Blaisdell FW, Schlobohm RM. The respiratory distress syndrome: a review. *Surgery* 1973; 74: 251.

329 Bernard GR, Luce JM *et al*. High-dose corticosteroids in patients with adult respiratory distress syndrome. *N Engl J Med* 1987; 317: 1565–70.

330 Shanies HM. Non-cardiogenic pulmonary oedema. *Med Clin North Am* 1977; 61: 1319.

331 Burgener L, Solmes JG. Spontaneous pneumothorax and pregnancy. *Can Med Assoc J* 1979; 120: 19.

332 Spellacy WN, Prem KA. Subcutaneous emphysema and pregnancy. Report of three cases. *Obstet Gynecol* 1963; 22: 521–3.

333 Hague WM. Mediastinal and subcutaneous emphysema in a pregnant asthmatic. *Br J Obstet Gynaecol* 1980; 87: 440–3.

334 Henry RJW, Vadas RA. Spontaneous rupture of the oesophagus following severe vomiting in early pregnancy. Case report. *Br J Obstet Gynecol* 1986; 93: 392–4.

335 Griffith HB, Barnes JC. Severe sarcoidosis in pregnancy. *Obstet Gynecol* 1987; 7: 272–3.

336 Luby BJ, Georgiev M, Warren SG, Capito R. Postpartum pneumopericardium. *Obstet Gynaecol* 1978; 62: 46S–50S.

337 Hamman L. Mediastinal emphysema. *J Am Med Assoc* 1945; 128: 1.

338 Farrell SJ. Spontaneous pneumothorax in pregnancy: a case report and review of the literature. *Obstet Gynecol* 1983; 62: 43S–45S.

339 Gray JM, Hanson CC. Mediastinal emphysema: Aetiology, diagnosis and treatment. *Thorax* 1966; 21: 325–31.

340 Hughson WG, Friedman PJ *et al*. Postpartum pleural effusion: a common radiologic finding. *Ann Intern Med* 1982; 97: 856–8.

341 Spring JE, Winston RML. Congenital lymphoedema and its complications in pregnancy and the puerperium. *J Obstet Gynaecol* 1985; 5: 170–3.

342 Udeshi UL, McHugo JM, Crawford JS. Postpartum pleural effusion. *Br J Obstet Gynaecol* 1988; 95: 894–7.

343 Suonio S, Saaranen M, Saarikoski S. Left-sided hydrothorax in connection with severe pre-eclampsia: case reports. *Int J Gynaecol Obstet* 1984; 22: 357–61.

344 Department of Health and Social Security. *Report on Confidential Enquiries into Maternal Deaths in England and Wales*. HMSO, London, 1991.

345 Department of Health. *Report on Confidential Enquiries into Maternal Deaths in the United Kingdom, 1988–90*. HMSO, London, 1994.

346 Department of Health and Social Security. *Report on Confidental Enquiries into Maternal Deaths in England and Wales, 1979–1981*. HMSO, London, 1986.

347 Pedersen H, Finster M. Anesthetic risk in the pregnant surgical patient. *Anesthesiology* 1979; 51: 439–51.

348 Scott DB. Mendelson's syndrome. *Br J Anaesth* 1978; 50: 81–2.

349 Bond VK, Stoetling RK, Cupta CD. Pulmonary aspiration syndrome after inhalation of gastric fluid containing antacids. *Anesthesiology* 1979; 51: 452–3.

350 Tatersall MP. Prescribing drugs in pregnancy. *Br J Hosp Med* 1983; 29: 382.

351 Dundee JW, Moore J, Johnston JF, McCaughey W. Cimetidine and obstetric anaesthesia. *Lancet* 1981; ii: 252.

352 McAvley DM, Halliday HL, Johnston JR, Dundee JW. Cimetidine in labour: absence of adverse effect on the high-risk fetus. *Br J Obstet Gynaecol* 1985; 92: 350–5.

353 McCaughey W, Howe JP, Moore J, Dundee JW. Cimetidine in elective Caesarean section: effect on gastric acidity. *Anaesthesia* 1981; 36: 167–72.

354 Howard FA, Sharp DS. Effect of metoclopramide on gastric emptying during labour. *Br Med J* 1973; 1: 446–8.

355 Drug and Therapeutics Bulletin. Prophylaxis against Mendelson's syndrome. *Drug Ther Bull* 1986; 24: 31–2.

356 Albright GA. *Anesthesia in Obstetrics, Maternal, Fetal and Neonatal Aspects*. Addison-Wesley, Massachussetts, 1978.

357 Sangoul F, Fox GS, Houle GL. Effect of regional analgesia on maternal oxygen consumption during the first stage of labour. *Am J Obstet Gynecol* 1975; 121: 1080.

358 Nava S, Zanotti E *et al*. Evidence of acute diaphragmatic fatigue in a 'natural' condition: the diaphragm during labour. *Annu Rev Respir Dis* 1992; 146: 1226–30.

359 Conn DA, Moffat AC, McCallum GDR, Thorburn J. Changes in pulmonary function test during spinal anaesthesia for caesarean section. *Int J Obstet Anesth* 1993; 2: 12–4.

360 Harrop-Griffiths AW, Ravalia A, Browne DA, Robinson PN. Regional anaesthesia and cough effectiveness. A study of patients undergoing caesarean section. *Anaesthesia* 1991; 46: 11–13.

2 Blood volume, haematinics, anaemia

Elizabeth A. Letsky

Blood volume

Although the 'plethora' of pregnancy was recognized early in the 19th century and German work as far back as 1854 showed a rise of blood volume in pregnant laboratory animals, the evidence for plethora in pregnant women rested primarily on the demonstration of reduced concentration of solids and cells in the blood until the early 20th century [1]. The best estimate of total blood volume is obtained when plasma volume and red cell mass are measured simultaneously; however, the majority of published reports of blood volume in pregnancy are based on either measured plasma volume or total red cell mass, the fraction not directly estimated being calculated from whole blood haematocrit.

Plasma volume

The measurement of plasma volume in pregnancy has a long history, which was comprehensively reviewed by Hytten and Leitch [2], later summarized and updated [3]. Plasma volume rises progressively throughout pregnancy, with a tendency to plateau in the last 8 weeks [4]. The terminal fall in plasma volume described by almost all investigators previously, occurs only when measurements are made in the supine position. The underestimation in the supine position is due to the bulky uterus obstructing venous return from the lower limbs resulting in incomplete mixing of dye [5]—a similar condition to the reduction in cardiac output seen in patients in the supine position (see Chapter 5).

There is little doubt that the amount of increase in plasma volume is correlated with obstetric outcome and the birthweight of the baby [2,4,6]. Because second and subsequent pregnancies tend to be more successful than the first, with bigger babies, a larger plasma volume increase in multigravidae would be expected; however, the evidence for this is not entirely satisfactory [2].

Women with multiple pregnancy have proportionately higher increments of plasma volume. The plasma volume at term was found to be approximately 1940 mL above control in eight women with twins and 2400 mL above control in eight women with twins and 2400 mL above control in two women with triplets [7]. One woman with a quadruplet pregnancy had raised her plasma volume by 2400 mL above her non-pregnant value by 34 weeks [8].

In contrast, women with poorly growing fetuses (particularly multigravidae with a history of poor reproductive performance) have a correspondingly poor plasma response [9].

In summary, healthy women in a normal first pregnancy increase their plasma volume from a non-pregnant level of almost 2600 mL by about 1250 mL. Most of the rise takes place before 32–34 weeks' gestation; thereafter there is relatively little change. In subsequent pregnancies, the increase is greater. The increase is related to the size of the fetus and there are particularly large increases in association with multiple pregnancy.

Red cell mass

The red cell 'mass' is a confusing term that expresses the total volume of red cells in the circulation. The more logical alternative of red cell volume cannot be used because of its specific meaning in haematology of the volume of a single erythrocyte.

There is less published information on red cell mass than plasma volume and the results are more variable. There is still disagreement as to how much the red cell mass increases in normal pregnancy. The extent of the increase is considerably influenced by iron medication, which will cause the red cell mass to rise in apparently healthy women even if they have no clinical evidence of iron deficiency. The stimulus for increased red cell production is due in part to the rise in erythropoietin levels that occurs from early pregnancy [10].

The early literature is summarized by Hytten and Leitch [2]. If one accepts a figure of about 1400 mL for the volume of red cells in average healthy women before pregnancy, then the rise in pregnancy for women not given iron supplements is about 240 mL (18%) and for those given iron is 400 mL (30%). The red cell mass increases steadily between the end of the first trimester and term. As with plasma volume, the extent of the increase is related to the size of the conceptus, particularly large increases being seen in association with multiple pregnancy [7,8].

The red cell mass falls immediately at delivery as a result of blood loss [11]. Non-pregnant blood volumes are reached around 3 weeks after delivery.

Changes in blood volume at parturition and during the puerperium

Acute blood loss causes dramatic changes in maternal blood volume at both vaginal delivery and caesarean section. If the blood loss at vaginal delivery is meticulously measured it is more than 500 mL of blood associated with singleton delivery and almost 1000 mL at delivery of twins. Caesarean section is associated with an average loss of 1000 mL.

In the normal pregnant female at term, hypervolaemia modifies the response to blood loss considerably. The blood volume drops following the acute loss at delivery but remains relatively stable unless the blood loss exceeds 25% of the predelivery volume. There is no compensatory increase in blood volume and there is a gradual fall in plasma volume, due primarily to diuresis. The red cell mass increase during pregnancy not lost at delivery is slowly reduced as the red cells come to the end of their lifespan. The overall result is that the haematocrit gradually increases and the blood volume returns to non-pregnant levels.

In the first few days following delivery there are fluctuations in plasma volume and haematocrit due to individual responses to dehydration, pregnancy hypervolaemia and the rapidity of blood loss. The average blood loss that can be tolerated without causing a significant fall in haemoglobin concentration is about 1000 mL but this depends in turn on a healthy increase in blood volume prior to delivery. Almost all the blood loss occurs within the first hour following delivery under normal circumstances. In the following 72 h only approximately 80 mL are lost vaginally. Patients with uterine atony, extended episiotomy or lacerations will, of course, lose much more. If the haematocrit or haemoglobin concentration at 5–7 days after delivery proves to be significantly less than before delivery, either there was pathological blood loss at delivery, or there was a poor increase in blood volume during pregnancy or both [12,13].

Benefits of hypervolaemia in pregnancy

The widely differing responses in plasma volume and red cell mass should have an explanation that makes biological sense.

Hypervolaemia *per se* combats the hazard of haemorrhage for the mother at delivery, as described above. It also helps to protect the mother from hypotension in the last trimester when sequestration occurs in the lower extremities on standing, sitting or lying supine (see Chapter 5).

The red cell mass should increase in line with the need for extra oxygen. It has been calculated that by the end of pregnancy the increase in oxygen requirement is about 15–16% [3]. This is met adequately by the increase in red cell mass of 18–25% [3].

The role of the much greater increase in plasma volume becomes clear when the distribution of the raised cardiac output is defined. Most of the extra cardiac output is directed to the skin and kidneys. Both serve as organs of excretion during pregnancy; the skin to allow for heat loss. For excretion they require plasma rather than the red cells. Also the decrease in viscosity caused by a low haematocrit causes decreased resistance to blood flow and also an increase in cardiac output with relatively less increase in cardiac work. These factors make biological sense of what is often seen as a disproportionate increase in plasma volume.

Total haemoglobin

The haemoglobin concentration, haematocrit and red cell count fall during pregnancy because the expansion of the plasma volume is greater than that of the red cell mass. However, there is a rise in total circulating haemoglobin directly related to the increase in red cell mass. This in turn is dependent partly on the iron status of the individual. Published evidence for the rise in total haemoglobin is unsatisfactory and is confused by the varying iron status of the women studied. It is impossible to give physiological limits for the expected rise in total haemoglobin until better figures are available.

The lowest normal haemoglobin in the healthy adult *non-pregnant* woman living at sea level is defined as 12 g/dL [14]. In most published studies the mean minimum in pregnancy is between 11 and 12 g/dL. The lowest haemoglobin observed in a carefully studied iron supplemented group was 10.44 g/dL [15]. The World Health Organization (WHO) recommends that haemoglobin ideally should be maintained at or above 11.0 g/dL and should not be allowed to fall below 10.5 g/dL in the second trimester [14,16,17].

Iron metabolism

In pregnancy the demand for iron is increased to meet the needs of the expanding red cell mass and requirements of the developing fetus and placenta. By far the greatest single demand for iron is that for the expansion of the red cell mass. The fetus derives its iron from the maternal serum by active transport across the placenta mainly in the last 4 weeks of pregnancy [18]. The total requirement for iron is of the order of 700–1400 mg. Overall the requirement is 4 mg/day, but this rises to 6.6 mg/day in the last few weeks of pregnancy. This can be met only by mobilizing iron stores in addition to achieving maximum absorption of dietary iron, because a normal mixed diet supplies about 14 mg of iron each day of which only 1–2 mg (5–15%) is absorbed.

Iron absorption is increased when there is erythroid hyperplasia—rapid iron turnover—and a high concentration of unsaturated transferrin all of which are part of the physiological response of the healthy pregnant woman. There is evidence that absorption of dietary iron is enhanced in the latter half of pregnancy [2] but this would still not provide enough iron for the needs of pregnancy and the puerperium for a woman on a normal mixed diet.

Iron absorption

There are at least two distinct pathways for iron absorption: one for inorganic iron and one for iron attached to haem. The availability of dietary iron is quite variable. In most foods inorganic iron is in the 'ferric' form and has to be converted to the ferrous form before absorption can take place. In foods derived from grain, iron often forms a stable complex with phylates and only small amounts can be converted to a soluble form. The iron in eggs is poorly absorbed because of binding with phosphates present in the yolk. Milk, particularly cows' milk, is poor in iron content. Tea inhibits the absorption of iron. The traditional Scottish breakfast of porridge and eggs washed down with milky tea is rich in protein but provides very little, if any, absorbable iron!

The intestinal mucosal control of iron absorption is complex and incompletely understood; however, in general, absorption is enhanced in times of increased need and deficiency. Haem iron derived from the haemoglobin and myoglobin of animal origin is more effectively absorbed than non-haem iron. Factors interfering with or promoting the absorption of inorganic iron have no effect on the absorption of haem iron. This puts vegetarians at a disadvantage in terms of iron sufficiency. The amount of iron absorbed will depend very much on the extent of the iron stores, the content of the diet and whether or not iron supplements are given. It was found, in a carefully controlled study in Sweden [19], that absorption rates differed markedly between those pregnant women receiving 100-mg ferrous iron supplements daily and those receiving a placebo. Iron absorption increased steadily throughout pregnancy in the placebo group. In the supplemented group there was no increase between the 12th and 24th week of gestation and thereafter the increase was only 60% of the placebo group. After delivery the mean absorption in the placebo group was markedly higher. These differences can be explained by the difference in storage iron between the two groups [19].

The commonest haematological problem in pregnancy is anaemia resulting from iron deficiency. The bulk of iron in the body is contained in the haemoglobin of the circulating red cells. Because many women enter pregnancy with depleted stores, it is not surprising that iron deficiency in pregnancy and the puerperium is so common when, in addition to the demands of the fetus and blood loss at delivery, the absolute red cell mass increases by approximately 25%.

Over the years there have been many studies that have proved without doubt that iron supplements prevent the development of anaemia [20–26] and that even in women taking a good diet who are not apparently anaemic at booking, the mean haemoglobin level can be raised by oral iron therapy throughout pregnancy. The difference in favour of those so treated is most marked at term when the need for haemoglobin is maximal [12,15,25].

Iron deficiency

Non-haematological effects of iron deficiency

Overt symptoms of iron deficiency are generally not prominent. Defects in oxygen carrying capacity are compensated for but the health implications of iron deficiency have been examined in a more detailed manner. Of particular interest are effects produced by impairment of the function of iron-dependent tissue enzymes. These are not the ultimate manifestation of severe untreated iron deficiency, but develop along with the fall in haemoglobin concentration [27].

It has been possible to demonstrate a marked decrease in work capacity in the iron-depleted but non-anaemic rat due to impaired mitochondrial function. There is also impairment in temperature maintenance, which has been shown in human subjects. Studies have suggested there are behavioural abnormalities in children with iron deficiency related to changes in concentration of chemical mediators in the brain [28]. Iron deficiency in the absence of anaemia is also associated with poor performance on the Bayley Mental Development Index [29]. It has also been shown that children with iron-deficiency anaemia in infancy are at risk for long-lasting developmental disadvantage compared with their peers who have better iron status [30]. These developmental delays in iron-deficient infants can be reversed by treatment with iron [31]. Performance as assessed by cognitive functioning has been shown to be improved by iron supplementation in non-anaemic iron-deficient adolescent girls in a randomized study [32].

Progress is being made in defining the biochemical abnormalities produced by iron deficiency in the central nervous system. It is well known that parenteral treatment of megaloblastic anaemia with appropriate haematinics, either folic acid or vitamin B_{12}, results in an immediate subjective feeling of improvement and well-being in the patient long before the haemoglobin level starts to rise. This is because of the non-haematological effects of depletion of these vitamins on various tissues. I have observed a similar immediate subjective feeling of well-being in those few patients under my care who have received a total dose infusion of iron, presumably for similar reasons (E.A. Letsky, personal observations). Women taking oral iron supplements often volunteer that they feel better long before the haemoglobin begins to rise significantly. Tissue enzyme malfunction undoubtedly occurs even in the very first stages of iron deficiency. Effects of iron deficiency on neuromuscular transmission may be responsible for anecdotal reports of increased blood loss at delivery in anaemic women given the importance of a well-contracted uterus to achieve haemostasis at the placental site postpartum. Various effects of iron deficiency may be responsible for the reported association between anaemia and preterm birth [33,34]. It is obvious that the prevention of nutritional iron deficiency is a desirable objective, especially when there is maximal stress on the haemopoietic system in pregnancy.

Even more far-reaching effects of maternal iron deficiency during pregnancy have been suggested. A retrospective study of 8000 deliveries at a busy obstetric unit in Oxford showed a correlation between maternal iron deficiency, high placental weight and an increased ratio of placental weight to birthweight [35]. High blood pressure in adult life has been linked with lower birthweight and high placental/birthweight ratios. More recently, in a prospective study of 1650 low-risk singleton pregnancies, placental size at term was inversely related to serum ferritin concentration at booking, supporting the previous findings [35a]. Prophylaxis of iron deficiency during pregnancy may therefore have important implications for the prevention of adult hypertension which appears to have its origin in fetal life [35–38].

Haemoglobin concentration

A reduction in concentration of circulating haemoglobin is a relatively late development in iron deficiency. This is preceded by a depletion of iron stores and then a reduction in serum iron before there is any detectable change in haemoglobin level. However, measurement of haemoglobin is the simplest, non-invasive practical test at our disposal and is the one investigation on which further action is usually taken.

The changes in blood volume and haemodilution are so variable that the normal range of haemoglobin concentration in healthy pregnancy at 30 weeks' gestation in women who have received parenteral iron is from 10 to 14.5 g/dL. However, haemoglobin values of <10.5 g/dL in the second and third trimesters are probably abnormal and require further investigation.

Red cell indices

The appearance of red cells on a stained film is a relatively insensitive gauge of iron status in pregnancy. The size of the red cell (mean corpuscular volume (MCV)), its haemoglobin content (mean corpuscular haemoglobin (MCH)) and haemoglobin concentration (mean corpuscular haemoglobin concentration (MCHC)) can be calculated from the red cell count (RBC), haemoglobin concentration and packed cell volume (PCV). A better guide to the diagnosis of iron deficiency is the examination of these red cell indices (Table 2.1).

Outside pregnancy, the earliest effect of iron-deficiency anaemia on the erythrocyte is a reduction in cell size (MCV). However, with the dramatic changes in red cell mass and plasma volume that occur during pregnancy, this does *not* appear to be the most sensitive indicator of underlying iron deficiency, and the MCV may still remain normal when stores first become depleted in the early stages of development of anaemia [39,40]. Hypochromia and a fall in MCV only appear with more severe established iron depletion.

Of course some women enter pregnancy with already established anaemia due to iron deficiency or with grossly depleted iron stores and they will quickly develop florid anaemia with reduced MCV, MCH and MCHC. These do not present any problems in diagnosis. It is those women who enter pregnancy in precarious iron balance with a normal haemoglobin concentration who present the most difficult diagnostic problems.

Serum iron and total iron-binding capacity

In health, the serum iron concentration of adult non-pregnant women lies between 13 and 27 μmol/L. It shows marked individual diurnal variation and fluctuates even from hour to hour. The total iron-binding capacity (TIBC) in the non-pregnant state lies in the range 45–72 μmol/L. It is raised in association with iron-deficiency and found to be low in chronic inflammatory states. In the non-anaemic person the TIBC is approximately one-third saturated with iron.

Most workers report a fall in the serum iron and percentage saturation of the TIBC in pregnancy; the fall in serum iron can largely be prevented by iron supplements. Serum iron even in combination with TIBC is not a reliable indication of iron stores because it fluctuates so widely and is also affected by recent ingestion of iron and other factors such as infection not directly involved with iron metabolism. With these considerable reservations, a serum iron of <12 μmol/L and a TIBC saturation of <15% indicate deficiency of iron during pregnancy.

Free erythrocyte protoporphyrin

Erythroblast protoporphyrin represents the substrate unused for haem synthesis, and levels rise when there is defective iron supply for the developing red cell. However, the use of this estimation is limited in that a misleading rise in free erythrocyte protoporphyrin (FEP) levels is observed in patients with chronic inflammatory disease, malignancy or infection. It has been dropped from the routine investigation of iron status in most laboratories.

Ferritin

Ferritin, a high molecular weight glycoprotein previously thought to be a totally intracellular iron storage compound, circulates in the plasma of healthy adults at concentrations in the range of 15–300 pg/L [41]. It is stable, not affected by recent ingestion of iron, and appears to reflect the iron stores accurately and quantitatively—particularly in the lower range associated with iron deficiency which is so important in pregnancy [39]. A study of serum ferritin during the course of pregnancy in 154 women was carried out in Cardiff [42]. The patients were divided randomly into roughly equal groups, one of which received oral iron supplements. Although there was a rapid decrease in iron stores during early pregnancy in all women studied, the stores (as assessed by serum ferritin levels) were prevented from reaching iron-deficient levels during the latter half of pregnancy in the supplemented group. This pattern has been demonstrated previously in an examination of the stainable iron in bone marrow at term [15]. Interestingly, the concentration of ferritin in the cord blood was substantially greater than the maternal level at term in all cases; but the babies born to iron-deficient mothers had significantly decreased cord ferritin levels compared to the others.

This trend was apparent in the data of another study of maternal and infant iron stores [43], although the authors interpreted their data without reference to it. There is a reduction in the iron accumulated by the fetuses of mothers with depleted iron stores and this may have an important bearing on the iron stores of the child during the first year of life.

	Normal range	Iron deficiency	Thalassaemia
PCV/RBC = MCV	75–99 fL	↓	↓
Hb/RBC = MCH	37–31 pg	↓	↓
Hb/PCV = MCHC	32–36 g/dL	↓	→

Table 2.1 Red cell indices in thalassaemia and iron deficiency.

PCV, packed cell volume; RBC, red cell count; Hb, haemoglobin; MCV, mean corpuscular volume; MCH, mean corpuscular haemoglobin; MCHC, mean corpuscular haemoglobin concentration.

Serum ferritin is estimated by a sensitive immunoradiometric assay. Even if there is delay in obtaining the result, it is valuable to have an accurate assessment of iron stores before therapy is started. In the development of iron deficiency, reduction in serum ferritin is the first test to become abnormal.

Serum transferrin receptor

Transferrin receptor (TfR) is present in all cells as a transmembrane protein that binds transferrin iron and transports it to the cell interior. Serum TfR provides a new and allegedly reliable method for assessing cellular iron status [44]. Any reduction in iron supply results in an increase in TfR synthesis and, like ferritin, TfR has been shown to circulate in the plasma in small amounts, which reflect the total body mass of TfR. In patients with iron-deficiency anaemia there is an increase in the density of surface TfR in iron-deficient cells. In these circumstances, the plasma TfR is elevated some threefold.

There is little or no change in serum TfR in the early stages of storage iron depletion but as soon as cellular iron deficiency is established, the serum TfR rises in direct proportion to the degree of iron lack. This rise precedes the reduction in MCV or the rise in FEP. It is particularly valuable in identifying iron deficiency in pregnancy [45].

TfR will give a true reflection of *tissue* iron deficiency in pregnancy when the ferritin may be low because of mobilization and in chronic inflammatory disease when ferritin is inappropriately elevated because of release from cells. In combination with serum ferritin, serum TfR will give a complete picture of iron status, the serum ferritin reflecting iron stores (in the absence of chronic inflammatory disease) and the TfR tissue iron status [40].

Marrow iron

Before serum ferritin and TfR were available, the only reliable method of assessing iron stores in pregnancy was by examination of an appropriately stained preparation of a bone-marrow sample. This will still give the most rapid answer. In the absence of iron supplementation there is no detectable stainable iron in over 80% of women at term [15]. No stainable iron (haemosiderin) may be visible once serum ferritin has fallen to below 30 μg/L, but other stigmata of iron deficiency in the developing erythroblasts, particularly the late normoblasts, will confirm that the anaemia is indeed due to iron deficiency in the absence of stainable iron. Arrested incorporation of stainable iron from reticuloendothelial cells into erythroblasts during chronic inflammatory states will also be demonstrated. The effects of frequently accompanying folate deficiency will also be apparent (see below).

Management of iron deficiency

In the UK the management of iron deficiency in pregnancy was largely one of prevention by daily oral supplements. Oral supplementation of 60–80 mg elemental iron per day from early pregnancy maintains the haemoglobin in the recognized normal range for pregnancy but does not maintain or restore the iron stores [15,46]. WHO recommends that supplements of 30–60 mg/day be given to those pregnant women who have normal iron stores and 120–240 mg to those women with none. Whether all pregnant women need iron is controversial and is discussed below, but if it is accepted that iron is necessary, a bewildering number of preparations of varying expense are available for use. In those women to whom additional iron cannot be given by the oral route either because of non-compliance or because of unacceptable side-effects, intramuscular injection of 1000 mg iron more than ensures iron sufficiency for the remainder of pregnancy. The injections are painful and can stain the skin but there is not the risk of incurring malignancy at the injection site in humans [47, 47a] that there is in rats [48].

There is no haematological benefit in giving parenteral as opposed to oral iron, but some women will not take oral preparations. The sole advantage of parenteral therapy is that the physician can be sure that such patients have received adequate supplementation.

The side-effects of oral administration of iron have been shown to be related to the quantity administered [49]; if the daily dose is reduced to 100 mg they are rare with any preparation. Although some women do have gastric symptoms the most common complaint is constipation, which is usually easily overcome by simple measures. Slow-release preparations, which are generally more expensive, are said to be relatively free of side-effects. This is only so because much of the iron is not released at all, is unabsorbed and excreted unchanged. This means that increased doses may have to be given to cover requirements, thereby further increasing expense. The majority of women tolerate the cheaper preparations with no significant side-effects and in the interests of economy these should be tried first. All the preparations used routinely in pregnancy are now combined with an appropriate dose of folic acid (see below). Prophylaxis of iron deficiency therefore depends partly on good antenatal care, but ultimately on regular attendance at the antenatal clinic and cooperation in taking the prescribed medication. In spite of suggestive evidence to the contrary (see below), not all obstetricians are convinced of the value of prophylaxis with haematinics.

The management of iron-deficiency anaemia diagnosed late in pregnancy presents a particular challenge to the obstetrician because a satisfactory response must be obtained in a limited time. Parenteral iron is useful in this situation particularly if the woman cannot be relied upon to take oral medication. Iron sorbitol citrate can be given as a series of intramuscular injections but it is associated with toxic reactions such as headache, nausea and vomiting if given simultaneously with oral iron [50].

Iron dextran is a preparation that was used extensively and may be administered as a series of intramuscular injections. Unfortunately, this preparation is no longer supplied by the manufacturers for intravenous use in the UK. This preparation does not appear to be associated with toxicity if given simultaneously with oral iron [51,52].

Preparations of iron–sucrose complex for intravenous use, which are not licensed for total dose infusions and have to be given in 5–10 mL aliquots up to three times weekly, have been used with success in pregnancy [53]. At Queen Charlotte's Hospital, London, we have used iron saccharate in selected cases with adequate responses in all and no adverse reactions.

In the absence of any other abnormality, an increase in haemoglobin concentration of 1 g/dL/week in the non-pregnant state, 0.8 g/dL/week in pregnancy can be reasonably expected with adequate iron treatment, whether oral or parenteral. If there is not time to achieve a reasonable haemoglobin concentration before delivery, blood transfusion with all its hazards has to be considered.

The case for prophylactic iron therapy

There is still considerable controversy about whether the fall in haemoglobin concentration that occurs in healthy women during pregnancy is an indication of iron deficiency and whether raising the haemoglobin with iron confers any benefit [54,55]. Many authors are not able to accept that the physiological requirements for iron in pregnancy are considerably higher than the usual intake of most healthy women with apparently good diets in industrialized countries. Arguments about policy among nutritionalists wishing to prevent iron deficiency are complicated by the problem of applying the same strategy in countries with differing standards of living. Paradoxically the greatest experience in prevention comes from those countries where iron deficiency is least common and least severe [56].

There is no doubt that in developing countries the incidence of anaemia and iron deficiency is high and many women enter pregnancy who are either anaemic or who have grossly depleted iron stores. A small but careful study of anaemia in pregnancy from Nigeria showed that once the major problems of malaria and the haemoglobinopathies had been partially solved by giving antimalarials and folic acid routinely throughout pregnancy, iron deficiency was also present in many of the patients with pregnancy anaemia. The conclusion was that the deficiency was primarily due to poor iron content in the diet, and routine iron supplementation was recommended [57]. Another larger controlled trial from the Philippines [58] showed clearly that those women with normal haemoglobin concentrations who had been given iron throughout pregnancy were able to maintain their haemoglobin levels; anaemic women on a larger dose of iron raised their haemoglobin concentrations when compared to those taking placebo or ascorbic acid alone.

One of the earliest large studies in the UK came from Manchester [24] in over 2000 pregnant women. In those not taking iron, a progressive drop in the haemoglobin concentration was observed—the lowest level being reached at 32 weeks' gestation—but it took more than a year after delivery before the pre-pregnancy haemoglobin level was re-achieved. Those women who took iron had consistently higher haemoglobin concentrations and the effects persisted into the postnatal period—pre-pregnancy haemoglobin levels being much more rapidly re-achieved. However, the majority of the women, whether taking iron or not, were perfectly healthy and had no complaints. This raises the question of whether a haemoglobin level raised by iron therapy is in itself an advantage. There was no advantage in terms of subjective health conferred by iron treatment in another double-blind study [59] in Aberdeen.

In general over the years there has been no convincing evidence for the obstetrician that the normal pregnant woman is at an advantage if she takes extra iron [60]. The fact that the fall of haemoglobin concentration in normal multigravidae is greater than that in primigravidae has been interpreted as indirect evidence of depletion of iron concentration by repeated pregnancy; however, multigravidae have a greater rise of plasma volume than primigravidae and therefore a correspondingly lower haemoglobin is to be expected. All these findings emphasize the important principle that 'normality' in pregnancy cannot be judged by reference to non-pregnant standards. Fall in haemoglobin concentration due to haemodilution seems to cause no anxiety in the mind of the obstetrician although a satisfactory level of haemoglobin concentration may indicate an unsatisfactory increase of plasma volume. The association of high maternal haemoglobin concentration with poor outcome of pregnancy in pre-eclampsia is, of course, due to inadequate plasma volume increase [6] and should not be taken as an argument against iron supplements [61]. Plasma volume and red cell mass are under separate control (see above). Fears that the haemochromatosis mutations may lead to iron overload if all women are offered iron supplements regardless of haemoglobin concentrations at booking, have not been realized. Indeed a study of iron stores in pregnancy including women with haemochromatosis mutations suggested that heterozygosity for the common Cys282Tyr mutation of the HFE gene has little influence on iron storage levels of young women in the reproductive years; of the two subjects homozygous for the gene, one had totally depleted iron stores with a serum ferritin of $7\,\mu g/L$ [62].

Hemminki and Starfield [63] have reviewed controlled clinical trials of iron administration during pregnancy in developed Western countries. Seventeen trials were found which fulfilled their criteria. Their analysis showed that there was no benefit in terms of birthweight, length of gestation, maternal and infant morbidity, and mortality in those women receiving iron compared with controls. They maintain that while age, economic status and poor nutrition affect the outcome of pregnancy, pregnancy anaemia is not related and is simply associated with other risk factors. They did not take into account the withdrawal of anaemic patients from the trials they reviewed. Their analysis may be correct but anaemia remains a potential danger in pregnancy especially in the face of haemorrhage. The most recent Cochrane review [60] of treatments for iron-deficiency anaemia during pregnancy is based on relevant randomized controlled trials in order to give guidance based on real evidence rather than on expert opinion.

Fifty-four studies were identified but only five provided sufficient data of appropriate quality to be included. In general, outcomes had been evaluated from laboratory data, clinical outcomes not being included in the majority (four out of five). The trials came from Australia, Singapore, Tanzania, UK and Java. Sadly the most important question of whether anaemia treatment modifies maternal and neonatal morbidity and mortality was not addressed by those studies that were considered appropriate for inclusion in the review [60]. The conclusions drawn were that with the available evidence it was not possible to give evidence-based guidelines for administration of iron supplements in pregnancy. The review is an 'invitation for researchers to produce relevant good quality research able to fill the gaps in knowledge of a condition faced daily in clinical practice'. The majority of women who do not receive iron supplements have no stores at all at the end of pregnancy [15,42]. Also offspring of non-anaemic women who have not received supplements have less storage iron than those of iron-replete women [42]. An analysis of factors leading to a 20% reduction in iron deficiency in Swedish women of childbearing age in the 10-year period 1965–75 attributed this to greater prescribing of iron tablets (10%) and fortification of food (7–8%); oral contraception also played a part (2–3%) [64].

The crucial information needed to interpret the physiological anaemia of pregnancy is whether or not the average young woman has sufficient storage iron. Svanberg [19] comments that the absence of iron stores in women of fertile age is not physiological and that the increased iron demand during pregnancy cannot be met by increased absorption. The conclusion is that, even with maximum iron content in the diet, the immediate demands of pregnancy cannot be covered by an increased absorption from the diet. From the evidence that is available it would appear that a high proportion of women in their reproductive years do lack storage iron [15,42].

A study from South Africa [65] reports the findings in Indian and black women attending antenatal clinics. Anaemia, by WHO standards, was found in 13% of the Asian women in the first trimester, increasing to 28 and 47% in the second and third trimesters, respectively, but iron deficiency (serum ferritin $<12\,\mu g/L$) was found to be far greater, i.e. 35% in the first trimester rising to 86% in the third.

The pregnant black women underwent similar investigations. Anaemia was detected in 19% rising to 29% later in pregnancy. However, the proportion with iron deficiency was not so dramatically increased as in the Asian counterparts—19% rising to 40% in the last trimester. This probably reflects the greater number of vegetarians among the Asian populations who will not have sufficient reserves of storage iron to meet the needs of pregnancy.

The finding that oral iron supplements may reduce both the bioavailability of zinc [66] and maternal zinc levels during pregnancy [66] has led to speculation about the relationship of these observations. There have also been reports suggesting that maternal tissue zinc depletion is associated with fetal growth restriction [67]. The results of a study of serial changes in serum zinc and magnesium concentrations before conception, throughout pregnancy to 12 weeks postpartum, indicates that the decrease in concentrations of both elements is a normal physiological adjustment to pregnancy and that oral iron supplementation does not influence these changes [68].

It has been suggested that women at risk from iron-deficiency anaemia could be identified by estimating the serum ferritin concentration in the first trimester. A serum ferritin of $<50 \mu g/L$ in early pregnancy is an indication for daily iron supplements. Women with serum ferritin concentrations of $>80 \mu g/L$ are unlikely to require iron supplements. Unnecessary routine supplementation would thus be avoided in women enjoying good nutrition, and any risk to the pregnancy arising from severe maternal anaemia would be avoided by prophylaxis and prompt treatment [69].

A study carried out at Queen Charlotte's Maternity Hospital, London, is of interest in this respect. Serum ferritin levels were estimated in 669 consecutive women who booked at 16 weeks' gestation or earlier with a haemoglobin concentration of 11 g/dL or above. As many as 552 women (82%) had serum ferritin levels of $50 \mu g/L$ or below, and would therefore qualify for routine daily iron supplements by the above criteria. These women were drawn from a cosmopolitan, largely well-nourished population; 12% had serum ferritin levels of $<12 \mu g/L$ and were therefore already iron deficient at booking, in spite of having a haemoglobin of 11 g/dL or more. Only 51 (8%) had ferritin levels of $80 \mu g/L$ or above [70].

The most recent guidelines for the use of iron supplements to prevent and treat iron-deficiency anaemia have been issued jointly by the International Nutritional Anaemia Consultative Group (INACG), WHO and UNICEF. For pregnancy it is suggested that where the prevalence of anaemia is $<40\%$ (e.g. UK) 60 mg iron plus 400 μg folic acid should be given daily for 6 months during pregnancy, and for those communities where the prevalence is $>40\%$ then these supplements should continue for 3 months postpartum [71].

In summary, negative iron balance throughout pregnancy, particularly in the latter half, may lead to iron-deficiency anaemia in the third trimester. This hazard—together with the increasing evidence of non-haematological effects of iron deficiency on exercise tolerance, cerebral function and temperature control—leads me to the conclusion that it is safer, more practical, and in the long term less expensive in terms of investigation, hospital admission and treatment, to give all women iron supplements from 16 weeks' gestation—especially as this would appear to do no harm [68,72], not to mention the advantages for the offspring, particularly in the first year of life [72a].

Folic acid and folate metabolism

Folic acid and iron are particularly important in nutrition during pregnancy. At a cellular level folic acid is reduced first to dihydrofolic (DHF) acid and then to tetrahydrofolic (THF) acid, which forms the pivot of cellular folate metabolism because it is fundamental (through linkage with L-carbon fragments) both to cell growth and cell division. The more active a tissue is in reproduction and growth, the more dependent it will be on the efficient turnover and supply of folate coenzymes. Bone marrow and epithelial linings are therefore particularly at risk.

Requirements for folate are increased in pregnancy to meet the needs of the fetus, the placenta, uterine hypertrophy and the expanded maternal red cell mass. They are increased still further by multiple pregnancy (see below). The placenta transports folate actively to the fetus even in the face of maternal deficiency, but maternal folate metabolism is altered early in pregnancy like many other maternal functions, before fetal demands act directly.

Plasma folate

With the exception of haemoglobin concentration and plasma iron levels, folic acid must be one of the most studied substances in maternal blood, but there are comparatively few serial data available. Nevertheless, it is generally agreed that plasma folate levels fall as pregnancy advances so that at term they are about half the non-pregnant values [73–76]. Plasma clearance of folate by the kidneys is more than doubled by as early as the eighth week of gestation [76,77]. It has been suggested that urinary loss may be a major factor in the fall of serum folate. Although the glomerular filtration rate is raised (see Chapter 7), the marked contrast between the comparatively unchanging plasma levels and the wide variation in urinary loss suggests a change in tubular reabsorption. It is unlikely that this is a major drain on maternal resources and it cannot play more than a marginal role [76,77].

There have been conflicting reports about the part intestinal malabsorption may play in the aetiology of folate deficiency in pregnancy. Traditionally absorption has been assessed from plasma levels following an oral load. Earlier reports of decreased absorption [78] were probably due to the underestimation of the rapid clearance of folate following an oral dose. Placental and maternal tissues contribute from an early stage probably under the influence of oestrogens, as oral contraceptives also increase plasma clearance of folate [79]. There is no change in absorption of either folate monoglutamates or polyglutamates in healthy pregnancy [80,81], although there is a wide scatter of results. The incidence of abnormally low serum folate concentrations in late pregnancy varies with the population studied and presumably reflects the local nutritional standards.

Substantial day-to-day variation of plasma folate occurs and postprandial increases have been noted. This variability limits the diagnostic value of plasma folate estimation when occasional samples taken at a casual antenatal clinic visit are considered.

It could be argued that the changes noted in pregnancy are positively advantageous. There is no reason why reduced plasma levels of nutrients such as folate should necessarily indicate deficiency, particularly when the levels of other nutrients such as glucose and amino acids are disregarded. The reduced levels may aid conservation in the face of a raised glomerular filtration rate. It is possible that the placenta may be able to compete more effectively with maternal tissues for folate supplies at lower maternal plasma levels and that it compensates for its relatively small receptive area in this way [76].

Red cell folate

The estimation of red cell folate levels may provide more useful information than plasma folate concentration, as red cell folate levels do not reflect the daily and other short-term variations that affect plasma folate levels. Red cell folate concentration is thought to give a better indication of overall body tissue levels, but the turnover of red blood cells is slow and there will be delay before significant reductions in the folate concentrations of the red cells, due to folate deficiency, are evident.

A number of investigations of erythrocyte folate in pregnancy have shown a slight downward trend even though, as would be expected, the fall is not so marked as that noted for the change in plasma concentration [82,83]. There is evidence that patients who have a low red cell folate at the beginning of pregnancy are more likely to develop megaloblastic anaemia in the third trimester [83].

Excretion of formiminoglutamic acid

A loading dose of histidine leads to increased formiminoglutamic acid (FIGLU) excretion in the urine when there is folate deficiency (the FIGLU test). There is no longer much to recommend this as a screening test in pregnancy primarily because the metabolism of histidine is altered [74] and this results in increased FIGLU excretion in normal early pregnancy [84].

Folic acid postpartum

In the 6 weeks following delivery, all indices of folate metabolism tend to return to non-pregnant values. However, should any deficiency of folate have developed and remained untreated in pregnancy, it may present clinically for the first time in the puerperium and its consequences may be detected for many months after delivery. Lactation provides an added folate stress. A folate content of $5 \mu g / 100 \, mL$ of human milk and a yield of 500 mL daily implies a loss of $25 \mu g$ folate daily in breast milk. In the Bantu, megaloblastic anaemia appears frequently in the year following pregnancy in association with lactation. Dietary folate intake is poor and it has been shown that folate deficiency becomes more apparent, as demonstrated by using FIGLU excretion, as lactation continues [85]. Red cell folate levels in lactating mothers are significantly lower than those of their infants during the first year of life [74]. In the UK, as early as 1919, Osler described the severe anaemia of pregnancy that had a high colour index and a striking incidence in the postpartum period [86].

Interpretation of investigations

The value of these various investigations in predicting megaloblastic anaemia and assessing subclinical folate deficiency has been the subject of numerous reports. Using these various tests it appears that folate 'deficiency' in pregnancy is not always accompanied by significant haematological change [84,85].

Even in the absence of any significant haematological changes in the peripheral blood, megaloblastic haemopoiesis should be suspected when the expected response to adequate iron therapy is not achieved. Evidence of megaloblastic haemopoiesis may become apparent only after iron therapy even though the rise in haemoglobin concentration appears adequate. No help can be expected from the use of tests of folate status. 'Abnormal' results are obtained with most of the tests but these are not significantly different from results in healthy pregnant women. The decline of serum folic acid levels from a mean of $6.0 \mu g / L$ in the non-pregnant to $3.4 \mu g / L$ at term should be viewed only as the physiological consequence of maternal tissue uptake, urinary loss and placental transfer—not of evidence of folate deficiency. The delay in fall of red cell folate makes this too impractical a test for folate deficiency in pregnancy. Therefore the diagnosis of folate deficiency in pregnancy has to be made ultimately on morphological grounds; this usually involves examinations of a suitably prepared marrow aspirate.

Megaloblastic anaemia

Folic acid deficiency

The cause of megaloblastic anaemia in pregnancy is nearly always folate deficiency. Vitamin B_{12} is only very rarely implicated (see below). A survey of reports from the UK over past decades suggest an incidence ranging from 0.2 to 5%, but a considerably greater number of women have megaloblastic changes in their marrow that are not suspected on examination of the peripheral blood alone [74,87]. The incidence of megaloblastic anaemia in other parts of the world is considerably greater and is thought to reflect the nutritional standards of the population. Several workers have pointed to the poor socioeconomic status of their patients as the major aetiological factor contributing to anaemia [74,88], which may be further exacerbated by seasonal changes in the availability of stable foodstuffs. Food folates are only partially available and the amount of folate supplied in the diet is difficult to quantify. In the UK, analysis of daily folate intake in foodstuffs showed a range of 129–300 µg [89]. The folate content of 24-h food collections in various studies in Sweden and Canada proved to be about 200 µg, with a range as great as 70–600 µg [74].

Foods that are very rich in folate include broccoli, spinach and Brussel sprouts, but up to 90% of their folate content is lost within the first few minutes of cooking by boiling or steaming, and they are unlikely to be eaten raw. Asparagus, avocado pears and mushrooms also have a fairly high folate content but are expensive. Natural folates are protected from oxidation and degradation by the presence of reducing substances such as ascorbate. Analysis of the folate content of food will give very low results if ascorbate is not added to the assay system—as occurred in the very earliest studies [74]. Having established the content of folate in food, there is only indirect evidence about its absorption. Monoglutamates are almost completely absorbed. Polyglutamates from different sources are variably available, but in general are less well absorbed, so that total folate intake should be combined with information about the source of food folate to give a realistic appraisal of the available folate content. In general, dietary intake is likely to be greater, rather than small, during pregnancy, but obviously in certain areas of the world malnutrition is an essential aetiological factor in determining folate status.

The effects of dietary inadequacy may be further amplified by frequent childbirth and by multiple pregnancy.

Folate deficiency occurred in one in 11 twin pregnancies compared with the expected incidence of one in 80 in a survey of over 1000 patients with folate deficiency [74].

The normal dietary folate intake is inadequate to prevent megaloblastic changes in the bone marrow in approximately 25% of pregnant women. The falls in serum and red cell folate levels could be a physiological phenomenon in pregnancy but the incidence of megaloblastic change in the bone marrow is reduced only when the blood folate levels are maintained in a steady state by adequate oral supplements. There is much controversy about the requirement for folate, particularly during pregnancy. WHO recommendations for daily folate intake were as high as 800 µg in the antenatal period, 600 µg during lactation and 400 µg in the non-pregnant adult [14]. There is an increased need of about 100 µg folic acid daily during pregnancy which, without supplements, must be found from natural folates in the diet [74]. In the past intakes recommended by WHO clearly overestimated the need. The daily amount of folate that has been given prophylactically in pregnancy varies from 30 to 500 µg and even to pharmacological doses of 5–15 mg [74]. Thirty micrograms daily was found to be too small to influence folate status appreciably [20] but supplements of 100 µg or more all reduced the frequency of megaloblastic changes in the marrow and eliminated megaloblastic anaemia as a clinical entity [89]. The most recent publication recommends a supplement of 400 µg folic acid daily with 60 mg of iron for 6 months in pregnancy, continuing for 3 months postpartum in areas of high incidence of nutritional deficiency [71].

In order to meet the folate needs of those women with a dietary intake well below average, the daily supplement during pregnancy should be about 200–300 µg daily—still very much below the original WHO recommended daily intake. The case for giving prophylactic folate throughout pregnancy is strong [74,90], particularly in countries where overt megaloblastic anaemia is frequent.

The main point at issue over recent years, however, is whether the apparently intrinsic folate deficiency of pregnancy can predispose the mother to a wide variety of other obstetric abnormalities and complications, in particular abortion, fetal malformations, prematurity and antepartum haemorrhage [74,88,91,92]. The extensive literature would seem to be almost equally divided in its opinion, but there is virtually no evidence that the routine use of folic acid supplements *during* pregnancy has reduced the incidence of anything but megaloblastic anaemia [76,93] except in areas of malnutrition where an increase in birthweight has been noted [94]. The recent association demonstrated between hyperhomocysteinaemia, a condition that can be treated by folate supplements and adverse fetal outcome particularly abruption (see Chapter 4), does, however, strengthen the speculation that folate deficiency may be associated with bad pregnancy outcome.

The case for *preconception* prophylaxis with folate to prevent neural tube defect is well established and is discussed below.

Severe megaloblastic anaemia is now uncommon in the UK during pregnancy or the puerperium but may occasionally still occur. Two case histories of severe macrocytic anaemia presenting in the puerperium with pancytopenia have been published [95]. In both cases leukaemia was considered because of the increase in promyelocytes in the bone marrow as well as because of florid megaloblastic change. Both responded completely to therapy with folic acid. Two similar cases have been seen at Queen Charlotte's Maternity Hospital, London, having been treated with intravenous iron alone for severe anaemia developing late in pregnancy, without additional parenteral folate supplementation.

An argument against routine folate supplementation in pregnancy is unrecognized vitamin B_{12} deficiency. Folate can aggravate the neuropathy due to vitamin B_{12} deficiency. The risk of adverse effects from folate administered to a pregnant woman suffering from vitamin B_{12} deficiency is very small indeed (see below). In fact there is *no* report of this occurring amongst the many thousands of women who have received folate supplements in pregnancy [96].

Folic acid should never be given without supplemental iron. A wide variety of preparations supplying both iron and folate are available and, provided that the folate content is not less than $100 \mu g$ daily, all are satisfactory for prophylaxis in pregnancy.

Once megaloblastic haemopoiesis is established, treatment of folic acid deficiency becomes more difficult, presumably due to megaloblastic changes in the gastrointestinal tract resulting in impaired absorption. A small number of patients [90] fail to respond to parenteral folate therapy and only recover after delivery. It is far better to intervene before these difficulties arise and to give routine prophylaxis throughout pregnancy.

Other disorders associated with folate deficiency

Disorders that may affect folate requirement in pregnancy

Problems may be caused in pregnancy by disorders that are associated with an increased folate requirement in the non-pregnant state. Women with haemolytic anaemia, particularly hereditary haemolytic conditions such as haemoglobinopathies and hereditary spherocytosis, require extra supplements from early pregnancy if development of megaloblastic anaemia is to be avoided. The recommended supplement in this situation is 5–10 mg orally daily. The anaemia associated with thalassaemia trait is not strictly due to haemolysis but to ineffective erythropoiesis (see below). However, the increased, though abortive, marrow turnover still results in folate depletion and such women would probably benefit from the routine administration of oral folic acid 5 mg daily from early pregnancy.

Folate supplements are of particular importance in the management of sickle cell syndromes during pregnancy if aplastic crises and megaloblastic anaemia are to be avoided.

Anticonvulsant drugs and pregnancy

The additional demand for folate during pregnancy leads to a rapid fall in red cell folate and to a high incidence of megaloblastic anaemia in those women taking anticonvulsant drugs for control of epilepsy. This is not surprising because non-pregnant individuals taking anticonvulsants tend to become folate deficient [74].

The risk of interfering with the control of epilepsy by the regular administration of iron–folate preparations during pregnancy and the precipitation of status epilepticus [97] has been overestimated [98]. Anticonvulsant therapy during pregnancy is associated with an increased incidence of congenital abnormality [99], prematurity and low birthweight [100]. Therefore folate supplements should be given to all epileptic women taking anticonvulsants in pregnancy (see Chapter 15) as well as before conception (see below).

In addition, neonates born to women taking anticonvulsant drugs may have increased prothrombin times and are at risk of bleeding. This risk appears to be preventable by giving the mothers oral vitamin K 20 mg daily for 2 weeks before delivery is recommended [101] but 10 mg may be sufficient.

The fetus and folate deficiency

There is an increased risk of megaloblastic anaemia occurring in the neonate of a folate-deficient mother, especially if delivery is preterm.

The young infant's requirement for folate has been estimated at 20–50 μg/day (four to 10 times the adult requirement on a weight basis). Serum and red cell folate levels are consistently higher in cord than in maternal blood, but the preterm infant is in severe negative folate balance because of high growth rate and reduced intake. The usual fall in serum and red cell folate in the term neonate is yet greater in the preterm neonate and even in the absence of other complicating factors may result in megaloblastic anaemia. This can be prevented by giving supplements of folic acid 50 µg/day [102,103].

Data suggesting an association between periconceptional folic acid deficiency and harelip, cleft palate and most important of all, neural tube defects [104–106], which have been well reviewed in the past [107] have now been clarified by some important, more recent studies.

The association between periconceptional folate deficiency and *recurrence* of neural tube defects has been confirmed in a large multicentre controlled trial of pre-pregnancy folate supplementation [108]. It has also been shown in a large randomized controlled trial in Hungary [109] that periconceptional supplement of 800 µg of folic acid in a combined vitamin preparation prevented the *first* occurrence of neural tube defects. The prevalence of harelip with or without cleft palate was not reduced by this supplementation. A more recent survey from China [110] showed clearly that the incidence of neural tube defects was reduced by giving periconceptional folic acid supplements in both low- and high-risk communities.

Preconception prophylaxis

We do not yet understand the association between folic acid and neural tube closure, i.e. whether supplementation corrects a dietary deficiency, overcomes a defect in absorption or metabolism, provides some extra benefit at supraphysiological doses or even selectively causes the abortion of fetuses with birth defects (terathenesia) [111]. It is recommended that women contemplating pregnancy should take folate supplements of 400 µg daily [112,113]. This dose is currently marketed in the UK as an 'over the counter' preparation. Although women have been encouraged to take folate supplements when planning to conceive, a recent paper has reported no reduction in the incidence of neural tube defects in the UK [114] probably because relatively few women do take the recommended supplements. Therefore it has been suggested that folate should be added to basic foodstuffs [115]. A policy of targeted food fortification is under consideration both in the USA and UK.

Vitamin B$_{12}$ deficiency

Muscle, red cell and serum vitamin B$_{12}$ concentrations fall during pregnancy [73,74,116,117]. Non-pregnant serum levels of 205–1025 µg/L fall to 20–510 µg/L at term, with low levels in multiple pregnancy [117]. Women who smoke tend to have lower serum B$_{12}$ levels [118], which may account for the positive correlation between birth-weight and serum levels in non-deficient mothers.

Vitamin B$_{12}$ absorption is unaltered in pregnancy [74,119]. It is possible that tissue uptake is increased by the action of oestrogens as oral contraceptives which thus cause a fall in serum vitamin B$_{12}$ level. Cord blood serum vitamin B$_{12}$ is higher than that of maternal blood. The fall in serum vitamin B$_{12}$ in the mother is related to preferential transfer of absorbed B$_{12}$ to the fetus at the expense of maintaining the maternal serum concentration [74]. Nevertheless the placenta does not transfer vitamin B$_{12}$ with the same efficiency as it does folate. Low serum vitamin B$_{12}$ levels in early pregnancy in vegetarian Hindus do not fall further while their infants often have subnormal concentrations. The vitamin B$_{12}$ binding capacity of plasma increases in pregnancy analogous to the rise in iron-binding capacity. The rise is confined to the liver-derived transcobalamin II concerned with transport rather than the leucocyte-derived transcobalamin I which is raised in other myeloproliferative conditions [120].

Pregnancy does not make a great impact on maternal vitamin B$_{12}$ stores. Adult stores are of the order of 3000 µg or more and vitamin B$_{12}$ stores in the newborn infant are about 50 µg [120].

Addisonian pernicious anaemia does not usually occur during the reproductive years. Vitamin B$_{12}$ deficiency is associated with infertility and pregnancy is likely only if the deficiency is remedied [121]. Vitamin B$_{12}$ deficiency in pregnancy may be associated with chronic tropical sprue. The megaloblastic anaemia that develops is due to long-standing vitamin B$_{12}$ deficiency and superadded folate deficiency; the cord vitamin B$_{12}$ levels remain above the maternal levels in these cases, but the concentration in the breast milk follows the maternal serum levels [74].

The recommended intake of vitamin B$_{12}$ is 2 µg/day in the non-pregnant and 3 µg/day during pregnancy [14]. This will be met by almost any diet that contains animal products, however deficient it may be in other essential substances. Strict vegans who do not eat animal-derived substances may have a deficient intake of vitamin B$_{12}$ and their diet should be supplemented during pregnancy.

Recent studies of very poor populations in Africa have revealed significant numbers who are B$_{12}$ deficient due to a diet consisting mainly of maize and containing very little animal protein, not even milk or eggs. A significant proportion of women from Malawi developed megaloblastic haemopoiesis associated with extremely low serum B$_{12}$ levels [122].

Haemoglobinopathies

Following the influx of immigrants from all parts of the world, obstetricians in the UK frequently encounter women with genetic defects of haemoglobin and its synthesis that are seldom seen in the indigenous population. It is important to recognize the specific defects early in pregnancy for the following reasons.

1 The clinical effects may complicate obstetric management and appropriate precautions can be taken;

2 It is now possible to offer prenatal diagnosis to those women carrying a fetus at risk of a serious defect of haemoglobin synthesis or structure at a time when termination of pregnancy is feasible [123–126].

The haemoglobinopathies are inherited defects of haemoglobin, resulting from impaired globin synthesis (thalassaemia syndromes) or from structural abnormality of globin (haemoglobin variants). Only some of these anomalies are of practical importance, so particular emphasis will be placed on those where adverse effects may be aggravated by pregnancy. A proper appreciation of these defects requires some understanding of the structure of normal haemoglobin.

The haemoglobin molecule consists of four globin chains each of which is associated with a haem complex. There are three normal haemoglobins in humans; HbA, HbA$_2$ and HbF—each of which contains two pairs of polypeptide globin chains. The synthesis and structure of the four globin chains α, β, γ and δ are under separate control (Fig. 2.1).

The adult levels shown in Fig. 2.1 are those achieved by 6 months of age. It is obvious that only those conditions affecting the synthesis or structure of HbA (α$_2$β$_2$), which should comprise over 95% of the total circulating haemoglobin in the adult, will be of significance for the mother during pregnancy. α-chain production is under the control of four genes, two inherited from each parent; as can be seen the α chains are common to all three haemoglobins. β-chain production, on the other hand, is under the control of only two genes—one inherited from each parent.

The thalassaemia syndromes

The thalassaemia syndromes are the commonest genetic disorders of the blood and constitute a vast public health problem in many parts of the world. The basic defect is a reduced rate of globin chain synthesis, the red cells being formed with inadequate haemoglobin content. The syndromes are divided into two main groups, the α and the β thalassaemias depending on whether the α- or the β-globin chain synthesis of adult haemoglobin (HbAα$_2$β$_2$) is depressed.

α THALASSAEMIA

Normal individuals have four functional α globin genes. α thalassaemia, unlike β thalassaemia, is often, but not always, a gene deletion defect. There are two forms of α thalassaemia trait, the result of inheriting three or two normal α genes instead of the usual four. They are called α$^+$ and α^0 thalassaemia (Fig. 2.2).

HbH disease is an intermediate form of α thalassaemia in which there is only one functional α gene and is the name given to the unstable haemoglobin formed by tetramers of the β chain (β4), when there is a relative lack of α chains. α thalassaemia major in which there are no functional α genes (both parents having transmitted α^0 thalassaemia) is incompatible with life, and pregnancy ends usually prematurely in a hydropic fetus, which will only survive a matter of hours if born alive. This is a common condition in South-East Asia. The name Hb Bart's was given to tetramers of the γ chain of fetal haemoglobin (HbFα$_2$γ$_2$). The tetramer (γ$_4$) forms *in utero* when no α chains are made and was first identified in a Chinese baby born at St Bartholomew's Hospital, London.

Management of α thalassaemia

During pregnancy, with its stress on the haemopoietic system, carriers of α thalassaemia, particularly those with α^0 thalassaemia (two deleted genes on one chromosome) may become very anaemic. They can be identified for further tests at booking, by finding abnormal red cell indices (Table 2.1). They have smaller red cells (MCV) and

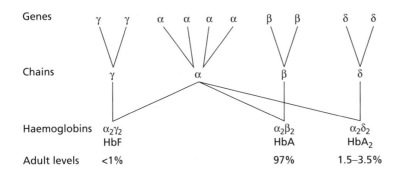

Fig 2.1 Genetic control of globin synthesis. The adult levels shown are those reached by 6 months of age.

a reduced individual MCH, although the MCHC is usually within the normal range (Table 2.1). These changes are often minimal in α^+ thalassaemia (one deleted gene) (Fig. 2.2) but this condition is not so important as is α^0 thalassaemia in terms of genetic counselling and prenatal diagnosis. This diagnosis can only be confirmed by DNA analysis of nucleated cells.

There is no abnormal haemoglobin made or excess or lack of one or other of the normal haemoglobins. These individuals need iron and folate oral supplements throughout the antenatal period. Sometimes intramuscular folic acid is helpful but parenteral iron should never be given (see below). If the haemoglobin level is not thought to be adequate for delivery at term, transfusion is indicated.

Patients with HbH disease have a chronic haemolytic anaemia and have 5–30% HbH in their peripheral blood, which can be identified by haemoglobin electrophoresis. They have a normal life expectancy but require daily oral folate supplements to cover the demands of increased marrow turnover. During pregnancy it is recommended to give 5 mg folate daily to women with HbH disease. They will transmit either α^0 or α^+ thalassaemia to their offspring.

Pregnancy with an α thalassaemia hydropic fetus may be associated with severe, sometimes life-threatening pre-eclampsia in the mother (cf. severe rhesus haemolytic disease), the so-called mirror syndrome. Vaginal deliveries are associated with obstetric complication, due to the large fetus and very bulky placenta. It has been estimated in Thailand that in the absence of obstetric care, up to 50% of mothers carrying an hydropic fetus may suffer lethal complications [127]. If routine screening of the parents (see below) indicates that the mother is at risk of carrying such a child, both parents having α^0 thalassaemia, she should be referred for prenatal diagnosis (see below).

β THALASSAEMIA

Thalassaemia major, homozygous β-thalassaemia resulting from the inheritance of a defective β-globin gene from each parent was the first identified form of the thalassaemia syndromes. It was described in the 1920s by Cooley, a physician in practice in the USA. The first few cases were found in the children of Greek and Italian immigrants. The name thalassaemia was derived from the Greek *thalassa* meaning the sea, or in the classical sense the Mediterranean sea, because it was thought to be confined to individuals of Mediterranean origin; however, we know now that the distribution is virtually worldwide, although the defect is concentrated in a broad geographical band, which excludes the UK. However, in the UK there are a fair number of heterozygotes, particularly in the immigrant Cypriot and Asian populations. The child of parents who are both carriers of β thalassaemia has a one in four chance of inheriting thalassaemia major. The carrier rate in the UK is about one in 10 000 compared with one in seven in Cyprus. There are between 300 and 400 patients with thalassaemia major in the UK today but worldwide there are over 100 000 babies born each year with the condition.

Although the majority of the 360 or so cases currently living in England are still to be found in and around the Greater London area, there is an increasing proportion of cases in the Midlands, Manchester, Bradford and Leeds. This is not only due to the fact that there have been an influx of Asian immigrants increasing the prevalence in specific areas outside London; but also the Cypriot population of Greater London is a homogeneous group who have taken advantage of the availability of prenatal diagnosis to reduce the number of homozygotes born in London to Cypriot couples at risk [128].

The Asian immigrant population, unlike the Cypriot, is very heterogeneous, with incidence of thalassaemia varying markedly from group to group. They continue to have a high incidence of first cousin marriages. A large group of rural Indians and Pakistanis have settled in the industrial towns of the Midlands and North-West. Few of this group make use of genetic counselling or fetal diagnosis, and the birth of thalassaemic children in this group continues to rise [129]. This is reflected in a recent audit of prenatal diagnosis in the UK [130].

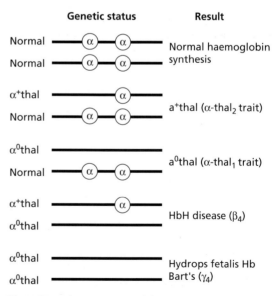

Fig 2.2 Normal α-gene status and the various changes observed in thalassaemia due to α-gene deletion.

Before the days of regular transfusion, a child born with homozygous β thalassaemia would die in the first few years of life from anaemia, congestive cardiac failure and intercurrent infection. Now that regular transfusion is routine where blood is freely available, survival is prolonged into the teens and early 20s. The management problem becomes one of iron overload derived mainly from the transfused red cells. This results in hepatic and endocrine dysfunction and, most important of all, myocardial damage—the cause of death being cardiac failure in the vast majority of cases. Puberty is delayed or incomplete. Successful pregnancy in a truly transfusion-dependent girl is very rare [131]. It remains to be seen how effective recently instituted intensive iron chelation programmes will be. The only way to cure this disease is to replace the defective gene with a healthy one. Bone-marrow transplantation (BMT) is having increasing success and the question is no longer whether, but when to transplant the patient with a histocompatible donor. Strategies for stem cell transplantation and gene therapy are being developed. However, it is important that the current group of patients with thalassaemia major is maintained in optimal clinical status if the patients are to avail themselves of these developments in BMT and genetic engineering [132,133].

Management of β thalassaemia

Sometimes survival is possible without regular transfusion in thalassaemia major but this usually results in severe bone deformities due to massive expansion of marrow tissue, the site of the largely ineffective erythropoiesis. Although iron loading still occurs from excessive gastrointestinal absorption, stimulated by the accelerated marrow turnover, it is much slower than in those who are transfused, and pregnancy may occur in this situation. Extra daily folate supplements should be given but iron in any form is contraindicated. The anaemia should be treated by transfusion during the antenatal period.

β-thalassaemia trait and pregnancy

Perhaps the commonest problem associated with haemoglobinopathies and pregnancy in the UK today is the anaemia developing in the antenatal period in women who have thalassaemia minor, heterozygous β thalassaemia. They can be identified for further examination of the booking blood by finding, as in α thalassaemia, low MCV and MCH together with near normal MCHC (see Table 2.1). The level of haemoglobin at booking may be normal or slightly below the normal range. The diagnosis will be confirmed by finding a raised concentration of HbA$_2$

($\alpha_2\delta_2$) with or without a raised HbF ($\alpha_2\gamma_2$), excess α chains combining with δ and γ chains because of the relative lack of β chains (see Fig. 2.1).

Women with β thalassaemia minor require the usual *oral* iron and folate supplements in the antenatal period. Oral iron for a limited period will not result in significant iron loading, even in the presence of replete iron stores, but parenteral iron should *never* be given. In our experience at Queen Charlotte's Maternity Hospital, London, many women with thalassaemia minor enter pregnancy with depleted iron stores as do many women with normal haemoglobin synthesis. Those women with β-thalassaemia trait particularly at risk of iron deficiency include Asian women on a traditional diet [134]. Iron deficiency has also been shown in non-pregnant women in the UK with thalassaemia minor in a study of serum ferritin levels [135]. If the anaemia does not respond to oral iron, and intramuscular folic acid has been tried, transfusion is indicated to achieve an adequate haemoglobin for delivery at term.

Haemoglobin variants

Over 250 structural variants of the globin chains of normal human haemoglobins have been described but the most important by far, both numerically and clinically, is sickle cell haemoglobin (HbS). This is a variant of the β-globin chain where there is one amino acid substitution at the sixth position, a glutamine replacing a valine residue. HbS has the unique physical property that, despite being a soluble protein in its oxygenated form, in its reduced state the molecules become stacked on one another, forming tactoids, which distort the red cells to the characteristic shape that gives the haemoglobin its name. Because of their rigid structure these sickled cells tend to block small blood vessels. The sickling phenomenon occurs particularly in conditions of lowered oxygen tension but may also be favoured by acidosis or dehydration and cooling, which cause stasis in small blood vessels (Fig. 2.3).

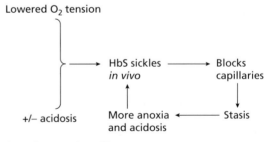

Fig 2.3 Intravascular sickling.

SICKLE CELL SYNDROMES

The sickling disorders include the heterozygous state for sickle cell haemoglobin, sickle cell trait (HbAS), homozygous sickle cell disease (HbSS), compound heterozygotes of haemoglobin variants, the most important of which is sickle cell/HbC disease (HbSC), and sickle cell thalassaemia. Although these disorders are more commonly seen in black people of African origin, they can be seen in Saudi Arabians, Indians and even in white Mediterraneans.

The characteristic feature of homozygous sickle cell anaemia (HbSS) is the occurrence of periods of health punctuated by periods of crisis. Between 3 and 6 months of age, when normal HbA production usually become predominant, a chronic haemolytic anaemia develops—the haemoglobin level being between 6 and 9 g/dL. Even if the haemoglobin concentration is in the lower part of the range, symptoms due to anaemia are surprisingly few; because of the low affinity of HbS for oxygen, oxygen delivery to the tissues is facilitated. The acute episodes due to intravascular sickling are of far greater practical importance because they cause vascular occlusion resulting in tissue infarction. The affected part is painful and the clinical manifestations are extremely variable, depending on the site at which sickling takes place. Sickling crises are often precipitated by infection and may be exacerbated by any accompanying dehydration. The majority of deaths are due to massive sickling following an acute infection. Prognosis depends in part on environmental factors such as availability of prompt treatment and prophylaxis of infection, but recent investigation of the variable clinical expression of sickle cell disease suggests that prognosis may largely be genetically determined [136]. Thirty per cent of young adults with sickle cell anaemia have a severe disorder, which mimics the 70-year-old with generalized vasculopathy. This may be clinically expressed as glomerulosclerosis, restrictive lung disease, retinopathy and repeat strokes. Sixty per cent have moderate disease while 10% run a benign course. Although high concentrations of fetal haemoglobin, HbF, inhibit polymerization of HbS, they do not necessarily confer protection against all manifestations.

Polymorphisms of the DNA that flank the sickle gene in the promoter or suppressor region of the β^s gene cluster and interaction with α^+ thalassaemia appear to modify the polymerization kinetics of HbS in a more consistent manner.

The rate of progression of disease and development of end-stage vasculopathy are thus genetically controlled. The most severe clinical problems such as renal failure, cerebral infarction, chronic lung disease, retinopathy and leg ulcers are observed in those with the Central African Republic (CAR) haplotype, although even this may be ameliorated by interaction with an α-thalassaemia gene [136].

Sickle cell haemoglobin C disease (HbSC) is a milder variant of HbSS with normal or near normal levels of haemoglobin. One of the dangers of this condition is that, owing to its mildness, neither the woman nor her obstetrician may be aware of its presence. These women are at risk of massive, sometimes fatal, sickling crises during pregnancy and particularly in the puerperium. It is therefore vital that the abnormality is detected, preferably before pregnancy, so that the appropriate precautions can be taken. Clinical manifestations of the doubly heterozygous condition, sickle cell thalassaemia, are usually indistinguishable from HbSS; those who make detectable amounts of HbA are usually less severely affected but they are still at risk from sickling crises during pregnancy.

Sickle cell trait (HbAS) results in no detectable abnormality under normal circumstances although it is easily diagnosed by specific investigations including haemoglobin electrophoresis (see below). Affected subjects are not anaemic even under the additional stress of pregnancy, unless there are additional complications, and sickling crises occur only in situations of extreme anoxia, dehydration and acidosis. A recent publication has demonstrated an increased incidence of pre-eclampsia in women with sickle cell trait [137].

Management of sickle cell syndromes

At present there is no routine long-term method of reducing the liability of red cells to sickle *in vivo* [138]. The role of BMT and gene therapy have yet to be established [138]. However, induction of HbF by the use of hydroxycarbamide (hydroxyurea) is now regarded by many as safe and effective therapy for sickle cell disease [139]. Although it is an antineoplastic agent there has been no suggestion of increase in birth defects among infants born to patients who were taking the drug at time of conception, though experience is limited. Very recently the introduction of pulse butyrate therapy has been shown to produce a sustained increase in HbF levels in more than two-thirds of adult sickle cell patients [140]. Like hydroxycarbamide (hydroxyurea), butyrate has been used as an antineoplastic agent, but neither anticancer drug causes direct modification of DNA and therefore neither should be expected to be mutagenic. Nevertheless, these drugs should only be used as a last resort in pregnancy when all other measures have failed.

Both drugs have a suppressive effect on erythropoiesis and myelopoiesis but result in significant increases in haemoglobin levels. This must be due to a reduction in haemolysis resulting in part from the protective effect of

HBF. With hydroxycarbamide (hydroxyurea), a marked decrease in adherence of patients' red blood cells to endothelial cells is observed long before HbF concentrations rise [139]. A larger prospective evaluation of the effects of pulse butyrate therapy on clinical outcome is obviously required [140]. Once a crisis is established, there is no evidence that alkalis, hyperbaric oxygen, vasodilators, plasma expanders, urea or anticoagulants are of any value. Where beneficial effects have been reported they can usually be attributed to the meticulous care and supportive therapy received by the patient, rather than to the specific measures themselves. Adequate fluid administration alone probably accounts for most of the benefit.

Contraception and sickle cell syndromes

There is much more longitudinal experience in the USA than there is as yet in the UK. Methods of contraception vary, but problems arise from the assumption that sicklers are at increased risk of thromboembolism if they use oral contraception. The patient's risk in taking the pill is less than that of pregnancy and there are almost no data to suggest that patients with sickle cell disease run a greater risk than any other patients using low-dose oestrogen preparations [141]. The usual contraindications hold true of course and patients should be monitored carefully for alterations in blood pressure and liver function.

Because patients' response to pregnancy varies, there should not be 'blanket' recommendations for all patients with sickle cell disease.

Sickle cell disease and pregnancy

Women with sickle cell disease present special problems in pregnancy [142–144]. Fetal loss is high, presumably due to sickling infarcts in the placental circulation [141,145]. Abortion, preterm labour and other complications are more common than in women who have normal haemoglobins. Although many women with sickle cell disease have no complications, the outcome in any individual case is always in doubt. The only consistently successful way of reducing the incidence of these complications due to sickling is by regular blood transfusion at approximately 6-week intervals, to maintain the proportion of HbA at 60–70% of the total [146]. Between 3 and 4 units of blood should be given at each transfusion. This regimen has two effects: it dilutes the circulating sickle haemoglobin and, by raising the haemoglobin, reduces the stimulus to the bone marrow and therefore the amount of sickle haemoglobin produced.

Sickle cells have a shorter life than normal red cells and so each successive transfusion is more effective. If this regimen has been instituted, a general anaesthetic may be given with safety, and sickling crises in the course of normal labour are much less likely. The management of sickle cell syndromes in pregnancy in the UK is a relatively recent problem, and longitudinal data are lacking. It is clear on review of the extensive US literature that although risks remain higher for pregnancy complicated by sickle cell disease, modern obstetric care alone, without transfusion, has reduced the maternal morbidity and mortality dramatically and also improved fetal outcome [142,147,148]. Some obstetric centres still use prophylactic transfusion regimens but the real benefit of such regimens remains to be proven by a large trial with contemporary controls [149]. A small multicentre trial in the USA suggests that the outcome is similar in women transfused prophylactically compared with those transfused only when indications arise [150].

A more recent multicentre retrospective study from the UK also showed that prophylactic transfusion did not improve obstetric outcome when compared with those pregnancies that were not transfused [151]. Both studies [150,151], however, highlighted serious sickling complications in twin pregnancies associated with sickle cell disease and suggest a case for *routine* prophylactic transfusion at least in women with twin pregnancy and sickle cell disease.

These regular transfusion protocols are not without complications. Of course there is a risk of transmitting infection, hepatitis B and C, and human immunodeficiency virus (HIV) to which the pregnant woman with her altered immunity is especially susceptible. Now that all blood donors are screened for exposure and response to HIV, the much-publicized and feared hazard of HIV infection resulting from 1-unit blood donations (non-pooled blood products) is extremely small. The risk of infected blood being undetected has been calculated to be 0.7 per million donations and that is if high-risk donors (paid donors, the promiscuous, drug addicts) are giving their blood. Such donors are asked not to give blood in the UK [152,153] and no donors are paid for giving blood.

The most worrying complication of transfusion has been the development of atypical red cell antibodies [154], resulting from the fact that the donor populations differ in ethnic origin from the recipients and carry different minor red cell antigens. This has resulted in extreme difficulties in finding compatible blood [144,155] and even in haemolytic disease of the newborn [144]. There is a real danger that regular top-up transfusions or partial exchange transfusion regimens may become accepted therapy in pregnancy complicated by sickle cell disease before their true benefits and hazards have been properly evaluated. The consensus from the USA is that transfusion should only be given in preparation for general anaesthesia or where there is evidence of maternal distress

[141,142,147,150]. If the disorder presents late in pregnancy and there is more urgency because, for instance, the woman is profoundly anaemic or is suffering a crisis, exchange transfusion can be used.

It is obvious that it would be far better to prevent the emergency situation during pregnancy by identification of women before pregnancy and early booking for antenatal care. However, even after preparation with regular transfusion, tissue hypoxia, acidosis and dehydration should be avoided because they will make the patient's own remaining red cells more likely to sickle. Also, perhaps due to the anti-aldosterone actions of progesterone, hyperkalaemia has been reported in pregnant women with sickle cell disease at levels of renal dysfunction below those observed in non-pregnant individuals with HbSS disease [156]. Tourniquets should not be used. To minimize pulmonary infection, prophylactic antibiotics are desirable to cover all anaesthetics. Recurrent pulmonary sickling crises may lead to chronic lung disease. One such case during pregnancy has been reported with maternal death at 31 weeks' gestation [157]. Severe painful crises or vascular necrosis of bone may be followed by embolism of bone marrow with fatty globules which may be seen in lungs, eyes, brain and urine. Most cases have occurred during pregnancy and this complication is associated with a high mortality [158].

The worry concerning aspiration pneumonitis, hypoxia and other perioperative pulmonary problems may be avoided by using regional anaesthesia but substitutes the risk of hypotension and venous pooling in the vessels of the lower extremities. Wrapping the legs in elastic bandages and elevating them will reduce venous pooling and subsequent hypotension. Epidural is preferred to spinal anaesthesia because there is less risk of hypotension if preoperative hydration regimens with left uterine displacement are adopted. Although a number of sicklers have been reported in the obstetric literature to have suffered pulmonary emboli [141,159], there is no good evidence to incriminate regional anaesthesia as a significant additional risk factor and indeed there are good physiological data to support it having a protective role. In an emergency, both regional and general anaesthesia may have to be undertaken without ideal preparation. Good communication and cooperation between anaesthetist, obstetrician and haematologist, together with meticulous postoperative care, are essential for a good outcome. Again, as with the controversy over blood transfusion, it is simple lack of awareness of potential problems and relaxation of vigilance that change the outcome [141] rather than lack of knowledge of the details of the measures adopted to deal with the many and varied hazards of sickle haemoglobin in pregnancy.

No special preparation with blood transfusion is required in pregnancy for women with sickle cell trait (HbAS). However, as in patients with HbSS, it is essential that hypoxia and dehydration are avoided during anaesthesia and labour, particularly in the immediate postdelivery period. In fact the majority of unexpected deaths associated with HbS have occurred in patients with sickle cell trait in the immediate postoperative or postpartum period.

The single most important pregnancy precaution is for the woman's partner to be screened, so that the couple can be advised of the risk of a serious haemoglobin defect in their offspring.

Detection of haemoglobin S

Any test designed to screen for the presence of HbS should detect not only sickle cell disease but also distinguish HbSC, HbS thalassaemia and sickle cell trait. The classic sickling test in which the red cell is suspended in a reducing agent is difficult to interpret and may occasionally give false-negative results. Furthermore, it is time consuming and its usefulness is limited when diagnosis is urgent. A proprietary product (Sickledex) is available that overcomes these drawbacks: it detects HbS by precipitation of deoxygenated HbS. It is rapid, reliable, and does not give false negatives. Definitive diagnosis of the particular sickle cell syndrome involved requires haemoglobin electrophoresis and sometimes, in the case of sickle cell thalassaemia, family studies. Screening early in pregnancy where there is no absolute urgency is probably best carried out by performing haemoglobin electrophoresis. The sickling test will then only have to be carried out on blood from those women with an abnormal band in the S region. Electrophoresis on cellulose acetate in tris buffer at pH 8.9 will distinguish it from HbD, which has similar mobility on conventional electrophoresis.

Screening for haemoglobinopathy

Unfortunately, at the moment, screening procedures are often not carried out until women are pregnant. In most cases this means that early prenatal diagnosis by DNA analysis of a chorion biopsy is not possible. Selection for screening in a busy antenatal clinic may be more time consuming than it is worth and, to be efficient, should involve detailed documentation of a woman's heritage before excluding her from testing. For this reason, and because of the remote possibility of missing such a defect in the non-immigrant population, general screening for haemoglobinopathies is carried out routinely on every woman's blood during pregnancy at Queen Charlotte's Maternity Hospital, London, which serves a cosmopolitan population. This involves examination of red cell indices (see Table 2.1), haemoglobin electrophoresis and quantification of HbA_2 and HbF on the booking sample of blood (Fig. 2.4).

If a haemoglobin variant or thalassaemia is found, the partner is requested to attend so that his blood can also be examined. By this means we are able to assess the chances of a serious haemoglobin defect in the fetus early in pregnancy in order to advise the parents of the potential hazard and to offer them prenatal diagnosis.

Although all cases of sickle cell disease and the vast majority of thalassaemia syndromes can be diagnosed by readily available DNA probes, the couples at risk would have to be identified before or within the first 8–10 weeks of fetal development for early prenatal diagnosis to be performed. With standard booking procedures this is unusual. We recognize that this inevitably results in late prenatal diagnosis and if indicated a painful, demoralizing, second-trimester termination, but unless couples at risk are identified *before* or during the first trimester of pregnancy, there is no other alternative.

Prenatal diagnosis of haemoglobinopathies

Fetal blood sampling

Until the mid-1970s the prenatal diagnosis of thalassaemia major and of sickle cell disease (also a β-globin chain defect) was thought to be a relatively unrealistic goal for two reasons. First, because information concerning β-chain synthesis in the first and second trimesters of human pregnancy was lacking, and secondly, because it was believed that any techniques necessary for acquisition of fetal blood would prove to be prohibitively dangerous with respect to the maintenance of the pregnancy.

Huehns *et al.* [160] at University College Hospital, London, showed that adult haemoglobin ($HbA\alpha_2\beta_2$) could be detected in the red cells of the fetus as early as 8–10 weeks' gestation (Fig. 2.5).

Prenatal diagnosis of these haemoglobinopathies was accomplished for the first time in the 1970s by the use of globin chain synthesis studies of fetal blood obtained by fetoscopy or 'blind' placental aspiration [161] at 18–22 weeks' gestation. The fetal loss rate using these techniques could be as high as 12–15% in those early days [162].

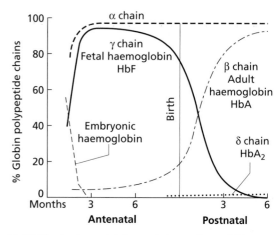

Fig 2.5 The developmental changes in human haemoglobin. (From [47]).

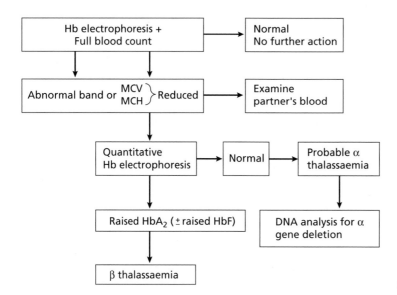

Fig 2.4 Screening for haemoglobinopathy.

Since the mid-1980s pure fetal blood has been obtained from the fetal cord by means of an ultrasound-guided needle introduced through the maternal abdominal wall [163]. The risks to the ongoing pregnancy of this procedure are considerably less than those associated with previous methods. Currently, fetal blood sampling overall carries a risk of fetal loss of 1–3% [164–166]. However, fetal blood sampling for the prenatal diagnosis of the haemoglobinopathies, for which it was originally introduced, has now largely been superseded [167].

It is now possible to detect genetic haemoglobin defects by DNA analysis of chorion villus samples and fetal cells in amniotic fluid. These samples can be obtained much earlier in gestation (see below) than fetal blood.

Globin gene analysis

The last few years have seen a remarkable advances in molecular biology and in particular the development of techniques for isolating and analysing DNA [124]. Normal globin genes have been examined using molecular hybridization and restriction endonuclease mapping techniques [167]. For the study of human genetic diseases, DNA is usually obtained from the nuclei of white blood cells in a peripheral blood sample. However, in the prenatal diagnosis of haemoglobinopathies there are two possible alternative sources of DNA for diagnosis of fetal disease, namely fetal cells in amniotic fluid and trophoblast tissue obtained by a transcervical chorion biopsy technique [123,124,168]. The use of these techniques depends on being able to identify an abnormality of the DNA of the globin gene involved in the haemoglobinopathy or a closely linked polymorphism, which is inherited with the relevant gene. Fetal DNA in maternal blood derived from cells [169] or plasma [170] can now be detected, and techniques are being developed for the prenatal diagnosis of genetic abnormalities. These will reduce the need for hazardous invasive procedures.

All cases of sickle cell disease can now be diagnosed prenatally by DNA analysis because of the identifiable base changes in the β-globin gene complex that synthesizes sickle haemoglobin. Most fetuses at risk for serious α-thalassaemia syndromes can be identified because the abnormalities result from α-gene deletion (see Fig. 2.2) [127,171]. Thalassaemias involving abnormal synthesis of both δ and β chains (δβ thalassaemias) are also diagnosable because they result from gene deletion [172]. A rapidly increasing number of cases of β thalassaemia have become identifiable by DNA analysis because of linked polymorphisms or partial gene deletions [173]. Unfortunately, however, in these cases, unless the couple has been identified and there is a large family available for study and plenty of time to perform the laboratory investiga-

tions required, the techniques have usually not been used until an affected child has been born.

A study of the Mediterranean population, which, of course, includes Cypriot migrants to the UK, suggests that in the vast majority of first pregnancies at risk for β thalassaemia, an affected fetus can be identified with oligonucleotide probes [126]. These are small, synthetic DNA fragments, which are constructed specifically to detect single base changes in DNA. Although oligonucleotide probe technology is still being developed, it has already been possible to construct probes that identify the single base changes that cause human single-gene disorders [125]. In those couples in which both partners carry a β-thalassaemia determinant, β-globin gene analysis is performed on amplified DNA in order to determine the molecular defect. The entire β-globin gene is amplified by using the polymerase chain reaction (PCR) with appropriate primers. Known mutations may be detected by gel electrophoresis, restriction endonuclease analysis, dot blot analysis with allele-specific probes, or primer-specific amplifications [173].

It is now possible to identify the base change in the β-globin gene complex that leads to the substitution of valine for glutamic acid and hence to the production of sickle haemoglobin. This means that all couples at risk of producing a child with sickle cell disease can have prenatal diagnosis using DNA analysis. The results of such analyses may be available on the same day that the fetal DNA is obtained [174].

Amniotic fluid cells

Amniocentesis is safer than fetal blood sampling and possibly safer than chorion villus sampling. Now that amplification of DNA is possible by PCR techniques, sufficient tissue is obtained for rapid prenatal diagnosis without the need for lengthy culturing procedures. Analysis of amniotic fetal cell DNA for prenatal diagnosis of α thalassaemia hydrops has been used for more than a decade in the Far East, but the recent improvements in detection and rapidity of tests have facilitated carrier detection and prenatal diagnosis of α-thalassaemia syndromes considerably [175,176].

It may be asked why prenatal diagnosis for α thalassaemia should be attempted when the major form of the disease is incompatible with life, and HbH disease probably does not adversely affect life expectancy. One reason is that pregnancy with an α thalassaemia hydrops is associated with severe, sometimes life-threatening, pre-eclampsia in the mother. Also, vaginal deliveries are associated with obstetric complications due to the large size of the fetus and placenta associated with the haemoglobinopathy (see above).

Chorion villus sampling

More than a decade ago, a report of 200 cases [177] of first-trimester fetal diagnosis for haemoglobinopathies carried out in the UK using chorionic villus sampling (CVS) and DNA analysis, suggested that provided CVS proves to be associated with an acceptably low fetal loss rate and that it has no significant long-term effects on fetal development, it would become the method of choice for fetal diagnosis of haemoglobinopathies and other single-gene disorders. The current CVS fetal loss rate is little more than 2%, which compares favourably with other methods used in prenatal diagnosis. However, limb reductions associated with this technique continue to give some cause for concern [178–180].

Initially transcervical villus sampling was carried out using an endoscope but this technique has largely been abandoned, and biopsy specimens are obtained using a fine-bore needle and cannula under ultrasound guidance. Even so the procedure still probably carries a risk of abortion at least two to three times greater than that of amniocentesis; there is also a maternal risk of endotoxic shock ascribed to penetration of a contaminated cervix. For these reasons, some workers have adopted the trans-abdominal approach [181]. They claim that this avoids the potentially infected endocervical canal, and also that needle-guided transabdominal CVS is more easily learned than transcervical techniques. Also it seemed that high abortion rates were associated with transcervical biopsy until the operator became skilled. In addition, the trans-abdominal method may be used over a wider gestational age range, i.e. 9–14 weeks as opposed to 9–12 weeks using the transcervical route. Maxwell *et al.* in 1986 [181] suggested that the technique should be widely evaluated in clinical practice possibly as part of a controlled trial comparing transabdominal with transcervical routes. There have now been many randomized trials comparing the two techniques. In the USA [182] the safety of both techniques was found to be similar. In Denmark [183] the unintentional fetal loss rate was much higher using the transcervical route (7.7%) compared with the transabdominal approach (3.7%).

The vast majority of the limb anomalies described in association with CVS have been in fetuses sampled before 10 weeks' gestation [178,180] and are thought to have a vascular aetiology related to either decreased fetal perfusion or thrombosis at the sampling site [178]. In the UK each fetal medicine unit has its preferred technique, but providing that the transcervical approach is avoided before 10 weeks' gestation (when there is an association with limb reduction) there appears to be no difference in outcome.

In summary, the prenatal diagnosis of the haemoglobinopathies originally performed by globin chain analysis of fetal blood samples taken in the second trimester has now largely been replaced by direct detection of the genetic defect by analysis of amplified DNA from fetal trophoblast or amniotic fluid cells obtained earlier in gestation.

Rationale for screening

The main reason why pre-pregnancy screening programmes for haemoglobinopathies should be set up is the handicap associated with homozygous β thalassaemia. The management of homozygous β thalassaemia by regular blood transfusion and chelating agents is extremely expensive and puts a major burden on the health services particularly in the developing countries where the disease is so common. Undoubtedly, the most cost-effective approach to the problem of thalassaemia is the development of programmes for the pre-pregnancy screening of potential mothers and, in cases where they are found to be carriers, of their partners [126]. Where both parents are affected they should be offered the possibility of antenatal diagnosis by fetal blood or trophoblast sampling and of abortion of homozygous fetuses. This type of programme is now well established in many parts of the world, but screening usually takes place in the antenatal period when conception has already occurred. Even if the couple is known to be at risk, having already had an affected child, there may not be time for proper investigation, so that advantage can be taken of the more acceptable trophoblast sampling technique for DNA analysis of the fetus, if indicated.

Implications for the future

Now that first-trimester fetal diagnosis has become possible for virtually all serious haemoglobinopathies and as the techniques become available in more centres over the world, screening should be extended beyond the antenatal clinic. It has been suggested [184] that education and counselling should be directed at three points in people's lives, namely, at school, at marriage and at family planning clinics. The information given should include details of where blood testing can be carried out and advice on when this should be done, although it should probably be left to the individual in possession of the information to request the test. This will involve education of the communities at risk and also—a component that is often forgotten—education of the medical practitioners caring for these communities.

The first audit of prenatal diagnosis for haemoglobin disorders in the UK covering the first 20 years has recently been published including an analysis of 2068 cases from 1974 to 1994. Over 50% of first prenatal diagnoses were performed in the second trimester. About 40% were retrospective after the birth of an affected child. Six such couples are known to have sued their obstetrician for negligence [128]. Overall, the extended findings point to serious shortcomings in present antenatal screening practices in the UK and to inadequate counselling resources, especially for British Asians with thalassaemia [129].

Miscellaneous anaemias

Many forms of anaemia, in particular the anaemia of renal failure, are exacerbated by pregnancy. However, supportive and prophylactic therapy for the various medical conditions concerned is improving, and maternal risks for the most part have been reduced, as have the risks to the fetus. Each case has to be considered individually: there are no general rules that can be applied in terms of management.

Aplastic anaemia

There have been sporadic case reports of refractory hypoplastic anaemia, sometimes recurrent, developing in pregnancy and appearing to be related in some way to the pregnancy [185,186]. Occasionally pregnancy occurs when chronic acquired aplastic anaemia is present as an underlying disease. It has been generally considered that in both these situations pregnancy exacerbates the marrow depression, results in rapid deterioration, and should be terminated. It is true that many cases do remit spontaneously after termination [187], but there is no record of excessive haemorrhage at delivery despite profound thrombocytopenia. Supportive measures in this situation are improving and pregnancy should be maintained as long as the health of the mother is not seriously impaired [188].

There are a few cases in the literature of reversible pure red cell aplasia (associated with pregnancy) following delivery. One report describes the course of relapsing pure red cell aplasia during three pregnancies [189]. Anaemia can be profound, and supportive red cell transfusions are necessary, but the outcome is generally good if there are no other interacting complications. The whole subject has been reviewed [190].

Autoimmune haemolytic anaemia and systemic lupus erythematosus

The rare combination of autoimmune haemolytic anaemia (AIHA) and pregnancy carries great risks to both the woman herself and the fetus. Very careful antenatal supervision and adjustment to steroid therapy are required [191].

Pregnancy may coincide with exacerbations of systemic lupus erythematosus (SLE), although up to 50% of women with this condition are reported to improve during pregnancy especially in the third trimester [192] (see also Chapter 8).

Haemolytic anaemia, leucopenia and thrombocytopenia (see Chapter 8) have all been observed in infants of women with active disease, presumably due to IgG antibody involved in the disease process crossing the placenta.

With regard to therapy, there have been a number of reports in which women have been treated with steroids [193] and other immune suppressives throughout pregnancy for a variety of conditions including immune thrombocytopenic purpura (ITP), SLE, AIHA and some forms of malignancy. Possible effects of steroids are considered in Chapter 1. The problems of their use are essentially the same as those outside pregnancy, but more frequent monitoring and adjustment are required due to the rapidly changing blood volume and changes in the circulating hormones during the antenatal and postnatal periods. There is also concern about the possible effects of azathioprine on the reproductive performance of female offspring (Chapter 8).

A rare form of haemolytic anaemia appears to be specific to pregnancy. It remits after delivery but tends to recur in subsequent pregnancies in about half of the women affected. Although no autoantibody has been identified, the anaemia responds to steroids and immunoglobulin. The fetus may be affected in about 20% of cases [194].

Polycythaemia rubra vera

Polycythaemia rubra vera (PRV) is a myeloproliferative disease involving a pluripotent haemopoietic stem cell. It is an uncommon disorder with an estimated incidence of one in 50 000. It affects women less often than men and is usually seen after the sixth decade of life and is therefore only rarely encountered in pregnant women.

Reports in the literature are very sparse, involving not many more than 15 pregnancies in nine women and were reviewed in 1983 [195].

Diagnosis of PRV depends on the demonstration of an increased red cell mass, which distinguishes the condition from 'stress' erythrocytosis characterized by an increased haematocrit but with a normal red cell mass. Differentiation from secondary polycythaemia is made by lack of increased erythropoietin levels in the urine. Also in PRV there is usually an absolute granulocytosis and thrombocytosis, which is not found in secondary poly-cythaemia. The maternal outcome in the few reports available is usually good, but there is an increased inci-dence of pregnancy-induced hypertension, and neonatal mortality is high due to frequent occurrence of abortion, stillbirth and preterm delivery.

Radioactive phosphorus ^{32}P has been the treatment of choice for older patients with PRV. Alkylating agents have been introduced more recently into treatment regi-mens. However, in younger patients these measures are usually avoided because of their leukaemogenic potential. During pregnancy the additional hazards of teratogeni-city and other harm to the fetus precludes their use.

Control of haematological parameters is best achieved by repeated phlebotomy. The haematocrit should be maintained at a value of <50% to reduce the associated hazards of abnormal bleeding, thrombosis and tissue hypoxia.

In PRV it has been recommended [195] that prophylac-tic antithrombotic measures should be taken during the intra- and postpartum period because of the associated hypercoagulability in uncomplicated pregnancy (see Chapter 4). Low-dose heparin appears to be the treatment of choice.

Surgery carries exceptional hazards of bleeding and thrombosis in the uncontrolled polycythaemic patient, and emergency phlebotomy is indicated in the uncon-trolled patient who needs an urgent caesarean section or other surgery.

Regional anaesthesia is the analgesic and anaesthetic of choice. During general anaesthesia alterations in pulmon-ary elasticity and ventilation–perfusion defects may lead to respiratory acidosis. Long-term prognosis is difficult to predict for any individual. An erythrocytic phase is often followed by an inactive phase, which may last as long as 25 years. As a rule, survival is longer in patients who are younger at the time of diagnosis. Maternal survival in older patients has been estimated at 16 years. Myeloid metaplasia is seen as the duration of the disease increases, and death usually results from terminal development of acute leukaemia or myelofibrosis.

Thrombocythaemia, thrombocytosis

Essential and primary thrombocythaemia (thrombocyto-sis) usually affects subjects beyond the childbearing age. A myeloproliferative disorder, characterized by an isol-ated high platelet count, it is associated with both haem-orrhagic and thromboembolic phenomena. Reports in the literature are sparse [196–198] and management strategies are therefore difficult to plan. If the thrombocythaemia is not accompanied by polycythaemia and there have been

no previous complications, then the treatment of choice should be aspirin (at least 75 mg/day) to inhibit platelet aggregation and thrombosis. This should be instituted when the platelet count exceeds 600×10^9/L [200]. Two asymptomatic women with platelet counts around 1000 $\times10^9$/L at our hospital were managed throughout preg-nancy with aspirin, and no complications occurred in either mother or fetus. Recurrent late abortion associated with thrombocythaemia has been managed successfully with aspirin. Cytotoxic agents have been used in this disease [199] but should be avoided in gestation.

Interferon α may be given where complications have not been prevented by therapy with aspirin [199]. It has been used without ill-effect in human pregnancy [200].

Paroxysmal nocturnal haemoglobinuria

This rare condition which occurs primarily in young adults is now known to be caused by a genetically deter-mined somatic mutation in a haemopoietic stem cell giving rise to populations of defective red cells, granulo-cytes and platelets [201,202]. The intrinsic defect in the red cell makes it particularly sensitive to lysis by complement. The disease varies widely in severity; it usually begins insidiously and haemoglobinuria, as a presenting symp-tom, is found in only 25% of all patients.

The laboratory diagnosis is made using a series of special tests that demonstrate the sensitivity of the patient's red cells to lysis by complement.

The main features of the disease are episodes of acute and chronic intravascular haemolysis with varying degrees of anaemia and haemoglobinuria. More important complica-tions arise from the defective platelets and granulocytes produced by the abnormal clone of stem cells.

Thrombosis accounts for approximately 50% of deaths in reported autopsies. The major morbidity also relates to venous thrombosis, which has been reported in periph-eral as well as in mesenteric, hepatic, portal and cerebral veins.

This hypercoagulable state has been attributed to the triggering effect of intravascular haemolysis and in-creased activity of coagulation factors, but the most rele-vant explanation for the enhanced thrombotic tendency is that the paroxysmal nocturnal haemoglobinuria (PNH) platelets can bind much greater amounts of complement (C3) than normal platelets. Activation of the complement pathway triggers PNH platelets to undergo the release reaction and aggregate, thus initiating thrombosis [203]. Similarly, poorly understood functional abnormalities of leucocyte function together with granulocytopenia are thought to contribute to the increased susceptibility to infection seen in patients with PNH.

As the disease progresses, the abnormal clone of cells takes over and normal bone marrow becomes increasingly hypoplastic and ultimately aplastic [204,205].

The most serious complications associated with PNH are thrombosis, infection and ultimately marrow aplasia.

The optimum treatment of PNH is replacement of the abnormal stem cell with cells producing normal cellular components by BMT, but this is not an option during pregnancy. Androgen therapy has been useful in suppressing haemolysis and increasing normal cell production in non-pregnant females and in males, but it has side-effects and its use is definitely contraindicated in pregnancy.

Prednisone 1 mg/kg may be useful in reducing haemolysis; if the patient responds to prednisone, this may safely be used throughout pregnancy (see Chapter 1).

Iron has been used to maintain the haematocrit and replace iron lost in the urine, but it has been shown in many studies to trigger acute haemolytic episodes and is therefore probably best avoided.

The fertility rate in this uncommon condition is thought to be low and experience of pregnancies associated with PNH is limited. To date fewer than 100 cases have been reported in the English literature. Awareness of the risks involved has led to the previous suggestion that conception should be avoided if possible. Although more recently there have been reports of successful maternal and fetal outcome of pregnancies associate with PNH [206–208], safe effective contraception needs to be considered. The hypercoagulable state in PNH rules out oral contraception and there has been a report of cerebral vein thrombosis in a woman with PNH associated with use of an oral contraceptive. The use of a conventional intrauterine device is contraindicated in the presence of thrombocytopenia and granulocytopenia. However, one of the newer hormone-coated intrauterine devices such as the Mirena coil that do not cause menorraghia or predispose to infection could be considered. Otherwise if couples at risk wish to delay pregnancy, barrier methods should be recommended and if they decide against further reproduction, either tubal ligation or vasectomy should be advised.

If pregnancy is embarked upon, the main hazards appear to be spontaneous abortion, often following acute haemolytic episodes, and serious thrombotic events mainly in the puerperium.

Prophylactic transfusions with washed red cells, which are not a source of extrinsic complement, maintaining the haematocrit between 25 and 30%, to suppress the production of abnormal cells, have been recommended in the first trimester [209]. The theory is that these transfusions will decrease the possibility of severe haemolytic episodes and therefore the risk of spontaneous abortion and the chance of a severe thrombotic episode early in pregnancy.

Hepatic vein thrombosis is the most common thrombotic complication, having a maximum incidence postpartum; antenatal pulmonary embolism has also been reported.

Low-dose heparin has been shown to be ineffective prophylaxis in at least one case in the antenatal period [210]. The maximum risk period is still after delivery. It has been suggested therefore that full anticoagulation should be used to treat any thrombotic episode in the antenatal period, and that full anticoagulation should be used prophylactically in the puerperium [209] (see Chapter 4).

'Nevertheless, despite the usual view that pregnancy is too hazardous in patients with PNH, a poor outcome may not be inevitable' [208].

Leukaemia

One in 1000 pregnancies is complicated by malignant disease [211,212]. The incidence of leukaemia in pregnancy should not exceed one in 75 000 pregnancies, but the information used to calculate this incidence is obtained from cases recorded in the literature—a method with serious limitations. Although peak incidence years for cancer do not coincide with the peak reproductive years, leukaemia was reported in 1969 as the second most common cause of death from malignant disease in females aged 15–34 in the USA. Several hundred cases of leukaemia in association with pregnancy have now been reported; most papers give an account of a specific case or cases and include a review of the published literature (e.g. [213–215]), and some include management considerations (e.g. [216]).

There is no objective evidence that pregnancy has a deleterious effect on leukaemia [213,216]. Survival times in pregnant women with leukaemia do not differ statistically from those of non-pregnant women. The application of modern treatment can result in remission of the disease, which is sometimes repeated, and more affected women may now have the opportunity to conceive or to survive until the fetus is viable.

The diagnosis during pregnancy is made most frequently in the second and third trimesters, although the disease may have been present earlier. This is because the early symptoms are non-specific, the most common being fatigue, which is often attributed by the woman and her obstetrician to the pregnancy itself. This emphasizes the importance of carrying out proper investigations, including bone-marrow examination of unexplained anaemia in pregnancy.

The occurrence of pregnancy in a woman suffering from or developing acute leukaemia creates special clinical problems, which fall into two main groups—those arising from the disease process and those arising from its treatment. There are increased risks of infection, haemorrhage and abortion arising from the disease process itself and from the effects of chemotherapy [217]. Fetal loss occurs in approximately 14% of women with chronic myeloid leukaemia and 33% of women with acute leukaemia. Haemorrhage may result from thrombocytopenia due to bone-marrow infiltration or from a consumption coagulopathy; this is a particularly common problem in acute myelomonocytic leukaemia. The powerful cytotoxic drugs that are often used to achieve remission in acute adult leukaemia include cytosine arabinoside, rubidomycin and thioguanine. Such agents have been shown to be toxic to fetal tissue in experimental animals. Malformations have occurred after treatment with cytotoxic drugs in the first trimester [215]. Methotrexate, a folic acid antagonist, is the most teratogenic drug known to man. Its administration early in pregnancy always results in either abortion or congenital malformation. Other published data have suggested that cytotoxic drugs might be given with safety in the second and third trimesters [214,215]. One more recently published study with follow-up of 43 children over a period of 3–19 years whose mothers had received chemotherapy for various malignancies including leukaemia, showed no adverse effect in the children. Nineteen of these mothers received treatment in the first trimester. A similar retrospective study also published in 1991 looked at 56 pregnancies in 48 women and found no increase in the incidence of complications during pregnancy compared with pregnancies in a healthy population [218].

Successful pregnancy has been reported in women receiving recombinant interferon α for management of chronic myeloid leukaemia [219].

It has been suggested [214] that a pregnant leukaemic woman should be treated with aggressive chemotherapy until a remission is achieved. The risk of a malformed fetus in a woman so treated in the first trimester is high, and termination should be considered once she is in remission and this can be performed with safety. Termination of pregnancy when therapy is started in the second or third trimester is only indicated on moral and medico-social grounds, as the fetus is likely to develop normally. Examination of chromosomes of fetal amniotic fluid cells and of fetal hair under the scanning electron microscope may provide evidence of fetal damage in those cases where treatment is started early in the second trimester [214]. An alternative approach later in the second trimester would be fetal blood sampling.

A more recent overview of leukaemia and lymphoma in pregnancy [220] tabulates published case reports of acute leukaemia since the comprehensive review of McLain [216]. Based on the combined data, the authors confirm the earlier conclusions that pregnancy itself has no adverse effect on the course of leukaemia unless specific chemotherapy is withheld for fear of damaging the fetus. However, the converse is not true. The greatest risks are maternal death before delivery and fetal damage or death related to maternal chemotherapy. Since 1989 there have been some reports of successful pregnancies in women who had prior allogeneic BMT, both in those whose conditioning therapy for BMT was by use of chemotherapy alone [221] and more recently in women who received total body irradiation [222].

Hodgkin's disease

The diagnosis of Hodgkin's disease depends upon the presence of the characteristic Reed–Sternberg cell in biopsy material. The various morphological subclasses of the Reed–Sternberg cell and the relative proportion of other cellular elements have no influence on the outcome of the disease unlike in the non-Hodgkin's lymphomata in which histology has a major influence on outcome [212,220,223]. Prognosis depends on the staging of the disease at presentation.

Treatment for Hodgkin's disease involves adequate radiotherapy for patients with relatively localized disease. A cure rate of over 90% can be expected in these cases. Combination chemotherapy regimens are used for those with more widespread disease and involvement both above and below the diaphragm. In cases with no systemic symptoms such as unexplained weight loss, pyrexia or night sweats, chemotherapy alone will produce a complete remission in 80–100% of patients with a probable cure in at least 50%.

Widespread disease with systemic manifestations has a poorer prognosis and is treated with aggressive repeated courses of combination chemotherapy often combined with radiotherapy.

Because the choice of treatment requires precise staging of the disease, pregnancy should always be ruled out before undertaking diagnostic studies and therapy.

The incidence of Hodgkin's disease in pregnancy is low, so it is most unlikely that there will ever be prospective randomized studies to resolve which is the optimum management strategy for the various stages of the disease that may occur during the antenatal period. The largely American retrospective experience has been reviewed [220,223]. A recently published British retrospective study of 48 women who had Hodgkin's disease compared with non-pregnant women at similar stages of disease matched for age and therapy showed that the 20-year survival of those women with a pregnancy was no different from their matched controls [224].

A communication from Italy reports a retrospective analysis of 219 female patients presenting between 1971 and 1982 with Hodgkin's disease [225]. Twenty-one patients were pregnant at the time of presentation. One hundred and fifty-five patients aged 15–45 years when Hodgkin's disease was diagnosed were selected as controls. The authors concluded, as have others [220], that pregnancy does not influence the symptoms or presentation of the disease. The slightly higher proportion of advanced stages among the pregnant patients in the study may be explained by the masking of the early signs and symptoms by pregnancy itself. Pregnancy does not affect prognosis, and the higher proportion of advanced stages has statistically negligible influence on survival. Pregnancy does not induce a higher relapse rate. A large proportion of treated patients whose menstruation is preserved are still fertile and can expect to produce apparently normal offspring especially in the younger age groups [225]. A more recent retrospective analysis of pregnancy outcome in 139 survivors of advanced Hodgkin's disease provided data on 302 pregnancies. There was an excess of low birthweights in women treated actively during the antenatal period but this was based on small numbers [226].

It would seem prudent to advise a patient to delay conception until 2 years after successful therapy has been completed because the risk of relapse falls off rapidly after that time. However, there is still concern about the long-term impact of ionizing radiation and chemotherapeutic agents on the ova and ultimately on the offspring of treated patients even if conception occurs well after therapy has been completed. It is known from animal studies that anomalies (induced in offspring) may not appear until later in life and it is even more difficult to evaluate the risk in the human.

Aborted fetuses, infants and children may not be adequately screened for defects. Applied therapy regimens differ from one treatment centre to another. Therapy-induced cases of mutagenesis tend to be emphasized in the literature making assessment of the true proportion of unfavourable outcome very difficult to estimate [227].

References

1 Miller JR, Keith NM, Rowntree LG. Plasma and blood volume in pregnancy. *J Am Med Assoc* 1915; 65: 779–882.
2 Hytten FE, Leitch I. The volume and composition of the blood. In: *The Physiology of Human Pregnancy*. Blackwell Scientific Publications, Oxford, 1971.
3 Hytten F. Blood volume changes in normal pregnancy. In: Letsky, EA, ed. *Haematological Disorders in Pregnancy*. W.B. Saunders, London, 1985: 601–12.
4 Pirani BB, Campbell DM, MacGillivray I. Plasma volume in normal first pregnancy. *J Obstet Gynaecol Br Commonwealth* 1973; 80 (10): 884–7.
5 Chesley LC, Duffus GM. Posture and apparent plasma volume in late pregnancy. *J Obstet Gynaecol Br Commonwealth* 1971; 78: 406–12.
6 Murphy JF, O'Riordan J, Newcombe RG, Coles EC, Pearson JF. Relation of haemoglobin levels in first and second trimesters to outcome of pregnancy. *Lancet* 1986; 1: 992–5.
7 Rovinsky JJ, Jaffin H. Cardiovascular hemodynamics in pregnancy. I. Blood and plasma volumes in multiple pregnancy. *Am J Obstet Gynecol* 1965; 93: 1.
8 Fullerton WT, Hytten FE, Klopper AI, McKay E. A case of quadruplet pregnancy. *J Obstet Gynaecol Br Commonwealth* 1965; 72: 791–6.
9 Gibson HM. Plasma volume and glomerular filtration rate in pregnancy and their relation to differences in fetal growth. *J Obstet Gynaecol Br Commonwealth* 1973; 80 (12): 1067–74.
10 Harstad TW, Mason RA, Cox SM. Serum erythropoietin quantitation in pregnancy using an enzyme-linked immunoassay. *Am J Perinatol* 1992; 9 (4): 233–5.
11 De Leeuw NK, Lowenstein L, Tucker EC, Dayal S. Correlation of red cell loss at delivery with changes in red cell mass. *Am J Obstet Gynecol* 1968; 100: 1092–101.
12 Peck TM, Arias F. Hematologic changes associated with pregnancy. *Clin Obstet Gynecol* 1979; 22 (4): 785–98.
13 Taylor DJ, Mallen C, McDougall N, Lind T. Effect of iron supplements on serum ferritin levels during and after pregnancy. *Br J Obstet Gynaecol* 1982; 89: 1011–17.
14 World Health Organization. *Nutritional Anaemias*. WHO, Geneva, 1972.
15 De Leeuw NK, Lowenstein L, Hsieh YS. Iron deficiency and hydremia in normal pregnancy. *Medicine (Baltimore)* 1966; 45: 291–315.
16 World Health Organization. *The Prevalence of Nutritional Anaemia in Women*. WHO, Geneva, 1992.
17 World Health Organization. Prevention and management of severe anaemia in pregnancy. Report of a Technical Working Group, Geneva, 20–22 May 1991. *Maternal Health and Safe Motherhood Programme*. WHO, Geneva, 1993.
18 Fletcher J, Suter PE. The transport of iron by the human placenta. *Clin Sci* 1969; 36: 209–20.
19 Svanberg B. Absorption of iron in pregnancy. *Acta Obstet Gynecol Scand (Suppl)* 1975; 48: 1–108.
20 Chanarin I, Rothman D, Berry V. Iron deficiency and its relation to folic acid status in pregnancy: Results of a clinical trial. *Br Med J* 1965; 1: 480–5.
21 Chisholm J. A controlled clinical trial of prophylactic folic acid and iron in pregnancy. *J Obstet Gynaecol* 1966; 73: 191–6.
22 Gatenby PBB. The anaemias of pregnancy in Dublin. *Proc Nutr Soc* 1956; 15: 115–19.
23 Lund CJ. Studies on the iron deficiency anemia of pregnancy including plasma volume, total hemoglobin, erythrocyte protoporphyrin in treated and untreated normal and anemic patients. *Am J Obstet Gynecol* 1951; 62: 947.
24 Magee HE, Milligan EHM. Haemoglobin levels before and after labour. *Br Med J* 1951; 2: 1307.
25 Morgan EH. Plasma iron and haemoglobin levels in pregnancy. The effect of oral iron. *Lancet* 1961; 1: 9–12.
26 Stott G. Anaemia in Mauritius. *Bull WHO* 1960; 23: 781–91.

27 Finch CA, Huebers H. Perspectives in iron metabolism. *N Engl J Med* 1982; 306: 1520–8.

28 Walter T. Effect of iron-deficiency anaemia on cognitive skills in infancy and childhood. *Baillieres Clin Haematol* 1994; 7: 815–27.

29 Oski FA. Iron deficiency—facts and fallacies. *Pediatr Clin North Am* 1985; 32: 493–7.

30 Lozoff B, Jimenez E, Wolf AW. Long-term developmental outcome of infants with iron deficiency. *N Engl J Med* 1991; 325: 687–94.

31 Idjradinata P, Pollitt E. Reversal of developmental delays in iron-deficient anaemic infants treated with iron. *Lancet* 1993; 341: 1–4.

32 Bruner AB, Joffe A, Duggan AK, Casella JF, Brandt J. Randomised study of cognitive effects of iron supplementation in non-anaemic iron-deficient adolescent girls. *Lancet* 1996; 348: 992–6.

33 Klebanoff MA, Shiono PH, Selby JV, Trachtenberg AI, Graubard BI. Anemia and spontaneous preterm birth. *Am J Obstet Gynecol* 1991; 164: 59–63.

34 Scholl TO, Hediger ML, Fischer RL, Shearer JW. Anemia vs iron deficiency. Increased risk of preterm delivery in a prospective study. *Am J Clin Nutr* 1992; 55: 985–8.

35 Godfrey KM, Redman CW, Barker DJ, Osmond C. The effect of maternal anaemia and iron deficiency on the ratio of fetal weight to placental weight. *Br J Obstet Gynaecol* 1991; 98: 886–91.

35a Hindmarsh PC, Geary MPP *et al.* Effect of early maternal iron stores on placental weight and structure. *Lancet* 2000; 356: 719–723.

36 Barker DJP, Bull AR, Osmond C, Golding J, Simmonds SJ. Fetal and placental size and risk of hypertension in adult life. *Br Med J* 1990; 301: 259–62.

37 Moore VM, Miller AG *et al.* Placental weight, birth measurements and blood pressure at age 8 years. *Arch Dis Childhood* 1996; 74: 538–41.

38 Paneth N, Susser M. Early origins of coronary heart disease (the 'Barker hypothesis'). *Br Med J* 1995; 310: 411–12.

39 Thompson WG. Comparison of tests for diagnosis of iron depletion in pregnancy. *Am J Obstet Gynecol* 1988; 159: 1132–4.

40 Van den Broek NR, Letsky EA, White SA, Shenkin A. Iron status in pregnant women: which measurements are valid? *Br J Haematol* 1998; 103: 817–24.

41 Jacobs A, Miller F, Worwood M, Beamish MR, Wardrop CA. Ferritin in the serum of normal subjects and patients with iron deficiency and iron overload. *Br Med J* 1972; 4: 206–8.

42 Fenton V, Cavill I, Fisher J. Iron stores in pregnancy. *Br J Haematol* 1977; 37: 145–9.

43 Rios E, Lipschitz DA, Cook JD, Smith NJ. Relationship of maternal and infant iron stores as assessed by determination of plasma ferritin. *Pediatrics* 1975; 55: 694–9.

44 Cook JD. Iron-deficiency anaemia. *Baillieres Clin Haematol* 1994; 7: 787–804.

45 Carriaga MT, Skikne BS, Finley B, Cutler B, Cook JD. Serum transferrin receptor for the detection of iron deficiency in pregnancy. *Am J Clin Nutr* 1991; 54: 1077–81.

46 Fleming AF, Martin JD, Hahnel R, Westlake AJ. Effects of iron and folic acid antenatal supplements on maternal haematology and fetal wellbeing. *Med J Aust* 1974; 2: 429–36.

47 Haddow A, Horning ES. On the carcinogenicity of an iron-dextran complex. *Br Med J* 1964; 1: 1593.

47a Fielding J. Does sarcoma occur in man after intramuscular iron? *Scand J Haematol* 1977; suppl. 32: 100–104.

48 Baker SB de C, Golberg, L *et al.* Tissue changes following injection of iron-dextran complex. *J Pathol Bacteriol* 1961; 82: 453–70.

49 Hallberg I, Ryttinger L, Solvell L. Side effects of oral iron therapy. *Acta Med Scand* 1966; 459 (Suppl): 3–10

50 Scott JM. Iron sorbitol citrate in pregnancy anaemia. *Br Med J* 1963; 2: 354–7.

51 Scott JM. Toxicity of iron sorbiton citrate. *Br Med J* 1962; ii: 480–1.

52 Stein ML, Gunston KD, May RM. Iron dextran in the treatment of iron-deficiency anaemia of pregnancy. Haematological response and incidence of side-effects. *S Afr Med J* 1991; 79: 195–6.

53 Al-Momen AK, Al-Meshari A *et al.* Intravenous iron sucrose complex in the treatment of iron deficiency anemia during pregnancy. *Eur J Obstet Gynecol Reprod Biol* 1996; 69: 121–4.

54 Anonymous. Do all pregnant women need iron? *Br Med J* 1978; ii: 1317.

55 Barrett JF, Whittaker PG, Williams JG, Lind T. Absorption of non-haem iron from food during normal pregnancy. *Br Med J* 1994; 309: 79–82.

56 Jacobs A, Worwood M. Iron metabolism, iron deficiency and iron overload. In: Hardisty, RM, Weatherall, DJ, eds. *Blood and its Disorders*, 2nd edn, pp. 149–197. Blackwell Scientific Publications, Oxford, 1982.

57 Ogunbode O, Akinyele IO, Hussain MA. Dietary iron intake of pregnant Nigerian women with anemia. *Int J Gynaecol Obstet* 1979; 17: 290–3.

58 Kuizon MD, Platon TP, Ancheta LP, Angeles JC, Nunez CB, Macapinlac MP. Iron supplementation studies among pregnant women. *Southeast Asian J Trop Med Publ Health* 1979; 10: 520–7.

59 Paintin DB, Thomson AM, Hytten FE. Iron and the haemoglobin level in pregnancy. *J Obstet Gynaecol Br Commonwealth* 1966; 73: 181–90.

60 Cuervo LG, Mahomed K. Treatments for iron deficiency anaemia during pregnancy (Protocol for a Cochrane Review). *The Cochrane Library*, 2000.

61 Steer P, Alam MA, Wadsworth J, Welch A. Relation between maternal haemoglobin concentration and birth weight in different ethnic groups. *Br Med J* 1995; 310: 489–91.

62 Jackson HA, Worwood M, Bentley DP. Haemochromatosis mutations and iron stores in pregnancy. *Br J Haematol* 1998; 101 (Suppl. 1): 25.

63 Hemminki E, Starfield B. Routine administration of iron and vitamins during pregnancy: review of controlled clinical trials. *Br J Obstet Gynaecol* 1978; 85: 404–10.

64 Hallberg L, Bengtsson C, Garby L, Lennartsson J, Rossander L, Tibblin E. An analysis of factors leading to a reduction in iron deficiency in Swedish women. *Bull WHO* 1979; 57 (6): 947–54.

65 Mayet FG. Anaemia of pregnancy. *S Afr Med J* 1985; 67: 804–9.

66 Meadows NJ, Grainger SL, Ruse W, Keeling PW, Thompson RP. Oral iron and the bioavailability of zinc. *Br Med J Clin Res Ed* 1983; 287: 1013–14.

67 Meadows NJ, Ruse W *et al.* Zinc and small babies. *Lancet* 1981; 2: 1135–7.

68 Sheldon WL, Aspillaga MO, Smith PA, Lind T. The effects of oral iron supplementation on zinc and magnesium levels during pregnancy. *Br J Obstet Gynaecol* 1985; 92 (9): 892–8.

69 Bentley DP. Iron metabolism and anaemia in pregnancy. *Clin Haematol* 1985; 14: 613–28.

70 Letsky EA. Anaemia in obstetrics. In: Studd, J, ed. *Progress in Obstetrics and Gynaecology*. Churchill Livingstone, Edinburgh, 1987: 23–58.

71 Stoltzfus RJ, Dreyfuss ML. *Guidelines for the Use of Iron Supplements to Prevent and Treat Iron Deficiency Anemia on Behalf of the International Nutritional Anemia Consultative Group (INACG).* International Life Sciences Institute Press, Washington, 1998.

72 Kullander S, Kallen B. A prospective study of drugs and pregnancy. 4. Miscellaneous drugs. *Acta Obstet Gynecol Scand* 1976; 55: 287–95.

72a Letsky EA. Maternal anaemia in pregnancy. Iron and pregnancy: a haematologist's view. *Fetal Matern Medi Rev* 2001; 12: 159–75.

73 Ball EW, Giles C. Folic acid and vitamin B_{12} levels in pregnancy and their relation to megaloblastic anaemia. *J Clin Pathol* 1964; 17: 165.

74 Chanarin I. Megaloblastic anaemia associated with pregnancy. In: *The Megaloblastic Anaemias.* Blackwell Scientific Publications, Oxford, 1979: 466.

75 Fleming AF, Martin JD, Stenhouse NS. Pregnancy anaemia, iron and folate deficiency in Western Australia. *Med J Aust* 1974; 2: 479–84.

76 Landon MJ. Folate metabolism in pregnancy. *Clin Obstet Gynaecol* 1975; 2: 413.

77 Fleming AF. Urinary excretion of folate in pregnancy. *J Obstet Gynaecol Br Commonwealth* 1972; 79: 916–20.

78 Chanarin J, MacGibbon BM, O'Sullivan WJ, Mollin DL. Folic acid deficiency in pregnancy; the pathogenesis of megaloblastic anaemia of pregnancy. *Lancet* 1959; ii: 634–9.

79 Stephens ME, Craft J, Peters TJ, Hoffbrand AV. Oral contraceptives and folate metabolism. *Clin Sci* 1972; 42: 405–14.

80 Landon MJ, Hytten FE. The excretion of folate in pregnancy. *J Obstet Gynaecol Br Commonwealth* 1971; 78: 769–75.

81 McLean FW, Heine MW, Held B, Streiff RB. Folic acid absorption in pregnancy. Comparison of the pteroylpolyglutamate and pteroylmonoglutamate. *Blood* 1970; 36: 628–31.

82 Avery B, Ledger WJ. Folic acid metabolism in well-nourished pregnant women. *Obstet Gynecol* 1970; 35: 616–24.

83 Chanarin I, Rothman D, Ward A, Perry J. Folate status and requirement in pregnancy. *Br Med J* 1968; 2: 390.

84 Stone ML, Luhby AL, Feldman R, Gordon M, Cooperman JM. Folic acid metabolism in pregnancy. *Am J Obstet Gynecol* 1967; 99: 638–48.

85 Shapiro J, Alberts HW, Welch P, Metz J. Folate and vitamin B_{12} deficiency associated with lactation. *Br J Haematol* 1965; 11: 498–504.

86 Osler W. Observations on the severe anaemias of pregnancy and the postpartum state. *Br Med J* 1919; u: 1–2.

87 Lowenstein L, Brunton L, Hsieh YS. Nutritional anemia and megaloblastosis in pregnancy. *Can Med Assoc J* 1966; 94: 636–45.

88 Coyle C, Geoghegan F. The problem of anaemia in a Dublin maternity hospital. *Proc R Soc Med* 1962; 55: 764–6.

89 Chanarin I. The folate content of food-stuffs and the availability of different folate analogues for absorption. In: *Getting the Most out of Food.* Van den Bergh and Jurgens, London, 1975: 41.

90 Giles C. An account of 335 cases of megaloblastic anaemia of pregnancy and the puerperium. *J Clin Pathol* 1966; 19: 1–11.

91 Gatenby PBB, Little EW. Clinical analysis of 100 cases of severe megaloblastic anaemia of pregnancy. *Br Med J* 1960; ii: 1111–14.

92 Rae PG, Robb PM. Megaloblastic anaemia of pregnancy, a clinical and laboratory study with particular reference to the total and labile serum folate levels. *J Clin Pathol* 1970; 23: 379–91.

93 Fletcher J, Gurr A, Fellingham FR, Prankerd TAJ, Brant HA, Menzies DN. The value of folic acid supplements in pregnancy. *J Obstet Gynaecol Br Commonwealth* 1971; 75: 781–5.

94 Baumslag N, Edelstein T, Metz J. Reduction of incidence of prematurity by folic acid supplementation in pregnancy. *Br Med J* 1970; 1: 16–17.

95 McCann SR, Lawlor E, McGovern M, Temperley IJ. Severe megaloblastic anaemia of pregnancy. *J Irish Med Assoc* 1980; 73: 197–8.

96 Chanarin I. Folate and cobalamin. *Clin Haematol* 1985; 14: 629–41.

97 Strauss RG, RB. Folic acid and dilantin antagonism in pregnancy. *Obstet Gynaecol* 1974; 44: 345–8.

98 Hiilesmaa VK, Teramo K, Granstrom ML, Bardy AH. Serum folate concentrations during pregnancy in women with epilepsy. Relation to anti-epileptic drug concentrations, numbers of seizures and fetal outcome. *Br Med J* 1983; 287: 577–9.

99 Hill RM, Verniaud WM, Horning MG, McCulley LB, Morgan NF. Infants exposed in utero to anti-epileptic drugs. *Am J Dis Child* 1974; 127: 645–53.

100 Bjerkedal T, Bahna SL. The course and outcome of pregnancy in women with epilepsy. *Obstet Gynaecol Scand* 1973; 52 (Suppl.): 245–8.

101 Deblay MF, Vert P, Andre M, Marchal F. Transplacental vitamin K prevents haemorrhagic disease of infant of epileptic mother. *Lancet* 1982; i: 1247.

102 Haworth C, Evans DIK. Nutritional aspects of blood disorders in the newborn. *J Hum Nutr* 1981; 35: 323–34.

103 Oski FA. Nutritional anemias. *Semin Perinatol* 1979; 3: 381–95.

104 Laurence KM, James N, Miller MH, Tennant GB, Campbell H. Double-blind randomised controlled trial of folate treatment before conception to prevent recurrence of neural-tube defects. *Br Med J Clin Res Ed* 1981; 282: 1509–11.

105 Smithells RW, Nevin NC *et al.* Further experience of vitamin supplementation for prevention of neural tube defect recurrences. *Lancet* 1983; 1: 1027–31.

106 Smithells RW, Sheppard S *et al.* Possible prevention of neural-tube defects by periconceptional vitamin supplementation. *Lancet* 1980; i: 339–40.

107 Elwood JM. Can vitamins prevent neural tube defects? *Can Med Assoc J* 1983; 129: 1088–92.

108 MRC. Prevention of neural tube defects: results of the Medical Research Council Vitamin Study. MRC Vitamin Study Research Group. *Lancet* 1991; 338: 131–7.

109 Czeizel AE, Dudas I. Prevention of the first occurrence of neural-tube defects by periconceptional vitamin supplementation. *N Engl J Med* 1992; 327: 1832–5.

110 Berry RJ, Li Z *et al.* Prevention of neural-tube defects with folic acid in China. *N Engl J Med* 1999; 341: 1485–90.

111 Hook EB, Czeizel AE. Can terathanasia explain the protective effect of folic acid supplements on birth defects? *Lancet* 1997; 350: 513–15.

112 Editorial. Folic acid and neural tube defects. *Lancet* 1991; 338: 153–4.

113 Rosenberg IH. Folic acid and neural-tube defects—time for action? *N Engl J Med* 1992; 327 (26): 1875–7.

114 Kadir RA, Sabin C, Whitlow B, Brockbank E, Economides D. Neural tube defects and periconceptional folic acid in England and Wales: retrospective study. *Br Med J* 1999; 319: 92–3.

115 Alberman E, Noble JM. Commentary: Food should be fortified with folic acid. *Br Med J* 1999; 319: 93.

116 Edelstein T, Metz J. Correlation between vitamin B_{12} concentration in serum and muscle in late pregnancy. *J Obstet Gynaecol Br Commonwealth* 1969; 76: 545–8.

117 Temperley IJ, Meehan MJ, Gatenby PB. Serum vitamin B_{12} levels in pregnant women. *J Obstet Gynaecol Br Commonwealth* 1968; 75: 511–16.

118 McGarry JM, Andrews J. Smoking in pregnancy and vitamin B 12 metabolism. *Br Med J* 1972; 2: 74–7.

119 Cooper BA. Folate and vitamin B_{12} in pregnancy. *Clin Haematol* 1973; 2: 461–6.

120 Fleming AF. Haematological changes in pregnancy. *Clin Obstet Gynaecol* 1975; 2: 269.

121 Jackson IMD, Doig WB, McDonald G. Pernicious anaemia as a cause of infertility. *Lancet* 1967; ii: 1159.

122 Van den Broek NR, Letsky EA. Etiology of anemia in pregnancy in South Malawi. *Am J Clin Nutr* 2000; 72: 247S–256S.

123 Nicolaides KH, Rodeck CH, Mibashan RS. Obstetric management and diagnosis of haematological disease in the fetus. *Clin Haematol* 1985; 14: 775–805.

124 Weatherall DJ. *The New Genetics and Clinical Practice*, 3rd edn. Oxford University Press, Oxford, 1991.

125 Weatherall DJ. Prenatal diagnosis of inherited blood disorders. In: Hann I, Gibson B, Letsky EA, eds. *Fetal and Neonatal Haematology*. Baillière Tindall, London, 1991: 285–314.

126 Weatherall DJ, Letsky EA. Genetic haematological disorders. In: Wald, NJ, Leck I, eds *Antenatal and Neonatal Screening*, 2nd edn, pp. 243–81. Oxford University Press, Oxford: 2000.

127 Higgs DR. Alpha thalassaemia in haemoglobinopathies. In: Higgs, DR, Weatherall, DJ, eds *Baillière's Clinical Haematology the Haemoglobinopathies*. Baillière Tindall: London, 1993: 117–50.

128 Modell B, Petrou M *et al.* Audit of prenatal diagnosis for haemoglobin disorders in the United Kingdom: the first 20 years. *Br Med J* 1997; 315: 779–84.

129 Gill PS, Modell B. Thalassaemia in Britain: a tale of two communities. *Br Med J* 1998; 317: 761–2.

130 Modell B, Harris R *et al.* Informed choice in genetic screening for thalassaemia during pregnancy: audit from a national confidential inquiry. *Br Med J* 2000; 320: 337–41.

131 Goldfarb AW, Hochner-Celnikier D *et al.* A successful pregnancy in transfusion dependent homozygous beta-thalassaemia: a case report. *Int J Gynaecol Obstet* 1982; 20: 319–22.

132 Oliveiri NF. Medical progress: The β-thalassemias. *N Engl J Med* 1999; 341: 99–109.

133 Roberts I. Current status of allogeneic transplantation for haemoglobinopathies. *Br J Haematol* 1997; 98: 1–7.

134 Bareford D. Thalassaemia in pregnancy (Letter). *Br Med J* 1991; 303: 120.

135 Hussein SS, Hoffbrand AV, Laulicht M, Attock B, Letsky EA. Serum ferritin levels in beta thalassaemia trait. *Br Med J* 1976; ii: 920.

136 Powars D, Chan LS, Schroeder WA. The variable expression of sickle cell disease is genetically determined. *Semin Hematol* 1990; 27: 360–76.

137 Larrabee KD, Monga M. Women with sickle cell trait are at increased risk for preeclampsia. *Am J Obstet Gynecol* 1997; 177: 425–8.

138 Steinberg MH. Management of sickle cell disease. *N Engl J Med* 1999; 340: 1021–30.

139 Bunn HF. Induction of fetal hemoglobin in sickle cell disease. *Blood* 1999; 93: 1787–9.

140 Atweh GF, Sutton M *et al.* Sustained induction of fetal hemoglobin by pulse butyrate therapy in sickle cell disease. *Blood* 1999; 93 (6): 1790–7.

141 Charache S, Niebyl JR. Pregnancy in sickle cell disease. In: Letsky, EA, ed. *Haematological Disorders in Pregnancy*. W.B. Saunders, London, 1985: 720–46.

142 Charache S, Scott J *et al.* Management of sickle cell disease in pregnant patients. *Obstet Gynecol* 1980; 55: 407–10.

143 Perry KG Jr, Morrison JC. The diagnosis and management of hemoglobinopathies during pregnancy. *Semin Perinatol* 1990; 14 (2): 90–102.

144 Tuck SM, Studd JWW, White JM. Pregnancy in sickle cell disease in the United Kingdom. *Br J Obstet Gynaecol* 1983; 90: 112–17.

145 Anyaegbunam A, Langer O, Brustman L, Whitty J, Merkatz IR. Third-trimester prediction of small-for-gestational-age infants in pregnant women with sickle cell disease: Development of the ultradop index. *J Reprod Med* 1991; 36: 577–80.

146 Huehns ER. The structure and function of haemoglobin: clinical disorders due to abnormal haemoglobin structure. In: Hardisty, RM, Weatherall, DJ, eds *Blood and its Disorders*. Blackwell Scientific Publications, Oxford, 1982: 323–400.

147 Koshy M, Burd L. Management of pregnancy in sickle cell syndromes. *Hematol Oncol Clin North Am* 1991; 5: 585–96.

148 Serjeant GR. Sickle haemoglobin and pregnancy. *Br Med J* 1983; 287: 628–30.

149 Tuck SM, James CE, Brewster EM, Pearson TC, Studd JW. Prophylactic blood transfusion in maternal sickle cell syndromes. *Br J Obstet Gynaecol* 1987; 94: 121–5.

150 Koshy M, Burd L, Wallace D, Moawad D, Baron J. Prophylactic red cell transfusions in pregnant patients with sickle cell disease. *N Engl J Med* 1988; 319: 1447–52.

151 Howard RJ, Tuck SM, Pearson TC. Pregnancy in sickle cell disease in the UK: results of a multicentre survey of the effect of prophylactic blood transfusion on maternal and fetal outcome. *Br J Obstet Gynaecol* 1995; 102: 947–51.

152 Acheson D. *Press Release 1*. Department of Health and Social Security, 1987, 87/5.

153 Williamson L, Heptonstall J, Soldan K. A SHOT in the arm for safer blood transfusion. *Br Med J* 1996; 313: 1221–2.

154 Rosse WF, Gallagher D *et al.* Transfusion and alloimmunization in sickle cell disease: The Cooperative Study of Sickle Cell Disease. *Blood* 1990; 76: 1431–7.

155 Miller JM, Horger EO *et al.* Management of sickle haemoglobinopathies in pregnant patients. *Am J Obstet Gynecol* 1981; 141: 237–41.

156 Lindheimer MD, Richardson DA, Ehrlich EN, Katz AI. Potassium homeostasis in pregnancy. *J Reprod Med* 1987; 32: 517–22.

157 Van Enk A, Visschers G *et al.* Maternal death due to sickle cell chronic lung disease. *Br J Obstet Gynaecol* 1992; 99: 162–3.

158 Serjeant GR. The clinical features of sickle cell disease. *Baillière's Clin Haematol* 1993; 6: 93–115.

159 Thomas AN, Pattison C, Serjeant GR. Causes of death in sickle cell disease in Jamaica. *Br Med J* 1982; 285: 633–55.

160 Huehns ER, Dance N, Beaven GH, Hecht F, Motulsky AG. Human embryonic haemoglobins. Cold Spring Harbor Symposium. *Quart Biol* 1964; 29: 327–31.

161 Kan YW, Trecartin RF, Golbus MS, Filly RA. Prenatal diagnosis of thalassaemia and sickle cell anaemia. Experience with 24 cases. *Lancet* 1977; i: 269–71.

162 Alter BP. Prenatal diagnosis of haemoglobinopathies and other haematologic diseases. *J Pediatr* 1979; 95: 501–13.

163 Nicolaides KH, Soothill PW, Rodeck CH, Campbell S. Ultrasound-guided sampling of umbilical cord and placental blood to assess fetal wellbeing. *Lancet* 1986; i: 1065–8.

164 Daffos F, Capella-Pavlosky M, Forestier F. Fetal blood sampling during pregnancy with use of a needle guided by ultrasound: a study of 606 consecutive cases. *Am J Obstet Gynecol* 1985; 153: 655–60.

165 Ghidini A, Sepulveda W, Lockwood CJ, Romero R. Complications of fetal blood sampling. *Am J Obstet Gynecol* 1993; 168: 1339–44.

166 Maxwell DJ, Johnson P, Hurley P, Neales K, Allan L, Knott P. Fetal blood sampling and pregnancy loss in relation to indication. *Br J Obstet Gynaecol* 1991; 98: 892–7.

167 Old JM, Thein SL, Weatherall DJ, Cao A, Loukopoulos D. Prenatal diagnosis of the major haemoglobin disorders. *Mol Biol Med* 1989; 6: 55–63.

168 Rodeck CH, Morsman JM. First trimester chorion biopsy. *Br Med Bull* 1983; 39: 338–42.

169 Lo YM, Bowell PJ *et al.* Prenatal determination of fetal RhD status by analysis of peripheral blood of rhesus negative mothers. *Lancet* 1993; 341: 1147–8.

170 Lo YMD, Corbetta N *et al.* Presence of fetal DNA in maternal plasma and serum. *Lancet* 1997; 350: 485–7.

171 Kan YW, Golbus MS, Dozy AM. Prenatal diagnosis of thalassaemia: Clinical application of molecular hybridization. *N Engl J Med* 1971; 295: 1165–7.

172 Orkin SH, Alter C *et al.* Application of endonuclease mapping to the analysis and prenatal diagnosis of thalassaemias caused by globin gene deletion. *N Engl J Med* 1978; 299: 166.

173 Cao A, Rosatelli MC. Screening and prenatal diagnosis of the haemoglobinopathies. *Baillière's Clin Haematol* 1993: 6: 263–86.

174 Embury SH, Scharf SJ *et al.* Rapid prenatal diagnosis of sickle cell anaemia by a new method of DNA analysis. *N Engl J Med* 1987; 316: 656–61.

175 Hsia YE. Detection and prevention of important alpha-thalassemia variants. *Semin Perinatol* 1991; 15: 35–42.

176 Ko TM, Tseng LH, Hsieh FJ, Hsu PM, Lee TY. Carrier detection and prenatal diagnosis of alpha-thalassaemia of Southeast Asian deletion by polymerase chain reaction. *Hum Genet* 1992; 88: 245–8.

177 Old JM, Fitches A *et al.* First-trimester fetal diagnosis for haemoglobinopathies. Report on 200 cases. *Lancet* 1986; ii: 763–7.

178 Burton BK, Schulz CJ, Burd LI. Limb anomalies associated with chorionic villus sampling. *Obstet Gynaecol* 1992; 79: 726–30.

179 Firth HV, Boyd PA, Chamberlain P, MacKenzie IZ, Lindenbaum RH, Huson SM. Severe limb abnormalities after chorion villus sampling at 56–66 days gestation. *Lancet* 1991; 337: 762–3.

180 Hurley PA, Rodeck CH. Fetal therapy. *Curr Opin Obstet Gynecol* 1992; 4: 4–9.

181 Maxwell D, Czepulkowski B, Clifford R, Heaton D, Coleman D. Transabdominal chorionic villus sampling. *Lancet* 1986; i: 123–6.

182 Jackson L, Zachary J *et al.* A randomized comparison of transcervical and transabdominal chorionic-villus sampling. *N Engl J Med* 1992; 327: 594–8.

183 Smidt-Jensen S, Permin M *et al.* Randomized comparison of amniocentesis and transabdominal and transcervical chorionic villus sampling. *Lancet* 1992; 340: 1237–44.

184 Modell B. Prevention of haemoglobinopathies. *Br Med Bull* 1983; 39: 386–91.

185 Taylor JJ, Studd JWW, Green ID. Primary refractory anaemia and pregnancy. *J Obstet Gynaecol Br Commonwealth* 1968; 75: 963–8.

186 van Besien K, Tricot G *et al.* Pregnancy-associated hypoplastic anemia—report of 3 cases. *Eur J Haematol* 1991; 47: 253–6.

187 Evans IL. Aplastic anaemia in pregnancy remitting after abortion. *Br Med J* 1968; 3: 166–7.

188 Lewis SM, Gordon-Smith, EC. Aplastic and dysplastic anaemias. In: Hardisty, RM, Weatherall, DJ, eds *Blood and its Disorders*. Blackwell Scientific Publications, Oxford, 1982: 1229–68.

189 Picot C, Triadou P, Lacombe C, Casadevall N, Girot R. Relapsing pure red-cell aplasia during pregnancy. *N Engl J Med* 1984; 311: 196.

190 Snyder TE, Lee LP, Lynch S. Pregnancy-associated hypoplastic anemia: a review. *Obstet Gynecol Surv* 1991; 46: 264–9.

191 Chaplin H, Cohen R, Bloomberg G, Kaplan HJ, Moore JA, Dorner L. Pregnancy and idiopathic auto-immune haemolytic anaemia. *Br J Haematol* 1973; 24: 219–39.

192 Dubois EL. *Lupus Erythematosus*. McGraw-Hill, New York, 1966.

193 Ng SC, Wong KK, Raman S, Bosco J. Autoimmune haemolytic anaemia in pregnancy: a case report. *Eur J Obstet Gynecol Reprod Biol* 1990; 37: 83–5.

194 Goodall HB, Ho Yen DO, Clark DM, Thomson MA, Browning MC, Crowder AM. Haemolytic anaemia of pregnancy. *Scand J Haematol* 1979; 22: 185–91.

195 Ferguson JE, Ueland K, Aronson WJ. Polycythemia rubra vera and pregnancy. *Obstet Gynecol* 1983; 62: 16S–20S.

196 Beard J, Hillmen P *et al.* Primary thrombocythaemia in pregnancy. *Br J Haematol* 1991; 77: 371–4.

197 Kaibra M, Kobayashi T, Matsusmoto S. Idiopathic thrombocythemia and pregnancy: Report of a case. *Obstet Gynecol* 1985; 65 (Suppl): 185–6.

198 Snethlage W, Tengate JW. Thrombocythaemia and recurrent late abortions. Normal outcome of pregnancies after antiaggregatory treatment. *Br J Obstet Gynaecol* 1986; 93: 386–8.

199 Pearson TC. Clinical annotation—primary thrombocythaemia. Diagnosis and management. *Br J Haematol* 1991; 78: 145–8.

200 Pearson T.C. Diagnosis and Classification of erythrocytoses and thrombocytoses. *Baillière's Clin Haematol* 1998; 11: 695–720.

201 Hillmen P, Bessler M *et al.* Specific defect in N-acetylglucosamine incorporation in the biosynthesis of the glycosylphosphatidylinositol anchor in cloned cell lines from patients with paroxysmal nocturnal hemoglobinuria. *Proc Natl Acad Sci USA* 1993; 90: 5272–6.

202 Miyata T, Takeda J *et al.* The cloning of PIG-A, a component in the early step of GPI-anchor biosynthesis. *Science* 1993; 259: 1318–20.

203 Vermylen J, Blockmans D *et al.* Thrombosis and immune disorders. *Clin Haematol* 1986; 15: 393–412.

204 Dacie JV, Lewis SM. Paroxysmal nocturnal haemoglobinuria. Clinical manifestations, haematology and nature of the disease. *Haematol Ser* 1972; 5: 3.

205 Rotoli B, Luzzatto L. Paroxysmal nocturnal haemoglobinuria. *Baillière's Clin Haematol* 1989; 2: 113–38.

206 Beresford CJ, Gudex DJ, Symmans WA. Paroxysmal nocturnal haemoglobinuria and pregnancy. *Lancet* 1986; 2: 1396–7.

207 De Gramont A, Krulik M, Debray J. Paroxysmal nocturnal haemoglobinuria and pregnancy. *Lancet* 1987; 1: 868.

208 Jacobs P, Wood L. Paroxysmal nocturnal haemoglobinuria and pregnancy. *Lancet* 1986; 2: (Letter) 1099.

209 Hurd WH, Miodovnik M, Stys SJ. Pregnancy associated with paroxysmal nocturnal hemoglobinuria. *Obstet Gynecol* 1982; 60: 742–6.

210 Spencer JAD. Paroxysmal nocturnal haemoglobinuria in pregnancy. *Br J Obstet Gynaecol* 1980; 87: 246–8.

211 Rothman LA, Cohen CJ, Astarloa J. Placental and fetal involvement by maternal malignancy: a report of rectal carcinoma and review of the literature. *Am J Obstet Gynecol* 1973; 116: 1023–33.

212 Slade R, James DK. Pregnancy and maternal malignant haematological disorders. In: Turner TL, ed. *Perinatal Haematological Problems*. John Wiley & Sons, Chichester, 1991: 23–38.

213 Ewing PA, Whittaker JA. Acute leukaemia in pregnancy. *Obstet Gynecol* 1973; 42: 245–51.

214 Gokal R, Durrant J, Baum JD, Bennett MJ. Successful pregnancy in acute monocyte leukaemia. *Br J Cancer* 1976; 34: 299–302.

215 Nicholson HO. Leukaemia and pregnancy. *J Obstet Gynaecol Br Commonwealth* 1968; 75: 517–20.

216 McLain CR. Leukemia in pregnancy. *Clin Obstet Gynecol* 1974; 17: 185–94.

217 Caliguri MA, Mayer RJ. Pregnancy and leukemia. *Semin Oncol* 1989; 16: 388–96.

218 Zuazu J, Julia A *et al*. Pregnancy outcome in hematologic malignancies. *Cancer* 1991; 67: 703–9.

219 Reichel RP, Linkesch W, Schetitska D. Therapy with recombinant interferon alpha-2c during unexpected pregnancy in a patient with chronic myeloid leukaemia. *Br J Haematol* 1992; 82: 472–3.

220 Lewis BJ, Laros RK. Leukaemia and lymphoma. In: Laros, RK, ed. *Blood Disorders in Pregnancy*. Lea & Febiger, Philadelphia, 1986: 85–101.

221 Milliken S, Powles R *et al*. Successful pregnancy following bone marrow transplantation for leukaemia. *Bone Marrow Transpl* 1990; 5: 135–7.

222 Giri N, Vowels MR, Barr AL, Mameghan H. Successful pregnancy after total body irradiation and bone marrow transplantation for acute leukaemia. *Bone Marrow Transpl* 1992; 10: 93–5.

223 Ward FT, Weiss RB. Lymphoma and pregnancy. *Semin Oncol* 1989; 16: 397–409.

224 Lishner M, Zemlickis D, Degendorfer P, Panzarella T, Sutcliffe SB, Koren G. Maternal and foetal outcome following Hodgkin's disease in pregnancy. *Br J Cancer* 1992; 65: 114–17.

225 Gobbi PG, Attardo-Parrinello G *et al*. Hodgkin's disease in pregnancy. *Haematologica* 1984; 69: 336–41.

226 Janov AJ, Anderson J *et al*. Pregnancy outcome in survivors of advanced Hodgkin's disease. *Cancer* 1992; 70: 688–92.

227 Blatt J, Mulvihill JJ *et al*. Pregnancy outcome following cancer chemotherapy. *Am J Med* 1980; 69: 828.

3 Coagulation defects
Elizabeth A. Letsky

Haemostasis and pregnancy

Healthy haemostasis depends on normal vasculature, platelets, coagulation factors and fibrinolysis. These act together to confine the circulating blood to the vascular bed and arrest bleeding after trauma. Normal pregnancy is accompanied by dramatic changes in the coagulation and fibrinolytic systems [1–3] where there is a marked increase in some of the coagulation factors, particularly fibrinogen. Fibrin is laid down in the uteroplacental vessel walls and fibrinolysis is suppressed. These changes, together with the increased blood volume, help to combat the hazard of haemorrhage at placental separation, but play only a secondary role to the unique process of myometrial contraction, which reduces the blood flow to the placental site. They also produce a vulnerable state for intravascular clotting, which is expressed as a whole spectrum of disorders in pregnancy ranging from thromboembolism (see Chapter 4) to bleeding due to disseminated intravascular coagulation (DIC) [4]. To make more understandable the pathophysiology and management of these disorders a short account follows of haemostasis during pregnancy and how it differs from that in the non-pregnant state.

Vascular integrity

It is not known how vascular integrity is normally maintained but it is clear that the platelets have a key role to play, because conditions in which their number is depleted or their function is abnormal are characterized by widespread spontaneous capillary haemorrhages. It is thought that the platelets in health are constantly sealing microdefects of the vasculature, by forming mini fibrin clots, the unwanted fibrin being removed by a process of fibrinolysis. Generation of prostacyclin appears to be the physiological mechanism that protects the vessel wall from excess deposition of platelet aggregates, and explains the fact that contact of platelets with healthy vascular endothelium is not a stimulus for thrombus formation [5].

Prostacyclin (prostaglandin I_2 (PGI_2)) is an unstable prostaglandin first discovered in 1976. It is the principal prostanoid that blood vessels synthesize, a powerful vasodilator and a potent inhibitor of platelet aggregation. Moncada and Vane [5] have proposed that there is a balance between the production of prostacyclin by the vessel wall, and the production of the vasoconstrictor and powerful aggregating agent thromboxane by the platelet. Prostacyclin prevents adhesion at much lower concentrations than are needed to prevent aggregation, therefore vascular damage leads to platelet adhesion but not necessarily to aggregation and thrombus formation.

In the blood vessel, prostacyclin synthetase is abundant in the intima and progressively decreases in concentration from the subendothelium to the adventitia. It follows that severe vessel damage or physical detachment of the endothelium will lead to the development of a large thrombus as opposed to simple platelet adherence.

There are several conditions in which the production of prostacyclin could be impaired, thereby upsetting the normal balance. Prostacyclin production has been shown to be reduced in fetal and placental tissue from pre-eclamptic pregnancies, and the current role of prostacyclin in the pathogenesis of pre-eclampsia continues to be investigated.

However, the endothelium is now regarded as an extremely important component of the haemostatic system, and endothelial cell injury leads to platelet activation and triggering of the coagulation system. It is possible that the changes in haemostatic components are purely a secondary response to underlying vascular disease.

Some studies have shown an increased oxygen free radical production in pre-eclampsia which will in turn decrease vascular prostacyclin and endothelial-dependent relaxing factor (i.e. nitric oxide, NO) release and increase thromboxane A_2 and endothelin release. The whole subject of endothelial function in pre-eclampsia has been well reviewed [6] (see also Chapter 6).

Platelets

Platelets are produced in the bone marrow by the megakaryocytes and have a lifespan of 9–12 days. At the end of their normal lifespan the effete cells are engulfed by cells of the reticuloendothelial system and most damaged platelets are sequestered in the spleen.

There have been conflicting reports concerning the platelet count during normal pregnancy. A review of publications over 25 years [7] revealed a majority consensus (of six), suggesting a small fall in the platelet count towards term, during normal pregnancy. However, few of these studies were longitudinal and in none of them was a within-patient analysis performed. Now that automated platelet counting is routine as part of the full blood count, more information is available about the platelet count in normal, uncomplicated pregnancy. It is becoming clear that, if mean values for platelet concentration are analysed throughout pregnancy, there is a downward trend [8] even though the majority fall within the accepted non-pregnant range [7,9,10].

There is also conflicting evidence [11,12] of increased platelet turnover and low-grade platelet activation as pregnancy advances resulting in a larger proportion of younger platelets with a greater mean platelet volume [7,8].

Most investigators agree that low-grade chronic intravascular coagulation within the uteroplacental circulation is a part of the physiological response of all women to pregnancy. This is partially compensated and therefore it is not surprising that the platelets should be involved giving either indices of increased turnover or in some cases a reduction in number.

A prospective study of 2263 healthy women delivering during 1 year at a Canadian obstetric centre [13] showed that 112 (8.3%) had mild thrombocytopenia at term (platelet counts $97 - 150 \times 10^9$/L). The frequency of thrombocytopenia in their offspring was no greater than that of babies born to women with platelet counts in the normal accepted range and no infant had a platelet count

$< 100 \times 10^9$/L. An extension of this study to include 6715 deliveries substantiates these original findings [14].

In one study patients with a normal pregnancy were compared with non-pregnant controls. They were shown to have a significantly lower platelet count and an increase in circulating platelet aggregates. *In vitro* the platelets were shown to be hypoaggregable. This was interpreted as suggesting platelet activation during pregnancy causing platelet aggregation and followed by exhaustion of platelets [15].

Earlier publications suggesting that there was no evidence of changes in platelet function or differences in platelet lifespan [11,16] between healthy non-pregnant and pregnant women have to be re-evaluated in the face of more recent investigations, but it is clear that *normal* pregnancy has little significant effect on the screening parameter that is usually measured, namely the platelet count.

The problem remains in defining a completely normal pregnancy. Certain disease states specific to pregnancy have profound effects on platelet consumption, lifespan and function. For example, a decrease in platelet count [17] and changes in platelet function [18] have been observed in pregnancies with fetal growth restriction, and the lifespan of platelets is shortened significantly even in mild pre-eclampsia [19,20].

Arrest of bleeding after trauma

An essential function of the haemostatic system is a rapid reaction to injury, which remains confined to the area of damage. This requires a control mechanism that will stimulate coagulation after trauma, and also limit the extent of the response. The substances involved in the formation of the haemostatic plug normally circulate in an inert form, until activated at the site of injury, or by some other factor released into the circulation that will trigger intravascular coagulation.

LOCAL RESPONSE

Platelets adhere to collagen on the injured basement membrane, which triggers a series of changes in the platelets themselves, including shape change and release of adenosine diphosphate (ADP) and other substances. Release of ADP stimulates further aggregation of platelets, which triggers the coagulation cascade generating thrombin; this in turn leads to the formation of fibrin which converts the platelet plug into a firm, stable wound seal. The role of platelets is of less importance in injury involving large vessels, because platelet aggregates are of insufficient size and strength to breach the defect. The coagulation mechanism is of major importance here, together with vascular contraction.

Coagulation system

The end result of blood coagulation is the formation of an insoluble fibrin clot from the soluble precursor fibrinogen in the plasma. This involves a complex interaction of clotting factors, and a sequential activation of a series of proenzymes, the coagulation cascade (Fig. 3.1). When a blood vessel is injured, blood coagulation is initiated by activation of Factor XII by collagen (intrinsic mechanism) and activation of Factor VII by thromboplastin release (extrinsic mechanism) from the damaged tissues. Both the intrinsic and extrinsic mechanisms are activated by components of the vessel wall and both are required for normal haemostasis. Strict divisions between the two pathways do not exist and interactions between activated factors in both pathways have been shown. They share a common pathway following the activation of Factor X.

The intrinsic pathway (or contact system) proceeds spontaneously and is relatively slow, requiring 5–20 min

for visible fibrin formation. All tissues contain a specific lipoprotein, thromboplastin (particularly concentrated in lung and brain), which markedly increases the rate at which blood clots. The placenta is also very rich in tissue factor (thromboplastin), which will produce fibrin formation within 12s; the acceleration of coagulation is brought about by bypassing the reactions involving the contact (intrinsic) system (Fig. 3.1). Because blood coagulation is strictly confined to the site of tissue injury in normal circumstances, powerful control mechanisms must be at work to prevent dissemination of coagulation.

Normal pregnancy is accompanied by major changes in the coagulation system, with increases in levels of Factors VII, VIII and X, and a particularly marked increase in the level of plasma fibrinogen [21] (Fig. 3.1). Elevated fibrinogen is probably the chief cause of the accelerated erythrocyte sedimentation rate (ESR) observed during pregnancy. In the second half of pregnancy, the 95th centile for ESR is

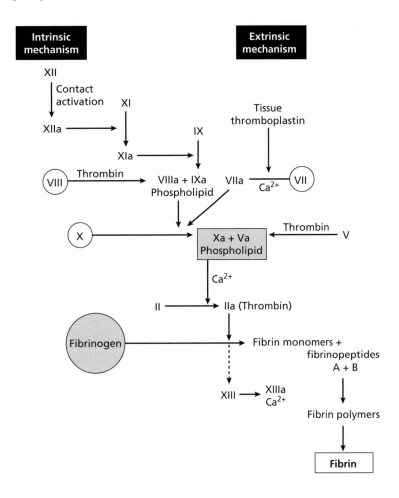

Fig 3.1 The factors involved in blood coagulation and their interactions. The circled factors show significant increases in pregnancy.

70 mm/h in a large group of healthy women studied at Queen Charlotte's Hospital, London [22]. The effect of pregnancy on the coagulation factors can be detected from about the third month of pregnancy, and the amount of fibrinogen in late pregnancy is at least double that of the non-pregnant state [21].

The naturally occurring anticoagulants

Mechanisms that limit and localize the clotting process at sites of trauma are critically important to protect against generalized thrombosis—and also to prevent spontaneous activation of those powerful procoagulant factors that circulate in normal plasma.

The recent investigation of healthy haemostasis, switched emphasis from the factors that promote clotting to those that prevent generalized and spontaneous activation of these factors. It is not appropriate to give an account of the complex interactions and biochemistry of all of these factors here. Only those of major importance in haemostasis and their relevance to pregnancy will be mentioned—the balance of procoagulant and inhibitory factors is discussed elsewhere [23].

ANTITHROMBIN

Antithrombin (AT) is considered to be the main physiological inhibitor of thrombin and Factor Xa. It is well known that heparin greatly enhances the reaction rate of enzyme AT interaction and this is the rationale for the use of low-dose heparin as prophylaxis in patients at risk for thromboembolism postoperatively, in pregnancy and the puerperium. An inherited deficiency of AT is one of several conditions in which a familial tendency to thrombosis has been described (see Chapter 4).

AT is synthesized in the liver. Its activity is low in cirrhosis and other chronic diseases of the liver, as well as in protein-losing renal disease, DIC and hypercoagulable states. The commonest cause of a small reduction in AT is the use of oral contraceptives; this effect is related to the oestrogen content of the pill.

During pregnancy there is little change in AT level but there is some decrease at parturition and an increase in the puerperium [24]. However, there must be increased synthesis in the antenatal period to maintain normal concentrations in the face of an increasing plasma volume.

PROTEIN C–THROMBOMODULIN–PROTEIN S

Protein C inactivates Factors V and VIII in conjunction with its cofactors thrombomodulin and protein S. Protein C is a vitamin K dependent anticoagulant synthesized in

the liver. To exert its effect it must be activated by an endothelial cell cofactor termed thrombomodulin. The importance of the protein C–thrombomodulin–protein S system is exemplified by the absence of thrombomodulin in the brain where the priority for haemostasis is higher than for anticoagulation.

Many kindreds with a deficiency or a functional deficit of protein C with associated recurrent thromboembolism have been described [25] (see Chapter 4). Purpura fulminans neonatalis is the homozygous expression of protein C deficiency with severe thrombosis and neonatal death [26].

Protein S, also a vitamin K dependent glycoprotein, acts as a cofactor for activated protein C by promoting its binding to lipid and platelet surface thus localizing the reaction.

Several families have been described with protein S deficiency and thromboembolic disease.

Data on protein C and protein S levels in healthy pregnancy are sparse. One study showed a significant reduction in functional protein S levels during pregnancy and the puerperium [27]. More recently, 14 patients followed longitudinally throughout gestation and postpartum, showed a rise of protein C within the normal non-pregnant range during the second trimester. In contrast, free protein S fell from the second trimester onwards but remained within the confines of the normal range [28].

Another study supported these findings and was extended to women using oral contraceptives in whom similar changes were found [29].

Although the investigation of natural anticoagulants had only just begun, the system has grown in complexity. There was always little doubt that in the future more components would be recognized as our ability to investigate objectively increased [30]. This allows a better and more thorough understanding of the mechanisms underlying the control of the delicate balance between procoagulant and anticoagulant factors [31] and enables us to manage these complex hypercoagulable states in pregnancy successfully [32].

The recognition of Factor V Leiden [33,34] the prothrombin gene variant together with other newly described genetic thrombophilia factors in pregnancy and their investigation and management [35] are discussed in Chapter 4.

Fibrinolysis

Fibrinolytic activity is an essential part of the dynamic, interacting haemostatic mechanism, and is dependent on plasminogen activator in the blood (Fig. 3.2). Fibrin and fibrinogen are digested by plasmin, a proenzyme derived from its inactive plasma precursor, plasminogen.

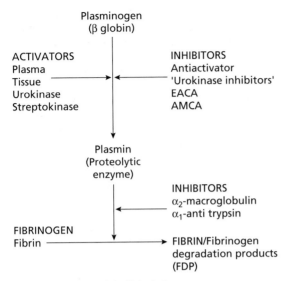

Fig 3.2 Components of the fibrinolytic system.

Increased amounts of activator are found in the plasma after strenuous exercise, emotional stress, surgical operations and other trauma. Tissue activator can be extracted from most human organs with the exception of the placenta. Tissues especially rich in activator include the uterus, ovaries, prostate, heart, lungs, thyroid, adrenals and lymph nodes. Activity in tissues is concentrated mainly around blood vessels, veins showing greater activity than arteries.

The inhibitors of fibrinolytic activity are of two types—antiactivator (antiplasminogens) and the antiplasmins. Inhibitors of plasminogen include ε amino caproic acid (EACA) and tranexamic acid (AMCA). Aprotinin (Trasy-lol) is another antiplasminogen that is commercially prepared from bovine lung.

Platelets, plasma and serum exert a strong inhibitory action on plasmin. Normally, plasma antiplasmin levels exceed levels of plasminogen and hence the levels of potential plasmin; otherwise we would dissolve away our connecting cement! When fibrinogen or fibrin is broken down by plasmin, fibrin degradation products are formed; these comprise the high molecular weight split products X and Y, and smaller fragments, A, B, C, D and E (Fig. 3.3). When a fibrin clot is formed, 70% of fragment X is retained in the clot, Y, D and E being retained to a somewhat lesser extent. Note that blood should be taken for estimation of fibrin degradation products (FDPs) by clean venepuncture. The tourniquet should not be left on too long because venous stasis also stimulates fibrinolytic activity. The blood should be allowed to clot in the presence of an antifibrinolytic agent such as EACA to stop the process of fibrinolysis, which would otherwise continue *in vitro*.

Plasma fibrinolytic activity is decreased during pregnancy, remains low during labour and delivery, and returns to normal within 1 h of delivery of the placenta [36]. This is thought to be due to the effect of placentally derived plasminogen activator inhibitor type 2 (PAI-2), which is present in abundance during pregnancy [37]. In addition the activity in the fibrinolytic system in response to stimulation has been found to be significantly reduced in pregnancy [38].

The changes in the coagulation system in normal pregnancy are consistent with a continuing low-grade process of coagulant activity. Using electron microscopy, fibrin deposition can be demonstrated in the intervillous space of the placenta and in the walls of the spiral arteries supplying the placenta [39]. As pregnancy advances, the

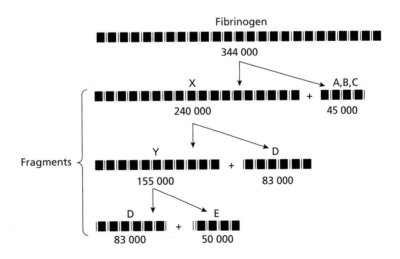

Fig 3.3 Fibrin degradation products (FDPs) produced by action of plasmin on fibrinogen. The molecular weights are shown.

elastic lamina and smooth muscle of these spiral arteries are replaced by a matrix containing fibrin. This allows expansion of the lumen to accommodate an increasing blood flow and reduces the vascular resistance of the placenta. At placental separation during normal childbirth, a blood flow of 500–800 mL/min has to be staunched within seconds, or serious haemorrhage will occur. Myometrial contraction plays a vital role in securing haemostasis by reducing the blood flow to the placental site. Rapid closure of the terminal part of the spiral artery will be further facilitated by removal of the elastic lamina. The placental site is rapidly covered by a fibrin mesh following delivery. The increased levels of fibrinogen and other coagulation factors will be advantageous to meet the sudden demand for haemostatic components.

The changes also produce a vulnerable state for intravascular clotting and a whole spectrum of disorders involving coagulation that occur in pregnancy.

Haemorrhage and coagulopathy

The changes in the haemostatic system and the local activation of the clotting system during parturition carry with them a risk, not only of thromboembolism but also of DIC. This results in consumption of clotting factors and platelets, leading in some cases to severe, particularly uterine and sometimes generalized, bleeding.

The first problem with DIC is in its definition. It is never primary, but always secondary to some general stimulation of coagulation activity by release of procoagulant substances into the blood (Fig. 3.4). Hypothetical triggers of this process in pregnancy include leakage of placental tissue fragments, amniotic fluid, incompatible red cells or bacterial products into the maternal circulation. There is a great spectrum of manifestations of the process of DIC (Fig. 3.4) ranging from a compensated state with no clinical manifestation but evidence of increased production and breakdown of coagulation factors, to the condition of massive uncontrollable haemorrhage with very low concentrations of plasma fibrinogen, pathological raised levels of FDPs and variable degrees of thrombocytopenia. Further cause for confusion is that there appears to be a transient state of intravascular coagulation during the whole of normal labour, maximal at the time of birth [3,40,41].

Fibrinolysis is stimulated by DIC, and the FDPs resulting from the process interfere with the formation of firm fibrin clots causing a vicious circle, which results in further disastrous bleeding.

FDPs also interfere with myometrial function and possibly cardiac function and therefore in themselves aggravate both haemorrhage and shock (Fig. 3.5).

Obstetric conditions associated with DIC include abruptio placentae, amniotic fluid embolism, septic abortion and intrauterine infection, retained dead fetus, hydatidiform mole, placenta accreta, pre-eclampsia and prolonged shock from any cause (see Fig. 3.4).

Despite the advances in obstetric care and the availability of highly developed blood transfusion services, haemorrhage still constitutes a major factor in maternal mortality and morbidity [42,43].

There have been many reports concerning small series of patients or individual patients with coagulation failure during pregnancy. However, no significant controlled trials of the value of the many possible therapeutic measures have been carried out. This is mainly because no one person or unit is likely to see enough cases to randomize patients into groups in which the numbers would achieve statistical significance. Also the complex and variable nature of the conditions associated with DIC, which are often self-correcting and treated with a variety of measures, make it difficult to draw helpful conclusions from the published reports.

Haematological management of the bleeding obstetric patient

The bleeding obstetric patient poses an acute and frightening problem. Because of the urgency of the situation there should be a planned routine agreed by haematologist, physician, anaesthetist, obstetrician and nursing staff in all maternity units, to deal with this situation whenever it arises. Good, reliable, continuing communication between the various clinicians, nursing paramedical and laboratory staff is essential. There should be frequent 'rehearsals'.

It is imperative that the source of bleeding, often an unsuspected uterine or genital laceration, be located and dealt with. Prolonged hypovolaemic shock, or indeed shock from any cause, may also trigger DIC and this may lead to haemostatic failure and further prolonged haemorrhage.

The management of haemorrhage is virtually the same whether the bleeding is initiated or augmented by coagulation failure. The clinical condition usually demands urgent treatment and there is no time to wait for results of coagulation factor assays or sophisticated tests of fibrinolytic system activity for precise definition of the extent of haemostatic failure (blood may be taken for this purpose and analysed later once the emergency is over).

The simple rapid tests recommended below will establish the competence or otherwise of the haemostatic system. In the vast majority of obstetric patients, coagulation failure results from a sudden transitory episode of DIC triggered by a variety of conditions (see Figs 3.4 & 3.5).

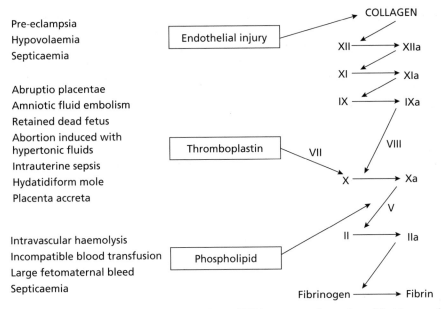

Pre-eclampsia
Hypovolaemia
Septicaemia

Abruptio placentae
Amniotic fluid embolism
Retained dead fetus
Abortion induced with
hypertonic fluids
Intrauterine sepsis
Hydatidiform mole
Placenta accreta

Intravascular haemolysis
Incompatible blood transfusion
Large fetomaternal bleed
Septicaemia

Fig 3.4 Trigger mechanisms of disseminated intravascular coagulation (DIC) in pregnancy. Interactions of the trigger mechanisms occur in many of these obstetric complications.

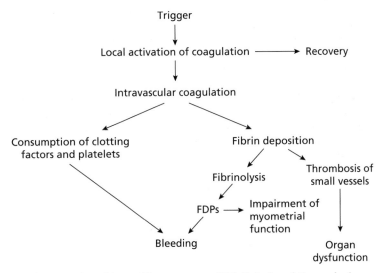

Fig 3.5 Stimulation of coagulation activity and its possible consequences (FDP, fibrin degradation product).

As soon as there is any concern about a patient bleeding from any cause, venous blood should be taken and delivered into a set of bottles kept in an emergency pack with a set of laboratory request forms previously made out which only require the patient's name and identification number to be added to them.

In order to avoid testing artefacts it is essential that the blood is obtained by a quick, efficient, non-traumatic technique.

Thromboplastin release from damaged tissues may contaminate the specimen and alter the results. This is likely to occur if difficulty is encountered in finding the vein, if the vein is only partly canalized and the flow is slow, or if there is excessive squeezing of tissues and repeated attempts to obtain a specimen with the same needle. In such circumstances the specimen may clot in the tube in spite of the presence of anticoagulant, or the coagulation times of the various tests will be altered and not reflect the true situation *in vivo*. The platelets may aggregate in clumps and give a falsely low count, be it automated or manual.

Heparin characteristically prolongs the partial thromboplastin time and thrombin time out of proportion to the prothrombin time. As little as 0.05 units of heparin per millilitre will prolong the coagulation test times. It is customary, although not desirable, to take blood for coagulation tests from lines that have been washed through with fluids containing heparin to keep them patent. I believe that it is almost impossible to overcome the effect of such fluids on the blood passing through such a line however much blood is taken and discarded before obtaining a sample for investigation. I would strongly recommend taking blood from another site not previously contaminated with heparin.

Any blood taken into a glass tube without anticoagulant will clot within a few minutes and natural fibrinolysis will continue *in vitro*. Unless the blood is taken into a fibrinolytic inhibitor such as EACA, a falsely high level of FDPs will be found, which bears no relationship to fibrinolysis *in vivo*. Similarly, leaving a tourniquet on too long before taking the specimen will stimulate local fibrinolytic activity *in vivo*.

Useful rapid screening tests for haemostatic failure include the platelet count, partial thromboplastin time, or accelerated whole-blood clotting time (which tests intrinsic coagulation), prothrombin time (which tests extrinsic coagulation), the thrombin time and estimation of fibrinogen (Fig. 3.6).

The measurement of FDPs provides an indirect test for fibrinolysis. In obstetric practice the measurement of FDPs is usually part of the investigation of suspected acute or chronic DIC. In the acute situation, raised FDPs only confirm the presence of DIC, but are not diagnostic, and once the specimen is taken the laboratory measurement should be delayed until after the emergency is over. In this way skilled laboratory workers can be performing a much more valuable service in providing results of coagulation screening tests and in providing blood and blood products suitable for transfusion. Of the tests of coagulation, probably the thrombin time, an estimation of the thrombin clottable fibrinogen in a citrated sample of plasma, is the most valuable overall rapid screen of haemostatic competence of coagulation factors in a previously haemostatically normal bleeding obstetric patient.

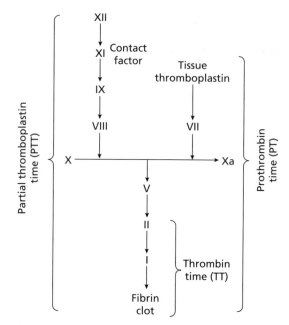

Fig 3.6 *In vitro* screening tests of coagulation competence and their relationship to the system involved.

The thrombin time of normal plasma is adjusted in the laboratory to 10–15 s, and the fibrin clot formed is firm and stable. In the most severe forms of DIC there is no clottable fibrinogen in the sample, and no fibrin clot appears even after 2–3 min. Indication of severe DIC is obtained usually by a prolonged thrombin time with a friable clot, which may dissolve on standing owing to fibrinolytic substances present in the plasma.

Prolongation of the thrombin time is observed not only with depleted fibrinogen but also in conditions where FDPs are increased.

There is no point whatsoever in the obstetrician, anaesthetist or nursing staff wasting time trying to perform bedside whole-blood clotting tests. Whole-blood clotting normally takes up to 7 min and should be performed in clean tubes in a 37°C water bath with suitable controls. Bedside (or other) estimation of whole-blood clotting time furnishes little information of practical value and only creates more panic. The valuable hands at the bedside are of more use doing the things they are trained to do in this emergency situation rather than wasting time performing a test that is time consuming, of little value or significance unless performed under strictly controlled conditions, and will not contribute much, if anything, to management. The alerted laboratory worker will be able to provide helpful results on which the obstetrician can act within 30 min at the most of receiving the specimen in the laboratory.

The tests referred to above are straightforward and should be available from any routine haematology laboratory. It is not necessary to have a specialist coagulation laboratory to perform these simple screening tests to confirm or refute a diagnosis of DIC.

Treatment of severe haemorrhage must include prompt and adequate fluid replacement in order to avoid complications such as renal shutdown. If effective circulation is restored without too much delay FDPs will be cleared from the blood mainly by the liver, which will further aid restoration of normal haemostasis. This is an aspect of management that is often not appropriately emphasized [44].

PLASMA SUBSTITUTES

There is much controversy around which plasma substitute to give to a bleeding patient. The remarks that follow relate to the supportive management of *acute haemorrhage from the placental site and birth canal* and should not be taken to apply to those situations in which hypovolaemia may be associated with severe hypoproteinaemia such as occurs in septic peritonitis, burns and bowel infarction. The choice lies between simple crystalloids, such as Hartman's solution or Ringer lactate, and artificial colloids, such as dextrans, hydroxyethyl starch and gelatin solution or the very expensive preparations of human albumin (albuminoids). If crystalloids are used, two to three times the volume of estimated blood loss should be administered because the crystalloid remains in the vascular compartment for a shorter time than colloids when renal function is maintained.

The infusion of plasma substitutes, i.e. plasma protein, dextran, gelatin and starch solutions may result in adverse reactions. Although the incidence of severe reactions is rare, they are diverse in nature, varying from allergic urticarial manifestations and mild fever to life-threatening anaphylactic reactions due to spasm of smooth muscle, with cardiac and respiratory arrest [45].

Dextrans adversely affect platelet function, may cause pseudoagglutination and interfere with interpretation of subsequent blood grouping and cross-matching tests. They are therefore contraindicated in the woman who is bleeding due to a complication associated with pregnancy where there is a high chance of there already being a serious haemostatic defect. The anaphylactoid reactions accompanying infusion of dextrans are probably related to IgG and IgM antidextran antibodies, which are found in high concentrations in all patients with severe reactions. Acute fetal distress has been reported in mothers giving Dextran 70 who suffered anaphylactoid reactions [46]. These Dextran-induced anaphylactoid reactions have

resulted in uterine hypertonia with subsequent severe fetal bradycardia even when immunoprophylaxis with Dextran Hapten has been administered [47]. There are many suitable superior alternatives for plasma expansion and the Royal College of Obstetricians recommends that Dextran should be avoided in obstetric practice [48].

Albuminoids are thought to be associated with fewer anaphylactoid reactions but they may be particularly harmful when transfused in the shocked patient by contributing to renal and particularly pulmonary failure, adversely affecting cardiac function and further impairing haemostasis [49].

Many previous studies suggested that the best way to deal with hypovolaemic shock initially is by transfusing simple balanced salt solutions (crystalloid) followed by red cells and fresh frozen plasma (FFP) [50–52]. More recent, but still dated work [53] has challenged this approach and suggests that albumin-containing solutions are superior to crystalloids for volume replacement in postoperative shocked patients with respiratory insufficiency. This aspect of management of shocked patients with blood loss still remains controversial pending the results of large clinical randomized controlled trials. I advocate the use of a derivative of bovine gelatin—polygeline (Haemaccel)—as a first-line fluid in resuscitation. It has a shelf-life of 8 years and can be stored at room temperature. It is iso-oncotic and does not interfere with platelet function or subsequent blood grouping or cross-matching. Renal function is improved when it is administered in hypovolaemic shock. Haemaccel is generally considered to be non-immunogenic and therefore does not trigger the production of antibodies in humans, even on repeated challenge. The reactions that occur related to Haemaccel infusion are thought to be due to histamine release [54], the incidence and severity of reactions being proportional to the extent of histamine release. There have been a few reports of severe reactions with bronchospasm and circulatory collapse but these are very rare and there has only been one report of a fatality [55]. Nevertheless, whatever substitute is used, this product is only a stopgap until suitable blood component therapy can be administered.

THE USE OF BLOOD AND COMPONENT THERAPY

Whole fresh blood might be the treatment of choice in coagulation failure associated with obstetric disorders, but whole fresh blood is not available from regional centres in the UK. To release blood components earlier than the usual 18–24 h would increase the risk of serologically incompatible transfusions, viral hepatitis and human immunodeficiency virus (HIV) [56]. Syphilis, cytomegalovirus and Epstein–Barr virus are examples of other infections that may be transmitted in fresh blood. Their viability diminishes rapidly on storage at 4°C. These infections, particularly in immunosuppressed or pregnant patients, can be particularly hazardous. The hypothetical hazard of transmission of new variant Creutzfeldt–Jakob disease (nvCJD) in blood products has had a profound impact on transfusion practice in recent years [57].

Fresh frozen plasma

FFP contains all the coagulation factors present in plasma obtained from whole blood within 6 h of donation. Frozen rapidly and stored at –30°C, the factors are well preserved for at least 1 year.

Cryoprecipitate

Although cryoprecipitate is richer in fibrinogen than FFP, it lacks AT which is rapidly consumed in obstetric bleeding associated with DIC. The use of cryoprecipitate also exposes the recipient to more donors with consequent potential associated hazards.

Platelets

Platelets, an essential haemostatic component, are not present in FFP and their functional activity rapidly deteriorates in stored blood. The platelet count reflects both the degree of intravascular coagulation and the amount of bank blood transfused. A patient with persistent bleeding and a very low platelet count ($< 20 \times 10^9/L$) may be given concentrated platelets, although they are seldom required in addition to FFP to achieve haemostasis in obstetric haemorrhage. A spontaneous recovery from the coagulation defect is to be expected once the uterus is empty and well contracted, provided that blood volume is maintained by adequate replacement monitored by central venous pressure and urinary output.

Problems arise when bleeding is difficult to control and the woman has a low haemoglobin before blood loss.

Red cell transfusion

Cross-matched blood should be available within 40 min of the maternal specimen reaching the laboratory. If the woman has had regular antenatal care her blood group will be documented. There is a good case for giving uncross-matched blood of her own group should the situation warrant it, provided that blood has been properly processed at the transfusion centre. If the blood group is unknown, uncross-matched group O Rh (D) negative

blood may be given if necessary. By this time laboratory screening tests of haemostatic function should be available. If these prove to be normal, but vaginal bleeding continues, the cause is nearly always concealed trauma or bleeding from the placental site due to failure of the myometrium to contract. It is imperative that the source of bleeding, often an unsuspected uterine or genital laceration, should be located and dealt with. Prolonged hypovolaemic shock or indeed shock from any cause may also trigger DIC and this may lead to haemostatic failure and further prolonged haemorrhage.

If the blood loss is replaced only by stored bank blood that is deficient in the labile clotting factors V, VIII and in platelets, then the circulation will rapidly become depleted in these essential components of haemostasis even if there is no DIC initially as the cause of haemorrhage. It is advisable to transfuse 2 units of FFP for every 4–6 units of bank red cells administered.

It seems sensible in any event, whatever the cause of bleeding, to change from the initial plasma substitute and transfuse 2 units of FFP (plasma from two donations) once it has thawed, while waiting for compatible blood to be available.

A spontaneous recovery from the coagulation defect is to be expected once the uterus is empty and well contracted, provided that blood volume is maintained by adequate replacement monitored by central venous pressure and urinary output.

Clinicians may be helped in the decision of which replacement fluid to give in an obstetric emergency by the knowledge that very few bleeding patients die from lack of circulating red cells, the oxygen-carrying moiety of the blood. Death in the majority of cases results from poor tissue perfusion due to hypovolaemia. Therefore every effort should be made to maintain a normal blood volume. Restoration of red cell mass can be delayed until suitable compatibility tests have been performed and bleeding is at least partially controlled [58].

The single most important component of haemostasis at delivery is contraction of the myometrium stemming the flow from the placental site. Massive transfusion of all clotting factors and platelets will not stop haemorrhage if the uterus remains flabby. Vaginal delivery will make less severe demand on the haemostatic mechanism than delivery by caesarean section, which requires the same haemostatic competence as any other major surgical procedure. Should DIC be established with the fetus *in utero*, rather than embark on heroic surgical delivery, it is better to correct the DIC and wait for spontaneous delivery if possible, or to stimulate vaginal delivery, avoiding soft-tissue damage.

ARTERIAL EMBOLIZATION FOR THE CONTROL OF OBSTETRIC HAEMORRHAGE

Transcatheter arterial embolization has been used for the control of pelvic haemorrhage resulting from trauma, malignancy and radiation since the late 1960s. During the last two decades there has been an increasing use of transcatheter embolization of the internal iliac or uterine artery for control of postpartum haemorrhage [59,60]. The general consensus is that selective emergency arterial embolization is an effective means of controlling severe intractable postpartum haemorrhage. High-risk surgery is avoided and reproductive ability is maintained.

Disseminated intravascular coagulation in clinical conditions

IN VITRO DETECTION OF LOW-GRADE DISSEMINATED INTRAVASCULAR COAGULATION

Rampant uncompensated DIC results in severe haemorrhage with the characteristic laboratory findings described above. However, low-grade DIC does not usually give rise to any clinical manifestations although the condition is a potentially hazardous one for both mother and fetus.

Many *in vitro* tests have been claimed to detect low-grade compensated DIC and space does not allow an account of all of these.

Fibrin degradation products

Estimation of FDPs will give some indication of low-grade DIC if these are significantly raised when fibrinogen, platelets and screening tests of haemostatic function appear to be within the normal range.

Soluble fibrin complexes

The action of thrombin on fibrinogen is crucial in DIC. Thrombin splits two molecules of fibrinopeptide A and two molecules of fibrinopeptide B from fibrinogen. The remaining molecule is called a fibrin monomer and polymerizes rapidly to fibrin (see Fig. 3.1). Free fibrinopeptides in the blood are a specific measure of thrombin activity, and high levels of fibrinopeptide A have been shown to be associated with compensated DIC in pregnancy [41].

Soluble fibrin complexes made up of fibrin–fibrinogen dimers are increased in conditions of low-grade DIC [61]. These complexes are generated during the process of thrombin generation and the conversion of soluble fibrinogen to insoluble fibrin (Fig. 3.7). Levels of soluble fibrin complexes are increased in patients with severe pre-eclampsia and with a retained dead fetus [62].

Factor VIII

During normal pregnancy the levels of both von Willebrand factor (vWF) and Factor VIII coagulation activity (VIIIC) rise in parallel [63,64]. An increase in the ratio of vWF to Factor VIIIC has been observed in conditions accompanied by low-grade DIC whether associated with pregnancy or not.

The stages in the spectrum of severity of DIC (Table 3.1) are not strictly delineated and there may be rapid progression from low-grade compensated DIC as diagnosed by paracoagulation tests described above, to the rampant form with haemostatic failure.

ABRUPTIO PLACENTAE

Premature separation of the placenta or abruptio placentae is the most frequent obstetric cause of coagulation failure. Many of the problems that confront the attendant in this situation are common to other conditions associated with DIC in pregnancy so that abruption will be used as the central focus to discuss management controversies.

Abruptio placentae can occur in apparently healthy women with no clinical warning or in the context of established pre-eclampsia. It is possible that clinically silent placental infarcts may predispose to placental separation by causing low-grade abnormalities of the haemostatic system such as increased Factor VIII consumption and raised FDPs [65].

There is a great spectrum in the severity of the haemostatic failure in this condition [66], which appears to be

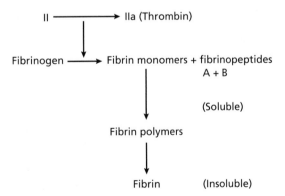

Fig 3.7 Generation of soluble complexes during the conversion of fibrinogen to insoluble fibrin.

	Severity of DIC	*In vitro* findings	Obstetric conditions commonly associated
Stage 1	Low-grade compensated	FDPs ↑ Increased soluble fibrin complexes Increased ratio vWF/Factor VIIIC	Pre-eclampsia Retained dead fetus
Stage 2	Uncompensated but no haemostatic failure	As above, plus fibrinogen ↓ Platelets ↓ Factors V and VIII ↓	Small abruptio Severe pre-eclampsia
Stage 3	Rampant with haemostatic failure	Platelets ↓↓ Gross depletion of coagulation factors, particularly fibrinogen FDPs ↑↑	Abruptio placentae Amniotic fluid embolism Eclampsia

Table 3.1 Spectrum of severity of disseminated intravascular coagulation (DIC): its relationship to specific complications in obstetrics.

Rapid progression from stage 1 to stage 3 is possible unless appropriate action is taken.
FDP, fibrin degradation product; vWF, von Willebrand factor.

related to the degree of placental separation. Only 10% of patients with abruptio placentae show significant coagulation abnormalities [67]. In some small abruptions there is a minor degree of failure of haemostatic processes and the fetus does not succumb (see Table 3.1). When the uterus is tense and tender and no fetal heart can be heard, the separation and retroplacental bleeding are extensive. No guide to the severity of the haemorrhage or coagulation failure will be given by the amount of vaginal bleeding. There may be no external vaginal blood loss, even when the placenta is completely separated, the fetus is dead, the circulating blood is incoagulable and there is up to 5 L of concealed blood loss resulting in hypovolaemic shock.

Haemostatic failure may be suspected if there is persistent oozing at the site of venepuncture or bleeding from the mucous membranes of the mouth or nose. Simple rapid screening tests, as described above and referred to below, will confirm the presence of DIC. There will be a low platelet count, greatly prolonged thrombin time, low fibrinogen, together with raised FDPs, due to secondary fibrinolysis stimulated by the intravascular deposition of fibrin [68]. A recent report [69], which linked elevated thrombomodulin with abruptio placentae, showed that the combination of thrombomodulin and ultrasound as a 'double-marker' detected all cases of abruption in this small series. The authors suggest that thrombomodulin may prove useful in the diagnosis of abruption associated with trauma or unexplained vaginal bleeding and may become a useful routine screening test.

The mainstay of treatment is to restore and maintain the circulating blood volume. This not only prevents renal shutdown and further haemostatic failure caused by hypovolaemic shock, but helps clearance of FDPs which in themselves act as potent anticoagulants. It has also been suggested that FDPs inhibit myometrial activity and serious postpartum haemorrhage in women with abruptio placentae was found to be associated with high levels of FDPs [70,71]. High levels of FDPs may also have a cardiotoxic effect decreasing contractility and resulting in low cardiac output and blood pressure despite a normal circulating blood volume.

If the fetus is dead the aim should be prompt vaginal delivery avoiding soft-tissue damage, once correction of hypovolaemia is underway. There is no evidence that the use of oxytocic agents aggravates thromboplastin release from the uterus [72].

Following emptying of the uterus, myometrial contraction will greatly reduce bleeding from the placental site and spontaneous correction of the haemostatic defect usually occurs shortly after delivery, if the measures recommended above have been taken. However, postpartum haemorrhage is a not infrequent complication and is the commonest cause of death in abruptio placentae [42].

In cases where the abruption is small and the fetus is still alive, prompt caesarean section may save the baby, if vaginal delivery is not imminent. FFP, bank red cells and platelet concentrates should be available to correct the potentially severe maternal coagulation defect.

In rare situations where vaginal delivery cannot be stimulated and haemorrhage continues, caesarean section is indicated even in the presence of a dead fetus. In these circumstances normal haemostasis should be restored as far as possible by the administration of FFP and platelet concentrates if necessary, as well as transfusing red cells before surgery is undertaken.

Despite extravasation of blood throughout the uterine muscle, myometrial function is not impaired and good contraction will follow removal of fetus, placenta and retroplacental clot. Regional anaesthesia or analgesia is contraindicated: expansion of the lower limb vascular bed resulting from regional block can add to the problem of uncorrected hypovolaemia; in the presence of haemostatic failure there is also the additional hazard of bleeding into the epidural space [21].

In recent years, heparin has been used to treat many cases of DIC, whatever their cause. There is, however, no objective evidence to demonstrate that its use in abruptio placentae decreased morbidity and mortality although anecdotal reports in the older literature continued to suggest this [73]. Very good results have been achieved without the use of heparin [44]. Its use, with an intact circulation, would be sensible and logical to break the vicious circle of DIC, but in the presence of already defective haemostasis with a large bleeding placental site, it may prolong massive local and generalized haemorrhage [74].

Treatment with antifibrinolytic agents such as EACA or Trasylol (aprotinin) can result in blockage of small vessels of vital organs, such as the kidney or brain, with fibrin. Such agents are therefore contraindicated, although Bonnar [21] suggests that delayed severe and prolonged haemorrhage from the placental site several hours post-delivery may respond to their use if all other measures fail.

It has been suggested [71,75] that Trasylol may be helpful in the management of abruptio placentae particularly in those cases with uterine inertia associated with high levels of FDPs. There is a high incidence (1.5%) of abruptio placentae in the obstetric admissions (18 000/ annum) at the Groote Schuur Obstetric Unit, Cape Town, where the first study was carried out. The selection of Trasylol depended on its alleged anticoagulant activity in addition to its well-known antifibrinolytic properties [76]. There has been a resurgence of use of Trasylol recently, particularly in cardiac surgery [77] where significant reduction in blood loss has been shown following cardiac bypass operations. This is thought to be due predominantly to platelet sparing. It is doubtful whether Trasylol would have any advantage in management of obstetric DIC.

Obstetricians appear unconvinced of the benefits of Trasylol in the treatment of DIC and abruptio placentae. Prompt supportive measures maintaining central venous pressure and replacing blood loss together with essential coagulation factors, will of course result in reduction in FDPs. This could improve myometrial function and contribute to the return of healthy haemostasis.

A report on reducing the frequency of severe abruption from Dallas, Texas [78], noted that the reduction in *fetal* death associated with abruption by 50% over a period covering more than 30 years (1958–90), could be accounted for by the decrease in women of very high parity and also by an increase in the proportion of Latin-American as opposed to black women in the population served. Abruption in the latter part of the study recurred in 12% of subsequent pregnancies and proved fatal to the fetus in 7 per cent, which was unchanged from earlier experience. With modern supportive measures, maternal death due directly to abruption is now extremely rare.

AMNIOTIC FLUID EMBOLISM [79]

This obstetric disaster usually occurs during or shortly after a vigorous labour with an intact amniotic sac, but can occur during a caesarean section. It is thought that amniotic fluid enters the maternal circulation via lacerations of membranes and placenta. Platelet fibrin thrombi are formed and trapped within the pulmonary blood vessels: profound shock follows, accompanied by respiratory distress and cyanosis. There is a high mortality at this stage from a combination of respiratory and cardiac failure [80]. If the mother survives long enough, massive intravascular coagulation with almost total consumption of coagulation factors invariably follows. There is bleeding from venepuncture sites and severe haemorrhage from the placental site after delivery.

Confirmation of diagnosis is usually made post mortem by finding histological evidence of amniotic fluid and fetal tissue within the substance of the maternal lungs; occasionally, similar material may be aspirated from a central venous pressure (CVP) catheter line—see below. It is therefore difficult to assess the value of therapeutic measures taken, in the few reports that have appeared, for the successful management of a clinical picture that can usually only be suggestive of amniotic fluid embolism [81–83].

The major differential diagnoses of amniotic fluid embolism in the collapsed patient are primary cardiovascular catastrophes such as pulmonary embolus or aspiration in the anaesthetized patient. Apart from the bleeding and evidence of DIC associated with amniotic fluid embolism, pulmonary embolus has specific features. These and other medical causes of shock in obstetric patients are considered in Table 3.1. Aspiration is usually associated with bronchospasm, which is very rare in amniotic fluid embolus [79]. At any time, if there is doubt about the diagnosis, the rapid fluid infusion necessary for the treatment of amniotic fluid embolus should be controlled by careful assessment of the CVP. Such rapid fluid infusion would cause a marked rise in CVP in patients with pulmonary embolus, and could well lead to fatal fluid overload. In addition, the present of the CVP line will allow aspiration of fetal material from the great veins, for confirmation of the diagnosis of amniotic fluid embolus [84]. Such material should also be sought in maternal sputum [85]. Because fetal material has been found in pulmonary arterial blood in some women who did not have amniotic fluid embolus [86], such a finding should not be considered pathognomonic for amniotic fluid embolus.

The object of the treatment is to sustain the circulation while the intravascular thrombin in the lungs is cleared by the fibrinolytic response of the endothelium of the pulmonary vessels. If bleeding from the placental site can be controlled by stimulation of uterine contraction, then the logical treatment is carefully monitored transfusion of FFP and packed red cells with heparin administration and, if necessary, ventilation.

RETENTION OF DEAD FETUS

The question of intrauterine fetal death and haemostatic failure has been reviewed in the past [87]. There is a gradual depletion of maternal coagulation factors following intrauterine fetal death and the changes are not usually detectable *in vitro* until after 3–4 weeks. Thromboplastic substances released from the dead tissues in the uterus into the maternal circulation are thought to be the trigger of DIC in this situation, which occurs in about one-third of patients who retain the dead fetus for more than 4–5 weeks. Problems arising from defective haemostasis are not observed in modern obstetric practice because labour is induced promptly following diagnosis of fetal death before clinically significant coagulation changes have developed.

Rupture of the membranes is recommended once induced labour has been established, as there is a risk of precipitate labour, and amniotic fluid embolism has been known to occur in these patients.

RETAINED DEAD FETUS AND LIVING TWIN

The occurrence of single fetal death in a preterm multiple pregnancy poses unique therapeutic dilemmas. The incidence of this problem is unknown but it is likely to be observed more frequently now that ultrasound is widely used in obstetrics. In addition, selective termination of the life of the affected twin is occasionally being offered in situations where only one fetus has been shown to be affected with a genetic disorder or to be involved in twin/twin transfusion syndrome. Haemostatic failure appears to be a hazard for the remaining fetus rather than for the mother.

INDUCED ABORTION

Changes in haemostatic components consistent with DIC have been demonstrated in patients undergoing abortion induced with hypertonic solutions of saline and urea [88–92]. This combination appears to be particularly hazardous [93] in comparison to the use of urea and prostaglandin or oxytocin [94]. The stimulus appears to be the release of tissue factor into the maternal circulation from the placenta, which is damaged by the hypertonic solutions.

In later pregnancy DIC has been described with both dilatation and evacuation [95] and also with prostaglandin and oxytocin termination [96].

The haemorrhage resulting may be massive and has resulted in maternal deaths. Prompt restoration of the blood volume and transfusions with red cells and FFP as described above should resolve the situation, which, once the uterus is empty, is self-limiting.

A unique case of DIC associated with chronic ectopic pregnancy has been reported [97].

INTRAUTERINE INFECTION [98]

Endotoxic shock associated with septic abortion and antepartum or postpartum intrauterine infection can trigger DIC [99,100]. Infection is usually with Gram-negative organisms. Fibrin is deposited in the microvasculature owing to endothelial damage caused by the endotoxin. Secondary red cell intravascular haemolysis with characteristic fragmentation, so-called microangiopathic haemolysis, is characteristic of the condition.

The patient is usually alert and flushed with a rapid pulse and low blood pressure. Transfusion has little or no effect on the hypotension in comparison to its benefit in the obstetric emergencies complicated by DIC triggered by hypovolaemic shock. Elimination of the uterine infection remains the most important aspect of management; this is probably best performed by a short intensive period of antibiotic therapy followed by evacuation of the uterine contents. A few European centres have used heparin in the management of septic abortion and have claimed a decrease in mortality. If the uterus is empty and contracted, there is no undue risk of severe bleeding from the placental site. If there is evidence of a consumptive coagulopathy, heparin may be useful as part of the management of this hazardous emergency [72] but this remains controversial [98,101].

PURPURA FULMINANS

This rare complication of infection sometimes occurs in the puerperium, precipitated by Gram-negative septicaemia.

Extensive haemorrhage occurs into the skin in association with DIC. The underlying mechanism is unknown but there appears to be an acute activation of the clotting system resulting in the deposition of fibrin thrombi within blood vessels of the skin and other organs [102]. The extremities and face are usually involved first, the purpuric patches having a jagged and erythematous border, which can be shown histologically to be the site of a leucocytoclastic vasculitis. Rapid enlargement of the lesions, which become necrotic and gangrenous, is associated with shock, tachycardia and fever. Without treatment the mortality rate is high, and among those who survive, digit or limb amputation may be necessary. The laboratory findings are those of DIC with leucocytosis. In this situation treatment with heparin should be started as soon as the diagnosis is apparent. It will prevent further consumption of platelets and coagulation factors. It should always be remembered however, that bleeding from any site in the presence of defective coagulation factors will be aggravated by the use of heparin. Survival in purpura fulminans is currently much improved because of better supportive treatment for the shocked patient and effective control of the triggering infection, together with heparin therapy.

ACUTE FATTY LIVER OF PREGNANCY

Acute fatty liver of pregnancy (AFLP) is a rare complication of pregnancy included in this section because it is often, if not always, associated with variable degrees of DIC, which contributes significantly to its morbidity and mortality [74,103]. Only the haematological aspects will be discussed here. For a full account of the disorder the reader is referred to Chapter 9.

Early diagnosis and subsequent delivery are essential for improving survival of both mother and child. Most patients have prodromal symptoms for at least 1 week before jaundice develops. The Royal Free series [104] draws attention to a characteristic blood picture of neutrophilia, thrombocytopenia and normoblasts. Some of the blood films available for review also showed basophilic stippling and giant platelets, and the authors suggest that these appearances might help towards an early diagnosis of AFLP. However, these features are not specific to AFLP and may be seen in any condition of additional stress on a bone marrow already working to capacity in the last trimester of pregnancy.

DIC complicating severe liver failure is an extremely complex topic. In AFLP the haemostatic defect is frequently resistant probably owing to prolonged activation of coagulation combined with very low to undetectable AT levels [74,105,106]. The replacement of AT with plasma or AT concentrate to shorten the period of DIC

and thereby decrease morbidity and mortality of AFLP has been suggested [74] and used successfully [43]. Heparin therapy can be very dangerous [107].

Low-grade disseminated intravascular coagulation, pre-eclampsia and related syndromes

PLATELETS IN PRE-ECLAMPSIA

There have been many reports and reviews showing that the circulating platelet count is reduced in pre-eclampsia [108,109]. The platelet count can be used to monitor severity of the disease process as well as for initial screening if there is concern about significant coagulation abnormalities [110]. A fall in the platelet count may precede any detectable rise in serum FDPs in women subsequently developing pre-eclampsia. The combination of a reduced platelet lifespan and a fall in the platelet count without platelet-associated antibodies (see below) indicates a low-grade coagulopathy. Platelets may either be consumed in thrombus formation or may suffer membrane damage from contact with abnormal surfaces and be prematurely removed from the circulation. Rarely, in very severe pre-eclampsia, the patient develops microangiopathic haemolytic anaemia. These patients have profound thrombocytopenia and this leads to confusion in the differential diagnosis between pre-eclampsia with or without HELLP (haemolysis, elevated liver enzymes, low platelets syndrome) and thrombotic thrombocytopenic purpura (TTP) (see below).

Activation of the haemostatic mechanisms in normal pregnancy has led to the view that the haematological manifestations of pre-eclampsia merely represent augmentation of the hypercoagulable state that accompanies normal pregnancy. In this respect many studies have been carried out on levels of individual coagulation factors. No clear pattern emerges but there appear to be some significant correlations of severity of the disease process with both the Factor VIII complex [111] and with AT [112].

A readily available and sensitive indicator of activation of the coagulation system is assay of fibrinopeptide A concentration in the plasma. Although in mild pre-eclampsia, patients may have a normal or only slight increase in fibrinopeptide A levels, marked increases occur in patients with severe pre-eclampsia [41].

Most studies in pre-eclampsia have shown increased levels of FDPs in serum and urine. Plasma levels of soluble fibrinogen–fibrin complexes are also raised in pre-eclampsia compared with normal pregnancy. Once the disease process is established, the most relevant coagulation abnormalities appear to be in the platelet count, Factor VIII and FDPs. Those women with the most marked abnormalities in these parameters suffer the greatest perinatal loss [113].

Following the reported association between thrombophilia factors, severe pre-eclampsia and intrauterine growth restriction (IUGR) [114] it has been suggested that investigation of pre-eclampsia should also include a search for defects in the naturally occurring anticoagulants so that future pregnancies can be managed appropriately (see Chapters 4 and 6).

Many investigators now believe that gestational hypertension with or without proteinuria, IUGR, HELLP syndrome, AFLP and eclampsia are part of the same disease process which presents with the related signs and symptoms depending on the organ targeted by small-vessel coagulopathy and varying degrees of DIC.

DISSEMINATED INTRAVASCULAR COAGULATION: SUMMARY

As emphasized, DIC is always a secondary phenomenon and the mainstay of management is therefore to remove the initiating stimulus if possible.

With rampant DIC and haemorrhage, recovery will usually follow delivery of the patient provided the blood volume is maintained and shock due to hypovolaemia is prevented. Myometrium that acts efficiently after delivery will stem haemorrhage from the placental site. Measures taken to achieve a firm contracted uterus are the major contribution to preventing continuing massive blood loss.

It is of interest that the maternal mortality of DIC associated with placental abruption is less than 1%, whereas that associated with infection and shock is 50–80%. The mortality rate reported in series of patients with DIC due to various aetiologies is 50–85% and the wide variation probably reflects the mortality rate of the underlying disorder, not of DIC itself [74]. There is no doubt that the major determinant of survival is our ability to identify the underlying trigger and manage it successfully.

Acquired primary defects of haemostasis

Thrombocytopenia

The commonest platelet abnormality encountered in clinical practice is thrombocytopenia. During the hundred years since platelets were first described, an increasing understanding of their role in haemostasis and thrombosis has taken place. At the same time there have been dramatic reductions in maternal and fetal mortality, but maternal thrombocytopenia remains a difficult management problem during pregnancy and can also have profound effects on fetal and neonatal well-being. The causes

and management of maternal and fetal thrombocytopenia have been reviewed [115,116]. Emphasis here will relate to those conditions that cause particular diagnostic and management problems in obstetric practice.

A low platelet count is seen most frequently in association with DIC (as already described). Sometimes severe megaloblastic anaemia of pregnancy is accompanied by thrombocytopenia, but the platelet count rapidly returns to normal after therapy with folic acid [21]. Toxic depression of bone-marrow megakaryocytes in pregnancy can occur in association with infection, certain drugs and alcoholism. Neoplastic infiltration may also result in thrombocytopenia. Probably the single most important cause of isolated thrombocytopenia is idiopathic (autoimmune) thrombocytopenic purpura (ITP), which is a disease primarily of young women in the reproductive years [117].

IDIOPATHIC (AUTOIMMUNE) THROMBOCYTOPENIC PURPURA

ITP has been found to have an incidence of one to two in 10 000 pregnancies [118]. Cases may present with skin bruising and platelet counts between 30 and $80 \times 10^9/L$ but it is rare to see severe bleeding associated with low platelet counts in the chronic form.

With the routine screening of pregnant women for anaemia and blood group antibodies, very mild thrombocytopenia may be discovered as an incidental finding and is not associated with risk to the mother or infant [13,119]. It may be that incidental thrombocytopenia represents a very mild ITP but as it is not associated with adverse effects it must be distinguished from cases of autoimmune thrombocytopenia, which can result in infants affected with severe thrombocytopenia [120–122]. There are no serological tests or clinical guidelines that reliably predict the hazard of thrombocytopenia in an individual fetus, the correlation between maternal and neonatal counts is poor [120,122] and the risk has been overestimated [123]. It has been assumed that caesarean section delivery is less traumatic to the fetus than vaginal delivery, and whilst that premise could be debated, the recognition in major centres that only a trivial minority of pregnancies are at risk of significant fetal thrombocytopenia has avoided many unnecessary fetal blood samples and caesarean sections.

Diagnosis

ITP is a diagnosis of exclusion with peripheral thrombocytopenia and normal or increased megakaryocytes in the bone marrow and the documented absence of other diseases. The red and white cells are essentially normal unless there is secondary anaemia. ITP requires the exclusion of systemic lupus erythematous (SLE), lupus anticoagulant and anticardiolipin antibody as they may co-exist with thrombocytopenia (see Chapter 8).

There have been a number of analyses of outcome of cases involving maternal ITP from the 1950s onwards. The findings may not be entirely applicable to current management because some of the documented poor fetal outcomes may have been associated with unrecognized maternal lupus, pre-eclampsia or alloimmune thrombocytopenia. Only symptomatic women and neonates were investigated because there was no general screening of the platelet count in healthy women. This resulted in an exaggerated reported incidence of both neonatal thrombocytopenia and the morbidity and mortality arising from it.

The majority of thrombocytopenic patients are asymptomatic and tests to estimate the bleeding risk in these patients would obviously be helpful.

In chronic platelet consumption disorders, a population of younger larger platelets is established which have enhanced function. Measurement of the mean platelet volume (MPV) or, if not available, examination of the stained blood film will detect the presence of these large platelets. The risk of bleeding at any given platelet count is less in those patients who have younger large platelets. The bleeding time, which has been severely criticized [124,125] as a predictor of bleeding at surgery, still has a place in this context according to some respected workers [126]. A bleeding time over 15 min indicates a greater risk than in those with a normal bleeding time.

The immune destruction of platelets has been shown to be due to autoantibodies directed against platelet surface antigens. This has special relevance in pregnancy because the placenta has receptors for the constant fragment (Fc) of the IgG immunoglobulin molecule facilitating active transport of immunoglobulin across the placenta to the fetal circulation. The immunoglobulin passage increases with advancing pregnancy [127,128] and may result in fetal thrombocytopenia.

The role of circulating immunoglobulin in the pathogenesis of immune thrombocytopenia was first documented in the 1950s [129,130]. However, the demonstration of antibody on the platelet membrane and in the plasma, by tests analogous to the direct and indirect Coombs' tests on red cells, has been slow to enter the routine repertoire of haematology laboratories. This is because these tests have been fraught with technological difficulties such as the intrinsic reactivity of platelets and the presence of some platelet-associated immunoglobulin (PAIgG) in normal individuals.

Antibody from some cases of ITP demonstrates a specificity for the platelet glycoprotein IIb/IIIa [131] or for glycoprotein Ib. In one study, the minority of cases of ITP demonstrating this specificity fared less well in their responses to splenectomy [132].

Whilst some cases of ITP have normal or increased amounts of immunoglobulin on the platelets or in the plasma [133,134], 10–35% of patients have no demonstrable PAIgG. The presence of IgG rather than IgM antibodies [135] has relevance to the pregnant patient because only IgG antibodies can be transported across the placenta and cause thrombocytopenia in the fetus. However, no currently available serological test can be used to reliably predict thrombocytopenia in the fetus [136].

In a study of 162 consecutive pregnant patients with platelet counts $< 150 \times 10^9/L$ gathered over 11 years, the absence of circulating IgG antiplatelet antibody at term, despite a history of thrombocytopenic purpura, was associated with minimal risk of thrombocytopenia in the fetus [122]. The absence of a history of ITP prior to the index pregnancy was also a low-risk indicator for neonatal thrombocytopenia [122]. In contrast, 18 neonates who were born with platelet counts $< 50 \times 10^9/L$, out of a total of 178, were all born to mothers with a history of ITP prior to pregnancy. In addition, 40% of mothers with a preceding history delivered infants with platelet counts $< 100 \times 10^9/L$. Of 162 infants delivered in the index pregnancy, 10 had bleeding complications of which five were serious. Intracranial haemorrhage (ICH) in infants born to women with a prior history of ITP and delivered vaginally, numbered two out of 17, whilst there were no cases of ICH in women with similar histories who were delivered by caesarean section [122]. A more recent review of the literature of ITP in pregnancy [126] shows a neonatal mortality rate of six in 1000 ITP patients, about the same or better than the overall perinatal mortality rate. All the deaths in this survey occurred in babies delivered by caesarean section, unlike in other reports, and all events appeared more than 24–48 h after delivery, the time of the platelet count nadir in the neonate.

Management of idiopathic (autoimmune) thrombocytopenic purpura in pregnancy

Management of ITP in pregnancy is directed at three aspects: (i) antenatal care of the mother; (ii) management of the mother and fetus during delivery; and (iii) the management of the neonate from the time of delivery.

The most important decision to make is whether the mother requires treatment at all. Many patients have significant thrombocytopenia (platelet count $< 100 \times 10^9/L$) but no evidence of an *in vivo* haemostatic disorder. In general the platelet count must be $< 50 \times 10^9/L$ for capillary bleeding and purpura to occur.

There is no need to treat asymptomatic women with mild to moderate thrombocytopenia (count $>50 \times 10^9/L$) and a normal bleeding time. However, the maternal platelet count should be monitored at every clinical visit and signs of haemostatic impairment looked for. The platelet count will show a downward trend during pregnancy with a nadir in the third trimester, and active treatment may have to be instituted to achieve safe haemostatic concentrations of platelets for delivery at term. The incidence of ante-partum haemorrhage is not increased in maternal ITP but there is a small increased risk of post-partum haemorrhagic complications not from the placental bed but from surgical incisions such as episiotomy and from soft-tissue lacerations.

Intervention in the antenatal period is based on clinical manifestations of thrombocytopenia. The woman with bruising or petechiae requires measures to raise the platelet count but the woman with mucous membrane bleeding that may be life threatening requires urgent treatment with platelet transfusions and intravenous IgG (see below) and occasionally emergency splenectomy.

The real dilemma in the pregnant woman with ITP is that nearly all patients have chronic disease. The long-term effects of treatment that is happily embarked on outside pregnancy have to be considered in the light of the possible complications during pregnancy in the mother and of any effects on the fetus. Hazards for the mother who is monitored carefully, and where appropriate measures have been taken, are negligible but most of her management is orientated towards what are thought to be optimal conditions for the delivery of the fetus who in turn may or may not be thrombocytopenic (see below).

Corticosteroids are a satisfactory short-term therapy but are unacceptable as long-term support unless the maintenance dose is very small [117,137]. Side-effects for the mother include weight gain, subcutaneous fat redistribution, acne and hypertension, the last of which is particularly undesirable during pregnancy. In addition, the incidence of gestational diabetes, postpartum psychosis and osteoporosis are all increased with the use of corticosteroids. Steroids are often used but they should be reserved as short-term therapy for patients with obvious risk of bleeding or to raise the platelet count of an asymptomatic woman at term allowing her to have epidural or spinal analgesia for delivery if desired or indicated.

The suggestion in the older literature of an association between steroid administration and cleft lip or palate has largely been refuted by more recent studies. Suppression of fetal adrenal glands is a theoretical hazard but approximately 90% of a dose of prednisolone or hydrocortisone is metabolized in the placenta and never reaches the fetus. This is in contrast to dexamethasone and β-methasone, which cross the placenta freely (see also Chapter 1). It has been suggested [135] that high doses of corticosteroids given to elevate platelet counts at or near term should be avoided because they may increase the transplacental passage of IgG antibody and thus expose the fetus to greater risk of severe thrombocytopenia. In my experience this is a theoretical hazard not seen in practice.

Intravenous IgG. The introduction of a highly successful treatment for ITP has altered the management options dramatically. It is known that intravenous administration of monomeric polyvalent human IgG in doses greater than those produced endogenously prolongs the clearance time of immune complexes by the reticuloendothelial system. It is thought that such a prolongation of clearance of IgG-coated platelets in ITP results in an increase in the number of circulating platelets but the mechanism is as yet unknown [138]. Used in the original recommended doses of 0.4 g/kg for 5 days by intravenous infusion, a persistent and predictable response was obtained in more than 80% of reported cases. More recently, alternative dosage regimens of this very expensive treatment have been suggested, which are just as effective, but easier to manage and use less total immunoglobulin [126]. A typical dose is 1 g/kg over 8 h in a single infusion. This dose will raise the platelet count to normal or safe levels in approximately half of the patients. In those in whom the platelet count does not rise, a similar dose can be repeated 2 days later. The advantages of this treatment are that it is safe, has very few side-effects and that the response to therapy is more rapid than with corticosteroids. The response usually occurs within 48 h and is maintained for 2–3 weeks. The main disadvantage is that it is very expensive and seldom produces a long-term cure of ITP.

It has been suggested that IgG given intravenously can cross the placenta and should provoke an identical response in the fetus [139] at risk but this has never been proved. Indeed, analysis of more recent literature indicates that the postulated transplacental effect is unreliable [127,128] and that exogenous IgG may not cross the placenta [140]. The use of IgG has been recommended [135,141] in all pregnant patients with platelet counts $<75 \times 10^9/L$ regardless of history or symptoms. There is no doubt about the value of IgG in selected cases of severe symptomatic thrombocytopenia where a rapid response is required but its indiscriminate use in all cases with significant thrombocytopenia would have to be shown to dramatically improve both maternal and fetal outcome to justify the high cost. Such improvement is unlikely to be demonstrated granted that the outcome is good in the vast majority of these patients.

Splenectomy will produce a cure or long-term drug-free remission in 60–80% of all patients with ITP. This is because the main site of antibody production is often the spleen and because many of the IgG-coated platelets are sequestered there. All patients should receive pneumococcal vaccine before splenectomy and twice daily oral penicillin for life following surgery to protect against pneumococcal infection. Reviews of past management of ITP have associated splenectomy during pregnancy with high fetal loss rates [137] and even an approximate 10% maternal mortality rate [142] but modern supportive measures and improved surgical practices have reduced the fetal loss rate considerably, and the risk of maternal mortality is negligible [143]. In current practice, splenectomy is hardly ever indicated in the pregnant patient and should be avoided given the success of medical management. However, removal of the spleen remains an option if all other attempts to increase the platelet count fail [144]. Splenectomy should be performed in the second trimester because surgery is best tolerated then and the size of the uterus will not make the operation technically difficult. If possible the platelet count should be raised to safe levels for surgery by intravenous IgG. Although transfused platelets will have a short life in the maternal circulation, they may help to achieve haemostasis at surgery. Platelet concentrates should be available but given only if abnormal bleeding occurs.

Other therapy. There are a number of other medications that have been used in ITP but most of them are contraindicated in pregnancy and in any case only have moderate success rates. Danazol, an attenuated anabolic steroid, has been used with moderate success in a few patients, although it should not be used in pregnancy. Vincristine has a transient beneficial effect in many patients but it is not recommended in pregnancy, and long-term associated neurotoxicity limits its usefulness.

Very occasionally immunosuppressives such as azathioprine and cyclophosphamide have to be used in severe intractable thrombocytopenia that does not respond to any other measures. Cyclophosphamide should be avoided in pregnancy if possible (although see Chapter 7 for an account of its use in renal transplant patients). Experience with relatively low doses of azathioprine in renal transplant patients who have negotiated pregnancy suggests that this drug is not associated with increased maternal or immediate fetal morbidity.

The most contentious issue in the management of ITP in pregnancy is the mode of delivery given that the fetus might be thrombocytopenic and may bleed from trauma during the birth process.

Assessment of the fetal platelet count. Hegde [135] analysed the reported cases in the literature from 1950 to 1983, which suggested an overall incidence of neonatal thrombocytopenia of 52% with significant morbidity in 12% of births. The probability of fetal thrombocytopenia increased according to the severity of maternal thrombocytopenia. For example the incidence increased to 70% of deliveries if maternal platelet counts were $< 100 \times 10^9/L$ at term. As a result of this and other analyses many strategies were developed to predict the fetal platelet count and to determine the optimal mode of delivery because it was believed that elective caesarean section was the best option for an affected fetus at risk from trauma during a vaginal delivery.

We now know that the incidence in these retrospective analyses was distorted because only symptomatic women were likely to have been investigated and reported (see above). A more recent report [122] studied the outcome of 162 consecutive pregnancies in women with presumed ITP presenting in the decade 1979–89. The overall incidence of thrombocytopenia (11%) in the offspring of these women was much lower than the earlier reported analyses, but two factors emerged of importance in predicting neonatal thrombocytopenia. In the absence of a history of ITP before pregnancy or in the absence of circulating platelet IgG antibodies in the index pregnancy in those with a history, the risk of severe thrombocytopenia in the fetus at term was negligible.

These findings are supported by other more recent reports [14,123]. In the study of Burrows and Kelton [14], 61 infants were born to 50 mothers with confirmed ITP. Only three (4.9%) had a cord platelet count $< 50 \times 10^9/L$. None of the infants had morbidity or mortality as a result of the thrombocytopenia. Two-thirds of the infants had a further fall in platelet count in the first 2 or 3 days after birth but in all the thrombocytopenia could easily be corrected. Some investigators have suggested that maternal splenectomy increases the probability of neonatal thrombocytopenia [137,145]. Closer scrutiny of published reports [126] shows that it is only in those women with splenectomy and persistent thrombocytopenia ($< 100 \times 10^9/L$) that the risk of neonatal thrombocytopenia is increased. What has become clear over the years is that analysis of the older literature gave an exaggerated incidence of neonatal thrombocytopenia and of the morbidity and mortality arising from it. However, even with benefit of accurate, automated, easily repeated platelet counts, estimation of IgG platelet antibodies and taking into consideration splenectomy status, it is still impossible to predict the fetal platelet count in any individual case [120] and to plan the mode of delivery based on any of these maternal parameters is not logical or sensible.

Fetal blood sampling. A method for direct measurement of the fetal platelet count in scalp blood obtained transcervically prior to or early in labour has been described [146–148]. The authors recommend that caesarean section be performed in all cases where the fetal platelet count is $< 50 \times 10^9/L$. This approach is more logical than a decision about the mode of delivery made on the basis of maternal platelet count, concentration of IgG or splenectomy status, but it is not without risk of significant haemorrhage in the truly thrombocytopenic fetus, often gives false-positive results [126] and demands urgent action to be taken on the results. Also the cervix must be sufficiently dilated to allow the fetal scalp to be sampled and the uterine contraction to achieve this may have caused the fetus to descend so far in the birth canal that caesarean section is technically difficult and also traumatic for the fetus.

The only way a reliable fetal platelet count can be obtained so that a decision concerning the optimal mode of delivery can be taken is by a percutaneous transabdominal fetal cord blood sample taken before term [149–151]. This gives time for discussion with the obstetrician, paediatrician, haematologist, anaesthetist and anyone else involved concerning delivery. It should be performed at 37–38 weeks' gestation under ultrasound guidance as the transfer of IgG increases in the last weeks of pregnancy: an earlier sample may give a higher fetal platelet count than one taken nearer term. There is no need for sampling earlier in gestation because the fetus is not at risk from spontaneous ICH *in utero* (cf. fetus with alloimmune thrombocytopenia).

There are the risks associated with the sampling of cord spasm and haemorrhage but in skilled hands the incidence of these is no more than 1% [127]. A caesarean section may be precipitated because of fetal distress during the procedure even if the platelet count proves to be normal. This is another good reason for performing a fetal blood sample (FBS) as late as possible in gestation if it is thought to be necessary. Given the low risk of identifying a problem and the risk of associated complications *in utero*, FBS can only be justified in very few ITP pregnancies. In the USA it would appear from a recently published survey that obstetricians have changed their policies of routine FBS and caesarean section in all ITP cases to follow a less interventional approach as now adopted in the UK [152].

Neonatal platelet count. After birth the platelet count will continue to fall for 2–5 days. If the cord platelet count shows severe thrombocytopenia and especially if there is evidence of skin or mucous membrane bleeding, measures can be taken to prevent this predicted fall. Intravenous hydrocortisone and platelet transfusion have been used with success but the recommended therapy nowadays should be intravenous IgG because of its relative safety and the rapidity with which a response is observed.

Mode of delivery in idiopathic (autoimmune) thrombocytopenic purpura. There is little risk to the mother whatever the mode of delivery. In most cases the maternal platelet count can be raised to haemostatic levels to cover the event. Even if the mother has to deliver in the face of a low platelet count, she is unlikely to bleed from the placental site once the uterus is empty but she is at risk of bleeding from any surgical incisions, soft-tissue injuries or tears. Platelets should be available but not given prophylactically. It should be remembered that the unnecessary transfusion of platelet concentrates in the absence of haemostatic failure may stimulate more autoantibody formation synthesis and thus increase maternal thrombocytopenia. Most anaesthetists require the platelet count to be at least $80 \times 10^9/L$ and preferably $>100 \times 10^9/L$ before they will administer an epidural anaesthetic but there is no good evidence that counts $>50 \times 10^9/L$ are insufficient to achieve haemostasis in ITP [153].

The major risk at delivery is to the fetus with thrombocytopenia who as the result of birth trauma may suffer ICH. If there is any question that a vaginal delivery will be difficult because of cephalopelvic disproportion, premature labour, previous history, etc., then elective caesarean section should be carried out.

For many centres the availability of planned or emergency transabdominal FBS is severely limited or nonexistent and so decisions concerning the mode of delivery will have to be taken without knowing the fetal platelet count.

As discussed earlier, maternal platelet count, maternal PAIgG, history and splenectomy status show trends regarding the incidence of fetal and neonatal thrombocytopenia but can never be used to predict fetal thrombocytopenia with absolute confidence in an individual case. It does appear, however, that it is very unlikely for the fetus to have severe thrombocytopenia if the mother has no previous history of ITP before the index pregnancy and if she has no detectable free IgG platelet antibody [122].

Many of the options proposed in the literature presuppose that caesarean section is less traumatic than uncomplicated vaginal delivery. There is no objective evidence to support this contention and there are undesirable associated complications of caesarean section *per se* for both mother and fetus. The only advantage is that there is more overall control of the delivery if it is by elective caesarean section and there are usually no unpredictable complications.

Based on an estimate of a 13–21% perinatal mortality associated with ITP, it was proposed [154] that all patients should be delivered by caesarean section. The mortality rate quoted is a gross overestimate, probably for reasons previously stated of selection of severe symptomatic cases for the analysis. As stated a recent review of the literature of ITP in pregnancy shows a neonatal mortality rate of six in 1000 ITP patients [126], about the same as or better than the overall perinatal mortality rate. All these deaths occurred in babies delivered by caesarean section and all events appeared more than 24–48h after delivery, the time of the platelet count nadir in the neonate.

The incidence of severe thrombocytopenia in the fetus of a woman with proven ITP is no more than 10%. Even if caesarean section is the optimal mode of delivery for the thrombocytopenic fetus, this does not justify this mode of delivery for the nine out of 10 fetuses without thrombocytopenia.

It is now thought to be optimal management not to deliver all fetuses with potential or identified thrombocytopenia by caesarean section. If delivery by caesarean section is indicated for obstetric reasons there is no point in performing FBS to obtain the platelet count and elective caesarean section should be performed.

In our hospital there is considerable expertise in intrauterine FBS but we only recommend this procedure in the following circumstances and then not always:

1 where the woman enters pregnancy with a history of ITP together with currently identifiable PAIgG antibodies; or

2 in those women who have to be treated for ITP during the index pregnancy.

Our obstetricians, like many others, prefer to deliver a fetus with significant thrombocytopenia (platelet count $<50 \times 10^9$/L) by caesarean section. However, individual units may need different policies depending on local expertise and practice.

Management of the neonate. An immediate cord platelet count should be performed following delivery in all neonates of mothers with ITP whenever or however diagnosed. The vast majority of babies will have platelet counts well above 50×10^9/L and will be symptom free. For those with low platelet counts, petechiae and purpura, steroids or preferably intravenous IgG should be administered. If there is mucous membrane bleeding, platelet concentrates should be administered also.

It should be remembered that the neonatal platelet count will fall further in the first few days of life and it is at the nadir that most complications occur, rather than at delivery. Measures should be taken to prevent the fall if the cord blood platelet count warrants this. The platelet count should be repeated daily for the first week in those neonates with thrombocytopenia at delivery.

The development of techniques to obtain fetal blood with relative safety to perform a fetal platelet count and

the widely held concept that caesarean section is less traumatic for the fetus than a normal vaginal delivery has led to often unnecessary intervention with risks to both mother and fetus.

At the time of writing the emphasis of management is to return to a non-intervention policy [155] of sensible monitoring, supportive therapy, and a mode of delivery determined mainly by obstetric indications and not primarily on either the maternal or fetal platelet count [152].

THROMBOCYTOPENIA ASSOCIATED WITH HUMAN IMMUNODEFICIENCY VIRUS INFECTION (see also Chapter 18)

Thrombocytopenia is a well-recognized complication of HIV infection and may be due to drugs and severe infection. The subject has been reviewed [156]. However, patients with the immune deficiency syndromes may have thrombocytopenia otherwise indistinguishable from ITP. This may be due to immune platelet destruction resulting from cross-reaction between HIV and the platelet glycoproteins IIb/IIA [157], which may explain acquired immune deficiency syndrome (AIDS)-free, HIV-associated ITP. It has also been suggested that disturbances in the B-cell subset, CD5, in HIV-infected patients may cause immunological changes correlating with the platelet count, and that non-specific deposition of complement and immune complexes on platelets leads to their removal from the circulation.

THROMBOCYTOPENIA AND SYSTEMIC LUPUS ERYTHEMATOSUS

SLE is frequently complicated by thrombocytopenia but this is seldom severe, fewer than 5% of cases having platelet counts $<30 \times 10^9$/L during the course of the disease [158]. Thrombocytopenia is often the first presenting feature and may antedate any other manifestations by months or even years. Such patients are often labelled as suffering from ITP, unless appropriate additional tests are carried out. PAIgG is often found on tasting but it is not clear whether this is due to antiplatelet antibody, immune complexes or both. The management of isolated thrombocytopenia associated with SLE in pregnancy does not differ substantially from that of ITP, but immunosuppressive therapy should not be reduced or discontinued during pregnancy [159]. The main management problem of SLE and pregnancy is the complication of the variably present *in vitro* lupus anticoagulant and its paradoxical association with *in vivo* thromboembolism and recurrent fetal loss. For fuller discussion of these complications, which have excited much current interest, see Chapter 8.

FETOMATERNAL ALLOIMMUNE THROMBOCYTOPENIA [160]

Fetomaternal alloimmune thrombocytopenia (FMAIT) is a syndrome that develops as a result of maternal sensitization to fetal platelet antigens. The mother is not thrombocytopenic herself but the fetal platelets are reduced and have altered function.

Severe alloimmune thrombocytopenia is a rare but important cause of fetal death and long-term neurological morbidity. The vast majority of clinically significant cases arise from fetomaternal incompatibility for the human platelet antigen HPA-1a.

Diagnosis and screening

It is important to identify FMAIT as a cause of fetal or neonatal thrombocytopenia because of the high risk of recurrence and of ICH in subsequent pregnancies.

Routine antenatal screening has been suggested as a perinatal health policy but has not been put into practice. Pilot studies have confirmed an incidence of one in 1000–2000 pregnancies [161], more common than in other conditions for which screening is carried out. However, HPA typing of platelets is not a routine hospital transfusion laboratory commitment and would require recently developed primer pairs for rapid HPA identification with allele-specific PCR.

Currently, the diagnosis of the maternal condition in the overwhelming number of cases is made after the birth of a thrombocytopenic infant or identification of a fetus (or neonate) with unexplained ICH. Serological testing of both parents is enough to establish the diagnosis. The importance of using one of a limited number of laboratories with the full range of capabilities required (including DNA-based typing) is emphasized.

Female relatives of the affected mother should be tested for HPA status in order to identify potential cases before the birth of a first affected infant.

Antenatal management

Unlike Rh(D) haemolytic disease of the newborn (HDN), first pregnancies may be severely affected and the maternal alloimmune platelet antibody has not proved useful in identifying or monitoring severity of the condition in the fetus.

The primary goal of antenatal management is to prevent *in utero* or perinatal ICH. Many fetal medicine centres in the UK give weekly transfusions of compatible platelets from as early as 22–24 weeks' gestation until 32 weeks or more [162]. The cumulative risk of loss during the possible 15 procedures (20–34 weeks) could be as high

as 13–23% and must be considered against the risk to the fetus from the disease [163]. The apparent success from many groups in the USA of weekly maternal infusions of intravenous immunoglobulin (IVIgG) in preventing fetal ICH has therefore been welcomed [164], but this success is still regarded with scepticism in the UK and Europe [165].

There is consensus that FBS and a platelet count is the only certain way to identify an affected fetus. Suitable platelet concentrates should be available to cover the procedure. The risk of exsanguination at FBS appears to be higher than in other conditions when cordocentesis is performed [166]. It has been suggested that function is disturbed by the antibody binding to a platelet membrane site involved in fibrinogen binding and aggregation and also to HPA-1a sites on the vascular endothelium.

Discrepancies between management approaches in North American and European centres reflect uncertainties regarding non-invasive monitoring and the hazards associated with invasive procedures. Optimal management is in the process of evolution, and the appropriate therapy in any individual case is uncertain. All approaches have drawbacks [166a]. Interventions are based on the balance of the assessed risk of the disease in the fetus exceeding the risk of the invasive procedures involved [167].

THROMBOTIC THROMBOCYTOPENIC PURPURA AND HAEMOLYTIC–URAEMIC SYNDROME

These conditions, extremely rare in pregnancy, share so many features that they have been considered as one disease with pathological effects confined largely to the kidney in haemolytic–uraemic syndrome (HUS) and being more generalized in TTP. Both are due to the presence of platelet thrombi in the microcirculation that cause ischaemic dysfunction and microangiopathic haemolysis.

In TTP, the focus shifts to multisystem disease, often with neurological involvement and fever. It has been associated with pregnancy and the postpartum period and in the non-pregnant state with the platelet anti-aggregating agent, ticlopidine [168]. It is associated with abnormal patterns of multimers of vWF in the plasma.

In the past few years the mechanisms of processing of vWF have been clarified. A proteolytic enzyme present in normal plasma cleaves peptide bonds in monomeric subunits of vWF thus degrading the large multimers. This proteolytic enzyme prevents the unusually large multimers from causing vWF-mediated adhesion of platelets to subendothelium after vascular damage [169].

Exciting new research by two groups of investigators has elucidated the role of vWF cleaving protease activity in TTP [170,171]. In all the patients studied with acute single episode TTP, there was little or no vWF-cleaving protease activity associated with an IgG autoantibody during the illness but the activity returned to normal following recovery [171]. However, in patients with chronic relapsing TTP unusually large multimers of vWF are found in the plasma even between acute episodes together with absence or low levels of vWF-cleaving protease activity [170]. What are the implications of these exciting new findings? First, the response of patients in the past to FFP component infusions that contain the vWF-cleaving protease activity is explained. The fact that plasmapheresis is often required in the acute phase to achieve a response is also clarified as this will remove autoantibodies as well as the abnormal large vWF multimers. Secondly, the diagnosis of TTP which has been confused with severe pre-eclampsia and HELLP syndrome may be clarified by a single laboratory test measuring the vWF-cleaving protease activity in the plasma and its inhibitor. This test will also help clinicians to distinguish between TTP and HUS, thought in the past to be a spectrum of clinical expression of the same disease. In HUS the levels of vWF-cleaving protease are normal or approaching normal and it also explains why plasma exchange has disappointing results in HUS. The possible role of microbial infections and steroid therapy in acute TTP remain unexplained but provide areas of research to explore the triggering of this condition in patients who do not have a genetic lack of vWF-cleaving protease activity.

The pentad of fever, normal coagulation tests with low platelets, haemolytic anaemia, neurological disorders and renal dysfunction are virtually pathognomonic of TTP. The thrombocytopenia may range from 50 to 100×10^9/L. The clinical picture is severe with a high maternal mortality. A crucial problem when dealing with TTP is to establish a correct diagnosis, because this condition can be confused with severe pre-eclampsia and placental abruption, especially if DIC (very uncommon in TTP) is triggered.

Unlike severe pre-eclampsia, HELLP and AFLP there is no evidence that prompt delivery affects the course of HUS or TTP. Most clinicians would recommend delivery if these conditions are present in late pregnancy so that the mother can be treated vigorously without fear of harming the fetus. Therapeutic strategies hinge on intensive plasma exchange or replacement.

In summary, objective diagnosis of TTP should now be facilitated by measurement of vWF-cleaving protease and its inhibitor. The basis of treatment depends on supplying the defective missing enzyme by infusion of plasma or cryosupernatant preferably in severe cases by exchange transfusion. It is reassuring that the vWF-cleaving protease is still present in all virally inactivated plasma products, whatever method is used.

Factor VIII antibody

An inhibitor of antihaemophilic factor is a rare cause of haemorrhage in previously healthy postpartum women [172–176]. There are less than 50 documented cases in the literature [175,176]. Women who may have had this type of haemorrhagic disorder were first reported in the late 1930s and the nature of the defect was first reported in 1946, when the plasma of two such patients was shown not only to resemble haemophilic plasma but also to have an inhibitory effect on normal clotting. In the late 1960s it was demonstrated that these inhibitors of Factor VIII were immunoglobulins, as are the Factor VIII antibodies found in treated haemophiliacs [176]. Of the postpartum coagulation defects of this type reported, nearly all were found on *in vitro* testing to be directed against Factor VIII. Only two were found to be anti-Factor IX antibodies.

AETIOLOGY

The aetiology of antibodies to Factor VIIIC is complex. The appearance of anti-VIII in non-haemophilic individuals is usually attributed to an autoimmune process, or in women postpartum to isoimmunization. However, no difference between maternal and fetal Factor VIII has been demonstrated, and neutralization of both maternal and fetal Factor VIII by the antibody is similar.

At present there is no definite evidence that Factor VIII antigen allotypes exist. If the bleeding tendency is to be explained, the antibody formed by stimulation of the maternal immune system by fetal Factor VIII has to cross-react with maternal Factor VIII. One would expect such an antibody to reappear after some of the subsequent pregnancies (by analogy with Rhesus sensitization). But relapses have not been reported. Assuming that these inhibitors are IgG antibodies, they are likely to cross the placenta and persist for several weeks in the neonate, as do antirhesus or antiviral antibodies. However, although Factor VIII antibody and reduced levels of Factor VIIIC have been found in neonates born to mothers with antibody there have been no case reports of haemorrhagic problems in their offspring. The variable nature of this disorder argues in favour of a more complex pathogenesis. There is an association between Factor VIII antibodies and autoimmune disorders such as rheumatoid arthritis and SLE. There is also a well-known alteration of immune reactivity in normal pregnancy. These two observations suggest that a likely explanation of postpartum Factor VIII antibodies is that of a temporary breakdown in the mother's tolerance to her own Factor VIII (or Factor IX). This rare disorder does resemble other autoimmune states in its variable onset and duration, its varying severity and in the fact that its aetiology is still a mystery [176].

CLINICAL MANIFESTATIONS

The patient usually presents within 3 months of delivery with severe and sometimes life-threatening bleeding, extensive painful bruising, bleeding from the gastrointestinal and genitourinary tract, and occasional haemarthroses. The reported confirmed cases presented in a period of 3 days to 17 months postpartum. The diagnosis is established on the basis of characteristic laboratory findings. The prothrombin time and thrombin time are normal but the partial thromboplastin time is very long. The partial thromboplastin time is not corrected by the addition of normal plasma or Factor VIII.

MANAGEMENT

Any woman who develops such an antibody should be under the care of an expert coagulation unit. Treatment of the acute bleeding episode is difficult because conventional amounts of Factor VIII may just enhance antibody formation and fail to control the bleeding. Immunosuppressive agents in combination with corticosteroids have been used to reduce the antibody production [172].

In one reported case [175] after failure of therapy with Factor VIII concentrate and fresh plasma, improvement in the clinical status was achieved by administration of an anti-inhibitor coagulation complex (Autoplex), a preparation of pooled fresh plasma containing precursors and activated clotting factors. The mechanism of action of Autoplex is unknown. It does not suppress or destroy the inhibitor but seems to control the acute haemorrhagic diathesis [175].

The natural history is for the antibody to disappear gradually, usually within 2 years. Women should be advised to avoid further pregnancy until coagulation returns to normal, although in the one documented case where conception occurred in the presence of clinically active antibody, it disappeared during the course of the pregnancy [176].

Inherited defects of haemostasis

It is important to recognize these uncommon conditions not only because the morbidity and mortality they cause

in the sufferer is almost completely preventable by correct diagnosis and treatment, but also because carriers of the most devastating of these conditions, particularly the X-linked haemophilias, can be identified and prenatal diagnosis offered if couples at risk so desire.

However, because of the profound changes in haemostasis during normal pregnancy, it is desirable to establish a correct diagnosis with appropriate family studies and DNA analysis where relevant before conception so that appropriate management and chorion villus sampling, in conditions where DNA prenatal diagnosis is feasible, can be planned in advance.

Severe congenital disorders of haemostasis are nearly always apparent early in life so that they will have been diagnosed before the obstetrician has to deal with the patient. Milder forms may go unrecognized until adult life and are more of a diagnostic challenge.

Patients with thrombocytopenia or platelet function abnormalities suffer primarily from mucosal bleeding, with epistaxis, gingival and gastrointestinal bleeding and menorrhagia. Bleeding occurs immediately after surgery or trauma and may not occur at all if primary haemostasis can be achieved surgically.

In contrast, patients with coagulation disorders typically suffer deep muscle haematoma and haemarthroses. Bleeding after trauma or surgery may be immediate or delayed.

A history of previous vaginal deliveries without undue bleeding does not exclude a significant coagulopathy because of the increase in coagulation factors, particularly Factor VIII, during normal pregnancy and the fact that a healthy myometrium is the most important haemostatic factor at parturition.

It is not uncommon for adult patients to have significant bleeding after surgery because of previously undiagnosed inherited haemostatic disorders. This is because surgery imposes a challenge to the haemostatic mechanisms that far exceeds anything encountered in everyday life.

Complete laboratory evaluation of a patient giving a history of 'easy bleeding or bruising' is time consuming and expensive and a history of significant previous haemostatic challenges should be obtained. For example, a patient who has undergone tonsillectomy, without transfusion or special treatment and lived to tell the tale, cannot possibly have an inherited haemostatic disorder!

Of more relevance perhaps is any history of dental extractions where haemorrhage can occur with both platelet disorders and coagulopathies. If prolonged bleeding has occurred and particularly if blood transfusion has been required, then a high index of suspicion of a congenital haemorrhagic disorder is justified. In such cases, even if initial laboratory screening tests—partial thromboplastin time, prothrombin time, platelet count and bleeding time are normal, the diagnosis should be vigorously pursued in consultation with an expert haematologist.

The most common congenital coagulation disorders are von Willebrand's disease, Factor VIII deficiency (haemophilia A) and Factor IX deficiency (haemophilia B). Less common disorders include Factor XI deficiency, abnormal or deficient fibrinogen and deficiency of Factor XIII (fibrin-stabilizing factor). All other coagulation factor disorders are extremely rare. The most frequent disorders of platelet function are von Willebrand's disease and storage pool disease [177].

Hereditary platelet abnormalities

FUNCTIONAL DEFECTS

Serious bleeding disorders due to inherited abnormalities of platelet function are rare, the inheritance being autosomal recessive. Clinically the signs and symptoms are similar to those of von Willebrand's disease (see below) with skin and mucosal haemorrhages. Spontaneous bruises are common but haemarthroses are not. Although these disorders can lead to life-threatening haemorrhage, particularly after surgery or trauma, the bleeding tendency is usually mild. The essential defect is intrinsic to the platelet. Bleeding time is prolonged and platelet function tests are abnormal, showing reduced aggregation and/or adhesions. In thrombasthenia (Glanzmann's disease), the platelets appear morphologically normal but they fail to aggregate with collagen, ADP or ristocetin. In the very rare Bernard–Soulier syndrome the aggregation defect is similar but the platelets have a characteristically abnormal giant appearance. Serious bleeding episodes are treated with fresh platelet concentrate infusions and plasmapheresis [178]. Families who have one or other of these rare defects may seek termination of pregnancy because of the severity of symptoms or the difficulties arising from management. It is theoretically possible to diagnose the condition prenatally from a pure FBS, because specific membrane glycoprotein defects have been identified in both syndromes. A sensitive monoclonal immunoassay applicable to small volumes of whole fetal blood, without the necessity of separating the platelets, greatly facilitates prenatal diagnoses in these conditions (see [179]).

THROMBOCYTOPENIA

Genetically determined thrombocytopenia may be associated with aplastic anaemia or isolated megakaryocytic aplasia. The syndrome of absent radii with thrombocytopenia is known as the TAR syndrome: these are thought to be autosomal recessive defects and have been successfully diagnosed prenatally by examination of fetal blood samples [149,180,181].

Patients with May–Hegglin anomaly, an autosomal dominant condition with variable thrombocytopenia and giant platelets, may receive platelet concentrates to achieve haemostasis at delivery and can be offered prenatal diagnosis [115]. More frequently, patients do not have a haemostatic disorder with May–Hegglin anomaly. If Dohle bodies (inclusions in white cells) are not prominent the patient might be labelled as chronic ITP—a difficult problem to resolve but examination of both parents' blood films may be helpful.

Another X-linked symptom complex is the Wiskott–Aldrich syndrome comprising severe immune deficiency with thrombocytopenia. It presents in the neonatal period but is probably expressed *in utero* and therefore susceptible to diagnosis prenatally. The five pregnancies at risk in one report were female and were not examined further [179]. Fanconi's anaemia, a familial autosomal recessively inherited condition, is a syndrome of aplastic anaemia with varying skeletal and other physical anomalies. Although thrombocytopenia is the earliest and dominant feature of marrow aplasia, presentation is usually delayed until at least 3 or 4 years of age, so that intrauterine diagnosis by detecting thrombocytopenia in fetal blood is precluded. However, the diagnosis has been made on the basis of excessive chromosomal breaks in chemically treated amniotic fluid fibroblast cultures [180]. A more rapid result could be obtained by using percutaneous transabdominal FBS for culture of fetal cells [179].

Hereditary coagulation disorders [182]

VON WILLEBRAND'S DISEASE

Von Willebrand's disease [183] is the most frequent of all inherited haemostatic disorders with an incidence of overt disease of more than one in 10 000, similar to that of haemophilia A; but because subclinical forms of the disorder are common the total incidence of von Willebrand's disease is greater than that of haemophilia.

In contrast to haemophilia (an X-linked condition) von Willebrand's disease has an autosomal inheritance and equal incidence in males and females. It therefore is the most frequent genetic haemostatic disorder encountered in obstetric practice.

Nature of the defect

Von Willebrand's disease is a disorder of the vWF portion of the human Factor VIII complex.

Factor VIII circulates as a complex of two proteins of unequal size (Table 3.2). There is a low molecular weight portion VIIIC (290 kDa) that promotes coagulation linked to a large multimer known as both vWF (VIIIWF) and VIIIRAg (VIII-related antigen). Factor VIII circulates as polymers ranging in size from 800 to more than 10 000 kDa. The biosynthesis of Factor VIIIC coded for by the X chromosome is reduced or abnormal in haemophilia A. The larger VIIIWF, which serves as a 'carrier' for VIIIC, is under separate autosomal control, is unaffected in haemophilia. vWF appears to stabilize the small coagulant protein or perhaps protect it from proteolytic digestion. Reduction in VIIIWF usually leads to comparable decrease in VIIIC activity.

vWF is the major protein in plasma that promotes platelet adhesion forming a bridge between the subendothelial collagen and a specific receptor on the platelet membrane. The large multimeric forms of VIIIWF appear to have the greatest physiological effect in promoting this adhesion, which is the first step in coagulation *in vivo*, followed by platelet aggregation. However, *in vitro* tests of platelet aggregation will be entirely normal in von Willebrand's disease because the initial step is bypassed and different platelet receptors are activated when they are exposed to collagen, ADP or thrombin in standard laboratory conditions. The platelet abnormality in von Willebrand's disease can be studied *in vitro* using the antibiotic ristocetin, which takes advantage of the fact that it will induce aggregation platelets, by a mechanism involving VIIIWF. The most sensitive test for detection of von Willebrand's disease is ristocetin cofactor assay—a functional assay for vWF. The ability of patients' plasma to induce aggregation of normal platelets in the presence

of ristocetin is assessed in this test. Ristocetin cofactor levels are normal in fewer than 10% of patients with von Willebrand's disease, and this test shows the best correlation with clinical manifestations of the disease. If the patient's own platelet-rich plasma is used in this test system the ristocetin aggregation is normal in more than one-third. However, the direct ristocetin platelet aggregation test may be useful in the diagnosis of one of the variants of von Willebrand's disease type IIb (see below).

Clinical manifestations are primarily those of a platelet defect, namely spontaneous mucous membrane and skin bleeding, with prolonged bleeding following trauma or surgery. In addition there is a variable secondary defect of Factor VIII coagulant activity and if this is severely depressed there may be clinical manifestations of a coagulation disorder. The most frequent problem encountered in the non-pregnant female is menorrhagia, which may be quite severe at times.

Patients with mild abnormalities may be asymptomatic and picked up only after excessive haemorrhage following trauma or related to surgery.

The severity of the disorder does not run true within families and fluctuates from time to time in the same individual.

Subtypes of von Willebrand's disease

The most common type of von Willebrand's disease accounting for 80% of all cases is type I. It is inherited as an autosomal dominant trait. The protein is qualitatively normal but there is a reduction in Factor VIII activity, both coagulation activity and platelet function being affected in roughly equal proportion. The manifestations

VIII	Molecular complex	Molecular weight $> 1 \times 10^6$
VIIIC	Procoagulant in plasma (detected in bioassay)	Molecular weight 293 000 X chromosome
VIIICAg	Antigen detectable by human antibody to VIIIC Immunoradiometric assay (IRMA)	
VIIIWF	von Willebrand factor Measured by bleeding time Ristocetin aggregation of platelets	Molecular weight (Polymers × 220 000) Chromosome 12
VIIIRAg	Antigen detectable by heterologous antibody raised in rabbit to human factor VIII (IRMA)	

Table 3.2 Factor VIII molecular complex.

result from a quantitative deficiency of a normal protein. The condition is usually mild.

A rare, apparently autosomal recessive form of the disorder is described in which there is absent *in vitro* Factor VIIIC, Factor VIIIRAg and ristocetin cofactor activity, which is accompanied by a severe bleeding disorder. It is in these cases that couples at risk may seek prenatal diagnosis (see below).

Type II von Willebrand's disease is characterized by an absence of large multimers of vWF, which seem to be essential for normal platelet function. In type IIa the large and intermediate size multimers are absent from both plasma and platelets and it accounts for fewer than 10% of all cases.

Approximately 5% of cases belong to the subtype IIb in which the large multimers are absent in the plasma but present in the platelets. Types IIc and IId and pseudo von Willebrand's disease have also been described on the basis of multimeric pattern and distribution of VIIIWF. It must be obvious from the discussion so far that any woman who is contemplating or has entered pregnancy with von Willebrand's disease or a history suggestive of this complex disorder must be managed by a unit that has access to expert haemostatic advice. The subtype must be correctly identified because this has serious implications in terms of the optimum management (see below).

Treatment

There are several forms of treatment of von Willebrand's disease in current use. In any given case the choice depends on the severity and type of the disease and also on the clinical setting. The aim is to correct the platelet and coagulation disorder by achieving normal levels of Factor VIII coagulant activity and a bleeding time within the normal range. The key feature in treatment is substitution with plasma concentrates containing functional vWF and VIIIC. In less severe cases the vasopressin analogue L-diamino-8-arginine-vasopressin (DDAVP) has been used with success. Contraceptive hormones have been used with success in treatment of menorrhagia in von Willebrand's disease [183]. It is extremely important that aspirin and related non-steroidal anti-inflammatory drugs should not be used in von Willebrand's disease. They will further compromise platelet function, and aspirin has been shown to prolong the bleeding time markedly in patients with platelet/coagulation disorders.

Substitution therapy. The main treatment in von Willebrand's disease used to be replacement therapy with cryoprecipitate or FFP. The latter is efficient, but large volumes may be required to secure haemostasis. In ob-

stetric practice, however, this did not cause any problems when covering delivery. Cryoprecipitate used to be the product of choice to cover elective surgery. Factor VIII concentrates were not used in the management of von Willebrand's disease because in commercial preparations the factor promoting platelet adhesion may be lost, and because of the increased risk of transmitting infection. However, the newer preparations of Factor VIII concentrate are now the treatment of choice. They retain some platelet-promoting activity and have the added advantage of being heat treated and therefore sterile. They now no longer carry the hazard of transmitting HIV and other viral infections. The use of cryoprecipitate and FFP is now contraindicated and cannot be recommended.

L-*diamino-8-arginine-vasopressin.* This vasopressin analogue has been shown to cause release of vWF from endothelial cells where it is synthesized and stored. This results in increased plasma levels of both ristocetin cofactor and of Factor VIIIC. It is therefore of benefit to patients with both von Willebrand's disease and haemophilia A. It is particularly effective in mildly affected patients and may in some cases replace the use of need for blood products in patients undergoing surgery. Toxicity associated with use of this product has been trivial. Occasional patients experience flushing and dizziness [183,184]. The theoretical risk of water intoxication and hyponatraemia due to the vasopressive effect has not been observed using the current dosage schedules. The recommended dose is an intravenous infusion of $0.3\,\mu g/kg$ of DDAVP given over 30 min with a total dose of $15-25\,\mu g$. This may be repeated every 12–24 h [185]. Patients with mild type I von Willebrand's disease would be expected to derive maximal benefit from this mode of treatment. VIIIC levels are dramatically increased provided that the baseline level is more than 10%. The effect of the use of DDAVP on the bleeding time is controversial but the overall consensus is that *in vitro* ristocetin cofactor levels increase and there is an overall reduction in clinical bleeding.

In patients with severe type I von Willebrand's disease, DDAVP will have no effect, and replacement therapy must be used.

In type IIB von Willebrand's disease the use of DDAVP is contraindicated. *In vivo* platelet aggregation and severe thrombocytopenia will follow the infusion although it does transiently improve the plasma multimeric pattern.

Von Willebrand's disease and pregnancy

A rise in both Factor VIIIC and vWF is observed in normal pregnancy. Patients with all but the severest forms of von

Willebrand's disease show a similar but variable rise in both these factors, although there may not be a reduction in the bleeding time [177,186–188].

After delivery, normal women maintain an elevated Factor VIIIC level for at least 5 days. This is followed by a slow fall to baseline levels over 4–6 weeks. The duration of Factor VIII activity postpartum in women with von Willebrand's disease seems to be related to the severity of the disorder. Those women with more severe forms of the condition may have a rapid fall in Factor VIII pro-coagulant and platelet haemostatic activity. They are then at risk of quite severe secondary postpartum haemorrhage.

What is the haemorrhagic risk during pregnancy and delivery for women with von Willebrand's disease? An analysis of published reports of 33 pregnancies in 22 women showed abnormal bleeding in 27% of pregnancies at the time of abortion, delivery or postpartum [188].

The vast majority of women will have increased their Factor VIIIC production to within the normal range (50–150%) by late gestation, and although Factor VIII concentrate should be standing by at delivery it will probably not be needed to achieve haemostasis [189].

There is virtually no need to use DDAVP in obstetric practice except perhaps in the puerperium because if a rise in Factor VIII is possible under the influence of DDAVP (milder cases) then it will have been achieved because of the stimulus of pregnancy itself. However, DDAVP has an obvious valuable place in the management of women with von Willebrand's disease undergoing gynaecological surgery. There is extensive experience indicating safety of DDAVP in pregnancy obtained in pregnant patients with diabetes insipidus (see Chapter 13).

THE HAEMOPHILIAS

The haemophilias are inherited disorders associated with reduced or absent coagulation Factors VIII or IX. Their incidence is about one in 10 000 in developed countries [190]. The most common is haemophilia A, which is associated with deficiency of Factor VIII: about one-sixth of the 3000–4000 cases in the UK today have a condition known as Christmas disease due to a lack of coagulation Factor IX (haemophilia B). Clinical manifestations of the two conditions are indistinguishable, the symptoms and signs being variable and depending on the degree of lack of the coagulation factors concerned. Severe disease with frequent spontaneous bleeding (particularly haemarthroses) is associated with clotting factor levels of 0–1%. Less severe disease is found in subjects with clotting factors of 1–4%. Spontaneous bleeding and severe bleeding after minor trauma are rare in cases with coagulation

factor levels between 5 and 30%; the danger is that the condition may be clinically silent but during the course of major surgery or following trauma, such subjects behave as if they have the very severest forms of haemophilia. Unless the defect is recognized and the lacking coagulation factor is replaced, such patients will continue to bleed. The inheritance of both haemophilias is X-linked recessive, being expressed in the male and carried by the female.

The implications of pregnancy for a female carrier of haemophilia are twofold:
1 she may, by process of Lyonization, have a very low Factor VIII or IX level which puts her at risk of excessive bleeding, particularly following a traumatic or surgical delivery;
2 50% of her male offspring will inherit haemophilia and 50% of her daughters will be carriers like herself.
This has important considerations now that prenatal diagnosis of these conditions is possible (see below).

Management of haemophilia in pregnancy

Female carriers of haemophilia do not usually have clinical manifestations but in rare individuals in whom the Factor VIIIC or IX levels are unusually low (10–30% of normal) abnormal bleeding may occur after trauma or surgery [191]. It is important to identify carriers prior to pregnancy, not only to provide genetic counselling (see below) but also so that appropriate provision can be made for those cases with pathologically low coagulation factor activities. Fortunately the level of the deficient factor tends to increase during the course of pregnancy as it does in normal women. There have been anecdotal reports of female homozygotes for haemophilia A who have negotiated pregnancy successfully [191]. Haemorrhage postpartum does not appear to be a consistent feature, particularly if delivery is by the vaginal route at term with little or no soft-tissue damage. The effect of pregnancy on Factor VIIIC levels in these rare cases has not been studied.

If the Factor VIII level remains low in carriers of haemophilia A, Factor VIII concentrates should be administered to maintain Factor VIII levels above 50% and continued for 3–4 days postpartum following a normal vaginal delivery. This cover will have to be maintained for a longer period if delivery is by caesarean section or there has been extensive soft-tissue damage. Now that Factor VIII concentrates are virally inactivated the hazards of multiple donations are avoided.

DDAVP has been shown to be of benefit in patients with mild haemophilia as with von Willebrand's disease (see above). However, the storage pools of Factor VIII released during treatment may become exhausted and tachyphylaxis does occur [185]. There are no controlled studies concerning the use of DDAVP for bleeding disorders during pregnancy although as noted above it is safe in the treatment of diabetes insipidus (see Chapter 13).

However, as indicated previously if the stimulus of pregnancy has not raised the level of Factor VIII as an expected physiological response in mild haemophilia, it is unlikely that DDAVP will do so.

A clinical problem is more likely in carriers of Factor IX deficiency (Christmas disease) than in those women who carry Factor VIII deficiency [192].

In the exceptionally rare situations where Factor IX level is very low and remains low during pregnancy, the patient should be managed with high-purity Factor IX concentrates to cover delivery and for 3–4 days postpartum. Low-purity factor IX concentrate (prothrombin concentrate) contains Factors II, VII and X, as well as Factor IX, and therefore carry a much greater thrombogenic hazard adding to the innate risk of thromboembolism in pregnancy. FFP will carry the very remote hazard (in the UK) of transmitting HIV infection [193]. The product of choice is therefore high-purity Factor IX concentrate. These patients should be managed in a unit with access to expert advice, 24-h laboratory coagulation service and immediate access to the appropriate plasma components required for replacement therapy.

Prenatal diagnosis of the haemophilias

Haemophilia is a relatively uncommon disease. In the UK there are between 3000 and 4000 cases and one in 25 000 of the population has the disease in a severe form. The ratio of haemophilia A to Christmas disease is in the region of 5 : 1. Affected males within the same family have similar residual levels of coagulation factor activity (<1% severe, 1–5% moderate, >6% mild).

Antenatal screening for these conditions will be largely restricted to families in which there is a history of the disease. It is usually indicated if a woman wishes to undergo prenatal diagnosis to determine whether her male fetus has the disease. Approximately one-third of cases have no family history and are presumed to result from spontaneous mutations.

Obligate carriers [194] are:

1 all daughters of a haemophiliac father;

2 a woman with more than one haemophiliac son;

3 a woman with one haemophiliac son and a proven haemophiliac relative in her own family or her mother's;

4 the relative of a haemophilia sufferer, the male fetus of whom is found to be haemophiliac on prenatal testing.

Putative carriers are daughters of a known haemophiliac carrier who have a 50:50 chance of inheriting the abnormal X chromosome, as do their brothers. The homozygous male is easily identified, but the heterozygous female may have to be content with a statistical estimate of her genotype by discriminate analysis utilizing family data and haematological investigation (see below).

A further aid to carrier detection in a few females was the demonstration of a linkage between haemophilia A and glucose-6-phosphate dehydrogenase (G6PD) variant, another X-linked genetic marker. It cannot be overemphasized that the clarification of carrier status goes hand in hand with prenatal diagnosis. This is particularly so when using direct DNA analysis (see below) [195].

Although it has proved possible to diagnose carrier status during pregnancy [179], the need to make early plans for fetal sexing and to take the required blood samples means that the status should be established before pregnancy whenever practicable.

Female carriers of haemophilia have on average 50% of the normal mean level of the coagulation factor involved, but because of the wide range of normal and variability of Lyonization of the X chromosome, carriers often have levels within the normal range. As far as haemophilia A is concerned it is sometimes possible to improve discrimination by measuring the level of vWF, the autosomally coded carrier protein for Factor VIII. Carriers, unlike the normal population, have lower levels of VIIIC than vWF (reduced VIIIC/vWF ratio)—but firm diagnosis of carrier status is still not possible in about 15% of cases.

In recent years specialist centres managing these diseases are turning to DNA technology for diagnosis. The Factor VIII and IX genes have been isolated and sequenced and many of the mutations that underlie haemophilia and Christmas disease have been determined. They may result from point mutations or deletions involving these genes. In addition, many restriction fragment length polymorphisms (RFLPs) have been found both within and in the flanking regions of these genes.

The specialist studies involved can be undertaken by the regional haemophilia centre in collaboration with the regional genetics centre.

For identified female carriers, prenatal diagnosis can be carried out in the majority of cases by DNA analysis of chorion villus samples. In the few families where DNA analysis is not currently informative, assay of plasma Factor VIIIC or Factor IXC in a fetal blood sample taken from 18 weeks' gestation onwards will provide an accurate but undesirable late prenatal diagnosis.

FACTOR XI DEFICIENCY (PLASMA
THROMBOPLASTIN ANTECEDENT DEFICIENCY)

This is a rare coagulation disorder that is less common than
the haemophilias but more common than the very rare
inherited deficiencies of the remaining coagulation factors.
It is inherited as an autosomal recessive, predominantly in
Ashkenazi Jews, and both men and women may be
affected. Usually only homozygotes have clinical evidence
of a coagulation disorder, although occasionally carriers
may have a bleeding tendency. It is a mild condition in
which spontaneous haemorrhages and haemarthroses are
rare but the danger lies in the fact that profuse bleeding
may follow major trauma or surgery if no prophylactic
Factor XI concentrate is given. Indeed it is often diagnosed
late in life following surgery in an individual who was
previously unaware of a serious haemostatic defect. The
diagnosis is made by finding a prolonged partial thromboplastin time, with a low Factor XI level in a coagulation
assay system in which all other coagulation tests are
normal. Management consists of replacement with Factor
XI concentrates as prophylaxis for surgery or to treat bleeding and to cover operative delivery.

Occasionally women with postpartum haemorrhage
are found to have this abnormality which may or may
not have contributed to the blood loss [196]. The effective
haemostatic level of Factor XI has a half-life of around
2 days. To cover surgery or delivery, women can be
treated with one infusion of Factor XI concentrate to
raise the level to 80–100% and until primary healing is
established.

Fortunately the condition rarely causes problems either
during pregnancy and labour or in the child: in particular,
prolonged bleeding at ritual circumcision is unusual.
There is therefore no justification in screening routinely
for this condition in the mother, fetus or neonate. Women
with Factor XI deficiency should be given documentation
of their defect so that appropriate measures can be taken
to cover surgery or accidental trauma [197].

GENETIC DISORDERS OF FIBRINOGEN (FACTOR I)

Fibrinogen is synthesized in the liver, has a molecular
weight of 340 000 and circulates in plasma at a concentration of 300 mg/dL. Both quantitative and qualitative
genetic abnormalities are described.

Afibrinogenaemia or hypofibrinogenaemia

These are rare autosomal recessive disorders resulting
from reduced fibrinogen synthesis. Most patients with
hypofibrinogenaemia are heterozygous.

Afibrinogenaemia is characterized by a lifelong bleeding tendency of variable severity. Prolonged bleeding
after minor injury and easy bruising are frequent symptoms. Menorrhagia can be very severe. Spontaneous
deep tissue bleeding and haemarthroses are rare, but
severe bleeding can occur after trauma or surgery and
several patients have suffered intracerebral haemorrhages.

In afibrinogenaemia all screening tests of coagulation
are prolonged, but corrected by addition of normal
plasma or fibrinogen. A prolonged bleeding time may
be present. The final diagnosis is made by quantitating
the concentration of circulating fibrinogen.

There are no fibrinogen concentrates available, and
plasma or cryoprecipitate have to be used as replacement
therapy to treat bleeding, or to cover surgery or delivery.
The *in vivo* half-life of fibrinogen is between 3 and 5 days.
Initial replacement should be achieved with 25 mL
plasma/kg and daily maintenance with 50–10 mL/kg for
7 days.

Congenital hypofibrinogenaemia has been associated
with recurrent early miscarriages and with recurrent placental abruption [198].

Dysfibrinogenaemia

Congenital dysfibrinogenaemia is an autosomal dominant
disorder. In contrast to patients with afibrinogenaemia,
patients with this disorder are often symptom free. Some
have a bleeding tendency; others have been shown to
have thromboembolic disease. The diagnosis is made by
demonstrating a prolonged thrombin time with a normal
immunological fibrinogen level.

Affected women, like those with hypofibrinogenaemia,
may have recurrent spontaneous abortion or repeated
placental abruption [198].

FACTOR XIII DEFICIENCY (FIBRIN STABILIZING
FACTOR DEFICIENCY)

This is an autosomal recessive disorder classically characterized by bleeding from the umbilical cord during the
first few days of life and later by ecchymoses, prolonged
post-traumatic haemorrhage and poor wound healing.
Bleeding is usually delayed and characteristically of a
slow oozing nature. ICH has been described in a significant proportion of reported cases. Spontaneous recurrent
abortion with excessive bleeding occurs in association
with Factor XIII deficiency [199]. All standard coagulation
tests are normal. Diagnosis of severe Factor XIII deficiency is made by the clot solubility test. Normal fibrin
clots will not dissolve when incubated overnight in

5 mol/L urea solutions, whereas the unstable clots formed in the absence of Factor XIII will be dissolved.

Factor XIII has a half-life of 6 days to 2 weeks and only 5% of normal Factor XIII levels are needed for effective haemostasis; therefore patients can be treated with FFP in doses of 5 mL/kg, which can be repeated every 3 weeks. Using this therapy, pregnancy has progressed safely to term in a woman who had previously suffered repeated abortions. Because of the high incidence of ICH, replacement therapy should be recommended for all individuals who are known to have Factor XIII deficiency [199].

OTHER PLASMA FACTOR DISORDERS

Congenital deficiencies of Factors II, V, VII and X are extremely rare and the reader is referred to a more detailed review of hereditary coagulopathies in pregnancy for an account of their diagnosis and special management problems [186].

Genetic collagen vascular disease

EHLERS–DANLOS SYNDROME (see also Chapter 5)

It is often forgotten that an essential part of the haemostatic system is healthy vasculature. The Ehlers–Danlos syndrome may be associated with bleeding because of increased fragility of vessels due to defects in collagen synthesis. It is also associated with hyperextensible joints and excess skin elasticity as a result of a connective tissue disorder. The disease has an autosomal dominant inheritance and has been subdivided into 10 subtypes of which type IV is the most severe and may have lethal complications. The bleeding symptoms include ease of bruising, gastrointestinal bleeding, haemoptysis and most important of all, rupture of the long arteries. The diagnosis may be suspected if the patient has papyraceous scars and pseudo-tumours over bony prominences. There may be calcified subcutaneous nodules. Ehlers–Danlos syndrome (type) IV is associated with an abnormality of collagen type III as a result of mutations in the corresponding gene COL3A1 but this abnormality can also be detected in milder subtypes of Ehlers–Danlos Syndrome. Attention is drawn to a recent review of the spectrum of severity of this condition [200].

Surgical procedures should be avoided unless essential because the tissues are friable and massive bleeding may occur and healing of incisions may be delayed. Pregnancy and delivery will be involved with obvious potential hazards. I draw this to the attention of readers because the diagnosis of this condition may be missed, especially in an obstetric/gynaecological scenario where many women complain of easy bruising, which is one of the main presenting symptoms. To further confuse the situation, platelet and coagulation screening tests will all yield results within the normal range.

References

1 Forbes CD, Greer IA. Physiology of haemostasis and the effect of pregnancy. In: Greer IA, Turpie AGG, Forbes CD, eds. *Haemostasis and Thrombosis in Obstetrics and Gynaecology*. Chapman & Hall, London, 1992: 1–25.

2 Letsky EA. Mechanisms of coagulation and the changes induced by pregnancy. *Curr Obstet Gynaecol*, 1991; 1: 203–9.

3 Stirling Y, Woolf L, North WR, Seghatchian MJ, Meade TW. Haemostasis in normal pregnancy. *Thromb Haemost* 1984; 52 (2): 176–82.

4 Levi M, Ten Cate H. Disseminated intravascular coagulation. *N Engl J Med* 1999; 341 (8): 586–92.

5 Moncada S, Vane JR. Arachidonic acid metabolites and the interactions between platelets and blood-vessel walls. *N Engl J Med* 1979; 300 (20): 1142–7.

6 Zeeman GG, Dekker GA, van Geijn HP, Kraayenbrink AA. Endothelial function in normal and pre-eclamptic pregnancy: a hypothesis. *Eur J Obstet Gynecol Reprod Biol* 1992; 43 (2): 113–22.

7 Sill PR, Lind T, Walker W. Platelet values during normal pregnancy. *Br J Obstet Gynaecol* 1985; 92 (5): 480–3.

8 Fay RA, Hughes AO, Farron NT. Platelets in pregnancy: hyperdestruction in pregnancy. *Obstet Gynecol* 1983; 61 (2): 238–40.

9 Beal DW, DeMasi AD. Role of the platelet count in management of the high-risk obstetric patient. *J Am Osteopath Assoc* 1985; 85 (4): 252–5.

10 Fenton V, Saunders K, Cavill I. The platelet count in pregnancy. *J Clin Pathol* 1977; 30 (1): 68–9.

11 Rakoczi I, Tallian F, Bagdany S, Gati I. Platelet life-span in normal pregnancy and pre-eclampsia as determined by a nonradioisotope technique. *Thromb Res* 1979; 15 (3–4): 553–6.

12 Wallenburg HC, van Kessel PH. Platelet lifespan in normal pregnancy as determined by a nonradioisotopic technique. *Br J Obstet Gynaecol* 1978; 85 (1): 33–6.

13 Burrows RF, Kelton JG. Incidentally detected thrombocytopenia in healthy mothers and their infants. *N Engl J Med* 1988; 319 (3): 142–5.

14 Burrows RF, Kelton JG. Thrombocytopenia at delivery. A prospective survey of 6715 deliveries. *Am J Obstet Gynecol*, 1990; 162 (3): 731–4.

15 O'Brien WF, Saba HI, Knuppel RA, Scerbo JC, Cohen GR. Alterations in platelet concentration and aggregation in normal pregnancy and preeclampsia. *Am J Obstet Gynecol* 1986; 155 (3): 486–90.

16 Romero R, Duffy TP. Platelet disorders in pregnancy. *Clin Perinatol* 1980; 7 (2): 327–48.

17 Redman CW, Bonnar J, Beilin L. Early platelet consumption in pre-eclampsia. *Br Med J* 1978; 1 (6111): 467–9.

18 Ahmed Y, Sullivan MH, Pearce JM, Elder MG. Changes in platelet function in pregnancies complicated by fetal growth restriction. *Eur J Obstet Gynecol Reprod Biol* 1991; 42 (3): 171–5.

19 Ballegeer VC, Spitz B et al. Platelet activation and vascular damage in gestational hypertension. *Am J Obstet Gynecol* 1992; 166 (2): 629–33.

20 Lin KC, Chou TC, Yin CS, Ding YA. The role of aggregation of platelets in pregnancy-induced hypertension: a comprehensive and longitudinal study. *Int J Cardiol* 1991; 33 (1): 125–31.

21 Bonnar J. Haemostasis and coagulation disorders in pregnancy. In: Bloom, AL Thomas, DP, eds. *Haemostasis and Thrombosis*. Churchill Livingstone, Edinburgh, 1987: 570–84.

22 Van den Broek NR, Letsky EA. Pregnancy and the erythrocyte sedimentation rate. *Br J Obstet Gynaecol* (2001; 108: 1164–67)

23 Lammle B, Griffin JH. Formation of the fibrin clot: the balance of procoagulant and inhibitory factors. *Clin Haematol* 1985; 14 (2): 281–342.

24 Hellgren M, Blomback M. Studies on blood coagulation and fibrinolysis in pregnancy, during delivery and in the puerperium. I. Normal condition. *Gynecologic Obstetric Invest* 1981; 12 (3): 141–54.

25 Bertina RM, Briet E, Engesser L, Reitsma PH. Protein C deficiency and the risk of venous thrombosis. *N Engl J Med* 1988; 318: 930–1.

26 Seligsohn U, Berger A *et al.* Homozygous protein C deficiency manifested by massive venous thrombosis in the newborn. *N Engl J Med*, 1984; 310 (9): 559–62.

27 Comp PC, Thurnau GR, Welsh J, Esmon CT. Functional and immunologic protein S levels are decreased during pregnancy. *Blood* 1986; 68 (4): 881–5.

28 Warwick R, Hutton RA, Goff L, Letsky E, Heard M. Changes in protein C and free protein S during pregnancy and following hysterectomy. *J R Soc Med*, 1989; 82 (10): 591–4.

29 Malm J, Laurell M, Dahlback B. Changes in the plasma levels of vitamin K-dependent proteins C and S and of C4b-binding protein during pregnancy and oral contraception. *Br J Haematol* 1988; 68 (4): 437–43.

30 Alving BM, Comp PC. Recent advances in understanding clotting and evaluating patients with recurrent thrombosis. *Am J Obstet Gynecol* 1992; 167 (4 Part 2): 1184–91.

31 Salem HH. The natural anticoagulants. In: Chesterman, CN, ed. *Thrombosis and the Vessel Wall. Clinics in Haematology*. W.B. Saunders, London, 1986: 371–91.

32 Walker ID. Management of thrombophilia in pregnancy. *Blood Rev* 1991; 5 (4): 227–33.

33 Bertina RM, Koeleman RPC *et al.* Mutation in blood coagulation factor V associated with resistance to activated protein C. *Nature* 1994; 369: 64–7.

34 Svensson PJ, Dahlback B. Resistance to activated protein C as a basis for venous thrombosis [see comments]. *N Engl J Med* 1994; 330 (8): 517–22.

35 Haemostasis and Thrombosis Task Force, British Committee for Standards in Haematology. Guideline: Investigation and Management of Heritable Thrombophilia. *Br J Haematol* 2001; 114: 512–528.

36 Bonnar J, Prentice CRM *et al.* Haemostatic mechanism in uterine circulation during placental separation. *Br Med J* 1971; 2: 564–7.

37 Booth NA, Reith A, Bennett B. A plasminogen activator inhibitor (PAI-2) circulates in two molecular forms during pregnancy. *Thromb Haemost* 1988; 59 (1): 77–9.

38 Ballegeer V, Mombaerts P *et al.* Fibrinolytic response to venous occlusion and fibrin fragment D-Dimer levels in normal and complicated pregnancy. *Thromb Haemost* 1987; 58 (4): 1030–2.

39 Sheppard BL, Bonnar J. The ultrastructure of the arterial supply of the human placenta in early and late pregnancy. *J Obstet Gynaecol Br Commonwealth* 1974; 81 (7): 497–511.

40 Gilabert J, Aznar J *et al.* Alteration in the coagulation and fibrinolysis system in pregnancy, labour and puerperium, with special reference to a possible transitory state of intravascular coagulation during labour. *Thromb Haemost* 1978; 40: 387–96.

41 Wallmo L, Karlsson K, Teger Nilsson AC. Fibrinopeptide A and intravascular coagulation in normotensive and hypertensive pregnancy and parturition. *Acta Obstet Gynecol Scand* 1984; 63 (7): 637–40.

42 Department of Health. *Why Mothers Die. Report on Confidential Enquiries into Maternal Deaths in the United Kingdom, 1994–6*. HMSO, London, 1998.

43 Letsky EA. Management of massive haemorrhage—the haematologist's role. In: Patel N, ed. *Maternal Mortality—the Way Forward*. Royal College of Obstetricians and Gynaecologists, London, 1992: 63–71.

44 Pritchard JA. Haematological problems associated with delivery, placental abruption, retained dead fetus and amniotic fluid embolism. *Clin Haematol* 1973; 2: 563–80.

45 Doenicke A, Grote B, Lorenz W. Blood and blood substitutes in management of the injured patient. *Br J Anaesth* 1977; 49: 681–8.

46 Barbier P, Jonville AP, Autret E, Coureau C. Fetal risks with dextrans during delivery. *Drug Saf* 1992; 7 (1): 71–3.

47 Berg EM, Fasting S, Sellevold OF. Serious complications with dextran-70 despite hapten prophylaxis. Is it best avoided prior to delivery? *Anaesthesia*, 1991; 46 (12): 1033–5.

48 RCOG Working Party. *Report of the RCOG Working Party on Prophylaxis against Thromboembolism in Gynaecology and Obstetrics*. The Royal College of Obstetricians and Gynaecologists, London, 1995.

49 Cash J. Blood replacement therapy. In: Bloom AL Thomas DP, eds. *Haemostasis and Thrombosis*. Churchill Livingstone, Edinburgh, 1987: 585–606.

50 Carey LC, Cloutier CT, Lowery BD. The use of balanced electrolyte solution for resuscitation. In: Fox CL, Nahas GG, eds. *Body Fluid Replacement in the Surgical Patient*. Grune & Stratton, New York, 1970.

51 Moss G. An argument in favour of electrolyte solutions for early resuscitation. *Surg Clin North Am* 1972; 52: 3–17.

52 Virgilio RWK, Rice CL *et al.* Crystalloid versus colloid resuscitation: is one better? *Surgery* 1979; 85: 129–39.

53 Hauser CJ, Shoemaker WC, Turpin I, Goldberg SJ. Oxygen transport responses to colloids and crystalloids in critically ill surgical patients. *Surg Gynecol Obstet* 1980; 159: 181–6.

54 Lorenz W, Doenicke A *et al.* Histamine release in human subjects by modified gelatin (Haemaccel) and dextran: An explanation for anaphylactoid reactions observed under clinical conditions. *Br J Anaesth* 1976; 48: 151–65.

55 Freeman M. Fatal reaction to haemaccel. *Anaesthesia* 1979; 34: 341–3.

56 Williamson LM, Lowe S *et al.* Serious hazards of transfusion (SHOT) initiative: analysis of the first two annual reports. *Br Med J* 1999; 319: 16–19.

57 Turner M. Review. The impact of new-variant Creutzfeldt–Jakob disease on blood transfusion practice. *Br J Haematol* 1999; 106: 842–50.

58 Marshall M, Bird T. *Blood Loss and Replacement*. Edward Arnold, London, 1983.

59 Hansch E, Chitkara U *et al.* Pelvic arterial embolization for control of obstetric hemorrhage: A five-year experience. *Am J Obstet Gynecol* 1999; 180(6): 1454–60.

60 Pelage J P, Le Dref O *et al.* Selective arterial embolization of the uterine arteries in the management of intractable post-partum hemorrhage. *Acta Obstet Gynecol Scand* 1999; 78: 698–703.

61 Aznar J, Gilabert J *et al*. Evaluation of the soluble fibrin monomer complexes and other coagulation parameters in obstetric patients. *Thromb Res* 1982; 27: 691–701.

62 Hafter R, Graeff H. Molecular aspects of defibrination in a reptilase treated case of 'dead fetus syndrome'. *Thromb Res*, 1975; 7: 391–9.

63 Fournie A, Monrozies M, Pontonnier G, Boneu B, Bierne R. Factor VIII complex in normal pregnancy, pre-eclampsia and fetal growth restriction. *Br J Obstet Gynaecol* 1981; 88: 250–4.

64 Whigham KAE, Howie PW, Shaf MM, Prentice CRM. Factor VIII related antigen and coagulant activity in intrauterine growth restriction. *Thromb Res* 1979; 16: 629–38.

65 Redman CWG. Coagulation problems in human pregnancy. *Postgrad Med J* 1979; 55: 367–71.

66 Gilabert J, Estelles A, Aznar J, Galbis M. Abruptio placentae and disseminated intravascular coagulation. *Acta Obstet Gynecol Scand* 1985; 64: 35–9.

67 Naumann RO, Weinstein L. Disseminated intravascular coagulation—the clinician's dilemma. *Obstetr Gynecol Surv* 1985; 40: 487–92.

68 Estelles A, Gilabert J, Espana F, Aznar J, Gómez-Lechón M. Fibrinolysis in preeclampsia. *Fibrinolysis*, 1987; 1: 209–14.

69 Magriples U, Chan DW, Bruzek D, Copel JA, Hsu C-D. Thrombomodulin. A new marker for placental abruption. *Thromb Haemost* 1999; 81: 32–4.

70 Basu HK. Fibrinolysis and abruptio placentae. *J Obstet Gynaecol Br Commonwealth* 1969; 76 (6): 481–96.

71 Sher G. Pathogenesis and management of uterine inertia complicating abruptio placentae with consumption coagulopathy. *Am J Obstet Gynecol*, 1977; 129: 164–70.

72 Bonnar J. Haemorrhagic disorders during pregnancy. In: Hathaway WE Bonnar J, eds. *Perinatal Coagulation Monographs in Neonatology*. Grune & Stratton, New York, 1978.

73 Thragarajah S, Wheby MS *et al*. Disseminated intravascular coagulation in pregnancy. The role of heparin therapy. *J Reprod Med* 1981; 26: 17–24.

74 Feinstein DI. Diagnosis and management of disseminated intravascular coagulation: The role of heparin therapy. *Blood* 1982; 60: 284–7.

75 Sher GI, Statland BE. Abruptio placentae with coagulopathy: a rational basis for management. *Clin Obstet Gynecol* 1985; 28: 15–23.

76 Amris CJ, Hilden M. Anticoagulant effects of Trasylol: *In vitro* and *in vivo* studies. *Ann NY Acad Sci* 1968; 146: 612–94.

77 Bidstrup BP, Royston D, Sapsford RN, Taylor KM. Reduction in blood loss and blood use after cardiopulmonary bypass with high dose aprotinin (Trasylol). *J Thorac Cardiovasc Surg* 1989; 97 (3): 364–72.

78 Pritchard JA, Cunningham FG, Pritchard SA, Mason RA. On reducing the frequency of severe abruptio placentae. *Am J Obstet Gynecol* 1991; 165 (5 Part 1): 1345–51.

79 Morgan M. Amniotic fluid embolism. *Anaesthesia* 1979; 34: 20–32.

80 Herbert WNP. Complications of the immediate puerperium. *Clin Obstet Gynecol* 1982; 25: 219–32.

81 Bonnar J. Blood coagulation and fibrinolysis in obstetrics. *Clin Haematol* 1973; 2: 213–33.

82 Chung AF, Merkatz IR. Survival following amniotic fluid embolism with early heparinisation. *Obstet Gynecol* 1973; 42: 809–14.

83 Skjodt P. Amniotic fluid embolism—a case investigated by coagulation and fibrinolysis studies. *Acta Obstet Gynecol Scand* 1965; 44: 437–57.

84 Resnik R, Swartz WH, Plumer MH, Bernirske K, Stratthaus ME. Amniotic fluid embolism with survival. *Obstet Gynecol* 1976; 47: 395–8.

85 Tuck CS. Amniotic fluid embolus. *Proc R Soc Med* 1972; 65: 94–5.

86 Clark SL, Pavlova Z, Greenspoon J, Horenstein J, Phelan JP. Squamous cells in the maternal pulmonary circulation. *Am J Obstet Gynecol* 1986; 154 (1): 104–6.

87 Romero R, Copel JA, Hobbins JC. Intrauterine fetal demise and hemostatic failure: the fetal death syndrome. *Clin Obstet Gynecol* 1985; 28: 24–31.

88 Grundy MFB, Craven ER. Consumption coagulopathy after intra-amniotic urea. *Br Med J* 1976; 2: 677–8.

89 Mackenzie IZ, Sayers L *et al*. Coagulation changes during second trimester abortion induced by intra-amniotic prostaglandin E_{2+} and hypertonic solutions. *Lancet* 1975; 2: 1066–9.

90 Spivak JL, Sprangler DB, Bell WR. Defibrination after intraamniotic injection of hypertonic saline. *N Engl J Med* 1972; 287: 321–3.

91 Stander RW, Flessa HC *et al*. Changes in maternal coagulation factors after intraamniotic injection of hypertonic saline. *Obstet Gynecol* 1971; 37: 321–3.

92 Van Royen EA. *Haemostasis in Human Pregnancy and Delivery*. MD Thesis University of Amsterdam, Amsterdam, 1974.

93 Clarkson AR, Sage RE, Lawrence JR. Consumption coagulopathy and acute renal failure due to Gram negative septicaemia after abortion. Complete recovery with heparin therapy. *Ann Intern Med* 1969; 70: 1191–9.

94 Burkman RT, Bell WR *et al*. Coagulopathy with midtrimester induced abortion. Association with hyperosmolar urea administration. *Am J Obstet Gynecol* 1977; 127: 533–6.

95 Davis G. Midtrimester abortion. Late dilation and evacuation and DIC. *Lancet* 1972; 2: 1026.

96 Savage W. Abortion. Methods and sequelae. *Br J Hosp Med* 1982; 27: 364–84.

97 Collier CB, Birrell WRS. Chronic ectopic pregnancy complicated by shock and disseminated intravascular coagulation. *Anaesth Intens Care* 1983; 11: 246–8.

98 Beller FK. Sepsis and coagulation. *Clin Obstet Gynecol* 1985; 28: 46–52.

99 Graeff H, Ernst E, Bocaz JA. Evaluation of hypercoagulability in septic abortion. *Haemostasis* 1976; 5: 285–94.

100 Steichele DF, Herschlein HJ. Intravascular coagulation in bacterial shock. Consumption coagulopathy and fibrinolysis after febrile abortion. *Med Welt* 1968; 1: 24–30.

101 Beller FK, Uszynski M. Disseminated intravascular coagulation in pregnancy. *Clin Obstet Gynecol* 1974; 17: 264–78.

102 McGibbon DH. Dermatological purpura. In: Ingram, GIC, Brozovic, M, Slater, NCP, eds. *Bleeding Disorders—Investigation and Management*. Blackwell Scientific Publications, Oxford, 1982: 220–42.

103 Laursen B, Frost L *et al*. Acute fatty liver of pregnancy with complicating disseminated intravascular coagulation. *Acta Obstet Gynecol Scand* 1983; 62: 403–7.

104 Burroughs AK, Seong NG *et al*. Idiopathic acute fatty liver of pregnancy in 12 patients. *Q J Med* 1982; 51: 481–97.

105 Hellgren M, Hagnevik K *et al*. Severe acquired antithrombin III deficiency in relation to hepatic and renal insufficiency and intra-uterine death in late pregnancy. *Gynecol Obstet Invest* 1983; 16: 107–8.

106 Laursen B, Mortensen J, Frost L, Hansen KB. Disseminated intravascular coagulation in hepatic failure treated with antithrombin III. *Thromb Res* 1981; 22: 701–4.

107 Goodin RC. Acute fatty liver of pregnancy. *Acta Obstet Gynecol Scand* 1984; 63: 379–80.

108 Baker P, Cunningham F. Platelet and coagulation abnormalities. In: Lindheimer M, Roberts J, Cunningham F, eds. *Chesley's Hypertensive Disorders in Pregnancy*. Appleton Lange, Stanford, CN, 1999: 349–73.

109 Romero R, Mazor M *et al*. Clinical significance, prevalence, and natural history of thrombocytopenia in pregnancy-induced hypertension. *Am J Perinatol* 1989; 6 (1): 32–8.

110 Leduc L, Wheeler JM, Kirshon B, Mitchell P, Cotton DB. Coagulation profile in severe preeclampsia. *Obstet Gynecol* 1992; 79 (1): 14–18.

111 Redman CW, Denson KW, Beilin LJ, Bolton FG, Stirrat GM. Factor VIII consumption in pre-eclampsia. *Lancet* 1977; 2 (8051): 1249–52.

112 Weiner CP, Kwaan HC *et al*. Antithrombin III activity in women with hypertension during pregnancy. *Obstet Gynecol* 1985; 65 (3): 301–6.

113 Thornton JG, Molloy BJ *et al*. A prospective study of haemostatic tests at 28 weeks gestation as predictors of pre-eclampsia and growth restriction. *Thromb Haemost* 1989; 61 (2): 243–5.

114 Kupferminc MJ, Eldor A *et al*. Increased frequency of genetic thrombophilia in women with complications of pregnancy. *N Engl J Med* 1999; 340: 9–13.

115 Colvin BT. Thrombocytopenia. In: Letsky EA, eds. *Haematological Disorders in Pregnancy*. W.B. Saunders, London, 1985: 661–81.

116 Pillai M. Platelets and pregnancy. *Br J Obstet Gynaecol* 1993; 100: 201–4.

117 McMillan R. Chronic idiopathic thrombocytopenic purpura. *N Engl J Med* 1981; 304: 1135–7.

118 Kessler I, Lancet M, Borenstein R, Berrebi A, Mogilner BM. The obstetrical management of patients with immunologic thrombocytopenic purpura. *Int J Gynaecol Obstet* 1982; 20 (1): 23–8.

119 Hart D, Dunetz C *et al*. An epidemic of maternal thrombocytopenia associated with elevated antiplatelet antibody. Platelet count and antiplatelet antibody in 116 consecutive pregnancies: relationship to neonatal platelet count. *Am J Obstet Gynecol* 1986; 154 (4): 878–83.

120 Kaplan C, Daffos F *et al*. Fetal platelet counts in thrombocytopenic pregnancy [see comments]. *Lancet* 1990; 336 (8721): 979–82.

121 Kelton JG. Management of the pregnant patient with idiopathic thrombocytopenic purpura. *Ann Intern Med* 1983; 99 (6): 796–800.

122 Samuels P, Bussel JB *et al*. Estimation of the risk of thrombocytopenia in the offspring of pregnant women with presumed immune thrombocytopenic purpura [see comments]. *N Engl J Med* 1990; 323 (4): 229–35.

123 Burrows RF, Kelton JG. Fetal thrombocytopenia and its relation to maternal thrombocytopenia. *N Engl J Med* 1993; 329: 1463–6.

124 Channing Rodgers RP, Levin J. A critical reappraisal of the bleeding time. *Semin Thromb Hemost* 1990; 16: 1–20.

125 Lind SE. The bleeding time does not predict surgical bleeding. *Blood* 1991; 77 (12): 2547–52.

126 Burrows RF, Kelton JG. Thrombocytopenia during pregnancy. In: Greer, IA, Turpie, AG, Forbes, CD, eds. *Haemostatis and Thrombosis in Obstetrics and Gynaecology*. Chapman & Hall, London, 1992: 407–29.

127 Nicolini U, Tannirandorn Y *et al*. Continuing controversy in alloimmune thrombocytopenia: fetal hyperimmunoglobulinemia fails to prevent thrombocytopenia. *Am J Obstet Gynecol* 1990; 163 (4 Part 1): 1144–6.

128 Tchernia G, Dreyfus M *et al*. Management of immune thrombocytopenia in pregnancy: Response of infusions of immunoglobulins. *Am J Obstet Gynecol* 1984; 148: 225–6.

129 Evans RS, Takahashi K *et al*. Primary thrombocytopenic purpura and acquired hemolytic anemia: Evidence for a common etiology. *Arch Intern Med* 1951; 87: 48–65.

130 Harrington WJ, Sprague CC *et al*. Immunologic mechanisms in idiopathic and neonatal thrombocytopenic purpura. *Ann Intern Med* 1953; 38: 433–69.

131 van Leeuwen EF, van der Ven JT, Engelfriet CP, von dem Borne AE. Specificity of autoantibodies in autoimmune thrombocytopenia. *Blood* 1982; 59 (1): 23–6.

132 Woods VL Jr, McMillan R. Platelet autoantigens in chronic ITP. *Br J Haematol* 1984; 57 (1): 1–4.

133 Cines DB, Dusak B, Tomaski A, Mennuti M, Schreiber AD. Immune thrombocytopenic purpura and pregnancy. *N Engl J Med* 1982; 306: 826–31.

134 Mueller Eckhardt C, Kayser W *et al*. The clinical significance of platelet-associated IgG: a study on 298 patients with various disorders. *Br J Haematol* 1980; 46 (1): 123–31.

135 Hegde UM. Immune thrombocytopenia in pregnancy and the newborn [editorial]. *Br J Obstet Gynaecol* 1985; 92 (7): 657–9.

136 Harrington WJ. Are platelet-antibody tests worthwhile? [editorial]. *N Engl J Med* 1987; 316 (4): 211–12.

137 Carloss HW, McMillan R, Crosby WH. Management of pregnancy in women with immune thrombocytopenic purpura. *J Am Med Assoc* 1980; 144: 2756–8.

138 Dwyer JM. Manipulating the immune system with immune globulin. *N Engl J Med* 1992; 326 (2): 107–16.

139 Morgenstern GR, Measday B, Hegde UM. Auto-immune thrombocytopenia in pregnancy. New approach to management. *Br Med J* 1983; 288: 584.

140 Pappas C. Placental transfer of immunoglobulins in immune thrombocytopenic purpura [letter]. *Lancet* 1986; 1 (8477): 389.

141 Hegde UM. Immune thrombocytopenia in pregnancy and the newborn: a review. *J Infect* 1987; 1: 55–8.

142 Bell WR. Hematologic abnormalities in pregnancy. *Med Clin North Am* 1977; 61: 165–203.

143 Martin JN Jr, Morrison JC, Files JC. Autoimmune thrombocytopenic purpura. current concepts and recommended practices. *Am J Obstet Gynecol* 1984; 150 (1): 86–96.

144 Gottlieb P, Axelsson O, Bakos O, Rastad J. Splenectomy during pregnancy: an option in the treatment of autoimmune thrombocytopenic purpura. *Br J Obstet Gynaecol* 1999; 106: 373–5.

145 Van Leeuwen EF, Helmerhorst FM *et al*. Maternal autoimmune thrombocytopenia and the newborn. *Br Med J* 1981; 283: 104.

146 Ayromlooi J. A new approach to the management of immunologic thrombocytopenic purpura in pregnancy. *Am J Obstet Gynecol* 1978; 130 (2): 235–6.

147 Scott JR, Cruikshank DP *et al*. Fetal platelet counts in the obstetric management of immunologic thrombocytopenic purpura. *Am J Obstet Gynecol* 1980; 136: 495–9.

148 Tchernia G. Immune thrombocytopenic purpura and pregnancy. *Curr Stud Hematol Blood Transfus* 1988; 55: 81–9.

149 Daffos F, Forestier F, Kaplan C, Cox W. Prenatal diagnosis and management of bleeding disorders with fetal blood sampling [see comments]. *Am J Obstet Gynecol* 1988; 158 (4): 939–46.

150 Moise KJ Jr, Carpenter RJ Jr, Cotton DB, Wasserstrum N, Kirshon B, Cano L. Percutaneous umbilical cord blood

sampling in the evaluation of fetal platelet counts in pregnant patients with autoimmune thrombocytopenia purpura. *Obstet Gynecol* 1988; 72 (3 Part 1): 346–50.

151 Scioscia AL, Grannum PA, Copel JA, Hobbins JC. The use of percutaneous umbilical blood sampling in immune thrombocytopenic purpura [see comments]. *Am J Obstet Gynecol* 1988; 159 (5): 1066–8.

152 Peleg D, Hunter SK. Perinatal management of women with immune thrombocytopenic purpura: Survey of United States perinatologists. *Am J Obstet Gynecol* 1999; 180: 645–9.

153 Letsky E. Haemostasis and epidural anesthesia. *Int J Obstet Anesth* 1991; 1: 51–4.

154 Murray JM, Harris RE. The management of the pregnant patient with idiopathic thrombocytopenic purpura. *Am J Obstet Gynecol* 1976; 126 (4): 449–51.

155 Aster RH. Gestational thrombocytopenia: a plea for conservative management [editorial]. *N Engl J Med* 1990; 323 (4): 264–6.

156 Costello C. Haematological abnormalities in human immunodeficiency virus (HIV) disease. *J Clin Pathol* 1988; 41 (7): 711–15.

157 Bettaieb A, Fromont P *et al.* Presence of cross-reactive antibody between human immunodeficiency virus (HIV) and platelet glycoproteins in HIV-related immune thrombocytopenic purpura. *Blood* 1992; 80 (1): 162–9.

158 Hughes GRV. Systemic lupus erythematosus. In: Hughes GRV, eds. *Connective Tissue Diseases*. Blackwell Scientific Publications, Oxford, 1987: 3–71.

159 Varner MW, Meehan RT, Syrop CH, Strottmann MP, Goplerud CP. Pregnancy in patients with systemic lupus erythematosus. *Am J Obstet Gynecol* 1983; 145: 1025–37.

160 Levine AB, Berkowitz RL. Neonatal alloimmune thrombocytopenia. *Semin Perinatol* 1991; 15 (3 Suppl. 2): 35–40.

161 Williamson LM, Hackett G *et al.* The natural history of fetomaternal alloimmunization to the platelet-specific antigen HPA-1a (PL^{A1}, Zw^a) as determined by antenatal screening. *Blood* 1998; 92 (7): 2280–7.

162 Murphy MF, Waters AH *et al.* Antenatal management of fetomaternal alloimmune thrombocytopenia (FMAIT): report of 15 affected pregnancies. *Transfus Med* 1994; 4: 281–92.

163 Burrows RF, Kelton JG. Perinatal thrombocytopenia. *Clin Perinatol* 1995; 22 (3): 779–801.

164 Bussel JB, Berkowitz RL *et al.* Antenatal management of alloimmune thrombocytopenia with intravenous γ-globulin: a randomized trial of the addition of low-dose steroid to intravenous γ-globulin. *Am J Obstet Gynecol* 1996; 174 (5): 1414–23.

165 Kaplan C, Murphy MF, Kroll H, Water AH. For the European Working group on FMAIT, Feto-maternal alloimmune thrombocytopenia: antenatal therapy with IvIgG and steroids—more questions than answers. *Br J Haematol* 1998; 100: 62–5.

166 Paidas MJ, Berkowitz RL *et al.* Alloimmune thrombocytopenia: fetal and neonatal losses related to cordocentesis. *Am J Obstet Gynecol*, 1995; 172: 475–9.

166a Overton TE, Duncan KR, Jolly M, Letsky EA, Fisk NM. Serial aggressive platelet transfusions for fetel allo-immune thrombocytopenis: platelet dynamics and perinatal outcome. *Am J Obset Gynecol* (In Press).

167 Bussel JB, Skupski DW, MacFarland JG. Fetal alloimmune thrombocytopenia. Consensus and controversy. *J Matern Fetal Med* 1996; 5: 281–92.

168 Page Y, Tardy B *et al.* Thrombotic thrombocytopenic purpura related to ticlopidine. *Lancet* 1991; 337: 774–6.

169 Moake JL. Moschcowitz, multimers, and metalloprotease (Editorial). *N Engl J Med* 1998; 339 (22): 1629–31.

170 Furlan M, Robles R *et al.* Von Willebrand factor-cleaving protease in thrombotic thrombocytopenic purpura and the hemolytic–uremic syndrome. *N Engl J Med* 1998; 339 (22): 1578–84.

171 Tsai H, Lian E-Y. Antibodies to von Willebrand factor-cleaving protease in acute thrombotic thrombocytopenic purpura. *N Engl J Med* 1998; 339 (22): 1585–94.

172 Coller BS, Hultin MB *et al.* Normal pregnancy in a patient with a prior post partum factor VIII inhibitor: With observations on pathogenesis and prognosis. *Blood* 1981; 58: 619–24.

173 Marengo-Rowe AJ, Murff G *et al.* Haemophilia-like disease associated with pregnancy. *Obstet Gynecol* 1972; 40: 56–64.

174 O'Brien JR. An acquired coagulation defect in a woman. *J Clin Pathol* 1954; 7: 22–5.

175 Reece EA, Fox HE, Rapoport F. Factor VIII inhibitor. A cause of severe postpartum hemorrhage. *Am J Obstet Gynecol* 1982; 144: 985–7.

176 Voke J, Letsky E. Pregnancy and antibody to factor VIII. *J Clin Pathol* 1977; 30: 928–32.

177 How HY, Bergmann F *et al.* Quantitative and qualitative platelet abnormalities during pregnancy. *Am J Obstet Gynecol* 1991; 164 (1 Part 1): 92–8.

178 Peaceman AM, Katz AR, Laville M. Bernard–Soulier syndrome complicating pregnancy: a case report. *Obstet Gynecol* 1989; 73 (3 Part 2): 457–9.

179 Mibashan RS, Millar DA. Fetal haemophilia and allied bleeding disorders. *Br Med Bull* 1983; 39: 392–8.

180 Auerbach AD, Adler B, Chaganti RSK. Prenatal and postnatal diagnosis and carrier detection of Fanconi anaemia by a cytogenetic method. *Paediatrics* 1981; 67: 128–35.

181 Nicolaides KH, Rodeck CH, Mibashan RS. Obstetric management and diagnosis of haematological disease in the fetus. *Clin Haematol* 1985; 14 (3): 775–805.

182 Kadir RA. Women and inherited bleeding disorders: pregnancy and delivery. *Sem Hematol* 1999; 36 (3 Part 4): 28–35.

183 Holmberg L, Nilsson IM. Von Willebrand disease. *Clin Haematol* 1985; 14 (2): 461–88.

184 Davison JM, Sheills EA, Philips PR, Barron WM, Lindheimer MD. Metabolic clearance of vasopressin and an analogue resistant to vasopressinase in human pregnancy. *Am J Physiol* 1993; 264 (2 Part 2): F348–53.

185 Linkler CA. Congenital disorders of haemostasis. In: Laros RK, eds. *Blood Disorders in Pregnancy*. Lea & Febiger, Philadelphia, 1986: 160.

186 Caldwell DC, Williamson RA, Goldsmith JC. Hereditary coagulopathies in pregnancy. *Clin Obstet Gynecol* 1985; 28: 53–72.

187 Chediak JR, Alban CM, Maxey B. Von Willebrand's disease and pregnancy: Management during delivery and outcome of offspring. *Am J Obstet Gynecol* 1986; 155: 618–24.

188 Conti M, Mari D *et al.* Pregnancy in women with different types of von Willebrand disease. *Obstet Gynecol* 1986; 68: 282–5.

189 Milaskiewicz RM, Holdcroft A, Letsky E. Epidural anaesthesia and von Willebrand's disease. *Anaesthesia* 1990; 45 (6): 462–4.

190 Jones P. Developments and problems in the management of hemophilia. *Semin Hematol* 1977; 14: 375–90.

191 Luscher JM, McMillan CW. Severe factor VIII and IX deficiency in females. *Am J Med* 1978; 65 (637).

192 Levin J. Disorders of blood coagulation and platelets. In: Barrow GN, Ferris TF, eds. *Medical Complications During Pregnancy*. W.B. Saunders, London, 1982: 70–3.

193 Williamson L, Heptonstall J, Soldan K. A SHOT in the arm for safer blood transfusion. *Br Med J* 1996; 313: 1221–2.

194 Mibashan RS, Rodeck CH *et al*. Dual diagnosis of prenatal haemophilia A by measurement of fetal Factor VIIIC and VIIIC antigen (VIIICAg). *Lancet* 1980; ii: 994–7.

195 Pembury ME, Mibashan RS. Prenatal diagnosis of haemophilia A. In: Seghatchian MJ, Savidge VF, eds. *Factor VIII Von Willebrand Factor*. CRC Press, Boca Raton, Florida, 1987.

196 David A, Letsky EA, Paterson-Brown S. Factor XI deficiency presenting in pregnancy: diagnosis and management. *Br J Obstet Gynaecol* (in press).

197 Kadir RA, Economides DL *et al*. Factor XI deficiency in women. *Am J Hematol* 2001; 60: 48–54.

198 Ness PM, Budzynski AZ *et al*. Congenital hypofibrinogenemia and recurrent placental abruption. *Obstet Gynecol* 1983; 61: 519–23.

199 Kitchens CS, Newcomb TF. Factor XIII. *Medicine (Baltimore)* 1979; 658: 413–29.

200 Hamel BCJ, Pals G *et al*. Ehlers–Danlos syndrome and type III collagen abnormalities: a variable clinical spectrum. *Clin Genet* 1998; 53: 440–6

4 Thromboembolism

Michael de Swiet

In this chapter we will consider deep vein thrombosis (DVT) and pulmonary embolus complicating pregnancy, and inherited abnormalities of the clotting and fibrinolytic systems such as the factor V Leiden mutation and antithrombin deficiency. For other general reviews see Ginsberg and Hirsh [1], Girling and de Swiet [2], Greer [3] and Letsky [4].

Cerebral vein thrombosis is described in Chapter 15 and systemic thromboembolism arising from mitral valve disease and artificial heart valves is considered in Chapter 5. See Chapter 8 for more discussion of the association between antiphospholipid syndrome and thromboembolism and Chapter 3 for the physiology of the clotting system. Thrombocytosis and paroxysmal nocturnal haemoglobinuria where there are also risks of thromboembolism are considered in Chapter 2.

Significance and incidence

The importance of pulmonary embolus is as a cause of maternal mortality. If the patient does not die, she usually recovers completely, although a few patients subsequently have symptomatic pulmonary hypertension and rather more than might be expected have abnormal lung function tests [5]. The mortality from pulmonary embolus in the non-pregnant population varies between 1% and 8% depending on patient selection [6]. This would be in keeping with the data of the Confidential Enquiry into Maternal Mortality [7] surveying the 3-year period from 1994 to 1996 in the UK: treatment for thromboembolism was only given in six of the 46 women who died,

i.e. death usually occurs in untreated patients and it is likely that the majority of women who are treated survive.

DVT is important because it predisposes to pulmonary embolus. But in addition only 20–25% of patients with DVT are symptom free when followed up 7–13 years after having had DVT [8,9] and 4% even have skin ulceration [8]. The long-term occurrence of leg symptoms following DVT seems to be a particular problem of those who have had the original episode in pregnancy [97].

Pulmonary embolism is now the most frequent cause of maternal mortality in the UK and is responsible for the deaths of about 16 women per year before or immediately after delivery (21 in every million maternities, total maternal mortality 12 per 100*000) [7]. We can be reasonably confident of these data because death from pulmonary embolus is relatively easy to diagnose. Also, at least 90% of all maternal deaths in the UK were analysed in the recent report [7]. Similarly pulmonary embolus was the second most common cause of maternal death in Massachusetts, USA, between 1982 and 1985 (mortality rate 12 per million) [10]. In general, as standards of living rise and the overall maternal mortality rate falls, pulmonary embolism becomes relatively more important as a cause of maternal death. So in a Mexican study where the overall maternal mortality rate was 64 per 100 000 the principal causes of death were hypertension and haemorrhage, and pulmonary embolism was only third as a cause of maternal mortality. Looking again at the data of the Confidential Enquiry into Maternal Mortality, it could be that the absolute death rate from pulmonary embolism is rising in the UK, 2.1 deaths per 100 000 maternities in 1994–96 compared to about 1.3 between 1985 and 1993 [7]. Although increased ascertainment may account for some of this rise it would not explain it all, and increasing maternal age and obesity may also be factors.

It is believed that thromboembolism and hence pulmonary embolism mortality is low in some racial groups such as the Africans and Chinese. However, it may be that under-ascertainment is part of the explanation. For example, in Hong Kong between 1961 and 1985, 3.6% of 438 maternal deaths were thought to be due to pulmonary embolus. But from 1986 all maternal deaths were investigated by coroner's post mortem and the pulmonary embolus rate rose to 53% of 15 deaths [11].

By contrast, in non-fatal cases pulmonary embolism and DVT are not easy to diagnose, particularly in pregnancy (see below). It is therefore difficult to obtain accurate data for the incidences of non-fatal DVT and pulmonary embolism. However, it does appear that pregnancy increases the risk of thromboembolism sixfold [12]. The absolute incidence varies widely between 0.1% [13] and 1.2% [14] of all pregnancies. In general the lower figures come from later studies where a whole population has been surveyed by contrast with data derived from specialist referral centres. Also lower incidences are found in later studies where the diagnosis has been made objectively (see below), although this is not invariably the case. For example in Denmark the incidence rose from 0.5 to 1.2 per 1000 after the introduction of ultrasound for the diagnosis of DVT [15]. DVT is about twice as common as pulmonary embolism.

Between one-fifth and one-half of the cases occur antenatally [16–18], although note that in a recent 3-year Confidential Enquiry into Maternal Mortality in the UK, 18 of 46 deaths occurred before delivery and 10 of these occurred in the first trimester [7]. The possibility of pulmonary embolism very early in pregnancy must not be ignored. Nevertheless, the postpartum period as defined in most of these studies was only 6 weeks, so the risk of thromboembolism per week is much greater after delivery than before.

Risk factors

Clotting factors (see also Chapter 3)

Any alteration in the balance between thrombosis due to activated clotting factors, and clot lysis due to fibrinolytic mechanisms and/or thrombin inhibitors, can precipitate blood clotting. During pregnancy, each of these systems is altered to change the balance towards clotting. After the first trimester, levels of Factors I (fibrinogen), II (prothrombin), VII, VIII, IX and X are increased [19,20] and a further increase in the levels of Factors V, VII and X occurs in the first few days after delivery, even in normal pregnancy [19]; this further postnatal rise could account for the extra risk of thromboembolism at this time. Yoshimura et al. [21] and Andersson et al. [22] confirmed these data by showing increased levels of fibrinopeptide A and thrombin–antithrombin III complexes (indicating increased blood clotting) at the time of placental separation; however, this effect is balanced by increased thrombolysis (raised tissue plasminogen activator and α_2-plasmin inhibitor–plasmin complexes), which starts during the first stage of labour.

The rise in Factor VIII may be particularly important because high levels of Factor VIII are thought to be an independent risk factor for thromboembolism [23].

Abnormal forms of fibrinogen have also been implicated as causes of thromboembolism in pregnancy [24] but usually in association with better established cause of thrombophilia such as protein C deficiency (see below) [25].

Dalaker [26] has shown that Factor VII levels rise to about 250% of non-pregnant values from 17 weeks' gestation due to the formation of a phospholipid–Factor VII complex. The placenta possibly induces this complex, since its level falls very rapidly after delivery. Dalaker documented an increase of Factors II and X to 136% and 171%, respectively [26]. Weiner et al. [27] suggest that an extra 400 mg of fibrinogen are consumed each day at the end of normal pregnancy on the basis of elevated levels of fibrinopeptide A, the first peptide split from fibrinogen during thrombin-mediated fibrin formation. The effect of an increase in clotting factors is added to by a decrease in the activity of some components of the fibrinolytic system [20].

For example the globulin lysis time decreases in pregnancy [28] as does the level of tissue plasminogen activator [29]. But other fibrinolytic indices such as plasminogen α_2-antiplasmin increase [29]. On balance it seems likely that both thrombosis and fibrinolysis increase in pregnancy. Certainly both thrombosis and fibrinolysis are under endocrine control at a cellular level [30] so that DVT has been reported in association with ovarian hyperstimulation [31]. However, although studies demonstrate an increased tendency of blood to clot in pregnancy it is difficult to define which patients are at risk of thrombosis on the basis of tests of coagulation [32]. For example one study, where clotting factors were estimated 6–12 months after delivery in 43 patients who had had thromboembolism in pregnancy, showed no excess clotting activity compared to controls and only a slight decrease in fibrinolysis [33].

Venous stasis

Although the hyperdynamic circulation of pregnancy reduces the overall circulation time, venous return from the lower limbs is reduced because the pregnant uterus obstructs the inferior vena cava [34, 35]. The effect on flow velocity is much greater in the left than in the right leg [36], which could account for the fact that 85% of leg deep vein thromboses occur on the left side [33, 37, 38]. A decrease in venous tone [39, 40] may be another factor promoting venous stasis and thus increasing the risk of DVT. Not surprisingly, compression stockings applied in pregnancy improve venous haemodynamics and subjective symptoms in the legs [41].

Bed rest

Venous stasis is the presumed mechanism whereby bed rest is thought to be associated with an increase in the risk of thromboembolism. This was noted in pregnancy by the Confidential Maternal Mortality reports [42], which also drew attention to the particular risk in patients with severe pre-eclampsia who are first rested in bed and then delivered by caesarean section [43]. Nevertheless most women with thromboembolism in pregnancy have not now had previous prolonged bed rest[44].

Air travel

Because women are particularly at risk from venous thromboembolism in association with air travel [45, 46] pregnant patients should be careful to keep mobile and well hydrated in any plane journey lasting >3 h [45].

Operative delivery

The 1979–81 maternal mortality series [43] suggested that the risk of fatal thromboembolism following caesarean section was markedly increased compared to that after vaginal delivery. In the 1994–96 series, there were 15 deaths following caesarean section, compared to 10 following vaginal delivery. The overall caesarean section rate was likely to have been about 15%; therefore the extra mortality risk associated with caesarean section was about 10-fold in the patients of the confidential series. Finnerty and MacKay [47] found that caesarean section increases the overall risk of thromboembolism to 0.66 in 100 deliveries compared to 0.26 in 100 deliveries for vaginal delivery. Hiilesma [48] showed a similar increase from 1.1 to 2.2%. Bergqvist *et al.* [49] performed strain gauge plethysmography on 169 women following caesarean section and showed that the incidence of DVT was 1.8%. However, in a series of over 1000 patients delivered by caesarean section the incidence of thromboembolism detected clinically was <1% [50]. It is likely that the increased risk of operative delivery is not specific to caesarean section, because Aaro and Juergens [51] found that 25% of cases of thromboembolism occurred in complications of pregnancy that included difficult forceps deliveries and prolonged labour, as well as caesarean section, pre-eclamptic toxaemia and haemorrhage. The cause of these increased risks will be multifactorial; one interesting observation relates to reactive thrombocytosis, the tendency for the platelet count to rise after trauma. A recent study found that 8 days after vaginal delivery, the platelet count had risen to 365, but following caesarean section it rose to 525; and the rise following caesarean section was maintained for more than 24 days after delivery [52]. This would certainly be a factor relating to late thromboembolism following caesarean section.

Age and parity

Age and parity operate independently of each other. The risk of fatal thromboembolism is 20 times greater in women over the age of 40 having their fifth or more pregnancy, compared with women of 20 in their first pregnancy [53]. The Scottish study found the overall incidence of thromboembolism in pregnancy to be over twice as high in those over 35 years old compared to those under 35 (1.02/1000 vs. 2.37/1000) [13].

Other factors

Other risk factors include oestrogen treatment to suppress lactation, which was shown to increase the risk of thromboembolism by Daniel *et al.* [54] and Jeffcoate *et al.* [55]; if any drug treatment is necessary for suppression of lactation, bromocriptine should be used rather than oestrogen.

Sickle cell anaemia is probably a risk factor for pulmonary embolus, because a high proportion of mortalities, due to sickle cell disease, have been reported to occur in pregnancy, usually due to pulmonary embolus [56]. Van Dinh *et al.* [57] have also reported massive pulmonary embolus in a patient with sickle cell trait. Although β thalassaemia major and intermedia have been associated with thromboembolism, the risk in pregnancy is uncertain [58].

A recent Confidential Maternal Mortality report demonstrates the importance of obesity [59]. This was also shown in a non-pregnant study of risk factors for pulmonary embolism in women. Obese women with body mass index (BMI) >29 had a threefold increased risk [60]. In the same study, smoking increased the risk by a similar amount. In pregnancy, smoking could increase the risk by causing a relative inhibition of fibrinolysis [61].

Congestive heart failure, dehydration, cancer [62] and anaemia are all said to increase the risk of thromboembolism [63] and probably do; but in general these risks have not been documented in obstetric practice. Similar risk factors have been demonstrated by Kimball *et al.* [64] for deaths caused by pulmonary embolus following legally induced abortion.

The presence of blood group O is associated with a decreased incidence of thromboembolism. To have a blood group other than O is therefore a positive risk factor [65]. This too is confirmed in the Confidential Maternal Mortality series from 1963 to 1975: the expected frequency of blood group O in the general population in England and Wales is 46%, but only 38% of those with pulmonary emboli had blood group O [53].

Behçet's disease, a form of vasculitis characterized by recurrent apthous and genital ulcers, uveitis and skin lesions is also associated with venous and arterial thromboembolism, although this is rarely a problem in pregnancy.

The risk of repeated thromboembolism in pregnancy in patients who have had thromboembolism in the past is considered below.

Thrombophilia

Thrombophilia is the term applied to the condition in which patients have defects or abnormalities that alter the physiological haemostatic balance in favour of fibrin formation or persistence, and hence that increase the risk of thrombosis. Although the abnormalities that were first described (antithrombin, protein C and protein S deficiencies) have been known for some time there has been an explosion of knowledge in this field recently. The abnormalities can be acquired or inherited. The most important of the acquired abnormalities is antiphospholipid syndrome; this is considered in more detail in Chapter 8. But many patients with the laboratory abnormalities of thrombophilia do not suffer with thromboses and many patients who from their histories appear to have a familial tendency to thrombosis, have no demonstrable haematological abnormality. So there appears to be a graded risk. Those who themselves have had an episode of thromboembolism and who have demonstrable thrombophilia are at greatest risk of recurrence either during pregnancy or at other times. Those who have had thrombophilia discovered because of a family history but who themselves have not had an episode of thromboembolism are at less risk and those with no family history but where thrombophilia has been discovered by population testing are at least risk, i.e. the presence of family history adds extra risk presumably because of other co-segregating

genetic factors that have not yet been elucidated. This would be in keeping with the observation that the risk of thromboembolism where multiple thrombophilia factors are present is greater than the arithmetic sum of the separate individual risks [66].

In general the risk of thrombosis increases with age and exposure to risk factors such as pregnancy and oestrogen. The presence of thrombophilia raises specific problems regarding treatment and prophylaxis of thromboembolism [70] that are also considered in the relevant sections later as well as in the general following description. A separate issue is the relation of thrombophilia to pregnancy outcome (see below).

Antithrombin deficiency

Antithrombin is a naturally occurring substance produced by the liver that inhibits the actions of thrombin and other clotting factors [67]. Because thrombin promotes blood clotting by forming fibrin from fibrinogen, antithrombin decreases the tendency of blood to clot. Antithrombin deficiency, where the level of antithrombin activity is 25–70% of normal, is therefore associated with an increased risk of blood clotting. Antithrombin activity can be measured by a functional test in laboratories that take a particular interest in blood clotting. Note that antithrombin levels are decreased by heparin therapy making it difficult to diagnose the condition once heparin therapy has been started. The condition is inherited as a Mendelian dominant trait [68] in the 40 or so families that have been described [69]. It is rare; Bergqvist [33] did not find a single case in over 500 patients screened for antithrombin deficiency following severe thrombotic disease. Only three cases were found in a Dutch study of 277 patients with DVT [71].

In some families the condition is due to gene deletion [72]. Antithrombin deficiency may either be expressed as the more severe type 1 quantitative deficiency of a qualitatively normal molecule or in type 2 the molecule itself may be abnormal (qualitative antithrombin deficiency) [73]. Characterization of the form of antithrombin deficiency is important in defining the risk of thromboembolism [74]. It is clear that antithrombin deficiency is quite heterogeneous because some abnormal forms of antithrombin have been described that are also inherited in Mendelian dominant fashion but where coagulation studies are normal [75]. Note that antithrombin levels are also reduced in liver disease and in all forms of consumption coagulopathy including pre-eclampsia (see Chapter 6), i.e. antithrombin deficiency may also be acquired. However, most clinical relevance relates to the inherited forms.

Table 4.1 Risk of thromboembolism by thrombophilia in 72 000 pregnancies in Scotland [303] and in 119 women with thromboembolism in pregnancy and 233 controls in Germany [66].

	Risk of thromboembolism in pregnancy (Scotland)%	Risk of thromboembolism in pregnancy (Germany)%
Controls	0.03	
Antithrombin deficiency type 1	36	
Antithrombin deficiency type 2	2.4	0.4
Protein C deficiency	0.88	0.1
Factor V Leiden	0.23	0.25
Prothrombin gene mutation		0.5

In common with other forms of thrombophilia, antithrombin deficiency often presents for the first time after oestrogen exposure either taking the contraceptive pill or in pregnancy. The best estimate of risk comes from a population study carried out by McColl, in Scotland, of 62 episodes of thromboembolism in about 72 000 pregnancies. The risks were found to be one in 2.8 for type 1 (quantitative) deficiency and one in 42 for type 2 qualitative deficiency (Table 4.1). Other studies where the nature of the deficit has not necessarily been quantified suggest a risk of thromboembolism of 40–70% [76, 77]. Winter *et al.* [78] found an even higher risk in three Scottish families (thrombosis in 15 of 16 pregnancies). The risk is so great that some form of prophylaxis must be considered particularly for type 1 disease. These patients are usually treated for life with warfarin because of the risk of fatal pulmonary embolism [79]. However, for the reasons given below, warfarin should be avoided in pregnancy. Although subcutaneous heparin treatment may be associated with a paradoxical decrease in antithrombin levels [80], Hellgren *et al.* [77] have shown that only one of seven patients adequately treated with subcutaneous heparin and antithrombin concentrate in pregnancy had an episode of thromboembolism; this must therefore be the treatment plan of choice.

Hellgren used high-dose unfractionated heparin, 20 000–45 000 units every 24 h to give a 5–10-s prolongation of the activated partial thromboplastin time, equivalent to 0.8–1.0 units of heparin/mL of plasma. The availability of high-dose low molecular weight heparins (LMWHs) is a particular advantage for patients with antithrombin deficiency where this high level of anticoagulation is desirable. Certainly for patients with type 1 deficiency the target anti-Xa level 4 h after dosing should be 0.8 units/mL, i.e. a therapeutic rather than a prophylactic blood level (see below). It could be argued that even patients with type 2 deficiency should receive similar therapeutic treatment rather than treatment at prophylactic levels particularly in the presence of other risk factors such as previous thromboembolism or increasing age. Heparin should be started instead of warfarin as soon as the patient knows that she is pregnant. The patient should have been counselled about the risk of bone demineralization from long-term heparin therapy before she became pregnant.

In addition Hellgren gave antithrombin concentrate at the time of labour [81] when heparin levels should be reduced to avoid the risk of bleeding. A similar approach was suggested by Brandt and Stenbjerg [69] and by Samson *et al.* [82]. Although it appears more elegant to perform a dose-finding exercise in order to give the correct dose of antithrombin to normalize antithrombin levels at the time of delivery, this is quite difficult to achieve in practice. It is not easy for busy laboratories to perform repeat assays of antithrombin over a period of days. We have successfully managed patients with antithrombin deficiency by empirically giving an infusion of 50 units/kg of antithrombin on the day of delivery having stopped subcutaneous heparin on the previous day. After delivery, heparin levels should be increased again to give the same degree of anticoagulation as was recommended for the antenatal period. One week after delivery, the patient can be fully warfarinized as in the non-pregnant state. Fresh frozen plasma may be a suitable alternative source of antithrombin rather than antithrombin concentrate [83]. As in most topics relating to the management of thromboembolism in pregnancy, the value of treatment with antithrombin concentrate has not been proven by clinical trial [84]. Patients have been managed successfully both with [85] and without [86] antithrombin concentrate. There certainly does not seem to be any place for its use in acquired antithrombin deficiency.

Thrombosis is a recognized complication of venography to which patients with antithrombin deficiency are particularly susceptible [87]. Fortunately, venography is used much less now than formerly. But if it is necessary, the less thrombogenic but more expensive contrast medium, metrizamide [88], should be used [87] washed through with heparin.

If thrombosis does occur in patients with antithrombin deficiency they should be treated with heparin and antithrombin concentrate [89, 90]. Thrombolytic therapy has also been used in pregnancy in these circumstances [91].

Because thrombosis has occurred in the neonatal period [92] antithrombin levels should be assayed in the neonate in at-risk cases. Parents will also be anxious to know the status of their child. However, note that normal neonatal antithrombin levels are about 50% those of the adult level [93]. The neonate may be protected from the thrombotic effect of physiological antithrombin deficiency by relatively high levels of α_2-macroglobulin, which also has antithrombin activity [94]. As the α_2-macroglobulin declines with age the infant with antithrombin deficiency becomes more susceptible to blood clotting as he or she grows up. Nevertheless, if the antithrombin level is less than 30%, antithrombin concentrate should be given in the neonatal period because of the risk of thrombosis [82]. Antithrombin levels should be checked again when the child is at least 6 months old before finalizing the diagnosis.

Protein C deficiency

Protein C, after activation to protein Ca selectively inhibits Factors V and VIII [95]. Therefore a deficiency of protein C increases the risk of thromboembolism particularly in pregnancy [96]. Nevertheless, large family studies have demonstrated no excess mortality in individuals with heterozygous protein C deficiency [97]. Resistance to activated protein C (APCR), is a screening test for other thrombophilias, in particular Factor V Leiden (see below).

Protein C deficiency may be inherited either as an autosomal dominant [98] or as a recessive [99], and functional abnormalities as well as deficiencies have been described [100]. Homozygous protein C deficiency is a very severe form of thrombophilia that is usually fatal in the infant period. Patients who survive are usually dependent on infusions of protein C concentrate.

Assay of protein C is only available in specialist laboratories. The levels of both functional and immunological protein C do not change in pregnancy [101].

Protein C deficiency is probably more common than antithrombin III deficiency, being present in 8% of patients with a first episode of thromboembolism before age 40 and 7% of patients with recurrent episodes [102]. In an unselected group of patients with DVT the prevalence was 3% [71]. Pregnancy was an associated factor in seven of 14 female cases of thromboembolism associated with protein C deficiency [102]. The risk of thromboembolism in pregnancy is one in 113 pregnancies (Table 4.1). Thrombosis is more common after delivery than before.

There is less experience than there is with antithrombin III deficiency concerning prophylaxis in pregnancy. On the basis of the above figures most would only offer heparin prophylaxis after delivery rather than throughout pregnancy unless there were additional risk factors such as previous thromboembolism. In pregnant women with protein C deficiency, consideration should be given to testing the father because homozygous protein C deficiency is such a serious condition.

Heparin treatment is effective in the acute phase of thromboembolism and therefore subcutaneous heparin may provide adequate prophylaxis. Care should be taken with warfarin therapy because this has caused skin necrosis [103]. Warfarin should not be used in homozygous protein C deficiency because of the risk of purpura fulminans [104]. Protein C concentrate is now available for the treatment of purpura fulminans (see below) [105]. It could be used for the treatment of thrombotic episodes and has been used in pregnancy [106].

Protein C deficiency is amenable to perinatal diagnosis by fetal blood sampling in the second trimester [107].

Protein S deficiency

Protein S is a cofactor for protein C. It exists in both free and bound forms. The level of free protein S is thought to be more important. By contrast with protein C, the level of free protein S falls by about 20% by the end of the third trimester [101, 108]. This makes diagnosis of protein S deficiency difficult in pregnancy. Families that are deficient in this protein have been described [109] and they have an increased risk of thromboembolism. Protein S deficiency occurs more frequently in patients with antiphospholipid syndrome than one would expect by chance. The reason for this is not clear but anticardiolipin antibodies may inactivate protein S as well [110].

In an unselected group of patients with DVT the prevalence of protein S deficiency was 2% [71]. The risk of developing thromboembolism throughout pregnancy is between 0 and 6%. After delivery the risk is between 7% and 22% [111–114]. These widely differing figures underline the lack of precision in assessing the risks of actual clot in patients with known thrombophilia. Because of the possible very low incidence of antenatal thromboembolism, most would not use heparin prophylaxis throughout pregnancy in patients with protein S deficiency unless there were some other risk factor.

Skin necrosis may also occur with warfarin treatment in protein S deficiency [115] but it is less common than in protein C deficiency. The neonate with homozygous protein S deficiency [116] is also at risk of massive bleeding into the skin, purpura fulminans.

Activated protein C resistance and Factor V Leiden

The first of the recent developments in thrombophilia was the discovery of APCR [117]. Activated protein C in conjunction with its cofactor protein S, inactivates Factor V. Most patients with APCR inherit an abnormal form of Factor V, Factor V Leiden, which is resistant to activated protein C. Factor V Leiden is caused by a single point mutation at position 506 in the Factor V gene that codes for glycine rather than arginine (R506Q). The abnormality is expressed in the heterozygote. Occasional individuals have been described who are homozygous for the abnormality. Their risk of thromboembolism is believed to be considerably greater [118].

There are other reasons for APCR including much rarer abnormalities in factor V, but factor V Leiden is by far the commonest. APCR may also be acquired either in pregnancy or when exposed to exogenous oestrogens; indeed it has been claimed that APCR is the mechanism of increased risk of thromboembolism in these circumstances.

APCR is usually expressed as a ratio, normal value 2, although this value varies between laboratories. Decreasing values of the ratio indicate increasing APCR. APCR values fall in pregnancy [119, 120] and therefore low values are not necessarily pathognomonic. However, APCR is usually checked as a screening test for Factor V Leiden. This is diagnosed by a genetic test, the polymerase chain reaction (PCR) which is unaffected by pregnancy. Therefore abnormally low values of APCR in pregnancy need to be evaluated further by genetic studies of Factor V Leiden.

The prevalence of Factor V Leiden varies markedly between populations. The original studies indicated a prevalence of 4.4% in European populations with the highest level in Greeks (7%). No cases were found in subjects from Africa, the Middle East or South-East Asia possibly accounting for the low incidence of thromboembolism in these populations [121]. Since then the prevalence of Factor V Leiden has been shown to be high in Sweden and isolated cases have been found in the Middle East [122]. It would be surprising if the mutation were totally absent from any population group.

In patients who are heterozygous for Factor V Leiden the risk of thromboembolism in pregnancy is about 0.25% (Table 4.1). Therefore, although the prevalence of the abnormality is high, routine screening in pregnancy (or before starting the combined oral contraceptive) is not advocated [123]. Similarly most would not suggest heparin prophylaxis throughout pregnancy for aysymptomatic heterozygous carriers of Factor V Leiden unless some additional risk factor were present. Studies in non-pregnant patients suggest that homozygotes for Factor V Leiden have a risk of thrombosis 50–80 times that of non-carriers [118], i.e. about a 2.5% risk given a background risk of 0.03% (Table 4.1). Until more data are available concerning the precise risk of thromboembolism in pregnancy in homozygotes, it would seem prudent to use heparin in prophylactic doses (see below) throughout pregnancy in such patients.

Prothrombin gene mutation

More recently a genetic variation in the proththrombin gene (G20210A mutation) has been associated with increased risk of thromboembolism in pregnancy [124]. Prothrombin gene mutation accounts for about 17% of all thromboembolism in pregnancy and confers a relative risk of 15 compared to the wild type. The absolute risk of thromboembolism is about 0.5%, i.e. greater than that of Factor V Leiden [66]. Prothrombin gene mutation often cosegregates with Factor V Leiden when the relative risk of thromboembolism increases to 107, absolute risk in pregnancy is 4.2%. The place of heparin prophylaxis throughout pregnancy for those with the uncomplicated defect in those without other risk factors is again uncertain. However, in view of the very high risk, those who have both Factor V Leiden and prothrombin gene mutation should have heparin throughout pregnancy.

Hyperhomocysteinaemia and homocysteinuria

For some time it has been known that patients with the inborn error of metabolism causing homocystinuria are at increased risk from arterial and venous thromboembolism [125]. This risk has been demonstrated in pregnancy [126,127] and relates to increased blood levels of homocysteine. (See Chapter 14 for further details on homocystinuria in pregnancy.) But homocystinuria is uncommon. Much more common is a milder abnormality whereby mutations in the gene coding for methylenetetrahydrofolate reductase (MTHFR) when present in homozygous form also lead to elevated blood levels of hyperhomocysteine, hyperhomocysteinaemia. These high levels of homocysteine appear to cause damage to both arteries and veins leading to thrombosis in both systems. Folic acid and vitamin B_{12} are cofactors for MTHFR and the levels of both decrease in pregnancy, but the contribution of hyperhomocysteinaemia to thrombosis in pregnancy and the non-pregnant state is at present unclear. For example one study comparing homocysteine levels in patients with DVT compared to controls showed that homocysteine levels above the 95th centile gave an odds ratio for DVT of 2.5 independent of other risk factors [128]. Another similar study showed that hyperhomocysteinaemia only conferred risk when associated with Factor V Leiden [129]. Further problems arise in diagnosing hyperhomocysteinaemia particularly in pregnancy when folate supplementation is common. Options are to estimate a random level of homocysteine, to measure homocysteine after methionine loading, or to test for the MTHFR mutation genetically. Homocysteine measurement is not widely available and is difficult. Methionine loading should not be performed in pregnancy because the acute rise in homocysteine that occurs may itself cause DVT or placental damage; so most would opt for genetic tests even though these do not predict the exact level of homocysteine; and it is likely that it is the level of homocysteine that is the determinant of thromboembolism risk. With regard to prophylaxis in those who are believed to suffer from hyperhomocysteinaemia, folic acid supplementation 5 mg daily should be sufficient, granted the uncertainty about the degree of risk.

Pregnancy outcome in thrombophilia

Adverse pregnancy outcomes have been described for some time in patients with antiphospholipid syndrome. Intrauterine death and severe pre-eclampsia were the first abnormalities to be noted; more recently the association with recurrent miscarriage became apparent (see Chapter 8 for more details). Granted the possibility of impaired maternal placental blood flow caused by thrombosis to account for the placental infarction that was also noted, it seemed natural to consider pregnancy outcome in other conditions predisposing to thrombosis. One early large study was that of Preston *et al.* who compared the outcome of pregnancy in 1384 women with known thrombophilia (1524 pregnancies) with that in controls where the putative father had thrombophilia (1019 pregnancies) [130]. If stillbirth alone was considered, antithrombin deficiency increased the risk fivefold and protein S deficiency increased the risk threefold; Factor V Leiden and protein C deficiency did not significantly increase risk on their own but when combined defects were present the risk increased 14-fold. With regard to miscarriage, only antithrombin deficiency was associated with increased risk (twofold) [130]. More recently Kupferminc *et al.* [131] studied a strictly defined community in Israel and found that over half (52%) of a group of adverse pregnancy outcomes, severe pre-eclampsia, intrauterine growth restriction, abruption and stillbirth were associated with Factor V Leiden, homozygosity for the 677 MTHFR mutation, or the prothrombin gene mutation.

These abnormalities were only present in 17% of women with a normal outcome. Numerous other studies have been performed or are in progress to assess the real significance of these findings. Thrombophilia cannot 'explain' half of all cases of pre-eclampsia granted the frequent occurrence of pre-eclampsia in black nations where the prevalence of thrombophilia is low. Yet the findings cannot be ignored; once the precise significance of thrombophilia in each population has been established, randomized controlled trials of antithrombotic therapy could be planned.

A separate issue is the consequence of thrombophilia in the neonate. A high prevalence of thrombophilia in particular Factor V Leiden has been found in neonates with cerebral infarction [132].

Diagnosis

Deep vein thrombosis

The history and physical signs of this condition are well described in standard textbooks of general medicine. However, pregnant women in particular seem to be prone to present with abdominal pain, perhaps because the DVTs are so often proximal. It is probable that women who do not have a typical history are unlikely to have a DVT, and aysymptomatic DVT is probably much rarer in pregnancy than in other gynaecological surgery. This is supported by the study of Bergqvist *et al.* [49] who showed by occlusion plethysmography that the incidence of DVT was only 1.8% even after caesarean section in comparison to 10–20% found after major gynaecological surgery [133, 134]. It is clear that it is very difficult to make an accurate diagnosis based on physical signs alone [135], because perhaps 50% of patients who have an acutely tender swollen calf do not have DVT. If an objective test such as ultrasound, plethysmography or venography is not used for the diagnosis of DVT, one to two patients are treated unnecessarily for every one treated correctly [136, 137]. Therefore, some form of investigation(s) must be performed to support a clinical diagnosis.

The non-invasive investigations available are based on the demonstration of blood clotting by D-dimer or β-thromboglobulin elevation [138], the measurement of blood flow and most recently by imaging of the blood clot by ultrasound [139]. Simple measurement of C-reactive protein has been shown to have a sensitivity of 100% in a small series of non-pregnant patients [140], i.e. a normal C-reactive protein excluded DVT in this study. The C-reactive protein level is not affected by pregnancy and this study should be repeated in a series of pregnant patients. Also there are inadequate data to evaluate D-dimer changes in pregnancy-associated DVT. This is particularly unfortunate, granted the value of D-dimer testing in excluding DVT [141].

Reduced blood flow in the affected limb may be shown by Doppler flow studies [142], impedance plethysmography [143] and thermography [144]. Using liquid crystal thermography to document the increased warmth of the affected leg, Sandler and Martin [144] showed that thermography had a sensitivity of 97% but rather low specificity (62%) in non-pregnant patients. The predictive value of a negative thermogram was helpful (96%). The technique could be improved by using ^{99m}Tc venoscanning in positive cases but this would need to be evaluated in pregnancy.

Radioactive iodine, the tracer element of iodine labelled albumin, should not be used in pregnancy. In the antenatal period it is trapped by the fetal thyroid and may cause hypothyroidism [145] or subsequent carcinoma. It is also secreted in high concentration in breast milk and the same risks apply to the breastfed infant.

Because of the problems of treatment in the index and future pregnancies (see below), an objective form of diagnosis is recommended in all patients who are considered to have DVT in pregnancy, unless the clinical diagnosis seems overwhelmingly certain. This occurs in severe proximal iliac vein thrombosis where the whole limb is markedly swollen.

The three techniques that are most appropriate for use in pregnancy are plethysmography, ultrasound and venography. Because of the radiation involved and the pain of the procedure, venography should now be reserved for use in those centres where plethysmography or ultrasound cannot be used, when there are technical difficulties or uncertainties with these procedures [146] or to confirm a positive plethysmograph test.

Plethysmography has been very carefully evaluated in non-pregnant subjects [147,148]. Studies should be performed in the left lateral position before delivery in order to reduce the reduction in venous return caused by the obstruction of the gravid uterus. Because blood flow from the leg is reduced in pregnancy [36], a normal (by non-pregnant standards) plethysmograph probably excludes significant DVT. A normal plethysmograph repeated over a 10-day period would also exclude a calf vein thrombosis extending to the thigh, and therefore becoming clinically significant. This approach has been vindicated in pregnancy by withholding anticoagulant therapy from 139 patients clinically suspected of having DVT but who had negative plethysmograph studies. None had symptomatic pulmonary embolus or recurrent venous thrombosis [149]. However, we do not yet know what constitutes a positive plethysmograph in pregnancy, and positive tests should therefore be confirmed by ultrasound or venography.

Ultrasound is the technique that is most widely used; it has been shown to be highly effective in the diagnosis of symptomatic proximal DVT by comparison with venography (but in non-pregnant patients). Also note that ultrasound lacks sensitivity for the diagnosis of asymptomatic DVT. The veins may be identified by Doppler and then imaged. If a clot is present, the vein is incompressible and it also does not dilate when venous pressure is raised during a Valsalva manoeuvre. The clot itself may also be imaged. The sensitivity and specificity of this technique have been reported to be over 97% for proximal vein thrombosis [150], but a formal comparison of ultrasound and venography has not been made in pregnancy. However, studies performed in pregnancy have been encouraging [151,152] and there is no reason to believe that ultrasonography would be any less accurate in pregnancy than in the non-pregnant state. If the initial test is negative and clinical suspicion is high, the test should be repeated after a few days. Treatment can always be started on clinical suspicion and before diagnosis is confirmed, particularly now that LMWH can be used in therapeutic doses (see below). But if the diagnosis is not confirmed, there should be no hesitation in stopping treatment.

Neither ultrasound nor impedance plethysmography is suitable for diagnosis of calf vein thrombosis, but because calf vein thrombi very rarely cause pulmonary emboli and because the tests being non-invasive can be repeated in worrying cases, this is not a problem. By contrast with plethysmography, ultrasound cannot be used for diagnosis of isolated thrombosis above the inguinal ligament. However, such thrombi are very rare in symptomatic patients [153]. At present ultrasound is the initial diagnostic technique of choice for pregnancy: it does not require the particular expertise and equipment of plethysmography and the apparatus should be available in all major obstetric centres.

Venography of the femoral and more distal veins can be performed in pregnancy. With adequate shielding of the uterus, the direct radiation dose is small, varying between $<500\,\mu$Gy for a limited study with shielding and $3140\,\mu$Gy for a unilateral study without shielding. Most studies have shown no risk of fetal injury at exposures of less than $50\,000\,\mu$Gy [154]. The use of less irritant, water-soluble, non-ionic contrast media makes it much less likely that venography itself will provoke thromboembolism [155].

Pulmonary embolus

Patients with major pulmonary emboli collapse with hypotension, chest pain, breathlessness and cyanosis. Occasionally they may present with abdominal pain only, due presumably to irritation of the diaphragm [156]. On further examination, they are also found to have a third heart sound, parasternal heave and elevated jugular venous pressure. It is the latter that helps to distinguish them from most of the other relatively common causes of collapse in pregnancy, where the diagnosis is not obvious, as it is in ante- and postpartum haemorrhage or ruptured

or inverted uterus. These causes of collapse and some differentiating features are shown in Table 4.2. Most of the other causes are also considered elsewhere: pulmonary aspiration in Chapter 1, amniotic fluid embolus in Chapter 3, myocardial infarction in Chapter 5 and Gram-negative septicaemia in Chapters 3, 7 and 16.

The diagnosis of major pulmonary embolus is rarely in doubt. However, pulmonary embolus is often preceded by smaller emboli, and a high index of clinical suspicion is essential to diagnose these. Warning signs and symptoms of small pulmonary emboli that are often ignored are unexplained pyrexia, syncope, cough, chest pain and

Table 4.2 Features of some 'occult' causes of collapse in pregnancy. This table excludes more obvious causes, such as ante- or postpartum haemorrhage, and ruptured or inverted uterus.

	Predisposing circumstances	Common presenting features	Helpful diagnostic features in acute stage*	
			Clinical	Investigations
Amniotic fluid embolism (Chapter 3)	Labour, not necessarily precipitate	Respiratory distress, cyanosis		Squames in SVC or sputum
Pulmonary embolus (Chapter 4)	Increasing age, multiparity, thromboembolism, operative delivery, bed rest, oestrogens, haemoglobinopathy	Respiratory distress, chest pain	JVP +; third heart sound, parasternal heave	ECG, chest radiograph, lung scan, blood gas, pulmonary angiography
Myocardial infarction (Chapter 5)	Increasing age	Chest pain, respiratory distress, cyanosis	Pain character, JVP +; crepitations	ECG
Dysrrhythmia (Chapter 5)	Pre-existing heart disease	Tachycardia/bradycardia	Pulse	ECG
Aspiration of gastric contents (Chapter 1)	Anaesthesia, not necessarily with vomiting	Respiratory distress, cyanosis	Bronchospasm	
Pneumothorax and pneumomediastinum	Previous history, labour	Chest pain	Chest signs	Chest radiograph
Intra-abdominal bleeding	Labour, although may occur spontaneously	Abdominal pain	JVP not +; signs in abdomen, laparotomy, paracentesis, culdocentesis	
Septicaemia (Chapters 3, 7, 16)	Previous infection (not necessarily)	Fever, rigors	Fever, rigors	Gram stain on blood sample. Blood culture positive
Intracerebral catastrophe	Pre-eclampsia/eclampsia A-V malformation	Seizures	CNS signs, neck stiffness	CT scan
Hypoglycaemia	Diabetes mellitus Addison's disease Hypopituitarism Hypothyroidism	Sweating, loss of consciousness		Blood glucose
Hyperglycaemia	Diabetes mellitus	Hyperventilation		Blood glucose, blood gas

*These features are not absolute. For example, it is possible to have pulmonary crepitations in patients with pulmonary embolus, and septicaemia without fever or rigors.
SVC, superior vena cava; JVP, jugular venous pressure; ECG, electrocardiogram; A-V, arteriovenous; CNS, central nervous system.

breathlessness. Unless the patient has a high temperature or is producing quantities of purulent sputum, pleurisy should not be considered to be due to infection until pulmonary embolism has been excluded. It may be necessary to treat the patient with both antibiotics and anticoagulants until diagnosis becomes clear.

CHEST RADIOGRAPH, ELECTROCARDIOGRAM AND BLOOD GASES

In considering the diagnosis of pulmonary embolus, it should be emphasized that the chest radiography may be normal and that the electrocardiogram may be normal or may show features such as a deep S wave in lead I and Q wave and inverted T wave in lead III that can be caused by pregnancy alone. Nevertheless, the chest radiograph should not be omitted if only because of its value in diagnosing chest pathology other than pulmonary embolus. Note that the radiation to the fetus from one chest radiograph is $<10\,\mu Gy$, very considerably less than the $50\,000\,\mu Gy$ at which fetal damage occurs [154] and about equal to that received from cosmic sources in one transatlantic flight.

Blood gas measurement can be helpful, although false-positive and false-negative results may occur [157]. If the patient is hypoxaemic, with PaO_2 $<11.3\,kPa$ ($85\,mmHg$) and $PaCO_2$ normal or reduced, it is likely that pulmonary embolus is the cause of chest symptoms, providing there is no radiological evidence of diffuse pulmonary disease or any other cause of reduced cardiac output. Such arterial samples should always be taken with the patient sitting, not supine (see Chapter 1).

LUNG SCANS

Because it is so important to make an accurate diagnosis of thromboembolism in pregnancy, lung scans should be obtained, preferably with ventilation/perfusion imaging in all suspicious cases. The isotopes used in these scans, krypton 81 m for ventilation and technetium 99 m for perfusion, have very short half-lives. The radiation to the fetus is therefore minimal, no more than $400\,\mu Gy$ [154]. Even if the mother is breastfeeding the quantities of technetium secreted in milk after the injection of technetium 99 m macroaggregated albumen are negligible [158]. The lung scan is particularly helpful in cases where the chest radiograph is normal. A normal lung scan then excludes a pulmonary embolus because false-negative results are very rare [149]. For example anticoagulants were withheld from 515 patients with suspected pulmonary embolus and negative lung scan unless they had DVT. Only one had symptomatic pulmonary embolus on follow-up [149].

Although false positives may occur, a large perfusion defect in the presence of a normal chest radiograph is likely to be due to pulmonary embolus. If the chest radiograph is abnormal, ventilation scanning is helpful. A reduction in perfusion with maintenance of ventilation indicates pulmonary embolus. If ventilation is reduced as well as perfusion, the condition is likely to be infective if the radiograph changes are acute. If the lung scan is equivocal it is helpful to examine the legs for DVT [159] by any of the techniques described above. If there is no evidence of DVT, the chance of subsequent or future clinical pulmonary emboli is small [159].

Spiral computed tomography (CT) scanning has high sensitivity and specificity for proximal pulmonary embolus [160]. In pregnancy the application is likely to be in the collapsed patient where diagnosis is required urgently notwithstanding the relatively high radiation dose. In the future, magnetic resonance imaging (MRI) may replace spiral CT in pregnancy in particular because of the lack of radiation. Pulmonary angiography is the 'gold standard' for diagnosis of pulmonary embolus but this is very rarely required in pregnancy.

Treatment

Patients with massive pulmonary embolus present with a catastrophic reduction in cardiac output, and the immediate treatment should be the standard cardiac arrest procedure. If it is thought likely that the cause of the arrest is pulmonary embolus, intravenous unfractionated heparin 20 000 units should be given to reverse the bronchoconstriction and vasoconstriction caused by the release of serotonin from platelets [161]. In addition, prolonged cardiac massage is advisable because this may break up the original clot, permitting an increase in pulmonary blood flow [162]. After emergency resuscitation for pulmonary embolus, the treatment of both DVT and pulmonary embolus may be divided into an initial acute phase, which lasts for up to a week, and a subsequent chronic phase lasting for several months, where the aim of therapy is to prevent further incidents of thromboembolism (see also chronic phase therapy heparin, below).

Uncontrolled studies by Villasanta [163] indicate that the maternal mortality associated with pulmonary embolus and DVT in pregnancy is reduced from 13% to 1% by anticoagulant therapy. A similar mortality (one in 113 patients) was found by Moseley and Kerstein [164] in a literature search of anticoagulant-treated patients. It is generally accepted that anticoagulation is the treatment of choice in pulmonary embolism without shock [165] and that it is highly efficacious [166]. Therefore it would now be unethical to compare anticoagulant and placebo treatment in thromboembolism, whether associated with pregnancy or not. The only controlled trial of anticoagulant vs. placebo therapy in pulmonary embolus was abandoned because of the high mortality in the placebo group [167].

Treatments used in the acute phase are heparin, surgery and thrombolytic agents such as streptokinase [168]. Treatment in the chronic phase is with warfarin or heparin.

Acute phase

UNFRACTIONATED HEPARIN

The majority of cases of venous thromboembolism are treated initially with heparin. Heparin, because it is so strongly polar, has particular advantages in pregnancy, because both unfractionated and LMWHs do not cross the placenta [169]. The object of heparin therapy in the initial phase of treatment of venous thromboembolism is to prevent further, possibly fatal, episodes. It is not believed that heparin increases the reabsorption of the original thrombus. In order to prevent further clot formation, relatively high blood levels of heparin must be achieved; it has been suggested that particularly large doses are necessary in the presence of a large initial thrombus [170]. Although up to 40 000 units/day of heparin have been given subcutaneously [171], this is not usually practical because of bruising and irregular absorption, and the initial treatment should be with intravenous heparin: initially a 5000-unit bolus followed by 40 000 units/day (approximately 1600 units/h) by continuous infusion, aiming to double the activated partial thromboplastin time (APTT).

In the acute phase, the heparin should be given by intravenous infusion [172]. Heparin is not stable in dextrose and should therefore be given in saline [173] preferably made up in a small volume of 10–20 mL and very slowly infused with a constant infusion pump. If this is not practical, the same total dose of heparin may be given by repeated intravenous injections, but no less frequently than every 3 h. The half-life of heparin is only about 1.5 h [174] and if the drug is given by large, infrequent intravenous injections, this produces unacceptable swings between hyper- and hypocoagulability [175]. The only side-effect of acute heparin administration is bleeding (see below for side-effects of prolonged therapy), although its preservative, cholorbutol, may cause hypotension [176].

If it is necessary to reverse heparin therapy, cessation of infusion alone will be sufficient for most patients given intravenous heparin. There will be undetectable levels in the blood 6 h after therapy has stopped. In the more urgent situation the patient can be given protamine 1 mg per 1090 units of administered heparin. When using a continuous infusion of heparin, twice the quantity of protamine should be given to neutralize the hourly dose. No more than 50 mg of protamine should be given in a 10-min period, because protamine itself can cause bleeding [63]. A better alternative is to calculate the quantity of protamine needed from the protamine sulphate neutralization test [177]. The neutralizing dose of protamine sulphate may be calculated as follows [178]:

Protamine sulphate required (mg) to neutralize heparin = plasma heparin concentration IU/mL × plasma volume × 0.01

Plasma volume in pregnancy is 50 mL/kg bodyweight; so, for example, a 70-kg woman with plasma heparin concentration 1.2 IU would require $1.2 \times (70 \times 50) \times 0.01 = 42$ mg protamine sulphate. If there is any doubt about the efficacy or desirability of protamine reversal, fresh frozen plasma should restore blood clotting to normal.

Because of the risk of haematoma formation in patients who are fully anticoagulated, other injections such as antibiotics should be given intravenously rather than intramuscularly. Arterial blood sampling should be from an intra-arterial cannula or by needling a superficial artery, such as the radial artery rather than the deeper femoral artery.

Initial phase, high-dose intravenous heparin therapy is continued for an arbitrary period of 7–14 days; the length of treatment depends on the severity of the initial episode of venous thromboembolism and whether there is any evidence of recurrence. Studies using intravenous heparin for 5 days rather than 10 days [179] have not been performed in pregnancy and have only been performed in the non-pregnant state in patients with DVT, not pulmonary embolus.

LOW MOLECULAR WEIGHT HEPARIN

In the non-pregnant state, fixed high-dose subcutaneous LMWH has become popular for the treatment of both DVT and to a lesser extent pulmonary embolus. The advantages are obvious and considerable: there is no need for dose adjustment on the basis of repeated APTT measurements and these were/are notoriously unreliable. The APTT has a 45% between-occasion variability even in patients on a continuous and steady infusion of heparin. This variation may be diurnal in nature, higher values occurring at night [180]. In addition, infusion pumps may not run steadily and the partial thromboplastin time also varies depending on the time between testing and drawing blood [181]. LMWH is given subcutaneously and does not require the extra labour and risk of an intravenous infusion. The patients may be treated in ambulatory setting or even at home.

The rationale for high-dose LMWH comes from trials such as those of logiparin [182], fraxiparin [183] and tinzaparine [184] in the initial phase of treatment of non-pregnant patients with DVT [182,183] and pulmonary embolus [184]. In the study of Hull *et al.* [182] there was less bleeding in the acute phase and fewer recurrences. But it should be emphasized that these studies were comparisons of unfractionated heparin and LMWH both supplemented with warfarin within a few days of initiating therapy. In pregnancy warfarin is not generally used for the treatment of thromboembolism (see below). Furthermore, the fixed dose may not be appropriate for pregnancy where in general heparin requirements are greater than in the non-pregnant state. At the very least, if LMWH is to be used in significant proven thromboembolism, dosing efficacy should be confirmed by anti-Xa measurements as has been done in the few case reports so far available [185]. Dose ranges suggested by the manufacturers are given in Table 4.3 but note that these do not relate to pregnancy. A reasonable target anti-Xa level would be 0.6–1.0 units 4h after dosing.

At present we reserve high-dose LMWH treatment for equivocal cases of both DVT and pulmonary embolus in the period before the diagnosis can be confirmed or refuted. This usually occurs at holiday periods or at weekends when there is not immediate availability of ventilation/perfusion scanning or Duplex ultrasound. Nevertheless it is likely that high-dose LMWH will become standard treatment for the acute episode of thromboembolism in pregnancy as more experience becomes available.

The alternatives or adjuvants to heparin in the initial phase of treatment are surgery and thrombolytic therapy.

Both these alternatives have the advantage of therapy directed towards removing the initial clot. Both should be considered in the non-pregnant state for initial treatment in patients with major pulmonary embolus or massive iliofemoral DVT.

THROMBOLYTIC THERAPY

Thrombolytic agents are probably underused in the non-pregnant state because there is evidence that patients who have had a DVT are much less likely to develop postphlebitic leg symptoms after being given thrombolytic therapy than after conventional treatment with heparin and warfarin [186]. Browse [187] also suggests that thrombolytic therapy is preferable to conventional anticoagulation to minimize the risk of massive pulmonary embolus in patients with extensive iliofemoral thrombosis where the proximal end of the clot is floating free; but this has not been proven.

In a comparison of heparin and oral anticoagulants with urokinase in the treatment of pulmonary embolus in the non-pregnant state, urokinase therapy was associated with earlier resolution as shown by pulmonary angiography [188]. Overviews suggest that there should be trials of streptokinase not only in (non-pregnant) patients with major pulmonary embolus, but also in those with minor emboli [189].

It has also been shown that, after a pulmonary embolus, the pulmonary capillary blood volume and pulmonary diffusing capacity are normal in patients treated with thrombolytic therapy, whereas they usually remain abnormal in patients treated with heparin and warfarin, even if they are asymptomatic at follow-up 1 year later [5].

Pfeiffer [190] claimed successful treatment of DVT in 12 pregnant patients with streptokinase given as a loading dose (250 000 units by intravenous infusion over 20 min) followed by an infusion of 160 000 units/h for 4h, with

	Dalteparin (Fragmin)	Enoxaparin (Clexane)[+]	Tinzaparin (Innohep)
Treatment	200 units/kg once daily or 100 units/kg twice daily[*]	1.5 mg (150 units)/kg once daily	175 units/kg once daily
Prophylaxis	2500 or 5000 units once daily	20 mg (2000 units) or 40 mg (4000 units) once daily	3500 or 4500 units once daily

Table 4.3 Recommended doses of low molecular weight heparins for the prophylaxis and treatment of deep vein thrombosis and pulmonary embolism (note these recommendations are only established for the non-pregnant state). (From *British National Formulary* 41: March 2001. Published by the British Medical Association and the Royal Pharmaceutical Society of Great Britain, London, 2001.)

*Twice-daily dosing recommended for those at risk of haemorrhage and generally in pregnancy. Maximum 18 000 units daily.
†There is probably greatest experience with enoxaparin in high dose for treatment of thromboembolism in pregnancy (see Thomson AJ *et al. J Obstet Gynaecol* 2001; 21 (Suppl. 1): S42).

subsequent alteration of the infusion rate depending on the plasma thrombin time. Bell and Meek [191] discount the necessity for adjusting the dosage schedule and would recommend a maintenance therapy of 100 000 units/h for 24–72 h after the initial loading dose. Although Pfeiffer [192] suggests that very little streptokinase crosses the human placenta, pregnancy is considered a minor contra-indication to the use of thrombolytic therapy, and subsequent delivery within 10 days is a major contraindication to thrombolytic therapy [193]. Because it is possible that thrombolytic therapy may precipitate premature labour by causing an increase in circulating plasminogen levels [194], there is a risk that the relatively minor contraindication will become a major contraindication. However, it has also been suggested that streptokinase therapy will cause relative uterine atony because of the interference of fibrin degradation products with uterine contraction [195].

If it is necessary to reverse thrombolytic therapy in pregnancy, aprotinin, which has large molecules and does not cross the placenta, should be used rather than aminocaproic acid. However, apart from the 12 patients treated in pregnancy by Pfeiffer [190], other studies are only case reports [194–196] reviewed by Turrentine *et al.* [197]. Since 1961, 36 reports have been published describing the use of thrombolytic agents in 172 pregnant women. The maternal mortality rate was relatively low (1.2%) considering the likely severity of the conditions treated. There were about 10 pregnancy losses and 8.1% of patients had serious bleeding problems. There is really still not sufficient experience to recommend the use of thrombolytic agents in pregnancy except in exceptional circumstances [198] such as life-threatening pulmonary embolus (see below).

SURGERY

Surgical removal of the thrombus (thrombectomy) may be indicated in massive iliofemoral DVT because of the suggestion that this too reduces the incidence of postphlebitic leg symptoms [199]; however, this has not been substantiated in follow-up studies [200] and thrombectomy is a technically difficult operation involving considerable blood loss. Thrombectomy had been advocated where limb swelling is so great as to cause venous gangrene [201, 202]. In pregnancy such patients should be delivered because the reduction of additional obstruction by the enlarged uterus often reduces limb swelling. Surgery (venous plication or insertion of a vena caval filter or umbrella) has also been advocated to prevent pulmonary embolus in cases of iliofemoral thrombosis [202]. With adequate anticoagulation this is rarely necessary [203] and in any case devices to filter large clots in the inferior vena cava are now

usually placed percutaneously via the other patent femoral vein or via the jugular vein rather than at open surgery [204]. This is discussed below under recurrent thromboembolism.

In cases of pulmonary embolus, patients who are shocked at the time of the initial event have traditionally been considered for pulmonary embolectomy using cardiopulmonary bypass [62, 205], as have those with any of the following features 1 h later: (i) systolic blood pressure <90 mmHg; (ii) Pao_2 <60 mmHg; or (iii) urine output <20 mL/h [175]. The decision whether to operate would usually be supported by pulmonary angiography or spiral CT to localize the embolus. At pulmonary angiography it may be possible to fragment the clot using a guide wire to advance the catheter through the clot [206]. This may obviate the necessity for pulmonary embolectomy.

However, it is currently believed that surgery for pulmonary embolus in non-pregnant patients should be reserved for those who deteriorate following thrombolytic therapy or who present with such haemodynamic compromise that the thrombolytic therapy is not justifiable [207]. The risks of thrombolytic therapy that are specific to pregnancy are the initiation of incoordinate preterm labour and subsequent postpartum haemorrhage. I think it reasonable to accept these risks in life-threatening massive pulmonary embolus. In the severely compromised patient, I would therefore suggest pulmonary angiography, an attempt to disperse the clot once it has been demonstrated, thrombolytic therapy if this fails or does not improve the haemodynamic status of the patient and then possibly surgery according to the criteria described above [207]. If pulmonary angiography and surgery are not available try thrombolytic therapy. There may not be much difference in the outcome between surgery and thrombolytic therapies [208]: clearly randomized trials are needed but it is difficult to see how these will be organized.

Chronic phase

WARFARIN

It is established that there is a definite, although low, incidence of teratogenesis associated with the use of warfarin in the first trimester of pregnancy [209–212]. The most common syndrome is *chondrodysplasia punctata*, in which cartilage and bone formation is abnormal [210, 213]; warfarin is not the only cause of this abnormality [214], which may also be inherited [215]. The asplenia syndrome [216] and diaphragmatic herniae have also been reported [217].

It has also been recognized that the use of warfarin in late pregnancy after 36 weeks' gestation is associated with serious retroplacental and intracerebral fetal bleeding

[163] because, unlike heparin, warfarin does cross the placenta. As premature infants have low levels of Factors XI and XII [217a], it is likely that the fetus has low levels of clotting factors; therefore the fetus will be excessively anticoagulated if the mother's prothrombin time is within the normal therapeutic range. For these reasons Hirsh *et al.* [169] used to recommend that after the initial period of heparinization in the acute attack, heparin should continue to be used for the first trimester, followed by warfarin between 13 and 36 weeks, reverting to heparin for the last weeks of pregnancy. These recommendations were widely followed at one time [16,218–221] and indeed in 1980 73% of practising obstetricians in the UK would have followed them [219]. However, by 1993 only 35% of obstetricians in the UK used warfarin for thromboprophylaxis [222] and the question has arisen as to whether oral anticoagulants should be used even after the first trimester [218] because of the risk of fetal malformation. Sherman and Hall [223] described a case of microcephaly in a patient who had taken warfarin for the last 6 months of pregnancy, and this stimulated further reports [224, 225], including one by Holzgreve *et al.* [226] in which five cases of microcephaly occurring in California were described. It has been suggested that warfarin causes repeated small intracerebral haemorrhages and that these are the causes of the optic atrophy, microcephaly and mental retardation that have been described [227]. Gross subdural haemorrhage may also occur in the fetus before 36 weeks' gestation [228].

These risks to the fetus may not be so great as anecdotal reports would suggest. Chen *et al.* [229] studied the outcome of 22 pregnancies, where the mother had taken warfarin in the first trimester, and 20 pregnancies where warfarin had been taken between 13 and 36 weeks. Warfarin was being used in the management of artificial heart valves. Although the spontaneous abortion rate was high (36% in those taking warfarin) there were no cases of chondrodysplasia punctata or microcephaly. In another study in which we compared the infants of 20 patients who had taken warfarin in the second and third trimesters with those of well-matched controls, there was no difference in intellectual attainment at a mean age of 4 years [230]. Microcephaly is therefore unlikely to be common in the children of women taking warfarin. It may relate to the method of control used for warfarin therapy and therefore to the amount of warfarin taken. Central nervous system (CNS) malformations do seem more common in those taking higher doses of warfarin. This was studied more formally by Vitale *et al.* [231] in a series of heart valve patients. They found fetal complications in 22 of 25 pregnancies where the mother was taking more than 5 mg warfarin daily. Eighteen of these complications were miscarriages. By comparison there were only five complications (four miscarriages) in 33 women taking 5 mg or less daily. In all cases the international normalized ratio (INR) was being kept between 2.5 and 3.5.

Bleeding also appears to be more of a problem in pregnant women treated with warfarin than in those treated with heparin, even if the patients have prothrombin times within the normal therapeutic range [232]. Even if patients are not anticoagulated, they are at risk from ante- and postpartum haemorrhages in pregnancy, and this risk seems to be increased by warfarin therapy. Fetomaternal haemorrhage has also been reported [233].

Finally there is an increased miscarriage rate in women taking warfarin; this is best established in those taking warfarin for artificial heart valves; it appears to be dose dependent becoming apparent in those taking more than 5 mg of warfarin daily. In my experience successful pregnancy is very uncommon in those taking more than 15 mg of warfarin daily.

For all the above reasons I, and others [63], believe that warfarin should not be used in the chronic phase of treatment of venous thromboembolism in pregnancy, or in the first week of the puerperium. The only situation where warfarin therapy is recommended in pregnancy is in the management of some patients with artificial heart valves or mitral valve disease (see Chapter 5).

The risk of genital tract bleeding is much less by 7 days after delivery, and it is therefore reasonable to use warfarin at that time as an alternative to subcutaneous heparin. Moreover, patients may continue to breastfeed [234] because there is no detectable secretion of warfarin in breast milk [235]. This is not so for phenindione where maternal therapy has caused severe haemorrhage in a breastfed infant [236]. However, phenindione may not be so teratogenic as warfarin [237]; unfortunately there is not sufficient experience to confirm this.

HEPARIN

Subcutaneous, self-administered heparin is the preferred chronic phase treatment for venous thromboembolism in pregnancy [238], because it does not have the risks of warfarin. (The possible complications of long-term heparin therapy are described below.)

When we relied entirely on unfractionated heparin and LMWH was not available we contrasted the acute phase of treatment requiring high-dose intravenous heparin for up to 14 days with a subsequent chronic phase of treatment lasting until at least 6 weeks after delivery when anticoagulation did not need to be so intense. In the chronic phase sufficient anticoagulation could be achieved by prophylactic doses of subcutaneous unfractionated heparin, 10 000 units twice daily. We did not believe it possible to achieve full anticoagulation, i.e. sufficient to double the APTT using subcutaneous heparin without causing intolerable bruising. It would have been impractical to continue full intravenous anticoagulation for the long periods required in pregnancy. Our regimen based on acute therapy with intravenous heparin followed by chronic therapy with subcutaneous lower-dose heparin (either unfractionated heparin 10 000 units twice daily or LMWH in prophylactic doses) worked and we did not have problems with recurrent thrombosis in the chronic phase [239]. Nevertheless, there was a degree of uneasiness because that level of anticoagulation achieved by subcutaneous unfractionated heparin 10 000 units twice daily was considerably less than that which would have been provided by standard therapy in the non-pregnant state, i.e. warfarin given in doses to achieve an INR of 2. Also the distinction between acute and chronic phase therapy is now blurred by the increasing availability of high-dose LMWH for both acute and longer-term therapy.

Most centres would now use LMWH rather than unfractionated because in prophylactic doses LMWH is only given once rather than twice daily; also LMWH probably has a better side-effect profile with less bleeding for a given degree of thromboprophylaxis, less heparin-induced thrombocytopenia (HIT) (see below) and less bone demineralization (see below). Also one of the LMWHs (enoxaparin) when given once daily in 20- or 40-mg doses has been shown to have a superior anti-Xa profile measured over a 24-h period compared to unfractionated heparin 7500 units given 12 hourly [240].

CHRONIC THERAPY, UNFRACTIONATED HEPARIN TREATMENT

If subcutaneous unfractionated heparin is to be given in the chronic phase, the dose should be 10 000 units twice daily. This small dose of heparin used in chronic therapy does not affect the whole blood-clotting system, and is below the limits of detection of conventional tests, such as the partial thromboplastin time or protamine sulphate neutralization test. Our policy was to monitor such chronic phase therapy with anti-Xa heparin levels to ensure that the level was less than 0.2 units/mL—the level at which there might be a bleeding risk. In practice this never happened and I see no evidence for the need to monitor anti-Xa levels during prophylactic therapy with unfractionated or LMWH treatment. Instead the platelet count should be checked within a few days of starting heparin therapy because of the possibility of HIT (see below) and at that same time a clotting screen should be performed. This, by prolongation of the thrombin time, will detect the very occasional patient who is particularly sensitive to heparin. The platelet count and

clotting screen should be repeated about every 6 weeks through pregnancy and preferably within a week of delivery. Anti-Xa assays should be reserved for the very occasional patient who bleeds unexpectedly. The anti-Xa heparin assay is quite difficult to perform and is unlikely to be rapidly available.

Although patients often show initial reluctance, the majority can be taught to give themselves subcutaneous heparin and can therefore be discharged home. Patients should use the concentrated heparin solution of 50 000 units/mL. We have not found any difference in bruising between sodium and calcium heparins. The heparin should be drawn up in a tuberculin syringe because of the small volumes used, and injected subcutaneously through a short (16 mm) 25-gauge needle. The injections should be made perpendicular to the skin surface to minimize the risk of trauma to skin blood vessels. Possible sites are the thighs and abdominal wall.

Because of the high incidence of thromboembolism in the days following labour and delivery [42], subcutaneous heparin administration should be continued through labour. There is no increased risk of intra- or postpartum haemorrhage in these patients [241,242], although those patients who inadvertently take too much heparin are at risk of bleeding [243]. Providing that the thrombin time is normal, it is now believed the epidural block is not contraindicated [244] for patients taking unfractionated heparin or LMWH, although formerly it was thought that there was an excessive risk of epidural haematoma [245]. Nevertheless, this is a continuing area of dispute with anaesthetists. One compromise is to delay the injection of heparin until after insertion or removal of the epidural catheter, thus avoiding peak blood levels at the time of greatest trauma.

At delivery, the dose of subcutaneous heparin is empirically reduced to 7500 units twice daily because of the contraction in circulating blood volume and because the clotting factors return towards normal levels during the puerperium. The platelet count and clotting screen are checked at least once after delivery if the patient continues to take subcutaneous heparin for the recommended 6 weeks postpartum.

CHRONIC THERAPY, LOW MOLECULAR WEIGHT HEPARIN TREATMENT

As indicated above, if LMWH has been used in acute therapy and/or is to be used in chronic phase therapy there is now more flexibility with regard to dosing. The doses recommended for therapeutic and prophylactic therapy for the various LMWH licensed in the UK at the time of writing are given in Table 4.3. Using enoxaparin as an example, the recommended therapeutic dose is

1.5mg/kg once daily; (though because of the prothrombotic state of pregnancy, many would prefer to give 1mg/1kg twice daily) depending on the patient's weight, the prophylactic dose for pregnancy is about a quarter of the therapeutic dose, 40 mg once daily. One option would be to continue with therapeutic doses of enoxaparin for at least 6 weeks after the initial event and then reduce to a lower dose, either the prophylactic dose or an intermediate dose, thereafter. Alternatively this dose reduction could take place as usual after the initial 7- to 14-day period of acute high-dose treatment. Unfortunately there are no trial data and all depends on clinical judgement with regard to individual patients and the perceived degree of risk.

If the patient is to remain on therapeutic doses of LMWH the anti-Xa assay (which must be set up for each of the different LMWH) should be checked at least every 4 weeks and more frequently depending on the clinical circumstances. At lower doses of LMWH treatment, anti-Xa monitoring is not necessary though the platelet count should be checked regularly because of the possibility of HIT. Patients should not be delivered taking therapeutic doses of LMWH because of the bleeding risk. The options are to stop LMWH at the time of delivery in the knowledge that the effect lasts about 24h; or to switch to prophylactic doses or to switch to unfractionated heparin. Again these decisions depend on local circumstances and clinical judgement.

There is very little experience with regard to reversal of LMWH. If simply stopping the drug does not give a sufficiently rapid response granted that the effect of LMWH lasts for up to 24h, protamine can be used but the correct dose and frequency of dosing are not clear. A haematologist must be consulted, as would always be the case for pregnant patients bleeding on heparin treatment.

CHRONIC THERAPY AFTER DELIVERY

One week after delivery, when the risk of secondary postpartum haemorrhage is much less, the patient may take warfarin rather than heparin, either unfractionated or LMWH. In either case breastfeeding is safe. Heparin is not secreted in breast milk and would not be absorbed from the infant's stomach. Warfarin is not excreted in breast milk [235]. The option as to whether to continue heparin or to switch to warfarin depends on which the patient finds less inconvenient. Heparin has the disadvantage of multiple injections but does not require laboratory control after the first week. Warfarin therapy has the disadvantage of needing repeated prothrombin estimations but is given orally. Most patients seem to favour continuing heparin because they do not want the frequent attendances necessary for establishing the correct dose of warfarin.

If the patient does opt to switch to warfarin the drug is given daily; the first two doses should be 10 mg each; the INR is checked before giving the third dose: and dosing then depends on the value of the INR. The target INR for the treatment of DVT is 2–3 [246]. Treatment with heparin should be continued until the target level is achieved (or exceeded). Heparin treatment does not interfere with estimation of the INR, providing that the activated partial thromboplastin time ratio is <2.5 or heparin level is <1.5 units/mL.

Therapy with heparin initiated in pregnancy or warfarin if introduced after 7 days postpartum, is continued for an arbitrary period of 6 weeks postpartum, at which time the extra risk of thromboembolism associated with pregnancy is considered to have passed. Patients who develop venous thromboembolism in the puerperium should be treated as above, except that, after the acute phase, warfarin may be used alone in chronic phase treatment though warfarin should not be given in the first 7 days after delivery because of the bleeding risk. The total length of anticoagulant treatment should be at least 3 months.

POSTPHLEBITIC LIMB SYNDROME

As indicated above postphlebitic limb syndrome is particularly common following DVT in pregnancy. Apart from routine anticoagulant therapy little is usually done to avoid it. Sensible measures include raising the leg until the swelling has subsided and wearing class II elastic stockings (20–25 mmHg at the ankle) from diagnosis for a prolonged period afterwards [247]; this could be life long or until repeat Duplex ultrasound shows that the venous system has retuned to normal.

Recurrent thromboembolism

All patients who have thromboembolism in pregnancy should be screened for thrombophilia but this is usually performed after delivery because of the effect of pregnancy on the various tests (see above). However if there is recurrent thromboembolism or there are other reasons to suspect thrombophilia (previous or family history of thromboembolism, bad obstetric history) the tests should be performed in pregnancy as far as possible.

In patients who develop recurrent thromboembolism during acute or chronic phase treatment, the diagnosis should again be established by objective criteria. The adequacy of anticoagulant treatment up to the time of recurrence should be reviewed. Patients should be screened for causes of recurrent thromboembolism as described above, although the diagnosis may be difficult in patients who are already taking anticoagulants as well as because of the pregnancy effect. If there really has been recurrent thromboembolism despite adequate anticoagulation, the patient should receive long-term intravenous unfractionated heparin [248] preferably by a Hickman line [249]; the dose should be adjusted to achieve a heparin level (anti-Xa assay) of 0.8–1.0 units/mL or APTT twice control. This dose will need to be reduced at the time of delivery in the same way as for patients with artificial heart valves (see Chapter 5). If the source appears to be in the legs or pelvic veins surgical interruption of the inferior vena cava or iliac veins with a sieve or filter [204, 250, 251] could be considered. Note that clinical trials do not support the use of filters merely because of the presence of proximal DVT [252].

Prophylaxis

There are three groups of patients in whom prophylaxis might be considered: (i) those who have had thromboembolism in the past [253]; (ii) those who are known to have thrombophilia because of family studies but who have not yet themselves had an episode of thromboembolism; and (iii) those who are at high risk because of age, parity, obesity or operative delivery [42, 59].

The first group of patients are those who have had thromboembolism in the past; they are considered to be at risk throughout pregnancy. Badaracco and Vessey [253] in a retrospective study estimated that there was about a 12% risk of developing pulmonary embolism or DVT in pregnancy if a patient had had thromboembolism in the past. The risk was not affected by the circumstances of the original event, i.e. whether it was associated with the contraceptive pill or not. The risk is likely to be exaggerated (see below): the study was based on a postal survey, and information is not available as to how the thromboembolism was diagnosed in pregnancy. If a patient has had thromboembolism in the past, there is a particularly strong tendency to diagnose it again on rather flimsy evidence.

In a previous survey, most British obstetricians (88%) would have used prophylactic anticoagulants for such patients if the index thromboembolism had previously occurred during pregnancy. Some (73%) would have used prophylaxis if the thromboembolism had occurred when taking the pill, and fewer (50%) would have used prophylaxis if the original thromboembolism had occurred 10 years previously when the patients were neither taking the pill nor were pregnant [219]. These figures were not substantially changed in a later survey [222].

The majority of obstetricians no longer use the modified Hirsh regime of warfarin [169] until 36 weeks' gestation

for venous thromboembolism prophylaxis [222], and this now seems unacceptable because of the maternal and fetal complications of warfarin therapy outlined above. The alternative is to use subcutaneous heparin throughout pregnancy and as indicated above LMWH is more attractive than unfractionated heparin. However, since these patients are asymptomatic at the beginning of treatment and because the treatment is only being used prophylactically, the safety of such therapy for mother and fetus must be established even more rigorously than in the treatment of established venous thromboembolism.

Hall *et al.* [225] performed a retrospective study of the outcome of pregnancies associated with anticoagulant therapy, based on literature reports. Such a study is likely to be biased towards the reporting of complications, but they found that of 135 fetuses, 13% were stillborn, 14% were born prematurely and 7% died in the neonatal period. It is likely that the bad pregnancy outcome related to the indication for treatment rather than the treatment itself. A comparative study performed at Queen Charlotte's Maternity Hospital of antenatal heparin prophylaxis compared to no antenatal prophylaxis did not show such a high perinatal mortality [254]. A further study at Queen Charlotte's Hospital confirmed that the majority of fetal losses in 69 pregnancies where mothers took LMWH were in the patients who had antiphospholipid syndrome [239]. Meta-analysis of all reports in 1999 of LMWH treatment in pregnancy suggests that the adverse pregnancy outcome rate (3.1%) was no greater in patients taking LMWH than in controls providing they did not have comorbid conditions; if they did it was much greater (13.4%) [255].

The most obvious maternal complication is bruising at the injection site. This can be reduced by good injection technique but rarely eliminated. Although this is undoubtedly an inconvenience, and at times painful, most mothers tolerate a degree of bruising.

A further maternal complication of prolonged heparin therapy is a form of bone demineralization described as osteopenia [256–258]. This occurred in one of our patients, and presented as severe backache, which was much worse in the puerperium [259]. Radiography in the puerperium showed that the patient had three collapsed vertebrae. Griffith *et al.* [260] reported that heparin-induced osteopenia only occurs in patients receiving more than 15 000 units/day for at least 6 months but bone demineralization has been reported following the administration of only 10 000 units of heparin per day in pregnancy for 19 weeks [261]. The incidence of symptomatic bone demineralization in those receiving heparin thromboprophylaxis had been estimated to be about 2% in a series of 184 pregnant women [262] but a more recent meta-analysis of 486 pregnancies in which LMWH was used estimated the risk to be about one in 500 [255]. This could be a real advantage of LMWH over unfractionated heparin.

The cause of the osteopenia is unknown. It had been attributed to a deficiency of 1,25-dihydroxytachysterol [263, 264] but this has not been confirmed in subsequent studies. Since heparin-induced osteopenia is much more common in pregnancy, it is likely that the enhanced bone turnover of pregnancy [265] and the fetal demand for calcium [266] are contributing factors. A follow-up study of those patients who are taking subcutaneous heparin suggests that even those patients who are asymptomatic may have some degree of bone demineralization [267]. Fortunately a follow-up study from Sweden based on radiological assessment of the spine suggests that heparin-induced osteopenia does regress once heparin treatment has been stopped [268]. Also Ginsberg *et al.* [269] studied 61 patients, 2 years after stopping long-term heparin treatment and found no difference in bone density when they were compared with controls. Both of these studies suggest that heparin-induced osteoporosis regresses on cessation of therapy. Furthermore no change in bone density was found before and after treatment with LMWH in 43 women treated throughout pregnancy [270].

Heparin may cause thrombocytopenia [271] (HIT) with subsequent thrombotic [272] or bleeding complications [273, 274]. Thrombocytopenia either presents acutely as a result of platelet aggregation or occurs 7–10 days after treatment starts because of an interaction between platelets, heparin and a specific IgG autoantibody [275, 276]. The latter form of HIT is the more serious and the major risk is of clotting not bleeding. It is caused by antibodies to a complex of heparin and platelet factor 4 and these antibodies may be assayed to diagnose the condition. However, these additional complications have not been problems in our experience using heparin in pregnancy. Although HIT undoubtedly occurs in pregnant women taking heparin, it is uncommon. The risk of HIT seems to be reduced but not eliminated [277, 278] by the use of LMWHs. There were no cases in the 486 pregnancies treated with LMWH reviewed by Sanson *et al.* [255]. Nevertheless patients who have had HIT in the past with unfractionated heparin should not take LMWH since a substantial number will get HIT again. Instead it is possible to use the heparinoid, danaproid which also does not cross the placenta. Hirudin should be avoided in pregnancy since it does cross the placenta [3] but it could be used after delivery and it is not secreted in breast milk [279].

Heparin may also cause alopecia and allergic reactions at the site of injection. The latter occurred in 0.6% of patients who had to stop or change therapy in the recent meta-analysis of LMWH treatment [255]. Such allergic reactions may be associated with eosinophilia which can be a presenting feature [280]. If allergic reactions do occur it is worth trying a different preparation of either unfractionated heparin or LMWH though this only occasionally cures the problem. If patients have had allergic reactions to subcutaneous heparin there will always be concern about anaphylaxis should they require intravenous heparin. This has not been a problem in our experience though we have usually added small amounts of hydrocortisone to the intravenous infusion in patients who have had previous reactions to subcutaneous heparin [281]. Other uncommon side-effects of LMWH are aldosterone suppression leading to hyperkalaemia [282] and hyperlipidaemia [283].

Even though long-term LMWH treatment is probably safer for women than unfractionated heparin it is still not without risk and puts the patient to considerable inconvenience. In patients who have previous thromboembolism there must be a gradation of recurrence risk depending on the presence or absence of other risk factors.

Our present approach [284] is to counsel patients about the relative risks of prophylactic therapy and recurrence of thromboembolism in the antenatal period. We only use subcutaneous heparin before labour in those patients who are considered particularly at risk, having had thromboembolism more than once in the past, having thrombophilia or having a family history of thromboembolism suggesting thrombophilia as yet undetectable. A less specific high-risk group would include the elderly or very obese. Subcutaneous heparin is also used in those patients who themselves are particularly concerned about the risk of repeated thromboembolism. In addition we use subcutaneous heparin in low-risk patients who have only had a single episode of thromboembolism at times when they are most at risk, such as during admission to hospital for surgery or bed rest.

High-risk patients take heparin throughout pregnancy, either LMWH or unfractionated heparin 10 000 units subcutaneously twice daily as described above regarding chronic phase therapy for the management of established thromboembolism. Granted the frequency of fatal thromboembolism in the first trimester (see above), this treatment should start as soon as the woman knows that she is pregnant. In practice all patients now take LMWH rather than unfractionated heparin. After delivery the patients receive LMWH for at least 1 week and either subcutaneous heparin or warfarin for a further 5 weeks making a total of 6 weeks' postnatal treatment. The choice between warfarin and heparin again depends on which treatment the patient finds less inconvenient (see above). As in the treatment of an established case of thromboembolism in pregnancy (see above) the length of time for which prophylaxis is continued after delivery is arbitrary.

Breastfeeding is safe in patients taking warfarin [235]. The efficacy of this regime was shown in our study of 69 pregnancies where 34 women with previous thromboembolism or thrombophilia took prophylactic enoxaparin throughout pregnancy as described above. There was only one case of recurrent thromboembolism and that occurred postnatally in a woman taking enoxaparin 20 mg daily early in the series and before we used what is now the generally accepted prophylactic dose for pregnancy, 40 mg once daily [239]. This was not a controlled trial and undoubtedly there will be failures with this method of prophylaxis as there are with any form of therapy; but from the figures given above, it is likely that the failure rate will be low.

Patients who have only had a single episode of thromboembolism in the past, no matter what the associated circumstances, are considered at low risk of recurrence in pregnancy if they do not have other risk factors. They are given aspirin 75 mg daily for thromboprophylaxis as soon as they know that they are pregnant. They then start LMWH in prophylactic doses when they present in labour or at elective delivery. Thereafter they are managed in the same way as the high-risk patients. Support for aspirin prophylaxis comes from large studies performed outside pregnancy where it has been shown to reduce the risk of pulmonary embolus and DVT by at least one third [285, 286]. The safety of low-dose aspirin in pregnancy has been demonstrated by the many studies such as CLASP (Collaborative Low-dose Aspirin Study in Pregnancy) where aspirin was evaluated for pre-eclampsia prophylaxis [287]. Our results using this form of low-risk prophylaxis in pregnancy have also been evaluated. There were no cases of thromboembolism in 35 low-risk patients treated in this way [288]. Again this was not a controlled trial but the failure rate of this form of prophylaxis is also unlikely to be very high. It seems likely that the study of Badaracco and Vessey [253] which suggests a 12% risk of thromboembolism in patients who have had DVT or pulmonary embolism in the past, very much overestimates the risk of antenatal thromboembolism; the risk appears to be of the order of 2% or less.

Another option would be to use heparin adjusting the dose to maintain a specific heparin level (0.08–0.15 unit/mL). This is attractive since it allows lower heparin doses [289] but there is no evidence that it is beneficial. The incidence of heparin-induced osteoporosis is independent of the doses that have been used [268] and in any case the incidence of bone demineralization with LMWH is low (see above); we have found heparin prophylaxis to be effective with a fixed dose regime and there is a lot more inconvenience for the patient and potential error adjusting the dose of heparin on the basis of frequent anti-Xa heparin assays.

At one time Dextran was advocated for peripartum thromboprophylaxis. Aside from subsequent problems with cross-matching, the major worry is anaphylaxis. This is a particular problem in pregnancy where Dextran-induced anaphylaxis has caused uterine hypertonus and hypoxic damage to the fetus (see Chapter 3).

A further alternative for management of the antenatal period would be to develop more accurate models to determine precisely which patients are at risk of repeat thromboembolism. Although it is difficult to define the prothrombotic state on the basis of coagulation tests (see above), Clayton *et al.* and others [290, 291] were able correctly to identify 95% of gynaecological patients who had postoperative DVT on the basis of four items of clinical information and measurement of fibrin degradation products and plasminogen activator activity. Hellgren [81] has used discriminant analysis and shown that a combination of fibrinopeptide A, fibrinogen, Factor VIIIC, antithrombin III and plasmin activator estimation will help detect women at risk of thromboembolism in pregnancy. But these techniques are time consuming and also do not predict the individual risk with sufficient precision. More advances are likely in this field.

The second group of patients to be considered for thromboprophylaxis is in many ways the most problematic; this is because the group has only become apparent recently since testing for thrombophilia started, i.e. those who have been found to have thrombophilia by family studies but who have not had an episode themselves at the time of presentation. The options are: no additional therapy, aspirin throughout pregnancy, prophylactic heparin peripartum and for some time in the puerperium, prophylactic heparin throughout pregnancy and therapeutic heparin throughout pregnancy. Granted the safety of low-dose aspirin, it is easy to recommend this treatment throughout pregnancy for all patients with thrombophilia. Table 4.1 is helpful with regard to individual thrombophilias, which have also been considered above. The risk of thrombosis in type 1 antithrombin deficiency is so high that such patients should have therapeutic heparin monitored by anti-Xa throughout pregnancy. In type 2 antithrombin deficiency and homozygous Factor V Leiden the risk would seem to be high enough to justify prophylactic heparin treatment throughout pregnancy. In all other thrombophilias the risk does not seem to be high enough to justify more than prophylactic heparin at delivery in the patient who is asymptomatic with no other risk factors. It is not clear which of this last subgroup should be given prophylactic heparin at delivery nor for how long. These are personal opinions and hopefully more information will be forthcoming in the future.

With regard to the third group at high risk because of age, parity, obesity or operative delivery, it is generally believed (although not proven) that the risk of thromboembolism is greatest in the puerperium and therefore that any prophylaxis need only be used during this period and to cover labour. The Confidential Maternal Mortality series very clearly shows that the risks of thromboembolism are increased markedly with high parity and increasing age, and that these risks are partly independent of each other [53]. Applying these and other data, there is a case for using some form of prophylaxis in all patients who have had bed rest for at least 1 week before delivery, the obese, those undergoing operative delivery over the age of 30 years, and also in those over the age of 35 or in their fourth pregnancy (excluding abortion), even if they have a spontaneous vaginal delivery [292].

A consensus statement has evaluated the risk in association with caesarean section and recommends a variety of treatments ranging from none if the operation is uncomplicated to low-dose heparin and elastic stockings in very high-risk patients [293].

Thrombosis in unusual sites

Septic pelvic thrombophlebitis

This is a diagnosis made by exclusion and then only infrequently. The patient has fever, usually following caesarean section, for which no cause can be found and which does not remit with appropriate antibiotic therapy. The more diligently the cause of a fever is sought, and the better the judgment in choice of antibiotic, the lower the incidence of 'septic pelvic thrombophlebitis'. Malkamy [294] found 11 patients in 1263 caesarean deliveries (0.9%) over a 2.5-year period. In those cases where a laparotomy or venography has been performed, the thrombosis is often seen to start in the ovarian vein(s) and may extend into the inferior vena cava [295] and renal vein [296]. In these circumstances CT scanning to demonstrate clot in the inferior vena cava and renal vein may be helpful diagnostically [296].

Other sites

The Budd–Chiari syndrome, occlusion of the hepatic veins is most worrying because of the likelihood of death from hepatic failure. A case has been reported of Budd–Chiari syndrome in association with Factor V Leiden mutation treated successfully by liver transplantation [297]. Portal vein thrombosis in pregnancy has been associated with protein C deficiency [298].

DVT in the arm and subclavian veins has a similar natural history to that in the leg except that it is less common. It should be confirmed by ultrasonography and certainly has the possibility of causing pulmonary embolus; indeed it may present that way [299]. It may be associated with jugular venous catheterization, vigorous exercise with the arm or occlusion in particular laying the arm under a partner's head (Lover's arm) [300]. Jugular vein thrombosis has also been reported as part of ovarian stimulation syndrome [31, 301]. It certainly seems to be much more common when ovarian stimulation is the precipitating cause. Thrombophilia is rather uncommon [302]. Upper limb DVT should be managed in the same way as lower limb DVT.

References

1 Ginsberg JS, Hirsh J. Use of antithrombotic agents during pregnancy. *Chest* 1998; 114 (Suppl. 5): 524S–530S.

2 Girling J, de Swiet M. Acquired thrombophilia. *Bailliere's Clin Obstet Gynaecol* 1997; 11 (3): 447–62.

3 Greer IA. Thrombosis in pregnancy: maternal and fetal issues. *Lancet* 1999; 353: 1258–65.

4 Letsky EA. Peripartum prophylaxis of thrombo-embolism. *Bailliere's Clin Obstet Gynaecol* 1997; 11 (3): 523–43.

5 Sharma GVRK, Burlesco VA, Sasahara A. Effect of thrombolytic therapy on pulmonary capillary blood volume in patients with pulmonary embolism. *N Engl J Med* 1980; 303: 842–5.

6 Hirsh J, Bates SM. Prognosis in acute pulmonary embolism. *Lancet* 1999; 353: 1375–6.

7 Department of Health. *Why Mothers Die. Report on Confidential Enquiries into Maternal Deaths in the United Kingdom 1994–1996.* HMSO, London, 1998: 20–34.

8 Bergqvist A, Bergqvist D, Lindhagen A, Matzsch T. Late symptoms after pregnancy-related deep vein thrombosis. *Br J Obstet Gynaecol* 1990; 97: 338–41.

9 Janssen MCH, Haenen JH *et al.* Clinical and haemodynamic sequelae of deep vein thrombosis: retrospective evaluation after 7–13 years. *Clin Sci* 1997; 93: 7–12.

10 Sachs BP, Brown DAJ *et al.* Maternal mortality in Massachusetts. Trends and prevention. *N Engl J Med* 1987; 316: 667–72.

11 Duthie SJ, Lee CP, Ma HK. Maternal mortality in Hong Kong 1986–1990. *Br J Obstet Gynaecol* 1994 (101): 906–7.

12 Royal College of General Practitioners. Oral contraception and thrombo-embolic disease. *J R Coll Gen Pract* 1967; 13: 267–9.

13 Macklon NS, Greer IA. Venous thromboembolic disease in obstetrics and gynaecology: the Scottish experience. *Scott Med J* 1996; 41 (3): 83–6.

14 Hellgren M, Nygards EB. Long term therapy with subcutaneous heparin during pregnancy. *Gynecol Obstet Invest* 1981; 13: 76–89.

15 Andersen BS, Steffensen FH, Sorensen HT, Nielsen GL, Olsen J. The cumulative incidence of venous thromboembolism during pregnancy and puerperium—an 11 year Danish population based study of 63,300 pregnancies. *Acta Obstet Gynecol Scand* 1998; 77 (2): 170–3.

16 Henderson SR, Lund CJ, Creasman Wt. Antepartum pulmonary embolism. *Am J Obstet Gynecol* 1972; 112: 476–86.

17 Kierkegaard A. Incidence and diagnosis of deep vein thrombosis associated with pregnancy. *Acta Obstet Gynecol Scand* 1983; 62: 239–43.

18 Treffers PE, Huidekoper BL, Weenik GH, Kloosterman GJ. Epidemiological observations of thrombo-embolic disease during pregnancy and in the puerperium in 56,022 women. *Int J Gynaecol Obstet* 1983; 21: 327–31.

19 Bonnar J. The blood coagulation and fibrinolytic systems in the newborn and the mother at birth. *Br J Obstet Gynaecol* 1971; 78: 355.

20 Gallus AS. Venous thromboembolism; incidence and clinical risk factors. In: Madden JL, Hume M, eds. *Venous Thromboembolism*. Appleton-Century-Crofts, New York, 1976.

21 Yoshimura T, Ito M, Nakamura T, Okamura H. The influence of labour on thrombotic and fibrinolytic systems. *Eur J Obstet Reprod Biol* 1992; 44: 195–9.

22 Andersson T, Lorentzen B *et al.* Thrombin inhibitor complexes in the blood during after delivery. *Thromb Res* 1996; 82: 109–17.

23 Koster T, Blann AD, Briet E, Vandenbroucke JP, Rosendaal FR. Role of clotting factor VIII in effect of von Willebrand factor on occurrence of deep-vein thrombosis. *Lancet* 1995; 345: 152–5.

24 Bentolila S, Samama MM, Conard J, Horellou MH, Ffrench P. Association dysfibrinogenemie et thrombose. A propos d'une famille (Fibrinogene Melun) et revue de la litterature. [Association of dysfibrinogenemia and thrombosis. Apropos of a family (Fibrinogen Melun) and review of the literature.] *Ann Med Interne Paris* 1995; 146 (8): 575–80.

25 Haverkate F, Samama M. Familial dysfibrinogenemia and thrombophilia. Report on a study of the SSC Subcommittee on Fibrinogen. *Thromb Haemost* 1995; 73 (1): 151–61.

26 Dalaker K. Clotting factor VII during pregnancy, delivery and puerperium. *Br J Obstet Gynaecol* 1986; 93: 17–21.

27 Weiner CP, Kwaan H *et al.* Fibrin generation in normal pregnancy. *Obstet Gynecol* 1984; 64: 46–8.

28 Howie PW. Blood clotting and fibrinolysis in pregnancy. *Postgrad Med J* 1979; 55: 362–6.

29 van Wersch JWJ, Ubacks JMH. Blood coagulation and fibrinolysis during normal pregnancy. *Eur J Clin Chem Biochem* 1991; 29: 45–50.

30 Grant PJ, Medcalf RL. Hormonal regulation of haemostasis and the molecular biology of the fibrinolytic system. *Clin Sci* 1990; 78: 3–11.

31 Kaaja R, Seigberg R, Titinen A, Koskimies A. Severe ovarian hyperstimulation syndrome and deep venous thrombosis. *Lancet* 1989; ii: 1043.

32 Davies JA. The pre-thrombotic state. *Clin Sci* 1985; 69: 641–6.

33 Bergqvist D, Hedner U. Pregnancy and venous thromboembolism. *Acta Obstet Gynecol Scand* 1983; 62: 449–53.

34 Clarke Pearson DL, Jelovsek FR. Alternatives of occlusion cuff impedance plethysmography in the obstetric patient. *Surgery* 1981; 89: 594–8.

35 Wright HP, Osborn SB, Edmund DG. Changes in the rate of flow of venous blood in the leg during pregnancy, measured with radioactive sodium. *Surg Gynecol Obstet* 1950; 90: 481–5.

36 Macklon NS, Greer IA, Bowman AW. An ultrasound study of gestational and postural changes in the deep venous system of the leg in pregnancy. *Br J Obstet Gynaecol* 1997; 104: 191–7.

37 Bergqvist A, Bergqvist D, Hallbrook T. Deep vein thrombosis during pregnancy. A prospective study. *Acta Obstet Gynecol Scand* 1983; 62: 443–8.

38 Lindhagen A, Berqvist A, Berqvist D, Hallbrook T. Late venous function in the leg after deep venous thrombosis occurring in relation to pregnancy. *Br J Obstet Gynaecol* 1986; 93: 348–52.

39 Flessa HC, Glueck HI, Dritshilo A. Thromboembolic disorders in pregnancy. *Clin Obstet Gynaecol* 1974; 17: 195.

40 McCausland AM, Hyman C, Winsor T, Trotter AD. Venous distensibility during pregnancy. *Am J Obstet Gynecol* 1961; 81: 472–9.

41 Buchtemann AS, Steins A *et al.* The effect of compression therapy on venous haemodynamics in pregnant women. *Br J Obstet Gynaecol* 1999; 106: 563–9.

42 Department of Health and Social Security. *Report on Confidential Enquiries into Maternal Deaths in England and Wales, 1975–1978.* HMSO, London, 1982.

43 Department of Health and Social Security. *Report on Confidential Enquiries into Maternal Deaths in England and Wales 1979–1981.* HMSO, London, 1986.

44 Danilenko-Dixon DR, Heit JA *et al.* Risk factors for deep vein thrombosis and pulmonary embolism during pregnancy or post partum: a population-based, case-control study. *Am J Obstet Gynecol* 2001; 184: 104–10.

45 Milne R. Venous thromboembolism and travel: is there an association? *J R Coll Phys Lond* 1992; 26: 47–9.

46 Sarvesranan R. Sudden natural deaths associated with commercial air-travel. *Med Sci Law* 1986; 26: 35–8.

47 Finnerty JJ, MacKay BR. Antepartum thrombophlebitis and pulmonary embolism. *Obstet Gynecol* 1962; 19: 405.

48 Hiilesma VK. Occurrence and anticoagulant treatment of thromboembolism in gravidas, parturients and gynecologic patients. *Acta Obstet Gynecol Scand* 1960; 39: 5.

49 Bergqvist A, Bergqvist D, Hallbrook T. Acute deep vein thrombosis (DVT) after Caesarean section. *Acta Obstet Gynecol Scand* 1979; 58: 473–6.

50 Nielsen TF, Hokegard K-H. Postoperative caesarean section morbidity. A prospective study. *Am J Obstet Gynecol* 1983; 146: 911–16.

51 Aaro KA, Juergens JL. Thrombophlebitis and pulmonary embolism as a complication of pregnancy. *Med Clin North Am* 1974; 58: 829.

52 Atalla RK, Thompson JR, Oppenheimer CA, Bell SC, Taylor DJ. Reactive thrombocytosis after caesarean section and vaginal delivery: implications for maternal thromboembolism and its prevention. *Br J Obstet Gynaecol* 2000; 107: 411–14.

53 Department of Health and Social Security. *Report on Confidential Enquiries into Maternal Deaths in England and Wales, 1973–1975.* HMSO, London, 1979.

54 Daniel DG, Campbell H, Turnbull AC. Puerperal thromboembolism and suppression of lactation. *Lancet* 1967; ii: 287.

55 Jeffcoate TNA, Miller J, Ros RF, Tindall VR. Puerperal thromboembolism in relation to the inhibition of lactation by oestrogen therapy. *Br Med J* 1968; iv: 19.

56 Thomas AN, Pattison C, Serjeant GR. Causes of death in sickle-cell disease in Jamaica. *Br Med J* 1982; 285: 633–5.

57 Van Dinh T, Boor PJ, Garza JR. Massive pulmonary embolism following delivery of a patient with sickle cell trait. *Am J Obstet Gynecol* 1982; 143: 722–4.

58 Borgna Pignatti C, Carnelli V *et al.* Thromboembolic events in beta thalassemia major: an Italian multicenter study. *Acta Haematol* 1998; 99 (2): 76–9.

59 Department of Health. *Report on Confidential Enquiries into Maternal Deaths in the United Kingdom 1988–1990.* HMSO, London, 1994.

60 Golhaber SZ, Grodstein F et al. A prospective study of risk factors for pulmonary embolism in women. *J Am Med Assoc* 1997; 277: 642–5.

61 Mercelina Roumans PEAM, Ubachs JMH, van Wersch JWJ. Coagulation and fibrinolysis in smoking and nonsmoking pregnant women. *Br J Obstet Gynaecol* 1996; 103 (8): 789–94.

62 Duff P, Greene VP. Pregnancy complicated by solid papillary epithelial tumour of the pancreas, pulmonary embolism and pulmonary embolectomy. *Am J Obstet Gynecol* 1985; 1: 152–80.

63 Laros RK, Alger LS. Thromboembolism and pregnancy. *Clin Obstet Gynecol* 1979; 22: 871–88.

64 Kimball AM, Hallum AV, Cotes W. Deaths caused by pulmonary thromboembolism after legally induced abortion. *Am J Obstet Gynecol* 1978; 132: 169–74.

65 Jick H, Slone D et al. Venous thromboembolic disease and ABO blood group. A cooperative study. *Lancet* 1969; i: 539–42.

66 Gerhardt A, Eberhard R et al. Prothrombin and Factor V mutations in women with a history of thrombosis during pregnancy and the puerperium. *N Engl J Med* 2000; 342: 374–80.

67 Lancet editorial. Familial antithrombin III deficiency. *Lancet* 1983; i: 1021–2.

68 Mackie M, Bennett B, Ogston D, Douglas A. Familial thrombosis: inherited deficiency of antithrombin III. *Br Med J* 1978; i: 136–8.

69 Brandt P, Stenbjerg A. Subcutaneous heparin for thrombosis in pregnant women with hereditary antithrombin deficiency. *Lancet* 1979; i: 100–1.

70 Walker ID. Management of thrombophilia in pregnancy. *Blood Rev* 1991; 5: 1–7.

71 Heijboer H, Brandjes DPM, Buller HR, Sturk A, ten Cate WJ. Deficiencies of coagulation-inhibiting and fibrinolytic proteins in outpatients with deep-vein thrombosis. *N Engl Med* 1990; 323: 1512–16.

72 Prochownik EV, Antonarakis S et al. Molecular heterogenicity of inherited anti-thrombin III deficiency. *N Engl J Med* 1983; 308: 1549–52.

73 Sas G, Blasko G, Banhegy D, Jake L, Palos LA. Abnormal antithrombin III (antithrombin III 'Budapest') as a cause of familial thrombophilia. *Thromb Diathesis Haemorrh* 1974; 32: 105–15.

74 Finazzi C, Caccia R, Barboi T. Different prevalence of thromboembolism in the subtypes of congenital antithrombin III deficiency: Review of 404 cases. *Thromb Haemost* 1987; 58: 1094.

75 Daly M, O'Meara A, Hallinan F. Characterisation of a novel mutant form of antithrombin III (antithrombin 'Dubin'). *Clin Sci* 1986; 71: 84P.

76 Conard J, Horellou MH, van Dreden P, LeCompte T, Samarna M. Thrombosis and pregnancy in congenital deficiencies in ATIII, protein C or protein S. Study of 78 women. *Thromb Haemost* 1990; 63: 319–20.

77 Hellgren M, Tengborn L, Abildgaard U. Pregnancy in women with congenital antithrombin III deficiency: Experience of treatment with heparin and antithrombin. *Gynecol Obstet Invest* 1982; 14: 127–41.

78 Winter JH, Fenech A et al. Familial antithrombin III deficiency. *Q J Med* 1982; 204: 373–95.

79 Vellenga E, van Imhoff GW, Aarnoudse JG. Effective prophylaxis with oral anticoagulants and low-dose heparin during pregnancy in an antithrombin III deficient woman. *Lancet* 1983; ii: 224.

80 Marciniak E, Gockerman JP. Heparin-induced decrease in circulating antithrombin III. *Lancet* 1977; ii: 581–4.

81 Hellgren M. *Thromboembolism and pregnancy.* MD Thesis, Karolinska Institute, Stockholm, 1981.

82 Samson D, Stirling Y et al. Management of planned pregnancy in a patient with congenital antithrombin III deficiency. *Br J Haematol* 1984; 56: 243–9.

83 Zucker ML, Comperts ED, Marcus RG. Prophylactic and therapeutic use of anticoagulants in inherited antithrombin III deficiency. *S Afr Med J* 1976; 50: 1743–8.

84 Lechner K, Kyrle PA. Antithrombin III concentrates—are they clinically useful? *Thromb Haemost* 1995; 73 (3): 340–81.

85 Mohapeloa HL, Wellnitz H, Laursen B. Medfodt antitrombindefekt og graviditet. Graviditetsforlobet hos seks kvinder med kendt medfodt antitrombindefekt. [Hereditary antithrombin deficiency and pregnancy. Pregnancy course in six women with known hereditary antithrombin deficiency.] *Ugeskr Laeger* 1998; 160 (49): 7130–4.

86 Neerhof MG, Krewson DP, Haut M, Librizzi Rj. Heparin therapy for congenital antithrombin III deficiency in pregnancy. *Am J Perinatol* 1993; 10 (4): 311–12.

87 Winter JH, Fenech A, Bennett B, Douglas AS. Thrombosis after venography in familial antithrombin III deficiency. *Br Med J* 1981; 283: 1436–7.

88 Albrechtsson U, Olsson CG. Thrombosis after phlebography: a comparison of two contrast media. *Cardiovasc Radiol* 1979; 2: 9–18.

89 Megha A, Finzi Q, Poli T, Manotti C, Dettori AG. Bilateral deep vein thrombosis in a pregnant woman with antithrombin III deficiency: treatment of acute episodes and preparation for delivery with replacement treatment. *J Obstet Gynecol* 1990; 10: 220–1.

90 Winter JH, Fenech A, Mackie M, Bennett B, Douglas AS. Treatment of venous thrombosis in antithrombin III deficient patients with concentrates of antithrombin III. *Clin Lab Haematol* 1982; 4: 101–8.

91 Baudo F, Caimi TM et al. Emergency treatment by recombinant tissue plasminogen activator of pulmonary embolism in a pregnant woman with antithrombin III deficiency. *Am J Obstet Gynecol* 1990; 163: 1274–5.

92 Bjarte B, Herin P, Blomback M. Neonatal aortic thrombosis, a possible clinical manifestation of congenital antithrombin III deficiency. *Acta Paediatr Scand* 1974; 63: 247–301.

93 Peters M, Jansen E et al. Neonatal antithrombin III. *Br J Haematol* 1984; 58: 579–87.

94 Mitchell L, Piovella F, Andrew M. Alpha 2 macroglobulin may provide protection from the thromboembolic events in antithrombin III deficient children. *Blood* 1991; 78 (2299): 304.

95 Clouse LH, Comp RC. The regulation of hemostasis: the protein C system. *N Engl J Med* 1986; 314: 1298–304.

96 Morrison AE, Walker ID, Black WP. Protein C deficiency presenting as deep venous thrombosis in pregnancy. Case report. *Br J Obstet Gynaecol* 1988; 95: 1077–80.

97 Allart CF, Rosendaal FR, Noteboom WNP, Vandenbroucke JP, Briet E. Survival in families with hereditary protein C deficiency. *Br Med J* 1995; 311: 910–13.

98 Broekmans AW, Veltkamp JJ, Bertina RM. Congenital protein C deficiency and venous thromboembolism. A study of three Dutch families. *N Engl J Med* 1983; 309: 340–4.

99 Seligsohn U, Berger A et al. Homozygous protein C deficiency manifested by massive venous thrombosis in the new born. *N Engl J Med* 1984; 310: 559–62.

100 Matsuda M, Sugo T et al. A thrombotic state due to an abnormal protein C. *N Engl J Med* 1988; 319: 1265–8.

101 Warwick R, Hutton RA, Coff L, Letsky E, Heard M. Changes in protein C and free protein S during pregnancy and following hysterectomy. *J R Soc Med* 1989; 82: 591–4.

102 Horellou MH, Conard J, Bertina RM, Samana M. Congenital protein C deficiency and thrombotic disease in nine French families. *Br Med J* 1984; 289: 1285–7.

103 Broekmans AW, Bertina RM, Loeliger EA, Hoffman V, Mingeman HG. Protein C and the development of skin necrosis during anticoagulant therapy. *Thromb Haemost* 1983; 49: 251.

104 Pescatore C, Horellou HM *et al.* Problems of oral anticoagulation in an adult with homozygous protein C deficiency and late onset of thrombosis. *Thromb Haemost* 1993; 69: 311–15.

105 Dreyfus M, Magny JF *et al.* Treatment of homozygous protein C deficiency and neonatal purpura fulminans with a purified protein C concentrate. *N Engl J Med* 1991; 325: 1565–8.

106 Richards EM, Makris M, Preston FE. The successful use of protein C concentrate during pregnancy in a patient with type 1 protein C deficiency, previous thrombosis and recurrent fetal loss. *Br J Haematol* 1997; 98 (3): 660–1.

107 Mibashan RS, Millar DS *et al.* Prenatal diagnosis of hereditary protein C deficiency. *N Engl J Med* 1985; 313: 1607.

108 Lao TT, Yuen PMP, Yin JA. Protein S and protein C levels in Chinese women during pregnancy, delivery and the puerperium. *Br J Obstet Gynaecol* 1989; 96: 167–70.

109 Comp PC, Esmon CT. Recurrent venous thromboembolism in patients with a partial deficiency of protein S. *N Engl J Med* 1984; 311: 1525–8.

110 Malnick SDH, Sthoeger ZM. Autoimmune protein S deficiency. *N Engl J Med* 1993; 329: 1898.

111 Conard J, Horellou MH, van Dreden P, Le Compte T, Samama M. Thrombosis in pregnancy and congenital defects in ATIII, protein C or protein S. Study of 78 women. *Thromb Haemost* 1990; 63: 319–20.

112 De Stefano V, Leone G *et al.* Thrombosis during pregnancy and surgery in patients with congenital deficiency of antithrombin III, protein C protein S. *Thromb Haemost* 1994; 71: 799–800.

113 Friederich PW, Sanson BJ *et al.* Frequency of pregnancy-related venous thromboembolism in anticoagulant factor-deficient women: implications for prophylaxis. *Ann Intern Med* 1996; 125: 955–60.

114 Pabinger I. A Study Group on natural Inhibitors. Thrombotic risk in hereditary anti thrombin III, protein C or protein S deficiency. *Arter Thromb Vasc Biol* 1996; 16: 742–8.

115 Grimaudo V, Gueissaz F *et al.* Necrosis of skin induced by coumarin in a patient deficient in protein S. *Br Med J* 1989; 298: 233–4.

116 Mahasandana C, Suvatte V *et al.* Neonatal purpura fulminans associated with homozygous protein S deficiency. *Lancet* 1990; 335: 61–2.

117 Svensson PJ, Dahlbick B. Resistance to activated protein C as a basis for venous thrombosis. *N Engl J Med* 1994; 330: 517–22.

118 Vandebroucke JP, Koster T *et al.* Increased risk of venous thombosis in oral contraceptive users who are carriers of factor V Leiden. *Lancet* 1994; 344: 1453–7.

119 Peek MJ, Nelson Piercy C, Manning R, de Swiet M, Letsky, EL. Activated protein C resistance in normal pregnancy. *Br J Obstet Gynaecol* 1997; 104: 1084–6.

120 Kjellberg U, Andersson NE, Rosen S, Tengborn L, Hellgren M. APC resistance and other haemostatic variables during pregnancy and puerperium. *Thromb Haemost* 1999; 81 (4): 527–31.

121 Rees DC, Cox M, Clegg JB. World distribution of factor V Leiden. *Lancet* 1995; 346: 1133–4.

122 Dzimiri N, Meyer B. World distribution of factor V Leiden. *Lancet* 1996; 347 (481): 2.

123 Vandenbroucke JP, van der Meer FJ *et al.* Factor V Leiden: should we screen oral contraceptive users and pregnant women? *BMJ* 1996; 313: 1127–30.

124 McColl MD, Walker ID, Greer IA. A mutation in the prothrombin gene contributing to venous thrombosis in pregnancy. *Br J Obstet Gynaecol* 1998; 105: 923–5.

125 Mudd SH, Skovby F *et al.* The natural history of homocystinemia due to cystathionine β-synthatase deficiency. *Am J Hum Genet* 1985; 37: 1–31.

126 Constantine G, Green A. Untreated homocystinuria: a maternal death in a woman with four pregnancies. *Br J Obstet Gynaecol* 1987; 94: 803–6.

127 Lamon JM, Lenke RR, Levy HL, Schulmann JD, Shih VE. Selected metabolic diseases. In: Schulmann JD, Simpson JL, eds. *Genetic Diseases in Pregnancy.* Academic Press, New York, 1980: 6–8.

128 den Heijer M, Koster T *et al.* Hyperhomocysteinaemia as a risk factor for deep-vein thrombosis. *N Engl J Med* 1996; 334: 759–62.

129 Mandel H, Brenner B *et al.* Coexistence of hereditary hyperhomocysteinaemia and factor V Leiden effect on thrombosis. *N Engl J Med* 1996; 334: 763–8.

130 Preston FE, Rosendaal FR *et al.* Increased fetal loss in women with heritable thrombophilia. *Lancet* 1996; 348: 913–16.

131 Kuperminc MJ, Eldor A *et al.* Increased frequency of genetic thrombophilia in women with complicated pregnancy. *N Engl J Med* 1999; 340: 9–13.

132 Becker S, Heller CH, Gropp F, Scharrer I, Kreuz W. Thrombophilic disorders in children with cerebral infarction. *Lancet* 1998; 352: 1756–7.

133 Bonnar J, Walsh J. Prevention of thrombosis after pelvic surgery by British dextran 70. *Lancet* 1972; ii: 614.

134 Friend JR, Kakkar VV. Deep vein thrombosis in obstetric and gynaecological patients. In: Kakkar W, AJ, ed. *Thromboembolism, Diagnosis and Treatment.* Churchill Livingstone, London, 1972: 131–8.

135 Simpson FG, Robinson PJ, Bark M, Losowsky MS. Prospective study of thrombophlebitis and pseudo thrombophlebitis. *Lancet* 1980; i: 331–3.

136 Ramsay LE. Impact of venography on the diagnosis and management of deep vein thrombosis. *Br Med J* 1983; 286: 698–9.

137 Sandler DA, Martin JF *et al.* Diagnosis of deep-vein thrombosis: comparison of clinical evaluation, ultrasound, plethysmograph and venoscan with X-ray venogram. *Lancet* 1984; ii: 716–19.

138 Ludlam CA, Bolton AE, Moore S, Cash JD. New rapid method of diagnosis of deep vein thrombosis. *Lancet* 1975; ii: 259–60.

139 Whitehouse C. Radiological diagnosis of deep vein thrombosis. *Br Med J* 1987; 295: 801–2.

140 Thomas EA, Cobby MJD, Rhys Davies E, Jeans WD, Whicher JT. Liquid crystal thermography and C reactive protein in the detection of deep venous thrombosis. *Br Med J* 1989; 299: 951–2.

141 Bernardi E, Prandoni P *et al.* D dimer testing as an adjunct to ultrasonography in patients with clinically suspected deep vein thrombosis: prospective cohort study. *Br Med J* 1998; 317: 1037–40.

142 Preston Flanigan D, Goodreau JJ, Burnham SJ, Bergan JJ, Yao JST. Vascular laboratory diagnosis of clinically suspected acute deep vein thrombosis. *Lancet* 1978; i: 331–4.

143 Hull R, Hirsh J, Sackett DL. Combined use of leg scanning and impedance plethysmography in suspected venous

thrombosis. An alternative to venography. *N Engl J Med* 1977; 296: 1497–500.

144 Sandler DA, Martin JF. Liquid crystal thermography as a screening test for deep-vein thrombosis. *Lancet* 1985; i: 665–8.

145 Excess R, Graeme B. Congenital athyroidism in the newborn infant from intrauterine radioactive iodine. *Biol Neonate* 1974; 24: 289–91.

146 Kearon C, Julian JA, Newman TE, Ginsberg JS. Non-invasive diagnosis of deep venous thrombosis. McMaster Diagnostic Imaging Practice Guidelines Initiative. *Ann Intern Med* 1998; 128 (8): 663–77.

147 Huisman MY, Buller HR, ten Cate JW, Vreeken J. Serial imped-ance plethysmography for suspected deep vein thrombosis in patients. The Amsterdam Research Practitioners Study. *N Engl J Med* 1986; 314: 823–8.

148 Hull RD, Hirsh J *et al.* Diagnostic efficacy of impedance plethysmography of clinically suspected deep-vein throm-bosis. *Ann Intern Med* 1985; 102: 21–8.

149 Hull RD, Raskob GE, Coates G, Panju AA. Clinical validity of a normal perfusion lung scan in patients with suspected pulmon-ary embolism. *Chest* 1990; 91: 23–6.

150 Lensing AWA, Prandoni P *et al.* Detection of deep vein thrombosis by real-time B-mode ultrasonography. *N Engl J Med* 1989; 320: 342–5.

151 Greer IA, Barry J, Mackon N, Allan PL. Diagnosis of deep venous thrombosis in pregnancy: a new role for diagnostic ultrasound. *Br J Obstet Gynaecol* 1990; 97: 53–7.

152 Polak JF, Wilkinson DL. Ultrasonographic diagnosis of symp-tomatic deep vein venous thrombosis in pregnancy. *Am J Obstet Gynecol* 1991; 165: 625–9.

153 Hull R, Hirsh J *et al.* Replacement of venography in suspected venous thrombosis by impedance plethysmography and 125I-fibrinogen leg scanning: a less invasive approach. *Ann Intern Med* 1981; 94: 12–15.

154 Toglia MR, Weg JG. Venous thromboembolism during preg-nancy. *N Engl J Med* 1996; 335: 108–14.

155 Thomas ML, Keeling FP, Piaggio RB, Treweeke PS. Contrast agent induced thrombophlebitis following leg phlebography: iopamidol versus meglumine iothalamate. *Br J Radiol* 1984; 57: 205–7.

156 Mussein IY, Critchey HOD. An unusual presentation of pul-monary thromboembolism in late pregnancy. Case report. *Br J Obstet Gynaecol* 1986; 93: 1161–2.

157 Robin ED. Overdiagnosis and overtreatment of pulmonary embolism: The emperor may have no clothes. *Ann Intern Med* 1977; 87: 775–81.

158 Tribukait B, Swedjemark GA. Secretion of 99TcM in breast milk after intravenous injection of marked macroaggregated albumin. *Acta Radiol Oncol* 1978; 17: 379–82.

159 Morrell NW, Seed WA. Diagnosing pulmonary embolism. *Br Med J* 1992; 304: 1126–7.

160 Hansell DM, Flower CDR. Imaging pulmonary embolism. *Br Med J* 1998; 16: 490–1.

161 Hume M, Sevitt S, Thomas DP. *Thrombosis and Pulmonary Embolism*. Harvard University Press, Cambridge, MA, 1970.

162 Heimbecker RO, Keon WJ, Richards KU. Massive pulmonary embolism: a new look at surgical management. *Arch Surg* 1973; 107: 740–6.

163 Villasanta U. Thromboembolic disease in pregnancy. *Am J Obstet Gynecol* 1965; 93: 142–60.

164 Moseley P, Kerstein MD. Pregnancy and thrombophlebitis. *Surg Gynecol Obstet* 1980; 150: 593–7.

165 Morris CK, Mitchell JRA. Clinical management of venous thromboembolism. *Br Med Bull* 1978; 34: 169–75.

166 Girard P, Mathieu M *et al.* Recurrence of pulmonary embol-ism during anticoagulant treatment: a prospective study. *Thorax* 1987; 42: 481–6.

167 Barritt DW, Jordan SC. Anticoagulant drugs in the treatment of pulmonary embolism: a controlled trial. *Lancet* 1960; i: 1309–12.

168 Ludwig H. Results of streptokinase therapy in deep vein thrombosis during pregnancy. *Postgrad Med J* 1973; 49 (Suppl. 5): 65–7.

169 Hirsh J, Cade JF, O'Sullivan EF. Clinical experience with anti-coagulant therapy during pregnancy. *Br Med J* 1970; i: 270–3.

170 Bonnar J. Thromboembolism in obstetric and gynaecological patients. In: Nicolaides AN, ed. *Thromboembolism Aetiology, Advances in Prevention and Management*. MTP Press, Lancaster, 1975: 311–34.

171 Bonnar J. Long-term self-administered heparin therapy for prevention and treatment of thromboembolic complications in pregnancy. In: Kakkar W, Thomas DP, eds. *Heparin Chem-istry and Clinical Usage*. Academic Press, London, 1976.

172 Salzman EW, Deykin D, Shapiro RM, Rosenberg R. Manage-ment of heparin therapy—controlled prospective trial. *N Engl J Med* 1975; 292: 1046–50.

173 Jacobs J, Kletter I *et al.* Intravenous infusions of heparin and penicillins. *J Clin Pathol* 1973; 26: 742–6.

174 Estes JW. Kinetics of the anticoagulation effect of heparin. *J Am Med Assoc* 1970; 212: 1492.

175 Sasahara AA. Therapy for pulmonary embolism. *J Am Med Assoc* 1974; 229: 1795.

176 Bowler GMR, Galloway DW, Meiklejohn BH, Macintyre CCA. Sharp fall in blood pressure after injection of heparin contain-ing chlorbutol. *Lancet* 1986; i: 848–9.

177 Dacie J. *Practical Haematology*. Churchill Livingstone, Edin-burgh, 1975: 413–14.

178 Letsky EA. *Coagulation Problems During Pregnancy*. Churchill Livingstone, Edinburgh, 1985.

179 Hull RD, Raskob GE *et al.* Heparin for 5 days as compared with 10 days in the initial treatment of proximal venous thrombosis. *N Engl J Med* 1990; 322: 1260–4.

180 Decousus HA, Croze M *et al.* Circadian changes in anticoagu-lant effect of heparin infused at a constant rate. *Br Med J* 1985; 290: 341–4.

181 Fennerty AG, Levine MN. Non-biological factors in day to day variation of heparin requirements. *Br Med J* 1989; 299: 1009–13.

182 Hull RD, Raskob GE *et al.* Subcutaneous low-molecular-weight heparin compared with continuous intravenous hep-arin in the treatment of proximal vein thrombosis. *N Engl J Med* 1992; 326: 975–82.

183 Prandoni P, Lensing AWA *et al.* Comparison of subcutaneous low-molecular-weight with intravenous standard heparin in proximal deep-vein thrombosis. *Lancet* 1992; 339: 441–5.

184 Simmoneau G, Sors H *et al.* A comparison of low molecular weight heparin with unfractionated heparin for acute pul-monary embolism. *N Engl J Med* 1997; 337: 663–9.

185 Thomson AJ, Walker ID, Greer IA. Low molecular weight heparin for immediate management of thromboembolic dis-ease in pregnancy. *Lancet* 1998; 352: 1904.

186 Elliot MS, Immelman EJ *et al.* A comparative trial of heparin versus streptokinase in the treatment of acute proximal venous thrombosis: an interim report of a prospective trial. *Br J Surg* 1979; 66: 838–43.

187 Browse N. Diagnosis of deep vein thrombosis. *Br Med Bull* 1978; 34: 163–7.

188 Urokinase Pulmonary Embolism Trial Study Group. Urokinase pulmonary embolism trial: Phase 1. *J Am Med Assoc* 1970; 214: 2163–72.

189 Editorial. Thrombolysis for pulmonary embolism. *Lancet* 1992; 340: 21–2.

190 Pfeiffer GW. The use of thrombolytic therapy in obstetrics and gynaecology. *Australas Ann Med* 1970; (Suppl): 28–31.

191 Bell WR, Meek AG. Guidelines for the use of thrombolytic agents. *N Engl J Med* 1979; 301: 1266–70.

192 Pfeiffer GW. Distribution and placental transfer of ^{141}I streptokinase. *Australas Ann Med* 1970; (Suppl): 17–18.

193 National Institute of Health. Consensus conference thrombolytic therapy in treatment of pulmonary embolus. *Br Med J* 1980; 280: 1585–7.

194 Amias AG. Streptokinase, cerebral vascular disease—and triplets. *Br Med J* 1977; i: 1414–15.

195 Hall RJC, Young C, Sutton GC, Cambell S. Treatment of acute massive pulmonary embolism by streptokinase during labour and delivery. *Br Med J* 1972; iv: 647–9.

196 McTaggart DR, Engram TC. Massive pulmonary embolism during pregnancy treated with streptokinase. *Med J Aust* 1977; 1: 18–20.

197 Turrentine MA, Braems G, Ramirez MM. Use of thrombolytics for the treatment of thromboembolic disease during pregnancy. *Obstet Gynecol Surv* 1995; 50 (7): 534–41.

198 Flute PT. Thrombolytic therapy. *Br J Hosp Med* 1976; 16: 135–42.

199 Mayor GE. Deep vein thrombosis—surgical management. *Br Med J* 1969; iv: 680–2.

200 Lansing AM, Davies WM. Five year follow-up study of ilio femoral venous thromboectomy. *Ann Surg* 1968; 168: 620–8.

201 Gurll W, Helfand Z, Salzman EF, Silen W. Peripheral venous thrombophlebitis during pregnancy. *Am J Surg* 1971; 121: 449–53.

202 Sautter RD. In: Fratantoni J, Wessler S, eds. *Prophylactic Therapy of Deep Vein Thrombosis and Pulmonary Embolism*. National Institutes of Health, Bethesada, 1975: 137–42.

203 Silver D, Sabiston DC. The role of vena caval interruption in the management of pulmonary embolism. *Surgery* 1975; 77: 3–10.

204 Banfield PJ, Pittam M, Marwood R. Recurrent pulmonary embolism in pregnancy managed with the Greenfield vena caval filter. *Int J Gynecol Obstet* 1990; 33: 275–8.

205 Gray HH, Miller GAH. Pulmonary embolectomy is still appropriate for a minority of patients with acute massive pulmonary embolism. *Br J Hosp Med* 1989; 41: 467–8.

206 Brady AJB, Crake T, Oakley CM. Percutaneous catheter fragmentation and distal dispersion of proximal pulmonary embolus. *Lancet* 1991; 338: 1186–9.

207 Gray HH, Miller GAH, Paneth M. Pulmonary embolectomy: Its place in the management of pulmonary embolism. *Lancet* 1988; i: 1441–4.

208 Gulb DC, Schmid C *et al*. Medical compared with surgical treatment for massive pulmonary embolism. *Lancet* 1994; 343: 576–7.

209 Abbott A, Sibert JR, Weaver JB. Chondrodysplasia punctata and maternal warfarin treatment. *Br Med J* 1977; i: 1639–40.

210 Becker MH, Genieser NB, Feingold M. Chondrodysplasia punctata: is maternal warfarin therapy a factor? *Am J Dis Child* 1975; 129: 356–7.

211 Kerber IJ, Warr OS III, Richardson C. Pregnancy in a patient with a prosthetic mitral valve associated with a fetal anomaly attributed to warfarin sodium. *J Am Med Assoc* 1968; 203: 223–5.

212 Pettifor JM, Benson R. Congenital malformations associated with the administration of oral anticoagulants during pregnancy. *J Pediatr* 1975; 86: 459–62.

213 Shaul WL, Emery H, Hall JG. Chondrodysplasia punctata and maternal warfarin use during pregnancy. *Am J Dis Child* 1975; 129: 360–2.

214 Sheffield LJ, Danks DM, Mayne V, Hutchinson LA. Chondrodysplasia punctata—23 cases of mild and relatively common variety. *J Pediatr* 1976; 89: 916–23.

215 Curry CJR, Magenis RE *et al*. Inherited chondrodysplasia punctata due to a deletion of the terminal short arm of X chromosome. *N Engl J Med* 1984; 311: 1010–15.

216 Cox DR, Martin L, Hall BD. Asplenia syndrome after fetal exposure to warfarin. *Lancet* 1977; ii: 1134.

217 O'Donnel D, Sevitz H *et al*. Pregnancy after renal transplantation. *Aust NZ J Med* 1985; 15: 320–5.

217a Andrew M, Bhogal M *et al*. Factors XI and XII and prekallikrein in sick and healthy premature infants. *N Engl J Med* 1981; 305: 1130–3.

218 Editorial. Venous thromboembolism and anticoagulants in pregnancy. *Br Med J* 1975; ii: 421–2.

219 de Swiet M, Bulpitt CJ, Lewis PJ. How obstetricians use anticoagulants in the prophylaxis of thromboembolism. *J Obstet Gynaecol* 1980; 1: 29–32.

220 Pridmore BR, Murray KH, McAllen PM. The management of anticoagulant therapy during and after pregnancy. *Br J Obstet Gynaecol* 1975; 82: 740–4.

221 Szekely P, Turner R, Snaith L. Pregnancy and the changing pattern of rheumatic heart disease. *Br Heart J* 1973; 35: 1293–303.

222 Greer IA, de Swiet M. Thrombosis prophylaxis in obstetrics and gynaecology. *Br J Obstet Gynaecol* 1993; 100: 37–9.

223 Sherman S, Hall BD. Warfarin and fetal abnormality. *Lancet* 1976; i: 692.

224 Hall JG. Warfarin and fetal abnormality. *Lancet* 1976; i: 1127.

225 Hall JG, Pauli RM, Wilson KM. Maternal and fetal sequelae of anticoagulation during pregnancy. *Am J Med* 1980; 68: 122–40.

226 Holzgreve W, Carey JC, Hall BD. Warfarin-induced fetal abnormalities. *Lancet* 1976; ii: 914–15.

227 Shaul WL, Hall JG. Multiple congenital anomalies associated with anticoagulants. *Am J Obstet Gynecol* 1977; 127: 191–8.

228 Smith MF, Cameron MD. Warfarin as teratogen. *Lancet* 1979; i: 727.

229 Chen WWC, Chan CS, Lee PR, Wang RYR, Wong VCW. Pregnancy in patients with prosthetic heart valves: An experience with 45 pregnancies. *Q J Med* 1982; 51: 358–65.

230 Chong MKB, Harvey D, de Swiet M. Follow-up study of children whose mothers were treated with warfarin during pregnancy. *Br J Obstet Gynaecol* 1984; 91: 1070–3.

231 Vitale N, De Feo M *et al*. Dose dependant fetal complications of warfarin in pregnant women with mechanical heart valves. *J Am Coll Cardiol* 1999; 33: 1637–41.

232 de Swiet M, Letsky E, Mellows H. Drug treatment and prophylaxis of thromboembolism in pregnancy. In: Lewis PJ, ed. *Therapentic Problems in Pregnancy*. MTP Press, Lancaster, 1977: 81–9.

233 Li TC, Smith ARB, Duncan SLB. Feto-maternal haemorrhage complicating warfarin therapy during pregnancy. *J Obstet Gynaecol* 1990; 10: 401–2.

234 Brambel CE, Hunter RE. Effect of dicoumarol on the nursing infant. *Am J Obstet Gynecol* 1950; 59: 1153–9.

235 Orme ML, Lewis PJ *et al.* May mothers given warfarin breast-feed their infants? *Br Med J* 1977; 1: 1564–5.

236 Eckstein H, Jack B. Breast feeding and anticoagulant therapy. *Lancet* 1970; i: 672–3.

237 Oakley CM, Hawkins DF. Pregnancy in patients with prosthetic heart valves. *Br Med J* 1983; 287: 358.

238 Hirsh J. Heparin. *N Engl J Med* 1991; 324: 1565–74.

239 Nelson-Piercy C, Letsky EA, de Swiet M. Low-molecular-weight heparin for obstetric thromboprophylaxis: Experience of sixty-nine pregnancies in sixty-one women at high risk. *Am J Obstet Gynecol* 1997; 176: 1062–8.

240 Gibson JL, Ekevall K, Walker I, Greer IA. Puerperal thromboprophylaxis: comparison of the anti Xa activity of enoxaparin and unfractionated heparin. *Br J Obstet Gynaecol* 1998; 105: 795–7.

241 de Swiet M, Fidler J, Howell R, Letsky E. Thromboembolism in pregnancy. In: Jewell DP, ed. *Advanced Medicine*. Pitman Medical, London, 1981: 309–17.

242 Hill NCW, Hill JG, Sargent JM, Taylor CG, Bush PV. Effect of low dose heparin on blood loss at caesarean section. *Br Med J* 1988; 296: 1505–6.

243 Anderson DR, Ginsberg JS, Burrows R, Brill-Edwards P. Subcutaneous heparin therapy during pregnancy: a need for concern at the time of delivery. *Thromb Haemost* 1991; 65: 248–50.

244 Letsky EA. Haemostasis and epidural anaesthesia. *Int J Obstet Anesth* 1991; 1: 51–4.

245 Crawford JS. *Principles and Practice of Obstetric Anaesthesia*, 4th edn. Blackwell Scientific Publications, Oxford, 1978: 182–3.

246 British Society for Haematology. British Committee for Standards of Haematology, Haemostasis and Thrombosis Task F. Guidelines on oral anticoagulation: second edition. *J Clin Pathol* 1990; 43: 177–83.

247 McCollum C. Avoiding the consequences of deep vein thrombosis. *Br Med J* 1998; 317: 696.

248 Cohen AW, Cabbe SG, Mennuti MT. Adjusted-dose heparin therapy by continuous intravenous infusion for recurrent pulmonary embolism during pregnancy. *Am J Obstet Gynecol* 1983; 146: 463–4.

249 Nelson DM, Stempel LE, Fabri PJ, Talbert M. Hickman catheter use in a pregnant patient requiring therapeutic heparin anticoagulation. *Am J Obstet Gynecol* 1984; 149: 461–2.

250 Adams E, Maguire N, Richmond D, Rowlands P. Retrievable inferior vena caval filter for thromboembolic disease in pregnancy. *Br J Obstet Gynaecol* 1998; 105: 1039 (letter).

251 Neill AM, Appleton DS, Richards P. Retrievable inferior vena caval filter for thromboembolic disease in pregnancy. *Br J Obstet Gynaecol* 1997; 104: 1416–18.

252 Decousus H, Leizorovicz A *et al.* A clinical trial of vena caval filters in the prevention of pulmonary embolism in patients with proximal deep vein thrombosis. *N Engl J Med* 1998; 338: 409–15.

253 Badaracco MA, Vessey M. Recurrence of venous thromboembolism disease and use of oral contraceptives. *Br Med J* 1974; i: 215–17.

254 Howell R, Fidler J, Letsky E, de Swiet M. The risks of antenatal subcutaneous heparin prophylaxis: a controlled trial. *Br J Obstet Gynaecol* 1983; 90: 1124–8.

255 Sanson B, Lensing AWA, Prins MH. Safety of low molecular weight heparin in pregnancy: a systematic review. *Thromb Haemost* 1999; 81: 668–72.

256 Avioli LV. Heparin-induced osteopenia: an appraisal. *Adv Exp Med Biol* 1975; 52: 375–87.

257 Jaffe MD, Willis PW. Multiple fractures associated with long-term sodium heparin therapy. *J Am Med Assoc* 1965; 193: 152–4.

258 Squires JW, Pinch LW. Heparin induced spinal fractures. *J Am Med Assoc* 1979; 241: 2417–18.

259 Wise PH, Hall AJ. Heparin induced osteopenia in pregnancy. *Br Med J* 1980; 281: 110–11.

260 Griffith GC, Nichols G, Asher JD, Hanagan B. Heparin osteoporosis. *J Am Med Assoc* 1965; 193: 91–4.

261 Griffiths HT, Liu DTY. Severe heparin osteoporosis in pregnancy. *Postgrad Med J* 1984; 60: 424–5.

262 Dahlmann TC. Osteoporotic fractures and the recurrence of thromboembolism during pregnancy and the puerperium in 184 women undergoing thromboprophylaxis with heparin. *Am J Obstet Gynecol* 1993; 168: 1265–70.

263 Aarskog D, Aksnes L, Lehmann V. Low 1,25-dihydoroxyvitamin D in heparin-induced osteopenia. *Lancet* 1980; ii: 650–1.

264 Aarskog D, Aksnes L, Markestad T, Ulstein M, Sagen N. Heparin-induced inhibition of 1, 25 dihydroxyvitamin D formation. *Am J Obstet Gynecology* 1984; 148: 1141–2.

265 Dahlman T, Sjoberg HE, Hellgren M, Bucht E. Calcium homeostasis in pregnancy during long-term heparin treatment. *Br J Obstet Gynaecol* 1992; 99: 412–16.

266 Misra R, Anderson DC. Providing the fetus with calcium. *Br Med J* 1991; 300: 1220–1.

267 de Swiet M, Dorrington Ward P *et al.* Prolonged heparin therapy in pregnancy causes bone demineralisation (heparin induced-osteopenia). *Br J Obstet Gynaecol* 1983; 90: 1129–34.

268 Dalhman T, Lindvall N, Hellgren M. Osteopenia in pregnancy during long-term heparin treatment: a radiological study post partum. *Br J Obstet Gynaecol* 1990; 97: 221–8.

269 Ginsberg JS, Kowah Ghuk G *et al.* Heparin effect on bone density. *Thromb Haemost* 1990; 64: 286–9.

270 Laskin C, Ginsberg JS *et al.* Low molecular weight heparin and ASA therapy in women with autoantibodies and unexplained recurrent fetal loss (U-RFL). *Am J Obstet Gynecol* 1997; 176: S125.

271 Hatjis CG. Heparin-induced thrombocytopenia in pregnancy. A case report. *J Reprod Med* 1984; 29: 337–8.

272 Cines DB, Kaywin P, Bina M, Tomaski A, Schreiber AD. Heparin-associated thrombocytopenia. *N Engl J Med* 1980; 303: 788–95.

273 Calhoun BC, Hesser JW. Heparin-associated antibody with pregnancy: Discussion of two cases. *Am J Obstet Gynecol* 1987; 156: 964–6.

274 Chong BH, Pitney WR, Castaldi PA. Heparin-induced thrombocytopenia: association of thrombotic complications with heparin-independent IgG antibody that induces thromboxane synthesis and platelet aggregation. *Lancet* 1982; ii: 1246–8.

275 Cines DB, Tornaski A, Tannenbaum S. Immune endothelial-cell injury in heparin-associated thrombocytopenia. *N Engl J Med* 1987; 316: 581–9.

276 Wolf H, Wick G. Antibodies interacting with, and corresponding binding site for heparin on human thrombocytes. *Lancet* 1986; ii: 222–3.

277 Eichinger S, Kyrie PA *et al.* Thrombocytopenia associated with low-molecular-weight heparin. *Lancet* 1991; 337: 1425–6.

278 LeCompte T, Luo SK, Stieltjes N, Lecrubier C, Samama MM. Thrombocytopenia associated with low-molecular-weight heparin. *Lancet* 1991; 338: 1217.

279 Lindhoff-Last E, Willeke A, Thalhammer C, Nowak G, Bauer-sachs R. Hirudin treatment in a breastfeeding woman. *Lancet* 2000; 355: 467–8.

280 Giustolisi R, Guglielmo P, di Raimondo F, Cacciola E, Stagno F. Hypereosinophilia and subcutaneous heparin. *Lancet* 1993; 342: 1371.

281 Ojukwu C, Jenkison SD, Obeid D. Deep vein thrombosis in pregnancy and heparin hypersensitivity. *Br J Obstet Gynaecol* 1996; 103: 934–6.

282 Canova CR, Fischler MP, Reinhart WH. Effect of low molecular weight heparin on serum potassium. *Lancet* 1997; 349: 1447–8.

283 Tomsu M, Preston F, Forrest ARW. Severe hyperlipidaemia in pregnancy related to the use of low-molecular-weight heparin-enoxaparin sodium (clexane). *J Obstet Gynaecol* 1998; 18: 83–4.

284 Lao TT, de Swiet M, Letsky E, Walters BNJ. Prophylaxis of thromboembolism in pregnancy: an alternative. *Br J Obstet Gynaecol* 1985; 92: 202–6.

285 Antiplatelet Trialists' Collaboration. Collaborative overview of randomised trials of antiplatelet therapy III. Reduction in venous thrombosis and pulmonary embolism by antiplatelet prophylaxis among surgical and medical patients. *Br Med J* 1994; 308: 235–46.

286 Pulmonary Embolism Prevention (PEP) Trial Collaborative Group. Prevention of pulmonary embolism and deep vein thrombosis with low-dose aspirin: Pulmonary Embolism Prevention (PEP) trial. *Lancet* 2000; 355: 1295–302.

287 CLASP Collaborative Group. A randomised trial of low-dose aspirin for the treatment of pre-eclampsia among 9364 pregnant women. *Lancet* 1994; b: 619–29.

288 Tan J, de Swiet M. Use of aspirin for obstetric thromboprophylaxis in low risk women. *J Obstet Gynaecol* 1998; 18 (Suppl. 1): S60.

289 Dahlman TC, Hellgren MSE, Blomback M. Thrombosis prophylaxis in pregnancy with use of subcutaneous heparin adjusted by monitoring heparin concentration in plasma. *Am J Obstet Gynecol* 1989; 161: 420–5.

290 Clayton JK, Anderson JA, McNicol GP. Preoperative prediction of postoperative deep vein thrombosis. *Br Med J* 1976; ii: 910–12.

291 Crandon AJ, Peel KR, Anderson JA, Thompson V, McNicol GP. Postoperative deep vein thrombosis: identifying high-risk patients. *Br Med J* 1980; 281: 343–4.

292 Lowe GDO, Cooke T *et al.* Thromboembolic risk factors (THRIFT) risks of and prophylaxis for venous thromboembolism in hospital patients. *Br Med J* 1992; 305: 567–74.

293 Working Party. *Report of the RCOG Working Party on Prophylaxis Against Thromboembolism in Gynaecology and Obstet.* The Royal College of Obstetricians and Gynaecologists, London, 1995.

294 Malkamy H. Heparin therapy in post Caesarean septic pelvic thrombophlebitis. *Int J Gynaecol Obstet* 1980; 17: 564–6.

295 Raja Rao AK, Zucker M, Sacks D. Right ovarian vein thrombosis with extension to the inferior vena cava. *Br J Radiol* 1980; 53: 160–1.

296 Bahnson RR, Wendel EF, Vogelzang RL. Renal vein thrombosis following puerperal ovarian vein thrombophlebitis. *Am J Obstet Gynecol* 1985; 1: 152–290.

297 Fickert P, Ramschak H *et al.* Acute Budd–chiari syndrome with fulminant hepatic failure in a pregnant woman with Factor V Leiden mutation. *Gastroenterology* 1996; 111: 1670–3.

298 Yapar EG, Bilge U, Dumanli H, Vural T, Gokmen O. Portal vein thrombosis concomitant with thrombophilia during pregnancy. *Eur J Obstet Gynecol Reprod Biol* 1996; 68: 213–17.

299 Elliott G. Upper extremity deep vein thrombosis. *Lancet* 1997; 349: 1188–9.

300 Koster T, van Boven HH, van Boom SSGE, Briet E. Lover's arm. *Lancet* 1992; 340: 1048 (letter).

301 Shibolet O, Schwaber MJ, Brezis M. Venous thromboembolism during pregnancy. *N Engl J Med* 1996; 335: 1846 (letter).

302 Martinelli I, Cattaneo M, Panzeri E, Taioli E, Mannucci PM. Risk factors for deep venous thrombosis of the upper extremities. *Ann Intern Medicine* 1997; 126: 707–11.

303 McColl MD, Walker ID, Greer IA. The role of inherited thrombophilia in venous thromboembolism associated with pregnancy. *Br J Obstet Gynaecol* 1999; 106: 756–66.

5 Heart disease in pregnancy

Michael de Swiet

Heart disease is a worrying problem to the obstetrician. As we shall see, it is uncommon, with an overall incidence of <1% of all pregnancies; thus, any one obstetrician is unlikely to acquire much experience in the management of heart disease in pregnancy. But heart disease is important, because it causes about 13 maternal deaths per year in the UK, making it second only to pulmonary embolism as a cause of maternal mortality[1]. However, although the overall incidence is <1%, symptoms such as breathlessness or signs such as an ejection systolic murmur that are suggestive of heart disease, may be present in up to 90% of the pregnant population as a consequence of the physiological changes induced by pregnancy itself. There is the problem of diagnosis therefore as well as that of management of a relatively rare condition. In this chapter, we review first the physiological changes that occur in pregnancy, and then consider the incidence, effects and management of heart disease in general. Sections follow, where relevant, on specific acquired and congenital conditions. For other reviews see [2–8, 336].

General considerations

Physiology

In normal individuals, pregnancy is associated with a rise in cardiac output of approximately 40%, i.e. from about 3.5 to 6.0 L/min when at rest [9]. Such data derived from the cardiac catheter laboratory must be viewed with objectivity, and too much reliability must not be placed on individual measurements. There is considerable variation between individuals, and the experimental conditions under which investigations have been made are not always relevant to the situations of clinical importance, such as labour or other forms of exercise. The time of this rise in cardiac output is also open to discussion. However, those investigators who have measured cardiac output early in pregnancy find that it is already markedly elevated in the first trimester.

What has been disputed is whether the cardiac output falls at the end of pregnancy and, if so by how much. It was originally thought that falls in cardiac output demonstrated in late pregnancy were spurious and associated with measurements made in the supine position [10]. However, the fall of cardiac output associated with lying in the supine position is very variable and may be no more than 3% [11].

More recently some non-invasive studies [12] using electrical impedance cardiography [10, 13] and Doppler estimation of aortic velocity [14] have also suggested that cardiac output falls to non-pregnant levels at term. Both these techniques are subject to criticism, the former [15] because of changes that may occur in pregnancy in the pulmonary blood vessels [16] that lead to underestimation of the cardiac output [17], and the latter because the aorta dilates in pregnancy [18]. However, Doppler studies that have also measured the cross-sectional area through which the blood is flowing at the pulmonary [19, 20], aortic [20] or mitral [20] valves or at the ascending aorta [21] are much more reliable and have shown a high correlation with cardiac output measured by thermodilution. The cardiac output is elevated at the onset of labour (mean 7 L/min), rising further within labour. A recent serial study performed by this technique has confirmed the early rise in cardiac output with no fall at the end of pregnancy [22]. In truth there may be some fall in cardiac output towards the end of pregnancy but the degree of fall, if it occurs, is likely to be very variable between subjects and much will depend on the measurement technique and the subject's state of mind at the time measurements are made.

Within the first 2 weeks after delivery, cardiac output falls considerably [19] and at 24 weeks after delivery the cardiac output has fallen further to 5 L/min [20], which is approximately normal for a non-pregnant woman.

The increase in cardiac output is caused partly by an increase in heart rate [23] and partly by an increase in stroke volume. Because blood pressure does not rise in pregnancy, and usually falls, the increase in cardiac output is associated with a marked fall in peripheral vascular resistance. Indeed, it is likely that the fall in peripheral resistance is one if not the major factor that causes the rise in cardiac output [24, 25]. Only part of the change in peripheral vascular resistance can be accounted for by blood flow through the low resistance shunt of the pregnant uterus because cardiac output is elevated during the first trimester, at a time when there is very little change in uterine blood flow.

Oestrogens [26], prostaglandins, including prostacyclin and other locally produced vasoactive substance such as nitric oxide, are likely mediators of the alterations in haemodynamics caused by pregnancy. Calcitonin gene-related peptide also increases in concentration in pregnancy and may contribute to the increase in cardiac output [27]; so too may relaxin, which has positive chronotropic and inotropic effects [28] and rises in concentration in the first trimester in particular. (For further reviews of these changes see [29, 30].)

In contrast to the considerable volume of studies of the haemodynamics of pregnancy in normal individuals, there is little information concerning patients with heart disease. Ueland *et al.* [31] showed that patients with asymptomatic mitral valve disease are unable to increase their cardiac output on exercise in pregnancy to the same level as normal patients at rest. More recently the application of Swan–Ganz catheterization to obstetric patients [32] has begun to yield further information. The usual indication has been the critically ill patient either with very severe pre-eclampsia [33] or septic shock [34]. Using this technique, Clarke *et al.* [35] demonstrated a sharp (10 mmHg) rise in left atrial pressure in patients with mitral stenosis immediately after delivery. These authors found that data from Swan–Ganz catheterizations were particularly helpful in the management of labour in such patients. Similar data have also been published in a patient in labour following myocardial infarction in pregnancy [36].

Natural history

INCIDENCE

The prevalence and incidence of all heart disease in pregnancy varies between 0.3 [37] and 3.5% [38]. Other studies include those of Etheridge [39] who found a prevalence of 0.5% in Australia, Rush *et al.* [40] of 0.8% in South Africa, Buemann and Kragelund [41] of 0.9% in Scandinavia, and recently Tan and de Swiet [42] 0.4% in 17 503 maternities in London. These figures probably do vary because of a genuine difference in the prevalence of heart disease in different communities. For example, the incidence of rheumatic fever varies considerably between countries, and is strongly and inversely related to their relative affluence. In addition, diagnostic criteria change with time and with the different referral populations of different hospitals.

Traditionally heart disease is divided into congenital and acquired; and acquired heart disease can be further subdivided into rheumatic, ischaemic and other.

It is surprising that we have not seen a marked change in the pattern of heart disease in pregnancy as a result of the marked increase in surgery for congenital heart diseases detected in infancy that occurred between 1965 and 1975. These patients should have become pregnant in significant numbers from the age of 18 years onwards so the change should be obvious by now. Yet even specialist centres serving referral hospitals that specialize in paediatric cardiology surgery still do not see more than 10–20 patients per year.

At present, the experience of congenital heart disease in pregnancy is still limited to relatively simple defects, which have usually not been corrected. Seven representative series are shown in Table 5.1. Although the total numbers in each series are different, the overall pattern is similar [43]. The most common lesions found are patent

Table 5.1 The prevalence (percentage) of various forms of congenital heart disease in pregnancy.

	Ohio (*n* = 125) [44]	Queensland (*n* = 93) [45]	Dublin (*n* = 74) [47]	Connecticut (*n* = 233) [65]	Leicester (*n* = 73) [37]	London (*n* = 50) [42]	Sri Lanka (*n* = 50) [48]	Total (*n* = 698)
Patent ductus arteriosus	24	27	9	51 (22)	11	3	3	(18)
Atrial septal defect	29	26	38	33 (14)	22	5	30	(26)
Pulmonary stenosis	4	12	6	23 (10)*	11	4		(9)
Ventricular septal defect	22	14	13	46 (20)	16	11	6	(18)
Tetralogy of Fallot	4	4	13	19 (8)	8	2	1	(7)
Coarctation of the aorta	10	6	6		7	2	1	(5)
Aortic valve disease	3	4	6	28 (12)	7	3	6	(8)
Mitral valve disease				16 (7)	14	17		(7)
Other	2	2		16 (7)	4	2	4	(4)
Unclassified	5	5				1		(1)

*Includes all pregnancies where mother had obstruction to right ventricular outflow.

ductus arteriosus, atrial septal defect and ventricular septal defect, together accounting for about 60% of cases; followed by pulmonary stenosis, ventricular septal defect, Fallot's tetralogy, aortic and mitral valve disease and coarctation of the aorta [44–47]. It is likely that these data reflect no more than the incidence of congenital heart disease in the general female population. However, three of the series are quite old, dating from 1963 to 1975. In the more recent series from Dublin (1981) [47], Leicester (1985) [37], London (1998) [42] and Sri Lanka (1995) [48] we see the effect of surgery, and more cases of patent ductus arteriosus have been corrected.

Studies of surgically corrected congenital heart disease generally indicate good results. For example 22 women who had surgical correction of transposition at the Mayo Clinic had 60 pregnancies that were in general uneventful. Although there is always concern about the ability of the morphological right ventricle to sustain systemic pressures, only one women developed congestive cardiac failure and that was due to systemic atrioventricular valve regurgitation. There were 11 unsuccessful pregnancies, although there was no clear pattern to the pregnancy loss [49].

With regard to acquired heart disease, the dominant lesion in rheumatic heart disease in all series has been mitral stenosis [6, 39, 47, 50–52]. In 1048 patients with rheumatic heart disease reported in Newcastle, Szekely *et al.* [6] found dominant mitral stenosis in 90%, mitral regurgitation in 6.6%, aortic regurgitation in 2.5% and aortic stenosis in 1%.

Other acquired conditions, such as coronary artery disease or symptomatic dysrhythmias, are rarely accurately documented in studies of heart disease in pregnancy. For example Rush *et al.* [40] reported coronary artery disease in 0.4% of 697 patients with heart disease in pregnancy. The same authors found an incidence of 17 cases of dysrhythmia in 679 patients with heart disease in pregnancy. Szekely *et al.* [6] found that 69 of 1048 cases of rheumatic heart disease are complicated by atrial fibrillation. However, ischaemic heart disease and dissection of the thoracic aorta are now important causes of maternal mortality in the UK [1] and this represents a considerable change in disease incidence.

MATERNAL MORTALITY

As we have seen above, heart disease is now the second most common cause of maternal mortality in the UK. Although sporadic fatalities will be seen in all forms of heart disease in pregnancy, maternal mortality is most likely in myocardial infarction, dissecting aneurysm and in those conditions where pulmonary blood flow cannot be increased [53]. For example in the recent Confidential Enquiry into Maternal Mortality in the UK for 1994–96, 60% of the deaths from congenital heart disease were due to pulmonary hypertension; and 52% of the deaths from acquired disease were due to myocardial infarction and dissection in approximately equal numbers [1] (Table 5.2).

Note that in normal pregnancy the pulmonary blood flow has to increase *pari passu* with systemic flow, and the pulmonary vascular resistance also falls [22]. The failure to increase pulmonary blood flow occurs because of obstruction, either within the pulmonary blood vessels or at the mitral valve.

The situation is documented clearly in Eisenmenger's syndrome, where up to now there has been no effective treatment and where the maternal mortality is between 30% and 50% [44, 52, 54, 55]. The maternal mortality (40%) had not improved in a recent UK survey of 15 pregnancies [56]. Only Batson [57] has reported a series of 23 pregnancies with no maternal deaths; the reason for this unusual success is not clear. Elevations in pulmonary vascular resistance are also found in pregnancy in cor pulmonale [40], patients with single ventricle [58], pulmonary venoocclusive disease [38] and in primary pulmonary hypertension. In the latter condition the maternal mortality is about 50% [54, 59–61].

In contrast, in Fallot's tetralogy where the pulmonary vascular resistance is normal, the reported maternal mortality varies between 4% and 20% [54, 62, 63]. Furthermore, the figure of 20% is only based on one maternal death in five pregnancies in the study of Jacoby [62]. Espino Vela and Alvarado-Toro [64] have reported a series of 105 patients with atrial septal defect (confirmed by catheter in 41 patients) who had up to 10 or more pregnancies with no maternal mortality.

Table 5.2 Deaths from heart disease in the UK 1994–6. (From [1].)

Congenital	
Aortic valve disease	2
Ventricular septal defect, Eisenmenger's syndrome	3
Primary pulmonary hypertension	3
Hypertrophic obstructive cardiomyopathy	1
Anomalous coronary arteries	1
Total	10
Acquired	
Puerperal cardiomyopathy	4
Cardiomyopathy and myocarditis	6
Aneurysm of thoracic aorta and its branches	7
Myocardial infarction	6
Pericarditis	1
Thrombosed mitral valve replacement	1
Left ventricular hypertrophy, cause unknown	1
Total	26

The Connecticut series [65] shows how good the results can be with obsessional care, because in 482 pregnancies from 233 women, including eight mothers with Eisenmenger's syndrome, there were no maternal deaths.

In Ehlers–Danlos syndrome the arterial and classic forms have also been associated with high mortality, due to arterial dissection and bleeding [66–68] (see also Chapter 3). More recently the Ehlers–Danlos syndrome has been characterized on the basis of the specific collagen defect [69] and in Ehlers–Danlos syndrome type IV, the maternal mortality is said to be as high as 25% in North America [70]. Further review of the literature based on 50 pregnancies in women with Ehlers–Danlos type IV has estimated the maternal mortality to be 20% per pregnancy [71]. This high mortality, which is largely due to haemorrhage from major blood vessels, has been disputed by Pope and Nicholls [72] in a different series from the UK implying a different referral population or genetic heterogeneity. (There is also a high fetal loss rate attributable to premature rupture of the membrane if either father or mother has Ehlers–Danlos syndrome [73]. This is presumably due to a collagen defect in the fetal membranes.)

In rheumatic heart disease maternal mortality can now be very low although rheumatic heart disease is still a major cause of mortality in developing countries [2]. Szekely *et al.* [6] reported 26 mortalities in 2856 pregnancies (about 1%) complicated by rheumatic heart disease between 1942 and 1969. Half of the deaths were due to pulmonary oedema, which became less common once mitral valvotomy was freely available. These authors reported no maternal deaths in about 1000 pregnancies occurring in 1960. Rush *et al.* [40] also reported a maternal mortality of 0.7% in 450 mothers with rheumatic heart disease in South Africa.

Although prognosis is good in patients with rheumatic heart disease in pregnancy, many clinicians still believe that '... every pregnancy was so many nails of a coffin of a woman with heart disease' [74]. Chesley [75] has reported a group of 38 patients with 51 pregnancies occurring after they were diagnosed as having severe rheumatic heart disease. These were compared with a group of 96 women with equally severe rheumatic heart disease who did not have any pregnancies after diagnosis. The mean survival time (14 years) was no less and, in fact, was greater in the group who did have further pregnancies compared to the group that did not (12 years). I would agree with Chesley [75] that pregnancy does not affect the long-term survival of a woman with rheumatic heart disease, providing that she survives pregnancy itself.

FETAL OUTCOME

The fetal outcome in rheumatic heart disease in pregnancy is usually good, and little different from that in patients who do not have heart disease [36, 39, 46]. However, the babies are likely to be lighter, by about 200 g in the study of Ho *et al.* [76].

In the seven series of patients with congenital heart disease in pregnancy cited in Table 5.1, there was no excess fetal mortality except in the group with cyanotic congenital heart disease, whether associated with pulmonary hypertension or not. Here the babies are generally growth restricted [57, 65, 77, 78], and the fetal loss including abortion may be as high as 45% [43, 51, 57, 65]. Even in the tetralogy of Fallot, which does not have a particularly high maternal mortality, the fetal loss rate may be as high as 57% [43] and the majority of the babies are growth restricted [62]. This is hardly surprising, in view of the mechanisms of placental exchange which cannot compensate for the maternal systemic hypoxaemia. It is likely that the fetus dies because of inadequate oxygen supply or because of prematurity [51] which may be iatrogenic due to elective preterm delivery. In contrast, the fetal results in 40 pregnancies following 27 cases of total correction of Fallot's tetralogy were excellent [79].

Uncorrected coarctation of the aorta has been associated with a 13% fetal loss rate [80] and intrauterine growth restriction [81], presumably because of inadequate placental perfusion. This has also been demonstrated by Doppler ultrasound in Takayasu's arteritis [82]. However, severe aortic occlusion requiring axillofemoral grafting may be compatible with a normally grown fetus [83].

Women or men who themselves have congenital heart disease are naturally concerned that their children may be similarly afflicted. Most studies suggested that for most forms of congenital heart disease the risk to the fetus was 2–4% if either parent was affected [84], at least double the risk in the normal population. A very large study of 393 offspring of 727 individuals with congenital heart disease was in keeping with this; the recurrence risk was 4.1% [85]. The defect is often concordant, i.e. of the same nature as that of the mother [86]. Surprisingly the risk to the fetus is much greater if the mother is affected than if the father is affected [87] suggesting the possibility of cytoplasmic inheritance [87] or some form of genomic imprinting [85].

However, congenital heart disease in the mother may have arisen because of environmental exposure when she herself was a fetus *in utero*. An obvious example is the maternal rubella syndrome. If the maternal abnormality can be shown to be due to an environmental factor, then the fetus probably has the same risk as that of a normal woman without congenital heart disease [88].

Many clinics refer patients who have already born a child with congenital heart disease or who themselves have congenital heart disease at about 20 weeks' gestation to an expert in fetal cardiology for detailed scanning additional to the standard anomaly scan. In the majority of cases the mothers' anxiety about having an abnormal baby will be allayed; in the minority who do have affected fetuses management of the infant including surgery can be planned but termination can also be considered [89].

Detection of heart disease in the fetus on the basis of routine obstetric anomaly scans is already making an impact. In a large UK series of 4799 pregnancies affected by congenital heart disease in the fetus or child a fetal diagnosis was made in 23% and there were 567 terminations of pregnancy for structural heart disease [90]: the precision of these scans will improve with increasing experience and better equipment [91]. In view of the above findings this would make a substantial impact on the pattern of congenital heart disease in surviving children.

Management

All pregnant patients with heart disease should be managed in a combined obstetric/cardiac clinic by obstetric and cardiology teams. In this way, the number of visits that the patient makes to the hospital is kept to a minimum, and the obstetricians and cardiologists obtain the maximum experience in the management of these relatively rare conditions.

HISTORY

As in all forms of medicine, the history is of paramount importance in the assessment of patients with heart disease. In the UK, most patients with heart disease know that they have it, or that they have a heart murmur. It is now rare to make a diagnosis of heart disease *de novo* in pregnancy. In all developed countries, women have frequent medical examinations from the time that they are babies, and attend infant welfare clinics, to when they visit family planning clinics or attend for examination prior to employment. The exceptions are recent immigrants and patients from deprived social classes. For example in a London cohort of 17 503 maternities there were 320 women referred for a cardiac opinion and of these 139 women were referred specifically because of a heart murmur. Only four women were found to have heart disease *de novo* (3% of those referred because of a murmur) and of these three were immigrants. The remaining woman had been known to have a murmur since childhood [42].

The most frequent symptom of heart disease in pregnancy is breathlessness. This is difficult to assess because it is a variable feature of normal pregnancy [92].

Some patients are aware of increasing their ventilation; others are not. Breathlessness arising in pregnancy does not therefore necessarily indicate heart disease, and it is important to consider whether the patients were breathless before they became pregnant. The New York Heart Association (NYHA) classification of heart disease is largely based on limitation of physical activity and associated symptoms of heart disease and is shown below.

Class 1: no resulting limitation of physical activity. Ordinary physical activity does not cause undue fatigue, palpitation, dyspnoea or anginal pain.

Class 2: slight limitation of physical activity. Patients are comfortable at rest. Ordinary physical activity results in fatigue, palpitation, dyspnoea or anginal pain.

Class 3: marked limitation of physical activity. Patients are comfortable at rest. Less than ordinary activity causes fatigue, palpitation, dyspnoea or anginal pain.

Class 4: inability to carry on any physical activity without discomfort. Symptoms of cardiac insufficiency or of anginal syndrome may be present even at rest. If any physical activity is undertaken, discomfort is increased [63].

However, such a classification is only of value if it indicates the severity of the condition at the time of classification, and if it is reliable in predicting the outcome of pregnancy. Both these criteria may not be met with regard to the NYHA classification. We have seen that symptoms of breathlessness are unreliable in pregnancy, and it is also well recognized that patients with mitral stenosis may have no symptoms at the beginning of pregnancy (class 1) and yet have pulmonary oedema by the end of pregnancy (class 4) [6,93]. Indeed, Sugrue *et al.* [47] reported that 39% of 38 patients with rheumatic heart disease, who developed heart failure in pregnancy, were originally classified as class 1; Szekely *et al.* reported that the majority of maternal deaths occurred in women who were initially in NYHA class 1 or 2 [6]. Therefore a precise anatomical diagnosis supported by a pathophysiological assessment of the severity of the condition is preferable.

Palpitations are very common in pregnancy and with syncope (see below) are frequent causes of referral for a medical opinion. Reassurance that such symptoms are common and that they convey no long-term threat to the mother or her child is usually all that is needed. Very often the cause of the palpitation is an increased awareness of the heart beating either regularly or in association with extra systoles; these symptoms presumably relate to the increased cardiac output in pregnancy. Shotan *et al.* [94] performed Holter monitoring in 110 women referred because of palpitations, dizziness and syncope in pregnancy and also in 52 controls who were referred with asymptomatic heart murmurs in pregnancy. Atrial and ventricular premature beats were common in both groups, more so in pregnancy than when the studies were repeated after delivery, and more in the symptomatic than in the asymptomatic group. However, there was no correlation between the incidence of dysrhythmias and symptoms, and only 10% of symptomatic episodes were accompanied by the presence of dysrhythmias. Even when dysrhythmia does occur it is often short in duration and does not necessarily need treatment.

Syncope occurs particularly in the middle trimester. Presumably in these patients peripheral vascular resistance transiently decreases more than cardiac output increases. However, syncope may also occur rarely in severe aortic stenosis, hypertrophic obstructive cardiomyopathy (HOCM, subaortic stenosis), Fallot's tetralogy and Eisenmenger's syndrome. Syncope, like chest pain, can occur because of dysrhythmias, but from the study of Shotan *et al.* [94] quoted above this is rarely the case.

Chest pain is usually a feature of ischaemic disease, but chest pain may also occur in severe aortic stenosis or, more commonly in pregnancy, in HOCM.

PHYSICAL SIGNS

The hyperdynamic circulation of pregnancy causes alterations in the cardiovascular system that mimic heart disease. Thus, 20% of patients originally thought in pregnancy to have rheumatic heart disease may have none at all, following a reassessment performed up to 30 years later.

Premature atrial and ventricular ectopic beats are common in pregnancy [47] and the peripheral pulse is increased in volume, suggesting aortic valve disease to the unwary. The neck veins pulsate more vigorously in pregnancy, but the mean right atrial pressure is unchanged (10 mmHg) and therefore the height of the jugular venous pressure is also unchanged. The heart apex beat is more forceful and because of the increase in cardiac output may suggest cardiomegaly in normal patients. However, if the apex heart beat is >2 cm outside the midclavicular line, this should be considered definitely abnormal.

Oedema is a non-specific sign of heart disease, even in non-pregnant patients. In pregnancy, oedema is a very common finding particularly in the lower limbs where obstruction to the venous return by the enlarging uterus is presumably an important factor. The fall in intravascular colloid osmotic pressure is another cause of oedema.

This may be exacerbated by injudicious administration of crystalloid solutions [96, 97], but it is offset by a concomitant fall in interstitial colloid osmotic pressure [98]. Oedema is so normal in pregnancy that by itself it should not be considered a sign of raised right atrial pressure and therefore of heart disease.

The auscultatory changes in normal pregnancy have been well documented in a phonocardiographic study by Cutford and MacDonald [99]. The first heart sound is loud and a third heart sound is audible in 84% of patients. This is the single greatest cause of confusion, because the third heart sound is interpreted as a diastolic murmur or opening snap. An ejection systolic sound can be heard in 96% of apparently normal pregnant women [99]. The murmur is widely conducted, and can even be heard over the back. Recent Doppler studies suggest that this murmur may often be due to tricuspid regurgitation [100]. In a UK population a systolic murmur discovered *de novo* in pregnancy is only indicative of heart disease in 3% of cases [42].

Although it is said that a diastolic murmur may be present in normal patients, due to blood flow across the tricuspid valve [99], this should be a diagnosis based on exclusion after echocardiography. In addition murmurs may be heard over the right and left second intercostal space, about 2 cm from the sternal edge. They may be systolic or continuous, and can be modified by pressure of the stethoscope. They are thought to be due to blood flow in mammary vessels [99]. Venous hums—continuous murmurs usually audible in the neck and modified by posture—may also be heard in pregnancy as in the non-pregnant state.

Any other murmurs or additional heart sounds should be considered significant. Particular difficulty occurs with systolic murmurs because they are so common in normal pregnancy. Those that are significant are:

1 pansystolic murmurs (ventricular septal defect, mitral regurgitation, tricuspid regurgitation);

2 late systolic murmurs (mitral regurgitation, mitral valve prolapse);

3 ejection systolic murmurs that are louder than grade 3/6 (aortic stenosis), or vary with respiration (pulmonary stenosis), or are associated with other abnormalities, e.g. ejection clicks (valvar pulmonary and aortic stenosis).

The clinical signs of heart disease are briefly discussed in some individual conditions below, but an assessment of the patient's cardiac status should also include the signs of heart failure, whether the patient is cyanosed or has finger clubbing, the presence of pulse deficits and other peripheral signs of endocarditis such as splinter haemorrhages.

INVESTIGATIONS

Chest radiography

The increase in cardiac output and pulmonary blood volume causes slight cardiomegaly, increased pulmonary vascular markings and distension of the pulmonary veins. These return to normal after delivery, and they do not necessarily indicate that the patient has heart disease. The chest radiograph is unhelpful in the diagnosis of minor degrees of heart disease but will, of course, show typical changes in those who have haemodynamically significant heart disease.

Electrocardiography

Oram and Holt [101], reported innocent depression of the ST segment and flattening of the T wave in the left-sided precordial leads in 14% of normal pregnant women. They state that such changes would normally lead one to suspect cardiomyopathy. Boyle and Lloyd-Jones [102] disputed these findings, but most cardiologists would accept that even T-wave inversion and Q waves in lead III [103], which would normally be considered pathological, may be seen in healthy pregnant women. ST segment changes are particularly common at caesarean section [104]. Although a change in the electrical axis of the heart during pregnancy may be part of the explanation [105], it does not account for all these findings. Indeed, pregnancy itself does not account for all the findings, and there may be more variability in the electrocardiogram of healthy non-pregnant women than had previously been realized [101]. As a consequence, in pregnancy the electrocardiogram is more helpful in the diagnosis of dysrhythmias and of rare cases of cardiomyopathy than in the demonstration of a structural abnormality of the heart.

Echocardiography

Studies in non-pregnant individuals have shown that the majority of structural cardiac abnormalities can be detected by echocardiography [106], and this is the technique of choice in pregnancy, because there is no radiation hazard, and because of the detailed information available in skilled hands. Certain abnormalities such as the presence of bacterial vegetations [107] or prosthetic valve dysfunction [108] are better demonstrated by transoesophageal echocardiography where the transducer is mounted on a flexible endoscope passed into the oesophagus at the level of the mediastinum.

Rubler et al. [109], in an echocardiographic study designed to look at changes in cardiac output, also established normal values for chamber size in pregnancy.

To establish the place of routine echocardiography in pregnancy, Northcoate et al. [110] studied 50 consecutive patients referred to a cardiac clinic because of murmurs in pregnancy. They found that echocardiography did not contribute anything further if the clinical assessment and electrocardiogram were normal. A similar study in 103 patients by Mishra et al. [111] had an identical outcome. Therefore, it is not necessary to perform echocardiography in patients who present to cardiologists in pregnancy with heart murmurs and where the cardiologist thinks the heart is normal.

Doppler may also be used to study flow patterns. In a study of 107 apparently normal women, Robson et al. [112] showed regurgitant flow across the tricuspid, mitral and pulmonary valves in 41–90% depending on the valve and gestational age. The prevalence of regurgitant flow across the right heart valves was significantly greater in normal women in pregnancy than in the non-pregnant state. These findings need to be considered when using Doppler to assess abnormal heart valves in pregnancy.

CLINICAL MANAGEMENT AND SURGERY

Patients should be seen in the combined clinic and the nature and severity of their heart lesion assessed. Many patients will have no evidence of any lesion at all, and no further follow-up will be required. Some may only have a mild lesion with no haemodynamic problems, such as congenital mitral valve prolapse, which has an excellent prognosis [113]. Again, no further follow-up is necessary although some may need antibiotic prophylaxis in labour (see below). The remainder do have a condition with real or potential haemodynamic implications. They must first be assessed as to the need for termination, if seen early enough in pregnancy, and secondly as to the need for surgery. In patients with well-managed heart disease, these decisions should have been made before the patient becomes pregnant [42,114], but inevitably some patients present for the first time in pregnancy or have been lost to follow-up before pregnancy.

Because of the mortality statistics indicated above, only Eisenmenger's syndrome, primary pulmonary hypertension and pulmonary veno-occlusive disease are absolute indications for termination of pregnancy. Termination may also be indicated very rarely in patients with such severe lung disease that they have pulmonary hypertension. Under these circumstances, pulmonary artery pressure, if not known, should be measured either directly by Swan–Ganz catheter (see Chapter 1) or indirectly by Doppler echocardiography measuring the tricuspid regurgitant flow velocity. The latter is probably sufficiently accurate providing due allowance is made for the increased tricuspid regurgitation that occurs because of pregnancy alone.

In all other cases, the decision of whether the pregnancy should continue depends on an individual assessment of the risk of pregnancy compared to the patient's desire to have children.

In general, the indications for surgery in pregnancy are similar to those in the non-pregnant state: failure of medical treatment with either intractable heart failure or intolerable symptoms. However, because of the bad reputation of severe mitral stenosis in pregnancy, closed mitral valvotomy [115] or valvuloplasty is performed relatively commonly in patients with suitable heart valves, whereas open-heart surgery is done with reluctance because of worries about the fetus. Szekely *et al.* [6] reported 69 mitral valvotomies during pregnancy after 1951, although only five were performed between 1966 and 1969; presumably after 1966 the majority of patients with mitral stenosis had their valvotomies performed before pregnancy. The indications for valvotomy are pulmonary congestion not responding rapidly to drugs, any episode of pulmonary oedema before pregnancy (likely to recur in pregnancy) and profuse haemoptysis. In patients considered for closed valvotomy or valvuloplasty, there should be no significant mitral regurgitation, the mitral valve should not be calcified, and there should be no other significant valve involvement. The operation is usually performed in the middle trimester, but may be performed at any time in pregnancy. Szekely *et al.* [6] reported only two operative deaths with good fetal results (although there were two spontaneous abortions and six perinatal deaths) in 69 valvotomies in pregnancy.

In a series of 110 closed mitral valvotomies from Sri Lanka there were no maternal deaths and only three fetal losses, all due to abortion [47]. Similar studies have been reported from South Africa (41 valvotomies) [117] and India (126 valvotomies) [118]. Nevertheless, mitral valvotomy has become a rare procedure in the UK. Only one has been performed in a patient referred to Queen Charlotte's Maternity Hospital, London, in the last 15 years, and Sugrue *et al.* reported only three cases from Dublin in 387 pregnancies complicated by rheumatic heart disease. Because very few cardiac surgeons now perform closed mitral valvotomies, preferring the improved control offered by open-heart surgery, this trend will continue. Furthermore, percutaneous balloon mitral valvuloplasty is now an accepted non-surgical technique for relieving mitral stenosis [32, 119] and this treatment could and should be used in many patients who previously would have had closed mitral valvotomies, i.e. those with pliable valves who do not have major mitral regurgitation. The

only potential problems in pregnancy are the extra radiation (which may be minimized by careful planning) and the need for the patient to remain supine for up to 1 h. The technique has been used successfully in pregnancy [120] and is likely to supersede closed mitral valvotomy.

In addition, aortic valvuloplasty has also been performed in pregnancy [121–123], and may avoid the problems of open-heart surgery in pregnancy (see below). The contraindications are again heavy valve calcification and significant regurgitation flow. Aortic valvuloplasty should probably be considered more of a palliative procedure than is mitral valvuloplasty, and these patients are likely to require aortic valve replacement after delivery.

A review of open-heart surgery during pregnancy by Zitnik *et al.* [124] indicated that, although maternal results are reasonable (5% mortality in a group of 22 women with severely affected hearts), the fetal results are not, with a perinatal mortality of 33%. There has been speculation that these poor figures are due to inadequate perfusion of the placenta during cardiopulmonary bypass, either because of relative hypotension or because of lack of pulsatile blood flow [125]. These speculations have been supported by several recent reports of lack of beat-to-beat variation and bradycardia recorded by external cardiotachography during cardiopulmonary bypass [124, 126–129]. Alternatively, some of these cardiotachographic findings may be accounted for by the artificially induced hypothermia occurring during cardiopulmonary bypass. It is likely that the fetus whose placental circulation is already compromised by maternal pre-eclampsia or growth retardation, will be particularly susceptible to the further insults of cardiopulmonary bypass [130]. The earlier reports summarized by Zitnik *et al.* [124] were all of surgery performed early in pregnancy with a high abortion rate. More recently, Eilen *et al.* [127] have reviewed the literature and found no fetal losses in patients operated on after the first trimester. Becker [131] found only 1% maternal and 20% fetal loss in 68 patients operated on at all stages of pregnancy. Nevertheless, the indication for open-heart surgery in pregnancy is usually life-threatening pulmonary oedema that cannot be managed medically.

Although the first case of open-heart surgery in pregnancy involved a woman with Fallot's tetralogy [21] cardiac surgery in pregnancy is rarely considered in congenital heart disease. In coarctation of the aorta, the risk of dissection in pregnancy has probably been exaggerated (see below). Repair would therefore not be advised unless hypertension could not be controlled medically. Valve replacement with an additional aortic prosthesis might be considered in some cases of Marfan's syndrome; the risks would be those already discussed of open-heart surgery.

Antenatal care

After initial assessment of the patient, the remainder of medical management during pregnancy is associated with avoiding, if possible, those factors that increase the risk of heart failure, and treating heart failure vigorously if it occurs. Risk factors for heart failure include infections (particularly urinary tract infection in pregnancy), hypertension (both pregnancy-associated and pregnancy-induced), obesity, multiple pregnancy, anaemia, the development of dysrhythmias and, very rarely, the development of hyperthyroidism. The increase in cardiac output in twin pregnancy, which is about 30% greater than in singleton pregnancy, is made by increasing heart rate and contractility rather than by increasing venous return. This suggests that cardiac reserve is particularly compromised in multiple pregnancy.

Obstetric management before labour includes early ultrasound examination of the conceptus to confirm gestational age and in women with congenital heart disease (see above) second-trimester examination of the fetal heart by ultrasound to exclude congenital malformations. In experienced hands this technique will diagnose or exclude all major congenital malformations by 18 weeks' gestation [132] allowing termination in selected cases, planning of paediatric care in less severely affected fetuses, and reassurance of the mother in the majority.

Those women who do not have haemodynamically significant heart disease require no special obstetric antenatal management. However, if there is haemodynamically significant heart disease and particularly if maternal arterial Po_2 is reduced as in cyanotic congenital heart disease, the fetus should be monitored for growth restriction and intra-uterine asphyxia. This would currently entail assessment of fetal growth and amniotic fluid volume clinically and by ultrasound, measurements of abnormalities in fetal heart rate by ultrasound (cardiotocography), measurement of fetal and maternal placental blood flow indices by Doppler ultrasound, and possibly fetal blood sampling for direct assessment of fetal hypoxia.

TREATMENT OF HEART FAILURE AND DYSRHYTHMIAS

The principles of treatment of heart failure in pregnancy are the same as in the non-pregnant state.

Digoxin

The indications for the use of digoxin are to control the heart rate in atrial fibrillation and some other supraventricular tachycardias, and to increase the force of contraction when given acutely in heart failure. Supraventricular tachycardia in the fetus arising *in utero* has also been managed by maternal digoxin therapy both successfully [133] and unsuccessfully [134–136]. Propranolol [137,138], procainamide [139], amiodarone, flecainide [134] and verapamil [140] have also been given to the mother for this purpose.

Dosage requirements for digoxin are believed to be the same in pregnancy as in the non-pregnant state [141]. Both digoxin [142] and digitoxin [143] cross the placenta, and produce similar drug levels in the fetus to those seen in the mother [142,144]. Digoxin enters the umbilical circulation within 5 min of intravenous administration to the mother [142]. In general, there is no evidence that therapeutic maternal drug levels of digoxin affect the neonatal electrocardiogram [63,144] or cause harm to the fetus. However, Szekely and Snaith [145] reported one case of transient junctional rhythm in the newborn infant of one of a series of mothers who had been digitalized in pregnancy. Although therapeutic maternal drug levels do not harm the fetus, toxic levels do, as was shown in one case of maternal digitoxin poisoning where electrocardiographic changes of digitalis toxicity were demonstrated in the neonate, which died aged 3 days [146].

The demonstration of the production of digoxin-like immunoreactive substance by the fetoplacental unit [147,148] particularly in hypertensive pregnancy [149] questions the validity of some the above statements. In addition digoxin may not cross the placenta so rapidly if fetal placental blood flow is impaired as in the hydropic fetus with congestive cardiac failure *in utero* [136].

Digoxin is also secreted in breast milk, but because the total daily excretion in the mother with therapeutic blood levels would not exceed 2 μg [150] this too is unlikely to cause any harm to the neonate unless it has any other predisposing causes of digitalis toxicity such as hypokalaemia.

Weaver and Pearson [151] have reported that the shorter labours generally believed to occur in patients with heart disease were confined to those patients who took digoxin and they postulated a direct stimulating effect of digoxin on the myometrium. But the babies born to the digoxin-treated mothers were small and born more prematurely and these factors may have been the cause of the more rapid labours.

There may be a place for prophylactic digoxin therapy in selected patients who are not in heart failure. This is most likely to be of value to those patients who are at risk from developing atrial fibrillation, i.e. those with rheumatic mitral valve disease who have an enlarged left atrium, and possibly those who have paroxysmal atrial fibrillation or frequent atrial ectopic beats. But this form of treatment had not been subjected to formal clinical trial, and there is certainly no case for digitalization of all patients with heart disease in pregnancy.

Diuretic therapy

Frusemide is the most commonly used and rapidly acting loop diuretic for the treatment of pulmonary oedema. Ethacrynic acid has also been used successfully in the management of pulmonary oedema associated with mitral stenosis in labour. In congestive cardiac failure where speed of action is not so important, oral thiazides are usually used in the first instance, although the extra potency of the loop diuretics may be necessary in a minority of cases. Anderson [152] showed that the use of thiazide in late pregnancy was not associated with any significant salt or water depletion in the neonate.

There are no risks to the use of diuretics in the treatment of heart failure that are specific to pregnancy, but, as in the non-pregnant state, hypokalaemia is an important complication in a patient who may also be taking digoxin.

Treatment of pulmonary oedema should also include opiates such as morphine, which reduce anxiety and decrease venous return by causing venodilatation. If the patient does not respond to these measures, vasodilating drugs should be used to unload the left ventricle. These include nitrates (cause venous dilatation and reduce preload) and hydrazaline (cause arteriolar dilatation and reduce afterload). Finally angiotensin-converting enzyme inhibitors such as captopril or enalapril should be considered. In this desperate situation the risks to the fetus of captopril (see Chapter 6) are not so important as the maternal risk. Life-threatening pulmonary oedema that does not respond to drug therapy may be helped by mechanical ventilation. If this is successful and in other cases that do not respond to medical treatment, cardiac surgery should be considered, if the patient has a potentially operable lesion.

Dysrhythmias

In general, most haemodynamically significant dysrhythmias are due to ischaemic heart disease, which usually presents in women after their childbearing years, and is rare in pregnancy [153,154]. Atrial fibrillation is of course common in rheumatic heart disease but that too is now very uncommon in the developed world. Therefore, there is limited experience in the treatment of dysrhythmias during pregnancy. Nevertheless, the problem does exist, particularly in patients who have non-ischaemic abnormalities of cardiac conducting tissue, such as occur in the Wolff–Parkinson–White and Lown–Ganong–Levine syndromes.

In addition paroxysmal atrial tachycardia is said to occur more frequently in pregnancy than in the non-pregnant state [155] and also persistent atrial tachycardia may be specific to pregnancy [156,157]. Association between paroxysmal supraventricular tachycardia incidence and the second half of the menstrual cycle has also been demonstrated [158]. In cases that do develop supraventricular tachycardia in pregnancy, hyperthyroidism should be excluded.

Patients who develop atrial fibrillation whether associated with rheumatic heart disease or not may need digoxin for rate control.

Requirements for anticoagulation depend on the presence or absence of additional risk factors. These are valve disease, heart failure and/or impaired left ventricular function demonstrated by echocardiography and thyroid disease. The presence of these risks is not so great as in patients with artificial heart valves (see below) and it would be reasonable to use low molecular weight heparin (LMWH) in prophylactic doses rather than warfarin with its attendant fetal risks. If there are no additional risk factors, low-dose aspirin, 75 mg/day could be used alone [159] although the additional thrombotic risk posed by pregnancy would make many wish to use low-dose subcutaneous heparin in addition. (See mitral stenosis below for comments about atrial fibrillation in this condition.)

The long QT syndrome, which predisposes to ventricular dysrhythmias, has been managed by pre-pregnancy removal of the left stellate ganglion [160]. Propranolol has also been used for the long QT syndrome in twin pregnancy [161].

The antidysrhythmic drugs that have been used most frequently in pregnancy are digoxin (discussed above), quinidine and β-adrenergic blocking agents, in particular propranolol, sotalol, atenolol and oxprenolol. The indications for use of these drugs are unaltered by pregnancy. Although there are isolated case reports of intrauterine growth restriction, acute fetal distress in labour and hypoglycaemia in the neonate, in patients taking β-adrenergic blocking agents [162–164] these have not been confirmed in clinical trials of oxprenolol [165,166], when used for hypertension in pregnancy (see Chapter 6). There is concern that atenolol in particular may cause growth restriction, when taken in the first half of pregnancy [167] although not when used in later pregnancy [167]. Therefore it is best to avoid atenolol if β blockers are needed for control of tachyarythmia in pregnancy. It would seem reasonable to use propranolol, sotalol or oxprenolol in both acute and long-term treatment of supraventricular and ventricular tachycardia in pregnancy.

The dose of oxprenolol received by infants breastfed by mothers taking oxprenolol is very small (0.1 mg/kg/24 h)

[168]. The concentrations of verapamil [169] and the calcium-blocking agent diltiazem [170] are approximately the same in breast milk as in maternal blood. The dose transferred to the infant would therefore be small, and breastfeeding should be encouraged in these circumstances [171].

Quinidine is used to maintain or induce sinus rhythm in patients either after DC conversion or when taking digoxin. It is well tolerated in pregnancy [12] and has only minimal oxytocic effect [38]. However, caution is necessary should the patient require succinylcholine for anaesthesia; pseudocholinesterase levels are depressed in pregnancy and quinidine reduces the enzyme activity still further [172]. Although there is little documentary evidence of the safety of verapamil in pregnancy, it has been widely used and should be considered safe in short-term therapy. There is much less experience of other antidysrhythmic drugs such as bretylium tosylate, disopyramide or amiodarone.

A case report has suggested that mexiletine is safe in pregnancy for the treatment of ventricular dysrhythmias and shown that mexiletine levels in cord blood are similar to those in maternal plasma [173]. However, mexiletine is secreted in fairly high proportions in breast milk where the concentration may be more than four times that in maternal plasma [174] so caution is necessary concerning breastfeeding. The use of disopyramide has been associated with hypertonic uterine activity on one occasion [175]; therefore disopyramide should be used in pregnancy with caution. The long-term risks of phenytoin are well known, and are described in Chapters 2 and 15; however, this drug is only likely to be used in acute treatment of dysrhythmias, particularly those induced by digitalis intoxication. Szekely and Snaith [145] have also used procainamide successfully to abolish atrial fibrillation in pregnancy.

Flecainide has been used for the treatment of supraventricular tachycardia in Wolff–Parkinson–White syndrome [177] and this could be a drug of choice in pregnancy granted that it is often used for the treatment of fetal dysrhythmias.

The use of amiodarone has been reviewed in at least 30 pregnancies [178, 179]. There is no evidence of teratogenicity in the relatively few pregnancies reported [180]. Amiodarone contains large quantities of iodine, is known to affect the maternal thyroid and might affect the fetal thyroid, producing hypo- or hyperthyroidism. Although neonatal hypothyroidism has been noted in one poorly documented case [181] other abnormalities have been mild and transient [182,183]. In addition, neonatal bradycardia and prolongation of QT intervals in the infant have also been found [182,184]. These abnormalities have also been transient and do not seem to have caused any harm. Amiodarone is a potentially dangerous drug, but on the basis of these reports it would seem reasonable to use amiodarone in dysrhythmias resistant to all other therapy in late pregnancy. Patients should not breastfeed when they are taking amiodarone.

Adenosine has become the agent of choice for the acute management of tachyarrythmias in preference to verapamil [185]. There is very little published experience with this drug in pregnancy but it is most unlikely to affect the fetus adversely because it has such a short plasma half-life, <2 s [185]. In any case adenosine has been given directly to the fetus to convert a fetal tachycardia associated with Wolff–Parkinson–White syndrome [186].

DC conversion for tachydysrhythmias is safe in pregnancy and does not harm the fetus [187].

The difficulty arises in considering long-term prophylactic treatment with antidysrhythmic drugs that have not been extensively used in pregnancy. Here each case must be considered on its own merits, paying particular attention to the frequency and severity of the attacks of the dysrhythmia. A single short episode of supraventricular tachycardia associated with no other symptoms does not require prophylactic treatment. Frequent attacks of ventricular tachycardia associated with syncope would require prophylaxis—whatever the outcome for the fetus.

Cardiopulmonary arrest

Cardiopulmonary arrest occurring in pregnancy should be managed initially in the same way as in the non-pregnant state with intubation, ventilation, external cardiac massage and treatment of dysrhythmia. However, very early consideration must be given to immediate delivery by caesarean section for both fetal and maternal reasons. The fetus is relatively resistant to maternal hypoxia, and healthy babies have been delivered 15–25 min after their mothers died or arrested [188–190]. In addition it can be difficult to perform effective external cardiac massage because of inadequate venous return due to obstruction of the inferior vena cava by the gravid uterus. Although this could in theory be overcome by placing the patient in the left lateral position, most maternity units do not have firm wedges that allow cardiopulmonary resuscitation in the left lateral position. Caesarean section is a more practical way of relieving the obstruction [188] and as indicated above may be of benefit for the fetus who would otherwise certainly have died.

ANTICOAGULANT THERAPY (see also section on artificial heart valves, below and Chapter 4)

This is a major problem in the management of patients with heart disease in pregnancy primarily in those who have mechanical heart valves. Anticoagulant therapy may also be necessary in patients with mitral stenosis, those who have pulmonary hypertension due to pulmonary vascular disease, and those with atrial fibrillation.

For conditions such as pulmonary embolus, heparin is safer than warfarin because of its lack of fetal effects relating to the fact that it does not cross the placenta (see Chapter 4). However, therapeutic levels of anticoagulation are required throughout pregnancy for mechanical heart valves. Heparin is conventionally given intravenously if dosing at therapeutic levels is required, and this is effectively impossible for the whole of pregnancy. Attempts have been made to achieve full anticoagulation with subcutaneous unfractionated heparin injections; they have not been successful in this very high-risk situation. It is possible that LMWHs given subcutaneously in therapeutic quantities (about four times prophylactic) will offer a safe alternative but this has not yet been established; nor is it yet known what should be therapeutic doses in pregnancy (see Chapter 4). Certainly high-dose LMWH is not without problems: valve thromboses and maternal deaths have occurred.

Other possible maternal side-effects of heparin therapy such as bone demineralization and heparin-induced thrombocytopenia are either very uncommon or trivial by comparison with those already considered.

Warfarin has no pregnancy-specific maternal risks apart from that of bleeding at delivery; and that problem is usually managed by switching to intravenous heparin treatment for a short time. The risks are all fetal. These risks have already been considered in Chapter 4. In brief they are miscarriage and congenital malformations such as chondrodysplasia punctata in the first trimester, fetal central nervous system (CNS) malformations ascribed to small fetal haemorrhages in the second and third trimesters, and gross fetal bleeding resulting in retroplacental and intracerebral haemorrhage in the third trimester.

The risks of warfarin therapy seem to be dose dependent being much greater at daily doses more than 5 mg [191]. Vitale *et al.* [191] found fetal complications in 22 of 25 pregnancies where the mother was taking more than 5 mg warfarin daily. Eighteen of these complications were miscarriages. By comparison there were only five complications (four miscarriages) in 33 women taking 5 mg or less daily. In all cases the international normalized ratio (INR) was being kept between 2.5 and 3.5.

The use of the minimum dose of warfarin maintaining an INR no greater than 3 rather than the generally recommended 3–4 [192] may decrease the teratogenic and abortion risks of warfarin [193] without any increase in the risk of thromboembolism [194].

It is also possible that the teratogenic effect of dindevan may be less than that of warfarin [176] but there are not the data to prove this; because there is more experience in general with warfarin, I would suggest that this drug should be used in preference.

Anticoagulation is considered further in the section below regarding mechanical heart valves.

LABOUR

Labour should not be induced because of heart disease; indeed, the risks of failed induction and of possible sepsis are relative contraindications. Nevertheless, these risks are slight, and induction should not be withheld if it is necessary for obstetric reasons. Furthermore, induction near term may be justified to plan delivery in daylight hours, in complicated cases requiring optimal medical support. A note of caution is necessary concerning the use of prostaglandin E_2 for the induction of labour in cardiac patients. Prostaglandin E_2 is a potent vasodilator and causes a marked rise in cardiac output [195]. In very high dosage when used for postpartum haemorrhage [196] and for termination of pregnancy [197], prostaglandin E has caused cardiac arrest in patients with normal hearts. Prostaglandins have also caused very severe deterioration in pulmonary oedema in a patient with pre-eclampsia [198]. Although there need not be a moratorium on the use of prostaglandins for induction of labour in cardiac patients, the minimum dose should be used, and prolonged treatment should not be attempted.

Patients with heart disease, particularly those with restrictive heart disease such as mitral stenosis, are at risk during labour because of the increase in cardiac output that occurs at this time [19]. This occurs for a number of reasons: physical exertion; pain; and the contractile effect of the uterus, which expels blood and increases left atrial pressure [199]. In addition many women in labour are given copious quantities of intravenous crystalloid fluids. If they have normal hearts, they can cope with the resultant increase in circulating blood volume and decrease in colloid osmotic pressure [97]. Patients with heart disease cannot, and may develop pulmonary oedema.

Patients with heart disease are also particularly sensitive to aortocaval compression by the gravid uterus in the supine position, causing marked hypotension with maternal and fetal distress. The risk of this is even greater after epidural anaesthesia [200]. Wedges to maintain the patient in the left lateral position can be helpful [201].

Some centres are gaining increasing experience in the use of elective central catheterization (Swan–Ganz technique) to measure the right atrial pressure, wedge pressure (indirect left atrial pressure) and the cardiac output in labour in patients with heart disease (see above). There is no doubt that this technique allows a much more rational use of fluid therapy, diuretics and inotropic agents. Preliminary results would also suggest that measurement of central venous pressure alone is so misleading as an index of left ventricular filling pressure that it should not be used for this purpose (although it is still invaluable in patients with bleeding problems). However, the technique of Swan–Ganz catheterization is quite difficult and it has a significant morbidity. Therefore, it should only be used in centres where there is sufficient experience.

Most patients with heart disease do have quite rapid uncomplicated labours. In the majority, analgesia is best given by epidural anaesthesia, which is a highly effective form of analgesic treatment. The effects of epidural block are complex and have not been fully evaluated. In normal patients having elective caesarean section where the cardiac output has not increased because of labour, epidural block in the left lateral position does not decrease cardiac output even though the systemic arterial pressure falls [202] (by contrast spinal anaesthesia causes a marked fall in cardiac output [203]). But in the labouring woman epidural block has the capacity to reduce the elevated cardiac output because of its efficacy as an analgesic and because of venodilatation and reduction of preload. But the effects of caval occlusion may be exaggerated by epidural block, which can also inhibit compensatory mechanisms for blood loss [204]. In some specific cardiac conditions such as Eisenmenger's syndrome and hypertrophic cardiomyopathy there is concern about the use of epidural block because of the reduction of afterload and preload. Also if epidural block is used rather than general anaesthesia for caesarean section, patients who are breathless may not be able to lie flat enough when awake.

However, in most centres regional block is now preferred to general anaesthesia for maternal and fetal reasons in uncomplicated pregnancy and there are therefore *a priori* reasons for preferring regional block in patients with heart disease. In the end the decision concerning the use of epidural block in patients with heart disease must be made jointly by the anaesthetist, obstetrician, cardiologist and the patient.

It would seem sensible to keep the second stage of labour short in order to decrease maternal effort in patients with heart disease, but there is obviously no advantage in performing a forceps delivery in a woman who is going to push her baby out quite easily herself.

The use of oxytocic drugs in the third stage of labour is debated. The theoretical disadvantage is that ergometrine and Syntocinon will cause a tonic contraction of the uterus, expressing about 500 mL of blood into a circulation whose capacitance has also been made smaller by associated venoconstriction. In patients with heart disease, left atrial pressure may rise by 10 mmHg at the third stage of labour. This is particularly obvious in patients with mitral stenosis (Fig. 5.1) [205]. However, the management of postpartum haemorrhage in a patient with heart disease is not easy. I would suggest using Syntocinon in all patients in the third stage, unless they are in heart failure when oxytocics should be withheld altogether. Syntocinon has less effect on blood vessels than ergometrine and can be given by infusion. This infusion can be accompanied by intravenous frusemide.

ENDOCARDITIS AND ITS PREVENTION

The Confidential Enquiries into Maternal Death in the UK report that 11 (10%) of the 115 cardiac deaths occurring between 1984 and 1996 were in association with endocarditis [1]. In the majority of the cases that have been reported in obstetric and gynaecological practice, the organism was a *Streptococcus* [206]. However, the case for antibiotic prophylaxis in labour has not been proven. There are several large series of patients with heart disease in pregnancy where no antibiotics have been given, and where no endocarditis has been observed [47,208]. It is difficult to document bacteraemia in labour [80,209]. Several authors have argued persuasively against antibiotic prophylaxis [6,7]. A British working party recommended antibiotic prophylaxis in labour only in women with

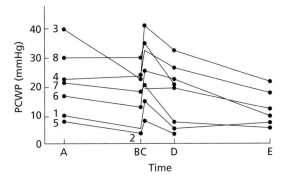

A First-stage labour
B Second-stage labour, 15–30 min before delivery
C 5–15 min postpartum
D 4–6 hours postpartum
E 18–25 hour postpartum [205]

Fig 5.1 Intrapartum alterations in pulmonary capillary wedge pressure (PCWP) in eight patients with mitral stenosis.

artificial heart valves, who are a particularly high-risk group if they do contract endocarditis [210].

Yet, from the data of the Confidential Maternal Mortality series, it would seem that women are at increased risk from endocarditis in pregnancy. What is not clear from some of these reports is whether endocarditis was contracted during labour, and was potentially preventable by peripartum antibiotic prophylaxis, or whether it arose at some other time. One case that is described in detail in the 1975–78 report [211] did appear to develop endocarditis during a normal delivery, and other similar non-fatal cases have been reported [212], in one associated with premature rupture of membranes as a possible source of sepsis [213]. Until more details are available, I will continue to advise antibiotic prophylaxis in all patients with structural heart disease except mitral valve prolapse without reflux where the risk of endocarditis is minimal. The antibiotics that we use are intramuscular ampicillin 500 mg and intramuscular gentamicin 80 mg; three injections are given every 8 h at the onset or induction of labour [214]. The patient who is penicillin sensitive receives one intravenous injection of vancomycin 1 g [214,215] followed by intravenous gentamicin 120 mg [216]. Vancomycin should be given over 60 min [217] because of the risk of idiosyncratic hypotensive reactions [218]. Because of these risks, intravenous teicoplanin 400 mg has been suggested as an alternative to vancomycin and gentamicin [219].

A compromise is to use prophylactic antibiotics only in those cases at high risk, i.e. those with previous endocarditis, valve replacement, instrumental delivery or delivery following prolonged rupture of membranes.

PULMONARY OEDEMA AND OTHER CARDIOVASCULAR SIDE-EFFECTS OF β-SYMPATHOMIMETIC DRUGS

Those obstetricians and physicians who practise in Western communities are more likely to see pulmonary oedema related to treatment of other conditions in pregnancy such as preterm labour and pre-eclampsia (see Chapter 6) or even malaria [135] than to structural heart disease. For example, in over 6000 obstetric admissions in Hamilton, Ontario, there were 12 cases of pulmonary oedema of which seven were related to parenteral tocolytic therapy. The incidence of pulmonary oedema in patients treated with isoxsuprine was 0.5% [220].

Whitehead *et al.* [221] reported the occurrence of chest pain and ischaemic electrocardiogram changes in one patient treated for 5 h with intravenous salbutamol (4.2 mg) and subsequently reported pulmonary oedema in another patient given salbutamol 2.2 mg intravenously over 6 h. Davies and Robertson [223] reported another case of

pulmonary oedema after the use of higher infusion rates of salbutamol (20 μg/min) over a longer period (56 h).

In North America, terbutaline (Bricanyl) is used to treat preterm labour. It has the advantage that it can be given subcutaneously. Stubblefield [224] reported one case of pulmonary oedema in which dexamethasone administration was an additional risk factor. Rogge *et al.* [225] reported three similar cases and cited knowledge of six other cases occurring in California. Pulmonary oedema has also been reported with the use of fenoterol [226] and ritodrine [227].

β-sympathomimetics are widely used for the treatment of premature labour [228] even though there are contradictory reports concerning their efficacy [229]. Possible mechanisms for pulmonary oedema include tachycardia, which occurs both directly and reflexly because of associated vasodilatation. Whitehead *et al.* suggested that vasodilatation might also be caused by concurrent administration of hydralazine and methyldopa for hypertension and cited one similar maternal death reported to the Committee of Safety of Medicine after use of salbutamol and methyldopa [221]. Glucocorticoids given for fetal lung maturation may further contribute to the increased circulating blood volume; so to, may the use of saline as an infusing fluid rather than dextrose [230].

Pulmonary oedema may be precipitated by the sudden reduction in vascular capacitance caused by giving ergometrine after delivery [223].

In addition, β-sympathomimetic agents have metabolic effects. They cause a rise in blood glucose by increasing glycogenolysis and decreasing glucose uptake. Free fatty acid and lactate concentrations increase, and hypokalaemia has also been reported [231]. These factors may further impair myocardial function in a situation that is already haemodynamically unfavourable. Although it has been suggested that tachycardia alone [232] and/or circulatory overload [223,233] are the real causes of pulmonary oedema in these patients, this seems unlikely. Pulmonary oedema is a rare complication of modern obstetrics, and its occurrence on so many occasions with the use of β-sympathomimetics suggests that there is specific interaction.

Because there is no universal belief in the efficacy of long-term β-sympathomimetics, and because of the maternal risk, the following guidelines are suggested concerning their use for the treatment of preterm labour. Use the minimum volume of infusate; this is best achieved by administering the drug with a syringe driver rather than a drip-set. Use dextrose as an infusate rather than saline. β-sympathomimetic infusions should not be given for more than 24 h, except in exceptional circumstances. The risk of cardiovascular side-effects increases in infusions given for more than 24 h. A delay in delivery of 24 h should allow sufficient time for glucocorticoids to enhance fetal lung maturation.

β-sympathomimetic drugs should be given with great care to patients with pre-existing heart disease. They may even unmask previously asymptomatic peripartum cardiomyopathy [234]. The nature and severity of the heart disease are obviously critical (e.g. there would probably be no additional risk of giving salbutamol to a patient with mild mitral regurgitation, whereas such therapy could be fatal in a patient with severe mitral stenosis).

β-sympathomimetics should not be used in conditions that predispose to supraventricular tachycardia such as Wolff–Parkinson–White and Lown–Ganong Levine syndromes [235]. β-sympathomimetic drugs should be stopped if any dysrhythmias develop, if the heart rate exceeds 120/min or if the patient develops chest pain or breathlessness.

However, non-specific electrocardiogram changes, ST depression, T-wave inversion and prolonged QT interval occur in about 75% [236,237] of patients given ritodrine. Similar data have been obtained in patients taking fenoterol. Therefore if β-sympathomimetics are used, these electrocardiogram changes occurring in isolation should not be criteria for stopping therapy.

Auscultation of the lung bases should be performed regularly in patients given parental β-sympathomimetics to detect early signs of pulmonary oedema. But this is a relatively insensitive technique. Transcutaneous monitoring of oxygen saturation is now widely available and will almost certainly detect hypoxaemia due to pulmonary oedema before any abnormalities can be found in the lungs clinically. Therefore continuous monitoring of oxygen saturation with a saturation meter should be employed in all patients receiving β-sympathomimetics for tocolysis [239]. The critical level appears to be an oxygen saturation of 94% corresponding to a Pao_2 of 10 kPa (75 mmHg). Above this level there is no threat to the mother (or fetus).

Following the widespread application of the above guidelines pulmonary oedema in association with tocolytic therapy has become much less common.

If β-sympathomimetic drugs are used, the obstetrician should also be aware of the risk of other therapies. Steroids will exacerbate hyperglycaemia as well as causing an increase in circulating blood volume. This will be exacerbated by vasodilator drugs, so scrupulous attention must be paid to fluid balance and the maternal heart rate.

Specific conditions occurring during pregnancy

Many specific conditions have already been mentioned. However, some give particular management problems and are considered below.

Acquired heart disease

CHRONIC RHEUMATIC HEART DISEASE, VALVULAR HEART DISEASE

This form of heart disease used to be the commonest in pregnancy in the UK and still is in many parts of the world. Szekely *et al.* have given exhaustive accounts from Newcastle of rheumatic heart disease in pregnancy [6,145]. By far the most important lesion is mitral stenosis, which may be the only lesion or the dominant abnormality amongst several others. Women with mitral stenosis are particularly likely to develop pulmonary oedema in pregnancy because of the increase in cardiac output, the increase in heart rate, preventing ventricular filling and the increase in pulmonary blood volume [80]. Mitral stenosis is the lesion that is most likely to require treatment for pulmonary oedema or heart failure (see above) and also to require surgery during pregnancy. Open and closed heart surgery and also mitral valvuloplasty have already been discussed (see above).

In patients with mitral stenosis who develop pulmonary oedema whether they are in sinus rhythm or have atrial fibrillation, the first line of treatment should be β blockade with propranolol to slow the heart rate. These women do not have heart failure and therefore the usual constraint not to use β blockade in heart failure does not apply. Instead they have a rate-dependent problem. At rapid heart rates the relative time for diastole is shortened and this prevents left atrial emptying. In patients who have atrial fibrillation, digoxin can be used as well to slow the ventricular rate but β blockade is more important in the first instance.

The risk of systemic thromboembolism in mitral stenosis in pregnancy is about 1–1.5% [6]. Patients with large left atria and those in atrial fibrillation have a greater risk. However, the risk is not so great as with artificial heart valves and it therefore seems reasonable to manage such patients with subcutaneous heparin in prophylactic doses supported by low-dose aspirin (75 mg daily).

The haemodynamic changes associated with labour in patients with mitral stenosis have been documented by Swan–Ganz catheterization. Patients entering labour with a wedge pressure (indirect left atrial pressure) <14 mmHg are unlikely to develop pulmonary oedema [240] (see Fig. 5.1).

Mitral regurgitation puts a volume load on the left atrium and left ventricle, but it does not cause pulmonary hypertension until late in the condition, and heart failure is rare in pregnancy; it usually occurs in older women. Endocarditis is more common in patients with mitral regurgitation, particularly if they are in sinus rhythm. It is now realized that many patients who were thought to have rheumatic mitral regurgitation do in fact have congenital abnormalities of the mitral valve. Although such abnormalities may be associated with dysrhythmias and endocarditis, this is uncommon, particularly in pregnancy. For practical purposes (i.e. endocarditis prophylaxis) patients with mitral valve prolapse are only at risk of endocarditis if they have mitral regurgitation.

Pregnancy may be associated with rupture of the chordae tendineae of the mitral valve [241] and the subsequent deterioration in cardiac function. This may occur in normal mitral valves or in those affected by rheumatic carditis or other disease (e.g. systemic lupus erythematosus) [242]. Very rarely, obstruction in the left atrium may be due to left atrial myxoma, which has been reported in pregnancy [243]. The echocardiogram is pathognomonic and the tumour should be removed surgically.

Rheumatic aortic valve disease is much less common in women than in men, and much less common than mitral valve disease in pregnancy. In young women (and now in the whole population) aortic valve disease is usually not rheumatic in origin. Severe aortic regurgitation causes pulmonary oedema; aortic stenosis may be associated with chest pain, syncope and sudden death. Although both conditions are usually not severe enough to be a problem in pregnancy, critical aortic stenosis may cause maternal death and should be relieved by aortic valve surgery or valvuloplasty (see above). In the non-pregnant state a 100-mmHg pressure gradient across the aortic valve is usually considered to indicate critical aortic stenosis. But the gradient depends on the cardiac output [244] and this is considerably increased in pregnancy. Therefore in pregnancy aortic gradients must be assessed with caution.

Disease of the tricuspid valve almost never occurs in isolation. Also, tricuspid valve disease rarely requires specific treatment; the patient improves when the rheumatic disease of the other valves is treated, either medically or surgically. Although there are case reports of successful pregnancy following triple valve replacement (aortic, mitral and tricuspid), it is unusual for such surgery to be necessary for patients within the reproductive age group [245].

ACUTE RHEUMATIC FEVER

In general there has been a steady decline in the incidence of rheumatic fever, although there was a resurgence in the USA between 1985 and 1988 [246]. Acute rheumatic fever is now very uncommon in pregnancy. The diagnosis may be missed in patients who only complain of non-specific malaise and joint pains, and who on investigation only have fever and anaemia that does not respond to haematinics. The more florid signs of swollen joints, rheumatic nodules and skin rashes do not necessarily occur in adults. The diagnosis may be made on the basis of a history of previous sore throat, elevated antistreptolysin O (ASO) titre, and electrocardiogram evidence of prolonged PR and QT intervals. The erythrocyte sedimentation rate (ESR) should be elevated to >80 mm/h, because levels of 40 mm/h are common in pregnancy. The level of C-reactive protein is also elevated and this is not affected by pregnancy.

If rheumatic fever does develop in pregnancy, it is likely to be severe with a high risk of heart failure due to myocarditis, which is part of the triad of pericarditis and endocarditis. Treatment should be bed rest, salicylates, steroids and penicillin (for any residual streptococcal infection). The patient should then receive a prolonged period of prophylactic penicillin therapy. Chorea, another manifestation of the rheumatic process, is described in Chapter 15.

PREGNANCY IN PATIENTS WITH MECHANICAL HEART VALVES, TISSUE VALVES OR PROSTHESES

Those patients who have successful isolated aortic or mitral valve replacement usually have near normal cardiac function and do not incur haemodynamic problems in pregnancy [247]. Even those patients with multiple valve replacements usually have sufficient cardiac reserve for a successful pregnancy [248].

As described earlier, anticoagulation is the major problem in these patients and the maternal need for a high level of anticoagulation has been stressed. A suggested target level using warfarin is INR 3–4 [192].

Maternal issues

One way of avoiding the problem of anticoagulation is to use bioprosthetic or homograft valves that do not require anticoagulation. Both these forms of biological graft are likely to have shorter lives and need to be replaced sooner than are mechanical valves. Homografts are usually only inserted in the aortic position; in the largest study to date (41 pregnancies) the maternal and fetal results from Auckland, New Zealand, were excellent with no evidence of valve deterioration [249]. In the same study the fetal results were also good in 41 pregnancies with bioprosthetic valves but structural deterioration of the valves occurred in 10% in the mitral position [249]. The same authors believe that pregnancy does not increase the rate of valve deterioration [250]. This is a contentious and important issue. If the New Zealand experience can be generally extrapolated, then it is tempting to suggest that young women who are likely to want children and who need valve replacement should have a bioprosthetic valve, have their children and accept the need for further surgery after childbearing. The contrary view is put by Oakley [251]. She argues that pregnancy does accelerate bioprosthetic valve deterioration, and that in any case patients with bioprosthetic valves may require anticoagulation for example when they develop atrial fibrillation. This important issue is unresolved at present.

Granted the fetal problems of warfarin therapy, some women with mechanical valves will refuse anticoagulation however they are advised. Limet and Crondin [253] have reported two patients with embolic problems following artificial valve replacement when the patients were either not anticoagulated or anticoagulated inadequately during pregnancy. They calculated from their own series that the risk of a woman having an embolic episode if she had an artificial valve and did not take anticoagulants was one in every 100 months of exposure. Their literature search suggested that the risk of thromboembolism in such patients is even higher (25% per pregnancy, one in 40 months). These embolic problems carry a high mortality from valve thrombosis and morbidity from stroke. Therefore patients with mechanical valves must be anticoagulated during pregnancy.

Ahmad et al. [254] and Biale et al. [255] have reported one and four cases, respectively, where patients with artificial heart valves have been treated with dipyridamole alone during pregnancy. There were no incidents of thromboembolism, but from the data above these series are too small to justify this form of therapy. Clinical experience suggests that dipyridamole alone will not have sufficient anticoagulant power in this very high-risk situation and this form of treatment is not recommended.

Heparin therapy is easier to control and there appears to be less maternal bleeding. However, where there is a risk of systemic thromboembolism as in heart disease, subcutaneous unfractionated heparin treatment does not seem to be adequate. Indeed there are reports of prosthetic valves that thrombosed during pregnancy when the mothers were either managed with subcutaneous unfractionated heparin [256,257] or were not anticoagulated [114]. Such disasters have been managed by thrombolysis or emergency cardiopulmonary bypass and caesarean section (assuming fetal maturity) followed by prosthetic valve replacement [258]. In the Auckland study [249, 250] there were nine pregnancies with cardiac complications including two valve thromboses in the 14 women with mechanical valves managed with heparin for the majority of their pregnancies; whereas there was only one such complication in 33 women managed with warfarin alone. The price to pay for warfarin treatment of women with mechanical valves in pregnancy is the very poor fetal outcome.

Fetal issues

As indicated elsewhere there is effectively no fetal risk from heparin because it does not cross the placenta. The principle risk from warfarin and one that is not generally realized is that of miscarriage. In the Auckland series of 33 pregnancies with mechanical valves treated by warfarin alone there were six terminations and 15 miscarriages amongst the remaining 27 pregnancies, a miscarriage rate of 55%; this should be compared with three miscarriages in 13 ongoing pregnancies (23%) where heparin was substituted in the first trimester.

The other well-described first-trimester effect of warfarin is the skeletal abnormality, chondrodysplasia punctata. The incidence of this varies from 0% [252] to 67% [259] in retrospective studies; one prospective study found an incidence of 29% [260]. This is difficult to assess because the severity of the abnormalities is so variable. They may consist of minor facial deformities [260] or a major syndrome resulting in death in the second trimester [249].

There are no good incidence data for the second trimester effects such as optic atrophy and microcephaly, thought to be due to repeated minor intracerebral haemorrhage. However, these are unlikely to be common because we found no difference in cognitive ability in 20 4-year-olds exposed to warfarin in the second and third trimesters compared to well-matched controls [261]. Nevertheless, the abnormalities are worrying because they are potentially very severe.

The fetal problem of anticoagulation is shown in four series from the Hammersmith Hospital, London [262], the National Maternity Hospital, Dublin [263], from Hong Kong [114] and from Barcelona [193] (Table 5.3). In the Dublin series of 18 pregnancies, all the patients were anticoagulated and there were eight fetal losses and one case of warfarin embryopathy. In the Hammersmith series, 24 pregnancies not treated with anticoagulants (usually because they had biological valves) resulted in 23 normal babies. Fifteen pregnancies treated with oral anticoagulants resulted in only seven healthy babies. In the Hong Kong series there were 10 fetal losses in 30 pregnancies treated with anticoagulants but only one fetal loss in the group not treated with anticoagulants. In a mixed series of 98 pregnancies Vitali et al. [264] confirmed that the risk of warfarin is increased fetal loss, particularly abortion.

Recommendations

There is no ideal solution to the problem. I would recommend that patients conceive taking warfarin; although it might be theoretically attractive to conceive taking some

Table 5.3 Fetal outcome of oral anticoagulation in pregnancy in mothers with artificial heart valves.

	Hammersmith [247]	Dublin [263]	Hong Kong [114]	Barcelona [193]
Number of pregnancies	39	18	41	46
Number anticoagulated and fetal mortality and morbidity (% of those anticoagulated)	15 (53)	18 (50)	30 (40)	42 (31–38)
Causes of fetal mortality and morbidity (% of those anticoagulated)				
Abortion	3 (20)	8 (44)	10 (33)	12 (21–29)*
Perinatal deaths	4 (27)	0 (0)	0 (0)	2 (0–5)*
Fetal malformation	1 (7)	1 (5)	2 (7)	2 (0–4)*
Number not anticoagulated and fetal mortality and morbidity (% of those not anticoagulated)	24 (4)	0 (0)	11 (9)	3†

*Not stated which of the fetal losses etc. were in the anticoagulated group so possible range is given.
† Fetal mortality and morbidity not known in the group who were not anticoagulated.

form of heparin, conception cannot be planned with precision and may take many months, thus exposing the woman unnecessarily to the extra risk of thromboembolism; let alone to the extra inconvenience of having to give herself heparin injections. If warfarin can be discontinued within the first 4 weeks following conception, there should be little risk of congenital malformation; fetal damage occurring at this time usually causes abortion.

If facilities exist the patient should then be admitted to hospital for an intravenous infusion of heparin aiming to double the activated partial thromboplastin time (APTT) from 6 weeks' to 12 weeks' gestation. This will protect the fetus the stage of pregnancy when it is at greatest risk from warfarin complications, particularly miscarriage. But the woman cannot take intravenous heparin throughout pregnancy so she should be restarted on warfarin after 12 weeks with target INR 3.

At 37 weeks when the risk of bleeding in the warfarinized fetus in association with labour seems to be too great, the patient should be admitted to hospital and given continuous intravenous heparin. The aim should be again to double the APTT. It is believed that the clotting system of the fetus will return to normal after warfarin has been withheld for about 1 week. At that time, maternal heparin therapy should be reduced to give a anti-X-a heparin level of <0.2 units/mL, and/or a thrombin time that is not prolonged and labour should be induced. If the patient inadvertently goes into labour taking warfarin, she should be given vitamin K to reverse the action of warfarin in the fetus and started on heparin therapy as above. In extreme cases, vitamin K has been given intramuscularly to the fetus

in utero by transamniotic injection [265]. It could now be given by cordocentesis.

After delivery, because of the risk of maternal postpartum haemorrhage, the patient should continue to receive heparin for about 7 days; then warfarin may be recommenced. This is not a contraindication to breastfeeding, because insignificant quantities of warfarin are secreted in breast milk [266]. However, dindevan is excreted in breast milk [267] and patients taking dindevan should not breastfeed.

The alternative that is now available is to take LMWH in therapeutic doses, accepting the current uncertain status of this treatment with regard to maternal thromboembolic risk. LMWH could be substituted in the 6–12-week intravenous heparin period or it could be given for the whole of pregnancy. Patients should not deliver taking therapeutic levels of LMWH because of the bleeding risk; the alternatives are just to stop LMWH 24 h before planned delivery and recommence afterwards; or to cover this period with prophylactic doses of LMWH or unfractionated heparin. There is insufficient experience of high-dose LMWH therapy in this and other circumstances to make firm recommendations [268].

Low-dose aspirin (75 mg daily) should be added to any subcutaneous heparin regimen because of its antithrombotic effect and relative safety.

The justification for the use of heparin in the first part of pregnancy comes from the study of Iturbe-Alessio *et al.* [260] in Mexico. They discontinued warfarin in 35 women as soon as they reported in pregnancy and substituted subcutaneous unfractionated heparin 5000 units twice daily until the end of the 12th week. At this stage warfarin was recommended to be replaced by heparin at the end of pregnancy. The results were compared with those in 37 controls who continued warfarin throughout the early part of pregnancy. In the control group there was an extraordinarily high rate of embryopathy (30%) mostly diagnosed on the basis of minor abnormalities of the face. There were no cases of embryopathy and only two abortions in 23 women who discontinued warfarin before 7 weeks; there were two cases of embryopathy in eight continuing pregnancies where warfarin was discontinued between 7 and 12 weeks.

The price to pay for this form of treatment was two massive valve thromboses in the heparin-treated group. Although the diagnosis of warfarin embryopathy must be questioned because of its very high incidence in the control group, it does appear that withholding warfarin between 7 and 12 weeks may prevent it. Ten thousand units of heparin per day is a very low dose in pregnancy and a more aggressive policy [269] with an adjusted dose continuous intravenous infusion [270] should reduce the incidence of embolism.

MYOCARDIAL INFARCTION

Myocardial infarction is rare in pregnancy and in young women in general. Only 1% of admissions for myocardial infarction occur in women younger than 45 years [271]. In 1996 Badui and Enciso [272] cited only 109 cases of myocardial infarction in pregnancy in the literature since 1922. Most of these cases were in women aged 30–40 years (mean age 32 years). However, the increasing incidence of myocardial infarction in women and the increasing age at which women become pregnant may result in an increased incidence of myocardial infarction in pregnancy. Table 5.2 shows that currently myocardial infarction and cardiomyopathy are second only to dissecting aneurysm as single causes of death from heart disease in pregnancy in the UK.

The immediate mortality from myocardial infarction in pregnancy is 19% [272]; some women die up to 4 years after the original event, making the overall mortality 32% [273]. The overall mortality from myocardial infarction rises during pregnancy from nil in the first trimester to 50% in the puerperium; surprisingly, younger patients are more likely to have myocardial infarction in the puerperium and therefore have a higher mortality [274]. Pregnancies in these younger patients have frequently been complicated by pre-eclampsia [275].

The precise mechanism of myocardial infarction is open to speculation. Women have a high incidence of coronary spasm, and atypical mechanisms seem to be common in pregnancy. Beary *et al.* [275] suggest that the group of patients with myocardial infarction occurring in the puerperium includes those who are most likely to have spasm or coronary artery thrombosis unassociated with atherosclerotic narrowing as described by Ciraulo and Markovitz [276]. The syndrome of myocardial infarction with normal coronary arteries occurring in young women is well documented [277]. In the non-pregnant state the prognosis is good if they survive the initial episode. Primary dissection of the coronary arteries is another cause of myocardial infarction particularly peripartum [278,279] when some cases have been associated with β-sympathomimetic tocolysis [280]. Coronary artery dissection in general is rare but more than 70% of cases occur in women and 25% of these cases have occurred at the end of or immediately after pregnancy [281]. This is presumably another example of the tendency for pregnancy-induced changes in vessel walls to cause any fault in arteries such as coronary, splenic [282, 283], adrenal or even the aorta [284] to rupture in pregnancy (see section on coarctation of the aorta, below) [285,286]. Iliac artery dissection has also been reported [287].

Because arteries do seem particularly 'fragile' in pregnancy, caution is necessary concerning angioplasty immediately following myocardial infarction in pregnancy [153] or even concerning coronary arteriography, which itself may precipitate dissection [288].

Anomalous origin of the coronary arteries [289] and arteritis due to systemic lupus or Kawasaki's disease [290] are other rare causes of myocardial infarction in pregnancy.

Left ventricular aneurysm formation may complicate myocardial infarction but is not an absolute contraindication to further pregnancies because a successful case has been reported [291]. Successful pregnancy is also possible following severe myocardial infarction which may include cardiac arrest [292]. Termination of pregnancy is therefore not mandatory under these circumstances.

The diagnosis of myocardial infarction in pregnancy will be made on the basis of chest pain, with possible pericardial friction rub and fever. Only serial electrocardiographic changes are meaningful, because of the electrocardiographic changes induced by pregnancy itself (see above); also regional anaesthesia (spinal or epidural block) is associated with 'ischaemic' electrocardiographic changes (ST depression) in about 60% of cases [293]. Moderate elevations of the white cell count and ESR are seen in normal pregnancy, when the level of lactic acid dehydrogenase may also be raised [294]. However, elevations of serum glutamic acid transaminase and creatinine phosphokinase levels would indicate myocardial infarction in the appropriate clinical setting [294]. During the puerperium interpretation of these enzymes levels must be cautious, because they are liberated by the associated tissue destruction of the involuting uterus. However, the MB isoenzyme of creatinine phosphokinase is specific to cardiac muscle. The differential diagnosis of other occult causes of collapse in pregnancy is considered on p. 106 and in Table 4.1, p. 101.

It is difficult to be confident about management, because there is little experience and the pathology may be diverse. It would be sensible to treat the initial episode in a coronary care unit, with conventional opiate analgesics and medication for complications such as dysrhythmias. Because of the possibility of coronary spasm, nitroglycerine or other vasodilators should be used early in patients with continuing pain. Once the patient has been delivered (again in an intensive care environment), there is a good case for coronary arteriography to delineate the pathology, which may be atypical (although note the caution above about the possibility of coronary artery dissection) [288]. The angiographic demonstration of coronary embolus would be an indication for anticoagulation, but otherwise the benefits of anticoagulation in myocardial infarction unassociated with pregnancy do not seem enough to justify the considerable extra risks imposed on the pregnancy. Similarly thrombolytic therapy, even though it improves mortality in non-pregnant patients, should not be used (except in early pregnancy) because of the possibility of precipitating preterm delivery and the bleeding hazards of delivery if it does occur (see Chapter 4). However, there is sufficient experience in the use of aspirin in pregnancy for the prophylaxis of pre-eclampsia; this drug has also been shown to decrease mortality in myocardial infarction and patients with myocardial infarction should therefore be given aspirin 300 mg at presentation and 150 mg daily thereafter unless there are any of the usual contraindications to aspirin therapy.

Patients should be allowed a spontaneous vaginal delivery, preferably with epidural anaesthesia, unless there are good obstetric reasons for interfering. However, as in other cases of heart disease, the second stage should be limited by forceps delivery. Syntocinon infusion should be used rather than ergometrine in the third stage, because ergometrine is more likely to cause coronary artery spasm.

There is no evidence that pregnancy predisposes to myocardial infarction. Unless it is thought that the patient has had a coronary embolus, pregnancy should not be discouraged in patients who have had myocardial infarction in the past.

CARDIOMYOPATHY

Hypertrophic obstructive cardiomyopathy

Cardiomyopathy may arise *de novo* during pregnancy, and there is probably at least one form of cardiomyopathy (puerperal cardiomyopathy, see below) that is specific to pregnancy. Alternatively, any form of cardiomyopathy due to other causes may complicate pregnancy [295]. By far the most common of these other causes is HOCM (subaortic stenosis) and even this condition is relatively rare. The precise cause is unknown though advances are being made very rapidly in the molecular genetics of the condition [296]. Some cases are familial. The pathological features are hypertrophy and disorganization of cardiac muscle, particularly that of the left ventricular outflow tract. The patient presents with chest pain, syncope, dysrhythmias, or the symptoms of heart failure; alternatively HOCM may be a chance finding at echocardiography performed because of a heart murmur in pregnancy [296]. The diagnosis can usually be made by echocardiography, which shows abnormally thickened and disorganized cardiac muscle.

Oakley *et al.* have reported extensive experience of the management of this condition in pregnancy from the Hammersmith Hospital [297]. These authors originally advocated β-adrenergic blockade in all cases to reduce the risk of syncope, due to obstruction of the left ventricular outflow tract; this is now reserved for symptomatic patients only. Patients should not be allowed to become hypovolaemic, because this too increases the risk of obstruction of the left ventricular outflow tract. They should not lie supine because of the risk of caval obstruction and subsequent decrease in venous return. Particular care should be taken to give adequate fluid replacement if there is antepartum haemorrhage and also to avoid postpartum haemorrhage. During labour, patients with HOCM should be given epidural anaesthesia with caution, because this causes relative hypovolaemia by increasing venous capacitance in the lower limbs.

Puerperal cardiomyopathy (peripartum cardiomyopathy, pregnancy cardiomyopathy)

This condition was first described by Hull and Hafkesbring [298] and was extensively reviewed by Stuart [299], Meadows [300] and others [295,301] whose papers should be consulted for further references. The incidence in the UK is probably less than one in 5000. The condition usually arises in the puerperium (Fig. 5.2).

The pathogenesis of this condition is unknown [301]; therefore, some authors have denied that puerperal cardiomyopathy is a specific entity [302] and considered the condition to be another form of congestive cardiomyopathy caused by hypertension [258]. Rand *et al.* [303] on the basis of antibodies to heart muscle present in cord blood and serum from the mother in a case of pregnancy cardiomyopathy, postulate an immunological cause. Alternatively, the combination of multiparity and low social class has suggested that the condition is due to an undefined nutritional defect. Melvin *et al.* [304] described three cases of puerperal cardiomyopathy due to myocarditis, proven by endomyocardial biopsy at cardiac catheterization, and these authors propose that infection may be an important cause. Cunningham *et al.* [305] reviewed 28 cases of obscure cardiomyopathy occurring in 106 000 pregnancies in Texas. In only seven cases was the condition really idiopathic, emphasizing the rarity of the condition, but these patients fared very badly. Four were dead within 8 years.

At presentation there is no other predisposing cause for the heart failure and the heart is grossly dilated. The patients are not necessarily multiparous, black, relatively elderly nor of poor social class in the sporadic cases seen in the UK. Pregnancy has often been complicated by hypertension. Multiple pregnancy is another risk factor [306]. Pulmonary, peripheral and particularly cerebral embolization is a major cause of morbidity and mortality, which is 25–50% [301]. The majority of deaths occur around the time of presentation but some women have protracted illnesses and die up to 8 years later. However, if the patient recovers fully from the initial episode, the long-term prognosis is good. The condition is likely to recur in future pregnancies [306], which are therefore contraindicated in view of the overall poor prognosis. For this reason any patient who develops pulmonary oedema peripartum should be investigated thoroughly in case the diagnosis of peripartum cardiomyopathy is made unjustifiably.

On investigation, the chest radiograph is not specific, showing pulmonary venous congestion and a large heart. The electrocardiogram may be normal or there may be widespread abnormalities. Rhythm disturbances are also common. The diagnosis of cardiomyopathy is confirmed by echocardiography which also excludes other subtle causes of raised left and/or right atrial blood pressure such as mitral valve disease, left atrial myxoma [243] and pericardial disease (see below). The distinction of puerperal cardiomyopathy from other forms of cardiomyopathy depends on the history and clinical features; the diagnosis is based on the exclusion of other known causes of cardiomyopathy. Apart from conventional antifailure treatment, which now includes angiotensin-converting inhibitors, these patients should also receive anticoagulant therapy until the heart size has returned to normal, and until they have no further dysrhythmias.

The place of immunosuppressive therapy with either prednisone or azathioprine is unclear. These have been used successfully in cases associated with acute myocarditis demonstrated by endomyocardial biopsy [307] but such treatment cannot be routinely recommended [308].

Those few patients who present before delivery (Fig. 5.2) should be electively delivered because the demand on their hearts will decrease after pregnancy is terminated. If the cervix is favourable, vaginal delivery should be chosen; if not, the patients should be delivered by caesarean section. Skilled epidural anaesthesia is preferred for both routes of delivery. There is no evidence that breast-feeding influences the course of puerperal cardiomyopathy.

Because of the poor prognosis of puerperal cardiomyopathy, the patients' young age and their social responsibilities having just been delivered, they should receive early consideration and high priority for cardiac transplantation [308]. The indication for transplantation is intractable pump failure despite optimal medical therapy.

In the few patients who have had pregnancies subsequent to one complicated by puerperal cardiomyopathy, the recurrence rate has been up to 50%. Recurrence may occur even if the heart appears to have returned to normal following the first episode [309]. Recurrence may also be demonstrated by echocardiography as a decrease in contractility even if this is not apparent clinically [310]. At present there are no prognostic indicators for who is at risk of recurrence, although it is likely that those who have permanent impairment of function are more at risk than those who do not. For these reasons patients who have had puerperal cardiomyopathy should be discouraged from further pregnancies. As already emphasized this means that the diagnosis of puerperal cardiomyopathy should not be made lightly.

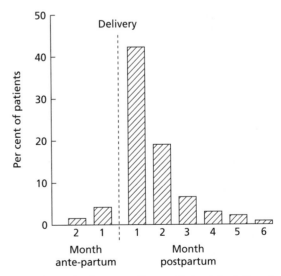

Fig 5.2 Onset of peripartum cardiomyopathy in relation to time of delivery. Total number of patients was 347 [301]. (Reproduced with permission of the Editor, *New England Journal of Medicine*.)

Davidson and Parry [311] have described a specific form of puerperal cardiac failure occurring in the Hausa tribe in Northern Nigeria. They were able to document 224 cases and claimed that in the peak season (summer) half the female medical beds in Zaria are occupied by patients with this condition. The peak incidence is 4 weeks postpartum. During this period, for up to 40 days after delivery, the Hausa woman spends 18 h/day lying on a mud bed, heated so that the ambient temperature reaches 40°C. She also increases her sodium intake to 450 mmol/day by eating kanwa salt from Lake Chad. Many of the patients are hypertensive, but the condition regresses rapidly with diuretic and digoxin therapy, which causes a weight loss of 29% in 15 days. Echocardiographic studies do not support ventricular dysfunction in this condition [312]. The contribution of hypertension to the heart failure is debated [313] but this would seem an extreme example of the instability of the cardiovascular system in the first weeks of the puerperium interacting with the particular susceptibility of Africans to dilated cardiomyopathy [314]. In all normal women, blood volume and cardiac output must fall while peripheral resistance rises after delivery. The practices of the Hausa tribe will cause a marked rise in circulating blood volume, which could be sufficient to produce clinical cardiac failure.

The high incidence of heart failure in the Hausa tribe demonstrates the vulnerability of the cardiovascular system in the puerperium and perhaps explains why so many of Stuart's cases presented at this time. In addition, if peripheral vascular resistance rises very rapidly, before cardiac output falls, systemic hypertension will ensue, as is occasionally seen in normal patients in the UK who have no history of antecedent hypertension in pregnancy before delivery [238] (see Chapter 6).

ENDOMYOCARDIAL FIBROSIS

In this uncommon condition, the endocardium is thickened and replaced by fibrous tissue. Haemodynamically the condition behaves like constrictive pericarditis (see below) because the heart cannot relax in diastole. The condition is more common in tropical climates; there have been three patients described in pregnancy. The most recent [315] developed congestive cardiac failure during pregnancy and died despite subsequent cardiac transplantation.

PERICARDIAL DISEASE

This is a rare complication of pregnancy but should be considered because of its specific haemodynamic problems [316]. Acute pericarditis is normally not of any haemodynamic consequence and is only of importance because it must be considered in patients presenting with chest pain and because of the necessity to diagnose the underlying cause. However, patients with significant pericardial effusion or more commonly with calcific pericarditis suffer because they cannot increase ventricular filling above the limit restricted by the pericardium. Therefore they can only increase cardiac output by increasing heart rate and they are dependent on maintaining both venous filling and heart rate in pregnancy.

Patients usually present with oedema, hepatomegaly, ascites and raised jugular venous pressure. Symptoms and signs of pulmonary oedema are a late finding. The diagnosis is often suggested by seeing calcification in the pericardium on radiography and is confirmed by echocardiography.

Patients should be treated with diuretics only if they develop pulmonary oedema or if peripheral oedema is a major problem. Digoxin is only indicated for atrial tachydysrhythmias. β-adrenergic blocking agents should not be used. Patients should not become hypovolaemic. The condition improves when circulating blood volume decreases after delivery. Definitive treatment is pericardiectomy, which can usually be deferred until after delivery [312]. Tuberculosis is an important cause of constrictive pericarditis.

Congenital heart disease

EISENMENGER'S SYNDROME AND OTHER CAUSES OF PULMONARY VASCULAR DISEASE (see maternal mortality, above)

As indicated above, Eisenmenger's syndrome has a very high maternal mortality. Only recently has there been any form of surgical treatment and the opportunities for this, heart and lung transplantation, arise infrequently [317]. A recent series of 28 cases of heart–lung transplantation had a perioperative mortality of 29% mainly due to obliterative bronchiolitis which was also a problem of the survivors [318].

Most patients with Eisenmenger's syndrome who die in pregnancy, do so in the puerperium. Although deaths are occasionally sudden, due to thromboembolism, this is not usually so. More frequently, these patients die due to a slowly falling systemic Pao_2 with associated decrease in cardiac output. A consideration of the haemodynamics involved (Fig. 5.3) suggests how this might occur and how it could be managed.

In a defect, such as a large ventricular septal defect, the blood is freely mixed in the right and left ventricles and the ratio of blood flow in the pulmonary circuit (Q_p) to that in the systemic circuit (Q_s) is inversely proportional

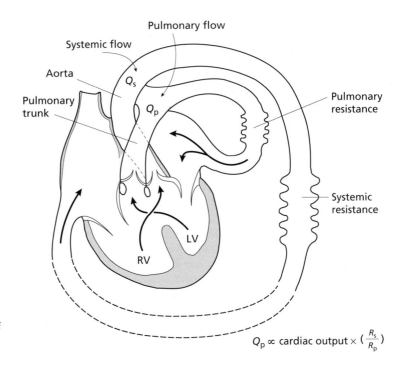

Systemic flow

Pulmonary flow

Aorta

Pulmonary trunk

Pulmonary resistance

Systemic resistance

Q_s

Q_p

LV

RV

Fig 5.3 Pulmonary and systemic blood flows and resistances in Eisenmenger's syndrome associated with ventricular septal defect [372] (see text). (Courtesy of the Editor, *Journal of the Royal College of Physicians*.)

$$Q_p \propto \text{cardiac output} \times \left(\frac{R_s}{R_p}\right)$$

to the ratio of the pulmonary resistance (R_p) to the systemic resistance (R_s), i.e.

$$Q_p / Q_s \propto R_s / R_p$$

Pulmonary blood flow is also proportional to cardiac output (CO) so

$$Q_p \propto \text{CO} \times R_s / R_p$$

Thus any fall in the ratio $R_s : R_p$ or in the cardiac output will cause a fall in pulmonary blood flow. For example, in pre-eclampsia, the pulmonary vascular resistance increases and the cardiac output falls [319]. These factors would therefore decrease pulmonary blood flow and this could account for the observed deterioration in Eisenmenger's syndrome, associated with hypertensive pregnancy [54].

What can be offered to the pregnant patient with Eisenmenger's syndrome? Unfortunately, abortion would appear to be the answer. The maternal mortality associated with abortion is only 7% in comparison to 30% for continuing pregnancy [52]. However, if the patient decides to continue with pregnancy, prophylactic anticoagulation, probably with subcutaneous heparin, should be offered, because of the risk of thromboembolism, both systemic and pulmonary. Labour should not be induced

unless there are good obstetric reasons. Induced labour carries a higher risk of caesarean section, which is associated with a particularly high maternal mortality in Eisenmenger's syndrome [52].

There is controversy concerning the place of epidural anaesthesia for the management of labour. Although epidural anaesthesia should decrease the $Q_p : Q_s$ ratio by decreasing the systemic vascular resistance, this may not occur, at least it did not in the one case studied by Midwall *et al.* [320]. On balance, a carefully administered elective epidural anaesthetic at the beginning of labour is probably preferable to emergency epidural or general anaesthesia if it is suddenly decided that instrumental delivery is necessary [52,321].

If the patient does become hypotensive with increasing cyanosis and decreasing cardiac output, it has been shown that high inspired oxygen concentrations can decrease pulmonary vascular resistance, increase the $Q_p : Q_s$ ratio and increase peripheral oxygen saturation [320]. In addition, α-sympathomimetic agents, such as phenylephrine, methoxamine and noradrenaline (norepinephrine), will increase R_s and thus increase pulmonary blood flow [322]. However, drugs such as tolazline, phentolamine, nitroprusside and isoprenaline, which have been used to decrease pulmonary vascular resistance in other clinical situations, probably should not be given, because they will also decrease the systemic vascular resistance [322]. If R_s

decreases more than R_p, pulmonary blood flow will decrease rather than increase. The same problem occurs with dopamine and β-sympathomimetic drugs, which have been given to increase cardiac output. They too will decrease R_s, and if R_s decreases more than the cardiac output increases, pulmonary blood flow will fall. Two other pulmonary vasodilators deserve mention. There is evidence of thromboxane/prostacyclin imbalance in primary pulmonary hypertension with too much thromboxane production and too little prostacyclin production [323]. In these circumstances prostacyclin infusion may act as a relatively selective pulmonary vasodilator [324]. The drug is expensive and has to be given by intravenous infusion, but it might just tip the balance in the deteriorating Eisenmenger patient to allow improved pulmonary blood flow and better myocardial oxygenation. Also, nitric oxide has now been identified as the endothelium-derived relaxing factor, which in turn is a very powerful vasodilator. When inhaled it could be a relatively selective pulmonary vasodilator and it has been shown to be effective both in the neonate [325] and in adults [326] with pulmonary hypertension. Unfortunately anecdotal experience with inhaled nitric oxide has not been favourable for patients with Eisenmenger's syndrome and fixed pulmonary resistance. In summary, the management of the deteriorating patient with Eisenmenger's syndrome depends on giving oxygen and α-sympathomimetic amines.

Cor pulmonale, pulmonary veno-occlusive disease, primary pulmonary hypertension

In cor pulmonale, pulmonary veno-occlusive disease and primary pulmonary hypertension where there is pulmonary hypertension and vascular disease in small blood vessels, the maternal mortality is still high and termination of pregnancy is still the management of choice [327].

Primary pulmonary hypertension is particularly worrying because although a rare condition it commonly presents in young women. Primary pulmonary hypertension (and valvular heart disease [328]) has been associated with taking appetite suppressant drugs [329].

Because of the risk of thrombotic microangiopathy, anticoagulation should be continued in pregnancy or instigated if the patient is not already on such therapy. The options are similar to those in patients with artificial heart valves (see above); either warfarin to maintain INR 2 or high-dose LMWH aiming for anti-X a level about 0.8 units/mL. Despite the thromboembolic risk, there does not seem to be any association between the development of primary pulmonary hypertension and combined oral contraceptive use [329]. On this basis, some would sanction the use of the combined pill in family members of those with primary

pulmonary hypertension unless there is an obvious Mendelian form of inheritance [330].

The problem in these conditions still appears to be one of maintaining adequate pulmonary blood flow for adequate oxygenation. Even though blood cannot be shunted directly from the pulmonary to the systemic circuit as in Eisenmenger's syndrome, excessive vasodilatation in the systemic circulation during epidural anaesthesia could still decrease preload to the right ventricle and therefore further decrease pulmonary blood flow.

Unfortunately, as in Eisenmenger's syndrome, selective pulmonary vasodilators are not available. The options include nifedipine, nitroprusside [331] and oxygen and the effects of prostacyclin infusion and nitric oxide inhalation are being investigated. Oral prostacyclin analogues are becoming available but have not yet been used in pregnancy [332]. Nifedipine may of course be taken on a long-term basis although the doses needed can be high, of the order of 240 mg/day [333]. Although nifedipine is used for control of systemic blood pressure in pregnancy (see Chapter 6), the effects of such high doses on the fetus are uncertain.

Manoeuvres that suddenly increase venous return (ergometrine injection, movement from supine to left lateral position) should be avoided, as should those that increase vagal tone (e.g. bladder catheterization). Several patients with primary pulmonary hypertension have died in association with bradycardia and atrioventricular block, which suggest vagally mediated mechanisms.

These patients should be delivered in an intensive care environment with elective insertion of a Swan–Ganz catheter (notwithstanding the risk in patients with pulmonary hypertension) and facilities for pacing [331]. If circumstances permit, there are arguments for elective testing of various potential pulmonary vasodilators on the day before delivery to see which (if any) will work in the event that the patient deteriorates [334]. To maintain haemodynamic stability Abboud *et al.* [59] used intrathecal morphine as an analgesic in labour in a patient with primary pulmonary hypertension. Intrathecal morphine gives very effective analgesia with little change in maternal haemodynamics and little transfer to the fetus. The most common side-effects are pruritus and late respiratory depression. The immediate results in this case were excellent as judged clinically and by Swan–Ganz monitoring. Unfortunately the patient died 7 days later from acute right ventricular strain. The theoretical advantage of epidural morphine over epidural block with local anaesthesia is the lack of haemodynamic effects. Yet conventional epidural anaesthesia when skilfully applied can be very beneficial in primary pulmonary hypertension [334] and fentanyl (an opiate) and bupivacaine have been combined with success for delivery in primary pulmonary hypertension [222]. Even if epidural block in any of its forms gives a superior haemodynamic profile it is also tempting to recommend caesarean section and general anaesthesia which offers a controlled process with less physical stress for the mother in the short term [335]. The anaesthetist's experience is likely to dictate which is the more suitable form of anaesthesia in these difficult and very uncommon situations.

By contrast two successful cases would suggest that proximal pulmonary stenosis like pulmonary valvular stenosis and Fallot's tetralogy where the small pulmonary blood vessels are not affected, should have a more successful outcome [147,336].

COARCTATION OF THE AORTA

In both coarctation of the aorta and Marfan's syndrome (see below), the maternal risk is dissection of the aorta associated with the hyperdynamic circulation of pregnancy and possibly with an increased risk of medial degeneration due to the hormonal environment of pregnancy [337]. These mechanisms could also explain the well-known pregnancy-associated risks in all patients, of rupture of aneurysms in the splenic, adrenal, renal, cerebral, coronary and ovarian arteries. Patients with coarctation also have the specific risk of cerebral haemorrhage due to ruptured berry aneurysm. The maternal mortality in coarctation has been stated to be as high as 17% [338]. It has therefore been suggested that all patients with coarctation presenting in pregnancy should either be aborted or have the defect repaired before delivery. However, Mendelson's series [338] dates from 1858 to 1939, and there have only been 14 maternal deaths reported in the whole of the literature, none of which occurred in the 83 patients studied since 1960 [339]. The risk of dissection has therefore probably been exaggerated, and good obstetric care and effective antihypertensive therapy would decrease the risk still further. It is probable that we no longer see the patients similar to those of Mendelson's series, because most patients with severe coarctation are operated on in infancy. In a series of 52 patients who had been operated on for coarctation, 18 had become pregnant 36 times. No adverse maternal cardiological events were recorded; pre-eclampsia was also uncommon [340]. Nevertheless there may be late problems following coarctation repair, in particular recoarctation and the development of aneurysms. These possibilities should be considered when assessing patients before or during pregnancy.

Only those patients who already have evidence of dissection should have the coarctation repaired in pregnancy. Percutaneous balloon angioplasty should be avoided because of the increased pregnancy risk of intimal tear provoking dissection.

Any upper limb hypertension should be treated aggressively with antihypertensive drugs [81]. If there is gross widening of the ascending aorta suggesting intrinsic disease of the aorta, the patient should be delivered by elective caesarean section to reduce the risk of dissection associated with labour. Associated mitral and aortic valve lesions (bicuspid aortic valve) rarely cause haemodynamic problems in pregnancy; they are an additional reason for endocarditis prophylaxis.

MARFAN'S SYNDROME (see also Chapter 14 for non-cardiological aspects)

Marfan's syndrome is due to a defect in fibrillin synthesis. In Marfan's syndrome (but not in some other marfanoid conditions such as contractural arachnodactyly) this defect is due to mutations of a fibrillin gene on chromosome 15 [341]. Patients contemplating pregnancy should be aware of the dominant inheritance of Marfan's syndrome as well as the haemodynamic risks. Definitive diagnosis in the index case and prenatal diagnosis in fetuses of patients with Marfan's disease is now possible in many families. Also it may be possible to explain the wide variation in phenotype on the basis of the many different mutations that have been shown to occur [342].

Some authors consider the risk of dissection to be so high in Marfan's syndrome that they advise avoidance of pregnancy or termination if there is any degree of aortic dilatation [343]. Again, this seems an extreme attitude, which Pyeritz had modified to suggest that dilatation of the aorta to >40 mm (as determined echocardiographically) should be the limit at which pregnancy is contraindicated [344]. Some patients and families with Marfan's syndrome have *formes frustes* of the condition where there may be arachnodactyly, a high arch palate, lens abnormalities and long patella tendons with no evidence of disease of the aorta or aortic valve; there may only be minor mitral valve abnormalities, if there is any cardiac disease at all. The families tend to 'breed true' and pregnancy would confer no extra risk.

Therefore, there cannot be an overall condemnation of pregnancy in all cases of Marfan's syndrome [345]. Pyeritz [344] has reported a series of pregnancies in 26 women with Marfan's syndrome. There was only one fatality and that patient died from endocarditis. However, in another UK series of 91 pregnancies in 36 women there were four aortic dissections relating to pregnancy two of which occurred with aortic roots only 4.0 and 4.2 cm [346]. So although the majority of pregnancies are uncomplicated, none is free from risk and these patients must be monitored closely.

Patients should have monthly transthoracic echocardiography to check aortic dimensions. As in coarctation of the aorta, any associated hypertension should be treated aggressively with β blockade to decrease the haemodynamic load on the ascending aorta. β-blocking drugs (propranolol) should also be used even in the absence of hypertension, if there is any dilatation of the aorta to protect the aorta [347]. Delivery should be by caesarean section if there is evidence of aortic disease.

Dissection of the aorta, even in labour and of the iliac artery [348] have been successfully managed with cardiopulmonary bypass in pregnancy. The treatment is surgical, either as an isolated procedure if the fetus is not yet viable [349] or following caesarean section if the fetus is viable [350,351].

Spontaneous uterine inversion has been reported in one case of Marfan's syndrome in pregnancy, possibly due to a generalized abnormality of connective tissue [352]; postpartum haemorrhage has been thought to be due to Marfanoid degeneration of the uterine blood vessels [353].

Once the aorta has dilated to 5.5 cm, elective replacement of the ascending aorta and aortic valve with a composite graft is a practical procedure [354] and should be considered even in symptom-free individuals [346]. Pregnancy might be considered after this has been performed.

CONGENITAL HEART BLOCK

Congenital heart block is usually no problem in pregnancy. Although part of the normal response to pregnancy includes an increase in heart rate to increase the cardiac output, this is not obligatory. There are many records of successful pregnancy in patients with heart block, both paced [355] and not paced. Presumably, patients are able to increase stroke volume sufficiently to cope with the increased demands of pregnancy. A few patients are unable to increase cardiac output sufficiently at the end of pregnancy or during labour [356]. Therefore, patients with heart block who are not paced, or those where there is any question of pacemaker failure, should be managed in obstetric units where there is access to pacing facilities.

TRICUSPID ATRESIA AND THE FONTAN PROCEDURE

In tricuspid atresia there is no communication between the right atrium and the right ventricle. If the child or fetus survives, blood exits the right atrium via an atrial septal defect and perfuses the lungs via a ventricular septal defect. In the Fontan procedure the right atrium is connected directly to the pulmonary artery to improve pulmonary blood flow and the atrial and ventricular septal defects are closed. There have been a number of reports of pregnancy in patients with tricuspid atresia, both corrected and uncorrected [357,358].

In general the maternal outcome depends on the patient's state of health at the beginning of pregnancy and the fetal outcome on the degree of maternal cyanosis. But in addition these patients have a high thromboembolic risk. In part this is due to the polycythaemia of cyanosis but in addition the Fontan procedure is associated with an acquired thrombotic state due in part to protein C, antithrombin and protein S deficiencies (see Chapter 4) [359]. It is likely that these deficiencies are due to impaired liver function possibly because of the high venous pressure resulting from the Fontan procedure. Protein C, antithrombin and protein S should be estimated in all patients following the Fontan procedure, particularly if they are contemplating pregnancy, and suitable thromboprophylaxis should be used if there are significant abnormalities. Subcutaneous heparin would be the obvious choice in pregnancy. Despite this concern, there were no thromboembolic complications in 33 pregnancies following the Fontan procedure in 14 women. Indeed there were no cardiological problems but the fetal loss rate was high with only 45% live births. The fetal losses were entirely accounted for by 13 spontaneous miscarriages and nine terminations [360]. Judging by the maternal outcome data, pregnancy does not need to be discouraged following the Fontan procedure.

MISCELLANEOUS

Pregnancy has been described in a number of patients with univentricular hearts, with or without transposition and usually after a surgical procedure [116,361–364]. The maternal outcome depends on the degree of pulmonary vascular disease, her symptoms, whether she has been in congestive cardiac failure and the nature of other abnormalities. The fetal outcome depends on the degree of maternal cyanosis.

In 41 pregnancies in a group of 15 women with pulmonary atresia, the outcome of pregnancy was as might be expected, better in the seven women who had had a radical repair. They were no longer cyanosed and had a much better fetal outcome. However, thromboembolism and dysrhythmias remained a problem even in the corrected group [365].

A woman has been successfully delivered following pregnancy complicated by uncorrected truncus arteriosus [366].

In Ebstein's malformation, the tricuspid valve is displaced into the right ventricle. The malformation, which can be diagnosed by echocardiography, is associated with maternal lithium therapy. The major risks are right-sided heart failure and dysrhythmias. In a large series from the Mayo Clinic in 46 women, 111 pregnancies complicated by Ebstein's anomaly were well tolerated. There were increased risks of prematurity, fetal loss and congenital heart disease in the offspring. In addition, a significantly lower birthweight was found in the offspring of cyanotic vs. acyanotic women with Ebstein's anomaly. Nevertheless, most pregnancies were successful [367].

Experience is increasing with pregnancy following heart transplantation. Guidelines for management have been published [368] and there has even been a successful case of twin pregnancy [369]. Hypertension, not necessarily pre-eclampsia, is common and the babies are likely to be growth restricted [370]. Peripartum cardiomyopathy did not reoccur in four women who had their hearts transplanted because of previous peripartum cardiomyopathy [371]. In general the problems are not haemodynamic but those of managing immunosuppressive therapy and for these we can draw on the much greater experience of renal transplants (see Chapter 7).

References

1 Department of Health. Why Mothers Die. *Report on Confidential Enquiries Into Maternal Deaths in the United Kingdom 1994–1996.* London, HMSO, 1998: 103–14.

2 Elkayam U, Gleicher N. *Cardiac Problems in Pregnancy. Diagnosis and Management of Maternal and Fetal Disease.* Alan R Liss, New York, 1982.

3 Patton DE, Lee W *et al.* Cyanotic maternal heart disease in pregnancy. *Obstet Gynaecol Surv* 1990; 45: 594–600.

4 Shine J, Mocarski EJM *et al.* Congenital heart disease in pregnancy: Short- and long-term implications. *Am J Obstet Gynecol* 1987; 156: 313–22.

5 Sullivan JM, Ramanathan KB. Management of medical problems in pregnancy–severe cardiac disease. *N Engl J Med* 1985; 313: 304–9.

6 Szekely P, Turner R *et al.* Pregnancy and the changing pattern of rheumatic heart disease. *Br Heart J* 1973; 35: 1293–303.

7 Tamari I, Eldar M, Rabinowitz B, Neufeld HN. Medical treatment of cardiovascular disorders during pregnancy. *Am Heart J* 1982; 104: 1357–63.

8 Oakley C, ed. *Heart Disease in Pregnancy.* BMJ Publishing Group, London, 1997.

9 Bader RA, Bader ME *et al.* Haemodynamics at rest and during exercise in normal pregnancy as studied by cardiac catheterization. *J Clin Invest* 1955; 34: 1524–36.

10 Davies P, Francis RI *et al.* Analysis of impedance cardiography longitudinally applied in pregnancy. *Br J Obstet Gynaecol* 1986; 93: 717–20.

11 Newman B, Derrington C *et al.* Cardiac output and the recumbent position in late pregnancy. *Anaesthesia* 1983; 38: 332–5.

12 Ueland K, McAnulty JH *et al.* Special considerations in the use of cardiovascular drugs. *Clin Obstet Gynecol* 1981; 24: 809–23.

13 Morton MJ, Paul MS *et al.* Exercise dynamics in late gestation: effects of physical training. *Am J Obstet Gynecol* 1985; 152: 91–7.

14 James CF, Banner T *et al.* Noninvasive determination of cardiac output throughout pregnancy. *Anaesthesiology* 1985; 63: A434.

15 Easterling TR, Benedetti TJ *et al.* Measurement of cardiac output in pregnancy by thermodilution and impedance techniques. *Br J Obstet Gynaecol* 1989; 96: 67–9.

16 de Swiet M, Talbert DG. The measurement of cardiac output by electrical impedance plethysmography in pregnancy. Are the assumptions valid? *Br J Obstet Gynaecol* 1986; 93: 721–6.

17 Milsom I, Forssman L *et al.* Measurement of cardiac stroke Volume by impedance cardiography in the last trimester of pregnancy. *Acta Obstet Gynecol Scand* 1983; 62: 473–9.

18 Hart MV, Morton MJ *et al.* Aortic function during normal pregnancy. *Am J Obstet Gynecol* 1986; 154: 887–91.

19 Robson SC, Dunlop W *et al.* Cardiac output during labour. *Br Med J* 1987; 295: 1169–72.

20 Robson SC, Hunter S *et al.* Serial study of factors influencing changes in cardiac output during human pregnancy. *Am J Physiol* 1989; 256: H1060–5.

21 Dubourg G. Correction complete d'une triade de Fallot en circulation extra-corporelle chez une femme enceinte. *Arch Mal Coeur Vaiss* 1959; 52: 1389–91.

22 Robson SC, Hunter S *et al.* Serial changes in pulmonary haemodynamics during human pregnancy: a non-invasive study using Doppler echocardiography. *Clin Sci* 1991; 80: 113–7.

23 Clapp JF III. Maternal heart rate in pregnancy. *Am J Obstet Gynecol* 1985; 152: 659–60.

24 Phippard AF, Horvath JS *et al.* Circulatory adaptation to pregnancy—serial studies of haemodynamics, blood volume, renin and aldosterone in the baboon (*Papio harmadryas*). *J Hypertens* 1986; 4: 773–9.

25 Schrier RW. A unifying hypothesis of body fluid volume regulation. *J R Coll Phys Lond* 1992; 26: 295–306.

26 Sanders SP, Levy RJ *et al.* Use of Hancock porcine xenografts in children and adolescents. *Am J Cardiol* 1980; 46: 429–38.

27 Stevenson JC, MacDonald DWR *et al.* Increased concentration of circulating calcitonin gene related peptide during normal human pregnancy. *Br Med J* 1986; 293: 1329–30.

28 Kakouris H, Eddie LW *et al.* Cardiac effects of relaxin in rats. *Lancet* 1992; 339: 1076–8.

29 de Swiet M. The cardiovascular svstem. In: Hytten F, Chamberlain GVP, eds. *Clinical Physiology in Obstetrics.* Blackwell Scientific Publications, Oxford, 1980.

30 de Swiet M. The physiology of normal pregnancy. In: Rubin PC, ed. *Hypertension in Pregnancy*, Vol. 12. *Handbook of Hypertension.* Elsevier, Amsterdam, 1988.

31 Ueland K, Novy MJ, Metcalfe S. Hemodynamic responses of patients with heart disease to pregnancy and exercise. *Am J Obstet Gynecol* 1972; 113: 47–59.

32 Cohen DJ, Kuntz RE *et al.* Predictors of long-term outcome after percutaneous balloon mitral valvuloplasty. *N Engl J Med* 1992; 327: 1329–35.

33 Visser W, Wallenburg HCS. Central haemodynamic observations in untreated pre-eclamptic toxaemia. *Hypertension* 1991; 17: 1072–7.

34 Lee W, Clark SL *et al.* Septic shock during pregnancy. *Am J Obstet Gynecol* 1988; 159: 410–16.

35 Clark SL, Phelan JP *et al.* Labour and delivery in the presence of mitral stenosis: Central hemodynamic observations. *Am J Obstet Gynecol* 1985; 8: 984–8.

36 Hawkins GBV, Wendel GB *et al*. Myocardial infarction during pregnancy: a review. *Obstet Gynecol* 1985; 65: 139–47.

37 MacNab C, MacAfee CAJ. A changing pattern of heart disease associated with pregnancy. *J Obstet Gynaecol* 1985; 5: 139–42.

38 Mendelson CL. Disorders of the heart beat during pregnancy. *Am J Obstet Gynecol* 1956; 72: 1268.

39 Etheridge MJ. Heart disease and pregnancy. *Aust NZ J Obstet Gynaecol* 1969; 9: 7–11.

40 Rush RW, Verjans M *et al*. Incidence of heart disease in pregnancy. A study done at Peninsular Maternity Services Hospital. *South Afr Med J* 1979; 55: 808–10.

41 Buemann B, Kragelund E. Clinical assessment of heart disease during pregnancy. *Acta Obstet Gynecol Scand* 1962; 41: 57.

42 Tan J, de Swiet M. Prevalence of heart disease diagnosed *de novo* in pregnancy in a West London population. *Br J Obstet Gynaecol* 1998; 105: 1185–8.

43 Pitkin RM, Perloff JK *et al*. Pregnancy and congenital heart disease. *Ann Intern Med* 1990; 112: 445–54.

44 Copeland WE, Wooley CF *et al*. Pregnancy and congenital heart disease. *Am J Obstet Gynecol* 1963; 86: 107–10.

45 Neilson G, Galea EG *et al*. Congenital heart disease and pregnancy. *Med J Aust* 1970; 1: 1086–8.

46 Ong HC, Puraviappan AP. Congenital heart disease and pregnancy in the tropics. *Aust NZ J Obstet Gynaecol* 1975; 15: 99–103.

47 Sugrue D, Blake S *et al*. Pregnancy complicated by maternal heart disease at the National Maternity Hospital, Dublin, Ireland 1969 to 1978. *Am J Obstet Gynecol* 1981; 139: 1–6.

48 Kaluarachchi A, Seneviratne HR. Heart disease in pregnancy— evaluation of disease pattern and outcome in Sri Lanka. *J Obstet Gynaecol* 1995; 15: 9–14.

49 Connolly HM, Grogan M *et al*. Pregnancy among women with congenitally corrected transposition of great arteries. *J Am Coll Cardiol* 1999; 33 (6): 1692–5.

50 Etheridge MJ. Heart disease and pregnancy. *Med J Aust* 1966; 2: 1172.

51 Gleicher N, Knutzen VK *et al*. Rheumatic heart disease diagnosed during pregnancy. A 30-year follow-up. *Int J Obstet Gynaecol* 1979; 17: 51–7.

52 Gleicher N, Midwall J *et al*. Eisenmenger's syndrome and pregnancy. *Obstet Gynecol Surv* 1979; 34: 721–41.

53 Jewett JF. Pulmonary hypertension and pre-eclampsia. *N Engl J Med* 1979; 301: 1063–4.

54 Morgan Jones A, Howitt G. Eisenmenger syndrome in pregnancy. *Br Med J* 1965; i: 1627–31.

55 Pitts JA, Crosby WM *et al*. Eisenmenger's syndrome in pregnancy. *Am Heart J* 1977; 93: 321–6.

56 Yentis SM, Steer PJ *et al*. Eisenmenger's syndrome in pregnancy: maternal and fetal mortality in the 1990s. *Br J Obstet Gynaecol* 1998; 105: 921–2.

57 Batson GA. Cyanotic congenital heart disease and pregnancy. *Br J Obstet Gynaecol* 1974; 81: 549–53.

58 Stiller RJ, Vintzileos AM *et al*. Single ventricle in pregnancy: Case report and review of the literature. *Obstet Gynecol* 1984; 64 (Suppl. 3): 19S–20S.

59 Abboud TK, Raya J *et al*. Intrathecal morphine for relief of labour pain in a parturient with severe pulmonary hypertension. *Anaesthesiology* 1983; 59: 477–9.

60 McCaffrey RM, Dunn LJ. Primary pulmonary hypertension and pregnancy. *Obstet Gynaecol Surv* 1964; 19: 567–91.

61 Sinnenberg RJ. Pulmonary hypertension in pregnancy. *South Med J* 1980; 73: 1529–31.

62 Jacoby WJ. Pregnancy with tetralogy and pentalogy of Fallot. *Am J Cardiol* 1964; 14: 866–73.

63 Mendelson CL. *Cardiac Disease in Pregnancy*. FA Davis, Philadelphia, PA, 1960.

64 Espino Vela J, Alvarado-Toro A. Natural history of atrial septal defect. *Cardiovasc Clin* 1971; 2: 104–25.

65 Whittemore R, Hobbins JC *et al*. Pregnancy and its outcome in women with and without surgical treatment of congenital heart disease. *Am J Cardiol* 1982; 50: 641–51.

66 Barabas AP. Heterogeneity of the Ehlers–Danlos syndrome: description of three clinical types and a hypothesis to explain the basic defect(s). *Br Med J* 1967; ii: 612–13.

67 Peaceman AM, Cruikshank DP. Ehlers–Danlos syndrome and pregnancy: association of type IV disease with maternal death. *Obstet Gynecol* 1987; 69: 428–31.

68 Pearl W, Spicer M. Ehlers–Danlos syndrome. *South Med J* 1981; 74: 80–1.

69 Smith R. The molecular genetics of collagen disorders. *Clin Sci* 1986; 17: 129–35.

70 Rudd NL, Nimrod C *et al*. Pregnancy complications in type IV Ehlers–Danlos syndrome. *Lancet* 1983; i: 50–3.

71 Lurie S, Manor M *et al*. The threat of type IV Ehlers–Danlos syndrome on maternal well-being during pregnancy: early delivery may make the difference. *J Obstet Gynaecol* 1998; 18: 245–8.

72 Pope FM, Nicholls AC. Pregnancy and Ehlers–Danlos syndrome type IV. *Lancet* 1983; i: 249–50.

73 Levick K. Pregnancy loss and fathers with Ehlers–Danlos syndrome. *Lancet* 1989; ii: 1151.

74 Webster JC. The conduct of pregnancy and labour in acute and chronic affections of the heart. *Trans Am Gynecol Soc* 1913; 38: 223.

75 Chesley LC. Severe rheumatic cardiac disease and pregnancy: the ultimate prognosis. *Am J Obstet Gynecol* 1980; 136: 552–8.

76 Ho PC, Chen TY *et al*. The effect of maternal cardiac disease and digoxin administration on labour, fetal weight and maturity at birth. *Aust NZ J Obstet Gynaecol* 1980; 20: 24–7.

77 Schaefer G, Arditi LI *et al*. Congenital heart disease and pregnancy. *Clin Obstet Gynecol* 1968; 11: 1048–63.

78 Presbitero P, Somerville J *et al*. Pregnancy in cyanotic congenital heart disease. Outcome of mother and fetus. *Circulation* 1994; 89 (6): 2673–6.

79 Singh H, Bolton PJ *et al*. Pregnancy after surgical correction of tetralogy of Fallot. *Br Med J* 1982; 285: 168–70.

80 Burwell CS, Metcalfe J. *Heart Disease and Pregnancy: Physiology and Management*. Little, Brown, Boston, MA, 1973.

81 Benny PS, Prasao J *et al*. Pregnancy and coarctation of the aorta. Case report. *Br J Obstet Gynaecol* 1980; 87: 1159–61.

82 Giles WB, Young AA *et al*. Doppler ultrasound features of stenosis of the aorta in a pregnancy complicated by Takayasu's arteritis. *Br J Obstet Gynaecol* 1987; 94: 902–9.

83 Socol NIL, Conn J *et al*. Pregnancy associated with partial aortic occlusion. *Am J Obstet Gynecol* 1981; 139: 965–7.

84 Nora JJ, Nora AH. The evolution of specific genetic and environmental counselling in congenital heart diseases. *Circulation* 1978; 57: 205–13.

85 Burn J, Brennan P *et al*. Recurrence risks in offspring of adults with major heart defects: results from first cohort of British collaborative study. *Lancet* 1998; 351: 311–16.

86 Emmanuel R, Somervill J *et al*. Evidence of congenital heart disease in the offspring of parents with atrioventricular defects. *Br Heart J* 1983; 49: 144–7.

87 Nora JJ, Nora AH. Maternal transmission of congenital heart diseases: New recurrent risk figures and the question of cytoplasmic inheritance and vulnerability to teratogens. *Am J Cardiol* 1987; 59: 459–63.

88 Burn J. The next lady has a heart defect. *Br J Obstet Gynaecol* 1987; 94: 97–9.

89 Crawford DC, Chita SK *et al.* Prenatal detection of congenital heart disease: Factors affecting obstetric management and survival. *Am J Obstet Gynecol* 1988; 159: 352–6.

90 Bull C, for the British Paediatric Cardiac Association. Current and potential impact of fetal diagnosis on prevalence and spectrum of serious congenital heart disease at term in the UK. *Lancet* 1999; 354: 1242–7.

91 Sharland GK, Allan LD. Screening for congenital heart disease prenatally. Results of a 2.5 year study in the South East Thames Region. *Br J Obstet Gynaecol* 1992; 99: 220–5.

92 Milne JA, Mowie AD *et al.* Dyspnoea during normal pregnancy. *Br J Obstet Gynaecol* 1978; 85: 260–3.

93 Howitt G. Heart disease and pregnancy. *Practitioner* 1971; 206: 765–72.

94 Shotan A, Ostrzega E *et al.* Incidence of arrhythmias in normal pregnancy and relation to palpitations, dizziness, and syncope. *Am J Cardiol* 1997; 79 (8): 1061–4.

95 Hart CW, Nauton RF. The ototoxicity of chloroquine phosphate. *Arch Otolaryngol* 1964; 80: 407.

96 Gonik B, Cotton DB. Peripartum colloid osmotic pressure changes: Influence of intravenous hydration. *Am J Obstet Gynecol* 1982; 150: 99–100.

97 Gonik B, Cotton D *et al.* Peripartum colloid osmotic pressure changes: effects of controlled fluid management. *Am J Obstet Gynecol* 1985; 151: 812–15.

98 Oian P, Malthau JM *et al.* Oedema-preventing mechanisms in subcutaneous tissue of normal pregnant women. *Br J Obstet Gynaecol* 1985; 92: 113–19.

99 Cutforth R, MacDonald CB. Heart sounds and murmurs in pregnancy. *Am Heart J* 1966; 71: 741–7.

100 Bell WR, Meek AG. Guidelines for the use of thrombolytic agents. *N Engl J Med* 1979; 301: 1266–70.

101 Oram HC, Holt M. Innocent depression of the ST segment and flattening of the T-wave during pregnancy. *J Obstet Gynaecol Br Commonwealth* 1961; 68: 765–70 May.

102 Boyle DMcC, Lloyd-Jones RL. The electrocardiographic S-T segment in pregnancy. *J Obstet Gynaecol Br Commonwealth* 1966; 73: 986–7.

103 Carr FB, Hamilton BE *et al.* The significance of large Q in lead III of the electrocardiogram during pregnancy. *Am Heart J* 1933; 8: 519.

104 Burton A, Camann W. Electrocardiographic changes during cesarean section: a review. *Int J Obstet Anesth* 1996; 5: 47–53.

105 Carruth SE, Mirvis SB *et al.* The electrocardiogram in normal pregnancy. *Am Heart J* 1981; 102: 1075–8.

106 St John Sutton MG, St John Sutton M *et al.* Valve replacement without preoperative cardiac catheterization. *N Engl J Med* 1981; 305: 1233–8.

107 Erbel R, Rohmann S *et al.* Improved diagnostic value of echocardiography in patients with infective endocarditis by transesophageal approach: a prospective study. *Eur Heart J* 1988; 9: 43–53.

108 Khanderia BK, Seward JB *et al.* Value and limitations of transesophageal echocardiography in assessment of mitral valve prostheses. *Circulation* 1991; 83: 1956–68.

109 Rubler S, Damani PM *et al.* Cardiac size and performance during pregnancy estimated with echocardiography. *Am J Cardiol* 1977; 40: 534–40.

110 Northcote RJ, Knight PV *et al.* Systolic murmurs in pregnancy: Value of echocardiographic assessment. *Clin Cardiol* 1985; 8: 327–8.

111 Mishra M, Chambers JB *et al.* Murmurs in pregnancy: an audit of echocardiography. *Br Med J* 1992; 304: 1413–14.

112 Robson SC, Richley D *et al.* Incidence of Doppler regurgitant flow velocities during normal pregnancy. *Eur Heart J* 1992; 13: 84–7.

113 Rayburn WF, Fontana ME. Mitral valve prolapse and pregnancy. *Am J Obstet Gynecol* 1981; 141: 9–11.

114 Chen WWC, Chan CS *et al.* Pregnancy in patients with prosthetic heart valves: An experience with 45 pregnancies. *Q J Med* 1982; 51: 358–65.

115 de Swiet M, Deverall PB. Pregnancy—still an indication for closed mitral valvotomy. *Int J Cardiol* 1990; 27: 323–4.

116 Leibbrand G, Muench U *et al.* Two successful pregnancies in a patient with single ventricle and transposition of the great arteries. *Int J Cardiol* 1982; 1: 257–62.

117 Vosloo S, Reichart B. The feasibility of closed mitral valvotomy in pregnancy. *J Thorac Cardiovasc Surg* 1987; 93: 675–9.

118 Pavankumar P, Venugopal P *et al.* Closed mitral valvotomy during pregnancy. *Scand J Thorac Cardiovasc Surg* 1988; 22: 11–5.

119 Hall R, Kirk R. Balloon dilatation of heart valves. *Br Med J* 1992; 305: 487–8.

120 Mangione JA, Zuliam MF *et al.* Percutaneous double balloon mitral valvuloplasty in pregnant women. *Am J Cardiol* 1989; 64: 99–102.

121 Angel JL, Chapman C *et al.* Percutaneous balloon aortic valvulopasty in pregnancy. *Obstet Gynecol* 1988; 72: 438–40.

122 Melvor RA. Percutaneous balloon aortic valvuloplasty during pregnancy. *Int J Cardiol* 1991; 32: 1–4.

123 Lao TT, Adelman AG *et al.* Balloon valvuloplasty for congenital aortic stenosis in pregnancy. *Br J Obstet Gynaecol* 1993; 100: 1141–2.

124 Zitnik RS, Brandenburg RO *et al.* Pregnancy and open heart surgery. *Circulation* 1969; 39 (Suppl.): 257.

125 Page PA, Toung TA. A new probe for measurement of muscle Po_2 and its use during cardiopulmonary bypass. *Surg Gynecol Obstet* 1975; 141: 579–81.

126 Bahary CM, Ninio A *et al.* Tococardiography in pregnancy during extra corporeal bypass for mitral valve replacement. *Israel J Med Sci* 1980; 16: 395–7.

127 Eilen B, Kaiser IH *et al.* Aortic valve replacement in the third trimester of pregnancy: case report and review of literature. *Obstet Gynecol* 1981; 57: 119–21.

128 Lamb MP, Ross K *et al.* Fetal heart monitoring during open heart surgery. *Br J Obstet Gynaecol* 1981; 88: 669–74.

129 Levy DL, Warringer RA *et al.* Fetal response to cardiopulmonary bypass. *Obstet Gynecol* 1980; 56: 112–15.

130 Izquierdo LA, Kushnir O *et al.* Effect of mitral valve prosthetic surgery on the outcome of a growth retarded fetus. A case report. *Am J Obstet Gynecol* 1990; 163: 584–6.

131 Becker RM. Intracardiac surgery in pregnant women. *Ann Thorac Surg* 1983; 36: 453–8.

132 Allan LD, Crawford DC *et al.* Familial recurrence of congenital heart disease in the prospective series of mothers referred for fetal echocardiography. *Am J Cardiol* 1986; 58: 334–7.

133 Harrigan JT, Kangos JJ *et al.* Successful treatment of fetal congestive heart failure secondary to tachycardia. *N Engl J Med* 1981; 304: 1527–9.

134 Macphail S, Walkinshaw SA. Fetal supraventricular tachycardia: detection by routine auscultation and successful in-utero management. Case report. *Br J Obstet Gynaecol* 1988; 95: 1073–6.

135 Newburger JW, Keane JF. Intrauterine supraventricular tachycardia. *J Pediatr* 1979; 95: 780–6.

136 Younis JS, Granat M. Insufficient transplacental digoxin transfer in severe hydrops fetalis. *Am J Obstet Gynecol* 1987; 157: 1268–9.

137 Klein AM, Holzman IR *et al.* Fetal tachycardia prior to the development of hydrops—attempted pharmacological cardinversion: Case report. *Am J Obstet Gynecol* 1979; 134: 347–8.

138 Teuscher A, Bossi E *et al.* Effect of propranolol on fetal tachycardia in diabetic pregnancy. *Am J Cardiol* 1978; 42: 304–7.

139 Dumesic DA, Silverman NH *et al.* Transplacental cardioversion of fetal supraventricular tachycardia with procainamide. *N Engl J Med* 1982; 307: 1128–31.

140 Rey E, Duperron L *et al.* Transplacental treatment of tachycardia-induced fetal heart failure with verapamil and amiodarone: a case report. *Am J Obstet Gynecol* 1985; 153: 311–12.

141 Conradsson TB, Werko L. Management of heart disease in pregnancy. *Prog Cardiovasc Dis* 1974; 16: 407–19.

142 Saarikoski S. Placental transfer and fetal uptake of 3H-digoxin in humans. *Br J Obstet Gynaecol* 1976; 83: 879–84.

143 Okita GT, Poltz EJ *et al.* Placental transfer of radioactive digitoxin in pregnant woman and its fetal distribution. *Circulation Res* 1956; 4: 376–80.

144 Rogers ME, Willerson JT *et al.* Serum digoxin concentrations in the human fetus, neonate and infant. *N Engl J Med* 1972; 287: 1010–13.

145 Szekely P, Snaith L. *Heart Disease and Pregnancy.* Churchill Livingstone, Edinburgh, 1974.

146 Sherman JL, Locke RV. Transplacental neonatal digitalis intoxication. *Am J Cardiol* 1960; 6: 834.

147 Togo T, Sugishita A *et al.* Uneventful pregnancy and delivery in a case of multiple peripheral pulmonary stenosis. *Acta Cardiol* 1983; 38: 143.

148 Wolfe CAD, Petruckevitch A *et al.* The rate of rise of corticotrophin releasing factor and endogenous digoxin-like immunoreactivity in normal and abnormal pregnancy. *Br J Obstet Gynaecol* 1990; 97: 832–7.

149 Poston L, Morris JF *et al.* Serum digoxin-like substances in pregnancy-induced hypertension. *Clin Sci* 1989; 77: 189–94.

150 Levy M, Grait L *et al.* Excretion of drugs in human milk. *N Engl J Med* 1977; 297: 789.

151 Weaver JB, Pearson JB. Influence of time of onset and duration of labour in women with cardiac disease. *Br Med J* 1973; ii: 519.

152 Anderson JB. The effect of diuretics in late pregnancy on the new born infant. *Acta Paediatr Scand* 1970; 59: 659–63.

153 Giudici MC, Artis AK *et al.* Postpartum myocardial infarction treated with percutaneous transluminal coronary angioplasty. *Am Heart J* 1989; 118: 614–16.

154 Husaini MH. Myocardial infarction during pregnancy: report of two cases and review of the literature. *Postgrad Med J* 1971; 47: 660.

155 Szekely P, Snaith L. Paroxysmal tachycardia in pregnancy. *Br Heart J* 1953; 15: 195.

156 Hubbard WN, Jenkins BAG *et al.* Persistent atrial tachycardia in pregnancy. *Br Med J* 1983; 287: 327.

157 Robards GJ, Saunders DM *et al.* Refractory supraventricular tachycardia complicating pregnancy. *Med J Aust* 1973; 2: 278–80.

158 Rosano GM, Leonardo F *et al.* Cyclical variation in paroxysmal supraventricular tachycardia in women. *Lancet* 1996; 347: 786–8.

159 Lip GYH. Thromboprophylaxis for atrial fibrillation. *Lancet* 1999; 353: 4–5.

160 Bruner JP, Barry MJ *et al.* Pregnancy in a patient with idiopathic long QT syndrome. *Am J Obstet Gynecol* 1984; 149: 690–1.

161 Wilkinson C, Gyaneshwar R *et al.* Twin pregnancy in a patient with idiopathic long QT syndrome. Case report. *Br J Obstet Gynaecol* 1991; 98: 1300–2.

162 Cotrill CM, McAllister RG Jr *et al.* Propranolol therapy during pregnancy, labour and delivery: evidence for transplacental drug transfer and impaired neonatal drug disposition. *J Pediatr* 1977; 91: 812–14.

163 Gladstone GR, Hordof A *et al.* Propranolol administration during pregnancy: effects on the fetus. *J Pediatr* 1975; 86: 962–4.

164 Habib A, McArthy JS. Effects on the neonate of propranolol administered during pregnancy. *J Pediatr* 1977; 91: 808–11.

165 Fidler J, Smith V *et al.* Randomised controlled comparative study of methyldopa and oxprenolol for the treatment of hypertension in pregnancy. *Br Med J* 1983; 286: 1927–30.

166 Gallery EDM, Saunders DM *et al.* Improvement in fetal growth with treatment of maternal hypertension in pregnancy. *Clin Sci Mol Med* 1978; 55: 359–61.

167 Rubin PC, Butters L *et al.* Placebo-controlled trial of atenolol in treatment of pregnancy associated hypertension. *Lancet* 1983; i: 431–4.

168 Fidler J, Smith V *et al.* The excretion of oxprenolol and timolol in breast milk. *Br J Obstet Gynaecol* 1983; 90: 961–5.

169 Inoue M, Unno N *et al.* Excretion of verapamil in breast milk. *Br Med J* 1983; 287: 1596.

170 Okada M, Inoue H *et al.* Excretion of diltiazem in human milk. *N Engl J Med* 1985; 312: 922–3.

171 de Swiet M. Excretion of verapamil in human milk. *Br Med J* 1984; 288: 644–5.

172 Kambam JR, Franks JJ *et al.* Inhibitory effect of quinidine on plasma pseudocholinesterase activity in pregnant women. *Am J Obstet Gynecol* 1987; 157: 897–9.

173 Timmis A'D, Jackson C *et al.* Mexiletine for control of ventricular dysrhythmias in pregnancy. *Lancet* 1980; ii: 647–8.

174 Lownes HE, Ives TJ. Mexiletine use in pregnancy and lactation. *Am J Obstet Gynecol* 1987; 157: 446–7.

175 Leonard RF, Braun TE *et al.* Initiation of uterine contractions by disopyramide during pregnancy. *N Engl J Med* 1978; 299: 84.

176 Finnerty JJ, MacKay BR. Antepartum thrombophlebitis and pulmonary embolism. *Obstet Gynecol* 1962; 19: 405.

177 Baroffio R, Tisi G *et al.* Tachicardia parossistica sopraventricolare reciprocante in gravidanza. A proposito di un caso. [Reciprocal supraventricular paroxysmal tachycardia in pregnancy. Apropos of a case.] *Minerva Ginecol* 1996; 48 (7–8): 327–30.

178 Barrett PA, Penn IM. Amiodarone in pregnancy. *Clin Prog Electrophysiol* 1986; 4: 158–9.

179 Foster CJ, Love HG. Amiodarone in pregnancy. Case report and review of literature. *Int J Cardiol* 1988; 20: 307–16.

180 Pitcher D, Leather HM *et al.* Amiodarone in pregnancy. *Lancet* 1983; i: 597–8.

181 Haffeje E. In discussion—amiodarone pharmacokinetics. *Am Heart J* 1983; 106: 847.

182 Penn IM, Barrett PA *et al* Amiodarone in pregnancy. *Am J Cardiol* 1985; 56: 196–7.

183 Robson DJ, Raj MVJ *et al*. Use of amiodarone in pregnancy. *Postgrad Med J* 1985; 61: 75–7.

184 McKenna WJ, Harris L *et al*. Amiodarone therapy during pregnancy. *Am J Cardiol* 1983; 51: 1231–3.

185 Camm AJ, Garratt CJ. Adenosine and supraventricular tachycardia. *N Engl J Med* 1991; 325: 1621–9.

186 Blanch G, Walkinshaw SA *et al*. Cardioversion of fetal tachyarrhythmia with adenosine. *Lancet* 1994; 344: 1646.

187 Finlay AY, Edmunds V. DC cardioversion in pregnancy. *Br J Clin Prac* 1979; 33: 8894.

188 Oates S, Williams GL *et al*. Cardiopulmonary resuscitation in late pregnancy. *Br Med J* 1988; 297: 404–5.

189 Weil AM, Graber VR. The management of the near term pregnant patient who dies undelivered. *Am J Obstet Gynecol* 1957; 73: 754–8.

190 Greiss GG, Steel MR *et al*. Caesarean section 26 minutes after cardiac arrest—a successful neonatal outcome. *J Obstet Gynaecol* 1994; 14: 432–3.

191 Vitale N, De Feo M *et al*. Dose-dependant fetal complications of warfarin in pregnant women with mechanical heart valves. *J Am Coll Cardiol* 1999; 33: 1637– 41.

192 Cannegeiter SC, Rosendaal FR *et al*. Optimal oral anticoagulant therapy in patients with mechanical heart valves. *N Engl J Med* 1995; 333: 11–17.

193 Javares T, Coto EC *et al*. Pregnancy after heart valve replacement. *Int J Cardiol* 1985; 5: 731–9.

194 Saour JN, Sieck JO *et al*. Trial of different intensities of anticoagulation in patients with prosthetic heart valves. *N Engl J Med* 1990; 322: 428–32.

195 Willis DC, Caton D *et al*. Cardiac output response to prostaglandin E2-induced abortion in the second trimester. *Am J Obstet Gynecol* 1987; 156: 170–3.

196 Lennox CE, Martin J. Cardiac arrest following intramyometrial prostaglandin E2. *J Obstet Gynaecol* 1991; 11: 263–4.

197 Katra PA, Litherland D *et al*. Cardiac standstill induced by prostaglandin pessaries. *Lancet* 1989; i: 1460–1.

198 Levy DM, Hinshaw K *et al*. Cardiogenic pulmonary oedema: presentation of pre-eclampsia exacerbated by prostaglandin abortifacients. *Br J Obstet Gynaecol* 1994; 101: 263–5.

199 Jakobi P, Adler Z *et al*. Effect of uterine contractions on left atrial pressure in a pregnant woman with rititral stenosis. *Br Med J* 1989; 298: 27.

200 Ueland K, Gills R *et al*. Maternal cardiovascular dynamics. 1. Caesarean section under subarachnoid block anesthesia. *Am J Obstet Gynecol* 1968; 100: 42–53.

201 Redick LF. An inflatable wedge for prevention of aortocaval compression during pregnancy. *Am J Obstet Gynecol* 1979; 133: 458–9.

202 Robson SC, Dunlop W *et al*. Haemodynamic changes associated with caesarean section under epidural anaesthesia. *Br J Obstet Gynaecol* 1989; 96: 642–7.

203 Robson SC, Boys R *et al*. Haemodynamic changes during epidural and spinal anaesthesia for elective caesarean section: correlation with umbilical artery pH. *Clin Sci* 1991; 11: 301.

204 Editorial. Epidural block for caesarean section and circulatory changes. *Lancet* 1989; ii: 1076–8.

205 Clark SL, Morenstein JM *et al*. Experience with pulmonary artery catheter. *Obstet Gynecol* 1985; 152: 374–80.

206 Seaworth BJ, Durack DT. Infective endocarditis in obstetric and gynecologic practice. *Am J Obstet Gynecol* 1986; 154: 180–8.

207 Fleming HA. Antibiotic prophylaxis against infective endocarditis after delivery. *Lancet* 1977; i: 144–5.

208 Smith RH, Radford DJ *et al*. Infective endocarditis: a summary of cases in the South-East region of Scotland 1969–72. *Thorax* 1976 (31): 373–9.

209 Redleaf PB, Farell EJ. Bacteremia during parturition—prevention of subacute bacterial endocarditis. *J Am Med Assoc* 1959; 169: 1284–5.

210 Report of a Working Party of the British Society for Antimicrobial Chemotherapy. The antibiotic prophylaxis of infective endocarditis. *Lancet* 1982; ii: 1323–6.

211 Department of Health and Social Security. *Report on Confidential Enquires into Maternal Deaths in United Kingdom, 1975–78*. HMSO, London, 1982.

212 de Swiet M, Louvois J *et al*. Failure of cephalosporins to prevent bacterial endocarditis during labour. *Lancet* 1975; ii: 186.

213 Hughes LO, McFadyen IR *et al*. Acute bacterial endocarditis on a normal aortic valve following vaginal delivery. *Int J Cardiol* 1988; 18: 261–2.

214 Durack DT. Current practice in prevention of bacterial endocarditis. *Br Heart J* 1975; 37: 478–81.

215 Garrod JP, Waterworth PM. The risks of dental extraction during penicillin treatment. *Br Heart J* 1962; 24: 39– 46.

216 Recommendations from the Endocarditis Working Party of the British Society for Antimicrobial Chemotherapy. Antibiotic prophylaxis of infective endocarditis. *Lancet* 1990; 335: 88–9.

217 Simmons NA, Cawson RA *et al*. Prophylaxis of infective endocarditis. *Lancet* 1986; i: 1267.

218 Hill LM. Fetal distress secondary to vancomycin induced maternal hypotension. *Am J Obstet Gynecol* 1985; 153: 74–5.

219 Simmons NA, Ball AP *et al*. Antibiotic prophylaxis and infective endocarditis. *Lancet* 1992; 339: 1292–3.

220 Nimrod C, Rambihar V *et al*. Pulmonary edema associated with isoxsuprine therapy. *Am J Obstet Gynecol* 1984; 148: 625–9.

221 Whitehead MI, Mander AM *et al*. Myocardial ischaemia after withdrawal of salbutamol for pre-term labour. *Lancet* 1979; ii: 904.

222 Voto LS, Agranatti D *et al*. Successful maternal and fetal outcome in a pregnant woman with primary pulmonary hypertension. *Curr Obstet Gynaecol* 1992; 2: 177–9.

223 Davies AE, Robertson MJS. Pulmonary oedema after the administration of intravenous salbutamol and ergometrine. *Br J Obstet Gynaecol* 1980; 87: 529– 41.

224 Stubblefield PG. Pulmonary edema occurring after therapy with dexamethasone and terbutaline for premature labour. A case report. *Am J Obstet Gynecol* 1978; 132: 341–2.

225 Rogge P, Young S *et al*. Post-partum pulmonary oedema associated with preventive therapy for premature labour. *Lancet* 1979; i: 1026–7.

226 Kubli F. Proceedings of the fifth study group of the Royal College of Obstetricians and Gynaecologists. In: Anderson A, Beard R, Brudenell M, Dunn PM, ed. *Preterm Labour*. Royal College of Obstetricians and Gynaecologists, London, 1977: 218–20.

227 Elliott HR, Abdulla U *et al*. Pulmonary oedema associated with ritodrine infusion and betamethasone administration in premature labour. *Br Med J* 1978; ii: 799–800.

228 Lewis PJ, de Swiet M *et al*. How obstetricians in the United Kingdom manage preterm labour. *Br J Obstet Gynaecol* 1980; 87: 574–7.

229 Hemminki E, Starfield B. Prevention and treatment of premature labour by drugs: review of clinical trials. *Br J Obstet Gynaecol* 1978; 85: 411–17.

230 Lamont RF. The pathophysiology of pulmonary oedema with the use of beta-agonists. *Br J Obstet Gynaecol* 2000; 107: 439–44.

231 Hastwell G, Lambert BE. The effect of oral salbutamol on serum potassium and blood sugar. *Br J Obstet Gynaecol* 1978; 85: 767–9.

232 Poole Wilson PA. Cardiac failure in hypertensive woman receiving salbutamol for premature labour. *Br Med J* 1980; 281: 226.

233 Fogarty AJ. Cardiac failure in a hypertensive woman receiving salbutamol for premature labour. *Br Med J* 1980; 281: 226.

234 Blickstein I, Zalel Y *et al.* Ritodrine-induced pulmonary edema unmasking underlying peripartum cardiomyopathy. *Am J Obstet Gynecol* 1988; 159: 332–3.

235 Carpenter RJ, Decuir P. Cardiovascular collapse associated with oral terbutaline tocolytic therapy. *Am J Obstet Gynecol* 1984; 148: 821–3.

236 Ben-Shlomo I, Zohar S *et al.* Myocardial ischaemia during intravenous ritodrine treatment: is it so rare? *Lancet* 1986; ii: 917–18.

237 Hendricks SK, Keroes J *et al.* Electrocardiographic changes associated with ritodrine-induced maternal tachycardia and hypokalemia. *Am J Obstet Gynecol* 1986; 154: 921–3.

238 Walters BNJ, Thompson ME *et al.* Blood pressure in the puerperium. *Clin Sci* 1986; 71: 589–94.

239 Watson NA, Morgan B. Pulmonary oedema and salbutamol in preterm labour. Case report and literature review. *Br J Obstet Gynaecol* 1989; 96: 1445–8.

240 Clark SL, Phelan JP *et al.* Labour and delivery in the presence of mitral stenosis: Central hemodynamic observations. *Am J Obstet Gynecol* 1985; 8: 984–8.

241 Caves PK, Paneth M. Acute mitral regurgitation in pregnancy due to ruptured chordae tendinae. *Br Heart J* 1972; 34: 541–4.

242 Olivera DBG, Dawkins KD *et al.* Chordal rupture 1: Aetiology and natural history. *Br Heart J* 1983; 50: 312–17.

243 Mann MS, Cossham PS *et al.* Left atrial myxoma in the second trimester of pregnancy. Case report. *Br J Obstet Gynaecol* 1987; 94: 592–3.

244 Burwash IG, Forbes AD *et al.* Echocardiographic volume flow and stenosis severity measures with changing flow in aortic stenosis. *Am J Physiol* 1993; 265: H1734–43.

245 Nagorney DM, Field CS. Successful pregnancy 10 years after triple cardiac valve replacement. *Obstet Gynecol* 1981; 57: 386–8.

246 Bisno AL. Group A streptococcal infections and acute rheumatic fever. *N Engl J Med* 1991; 325: 783–93.

247 Oakley CM. Pregnancy in patients with prosthetic heart valves. *Br Med J* 1983; 286: 1680–2.

248 Andrinopoulos GC, Arias F. Triple heart valve prosthesis and pregnancy. *Obstet Gynecol* 1980; 55: 762–4.

249 Sadler L, McCowanb L *et al.* Pregnancy outcomes and cardiac complications in women with mechanical, bioprosthetic and homograft valves. *Br J Obstet Gynaecol* 2000; 107: 245–53.

250 North RA, Sadler L *et al* Long-term survival and valve-related complications in young women with cardiac valve replacements. *Circulation* 1999; 99: 2669–76.

251 Oakley C, ed. *Heart Disease in Pregnancy.* BMJ Publishing Group, London, 1997: 135–46.

252 Sbarouni E, Oakley CM. Outcome of pregnancy in women with valve protheses. *Br Heart J* 1994; 71: 96–201.

253 Limet R, Crondin CM. Cardiac valve prosthesis, anticoagulation and pregnancy. *Ann Thorac Surg* 1977; 23: 337–431.

254 Ahmad R, Rajah SM *et al.* Dipyridamole in successful management of pregnant women with prosthetic heart valve. *Lancet* 1976; ii: 1414–15.

255 Biale Y, Cantor A *et al.* The course of pregnancy in patients with artificial heart valves treated with dipyridamole. *Int J Obstet Gynaecol* 1980; 18: 128–32.

256 Bennett GG, Oakley CM. Pregnancy in a patient with a mitral valve prosthesis. *Lancet* 1968; i: 616–19.

257 McLeod AA, Jennings KP *et al.* Near fatal puerperal thrombosis on Bjork–Shiley mitral valve prosthesis. *Br Heart J* 1978; 40: 934–7.

258 Benchimol AB, Carneiro RD *et al.* Postpartum heart disease. *Br Heart J* 1959; 21: 89.

259 Wong V, Cheng CH *et al.* Fetal and neonatal outcome of exposure to anticoagulants during pregnancy. *Am J Med Genet* 1993; 45: 17–21.

260 Iturbe-Alessio I, Fonseca M *et al.* Risks of anticoagulant therapy in pregnant women with artificial heart valves. *N Engl J Med* 1986; 315: 1390–3.

261 Chong MKB, Harvey DH *et al.* Follow-up study of children whose mothers were treated with warfarin during pregnancy. *Br J Obstet Gynaecol* 1984; 91: 1070–3.

262 Oakley CM, Doherty P. Pregnancy in patients with valve replacement. *Br Heart J* 1976; 38: 1040–8.

263 O'Neill H, Blake S *et al.* Problems in the management of patients with artificial heart valves during pregnancy. *Br J Obstet Gynaecol* 1982; 89: 940–3.

264 Vitali E, Donatelli F *et al.* Pregnancy in patients with mechanical prosthetic heart valves. *J Cardiovasc Surg* 1986; 27: 221–7.

265 Larsen JF, Jacobsen B *et al.* Intrauterine injection of vitamin K before delivery during anticoagulant treatment of the mother. *Acta Obstet Gynecol Scand* 1978; 57: 227–30.

266 Orme ML, Lewis PJ *et al.* May mothers given warfarin breast-feed their infants? *Br Med J* 1977; i: 1564–5.

267 Eckstein H, Jack B. Breast feeding and anticoagulant therapy. *Lancet* 1970; i: 672–3.

268 Elkayam U. Pregnancy through a prosthetic heart valve. *J Am Coll Cardiol* 1999; 33: 1642–5.

269 Rabinovici J, Mani A *et al.* Long term ambulatory anticoagulation by constant subcutaneous heparin infusion in pregnancy. *Br J Obstet Gynaecol* 1987; 94: 89–91.

270 Nelson DM, Stempel LE *et al.* Hickman catheter use in a pregnant patient requiring therapeutic heparin anticoagulation. *Am J Obstet Gynecol* 1984; 149: 461–2.

271 Peterson DR, Thompson DJ & Chinn N. Ischaemic heart disease prognosis. A community-made assessment (1966–1969). *J Am Med Assoc* 1972; 219: 1423–7.

272 Badui E, Enciso R. Acute myocardial infarction during pregnancy and puerperium: a review. *Angiology* 1996; 47: 739–56.

273 Cortis BS, Freese E *et al.* Precordial pain and myocardial infarction in pregnancy. *G Ital Cardiol* 1979; 9: 532–4.

274 Ginz B. Myocardial infarction in pregnancy. *J Obstet Gynaecol Br Commonwealth* 1970; 77: 610.

275 Beary JF, Summer WR *et al.* Postpartum acute myocardial infarction: a rare occurrence of uncertain etiology. *Am J Cardiol* 1979; 43: 158–60.

276 Ciraulo DA, Markovitz A. Myocardial infarction in pregnancy associated with a coronary artery thrombosis. *Arch Intern Med* 1979; 139: 1046–7.

277 Sonel A, Erol C *et al.* Acute myocardial infarction and normal coronary arteries in a pregnant woman. *Cardiology* 1988; 75: 218–20.

278 Bulkley BH, Roberts WC. Dissecting aneurysm (haematoma) limited to coronary artery. *Am J Med* 1973; 55: 747–56.

279 Jewett JF. Two dissecting coronary artery aneurysms post partum. *N Engl J Med* 1978; 278: 1255–6.

280 Hayden J, Mort T *et al.* Acute coronary artery dissection during pregnancy. Case report. *Int J Obstet Anesth* 1991; 1: 43–5.

281 Vicari R, Eybel C *et al.* Survival following spontaneous coronary artery dissection: Surgical repair by extrusion of intramural haematoma. *Am Heart J* 1986; 111: 593–4.

282 Wandsworth R, Devine A *et al.* Splenic aneurysm rupture as a cause of maternal collapse. *Int J Obstet Anesthesia* 1996; 5: 99–102

283 Cressey D, Reid MF. Splenic artery aneurysm rupture in pregnancy. *Int J Obstet Anesth* 1996; 5: 103–4.

284 Snir E, Levinsky L *et al.* Dissecting aortic aneurysm in pregnant women without Marfan disease. *Surg Gynecol Obstet* 1988; 167: 463–5.

285 Anderson RA, Fineron PW. Aortic dissection in pregnancy: importance of pregnancy-induced changes in the vessel wall and bicuspid aortic valve in pathogenesis. *Br J Obstet Gynaecol* 1994; 101: 1085–8.

286 Hartman JD, Eftychiadis AS. Medial smooth-muscle cell lesions and dissection of the aorta and muscular arteries. *Arch Pathol Lab Med* 1990; 114: 50–61.

287 Bosio PM, Barry-Kinsella C *et al.* Spontaneous iliac artery dissection in a healthy postpartum woman. *J Obstet Gynaecol* 1998; 18: 88–9.

288 Movsesian AM, Wray RB. Postpartum myocardial infarction. *Br Heart J* 1989; 62: 154–6.

289 Klein VR, Repke JT *et al.* The Bland–White–Garland syndrome in pregnancy. *Am J Obstet Gynecol* 1984; 150: 106–7.

290 Nolan TE, Savage RW. Peripartum myocardial infarction from presumed Kawasaki's disease. *South Med J* 1990; 83: 1360–1.

291 Roberts ADC, Low RAL *et al.* Left ventricular aneurysm complicating myocardial infarction occurring during pregnancy. Case report. *Br J Obstet Gynaecol* 1983; 90: 969–70.

292 Stokes IM, Evans J *et al.* Myocardial infarction and cardiac output in the second trimester followed by assisted vaginal delivery under epidural anaesthesia at 38 weeks gestation. Case report. *Br J Obstet Gynaecol* 1984; 91: 197–8.

293 McLintic AJ, Lilley S *et al.* Electrocardiographic changes during caesarean section under regional anaesthesia. *Int J Obstet Anesth* 1991; 1: 55–7.

294 Stone NIL, Lending M *et al.* Glutamine oxalacetic transaminase and lactic dehydrogenase in pregnancy. *Am J Obstet Gynecol* 1960; 80: 104.

295 Julian DC Szekely P. Peripartum cardiomyopathy. *Prog Cardiovasc Dis* 1985; 27: 223–40.

296 Spirito P, Seidman CE *et al.* The management of hypertrophic cardiomyopathy. *N Engl J Med* 1997; 336: 775–85.

297 Oakley GDG, McGarry K *et al.* Management of pregnancy in patients with hypertrophic cardiomyopathy. *Br Med J* 1979; i: 1749–50.

298 Hull E, Hafkesbring E. 'Toxic' postpartal heart disease. *New Orleans Med Surg J* 1937; 89: 550.

299 Stuart KL. Cardiomyopathy of pregnancy and the puerperium. *Q J Med* 1968; 37: 463–78.

300 Meadows WIZ. Myocardial failure in the last trimester of pregnancy and the puerperium. *Circulation* 1957; 15: 903–14.

301 Homans DC. Peripartum cardiomyopathy. *N Engl J Med* 1985; 312: 1432–7.

302 Brown AK, Doukas N *et al.* Cardiomyopathy and pregnancy. *Br Heart J* 1967; 29: 387–93.

303 Rand RH, Jenkins BM *et al.* Maternal cardiomyopathy in pregnancy causing stillbirth. *Br J Obstet Gynaecol* 1975; 82: 172–5.

304 Melvin KR, Richardson PJ *et al.* Peripartum cardiomyopathy due to myocarditis. *N Engl J Med* 1982; 307: 731–4.

305 Cunningham FG, Pritchard JA *et al.* Peripartum heart failure: Idiopathic cardiomyopathy of compounding cardiovascular events. *Obstet Gynecol* 1986; 67: 157–68.

306 Demarkis JG, Rahimtoola SM *et al.* Natural course of peripartum cardiomyopathy. *Circulation* 1971; 44: 1053–61.

307 Midei MG, DeMent SH *et al.* Peripartum myocarditis and cardiomyopathy. *Circulation* 1990; 81: 922–8.

308 Aravot DJ, Banner NR *et al.* Heart transplantation for peripartum cardiomyopathy. *Lancet* 1987; ii: 1024.

309 Ceci O, Berardesca C *et al.* Recurrent peripartum cardiomyopathy. *Eur J Obstet Gynecol Reprod Biol* 1998; 76 (1): 29–30.

310 Rutherford JM. Subsequent pregnancy in patients with previous peripartum cardiomyopathy *Curr Obstet Gynaecol* 1998; 8: 56–8.

311 Davidson NMcD, Parry EHO. Peri-partum cardiac failure. *Q J Med* 1978; 47: 431–61.

312 Sanderson JF, Adesanya CO *et al.* Post partum cardiac failure—heart failure due to volume overload. *Am Heart J* 1979; 97: 613–21.

313 Sanderson JE. Oedema and heart failure in the tropics. *Lancet* 1977; ii: 1159–61.

314 Editorial. Dilated cardiomyopathy in Africa. *Lancet* 1985; i: 557–8.

315 Nysenbaum AM. Pregnancy in a patient with endocardial fibroelastosis. *J Obstet Gynaecol* 1986; 7: 121–2.

316 Blake S, Bonar F *et al.* Pregnancy with constrictive pericarditis. *Br J Obstet Gynaecol* 1984; 91: 404–6.

317 Reitz BA, Wallwork JL *et al.* Heart–lung transplantation. Successful therapy with pulmonary vascular disease. *N Engl J Med* 1982; 306: 557–64.

318 Burke CM, Theodore J *et al.* Twenty-eight cases of human heart-lung transplantation. *Lancet* 1986; i: 517–19.

319 Littler WA, Redman CWC *et al.* Reduced pulmonary arterial compliance in hypertensive pregnancy. *Lancet* 1973; i: 1274–8.

320 Millwall J, Jaffin H *et al.* Shunt flow and pulmonary haemodynamics during labour and delivery in the Eisenmenger syndrome. *Am J Cardiol* 1978; 42: 299–303.

321 Crawford JS, Mills WG *et al.* A pregnant patient with Eisenmenger syndrome. *Br J Anaesth* 1971; 43: 1091–4.

322 Devitt JH, Noble WH. Eisenmenger's syndrome and pregnancy. *N Engl J Med* 1980; 302: 751.

323 Christman BW, McPherson CD *et al.* An imbalance between the excretion of thromboxane and prostacyclin metabolites in pulmonary hypertension. *N Engl J Med* 1992; 327: 70–5.

324 Jones K, Higenbottam T *et al.* Pulmonary vasodilation with prostacyclin in primary and secondary hypertension. *Chest* 1989; 96: 748–89.

325 Roberts JD, Polaner DM *et al.* Inhaled nitric oxide in persistent pulmonary hypertension of the newborn. *Lancet* 1992; 340: 818–19.

326 Pepke-Zaba J, Higenbottam TW *et al.* Inhaled nitric oxide as a cause of selective pulmonary vasodilatation in pulmonary hypertension. *Lancet* 1991; 338: 1173–4.

327 Bowers C, Devine PA *et al.* Dilation and evacuation during the second trimester of pregnancy in a woman with primary pulmonary hypertension. *J Reprod Med* 1988; 33: 787–8.

328 Connolly HMM, Crary JL *et al.* Valvular heart disease associated with fenluramine-phenteremine. *N Engl J Med* 1997; 337: 581–8.

329 Abenhaim L, Moride Y *et al*. Appetite suppressant drugs and risk of primary pulmonary hypertension hypertension. *N Engl J Med* 1996; 335: 609–16.

330 Bishop A, Oldershaw P. Thromboembolism in primary pulmonary hypertension. *Br Med J* 1996; 313: 1418–19.

331 Nelson DM, Main E *et al*. Peripartum heart failure due to primary pulmonary hypertension. *Obstet Gynecol* 1983; 62: 58S–63S.

332 Okano Y, Yoshioka T *et al*. Orally active prostacyclin analogue in primary pulmonary hypertension. *Lancet* 1997; 349: 1365.

333 Rich S, Kauffmann E *et al*. The effect of high doses of calcium channel blockers on survival in primary pulmonary hypertension. *N Engl J Med* 1992; 327: 76–81.

334 Slomka F, Salmeron S *et al*. Primary pulmonary hypertension and pregnancy: Anesthetic management of delivery. *Anesthesiology* 1988; 69: 959–61.

335 Oakley C, ed. *Heart Disease in Pregnancy*. BMJ Publishing Group, London, 1997: 94.

336 Landsberger EJ, Grossman II JH. Multiple peripheral pulmonic stenosis in pregnancy. *Am J Obstet Gynecol* 1986; 154: 152–3.

337 Konishi Y, Tatsuta N *et al*. Dissecting aneurysm during pregnancy and the puerperium. *Jap Circulation J* 1980; 44: 726–32.

338 Mendelson CL. Pregnancy and coarctation of the aorta. *Am J Obstet Gynecol* 1940; 39: 1014– 42.

339 Deal K, Wooley CF. Coarctation of the aorta and pregnancy. *Ann Intern Med* 1973; 78: 706–10.

340 Saidi AS, Bezold LI *et al*. Outcome of pregnancy following intervention for coarctation of the aorta. *Am J Cardiol* 1998; 82 (6): 786–8.

341 Tsipouras P, Del Mastro R *et al*. Genetic linkage of the Marfan syndrome, ectopia lentis and congenital contractural arachnodactyly to the fibrillin genes on chromosomes 15 and 5. *N Engl J Med* 1992; 326: 905–90.

342 Pereira L, Levran O *et al*. A molecular approach to the stratification of cardiovascular risk in families with Marfan's syndrome. *N Engl J Med* 1994; 331: 148–53.

343 Pyeritz RE, McKuisick VA. The Marfan syndrome: diagnosis and management. *N Engl J Med* 1979; 300: 772–7.

344 Pyeritz RE. Maternal and fetal complication of pregnancy in the Marfan syndrome. *Am J Med* 1981; 71: 784–90.

345 Beighton P. Pregnancy in the Marfan syndrome. *Br Med J* 1982; 285: 464.

346 Lipscomb KJ, Smith JC *et al*. Outcome of pregnancy in women with Marfan's syndrome. *Br J Obstet Gynaecol* 1997; 104: 210–16.

347 Shores J, Berger KR *et al*. Progression of aortic dilatation and the benefit of long-term β-adrenergic blockade in Marfan's syndrome. *N Engl J Med* 1994; 330: 1335–41.

348 Barker SG, Burnand KG. Retrograde iliac artery dissection in Marfan's syndrome. A case report. *J Cardiovasc Surg Torino* 1989; 30: 953– 4.

349 Coln LM, Lavin JP Jr. Pregnancy complicated by Marfan's syndrome with aortic arch dissection, subsequent aortic arch replacement and triple coronary artery bypass grafts. *J Reprod Med* 1985; 30: 685–8.

350 Ferguson JE, Veland K *et al*. Marfan's syndrome: acute aortic dissection during labor, resulting in fetal distress and cesarean section, followed by successful surgical repair. *Am J Obstet Gynecol* 1983; 147: 759–62.

351 Maruyama Y, Oguma F *et al*. Successful repair of an acute type A dissection during pregnancy. *Nippon Kyolia Geka Gakkai Zasshi* 1990; 38: 2296–9.

352 Quirm RJ, Mukerjee B. Spontaneous uterine inversion in association with Marfan's syndrome. *Aust NZ J Obstet Gynaecol* 1982; 22: 163–4.

353 Irons DW, Pollard KP. Postpartum haemorrhage secondary to Marfan's disease of the uterine vasculature. *Br J Obstet Gynaecol* 1993; 100: 279–81.

354 Gott VL, Pyeritz RE *et al*. Surgical treatment of aneurysms of the ascending aorta in the Marfan syndrome. Results of composite graft repair in 50 patients. *N Engl J Med* 1986; 314: 1070– 4.

355 Ginns HM, Holinrake K. Complete heart block in pregnancy treated with an internal cardiac pacemaker. *J Obstet Gynaecol Br Commonwealth* 1970; 77: 719.

356 Bowman PR, Millar-Craig MW. Congenital heart block and pregnancy: a further case report. *J Obstet Gynaecol* 1980; 1: 98–9.

357 Hatjis CG, Gibson M *et al*. Pregnancy in a patient with tricuspid atresia. *Am J Obstet Gynecol* 1983; 145: 114–15.

358 Novy MJ, Peterson EN *et al*. Respiratory characteristics of maternal and fetal blood in cyanotic congenital heart disease. *Am J Obstet Gynecol* 1968; 100: 821.

359 Cromme-Dijkhuis AH, Henkens CMA *et al*. Coagulation factor abnormalities as possible thrombotic risk factors after Fontan operations. *Lancet* 1990; 336: 1087–90.

360 Canobbio MM, Mair DD *et al*. Pregnancy outcomes after the Fontan repair. *J Am Coll Cardiol* 1996; 28 (3): 763–7.

361 Baumann H, Schneider H *et al*. Pregnancy and delivery by Caesarean section in a patient with transposition of the great arteries and single ventricle. Case report. *Br J Obstet Gynaecol* 1987; 94: 704–8.

362 Johnston TA, De Bono D. Single ventricle and pulmonary hypertension. A successful pregnancy. Case report. *Br J Obstet Gynaecol* 1989; 96: 731– 4.

363 Walsh T, Savage R *et al*. Successful pregnancy in a patient with a double inlet left ventricle treated with a septation procedure. *South Med J* 1990; 83: 358–9.

364 Yuzpe AA, Sanghvi VR *et al*. Successful pregnancy in a patient with single ventricle and other congenital cardiac anomalies. *Can Med Assoc J* 1970; 108: 1073–5.

365 Neumayer U, Somerville J. Outcome of pregnancies in patients with complex pulmonary atresia. *Heart* 1997; 78: 16–21.

366 Bosatra MG, Passarani S *et al*. Caesarean delivery of a patient with truncus arteriosus. *Int J Obstet Anesth* 1997; 6: 279–84.

367 Connolly HM, Warnes CA. Ebstein's anomaly: outcome of pregnancy. *J Am Coll Cardiol* 1994; 23 (5): 1194–8.

368 Kossoy LR, Herbert CM *et al*. Management of heart transplant recipients: Guidelines for the obstetrician-gynecologist. *Am J Obstet Gynecol* 1988; 159: 490–9.

369 Hedon B, Montoya F *et al*. Twin pregnancy and vaginal birth after heart transplantation. *Lancet* 1990; 335: 476–7.

370 Troche V, Ville Y *et al*. Pregnancy after heart or heart-lung transplantation: a series of 10 pregnancies. *Br J Obstet Gynaecol* 1998; 105: 454–8.

371 Scott JR, Wagoner LE *et al*. Pregnancy in heart transplant recipients: management and outcome. *Obstet Gynecol* 1993; 82: 324–7.

372 de Swiet M, Fidler J. Heart disease in pregnancy: some controversies. *J R Coll Physicians* 1981; 15: 183–6.

6 Hypertension

Christopher W. G. Redman

Terminology

In this chapter the term 'hypertension' is used to describe a blood pressure deemed to be higher than normal. Hypertension in pregnancy has three possible aetiologies: it may be caused by the pregnancy itself; it may be a long-term problem present before the pregnancy began; or much more rarely, it may be a new medical problem, by chance coinciding with pregnancy. Pregnancy-induced hypertension (PIH), transient hypertension of pregnancy or gestational hypertension are terms used to describe new hypertension, which appears after mid-term (20 weeks) and resolves after delivery. 'Chronic hypertension' is used to describe the condition of long-term high blood pressure. The usual cause is 'essential hypertension', meaning an inherited condition with no underlying pathology. There are other rarer causes, discussed later. Superimposed pre-eclampsia describes a mixed syndrome comprising pre-eclampsia in an individual with pre-existing or chronic hypertension (CHT).

Cardiovascular changes in pregnancy

Cardiovascular adaptations to pregnancy begin early, persist to an extent postpartum, and appear to be enhanced by a subsequent pregnancy (Clapp & Capeless 1997; Hennessy *et al.* 1996). Cardiac output increases by about 40% during the first trimester. According to most investigators it declines during the third trimester (van Oppen *et al.* 1996), partly because, in the supine position, the venous return to the heart is obstructed by the gravid uterus. This reduces cardiac output acutely by 20% or more (Lees *et al.* 1967). The primary maternal haemodynamic adaptation in early pregnancy is probably a fall in systemic vascular tone, a fall in preload and afterload, which leads to a compensatory increase in heart rate and activation of the volume-restoring mechanisms. Subsequently cardiac output increases because of a rise in stroke volume (Duvekot *et al.* 1993).

Arterial pressure falls during pregnancy (Fig. 6.1) (Chapman *et al.* 1998), beginning in the first trimester, when the cardiac output is already rising, and reaching a nadir in mid-pregnancy (MacGillivray *et al.* 1969). During the third trimester both systolic and diastolic readings slowly rise to about the pre-pregnant levels (MacGillivray *et al.* 1969). However, the measurements depend on posture. In the supine position, with vena-caval compression and reduced venous return, arterial pressure is maintained by reflex vasoconstriction (Lees *et al.* 1967), which causes a narrowing of the pulse pressure (Holmes 1960). The systolic pressure may fall nevertheless, by more than 30% in 10% of cases (Holmes 1960). Signs and symptoms of 'supine hypotension' may then occur including restlessness, faintness, hyperpnoea and pallor.

The reduced peripheral resistance of normal pregnancy is associated with relative arterial refractoriness to the constrictor actions of exogenous angiotensin II (Gant *et al.* 1973). Reduced reactivity to angiotensin II is already detectable at 8 weeks' gestation and maximal at mid-pregnancy (Gant *et al.* 1973). The mechanism of this

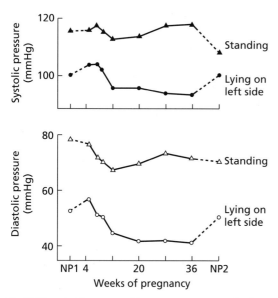

Fig 6.1 The arterial pressures of 10 women were measured using a London School of Hygiene sphygomanometer to reduce observer bias. Readings were taken in the right arm and phase IV of the Korotkoff sounds defined the diastolic pressures. Pressures taken before conception (NP1), during pregnancy, and 6 weeks after delivery (NP2) are shown, both standing (▲, △) and supine on the left side (●, ○) (C.W.G. Redman, unpublished observations).

blunted responsiveness has not been elucidated but may be prostaglandin dependent. The contribution of endothelial nitric oxide synthesis to the vasodilatation and vascular inertia of pregnancy is unresolved. In pregnant animals it plays a role but this is less certain in pregnant women (Sladek *et al.* 1997).

Factors affecting blood pressure in normal pregnancy

In non-gravid individuals, blood pressure levels are influenced by age, sex, race, body build and many other factors particularly the circumstances under which the measurement is taken, and the time of day. Pregnant women are usually young and fit. The range of blood pressures is therefore narrower than in the general population and distributed around mean levels which change at different stages of gestation but which in mid-pregnancy are lower than in a comparable non-pregnant population.

Errors in the measurement of blood pressure

The indirect method of measuring blood pressure gives an approximate estimate of the true intra-arterial pressure. There is no agreement as to the cause or magnitude

of the discrepancies between direct and indirect measurements in non-pregnant subjects (Pickering 1968). In two studies of simultaneous measurements in pregnant women the direct readings differed on average by −6/−15 and +5/−7 mmHg, respectively, from indirect readings (Raftery & Ward 1968; Ginsberg & Duncan 1969). The discrepancies were not related to the level of blood pressure, arm skinfold thickness or arm circumference (Raftery & Ward 1968). It is generally agreed that hypertension in obese individuals is overdiagnosed if the cuff is too small in relation to the arm circumference. When the latter exceeds 35 cm either a larger arm cuff (15 × 33 cm) or even a thigh cuff (18 × 36 cm) should be used rather than a regular cuff (12× 23 cm) (Maxwell *et al.* 1982).

The mean arm circumference of chronically hypertensive pregnant women is 27.5 cm, exceeding 35 cm in fewer than 5% of this group, so the problem of a large arm is not common. The effect of bodyweight on the booking blood pressure in pregnant women is shown in Fig. 6.2.

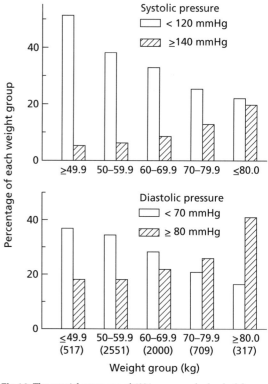

Fig 6.2 The arterial pressures of 6094 women who booked for antenatal care at 10–20 weeks have been studied. The effect of maternal weight is shown in terms of the preponderance of small women with low pressures, and heavy women with high pressures. The numbers in parentheses are the totals for each weight group (C.W.G. Redman, unpublished observations).

Indirect blood pressure measurements should be made with the cuff at the level of the heart. If it is above or below this position the pressure in the brachial artery will fall or rise because of hydrostatic forces. Thus, a pressure in the right (uppermost) arm with the patient lying on her left side will seem to be lower than the same reading when she lies flat on her back (Fig. 6.3). This is relevant when the lateral position is used in the third trimester to avoid the 'supine hypotension syndrome'. If the patient sits or stands, peripheral resistance increases by vasoconstriction in the lower extremities to maintain systolic pressure, with the effect of increasing diastolic pressure (Fig. 6.3). Thus, standardization of posture and arm position is crucial. The problem can be resolved by taking blood pressures in the sitting patient as recommended in the consensus report from the USA (National High Blood Pressure Education Program 1990).

Another problem is the interpretation of the Korotkoff sounds. Phase I of the Korotkoff sounds defines the systolic pressure. In non-gravid individuals phase V (extinction of Korotkoff sounds) is recommended as the diastolic end point rather than phase IV (muffling) (Kirkendall *et al.* 1981). In some pregnant women, the Korotkoff sounds are heard at zero cuff pressure. In these, phase IV has to be used as the diastolic end point even though phase V, when present, is slightly better correlated with the directly measured diastolic pressure (Raftery & Ward 1968). Previously it was recommended that diastolic pressure measurements in pregnancy were based on phase IV readings, but now phase V is preferred, to be consistent with practice in other branches of medicine (National High Blood Pressure Education Program 1990) and because it can be more consistently identified (Shennan *et al.* 1996). In pregnant women

the median difference between phase IV and phase V readings is 2.7 mmHg (Perry *et al.* 1990) compared with 0.7 mmHg in non-pregnant control subjects; in 5% the differences exceed 10 mmHg but in this survey the investigators did not find, as reported previously (MacGillivray *et al.* 1969), that Korotkoff sounds at zero cuff pressure are a problem.

Vibrations in the arterial wall (Wiggers 1956) produce the Korotkoff sounds. They are less distinct if the arterial wall is rigid—for example in shock (Cohn 1967) or eclampsia (Seligman 1971)—when the indirect readings may grossly underestimate the arterial pressure.

There are now several types of blood-pressure measuring devices including mercury or aneroid sphygmomanometers for direct auscultation and various automated devices that give electronic digital displays of the estimated blood pressure. Not all are accurate (Gupta *et al.* 1997). There are defined protocols for validating such instruments and it is important that criteria of accuracy have been met before they are used in clinical or research practice.

Ambulatory blood pressure measurements

The time of day is an important determinant of blood pressure. Figure 6.4 shows a 24-h blood pressure record of a hospitalized woman in the third trimester classified by conventional clinical criteria as having mild CHT. Her blood pressure varies from 130/85 to 70/40 at night. As in non-gravid individuals the major change occurs in sleep (Redman *et al.* 1976a). However, even whilst awake the patient's blood pressure fluctuates from 100/50 to 130/85. This well-known variability of blood pressure means that

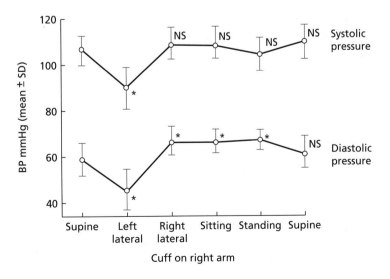

Fig 6.3 Twenty normal women were studied in mid-pregnancy. Their arterial pressures were taken in the right arm using a London School of Hygiene sphygomanometer. The readings were taken in the right arm using a London School of Hygiene sphygomanometer and phase IV of the Korotkoff sounds defined the diastolic pressures. The effect of different positions is clearly shown, particularly the reduced pressure in the uppermost arm when the subject lies on her left side. (Difference from supine position: NS, not significant; *p < 0.05) (C.W.G. Redman, unpublished observations.)

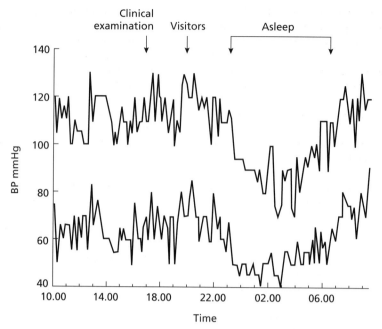

Fig 6.4 The circadian pattern of the arterial pressure of a pregnant woman at rest in bed during the third trimester is shown. The major change in the levels is the normal fall which occurs during sleep (C.W.G. Redman, unpublished observations).

any one reading, however carefully and accurately taken, may deviate significantly from what is typical for an individual. In other words there are large sampling errors, which are distinct from the possible technical errors of measurement, and which can be reduced by averaging a large number of readings. Ambulatory monitors can now be used for this purpose. A number of devices that have been validated have been tested in pregnancy and reference ranges have been published (Brown *et al*. 1998). In comparison with office or clinic readings and by contrast with the-non-pregnant state, 24-h ambulatory measurements are higher (Churchill & Beevers 1996) and therefore different criteria of judging normality may be needed.

Measurement of blood pressure in a clinic may, in some individuals, yield atypically high readings—'white coat' hypertension (Pickering 1996). Where this is suspected an ambulatory record may confirm the diagnosis (Bar *et al*. 1999), but it is doubtful whether this is a clinically useful procedure (Brown *et al*. 1999).

What is hypertension in pregnancy?

Arterial pressure is distributed continuously in the population at large; and the dividing line between normotension and hypertension is an artefact (Pickering 1968). This is as true for pregnant women as for the general population. Hypertension in pregnancy is an artificial concept. An arbitrary threshold is used which divides the population quantitatively but not qualitatively—an important but frequently forgotten distinction. A high blood pressure may be unusual, but not necessarily abnormal.

The average blood pressure of over 6000 women booking before 20 weeks for delivery in Oxford was 120/70. Two and three standard deviations above this mean were 144/87 and 156/95, respectively. The actual distribution of the readings is shown in Table 6.1. Later in pregnancy the blood pressure rises. A maximum antenatal reading (excluding those taken in labour) of 140/90 or more was found in 21.6% of all women; of 170/110

Table 6.1 Blood pressures of 6790 women in pregnancy. Cumulative frequency distributions.

Blood pressure (mmHg)	At booking before 20 weeks (%)	Maximum during antenatal period (%)
≥170/110	0.0	1.2
≥160/100	0.1	3.7
≥150/95	0.4	8.7
≥140/90	2.0	21.5
≥130/85	5.0	38.7
≥120/80	21.0	76.7

or more in 1.2%. These data describe the blood pressures observed in a unit serving an unselected obstetric population. By convention the threshold for 'diagnosing' hypertension in pregnancy is 140/90 mmHg. In the first half of pregnancy this identifies a small group (<2.0%) of hypertensive individuals. In the second half, a much greater proportion (21.6%) exceeds this limit at least once. So although 140/90 is an appropriate limit to begin with, in the second half of pregnancy it would be better to use a cut-off of 170/110 (maximum antenatal reading) to identify the extreme end of the distribution in populations that resemble the Oxford population. However, more usually, 170/110 or higher, is considered to be 'severe' hypertension (Davey & MacGillivray 1988).

Summary of the definition of hypertension in pregnancy

Blood pressure should be measured in the sitting position with a cuff, which is large enough for the patient's arm. Phases I and V of the Korotkoff sounds identify the systolic and diastolic pressures, respectively. A single reading cannot characterize an individual's blood pressure status accurately. Hypertension is not a disease but one end of the continuous distribution of all individuals' blood pressures. 140/90 is the conventional dividing line for obstetric hypertension. In the first half of pregnancy this is appropriate. In the second half of pregnancy a maximum reading of 170/110 or more would be better for defining a small hypertensive group. Classification of individuals as normotensive and hypertensive is a crude and, to some extent, arbitrary simplification.

Pre-eclampsia

Pre-eclampsia, pre-eclamptic toxaemia (PET) or gestosis are roughly synonymous terms, describing a common syndrome that becomes detectable in the second half of pregnancy (although the origins may lie in the first half) and which is defined in terms of the new development of hypertension and proteinuria. It is common, dangerous to both mother and baby, and of unknown cause. Toxaemia is an obsolete expression, previously used to describe any hypertension or proteinuria in pregnancy, whether pregnancy-induced or not.

Definition

The syndrome of pre-eclampsia has been defined in terms of PIH (see above) and proteinuria in various different ways (Davey & MacGillivray 1988; ACOG 1996). Because fluid retention is a common (but not invariable) symptom,

and easily detected, it has also featured in some of the older definitions (reviewed by Redman 1987). For reasons that are historical rather than logical and, to some extent arbitrary, PIH is deemed to be a mandatory part of the syndrome. But a syndrome requires at least two specific features before it can be recognized. Thus, PIH on its own (a common clinical presentation) is not pre-eclampsia; at least one more sign (by convention, pregnancy-induced proteinuria) is required. It is to be regretted that many clinicians and investigators fail to appreciate this fact and use PIH and pre-eclampsia interchangeably so muddling further an already muddled subject.

One definition of pre-eclampsia is given in Table 6.2. This and other definitions are chosen by consensus, for convenience. They describe outward appearances and embody no special truth about the underlying disease or diseases. When a syndrome such as pre-eclampsia is 'defined', rules are set that bring consistency to what is being discussed. The rules may be sensible, or not, but their validity cannot be tested because there is no standard to which to refer. All the definitions of pre-eclampsia suffer from these limitations; nor will there be progress, by making the definitions more elaborate, unless the mechanisms of the disease or diseases that contribute to the syndrome can be elucidated. Most definitions of pre-eclampsia have been devised for use in epidemiological studies (Nelson 1955; Chesley 1978). They are less useful for clinicians who have to make individual diagnoses. In different ways they emphasize three features: hypertension, proteinuria and sometimes oedema, not because these are known to be the most important, but because, historically, they were the first to be defined and happened to be easily accessible signs.

The cause of pre-eclampsia is not yet known but must lie within the gravid uterus. Hence, although pre-eclampsia is conventionally defined by hypertension it is

Table 6.2 Definition of pre-eclampsia accepted by the International Society for the Study of Hypertension (Davey & MacGillivray 1988).

Hypertension	Diastolic pressure: $\geq$90 mmHg or two or more consecutive occasions $\geq$4 h apart; or $\geq$110 mmHg once
Proteinuria	24-h urine collection: $\geq$300 mg protein; or two MSUs collected more than 4 h apart with $\geq$ +1 on stick test
Pre-eclampsia	New hypertension and new proteinuria developing after 20 weeks' gestational age and regressing remotely after delivery

not primarily a hypertensive disease. The raised blood pressure and other maternal signs by which it is recognized are secondary features, reflections of an intrauterine problem. Because pre-eclampsia is a disorder of pregnancy and not simply a maternal problem, the fetus is usually involved, although this may not always be clinically apparent. It can therefore suffer its own morbidity or mortality. The signs of pre-eclampsia are therefore best considered as secondary to a uteroplacental disorder, affecting specific maternal target systems. The targets include the maternal cardiovascular, renal, coagulation and hepatic systems. The widespread systemic nature of the maternal disturbances is all too often not recognized. Some clinicians still wrongly conceive of pre-eclampsia as only the aggregate of its conventionally defined signs of hypertension, oedema and proteinuria.

Incidence of pre-eclampsia and eclampsia

The incidence of pre-eclampsia depends on how it is defined and how assiduously the signs are sought. Thus, it is possible only to estimate the size of the problem. Just as the classification of hypertension has many observational problems so does that of proteinuria, which is the second defining feature of the syndrome. Urine testing is more often omitted than blood pressure measurements, particularly during labour or the early puerperium when significant pre-eclampsia may present for the first time. Or, if the test is done, a positive result may be discounted because it was not confirmed in a 24-h urine collection (for which, in the worst presentations, there is never time) or because a urine infection was not excluded.

In Aberdeen the incidence in primigravidae has fluctuated between 3.0% and 7.7% since 1950. In the same study the incidence in multiparae was 0.8–2.6% (Campbell & MacGillivray 1999). A comparable incidence of 3.1% was documented in the British national perinatal survey of 1970 (Chamberlain *et al.* 1978b). In the USA (1979–86) there was an incidence of 2.3%, using somewhat broader diagnostic criteria (Saftlas *et al.* 1990). The incidences will be affected by the proportions of primigravidae in the different populations. In addition there may be true regional differences (World Health Organization 1988). Hence, the incidence of proteinuric pre-eclampsia in the UK is of the order of one in 20–40 maternities.

Pre-eclampsia, once established, is relentlessly progressive until delivery. Throughout almost all its course the patient is symptomless—a critical feature where diagnosis and management are concerned. Terminally the patient may feel ill with headaches, visual disturbances, nausea, vomiting, epigastric pain and neurological irritability—including clonus and shaking. At this point con-

vulsions may occur and the illness has progressed to its end point of eclampsia.

Eclampsia complicates one in 2000 pregnancies in the UK (Douglas & Redman 1994). In about 10% of cases it is totally unheralded without prodromal signs or symptoms (Douglas & Redman 1994). In 10% of cases the only warning sign is proteinuria and in another 20% there is hypertension only (Douglas & Redman 1994). Hence, extreme hypertension is not a necessary (or indeed sufficient) predisposing factor. This said, eclampsia occurs 7–8 times more commonly in the context of proteinuric than of nonproteinuric pre-eclampsia (Nelson 1955) and the average blood pressures of women with eclampsia are higher than those with severe pre-eclampsia (Sibai *et al.* 1981).

In the UK (and probably other Western countries) the majority of cases occur during labour or after delivery. Such presentations are mostly at term and occur in hospital. Preterm eclampsia is more likely to be antepartum (Douglas & Redman 1994). Eclampsia has been observed as early as 16 weeks of pregnancy (Lindheimer *et al.* 1974). Most postpartum fits occur within 24 h of delivery (Porapakkham 1979), but they have been described up to 23 days postpartum (Samuels 1960). Perhaps as many as half the cases of postpartum eclampsia occur more than 48 h after delivery (Watson *et al.* 1983).

Aetiology and pathogenesis of pre-eclampsia

PRE-ECLAMPSIA IS A PLACENTAL DISEASE

Pre-eclampsia is not only relatively common but dangerous, unpredictable and highly variable in presentation. The presence of a placenta is necessary and sufficient to cause the disorder. A fetus is not required because pre-eclampsia can occur with hydatidiform mole (Chun *et al.* 1964). A uterus is probably not required because pre-eclampsia may develop with abdominal pregnancy (Piering *et al.* 1993). Central to management is delivery, which removes the causative organ, namely the placenta.

The problem with the placenta is generally considered to be an inadequate maternal or uteroplacental circulation leading to placental hypoxia, oxidative stress and infarction. The uteroplacental circulation is unlike any other in the adult. It lacks a microcirculation; there are no arterioles, capillaries or venules. Instead more than a hundred spiral arteries deliver the 500 mL/min of blood normally required at the end of term pregnancy, directly into the intervillous space. In pre-eclampsia, two lesions may affect the spiral arteries. The first, called deficient placentation, comprises a relative lack of the structural remodelling and dilatation that develops between weeks 8 and 18 (Brosens *et al* 1972; Robertson *et al*. 1975) so that in normal pregnancy the arteries can transmit the expanded utero-placental blood flow of the second half of gestation. At this time there is no clinical disease. The problem is not specific to pre-eclampsia; it is also found in some cases of intrauterine growth restriction without a maternal syndrome (Sheppard & Bonnar 1976).

The second lesion in the spiral arteries is 'acute atherosis'—aggregates of fibrin, platelets and lipid-loaded macrophages (lipophages), which partially or completely block the arteries (Zeek & Assali 1950; Robertson *et al*. 1967). The time course of development is obscure, but it is likely that acute atherosis is a late pathological feature. The cause is not known. The lesions are not the consequence of hypertensive injury. Acute atherosis and the associated thromboses are the cause of placental infarctions (Brosens & Renaer 1972), which are more common in pre-eclampsia (Little 1960). The two spiral artery pathologies also can explain the reduced uteroplacental blood flow of pre-eclampsia (Kaar *et al*. 1980) and the desaturation of intervillous blood (Howard *et al*. 1961) in the disorder. All these changes are consistent with an underlying placental ischaemia to which the maternal signs of pre-eclampsia are secondary. There are now several ways of inducing pre-eclampsia-like illnesses in pregnant rodents, dogs or primates. One involves surgical reduction of the blood supply to the uterus or placenta to generate placental ischaemia, of which there are several reports, for example, in baboons (Cavanagh *et al*. 1985) or rhesus monkeys (Combs *et al*. 1993).

Impairment of the uteroplacental circulation affects the placental functions that sustain the fetus. Pre-eclampsia is conventionally considered to be a maternal disorder in which the fetus is an incidental participant. A more complete perception is that the placental problem causes both maternal and fetal syndromes (Redman 1991). The balance of the two syndromes varies: in some cases there is a major fetal problem whereas the maternal features are relatively trivial; in others the converse picture may be seen.

THE MATERNAL SYNDROME OF PRE-ECLAMPSIA IS SECONDARY TO SYSTEMIC ENDOTHELIAL DYSFUNCTION

The maternal syndrome is surprisingly variable, in the time of onset, speed of progression and the extent to which it involves different systems. It can cause hypertension, renal impairment and proteinuria, convulsions, hepatic dysfunction and necrosis, jaundice, abdominal pain, disseminated intravascular coagulation (DIC) or normo-

> **Box 6.1 Complications of pre-eclampsia**
> *Central nervous system*
> - Eclamptic convulsions
> - Cerebral haemorrhage
> - Cerebral oedema
> - Cortical blindness
> - Retinal oedema
> - Retinal detachment
> *Renal system*
> - Renal cortical necrosis
> - Renal tubular necrosis
> *Respiratory system*
> - Laryngeal oedema
> - Pulmonary oedema
> *Liver*
> - Jaundice
> - Hepatic infarction
> - HELLP syndrome
> - Hepatic rupture
> *Coagulation system*
> - DIC
> - Microangiopathic haemolysis
> - HELLP syndrome
> *Placenta*
> - Placental infarction
> - Retroplacental bleeding and abruptio placentae

tensive proteinuria (among others—see Box 6.1). Until recently it was impossible to explain this astounding variability by a single underlying pathological process; certainly hypertension could not account for all these features.

But the concept that the maternal endothelium is the target organ for the pre-eclampsia process has resolved this difficulty (Roberts *et al*. 1989). In short the maternal syndrome can be explained if it is seen, not as a hypertensive problem, but as the sum of the consequences of diffuse endothelial dysfunction.

There is both structural and functional evidence for endothelial dysfunction in pre-eclampsia. One example is the renal lesion of glomerular endotheliosis (Pollak & Nettles 1960). Endothelial swelling is also seen in uterine venules (Shanklin & Sibai 1989) and myocardial vessels (Barton *et al*. 1991). When endothelium is injured, or activated, it releases certain products including cellular fibronectin, the von Willebrand factor and type 1 plasminogen activator inhibitor. All are increased in the plasma of pre-eclamptic women (Redman *et al*. 1977; Gilabert *et al*. 1990; Taylor *et al*. 1991). So these findings are consistent with the hypothesis.

IN PRE-ECLAMPSIA, THE ENDOTHELIAL DYSFUNCTION IS PART OF A MATERNAL SYSTEMIC INFLAMMATORY RESPONSE

Systemic inflammation comprises multiple changes. Apart from endothelial dysfunction, there is activation of circulating leucocytes (especially granulocytes and monocytes) and of the clotting and complement systems. All such changes have been demonstrated in pre-eclampsia (Redman *et al.* 1999). Hence, it has been concluded that the endothelial dysfunction is one aspect of a more generalized process (Sacks *et al.* 1998; Redman *et al.* 1999). Sepsis is often considered to be the paradigm of systemic inflammation. Two of its features are not encountered in pre-eclampsia, namely fever and hypotensive shock. However, the aetiology of the changes in pre-eclampsia is not from infection. A pre-eclampsia-like illness can be induced in experimental rats by stimulating a sterile inflammatory response (Faas *et al.* 1994; Faas *et al.* 2000). A single injection of a very small dose of endotoxin, which causes no changes in non-pregnant animals, is required. The cardiovascular response depends on the dose of the endotoxin. A large dose causes hypotension; an ultra-small dose causes hypertension.

PRE-ECLAMPSIA AND NORMAL PREGNANCY ARE PART OF THE SAME CONTINUUM

A maternal systemic inflammatory response is also detected in normal third-trimester pregnancy when it is not intrinsically different from that in pre-eclampsia except that it is milder (Sacks *et al.* 1998). It has been suggested that pre-eclampsia develops when the systemic inflammatory process causes one or other maternal system to decompensate (Redman *et al.* 1999). In other words, the disorder is not a separate condition but simply the extreme end of a range of maternal systemic inflammatory responses engendered by pregnancy itself. The problem is not the pre-eclampsia but pregnancy itself. This explains why, in clinical practice, it is often extraordinarily difficult to decide whether an atypical presentation is, or is not, pre-eclampsia.

PRE-ECLAMPSIA IS HETEROGENEOUS AND CANNOT BE DISTINGUISHED COMPLETELY FROM NORMAL PREGNANCY

This concept suggests that pre-eclampsia is the outcome of two opposing factors: of a pro-inflammatory stimulus released by the placenta and of a mother's ability to respond and accommodate to the stimulus. Excessive inflammatory stimuli from the placenta could vary with either its physical size or a change in the intensity of (unknown) pro-inflammatory signals from the placenta. The larger the placenta, the larger the inflammatory burden—as, for example, with multiple pregnancy, a well-known predisposition to pre-eclampsia. In addition: advancing gestational age, which increases the physical bulk of the placenta, is itself a major risk factor for pre-eclampsia. Near term, normal pregnancy is characterized by many changes that are so well known that they are taken for granted, for example a rising diastolic pressure (MacGillivray *et al.* 1969), which blur the distinction between normality and pre-eclampsia. In other words, during the last few weeks of normal pregnancy, more and more women appear to be driven towards the margin that distinguishes normal pregnancy from pre-eclamptic pregnancy.

Factors, other than placental size, must also be involved. With respect to the intensity of the pro-inflammatory stimulus of pregnancy there are situations when, even from a small placenta, the inflammatory stimulus is excessive. It is suggested that, in this case, placental hypoxia, secondary to uteroplacental arterial insufficiency, amplify release of inflammatory stimuli into the maternal circulation. These concepts imply that there cannot be a single cause of pre-eclampsia (Ness & Roberts 1996; Redman *et al.* 1999). Different factors, particularly genetic factors that alter maternal inflammatory responses, will contribute. If the mother is genetically unusually susceptible to inflammatory stimuli her constitution becomes the main determinant of the disorder (maternal pre-eclampsia). The other end of the spectrum is when the placenta is the main determinant (placental pre-eclampsia).

Heterogeneity of cause will lead to heterogeneity of clinical presentation. This is a main characteristic of the disorder that will be constantly emphasized in the ensuing sections. Furthermore these considerations also lead to the conclusion that there can be no single preventive measure. Different prophylactic strategies will need to be targeted to the needs of different women.

Secondary features of pre-eclampsia

INVOLVEMENT OF THE MATERNAL CARDIOVASCULAR SYSTEM

The hypertension of pre-eclampsia is an early feature, not associated with a single haemodynamic pattern. Some investigators find increased cardiac output (Mabie *et al.* 1989; Easterling *et al.* 1990) others the converse (Groenendijk *et al.* 1984; Lang *et al.* 1991; Visser & Wallenburg 1991). Some of the differences between studies may reflect drug use; for example, treatment with vasodilators stimulates cardiac output by reducing afterload (Groenindijk et al. 1984). It is, however, agreed that peripheral resistance is increased once the condition is clinically apparent.

The blood pressure is typically unstable at rest (Chesley 1978), possibly owing to reduced baroceptor sensitivity (Wasserstrum et al. 1989). Circadian variation is altered with, first, a loss of the normal fall in blood pressure at night (Seligman 1971) then, in the worst cases, a reversed pattern with the highest readings during sleep (Redman et al. 1976a). Arterial reactivity to exogenous vasopressor substances such as angiotensin II (Gant et al. 1973) is increased.

Pre-eclamptic hypertension is a form of secondary hypertension, arising from pathology in the placenta. Antihypertensive treatment is therefore not a cure; the definitive treatment is to remove the causative organ, the placenta; which means delivery. The hypertension is important because it is an accessible and early diagnostic sign of pre-eclampsia. In addition, if it is extreme, it may predispose to cerebral haemorrhage.

COMPLICATIONS OF THE HYPERTENSION

A sudden increase of blood pressure above a critical threshold causes acute arterial damage and loss of vascular autoregulation (Johansson et al. 1974). The central nervous system appears to be particularly sensitive to hypertensive pathology including cerebral haemorrhage, which antihypertensive treatment helps to prevent giving further proof of the aetiology (Pickering 1968).

Pre-eclampsia may cause blood pressures which are well above the threshold (i.e. a mean arterial pressure of about 140 mmHg) at which arterial damage would be expected. Until recently, cerebral haemorrhage was a prominent cause of maternal death from pre-eclampsia and eclampsia in England and Wales (Department of Health and Social Security 1979, 1982, 1986, 1989, 1991, 1994), with a similar pathology to other hypertensive states (Sheehan & Lynch 1973).

THE MATERNAL RENAL SYSTEM

Proteinuria is a defining sign of pre-eclampsia. Once present it indicates a poorer prognosis for both mother and baby than when it is absent (Butler & Bonham 1963; Naeye & Friedman 1979). On average it appears about 3 weeks before intrauterine death or mandatory delivery (Redman et al. 1976b). It may be heavy (greater than 5.0 g/day). Overall, pre-eclampsia is the commonest cause of nephrotic syndrome in pregnancy (Fisher et al. 1977).

Proteinuria is one of several signs of involvement of the renal glomerulus in pre-eclampsia. Renal biopsy has shown a characteristic non-inflammatory lesion, primarily of swelling of the glomerular endothelial cells (histopathological evidence of the endothelial pathology of pre-eclampsia), which encroach on and occlude the capillary lumina—'glomerular endotheliosis'. It should be noted that renal biopsy is never indicated to resolve the differential diagnosis of pre-eclampsia, however atypical or difficult the presentation. The investigation is reserved for those who continue to have significant proteinuria renal impairment at a remote time after delivery or very occasionally in early pregnancy where the specific diagnosis of renal disease will alter management (see Chapter 7). It has been claimed (Spargo et al. 1959) and denied (Fisher et al. 1969) that the glomerular lesions are pathognomonic. In some cases of eclampsia there is normal renal histology (Dennis et al. 1963).

Renal function is also impaired. Often the changes are biphasic involving first tubular function and later glomerular function. An early feature of pre-eclampsia is a reduced uric acid clearance, reflecting altered tubular function (Chesley & Williams 1945), and causing a reciprocal rise in plasma urate. Later, at about the time that proteinuria develops, glomerular filtration becomes impaired. At this point the plasma creatinine rises and clearance falls. A rising plasma urate is thus an early sign of pre-eclampsia (Redman et al. 1976c) but it is not always demonstrated, reflecting the heterogeneity of the disease (see above). It is also the biochemical change, which best correlates with the renal biopsy appearances of pre-eclampsia (Pollak & Nettles 1960). Another relatively early but inconsistent change in renal function is hypocalciuria (Taufield et al. 1987) which is not a feature of pregnant women with other forms of hypertension. The end stage of renal involvement is acute renal failure, with tubular, partial cortical or total cortical necrosis. The latter two events are more likely in the context of abruptio placentae complicating pre-eclampsia or eclampsia (Smith et al. 1968). In relation to management it is important to note that glomerular hypofiltration in pre-eclampsia does not have a haemodynamic basis, but results from structural changes of the glomeruli (Lafayette et al. 1998).

PLASMA VOLUME, COLLOID OSMOTIC PRESSURE AND OEDEMA

Maternal plasma volume increases during the second and third trimesters of normal pregnancy (Pirani et al. 1973). The extent of the increase depends on the size of the conceptus. It is greater in women with multiple pregnancy (Rovinsky & Jaffin 1965), and least in those with fetuses, which are small for gestational age (Duffus et al. 1971). Maternal plasma volume is reduced in pre-eclampsia in relation to normal pregnancy (Gallery *et al.* 1979). Pre-eclampsia is frequently associated with growth-restricted fetuses, which may account for some of the observed change in plasma volume. But whether the plasma volume is further decreased, even given fetal size, has not been determined. Hypertension itself may be a factor, because it is associated with reduced plasma volumes in non-pregnant subjects (Bing & Smith 1981). More important may be the hypoalbuminaemia characteristic of the disorder (Studd *et al.* 1970), which causes a lower colloid osmotic pressure (Zinaman *et al.* 1985). This alters fluid transport across the capillaries, so that the vascular system in pre-eclampsia becomes 'leaky', with a maldistribution of fluid: too much in the interstitial spaces (oedema) and too little in the vascular compartment (hypovolaemia).

Eighty-five per cent of women with proteinuric pre-eclampsia have oedema (Thomson *et al.* 1967). However, pre-eclampsia without oedema—'dry pre-eclampsia'—has long been recognized as a particularly dangerous variant (Eden 1922), for example the perinatal mortality is higher than if oedema is present (Chesley 1978). Complications of the fluid retention include ascites, which is not uncommon, for example affecting 13 of 99 women seen personally with severe pre-eclampsia. Pulmonary oedema is a rare but life-threatening complication presenting before or after delivery (Sibai *et al.* 1987a). Laryngeal oedema may cause respiratory obstruction as well as difficulties at intubation if a general anaesthetic is required (Jouppila *et al.* 1980).

INVOLVEMENT OF THE CLOTTING SYSTEM

During normal pregnancy the clotting system is activated such that pregnancy becomes a 'hypercoagulable' state (see Chapter 3). This would be expected as part of the systemic inflammatory response that is intrinsic to late normal pregnancy (see above). The blood response to clotting stimuli is brisker and the natural 'turnover' of the system is enhanced. Standard clinical tests do not detect these changes readily although many clotting factors including fibrinogen are increased and some inhibitors (such as protein S activity) are significantly reduced (Gatti *et al.* 1994). There is a very low-grade intravascular generation of thrombin, detected by the increased circulating levels of soluble fibrin monomer complexes and thrombin complexed to its inhibitor, antithrombin III (van Wersch & Ubachs 1991). The changes are in some regards as intense as those seen after acute thromboembolism (Eichinger *et al.* 1999). In parallel, circulating platelets are also progressively activated. The total platelet count alters little. But surface markers of activation are increased (Janes & Goodall

1994), the platelets are hyper-responsive to certain stimuli (Hayashi *et al.* 1999) and there are increased circulating concentrations of soluble products of activation such as β-thromboglobulin (Yoneyama *et al.* 2000).

Consistent with the continuum between normal pregnancy and pre-eclampsia the activation of the clotting system is exaggerated in pre-eclampsia and may, in severe cases, decompensate as DIC. Before decompensation the platelet count may be moderately reduced (Redman *et al.* 1978) owing to increased consumption with a reduced platelet lifespan (Boneu *et al.* 1980). Platelet activation has been confirmed by the higher circulating levels of the platelet-specific proteins, β-thromboglobulin (Douglas *et al.* 1982) and platelet factor 4 (Ayhan *et al.* 1990), which are products of the platelet release reaction. The platelets tend to be larger (that is, probably younger—Giles & Inglis 1981), even in the absence of thrombocytopenia (Stubbs *et al.* 1986). Thrombocytopenia is an inconsistent part of the syndrome: for example only 29% of one series of eclamptic women had platelet counts of less than 150×10^9 L (Pritchard *et al.* 1976). There is also increased intravascular thrombin generation shown by higher circulating levels of D-dimer (Trofatter *et al.* 1989)—a specific fibrin degradation product, fibrinopeptide-A (Douglas *et al.* 1982)—a product of the action of thrombin on fibrinogen, and thrombin–antithrombin III complexes (Reinthaller *et al.* 1990).

In the earlier stages this is a chronic, fully compensated process which cannot be labelled as a pathological DIC which is, however, the end stage of the process. DIC is a late and inconstant feature of preictal pre-eclampsia and eclampsia, first demonstrated in an autopsy series (McKay *et al.* 1953). It is particularly severe if there is concomitant hepatic involvement (Killam *et al.* 1975). The features and consequences of DIC are described in Chapter 3. Microangiopathic haemolysis is a complication of DIC, associated with haemoglobinaemia and a sudden fall in the haemoglobin concentration. Circulating haptoglobin levels are reduced (Schrocksnadel *et al.* 1992), because the haptoglobin binds to the free haemoglobin after which it is rapidly cleared. The haemolysis is associated with fragmented or distorted red cells in the peripheral blood film (Weinstein 1982). DIC and haemolysis are particularly associated with liver dysfunction, as described in the next section.

INVOLVEMENT OF THE LIVER (see also Chapter 9)

Liver dysfunction is a feature of pre-eclampsia detected by elevations of circulating hepatic enzymes (Sibai *et al.* 1993), which may progress to jaundice and severe hepatic impairment (Davies *et al.* 1980). Epigastric pain and vomiting are the typical symptoms but are not always present (Sheehan & Lynch 1973). About two-thirds of women dying from eclampsia have specific lesions in the liver (Sheehan & Lynch 1973), which are periportal 'lake' haemorrhages and various grades of ischaemic damage, including complete infarction (Sheehan & Lynch 1973). Most of this pathology has been defined postmortem, although it has been confirmed in biopsy studies.

Liver damage is particularly associated with DIC in pre-eclampsia. If this occurs together with haemolysis the acronym 'HELLP syndrome' has been used to label the concurrence of haemolysis, elevated liver enzymes and low platelet counts (Weinstein 1982). It is a dangerous complication that is often not associated with marked hypertension (Weinstein 1982; Sibai et al. 1993). Indeed liver damage and low platelet counts have been demonstrated in primigravidae, without hypertension or proteinuria, but with the typical hepatic histology of pre-eclampsia including fibrin deposition in the sinusoids (Aarnoudse et al. 1986).

Epigastric pain is the key symptom. It may be very severe and misinterpreted as a surgical emergency. Less severe pain is often mistreated as heartburn. Signs of pre-eclampsia may not be evident at first presentation (Sibai et al. 1993). Antepartum HELLP syndrome has been documented as early as 17 weeks but 30% of cases present after delivery, sometimes very suddenly. Eclampsia, pulmonary oedema and acute renal failure are associated complications. Maternal mortality is of the order of 1% (Sibai et al. 1993) and is most commonly associated with cerebral haemorrhage (Isler et al. 1999). Recovery from the primary problem may take up to 11 days (Martin et al. 1990), or longer if there is renal failure; and be complicated by rebound hypercoagulability, which can cause fatal thrombosis (Katz & Cefalo 1989).

In certain severe cases, typically of multiparae rather than primiparae, there may be bleeding under the liver capsule (Sheehan & Lynch 1973). Subsequently this may rupture to cause massive haemoperitoneum, shock and (usually) maternal death (Bis & Waxman 1976). There may well be an overlap between the liver involvement in pre-eclampsia and acute fatty liver of pregnancy (Lancet 1983) as described in Chapter 9.

ECLAMPTIC CONVULSIONS

Eclampsia is a form of hypertensive encephalopathy, an acute or subacute syndrome of diffuse rather than focal cerebral dysfunction, not ascribable to uraemia. In non-pregnant individuals, headaches, nausea and vomiting are typical associated symptoms of hypertensive en-cephalopathy (Chester et al. 1978), as are relatively low blood pressure levels. While gross papilloedema or retinopathy are rare in eclampsia, cortical blindness is a complication of both non-pregnant hypertensive encephalopathy (Jellinek et al. 1964), and severe pre-eclampsia or eclampsia (many reports, see for example Liebowitz 1984).

The cerebral pathology of eclampsia resembles that of other hypertensive encephalopathies and comprises thrombosis, fibrinoid necrosis of the cerebral arterioles, diffuse microinfarcts and petechial haemorrhages (Sheehan & Lynch 1973; Chester et al. 1978). These changes are not found in malignant hypertension. Whether or not cerebral oedema is a consistent feature of eclampsia is not clear. It is said to be the cause of death in about 20% of those dying from pre-eclampsia or eclampsia (Hibbard 1973). But whereas it was the only cerebral pathology documented in 20% of one series of deaths (Lopez Llera et al. 1976) it was not demonstrated at all in another (Sheehan & Lynch 1973). Diffuse or focal cerebral oedema has been documented by computed tomography (Beeson & Duda 1982; Kirby & Jaindl 1984) or magnetic resonance imaging (Hinchey et al. 1996) and was the clinical diagnosis in nearly 6% of cases in one series (Cunningham & Twickler 2000). Other lesions include haemorrhages (Milliez et al. 1990) and infarcts (Gaitz & Bamford 1982), which have also been demonstrated by computed tomography. Magnetic resonance imaging of the brains of eclamptic women reveals reversible focal changes characteristic of ischaemia (Sanders et al. 1991). Cerebral arterial constriction has been demonstrated by various methods including conventional angiography (Trommer et al. 1988), magnetic resonance angiography (Sengar et al. 1997) and, indirectly, by Doppler ultrasound examination of the cerebral circulation (Qureshi et al. 1996).

Despite these many observations the cause of the cerebral dysfunction in hypertensive encephalopathy is still not fully defined. One view is that the problem is of ischaemia secondary to intense vasoconstriction (Sheehan & Lynch 1973), which is compatible with evidence derived from cerebral imaging (Horn et al. 1990) and with the generalized endothelial dysfunction in pre-eclampsia. However, others argue that the vasoconstriction is an essential, protective response to extremes of arterial pressure (Johansson et al. 1974), which prevents an uncontrolled increase in tissue perfusion and damage to the microcirculation distal to the arterioles (Strandgaard et al. 1973). The occurrence of eclampsia at relatively low or even normal arterial blood pressures makes the latter unlikely. Recovery from the hypertensive encephalopathy is associated with control of the blood pressure, so that a cause and effect relationship has been imputed. However, this is not justified by the available evidence and certainly there is no direct evidence that eclampsia is caused by sudden increases in blood pressure or prevented by adequate blood pressure control.

The fetal syndrome of pre-eclampsia

The placental dysfunction of pre-eclampsia causes impaired transfer functions. The fetus is often malnourished and small for gestational age, particularly with early-onset disease (Moore & Redman 1983). Retroplacental bleeding and abruption are associated complications so that the fetus may become acutely hypoxic or, with progressive ischaemic damage to the placenta, chronically hypoxic. Pre-eclampsia is the commonest reason for iatrogenic preterm delivery, and it is in this context that most of the perinatal mortality occurs. In a substantial proportion of cases, early delivery is necessary only because of signs of severe fetal compromise.

Maternal mortality in pre-eclampsia

In the first Confidential Enquiry into Maternal Deaths (Ministry of Health 1957), more than 40 years ago, pre-eclampsia was the foremost cause of direct maternal deaths in the country. It remains a prime cause of maternal death in the UK as well as worldwide. It is often not realized that the most dangerous variety of pre-eclampsia is that occurring preterm, which is where maternal mortality is concentrated (Table 6.3). This needs to be considered when antenatal care is organized (see below). Previously, cerebral haemorrhage was the predominant cause of death. This has declined in relative importance perhaps because of the better use of antihypertensive agents. Now, respiratory complications, often associated with ventilatory management in intensive care units are becoming more important.

Table 6.3 Preterm pre-eclampsia and eclampsia have the highest maternal mortality. (Derived from reports on Confidential Enquiries into Maternal Deaths in the UK).

	1988–90[1]	1991–93[2]	1994–96[3]
Delivery at or before 37 weeks	19 (73%)*	15 (79%)	16 (94%)†
Delivery after 37 weeks	7 (27%)	4 (21%)	1 (6%)

*One woman died undelivered.
† Three women died undelivered; inadequate information in three deaths (date omitted).
Department of Health and Social Security 1994[1], 1996[2], Department of Health 1998[3].

Maternal risk factors for pre-eclampsia

Pre-eclampsia is diagnosed by screening symptomless women. It can occur at any time after 20 weeks' gestation and progress to a dangerous extent quickly (within 2 weeks or less in some cases). Current routines of care intensify the frequency of antenatal checks as full term approaches. But early-onset pre-eclampsia is the most dangerous for both mother and fetus. Antenatal screening needs to be more intensive at early gestational ages if the mother is known to have a high risk of developing pre-eclampsia. Hence the assessment of risk is an important part of management. Maternal and fetal risk factors are listed in Table 6.4.

Risk factors may be specific to the mother or the pregnancy. Some, such as primigravidity or a past history of pre-eclampsia are well known. Primigravidae are 15 times more likely to develop proteinuric pre-eclampsia than parous women (MacGillivray 1959). Even secundiparae with an affected first pregnancy have a lower overall incidence, which nevertheless is 10–15 times higher than for secundiparae with a previously normal pregnancy (Campbell *et al*. 1985). The concept of primigravidity may be better considered as one of primipaternity, which can account for the increased likelihood of pre-eclampsia with a new partner or sperm donor. The

Table 6.4 Risk factors for pre-eclampsia.

Maternal factors	Placental/fetal factors
Primigravidity	Advancing gestational age
Primipaternity*	Poor placentation‡
Short period of cohabitation†	Multiple pregnancy
Increasing maternal age	Hydatidiform mole
Previous pre-eclampsia	Triploidy
Obesity (syndrome X, polycystic	Trisomy 13
ovarian syndrome)	Trisomy 16 mosaic
Medical disorders	Placental hydrops
diabetes	
chronic hypertension	
chronic renal disease	
antiphospholipid antibody	
syndromes and thrombophilia	
migraine	
asthma	
Family history of pre-eclampsia	
Stressful job	

*There is a partner specificity about the occurrence of pre-eclampsia. Hence it is not simply the first pregnancy that is an important risk factor but the first by the current partner.
† Stable cohabitation with a single partner seems to reduce the risk of pre-eclampsia in the first pregnancy by that partner.
‡ See text for explanation of terminology.

protective effect of a longer duration of cohabitation (Robillard & Hulsey 1996) could explain at least part of the special predisposition of teenagers to the condition.

The risk increases slightly with age but is not affected by social class (Baird 1977). The predisposition to pre-eclampsia is, in part, inherited (Chesley & Cooper 1986) so that a positive family history is a risk factor (Cincotta & Brennecke 1998): the daughters of eclamptic women are eight times more likely to have pre-eclampsia than would be expected (Chesley et al. 1968). However, there is poor concordance between identical twin sisters (Thornton & MacDonald 1999) so that maternal genes are not a dominant factor.

Obese women are particularly susceptible (Sibai et al. 1997; Ros et al. 1998), although in one series of eclampsia the women tended to be underweight (Chesley 1984). Obesity is associated with a constellation of other medical problems including type 2 diabetes and hypertension (syndrome X). The separate parts of this constellation have all been associated with an increased tendency to pre-eclampsia (Kaaja et al. 1999). The importance of renal disease increases with the degree of renal dysfunction and hypertension. Migraines have been repeatedly associated with the condition (Moore & Redman 1983; Marcoux et al. 1992). The association with antiphospholipid antibodies is strong (Branch et al. 1989). Because of the very intense growth restriction that occurs it may be that the major part of the risk is generated by poor placentation. Antiphospholipid antibodies are an acquired cause of thrombophilia. This is a term used to describe a constitutional tendency to thromboembolism, some of which are genetically determined, for example possession of the Factor V Leiden gene or antithrombin III deficiency. Thrombophilia is associated with more pregnancy complications and perinatal losses, including pre-eclampsia (Kupferminc et al. 1999). Recently asthma has also been identified as a risk factor (Demissie et al. 1998), although there is evidence that this may be more associated with coincidental corticosteroid therapy than the disease itself (Schatz et al. 1997)

Chronically hypertensive women are 3–7 times more likely to develop higher blood pressure combined with proteinuria or 'superimposed pre-eclampsia' than are normotensive women (see for example Butler & Bonham 1963). If hypertension is combined with renal disease then the risk is particularly high (Felding 1969). Since the first report (Zabriskie 1963) it has been repeatedly shown that cigarette smoking, for unknown reasons, is associated with a reduced incidence of pre-eclampsia, albeit with an increased perinatal mortality from other causes (Cnattingius et al. 1997).

It is now known that non-pregnant individuals suffering obesity, syndrome X, type 2 diabetes or hypertension show evidence of endothelial dysfunction or systemic inflammation (Dalekos et al. 1996; Pickup et al. 1997; Visser et al. 1999). Thus, it is possible that these conditions all predispose to pre-eclampsia because they cause high susceptibility to processes that that are important in pre-eclampsia.

There are a number of reports (for example Klonoff Cohen et al. 1996) suggesting that stress at work may increase the risk of pre-eclampsia. This tends to become an issue after an episode of pre-eclampsia when women wish to review whether their lifestyle contributed to their problem.

Considering pre-eclampsia is primarily a placental disease (see above), it is not surprising that placental/fetal factors may increase risk. Some are associated with larger than average placentas. One example is advancing gestational age, which is such a basic feature of the disease that it is rarely considered in this context. There are also the associations with multiple pregnancy (MacGillivray 1959), placental hydrops (Jeffcoate & Scott 1959) or hydatidiform mole (Chun et al. 1964). Certain chromosomal anomalies such as triploidy (Rijhsinghani et al. 1997), trisomy 13 (Boyd et al. 1987) and trisomy 16 mosaicism (Brandenburg et al. 1996) presumably increase the risk of pre-eclampsia by placental mechanisms. If it is considered that poor placentation is a separate condition that may or may not be associated with pre-eclampsia, then it must be also considered to be a powerful predisposing factor (Redman et al. 1999).

It is not know whether all these risk factors can be formally combined to give clinically useful predictions of the onset of pre-eclampsia.

Prediction of pre-eclampsia

If the continuum theory of pre-eclampsia described above is accepted, then it is to be expected that there cannot be one reliable predictive test and indeed this is the case so far as is known, although numerous variables have been investigated. In brief, the maternal syndrome is too heterogeneous in its origins to be anticipated by a single test. Measurement of blood pressure and urine testing for proteinuria persist as the basic screening modes because they are relatively cheap, non-invasive and give an immediate result. As these are the basic diagnostic measurements, efforts to improve their precision may yield some advantages in earlier detection of incipient problems. Thus, 24-h blood pressure monitoring (see above) eliminates many of the sampling errors of single measurements and provides a better estimate of the true blood pressure (see, for example, Penny et al. 1998) and may detect the changes of pre-eclampsia earlier (Benedetto et al. 1998). However, it is neither cheap nor simple to use and not all investigators agree that the information obtained is useful (Higgins *et al.* 1997). An elevated blood pressure in mid-gestation has been proposed as a useful predictive test (Ales *et al.* 1989) but others cannot replicate these findings (Villar & Sibai 1989). An alternative strategy, to detect undue sensitivity to the pressor effects of infused angiotensin II (Gant *et al.* 1973), has long been considered to be the gold standard for predictive tests; but a very large, recent study failed to confirm the earlier claims (Kyle *et al.* 1995). It was hoped that by measuring microalbuminuria there would be greater precision in detecting or anticipating the disorder. But results have again been inconsistent (Lopez Espinoza *et al.* 1986; Rodriguez *et al.* 1988).

A marginally more effective and perhaps more logical predictive test is based on gaining ultrasound Doppler evidence of a high-resistance blood-flow pattern in the uterine arteries in mid-pregnancy (Bower *et al.* 1993). This can be expressed either quantitatively as conventional indices such as the resistance index or qualitatively as the presence or absence of diastolic notches (Mires *et al.* 1995). Although reports are consistent about the association of high-resistance patterns with a high risk of later pre-eclampsia, the test shares the limitations common to all 'predictive' procedures, with relatively low sensitivity (Mires *et al.* 1998).

Various blood tests can identify groups of women at significantly increased risk, but none can qualify as effective predictive tests (Stamilio *et al.* 2000). Elevated serum human chorionic gonadotrophin (hCG) in the second trimester has repeatedly been shown to be significantly associated with later pre-eclampsia (see, for example, Muller *et al.* 1996), although with low sensitivity (Pouta *et al.* 1998) and specificity (Luckas *et al.* 1998). Another placental product—inhibin A—which is elevated in established pre-eclampsia (Muttukrishna *et al.* 1997) is also elevated before the overt disorder in some women (Cuckle *et al.* 1998).

Markers of endothelial dysfunction plasma include fibronectin (see, for example, Taylor *et al.* 1991) and thrombomodulin (Boffa *et al.* 1998). The effectiveness of markers of inflammation has yet to be tested, but circulating levels of the soluble interleukin-2 receptor (a marker of immune activation) have been reported to be elevated as early as the first trimester in women later to develop pre-eclampsia (Eneroth *et al.* 1998). Increased circulating free fatty acids is a relatively early feature of pre-eclampsia antedating clinical signs in many cases (Lorentzen *et al.* 1995). Hyperlipidaemia is also a feature of the inflammatory response (Gouni *et al.* 1993) so this is consistent with the concepts presented above.

Some markers of platelet activation have been found to be significantly increased in women prior to the diagnosis

of pre-eclampsia (Janes *et al.* 1995; Felfernig *et al.* 2000). However, there is considerable overlap with normal, and none of the tests is accessible to general clinicians. The platelet count may fall as an early feature (Redman *et al.* 1978) but the time courses are inconsistent.

In summary, the reality is in line with the predictions outlined at the beginning of this section, namely that it is unlikely that a single test will ever predict pre-eclampsia reliably.

Diagnosis of pre-eclampsia

In general, none of the signs of pre-eclampsia is specific; even convulsions in pregnancy are, in modern practice, more likely to have causes other than eclampsia. Diagnosis therefore depends on finding a coincidence of several pre-eclamptic features. The final proof is their regression after delivery.

There are two ways to make the diagnosis. For research purposes the rules have to be followed which require the presence of PIH and pregnancy-induced proteinuria. In practice clinicians need to take a broader view and accept a wider range of combinations of the possible features of the syndrome, some of which are listed in Table 6.5. As with all syndromes, the more of the features that are clustered together the more certain is the diagnosis. But, and this important proviso is not fully appreciated by many clinicians, the absence of any one feature does not

Table 6.5 Recognition of the pre-eclampsia syndrome.

Maternal signs
Pregnancy-induced hypertension
Excessive weight gain (>1.0 kg/week)
Generalized oedema
Evidence for haemoconcentration
• increased haematocrit
Disturbances of renal function
• hyperuricaemia
• proteinuria
• raised plasma creatinine, reduced creatinine clearance
• hypocalciuria
Increased circulating markers of endothelial dysfunction
• plasma von Willebrand factor
• plasma cellular fibronectin
Laboratory evidence of excessive activation of the clotting system
• reduced plasma concentration of antithrombin III
• thrombocytopenia
• increased circulating fibrin D-dimer
Increased circulating concentrations of liver enzymes
Fetal syndrome
Intrauterine growth restriction
Intrauterine hypoxaemia

exclude the diagnosis. For example eclampsia can occur without proteinuria. Even hypertension seems not to be an essential component. To diagnose pre-eclampsia superimposed on long-term hypertension or renal disease, there are, as stated already, no clear rules. In these circumstances the diagnosis has to be made intuitively by judging the exacerbation of the long-term hypertension or proteinuria, in association with the appearance of other associated signs.

In practical terms, hypertension, proteinuria and excessive weight gain have to be the signs of interest for screening in routine antenatal clinics. Different definitions have been proposed as to what constitutes hypertension. The details are less important than the principle of an increment from a recording taken in the first half of pregnancy; this establishes the existence of PIH. Between weeks 20 and 30 the blood pressure is normally steady so that even a small consistent rise is clinically important. Between week 30 and term, the diastolic will rise by about 10 mmHg on average. A sustained rise of at least 25 mmHg to a threshold of 90 mmHg or more is typical of pre-eclampsia (Redman & Jefferies 1988). However, it needs to be remembered that these are guidelines; there is no clinical situation where rigid interpretation of the blood pressure is helpful.

The same applies to other measurements such as changes in the plasma urate. As a rough guide: abnormal levels are in excess of 0.30, 0.35, 0.40 and 0.45 mmol/L at 28, 32, 36 and 40 weeks, respectively; or, if a baseline taken before 20 weeks is available, then increases of 0.10, 0.15, 0.20 and 0.25 mmol/L at 28, 32, 36 and 40 weeks, respectively.

Proteinuria and evidence of a reduced glomerular filtration rate are later signs. The changes in the measurements of renal function are usually within the normal range for non-pregnant individuals. In general, abnormal concentrations of plasma creatinine and urea are above 100 μmol/L and 6.0 mmol/L, respectively. The proteinuria of pre-eclampsia ranges from 0.5 to 15 g/24 h depending on the individual and the stage of evolution of the disorder. In terms of stick testing, 0.5 g/24 h corresponds to at least '+' in every specimen of urine tested. When this point is reached the disease can be said to have entered its proteinuric phase.

Thrombocytopenia ($< 100 \times 10^9 /L$) and increased plasma fibrin/fibrinogen degradation products (or specific fragments thereof such as the D-dimer) tend to be late developments. The same is true for raised liver enzymes. In regard to the latter it should be noted that plasma alkaline phosphatase is often elevated in late pregnancy because of the contribution from the placental isoenzyme so that its measurement is not a useful guide to hepatic function. Serum bilirubin is rarely abnormal. γ-glutamyl transferase is increased only late in the evolution of the HELLP syndrome. Therefore the best simple tests are plasma aspartate amino-transferase or lactate dehydrogenase.

Pre-eclampsia is usually symptomless. Therefore its detection depends on signs or investigations. However, one symptom is crucially important, because it is so often misinterpreted. The epigastric pain, which reflects hepatic involvement and is the typical presentation of the HELLP syndrome, may easily be confused with heartburn, a very common problem of pregnancy. However, it is not burning in quality, does not spread upwards towards the throat, is associated with hepatic tenderness, may radiate through to the back, and is not relieved by antacid. It is often very severe—described by sufferers as the worst pain that they have ever experienced. Affected women are not uncommonly referred to general surgeons as suffering from an acute abdomen, for example, acute cholecystitis.

PIH on its own is *not* pre-eclampsia, although the term is commonly, but wrongly, used to mean mild or early pre-eclampsia. It is true that PIH may be the first indication of the onset of pre-eclampsia, but until other signs appear this remains unconfirmed. Often spontaneous or induced delivery prevents further developments so that a final certain diagnosis cannot be made.

HYPERTENSION AS A DIAGNOSTIC SIGN

A rise in the blood pressure during the second half of pregnancy, which is abnormal in magnitude relative to the time of pregnancy at which it occurs, is sought. Thus, a diastolic rise of about 10 mmHg is normal for the last 12 weeks of pregnancy (MacGillivray *et al.* 1969) (Fig. 6.5) but a rise of only 5 mmHg between weeks 20 and 30 is associated with significantly higher rates of maternal proteinuria, prematurity and perinatal death (MacGillivray 1961). In addition it is necessary to refer to a change from a baseline rather than an absolute level, for example if the systolic and diastolic pressures increase by at least 30 mmHg and 15 mmHg, respectively (National High Blood Pressure Education Program 1990).

Before 20 weeks, hypertension usually reflects a problem that preceded pregnancy. After 20 weeks it may represent a continuation of CHT or pre-eclampsia. Given the technical and sampling errors of blood pressure measurement, small increases of pre-eclamptic origin are difficult to detect. It may be possible to improve diagnostic accuracy by rigid standardization of the methods of measurement (Gallery *et al.* 1977) or by ambulatory monitoring (see above).

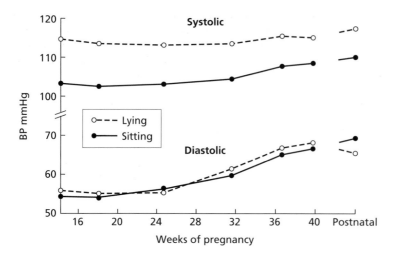

Fig 6.5 Serial arterial pressures in 226 primigravidae taken both lying and sitting (reproduced with permission MacGillivray *et al.* 1969).

A normal blood pressure in the first half of pregnancy does not necessarily mean long-term normotension because the fall in blood pressure induced in early pregnancy may be exaggerated in some women; many with relatively severe hypertension may have normal blood pressures by 12 weeks, without treatment. In other words some women enjoy the benefits of pregnancy-induced normotension just as others suffer the disadvantages of PIH. Pregnancy-induced normotension tends to be lost in the third trimester. If the pre-pregnancy blood pressures are unknown then this development may be misinterpreted as PIH. In an extreme case, a woman had pre-pregnancy readings of 224–280/140–180 mmHg; during pregnancy the pressure fell, without treatment, which was not available at that time, to normal levels of 110–130/60–80 mmHg (Chesley & Annitto. 1947) During the third trimester extreme hypertension developed as the woman's normal cardiovascular status reappeared. This case report demonstrates clearly how CHT can masquerade as PIH—a common problem in clinical practice, although its exact extent has never been assessed.

DIAGNOSTIC VALUE OF OEDEMA AND CHANGES IN RENAL FUNCTION

The pathological oedema of pre-eclampsia is easily confused with the physiological oedema found in 80% of normal pregnant women (Robertson 1971). Development of oedema is associated with a higher rate of weight gain; hence the numerous reports associating excessive weight gain with the development of pre-eclampsia (see, for example, Theron & Thompson 1993). But the clinical usefulness of routine weighing for antenatal care has been queried (Dawes & Grudzinskas 1991) and it is now no longer practised. This is a pity because it is cheap and non-invasive. In general an acceleration of weight gain to consistently more than 1 kg per week is suggestive of incipient pre-eclampsia.

A rising plasma uric acid may be a useful diagnostic feature of early pre-eclampsia (see, for example, McFarlane 1963). It can precede proteinuria and is a simple investigation, which can suggest the 'diagnosis' of non-proteinuric pre-eclampsia in the presence of PIH, an example of a clinical diagnosis not included in the formal definitions. Hyperuricaemia is both non-specific and variable in its time course in relation to other features. It may also result from long-term renal impairment, diuretic use, or merely reflect a long-term constitutional characteristic of the gravid woman. A raised plasma creatinine ($\geq 90\,\mu mol/L$) or blood urea ($\geq 6.0\,mmol/L$) is usual only with proteinuric pre-eclampsia. In this situation these measurements are essential not for diagnosis but to anticipate increasing renal impairment, which might precede acute renal failure.

DIAGNOSTIC VALUE OF CHANGES IN THE COAGULATION SYSTEM

Although a declining platelet count may be an early feature of pre-eclampsia (Redman *et al.* 1978), it has limited diagnostic value because of the large variability between individuals in normal pregnancy. Prospective serial counts in selected high-risk patients are more useful when the patient's own baseline is established early in pregnancy. An alternative technique is to monitor for falling plasma concentrations of antithrombin III (Weiner *et al.* 1985). Markers of endothelial cell activation may be increased early in the disease, for example von Willebrand factor (Redman *et al.* 1977) or fibronectin (Taylor *et al.* 1991). But there are no definitive studies that demonstrate the benefits or limitations of these measurements. It is probably still true that, in early disease it is easier to detect the renal changes rather than the clotting disturbances (Dunlop *et al.* 1978).

The clotting disturbances of advanced pre-eclampsia are more readily observed, correlate with an adverse outcome and can be used to monitor the course of the disease (Howie *et al.* 1976). A diminished platelet count and raised fibrin/fibrinogen degradation products are the most easily detected changes. In severe pre-eclampsia it is essential to know the degree of the clotting disturbance because if DIC is present it indicates a much more serious situation as well as posing specific management problems at delivery. It needs to be re-emphasized that 40% of cases of eclampsia present without fully developed signs of pre-eclampsia (partially heralded or unheralded eclampsia).

Management of pre-eclamptic hypertension and associated problems

Pre-eclampsia is probably the commonest cause of secondary hypertension in clinical practice; delivery always reverses the problem because it removes the causative organ—the placenta. The principles of management are screening of the symptomless patient, diagnosis and well-timed delivery. Interposed between diagnosis and delivery is the need for hospital admission to monitor a condition that may change rapidly and unpredictably. It is essential for the correct timing and management of pre-emptive delivery. The problem is to decide at what stage the pre-eclamptic patient should be admitted. In general, symptomatic pre-eclampsia (symptoms, hypertension and proteinuria) justifies an emergency admission. Symptomless proteinuric pre-eclampsia demands urgent admission on the day of diagnosis. Pre-eclampsia without proteinuria, which has been confirmed by biochemical testing (e.g. hyperuricaemia) is usually best managed in a day assessment unit where frequent detailed checks are routine. Mild hypertension with no other complicating factor can be managed conservatively from routine clinics.

ANTIHYPERTENSIVE DRUGS

Antihypertensive treatment will prevent only those problems directly caused by maternal hypertension. From the preceding discussion it will be apparent that pre-eclamptic hypertension is a secondary or peripheral feature of a more fundamental problem; that extreme pre-eclamptic hypertension causes direct arterial injury that predispose to the cerebral haemorrhages which make pre-eclampsia a potentially lethal disorder. Hence, pre-eclamptic women must be managed to avoid hypertension of a degree that can cause arterial injury. The threshold at which this occurs is at about a mean arterial pressure of 140 mmHg (180–190/120–130). Definitive treatment is delivery, but antihypertensive agents may need to be used to protect the mother before, during and after parturition. Our aim is to keep all blood pressure readings below 170/110; hence treatment is started if maximum blood pressures repeatedly reach these limits in any period. Other centres have slightly different thresholds; the exact levels are less important than the understanding of the principles that determine the need for treatment.

Treatment of extreme pre-eclamptic hypertension

The vasospasm responds best to the drugs that directly relax vascular smooth muscle. A smooth and sustained reduction is to be preferred to sudden short-term changes. A number of vasodilating agents given parenterally have been used, including hydralazine, labetalol, nitroglycerine or sodium nitroprusside. In addition, oral calcium-channel blocking agents are increasingly administered for this purpose.

Hydralazine has been the preferred antihypertensive agent for the treatment of acute severe pre-eclampsia (Chamberlain *et al.* 1978a). It is usually given intravenously by continuous infusion or intermittent boluses (Paterson Brown *et al.* 1994), or by intramuscular or subcutaneous injections (Redman 1980). After intravenous administration there is a substantial delay in the onset of action of 20–30 min. Hydralazine directly inhibits the contractile activity of smooth muscle (Jacobs 1984). In the cerebral circulation it first dilates the capacitance vessels causing an increase in the intracranial pressure (Overgaard & Skinhoj 1975), which probably accounts for the common side-effect of severe headaches. This is an undesirable action, particularly in the context of actual or impending eclampsia where intracranial pressure may already be increased. Subsequently the resistance vessels dilate and cerebrovascular flow increases (Overgaard & Skinhoj 1975). Cardiac output increases (Assali *et al.* 1953) because of the increased venous return. A marked tachycardia nearly always occurs. Originally this was thought to result from stimulation of baroceptor reflexes. But hydralazine also causes a prolonged release of noradrenaline (norepinephrine) (Lin *et al.* 1983), which correlates closely with the tachycardia, and could also explain the anxiety, restlessness and hyper-reflexia, which are common side-effects. These symptoms and signs, together with headaches, may affect 50% of women (Assali *et al.* 1953) and simulate the features of impending eclampsia. Then the symptoms of the disease cannot be disentangled from those caused by the treatment.

It is relevant that hydralazine stimulates the release of noradrenaline which is a potent vasoconstrictor of the uteroplacental circulation, for example in rhesus monkeys (Wallenburg & Hutchinson 1979), and therefore probably in humans. Thus, although it increases cardiac output, hydralazine fails to improve indices of uteroplacental perfusion in pre-eclamptic women (see, for example, Suonio *et al.* 1986). Signs of fetal distress (heart rate decelerations) have been noted after its use (Vink & Moodley 1982). Thus, hydralazine is not an ideal drug. A recent meta-analysis leads to the conclusion that it should not be the drug of first choice for acute hypertension in pregnancy (Magee *et al.* 1999). It is easier to use if the sympathetic nervous system is already inhibited by methyldopa or adrenergic-blocking agents. A continuous infusion is not a rational way to achieve control of the blood pressure for more than 4–6 h, for which purpose either methyldopa or labetalol should be given orally. In our own practice we give intermittent intramuscular hydralazine (10 mg) only when nifedipine has failed to achieve its effect (see below). Monitoring of the fetus is essential but in our experience fetal distress is rare, and more related to the severity of the pre-eclampsia than to the administration of the hydralazine.

Other drugs for the acute control of hypertension

Labetalol is a combined α- and β-adrenergic blocking agent, which can be given intravenously. It lowers the blood pressure smoothly but rapidly without the tachycardia characteristic of treatment with hydralazine, although collapse with atrioventricular tachycardia has been reported with postpartum use (Olsen & Beier Holgersen 1992b). A typical regimen starts with 20 mg/h, which is doubled every 30 min until control has been gained (Garden *et al.* 1982). As α-adrenergic stimulation is thought to constrict the uteroplacental circulation, labetalol (α blockade) would be expected to enhance flow; in fact, no effect, good or bad, has been observed (Lunell *et al.* 1983). A fetal death associated with a sudden drop in the blood pressure after labetalol has been reported (Olsen & Beier Holgersen 1992a). Other reports have described symptomatic neonatal β-adrenergic blockade after *in utero* exposure (Klarr *et al.* 1994; Crooks *et al.* 1998). Single case reports may be misleading and there are no adequate trials of its parenteral use in pregnancy to show how it might affect perinatal outcome.

Other vasodilators include sodium nitroprusside (Shoemaker & Meyers 1984) and nitroglycerine (Cotton *et al.* 1986), given intravenously to severely hypertensive pregnant women. Neither is to be recommended except in extreme circumstances and in specialist intensive care. Sodium nitroprusside is potentially toxic to the fetus but normal fetal survival has been associated with its use (Goodlin 1983). Nitroglycerine has been used to attenuate the pressor response to endolaryngeal intubation during caesarean section (Longmire *et al.* 1991).

The calcium-channel blocking agent, nifedipine, is an effective vasodilator that acts rapidly when given by mouth. Nifedipine capsules that act within 10–15 min have caused dangerously abrupt blood pressure reductions in non-pregnant individuals and should no longer be used. Slow-release tablets have an onset of action within about 60 min and a more prolonged effect. Nifedipine appears to be at least as safe as hydralazine and, in some aspects of neonatal complications of prematurity with severe pre-eclampsia, possibly superior (Fenakel *et al.* 1991). Tachycardia occurs but is less of a problem than with hydralazine. In theory there could be a problem if parenteral magnesium sulphate were also used for the prophylaxis or treatment of eclampsia because of the separate effect of the magnesium ion on calcium-channel functions (Iseri & French 1984); in practice there has only been a report of two cases of profound hypotension in this context (Waisman *et al.* 1988). The advantage of nifedipine over hydralazine is its ease of administration. It can also cause severe headaches like hydralazine. Reports of the effects of nifedipine on the fetal or uteroplacental circulations (assessed by Doppler ultrasonography) are so far reassuring (many reports; see, for example, Hanretty *et al.* 1989). An inhibitory effect of nifedipine on platelet function (Rubin *et al.* 1988) could be an advantage. An antitocolytic effect on uterine muscle (Ulmsten 1984) might predispose to postpartum haemorrhage, although this complication has not been reported. Nimodipine, another calcium-channel blocker, with a selective effect on the cerebral circulation, has been used to treat cerebral ischaemia in an eclamptic woman (Horn *et al.* 1990).

CONSERVATIVE MANAGEMENT OF SEVERE PRE-ECLAMPSIA (BLOOD PRESSURE >170/110)

There have to be compelling special reasons to leave women with proteinuric pre-eclampsia undelivered after 36 weeks' gestation. Indeed, after 34 weeks it becomes increasingly more difficult to justify conservative management. The same arguments can be transposed to women with definite non-proteinuric pre-eclampsia at 38–40 weeks.

The most difficult problems arise with proteinuric pre-eclampsia, without symptoms, presenting between 26 and 34 weeks of pregnancy. Although delivery is desirable, it is not essential. If it can be deferred for 2 weeks or longer, significant maturation of the fetus may be achieved to reduce the problems of immaturity after birth. Conservative management of proteinuric pre-eclampsia can only be undertaken by an experienced team offering continuous monitoring and care. It is not easy, and sometimes impossible, for this to be achieved in understaffed, busy units with heavy routine commitments. It is thus desirable that such patients are moved at an early stage to specialized regional centres and also desirable that there are such centres, which have adequate skilled staff and other resources.

The conservative approach needs to be used with discretion and in the knowledge that in some patients it will achieve little or no gain in time. To defer delivery safely it is essential to know how all the maternal systems are affected by the disorder. The fetal state must be reviewed continually also. Delivery is necessary if the maternal blood pressure cannot be controlled, if the platelet count is $<50 \times 10^9/L$, if the plasma creatinine has risen from normal levels to $>120\,\mu mol/L$, if there is evidence of liver damage or if the women has symptoms. In some cases, increasing fetal problems may make extrauterine life safer. These developments may happen unpredictably and suddenly, and will be missed unless the monitoring and care is maintained at a high level.

Of 122 cases of symptomless proteinuric pre-eclampsia presenting before 32 weeks in Oxford in 1980–85, conservative management extended the life of the pregnancy beyond the onset of proteinuria by an average time of 15 days. Thirty-one per cent were delivered because of maternal problems, 48% because of fetal problems, and 7% because of both. The remainder were delivered non-urgently because adequate maturation had been achieved, or because they went into spontaneous labour. Five infants all weighing less than 1000 g and all but one at less than 28 weeks died *in utero*. Two trials comparing conservative management with immediate delivery have confirmed the potential advantages of a cautiously expectant approach (Odendaal *et al.* 1990; Sibai *et al.* 1994).

LONGER-TERM CONTROL OF SEVERE PRE-ECLAMPTIC HYPERTENSION

Parenteral therapy is inappropriate if conservative management is being attempted, and oral agents need to be used. Methyldopa is the first choice. The safety of methyldopa in pregnancy has been established by case–controlled studies (Redman *et al.* 1976c). No serious adverse fetal effects have yet been documented. Methyldopa crosses the placenta and accumulates in relatively high concentrations in amniotic fluid (Jones & Cummings 1978). Neonatal blood pressure is transiently reduced for a short period after delivery (Whitelaw 1981). None of these effects is clinically important. Its use not only relieves the patient of the problems of parenteral therapy, but if, at a later time, hydralazine or another vasodilator is needed, their action is potentiated.

Oral administration can achieve an adequate therapeutic response within 12 h provided a large initial loading dose of 500–750 mg is used. This can be followed by 1–2 g/day, which may be increased to 3 g/day as needed. A satisfactory drop in the blood pressure tends to provoke transient oliguria, which may cause anxiety about renal failure—a complication discounted by measuring the plasma urea and creatinine. Despite good blood pressure control, the other changes of pre-eclampsia (abnormalities of renal, coagulation and placental function) remain unchanged. Thus, hypotensive treatment is merely suppressing one dangerous manifestation of this disorder. The treatment regimen of hypertension in pre-eclampsia may need to anticipate nocturnal hypertension (Redman *et al.* 1976a) by a variable schedule with the largest doses at night.

The β-adrenergic antagonists (β blockers) have the advantage of causing fewer subjective side-effects but their safety in pregnancy has not been so exhaustively investigated. A preparation such as atenolol has a slow onset of action and a flat dose–response curve, which make the day-to-day titration of blood pressure control almost impossible. However, its short-term safety for the fetus and neonate has been adequately demonstrated (Rubin *et al.* 1983). Oxprenolol and labetalol are faster-acting alternatives, labetalol being the antihypertensive agent most used in British obstetric practice (Hutton *et al.* 1992). Which agent is preferred probably matters less than the clinician's familiarity with its use.

ESCAPE FROM BLOOD PRESSURE CONTROL

So long as pregnancy continues, pre-eclampsia is a relentlessly progressive disorder, so that sooner or later escape from blood pressure control can be expected. In general, the maternal and fetal conditions deteriorate together and it is not difficult to see when the limits of conservative management have been reached and delivery is indicated. Oral vasodilators, however, may be usefully added to the medical regimen to prevent loss of blood pressure control. Oral hydralazine, which on its own is a weak hypotensive agent, effectively augments methyldopa given at doses of 25–75 mg every 6 h. An alternative is slow-release nifedipine, at doses of 10–30 mg up to four times per day. A recent study suggests that prazosin may be an alternative providing equally effective antihypertensive action, but at the possible expense of more fetal problems (Hall *et al.* 2000).

Antihypertensive treatment would be expected to help prevent cerebral haemorrhages but not eclampsia (see above).

MANAGEMENT OF FLUID BALANCE AND OLIGURIA

Pre-eclampsia is associated with hypovolaemia. It has been claimed that plasma volume expansion is beneficial (see, for example, Morris & O'Grady 1979) to correct poor renal and placental function. The evidence in favour is circumstantial and unvalidated. Belfort *et al.* (1989) find that plasma protein infusions do not lower blood pressure in pre-eclamptic women. The postulated improvement in uteroplacental circulation has not been demonstrated (Jouppila *et al.* 1982a). It has been claimed that infusion of colloid with haemodynamic monitoring with a Swan–Ganz catheter allows safe conservative management of complicated pre-eclampsia, including the HELLP syndrome or eclampsia (Visser & Wallenburg 1995a,b). Even if true, and the trials are yet to be done, most units would find it too expensive to provide the intensive monitoring needed for such management. In developing countries it is out of the question. The possibility that it could cause circulatory overload and pulmonary oedema makes the treatment potentially dangerous. It cannot therefore be considered to be a part of routine management.

Nearly half the women who die with pre-eclampsia in the UK die of pulmonary complications (Department of Health 1998). Fluid overload was a contributory factor in one-third of these cases. The management of reduced urine output and oliguria is therefore crucial in order to miminize the risk of pulmonary oedema. It is often forgotten that the renal problem that may cause oliguria and anuria in pre-eclampsia arises from structural disease in the glomeruli and not haemodynamic factors (Lafayette *et al.* 1998) so that the problems are not resolved by fluid administration. Hypovolaemia secondary to blood loss associated with bleeding at delivery clearly must be excluded, and for this a central venous line is essential. But once the cardiac return is assured by adequate venous filling, fluid replacement must be used with caution. In particular the intensive care unit convention that urine output must be seen to be at least 30 mL/h is inapplicable. With an adequate central venous pressure the most important information that determines management is the level of plasma creatinine and the degree of associated

systemic disturbances, particularly the haemolysis of the HELLP syndrome. If plasma creatinine is less than 100 mmol/L and there are no signs of HELLP, there is no problem even if the urine output drops to the range 10–20 mL/h providing there is no clinical evidence of blood loss. Such reduced urinary output will be transient and will correct itself. However, in the presence of a rising plasma creatinine (>100 mmol/L) with haemolysis, poor urine output is highly likely to be secondary to structural deficits in the kidneys, which are not going to be corrected by infusion of fluids. Indeed all that can happen is that the infusions will overflow into the lungs. Genuine anuria, even for as short a time as 1 h, is always abnormal and may herald total renal failure.

PREVENTION AND TREATMENT OF ECLAMPTIC CONVULSIONS

Eclampsia complicates one in 2000 maternities in the UK (Douglas & Redman 1994) so that few obstetricians have extensive experience of its presentation or management. About 40% of cases are either completely unheralded or only partially heralded. More cases occur in labour or after delivery than antepartum for which reason alone, the first eclamptic convulsion occurs after admission to hospital in the majority of women (Sibai *et al.* 1981). The aim of management is to protect the maternal airway, control convulsions, control extreme hypertension and expedite delivery.

If a patient needs anticonvulsant medication she also needs urgent delivery. Most eclamptic convulsions stop quickly and spontaneously without intervention. It is nevertheless customary to terminate the fit medically. Intravenous diazepam is the agent of choice and is that which is used most widely in the UK (Hutton *et al.* 1992). Aliquots of 5 mg can be given by slow intravenous injection with cautious attention to the avoidance of oversedation and respiratory depression. Diazepam is, however, inappropriate for longer-term prevention in which case magnesium sulphate should be used. This has been clearly shown to be superior to either parenteral phenytoin or long-term diazepam to prevent further convulsions (Collaborative Eclampsia Trial 1995). Magnesium sulphate can be given intravenously or by intramuscular injection, although with both regimens an initial loading dose (usually 4 g) is given by slow intravenous injection. The advantage of the former is more precise control of dosage. The disadvantage is the risk of overdose. This is highest if there is acute impairment of renal function when a continuous infusion causes rapid accumulation of magnesium and toxic side-effects. A serious side-effect of magnesium overdose is muscular weakness, which may cause respiratory paralysis, heart failure and death. Hence, there is the need to monitor blood levels of magnesium. Therapeutic levels are 2–3.5 mmol/L. A simple clinical test is to check the deep tendon reflexes. If they are suppressed, no more magnesium can be given pending more accurate knowledge of what the plasma concentrations are. The antidote for magnesium sulphate is calcium gluconate (1 g calcium gluconate i.v.; 10-mL ampoule of 10% calcium gluconate administered over 10 min).

Continuous monitoring of urine output from an indwelling catheter is essential, as is knowing the plasma creatinine. Oliguria (<10 mL/h) or anuria is a reason to stop administration of magnesium, as is a high plasma creatinine (>150 mmol/L). Extreme caution should be exercised if the urine output is 10–20 mL/h or the plasma creatinine is 100–150 mmol/L when the rate of infusion should be slowed if not stopped. To minimize the risk of accidental infusion of overdoses, 10g of magnesium sulphate in a 50-mL solution of 0.9% (5 mL) saline should be given by an infusion pump. In the USA the preferred rate of administration is 2 g/h whereas in the UK the regimen of the Collaborative Eclampsia Trial (1995), 1g/h, tends to be followed. Intramuscular magnesium sulphate is easier to manage but achieves a less precise dosage regimen. The major disadvantage is that it is painful and there is a risk of abscesses forming at the site of injection.

It is likely that magnesium sulphate acts by reversing cerebral vasoconstriction. This can be demonstrated in experimental animals (Kemp *et al.* 1999) and indirectly in pregnant women (Belfort & Moise 1992). Hence, it is a more logical treatment for eclampsia, where the underlying problem is thought to be cerebral ischaemia, than drugs that are given to suppress dysfunctional neurones.

There are many side-effects associated with magnesium sulphate, which are listed in Table 6.6. Because it is easy to administer overdoses and because these are potentially lethal, magnesium sulphate should be used in a targeted way. At the moment the only unequivocal indication is to prevent further convulsions in a woman who already has had one or more such fits.

It is standard practice in many parts of the world and in some units in the UK to use magnesium sulphate for prophylaxis in women with pre-eclampsia who have not had a convulsion. A large trial is in progress (MAGPIE – Duley and Neilson 1999) that is expected to provide evidence of efficacy, and two small trials already demonstrate favourable results (Lucas *et al.* 1995; Coetzee *et al.* 1998). It seems very likely that it will be proved beyond reasonable doubt that magnesium sulphate is effective. The problem is not its efficacy but who to treat. Lucas *et al.* (1995) had to treat 100 women to prevent one convulsion. In a South African black population, with severe pre-eclampsia requiring induction, 30 women had to be treated to prevent one convulsion (Coetzee *et al.* 1998). In the UK, in women with severe pre-eclampsia who are given no anticonvulsants, the eclampsia rate is of the order of 1% (Chua & Redman 1991). Hence even with these selection criteria it is likely that 100 women would need prophylaxis to prevent one case. In addition about 40% of cases could not be prevented because they are either partially or totally unheralded. More have only moderate pre-eclampsia before convulsing and others unexpectedly convulse at home without prior documentation of warning signs so, at best, less than half of all convulsions are preventable. In the UK there would be about 150 preventable cases, and prophylaxis would need to be given to 15 000 other women to reach this target. At this rate rare side-effects of magnesium sulphate are likely

Table 6.6 Side-effects of magnesium sulphate given for preventing or treating eclampsia.

Maternal death from accidental overdose	Hibbard (1973), Pritchard *et al.* (1984)
Cardiopulmonary arrest	McCubbin (1981); Swartjes *et al.* (1992)
Diminished pulmonary function	Herpolsheimer *et al.* (1991)
Paralysis in women with neuromuscular disorders	Bruner and Yeast (1990)
Recurrent convulsions	Pritchard and Stone (1967), Sibai *et al.* (1981)
Increased length of labour, increased caesarean delivery rate, increased postpartum bleeding	Witlin and Sibai (1998)
Hypotension	Bourgeouis *et al.* (1986)
Prolonged bleeding time	Fuentes *et al.* (1995)
Maternal hyperkalaemia	Spital and Greenwell (1991)
Maternal hypocalcaemia and tetany	Eisenbud and LoBue (1976); Cruikshank *et al.* (1993)
Neonatal hypotonia and lower APGAR scores	Lipsitz (1971); Riaz *et al.* (1998)
Reduced fetal heart rate variation	Atkinson *et al.* (1994); Hiett *et al.* (1995)

to be important. The case for prophylaxis would be stronger if those at highest risk could be identified accurately.

It is already known that not all fits can be prevented with magnesium sulphate (Pritchard & Stone 1967; Sibai *et al*. 1981). For example the evidence from all sources is that about 10% of women fit again after starting magnesium sulphate treatment (Pritchard *et al*. 1984; Collaborative Eclampsia Trial 1995; Sawhney *et al*. 1999).

OTHER MEASURES FOR THE TREATMENT OF
PRE-ECLAMPSIA AND ITS COMPLICATIONS

After their introduction, the thiazide diuretics were prescribed widely for the prevention and treatment of pre-eclampsia. Nearly 7000 women were randomized in 11 controlled trials of varying size and quality. In the pooled data the incidence of stillbirth was reduced by one-third, a difference that is not statistically significant (Collins *et al*. 1985). Otherwise there was no evidence of benefit. A number of serious side-effects have been associated with the use of thiazide diuretics. In addition they may cause hyperuricaemia, which obscures one of the more useful signs of early pre-eclampsia. For these reasons diuretics should not now be used in the management of pre-eclampsia, except for treating the rare complication of pulmonary oedema.

In general the only remedy for DIC is to correct the underlying problem. In pre-eclampsia this means delivery. With the knowledge that abnormal coagulation probably mediates at least some of the terminal complications of the disorder, various regimens of anticoagulation have been tried and are ineffective. The dangers of anticoagulation in patients at risk of cerebral haemorrhage need to be emphasized. The poor haemostasis of individuals recovering from severe DIC postpartum can cause intractable haemorrhage. Transfusions of platelets and fresh frozen plasma may be needed in addition to the replacement of whole blood as supportive treatment.

Management of labour and delivery

If premature delivery is necessary then the question arises as to whether corticosteroids should be given to accelerate fetal pulmonary maturation. Although the original trial of their use suggested that in the context of pre-eclampsia there was a significantly worse perinatal outcome, no further data on this subject have been presented and the current consensus is that they should be given as they would for any other preterm delivery.

The mode of delivery is determined amongst other variables by the speed with which it must be expedited,

the ability of the fetus to withstand labour, and the chances of successful induction of labour at early gestational ages. As in other circumstances, vaginal delivery is always to be preferred if it is safe.

Oxytocin (2–5 µg/min i.v.) has antidiuretic activity which is evident within 10–15 min of administration (Abdul-Karim & Rizk 1970); if given with large volumes of 5% dextrose and water, it can cause hyponatraemia and convulsions (McKenna & Shaw 1979). The drug causes peripheral vasodilatation with a reflex tachycardia that may stimulate significant increases in cardiac output. If cardiac function is already compromised, which happens in rare cases of severe pre-eclampsia, myocardial failure may occur (Tepperman *et al*. 1977).

Ergometrine may provoke extreme hypertension in the pre-eclamptic patient (Baillie 1963); it can cause headaches, convulsions or even death (Tepperman *et al*. 1977). For this reason syntocinon, not ergometrine, should be used in the management of the third stage (Forman & Sullivan 1952).

A woman with a shrunken intravascular compartment is less tolerant of blood loss than is the normal pregnant woman. Blood replacement must therefore be initiated sooner, at the same time very carefully, to guard against the dangers of underfilling or overfilling.

Pre-eclampsia is not a primary contraindication to epidural analgesia. Studies of epidural block in patients with pre-eclampsia have shown that maternal cardiac output is unaffected (Newsome *et al*. 1986), placental intervillous blood flow appears to be enhanced (Jouppila *et al*. 1982b), and control of maternal blood pressure is improved (Newsome *et al*. 1986), although there is no effect on the maximum recorded pressures (Greenwood & Lilford 1986). Vasodilatation and pooling of the blood in the veins of the lower extremities may cause hypovolaemia. This problem can be anticipated and avoided so that the benefits seem to outweigh the disadvantages. However, epidural analgesia is contraindicated if there is evidence of actual or incipient DIC. A knowledge of at least the platelet count is essential and, if $<100 \times 10^9$/L, the procedure may be too risky.

A caesarean section may have to be done too quickly to consider using epidural anaesthesia. Although general anaesthesia allows more precise control of the speed and timing of surgery, there are particular risks for pre-eclamptic women. Intubation may be difficult (Jouppila *et al*. 1980) or impossible (Heller *et al*. 1983) because of laryngeal oedema, which may also cause postoperative respiratory obstruction and cardiac arrest (Tillmann Hein 1984). Laryngoscopy is a well-known cause of extreme transient reflex hypertension in all individuals. The problem is aggravated in pre-eclamptic women (Hodgkinson *et al.* 1980) and may be so extreme as to cause acute pulmonary oedema (Fox *et al.* 1977). The blood pressure swings at laryngoscopy are ameliorated if adequate blood pressure control has been gained before the anaesthetic is given. Pretreatment with either nitroglycerine (Longmire *et al.* 1991) or labetalol (Ramanathan *et al.* 1988) has been given acutely to attenuate this problem. Laryngeal oedema is one of the few indications for the use of diuretics in pre-eclampsia; if it is anticipated, an experienced and well-briefed anaesthetist should do the intubation.

Prevention of pre-eclampsia

PRIMARY PREVENTION

No effective measure for the primary prevention of pre-eclampsia has been found (Sibai 1998). If the concepts of pathogenesis are correct (see above), it is unlikely that any single measure will ever be identified for all susceptible women. But specific measures of reducing the susceptibilities among subgroups of women may be identified. Measures, which may be effective or are probably or definitely ineffective, are summarized in Table 6.7.

Trials of antiplatelet agents, in particular low doses of aspirin, have given mixed results. Those that have shown antiplatelet therapy to be ineffective have tended to be the largest (ECPPA 1996; Golding 1998; Rotchell *et al.* 1998) with the least selective recruitment. Overall there is still evidence of benefit if all the trial results are pooled (Knight *et al.* 2000). Effectiveness may depend on both an adequate dose and use at an early enough stage of pregnancy (Dumont *et al.* 1999). The benefits of aspirin appear to be greatest in preventing early-onset pre-eclampsia (which is relatively rare) and least in preventing the disorder presenting at term (which is common) (CLASP 1994). If the condition is becoming overt early in the second half of pregnancy it is logical to predict that effective prevention will have to begin earlier than 16–20

weeks, which is the average time for most large trials. For example a large trial focused on high-risk women (Caritis *et al.* 1998) had an average time of randomization of 20.1 weeks for all women. Antiplatelet therapy does not benefit women if started after the signs of pre-eclampsia have appeared. A significant benefit was observed in one randomized trial where the serotonin antagonist, ketanserin, combined with low-dose aspirin was compared with low-dose aspirin alone when given to high-risk women (Steyn & Odendaal 1997).

As yet there has been no clear demonstration that perinatal survival is enhanced by the use of aspirin. However, its use in pregnancy seems to be safe: there may be a slight increase in maternal bleeding problems around the time of delivery. No adverse effect on the fetus has yet been identified.

SECONDARY PREVENTION

All the evidence is that, once it becomes overt, pre-eclampsia cannot be reversed except by delivery. Pre-eclampsia cannot be predicted accurately (see above). Hence, by far the most important part of secondary prevention is regular antenatal care to screen for asymptomatic incipient or early pre-eclampsia and therefore to allow timely delivery to be arranged before the disease becomes dangerous. Screening assessments have to be repeatedly updated during the second half of pregnancy because pre-eclampsia can evolve over a short time course, rarely 1 week or less, often within 2 weeks. The key feature is the regularity of repeated checks, the backbone of antenatal care. The longer the interval between one check and the next, the greater the risk of a serious episode of pre-eclampsia going undetected. The critical issue is therefore the duration of the screening interval. One longer than 4 weeks is always too long except for the lowest risk group, which comprises normal multiparae with singleton pregnancies, and no past history of hypertension in pregnancy.

Longer intervals at gestations between 20 and 28 weeks are a feature of routines of antenatal care. But early-onset pre-eclampsia and eclampsia at this time are the most dangerous, both for the mother and in terms of perinatal outcome. The disease is characterized by more intrauterine growth restriction, a substantially higher perinatal mortality and more maternal complications (Moller & Lindmark 1986; Douglas & Redman 1994; Department of Health 1998). More than 75% of the maternal deaths from the disease in the UK occur in this group (see Table 6.3).

Recently there have been proposals to reduce antenatal care (Department of Health 1993), which in practice, involve minimizing the number of visits between 20 and 36

Table 6.7 Primary prevention of pre-eclampsia.

Probably or definitely ineffective	May be effective for at least some women
Weight restriction	Low-dose aspirin and other antiplatelet agents
Salt restriction	
Diuretics	Anti-oxidant vitamins (vitamin C and E)
Antihypertensive agents	
Calcium supplements	
Fish oil supplements	

weeks, leading to even longer screening intervals at this time. Given the fact that most of antenatal care has been introduced explicitly to protect expectant mothers from pre-eclampsia it is illogical to leave them without care at precisely that time when it is most needed. The problem is addressed in the chapter on Hypertensive Disease of the Confidential Enquiries into Maternal Deaths in the United Kingdom 1991–93 (1996) where it is concluded: 'It may be necessary to treat with caution any local proposals to reduce the intensity of ante-natal screening, in whatever setting, from 24 weeks onwards, even in those women who are normotensive at booking'. Recently two analyses of risk factors for eclampsia have been published. Neither was addressing specifically the issue of antenatal care but no, or inadequate, care was included among the independent variables affecting outcome (eclampsia). In both, these were statistically significant and, in terms of magnitudes of increased risk, the most important (Abi Said *et al*. 1995; Ansari *et al*. 1995). This highlights the role of good antenatal care as the primary effective measure in secondary prevention.

Of the other measures, there is no evidence that blood pressure control attenuates the progression of early pre-eclampsia, nor that it prevents superimposition of pre-eclampsia in chronically hypertensive women, who otherwise are more susceptible to the disorder. The only clear advantage of antihypertensive treatment is where the hypertension is so severe that delivery is essential to preserve maternal safety. At early gestational ages, antihypertensive treatment can allow prolongation of pregnancy in this context. The benefit is not from prevention but palliation. The extent of the presumed benefit has not been measured because severe hypertension is a reason for exclusion from randomized trials of treatment. Hence, in all contexts antihypertensive treatment helps to protect the mother from the consequences of her problem, but not from the problem itself.

Undoubtedly treatment can lower the blood pressure in early pre-eclampsia; by so doing it can modify the medical interventions that are triggered when hypertension of a particular severity is observed. Some of the benefits claimed, for example fewer hospital admissions (Rubin *et al*. 1983), or fewer caesarean sections (Plouin *et al*. 1990), may reflect this fact rather than genuine alterations in disease severity. If the interventions are, in reality, unnecessary then all that the drug treatment achieves is to protect the patient from her doctors. Treatment has been associated with a reduced incidence of proteinuria in two trials (Rubin *et al*. 1983; Blake & Macdonald 1991). Had pre-eclamptic processes truly been prevented then perinatal outcome should have been improved. But it was not: in the former there was no difference and in the latter there was significantly more intrauterine growth restriction.

Most trials of antihypertensive treatment are not associated with an improved perinatal outcome, which has been reported only once (Redman *et al*. 1976c); in this study the excess of fetal losses in the control group, which included several mid-pregnancy losses, could not be ascribed to pre-eclampsia-related pathology. In general, antihypertensive treatment does not seem to modify the pre-eclamptic process. The evidence, in many regards imperfect, is most reliable with respect to the inability of treatment to prevent superimposed pre-eclampsia in women with CHT (Redman 1980; Sibai *et al*. 1990).

Some specific dietary supplements, for example calcium, appear to be more effective. It has been postulated that calcium deficiency predisposes to pre-eclampsia and PIH (Belizan & Villar 1980). Just as calcium supplements reduce the blood pressure in men and non-gravid women (McCarron & Morris 1985) so they lessen the incidence of PIH (Belizan *et al*. 1991). But a large trial to test their efficacy in a primigravid population showed no benefit (Levine *et al*. 1997). At the time of writing there is one small trial suggesting benefit from the prophylactic use of antioxidant vitamins C and E started in mid-gestation in carefully selected groups of at risk women (Chappell *et al*. 1999). It is too soon to know if this is likely to be confirmed as a safe and effective preventive regimen.

Postpartum hypertension

The arterial pressure progressively rises during the first 5 days after normal delivery (Walters *et al*. 1986). This trend may be exaggerated in hypertensive women, so that the highest readings of all can be recorded during this period. Concurrently, the signs and symptoms of severe pre-eclampsia can appear for the first time, with the onset of epigastric pain (McKay 1972) or eclampsia. A maternal death with an eclamptic convulsion on the sixth day after delivery has been reported (Chapman & Karimi 1973). It is relatively unusual for these potential problems to be anticipated after delivery, so that inappropriately early postpartum discharge has been identified as one preventable factor associated with maternal death from pre-eclampsia or eclampsia (Hibbard 1973).

Postpartum hypertension needs to be managed, as is antepartum hypertension, with treatment titrated to prevent severe hypertension. It is better not to use methyldopa because of the tiredness and depression that it causes. Of the β-blocking agents, labetalol has the advantage of a quick onset of action but postural hypotension can be a problem. For this reason the author prefers oxprenolol starting at 80 mg four times per day. Both atenolol and acebutolol (Boutroy *et al*. 1986; Schimmel *et al*. 1989) are secreted in breast milk, enough to cause occasional problems in the neonate and therefore to make oxprenolol a better choice. Women with a history of asthma should not be given these β-blocking drugs and offered nifedipine on its own. The patient can usually be discharged 6–8 days after delivery. Within 2–3 weeks of discharge antihypertensive treatment can usually be reduced or stopped—a decision that can be delegated to the general practitioner. Whereas angiotensin-converting enzyme (ACE) inhibitors are contraindicated in the second half of pregnancy, they can be used in the puerperium. There is no clear evidence that treatment interferes with breastfeeding. What is known is summarized in Table 6.8.

Remote postpartum assessment and recurrent pre-eclampsia

Women who have suffered pre-eclampsia and its complications always ask for information about the likelihood of recurrence. In general, if all grades of pre-eclampsia are considered, the recurrence rate is 7.5% (Campbell et al. 1985). The risk increases with the severity of the disease (Sibai et al. 1986), with early-onset disease (Sibai et al. 1986) and is particularly high, estimated at nearly 50%, in the predominantly black women suffering pre-eclampsia in the second trimester, studied by Sibai et al. (1991). Recurrent eclampsia is rare (Lopez Llera 1993) but an exceptionally high rate (15.6%) has been reported from Nigeria (Adelusi & Ojengbede 1986). The rate in the UK is not known but must be less than 1%. The HELLP syndrome recurs in about 3% of women, the rate being unaffected by whether the woman has underlying CHT or not (Sibai et al. 1995).

It is necessary to determine what if any long-term medical problems underlie an episode of severe pre-eclampsia. These include CHT, chronic renal disease, the antiphospholipid antibody syndrome and possibly thrombophilia. This is important not only to determine the risk of recurrence (higher if there are such underlying medical

Table 6.8 Antihypertensive drugs and breastfeeding.

Drug	Secretion in breast milk
Methyl dopa	Minimal secretion; too small to be harmful
Labetalol	Secreted in breast milk in small amounts
Atenolol, acebutolol	Secreted in breast milk
Nifedipine	Secreted in breast milk
ACE inhibitors	Secreted in breast milk but in small amounts that are unlikely to be harmful

ACE, angiotensin-converting enzyme.

problems), to advise about contraception options and to give advice about lifestyle and medical surveillance in relation to long-term medical health.

Since the first report (Brownrigg 1962), oral contraceptives have been implicated as a cause of hypertension which may be severe and very rarely malignant (Zech et al. 1975). For this reason CHT is a relative contraindication to their use. It has been suggested (Carmichael et al. 1970) but not confirmed (Pritchard & Pritchard 1977) that pre-eclampsia may be associated with hypertension induced by oral contraceptives. The advice given to postpartum women should therefore be guided by whether or not hypertension persists as a chronic problem. Women with thrombophilia including antiphospholipid antibodies should avoid oestrogen-containing oral contraceptives, although progestogen-only preparations are deemed to be safe. For the rest, if a pre-eclamptic woman's blood pressure returns to normal, there seems little reason to deny her the benefits of oral contraceptives provided adequate and continuing medical supervision is available. Likewise it is not known that an episode of HELLP syndrome is of itself a contraindication to use of oestrogen-containing oral contraceptives in the absence of CHT.

Severe pre-eclampsia and eclampsia can cause irreversible maternal damage, particularly acute renal cortical necrosis or cerebral haemorrhage. In the absence of these complications there is no clear information of the impact of a pre-eclamptic episode on long-term maternal health. In terms of later life, women with pre-eclampsia as a group have a higher incidence of CHT (Nisell et al. 1995) and ischaemic heart disease (Jonsdottir et al. 1995). Given the fact that many of the conditions that predispose to pre-eclampsia are those that predispose to later arterial disease, it is difficult to disentangle the relative contributions of an episode of pre-eclampsia itself from these underlying risk factors with regard to the long-term maternal risks. Those who have an episode in the first pregnancy only and become normotensive soon after delivery, have a normal life expectancy. Women who have had recurrent pre-eclampsia in several pregnancies, or blood pressures that remain elevated in the puerperium, have a higher incidence of later cardiovascular disorders and a reduced life expectancy compatible with the diagnosis that the initial episode of pre-eclampsia was superimposed on pre-existing hypertension.

There may be considerable residual distress and anxiety after a mother has endured a severe episode of pre-eclampsia. Events such as emergency caesarean deliveries (Ryding et al. 1997), perinatal death or severe perinatal complications such as prematurity or neonatal intensive care, even at term (De Mier et al. 1996), markedly increase the likelihood of puerperal post-traumatic stress reactions. There is no specific documentation of these problems in relation to pre-eclampsia itself but those who meet such women after the event will know that prolonged and debilitating post-traumatic distress syndromes can ensue. It is essential to recognize the problem, to offer appropriate counselling or to help the sufferers gain professional counselling.

Other causes of hypertension in pregnancy

This group comprises women with essential and renal hypertension, and hypertension caused by miscellaneous but rare conditions. Women with essential hypertension tend to be older, hence more likely to be parous, heavier and to have a family history of hypertension (Table 6.9).

Chronic (essential) hypertension

CHT is detected either by an antecedent medical history or by a raised blood pressure (140/90 mmHg or more) in the first half of pregnancy. The physiological decline in the blood pressure in early pregnancy is exaggerated in women with CHT (Chesley 1978) so that they may become normotensive. Conversely, in later pregnancy the normal rise in blood pressure is exaggerated. Thus, a woman with CHT may be normotensive when she starts antenatal care early in the second trimester but then develop hypertension in the third trimester; she thus presents as PIH. Not uncommonly the presentation is of mild hypertension alone in the second half of pregnancy without any antecedent readings at all. In these circumstances it is not possible to distinguish CHT from incipient pre-eclampsia with absolute certainty.

The specific problem of CHT in pregnancy is that it is one of the major predisposing factors to pre-eclampsia.

Pre-eclampsia superimposed on CHT tends to be recurrent in later pregnancies whereas in a normotensive individual, pre-eclampsia tends not to recur. Among women with a blood pressure of 140/90 mmHg or more in the first half of pregnancy the likelihood of developing pre-eclampsia is about five times more than in normotensive individuals (Butler & Bonham 1963). This association led earlier clinicians to conclude that CHT is extremely dangerous when combined with pregnancy (Browne & Dodds 1942).

The signs of pre-eclampsia in chronically hypertensive women are the same as in other women except that the blood pressure levels start from a higher baseline. Thus, the demonstration of a rise in the blood pressure (for example +30/+15 mmHg from baseline), a progressive hyperuricaemia, or abnormal activation of the clotting system is evidence of superimposed pre-eclampsia that will progress to proteinuria unless pre-empted by delivery. When proteinuria develops, intrauterine growth restriction is almost the rule. The easiest diagnostic guide is the maternal plasma urate level. Values below 0.30 mmol/L are not in favour of pre-eclampsia, and in a hypertensive woman would suggest the diagnosis of a chronic problem. Overall the differential diagnosis of chronic from pre-eclamptic hypertension rests on the demonstration of the absence of pre-eclamptic features. There is no change in the blood pressure from baseline, no increase in maternal plasma urate levels, no proteinuria and no activation of the clotting system.

Chronically hypertensive women who do not get pre-eclampsia can usually expect a normal and uncomplicated perinatal outcome (Chamberlain *et al.* 1978b). Opinion is divided as to whether CHT predisposes to abruptio placentae. Some find that it is (Williams *et al.* 1991),

	Normotensive	Chronic Hypertension	Pre-eclampsia
Number	14 109	485	1617
Age (years)*	27.5 + 5.0	28.5 + 5.2	26.6 + 4.9
Weight/height^2 (g/cm^2)*	24 ± 4	27 ± 6	24 ± 4
Primigravidae	40.6%	41.4%	60.7%
Proteinuria	0.5%	2.4%	5.5%
Birthweight (kg)*	3.34 ± 0.52	3.26 ± 0.63	3.17 ± 0.65
Maturity at delivery (days)*	279 ± 13	273 ± 17	274 ± 16
Perinatal deaths			
Primigravidae	51/5731 (0.89%)	6/201 (2.99%)	11/981 (1.12%)
Multigravidae	75/8378 (0.90%)	2/284 (0.70%)	8/636 (1.26%)

Table 6.9 Characteristics of women with and without hypertension: chronic and pre-eclamptic.

*Means ± SD.

All women presented for care in the John Radcliffe Hospital, Oxford, before 20 weeks' gestation in 1981–84. The classification of the diagnoses is that of Redman and Jefferies (1988).

Hypertension **185**

whereas others disagree (Paterson 1979; Ananth *et al.* 1997). The reported incidence of abruption has varied from 0.45% to 5.6% (reviewed by Sibai 1991). All that can be said is that it is a relatively rare complication (about 1%). There is some evidence for a modestly increased incidence of fetal growth restriction associated with CHT (Haelterman *et al.* 1997).

TREATMENT

If antihypertensive treatment has been started before conception, the patient may seek advice about the possible effects of her medication on the growth and development of her fetus. None of the commonly used antihypertensive drugs is known to be teratogenic. This does not exclude the possibility of subtle problems, which are as yet unknown. For this reason it is appropriate that women with no more than moderate hypertension should stop treatment before conception; so that only those whose hypertension is an immediate health hazard need continue on medication throughout the first trimester. By the 12th week the normal fall in blood pressure is such that the need for treatment in this group is either temporarily diminished or no longer present, so that at this stage all treatment can be temporarily reduced or stopped to be restarted as the blood pressure rises again during the third trimester.

If CHT is diagnosed for the first time in pregnancy, it is necessary to treat those in whom it presents an immediate (as opposed to a long-term) hazard. The precise levels for treatment have not been agreed upon; we take a cut-off point at or above 170/110 mmHg.

The problem of less severe CHT (i.e. 140–170/90–110 mmHg) needs to be considered. In general medical practice the purpose of treating this degree of hypertension is to prevent long-term complications, which are not relevant for the brief period of gestation. For this reason the only indication for antihypertensive treatment in these women would be if it could prevent the superimposition of pre-eclampsia, which is the major short-term problem. There is evidence from randomized controlled trials that the early control of moderate CHT does not lessen the eventual incidence of superimposed pre-eclampsia (Redman 1980; Sibai *et al.* 1990). Thus, there is no worthwhile fetal indication for the control of moderate hypertension in pregnancy, and consequently the medical management hinges entirely around considerations of maternal welfare.

The choice of drugs is dictated by fetal considerations. Methyldopa is preferred because its fetal effects have been defined much more clearly than those of any other drug. Its

antihypertensive action and side-effects are the same as in non-pregnant individuals. Detailed developmental follow-ups of drug-exposed fetuses to the age of 7 years confirm the absence of any significant adverse drug reaction (Mutch *et al.* 1977; Cockburn *et al.* 1982). The usual treatment schedule is 0.75–3 g/day in divided doses. Methyldopa can be supplemented with nifedipine for the treatment of pre-eclamptic hypertension. The use of other drugs such as labetalol and the conventional β blockers has been fully discussed above. There has been a tendency for β blockers to be associated with smaller fetuses (Sibai *et al.* 1987b; Butters *et al.* 1990) or placentas (Thorley 1984). The effect on fetal growth was so striking in one study (Butters *et al.* 1990) that β blockers are better avoided for the long-term treatment of hypertension in pregnancy. This does not preclude their short-term use in the third trimester, for the treatment of pre-eclampsia or PIH, which has not been associated with adverse effects on the fetus (see Rubin *et al.* 1983).

If diuretics are essential for good blood pressure control they can be continued throughout pregnancy but their use carries certain disadvantages if pre-eclampsia should supervene, as already discussed.

ACE inhibitors are widely used for the treatment of various forms of long-term hypertension. Although ACE inhibitors have been given to women who have had successful pregnancies (Kreft-Jais *et al.* 1988) there are anxieties about their safety for the fetus, based on animal experiments and the high incidence of fetal death and neonatal renal failure in the offspring of treated women (Rosa *et al.* 1989). For this reason although they seem to be safe in the first trimester and the puerperium, they should not be used during the second two trimesters.

Long-term use of antihypertensive agents of all sorts has been associated with modest fetal growth restriction (von Dadelszen *et al.* 2000). This may be because lowering the arterial pressure reduces placental perfusion; or that other effects of the drugs, all of which must be assumed to cross the placenta, have a separate effect on the growth rates of exposed fetuses. This is an excellent justification for the conservative criteria for using these agents, described in this chapter. They should be limited to the treatment of women with severe, rather than mild or moderate, hypertension.

The selection of antihypertensive drugs for use in pregnancy is summarized in Table 6.10.

Phaeochromocytoma

This is a rare but dangerous complication of pregnancy. Maternal mortality has previously been as high as 50% (Blair 1963) but more recently has been reported as 4%

Stage of pregnancy	Relatively contraindicated drugs	Absolutely contraindicated drugs	Drugs that may be used
First trimester	None known	None known	Avoid all if possible
Second trimester	β blockers Diuretics	ACE inhibitors	Methyldopa Nifedipine Labetalol
Third trimester	Diuretics	ACE inhibitors	Methyldopa Nifedipine Labetalol Doxazosin Prazosin
Puerperium	Methyldopa	None known	β blockers Nifedipine ACE inhibitors Diuretics

Table 6.10 Antihypertensive drugs in pregnancy.

ACE, angiotensin-converting enzyme.

(Ahlawat *et al.* 1999). The presentation frequently simulates severe pre-eclampsia (Lamming *et al.* 1990) with extreme but unstable hypertension, proteinuria and pre-eclamptic like symptoms such as headaches (Schenker & Chowers 1971). For this reason all patients with proteinuric hypertension in pregnancy should be screened for phaeochromocytoma, although even then the diagnosis can be missed by false-negative results (Coden 1972). In other situations the diagnosis should be suspected if there is hypertension with paroxysmal features including cold sweats or palpitations, or with unexplained collapse or heart failure. Provided the condition can be identified and treated before delivery, the maternal mortality is reduced, to zero in cases where α-adrenergic blockade has been used (Harper *et al.* 1989). Methods of diagnosis are the same as in non-pregnant individuals and include urinary excretion of vanillylmandelic acid (VMA) and/or catecholamines. The dietary contribution to urinary VMA is negligible and no special dietary precautions are needed. An excretion twice normal is highly suggestive of the diagnosis, and thrice normal is diagnostic. Other tests that may be needed in certain circumstances include plasma catecholamines and suppression tests using phentolamine or clonidine. The best methods for imaging an adrenal tumour are by computed tomography or magnetic resonance imaging (preferable in pregnancy). Ten per cent of phaeochromocytomas are extramedullary and these are the ones that are more likely to be or become malignant. Such have been reported in pregnancy (Fawcett & Kimbell 1971; Simanis *et al.* 1972). Treatment with α-adrenergic blockade with or without addition of β-adrenergic blockade is compatible with normal fetal

survival. Given adequate medical treatment, tumour resection can be successfully accomplished early in pregnancy (Harper *et al.* 1989) at delivery by caesarean section (Burgess 1979) or at a later elective date (Schenker & Chowers 1971).

Coarctation of the aorta (see also Chapter 5)

Previously this condition was associated with a high enough mortality in pregnancy for termination to be recommended (Deal & Wooley 1973). Maternal death was primarily from dissection or rupture of the aorta. Contemporary experience is more favourable, and decisions about the advisability of a pregnancy may depend more on related factors such as associated cardiac malformation. Surgical resection during pregnancy is not advisable (Goodwin 1961). A previous successful resection is not a contraindication to undertaking pregnancy.

Cushing's syndrome (see also Chapter 13)

Amenorrhoea and menstrual irregularities are common features of Cushing's syndrome so that the likelihood of conception is diminished. Many of the features of the syndrome—increased pigmentation, striae, weight gain, hyperglycaemia and hypertension—may occur during pregnancy in the absence of the disease. Congestive heart failure may be a presenting symptom. Difficulties of diagnosis are further compounded because normal pregnancy causes increased bound and unbound plasma cortisol with blunting of its diurnal variation, increased urinary free cortisol, and moderately increased 17-

hydroxysteroids and 17-ketosteroids (Ramsay 1980). Suppression of cortisol production by dexamethasone is the appropriate diagnostic test, although normally this is less complete than in non-pregnant subjects. There is a relatively high incidence of primary adrenal tumours including carcinoma in rare instances (Kreines & DeVaux 1971). For these reasons surgical exploration and removal should be considered once the diagnosis is made. Adrenalectomy during pregnancy with a later successful outcome has been reported (Bevan *et al*. 1987), as has trans-sphenoidal pituitary adenectomy (Casson *et al*. 1987). An uncomplicated pregnancy managed medically with ketocanazole has also been described (Berwaerts *et al*. 1999). Fetal loss is high in Cushing's syndrome and there may be neonatal adrenal insufficiency (Kreines & DeVaux 1971). The subject is reviewed in more detail in Chapter 13 and elsewhere (Sheeler 1994).

Primary aldosteronism (Conn's syndrome)

This is a rare cause of hypertension in pregnancy. It has usually been diagnosed either before or after pregnancy on the basis of hypokalaemia combined with hypertension (Crane *et al*. 1964; Gordon *et al*. 1967), which becomes particularly severe postpartum (Nezu *et al*. 2000). The hypokalaemia may cause muscle weakness (Fujiyama *et al*. 1999). During pregnancy both plasma concentrations and urinary excretion of aldosterone are increased, which makes diagnosis difficult. Remission of the disorder may occur during pregnancy possibly caused by progesterone, which antagonizes the renal action of aldosterone (Aoi *et al*. 1978). Successful pregnancies with and without medical treatment have been reported. If the adrenal adenoma can be identified, resection in the second trimester may be the treatment of choice (Aboud *et al*. 1995; Solomon *et al*. 1996).

Conclusions

1 Hypertension in pregnancy arises from the pregnancy-specific disorder of pre-eclampsia or a long-term maternal attribute, most commonly CHT.

2 PIH is not pre-eclampsia. It may signify a prodromal phase that evolves into pre-eclampsia or underlying long-term hypertension revealed by the pregnancy.

3 Pre-eclampsia arises from a systemic inflammatory response that causes endothelial dysfunction. The response is common to all pregnancies, and pre-eclampsia is simply the extreme end of the spectrum.

4 In pre-eclampsia the main differential diagnosis is from CHT which in its pure form does not share the renal, coagulation, hepatic and placental abnormalities of pre-eclampsia.

5 The principal perinatal risks of CHT in pregnancy result from superimposed pre-eclampsia.

6 Extreme hypertension in pregnancy ($\geq 170/110$ mmHg) is as dangerous as it is in any other medical situation and demands urgent treatment.

7 There is no case for antihypertensive treatment for mild to moderate hypertension (140–165/90–105 mmHg). There is evidence that long-term antihypertensive treatment in pregnancy causes a degree of fetal growth restriction.

8 Methyldopa is the most thoroughly tested antihypertensive agent in pregnancy. β-blocking agents are safe for short-term use but can cause significant fetal growth restriction if administered over longer periods (from the first half of pregnancy). Nifedipine appears to be safe.

9 Diuretics should primarily be reserved for the treatment of heart failure complicating pre-eclampsia.

10 ACE inhibitors are contraindicated for use in the second and third trimesters of pregnancy because of adverse effects on fetal renal function.

References

Aarnoudse, J.G., Houthoff, H.J., Weits, J., Vellenga, E. & Huisjes, H. (1986) A syndrome of liver damage and intravascular coagulation in the last trimester of normotensive pregnancy. *British Journal of Obstetrics and Gynaecology* **93**, 145–155.

Abdul-Karim, R.W. & Rizk, P.T. (1970) The effect of oxytocin on renal hemodynamics, water and electrolyte excretion. *Obstetrical and Gynecological Survey* **25**, 805–813.

Abi Said, D., Annegers, J.F., Combs Cantrell, D., Frankowski, R.F. & Willmore, L.J. (1995) Case-control study of the risk factors for eclampsia. *American Journal of Epidemiology* **142**, 437–441.

Aboud, E., de Swiet, M. & Gordon, H. (1995) Primary aldosteronism in pregnancy – should it be treated surgically? *Irish Journal of Medical Science* **164**, 279–280.

ACOG (1996) *Hypertension in Pregnancy*. Technical Bulletin Number 219. American College of Obstetricians and Gynecologists, Washington, DC.

Adelusi, B. & Ojengbede, O.A. (1986) Reproductive performance after eclampsia. *International Journal of Gynaecology and Obstetrics* **24**, 183–189.

Ahlawat, S.K., Jain, S., Kumari, S., Varma, S. & Sharma, B.K. (1999) Pheochromocytoma associated with pregnancy: case report and review of the literature. *Obstetrical and Gynecological Survey* **54**, 728–737.

Ales, K.L., Norton, M.E. & Druzin, M.L. (1989) Early prediction of antepartum hypertension. *Obstetrics and Gynecology* **73**, 928–933.

Ananth, C.V., Savitz, D.A., Bowes, W.A. & Luther, E.R. (1997) Influence of hypertensive disorders and cigarette smoking on placental abruption and uterine bleeding during pregnancy. *British Journal of Obstetrics and Gynaecology* **104**, 572–578.

Ansari, M.Z., Mueller, B.A. & Krohn, M.A. (1995) Epidemiology of eclampsia. *European Journal of Epidemiology* **11**, 447–451.

Aoi, W., Doi, Y., Tasaki, S., Mitsuoka, J., Suzuki, S. & Hashiba, K. (1978) Primary aldosteronism aggravated during peripartum period. *Japanese Heart Journal* **19**, 946–953.

Assali, N.S., Kaplan, S., Oighenstein, S. & Suyemoto, R. (1953) Hemodynamic effects of l-hydrazinophthalazine in human pregnancy; results of intravenous administration. *Journal of Clinical Investigations* **32**, 922–930.

Atkinson, M.W., Belfort, M.A., Saade, G.R. & Moise, K.J. Jr (1994) The relation between magnesium sulfate therapy and fetal heart rate variability. *Obstetrics and Gynecology* **83**, 967–970.

Ayhan, A., Akkok, E., Urman, B., Yarali, H., Dundar, S. & Kirazli, S. (1990) Beta-thromboglobulin and platelet factor 4 levels in pregnancy and preeclampsia. *Gynecological Obstetrics and Investigation* **30**, 12–14.

Baillie, T.W. (1963) Vasopressor activity of ergometrine maleate in anaesthetised parturient women. *British Medical Journal* **1**, 585–588.

Baird, D. (1977) Epidemiological aspects of hypertensive pregnancy. *Clinical Obstetrics and Gynaecology* **4**, 531–548.

Bar, J., Maymon, R. *et al.* (1999) White coat hypertension and pregnancy outcome. *Journal of Human Hypertension* **13**, 541–545.

Barton, J.R., Hiett, A.K., O'Connor, W.N., Nissen, S.E. & Greene, J.W.J. (1991) Endomyocardial ultrastructural findings in preeclampsia. *American Journal of Obstetrics and Gynecology* **165**, 389–391.

Beeson, J.H. & Duda, E.E. (1982) Computed axial tomography scan demonstration of cerebral edema in eclampsia preceded by blindness. *Obstetrics and Gynecology* **60**, 529–532.

Belfort, M.A. & Moise, K.J. (1992) Effect of magnesium sulfate on maternal brain blood flow in preeclampsia: a randomized, placebo-controlled Study. *American Journal of Obstetrics and Gynecology* **167**, 661–666.

Belfort, M.A., Uys, P., Dommisse, J. & Davey, D.A. (1989) Haemodynamic changes in gestational proteinuric hypertension: the effects of rapid volume expansion and vasodilator therapy. *British Journal of Obstetrics and Gynaecology* **96**, 634–641.

Belizan, J.M. & Villar, J. (1980) The relationship between calcium intake and edema-, proteinuria-, and hypertension-gestosis: an hypothesis. *American Journal of Clinical Nutrition* **33**, 2202–2210.

Belizan, J.M., Villar, J., Gonzalez, L., Campodonico, L. & Bergel, E. (1991) Calcium supplementation to prevent hypertensive disorders of pregnancy. *New England Journal of Medicine* **325**, 1399–1405.

Benedetto, C., Marozio, L., Giarola, M., Chiarolini, L., Maula, V. & Massobrio, M. (1998) Twenty-four hour blood pressure monitoring in early pregnancy: is it predictive of pregnancy-induced hypertension and preeclampsia? *Acta Obstetrica et Gynecologica Scandinavica* **77**, 14–21.

Berwaerts, J., Verhelst, J., Mahler, C. & Abstract, R. (1999) Cushing's syndrome in pregnancy treated by ketoconazole: case report and review of the literature. *Gynecological Endocrinology* **13**, 175–182.

Bevan, J.S., Gough, M.H., Gillmer, M.D.G. & Burke, C.W. (1987) Cushing's syndrome in pregnancy: The timing of definitive treatment. *Clinical Endocrinology (Oxford)* **27**, 225–233.

Bing, R.F. & Smith, A.J. (1981) Plasma and interstitial volumes in essential hypertension: relationship to blood pressure. *Clinical Science* **61**, 287–293.

Bis, K.A. & Waxman, B. (1976) Rupture of the liver associated with pregnancy: a review of the literature and report of 2 cases. *Obstetrical and Gynecological Survey* **31**, 763–773.

Blair, R.G. (1963) Phaeochromocytoma and pregnancy. *Journal of Obstetrics and Gynaecology of the British Commonwealth* **70**, 110–119.

Blake, S. & MacDonald, D.(1991) The prevention of the maternal manifestations of pre-eclampsia by intensive antihypertensive treatment. *British Journal of Obstetrics and Gynaecology* **98**, 244–248.

Boffa, M.C., Valsecchi, L. *et al.* (1998) Predictive value of plasma thrombomodulin in preeclampsia and gestational hypertension. *Thrombosis and Haemostasis* **79**, 1092–1095.

Boneu, B., Fournie, A., Sie, P., Grandjean, H., Bierme, R. & Pontonnier, G. (1980) Platelet production time, uricemia and some hemostasis tests in pre-eclampsia. *European Journal of Obstetrics, Gynecology, and Reproductive Biology* **11**, 85–94.

Bourgeois, F.J., Thiagarajah, S., Harbert, G.M.J. & Di Fazio, C. (1986) Profound hypotension complicating magnesium therapy. *American Journal of Obstetrics and Gynecology* **154**, 919–920.

Boutroy, M.J., Bianchetti, G., Dubruc, C., Vert, P. & Morselli, P.L. (1986) To nurse when receiving acebutolol. Is it dangerous for the neonate? *European Journal of Clinical Pharmacology* **30**, 737–739.

Bower, S., Bewley, S. & Campbell, S. (1993) Improved prediction of preeclampsia by two-stage screening of uterine arteries using the early diastolic notch and color Doppler imaging. *Obstetrics and Gynecology* **82**, 78–83.

Boyd, P.A., Lindenbaum, R.H. & Redman, C.W.G. (1987) Preeclampsia and trisomy 13: a possible association. *Lancet* **ii**, 425–427.

Branch, D.W., Andres, R., Digre, K.B., Rote, N.S. & Scott, J.R. (1989) The association of antiphospholipid antibodies with severe preeclampsia. *Obstetrics and Gynecology* **73**, 541–545.

Brandenburg, H., Los, F.J. & In't Veld, P. (1996) Clinical significance of placenta-confined non-mosaic trisomy 16. *American Journal of Obstetrics and Gynecology* **174**, 1663–1664.

Brosens, I. & Renaer, M. (1972) On the pathogenesis of placental infarcts in pre-eclampsia. *Journal of Obstetrics and Gynaecology of the British Commonwealth* **79**, 794–799.

Brosens, I.A., Robertson, W.B. & Dixon, H.G. (1972) The role of the spiral arteries in the pathogenesis of preeclampsia. *Obstetrics and Gynecological Annual* **1**, 177–191.

Brown, M.A., Robinson, A. *et al.* (1998) Ambulatory blood pressure monitoring in pregnancy: what is normal? *American Journal of Obstetrics and Gynecology* **178**, 836–842.

Brown, M.A., Robinson, A. & Jones, M. (1999) The white coat effect in hypertensive pregnancy: much ado about nothing? *British Journal of Obstetrics and Gynaecology* **106**, 474–480.

Browne, F.J. & Dodds, G.H. (1942) Pregnancy in the patient with chronic hypertension. *Journal of Obstetrics and Gynaecology of the British Empire* **49**, 1–17.

Brownrigg, G.M. (1962) Toxemia in hormone-induced pseudopregnancy. *Canadian Medical Association Journal* **87**, 408–409.

Bruner, J.P. & Yeast, J.D. (1990) Pregnancy associated with Friedreich ataxia. *Obstetrics and Gynecology* **76**, 976–977.

Burgess, G.E. (1979) Alpha blockade and surgical intervention of pheochromocytoma in pregnancy. *Obstetrics and Gynecology* **53**, 266–270.

Butler, N.R. & Bonham, D.G. (1963) Toxaemia in pregnancy. In: *Perinatal Mortality*. E and S Livingstone, Edinburgh: pp. 87–100.

Butters, L., Kennedy, S. & Rubin, P.C. (1990) Atenolol in essential hypertension during pregnancy. *British Medical Journal* **301**, 587–589.

Campbell, D.M. & MacGillivray, I. (1999) Preeclampsia in twin pregnancies: incidence and outcome. *Hypertension in Pregnancy* **18**, 197–207.

Campbell, D.M., MacGillivray, I. & Carr Hill, R. (1985) Preeclampsia in second pregnancy. *British Journal of Obstetrics and Gynaecology* **82**, 131–140.

Caritis, S., Sibai, B. *et al.* (1998) Low-dose aspirin to prevent preeclampsia in women at high risk. National Institute of Child Health and Human Development Network of Maternal-Fetal Medicine Units. *New England Journal of Medicine* **338**, 701–705.

Carmichael, S.M., Taylor, M.M. & Ayers, C.R. (1970) Oral contraceptives, hypertension and toxemia. *Obstetrics and Gynecology* **35**, 371–376.

Casson, I.F., Davis, J.C., Jeffreys, R.V., Silas, J.H., Williams, J. & Belchetz, P.E. (1987) Successful management of Cushing's disease during pregnancy by transsphenoidal adenectomy. *Clinical Endocrinology (Oxford)* **27**, 423–428.

Cavanagh, D., Rao, P.S., Knuppel, R.A., Desai, U. & Balis, J.U. (1985) Pregnancy-induced hypertension: development of a model in the pregnant primate (*Papio anubis*). *American Journal of Obstetrics and Gynecology* **151**, 987–999.

Chamberlain, G.V.P., Lewis, P.J., de Swiet, M. & Bulpitt, J.J. (1978a) How obstetricians manage hypertension in pregnancy. *British Medical Journal* **1**, 626–629.

Chamberlain, G., Philipp, E., Howlett, B. & Masters, K. (1978b) *British Births 1970, Vol. 2: Obstetric Care*. London.

Chapman, A.B., Abraham, W.T. *et al.* (1998) Temporal relationships between hormonal and hemodynamic changes in early human pregnancy. *Kidney International* **54**, 2056–2063.

Chapman, K. & Karimi, R. (1973) A case of post partum eclampsia of late onset confirmed by autopsy. *American Journal of Obstetrics and Gynecology* **117**, 858–861.

Chappell, L.C., Seed, P.T. *et al.* (1999) Effect of antioxidants on the occurrence of pre-eclampsia in women at increased risk: a randomised trial. *Lancet* **354**, 810–816.

Chesley, L.C. (1978) *Hypertensive Disorders in Pregnancy*. Appleton-Century-Crofts, New York.

Chesley, L.C. (1984) Habitus and eclampsia. *Obstetrics and Gynecology* **64**, 315–318.

Chesley, L.C. & Annitto, J.E. (1947) Pregnancy in the patient with hypertensive disease. *American Journal of Obstetrics and Gynecology* **53**, 372–381.

Chesley, L.C. & Cooper, D.W. (1986) Genetics of hypertension in pregnancy: possible single gene control of pre-eclampsia and eclampsia in the descendants of eclamptic women. *British Journal of Obstetrics and Gynaecology* **93**, 898–908.

Chesley, L.C. & Williams, L.O. (1945) Renal glomerular and tubular functions in relation to the hyperuricemia of pre-eclampsia and eclampsia. *American Journal of Obstetrics and Gynecology* **50**, 367–375.

Chesley, L.C., Annitto, J.E. & Cosgrove, R.A. (1968) The familial factor in toxemia of pregnancy. *Obstetrics and Gynecology* **32**, 303–311.

Chester, E.M., Agamanolis, D.P., Banker, B.Q. & Victor, M. (1978) Hypertensive encephalopathy: a clinicopathologic study of 20 cases. *Neurology* **28**, 928–939.

Chua, S. & Redman, C.W.G. (1991) Are prophylactic anticonvulsants required in severe pre-eclampsia? *Lancet* **337**, 250–251.

Chun, D., Braga, C., Chow, C. & Lok, L. (1964) Clinical observations on some aspects of hydatidiform moles. *Journal of Obstetrics and Gynaecology of the British Commonwealth* **71**, 180–184.

Churchill, D. & Beevers, D.G. (1996) Differences between office and 24-hour ambulatory blood pressure measurement during pregnancy. *Obstetrics and Gynecology* **88**, 455–461.

Cincotta, R.B. & Brennecke, S.P. (1998) Family history of preeclampsia as a predictor for pre-eclampsia in primigravidas. *International Journal of Gynaecology and Obstetrics* **60**, 23–27.

Clapp, J.F. & Capeless, E. (1997) Cardiovascular function before, during, and after the first and subsequent pregnancies. *American Journal of Cardiology* **80**, 1469–1473.

CLASP (1994) A randomised trial of low-dose aspirin for the prevention and treatment of pre-eclampsia among 9364 pregnant women. *Lancet* **343**, 619–629.

Cnattingius, S., Mills, J.L., Yuen, J., Eriksson, O. & Salonen, H. (1997) The paradoxical effect of smoking in preeclamptic pregnancies: smoking reduces the incidence but increases the rates of perinatal mortality, abruptio placentae, and intrauterine growth restriction. *American Journal of Obstetrics and Gynecology* **177**, 156–161.

Cockburn, J., Moar, V.A., Ounsted, M. & Redman, C.W.G. (1982) Final report of study on hypertension during pregnancy: the effects of specific treatment on the growth and development of the children. *Lancet* **1**, 647–649.

Coden, J. (1972) Phaeochromocytoma in pregnancy. *Journal of the Royal Society of Medicine* **65**, 863.

Coetzee, E.J., Dommisse, J. & Anthony, J. (1998) A randomised controlled trial of intravenous magnesium sulphate versus placebo in the management of women with severe pre-eclampsia. *British Journal of Obstetrics and Gynaecology* **105**, 300–303.

Cohn, J.N. (1967) Blood pressure measurement in shock. *Journal of the American Medical Association* **199**, 972–976.

Collaborative Eclampsia Trial (1995) Which anticonvulsant for women with eclampsia? Evidence from the Collaborative Eclampsia Trial. *Lancet* **345**, 1455–1463.

Collins, R., Yusuf, S. & Peto, R. (1985) Overview of randomised trials of diuretics in pregnancy. *British Medical Journal* **290**, 17–23.

Combs, C.A., Katz, M.A., Kitzmille, J.L. & Brescia, R.J. (1993) Experimental preeclampsia produced by chronic constriction of the lower aorta: validation with longitudinal blood pressure measurements in conscious rhesus monkeys. *American Journal of Obstetrics and Gynecology* **169**, 215–223.

Cotton, D.B., Longmire, S., Jones, M.M., Dorman, K.F., Tessem, J. & Joyce, T.H. (1986) Cardiovascular alterations in severe pregnancy-induced hypertension: effects of intravenous nitroglycerin coupled with blood volume expansion. *American Journal of Obstetrics and Gynecology* **154**, 1053–1059.

Crane, M.G., Andes, J.P., Harris, J.J. & Slate, W.G. (1964) Primary aldosteronism in pregnancy. *Obstetrics and Gynecology* **23**, 200–208.

Crooks, B.N., Deshpande, S.A., Hall, C., Platt, M.P. & Milligan, D.W. (1998) Adverse neonatal effects of maternal labetalol treatment. *Archives of Disease in Childhood. Fetal and Neonatal Edition* **79**, F150–F151.

Cruikshank, D.P., Chan, G.M. & Doerrfeld, D. (1993) Alterations in vitamin D and calcium metabolism with magnesium sulfate treatment of preeclampsia. *American Journal of Obstetrics and Gynecology* **168**, 1170–1176.

Cuckle, H., Sehmi, I. & Jones, R. (1998) Maternal serum inhibin A can predict pre-eclampsia. *British Journal of Obstetrics and Gynaecology* **105**, 1101–1103.

Cunningham, F.G. & Twickler, D. (2000) Cerebral edema complicating eclampsia. *American Journal of Obstetrics and Gynecology* **182**, 94–100.

von Dadelszen, P., Ornstein, M.P., Bull, S.B., Logan, A.G., Koren, G. & Magee, L.A. (2000) Fall in mean arterial pressure and fetal growth restriction in pregnancy hypertension: a meta-analysis. *Lancet* **355**, 87–92.

Dalekos, G.N., Elisaf, M.S., Papagalanis, N., Tzallas, C. & Siamopoulos, K.C. (1996) Elevated interleukin-1-beta in the circulation of patients with essential hypertension before any drug therapy: a pilot study. *European Journal of Clinical Investigation* **26**, 936–939.

Davey, D.A. & MacGillivray, I. (1988) The classification and definition of the hypertensive disorders of pregnancy. *American Journal of Obstetrics and Gynecology* **158**, 892–898.

Davies, M.H., Wilkinson, S.P *et al.* (1980) Acute liver disease with encephalopathy and renal failure in late pregnancy and the early puerperium: a study of fourteen patients. *British Journal of Obstetrics and Gynaecology* **87**, 1005–1014.

Dawes, M.G. & Grudzinskas, J.G. (1991) Repeated measurement of maternal weight during pregnancy. Is this a useful practice? *British Journal of Obstetrics and Gynaecology* **98**, 189–194.

De Mier, R.L., Hynan, M.T., Harris, H.B. & Manniello, R.L. (1996) Perinatal stressors as predictors of symptoms of post traumatic stress in mothers of infants at high risk. *Journal of Perinatology* **16**, 276–280.

Deal, K. & Wooley, C.F. (1973) Coarctation of the aorta and pregnancy. *Annals of International Medicine* **78**, 706–710.

Demissie, K., Breckenridge, M.B. & Rhoads, G.G. (1998) Infant and maternal outcomes in the pregnancies of asthmatic women. *American Journal of Respiratory and Critical Care Medicine* **158**, 1091–1095.

Dennis, E.J., Smythe, C.M., McIver, F.A. & Howe, H.G. (1963) Percutaneous renal biopsy in eclampsia. *American Journal of Obstetrics and Gynecology* **87**, 364–371.

Department of Health (1993) Changing childbirth. *Report of the Expert Maternity Group*, pp. 19–22. HMSO, London.

Department of Health (1998) Why mothers die. *Report on the Confidential Enquiries into Maternal Deaths in the United Kingdom 1994–96*. Stationery Office, London: 35–46.

Department of Health and Social Security. (1979) *Report on Confidential Enquiries into Maternal Deaths in England and Wales 1973–75*. HMSO, London: 21–29.

Department of Health and Social Security (1982) *Report on Confidential Enquiries into Maternal Deaths in England and Wales 1976–78*. HMSO, London: 19–25.

Department of Health and Social Security (1986) *Report on Confidential Enquiries into Maternal Deaths in England and Wales 1979–81*. HMSO, London: 13–21.

Department of Health and Social Security (1989) *Report on Confidential Enquiries into Maternal Deaths in England and Wales 1982–84*. HMSO, London: 10–19.

Department of Health and Social Security (1991) *Report on Confidential Enquiries into Maternal Deaths in the United Kingdom 1985–87*. HMSO, London: 17–27.

Department of Health and Social Security (1994) *Report on Confidential Enquiries into Maternal Deaths in the United Kingdom 1988–90*. HMSO, London: 22–33.

Department of Health and Social Security (1996) *Report on Confidential Enquiries into Maternal Deaths in the United Kingdom 1991–93*. HMSO, London: 20–31.

Douglas, J.T., Shah, M., Lowe, G.D.O., Belch, J.J.F., Forbes, C.D. & Prentice, C.R.M. (1982) Plasma fibrinopeptide A and beta-thromboglobulin in pre-eclampsia and pregnancy hypertension. *Thrombosis and Haemostasis* **47**, 54–55.

Douglas, K.A. & Redman, C.W.G. (1994) Eclampsia in the United Kingdom. *British Medical Journal* **309**, 1395–1400.

Duffus, G.M., MacGillivray, I. & Dennis, K.J. (1971) The relationship between baby weight and changes in maternal weight, total body water, plasma volume, electrolytes and proteins and urinary oestriol excretion. *Journal of Obstetrics and Gynaecology of the British Commonwealth* **78**, 97–104.

Duley, L. & Neilson, J.P. (1999) Magnesium sulphate and pre-eclampsia. *British Medical Journal* **319**, 3–4.

Dumont, A., Flahault, A., Beaufils, M., Verdy, E. & Uzan, S. (1999) Effect of aspirin in pregnant women is dependent on increase in bleeding time. *American Journal of Obstetrics and Gynecology* **180**, 135–140.

Dunlop, W., Hill, L.M., Landon, M.J., Oxley, A. & Jones, P. (1978) Clinical relevance of coagulation and renal changes in pre-eclampsia. *Lancet* **2**, 346–350.

Duvekot, J.J., Cheriex, E.C., Pieters, F.A., Menheere, P.P. & Peeters, L.H. (1993) Early pregnancy changes in hemodynamics and volume homeostasis are consecutive adjustments triggered by a primary fall in systemic vascular tone. *American Journal of Obstetrics and Gynecology* **169**, 1382–1392.

Easterling, T.R., Benedetti, T.J., Schmucker, B.C. & Millard, S.P. (1990) Maternal hemodynamics in normal and preeclamptic pregnancies: a longitudinal study. *Obstetrics and Gynecology* **76**, 1061–1069.

ECPPA (1996) Randomised trial of low dose aspirin for the prevention of maternal and fetal complications in high risk pregnant women ECPPA (Estudo Colaborativo para Prevencao da Pre-eclampsia com Aspirina) Collaborative Group. *British Journal of Obstetrics and Gynaecology* **103**, 39–47.

Eden, T.W. (1922) Eclampsia: a commentary on the reports presented to the British Congress of Obstetrics and Gynaecology. *Journal of Obstetrics and Gynaecology of the British Empire* **29**, 386–401.

Eichinger, S., Weltermann, A. *et al.* (1999) Prospective evaluation of hemostatic system activation and thrombin potential in healthy pregnant women with and without factor V Leiden. *Thrombosis and Haemostasis* **82**, 1232–1236.

Eisenbud, E. & Lobue, C.C. (1976) Hypocalcemia after therapeutic use of magnesium sulfate. *Archives of Internal Medicine* **136**, 688–691.

Eneroth, E., Remberger, M., Vahlne, A. & Ringden, O. (1998) Increased serum concentrations of interleukin-2 receptor in the first trimester in women who later developed severe preeclampsia. *Acta Obstetrica et Gynecologica Scandinavica* **77**, 591–593.

Faas, M.M., Schuiling, G.A., Baller, J.F., Visscher, C.A. & Bakker, W.W. (1994) A new animal model for human preeclampsia: ultra-low-dose endotoxin infusion in pregnant rats. *American Journal of Obstetrics and Gynecology* **171**, 158–164.

Faas, M.M., Schuiling, G.A., Linton, E.A., Sargent, I.L. & Redman, C.W.G. (2000) Activation of peripheral leukocytes in rat pregnancy and experimental pre-eclampsia. *American Journal of Obstetrics and Gynecology* **182**, 351–357.

Fawcett, F.J. & Kimbell, N.K.B. (1971) Phaeochromocytoma of the ovary. *British Journal of Obstetrics and Gynaecology* **78**, 458–459.

Felding, C.F. (1969) Obstetric aspects in women with histories of renal disease. *Acta Obstetrica et Gynecologica Scandinavica* **48** (Suppl. 2), 1–43.

Felfernig, B.D., Salat, A. *et al.* (2000) Early detection of preeclampsia by determination of platelet aggregability. *Thrombosis Research* **98**, 139–146.

Fenakel, K., Fenakel, G., Appelman, Z., Lurie, S., Katz, Z. & Shoham, Z. (1991) Nifedipine in the treatment of severe pre-eclampsia. *Obstetrics and Gynecology* **77**, 331–337.

Fisher, K.A., Ahuja, S., Luger, A., Spargo, B. & Lindheimer, M. (1977) Nephrotic proteinuria with pre-eclampsia. *American Journal of Obstetrics and Gynecology* **129**, 643–646.

Fisher, E.R., Pardo, V., Paul, R. & Hayashi, T.T. (1969) Ultrastructural studies in hypertension IV. Toxemia of pregnancy. *American Journal of Pathology* **55**, 109–131.

Forman, J.B. & Sullivan, R.L. (1952) The effects of intravenous injections of ergonovine and methergine on the post partum patient. *American Journal of Obstetrics and Gynecology* **63**, 640–644.

Fox, E.J., Sklar, G.J., Hill, C.H., Villanueva, R. & King, B.D. (1977) Complications related to the pressor response. *Anesthesiology* **47**, 524–525.

Fuentes, A., Rojas, A., Porter, K.B., Saviello, G. & O'Brien, W.F. (1995) The effect of magnesium sulfate on bleeding time in pregnancy. *American Journal of Obstetrics and Gynecology* **173**, 1246–1249.

Fujiyama, S., Mori, Y. *et al.* (1999) Primary aldosteronism with aldosterone-producing adrenal adenoma in a pregnant woman. *Internal Medicine* **38**, 36–39.

Gaitz, J.P. & Bamford, C.R. (1982) Unusual computed tomographic scan in eclampsia. *Archives of Neurology* **39**, 66.

Gallery, E.D.M., Ross, M., Hunyor, S.N. & Gyory, A.Z. (1977) Predicting the development of pregnancy-associated hypertension. *Lancet* **1**, 1273–1275.

Gallery, E.D.M., Saunders, D.M., Hunyor, S.N. & Gyory, A.Z. (1979) Randomised comparison of methyldopa and oxprenolol for treatment of hypertension in pregnancy. *British Medical Journal* **1**, 1591–1594.

Gant, N.F., Daley, G.L., Chand, S., Whalley, P.J. & MacDonald, P.C. (1973) A study of angiotensin II pressure response throughout primigravid pregnancy. *Journal of Clinical Investigation* **52**, 2682–2689.

Garden, A., Davey, D.A. & Dommisse, J. (1982) Intravenous labetalol and intravenous dihydralazine in severe hypertension in pregnancy. *Clinical and Experimental Hypertension, Part B* **1**, 371–383.

Gatti, L., Tenconi, P.M. *et al.* (1994) Hemostatic parameters and platelet activation by flow-cytometry in normal pregnancy: a longitudinal study. *International Journal of Clinical and Laboratory Research* **24**, 217–219.

Gilabert, J., Estelles, A., Ridocci, F., Espana, F., Aznar, J. & Galbis, M. (1990) Clinical and haemostatic parameters in the HELLP syndrome: relevance of plasminogen activator inhibitors. *Gynecologic and Obstetric Investigation* **30**, 81–86.

Giles, C. & Inglis, T.C.M. (1981) Thrombocytopenia and macrothrombocytosis in gestational hypertension. *British Journal of Obstetrics and Gynaecology* **88**, 1115–1119.

Ginsberg, J. & Duncan, S.B. (1969) Direct and indirect blood pressure measurement in pregnancy. *Journal of Obstetrics and Gynaecology of the British Commonwealth* **76**, 705–710.

Golding, J. (1998) A randomised trial of low dose aspirin for primiparae in pregnancy. The Jamaica Low Dose Aspirin study Group. *British Journal of Obstetrics and Gynaecology* **105**, 293–299.

Goodlin, R.C. (1983) Safety of sodium nitroprusside. *Obstetrics and Gynecology* **62**, 270.

Goodwin, J.F. (1961) Pregnancy and coarctation of the aorta. *Clinical Obstetrics and Gynaecology* **4**, 645–664.

Gordon, R.D., Fishman, L.M. & Liddle, G.W. (1967) Plasma renin activity and aldosterone secretion in a pregnant woman with primary aldosteronism. *Journal of Clinical Endocrinology and Metabolism* **27**, 385–388.

Gouni, I., Oka, K., Etienne, J. & Chan, L. (1993) Endotoxin-induced hypertriglyceridemia is mediated by suppression of lipoprotein lipase at a post-transcriptional level. *Journal of Lipid Research* **34**, 139–146.

Greenwood, P.A. & Lilford, R.J. (1986) Effect of epidural analgesia on maximum and minimum blood pressures during the first stage of labour in primigravidae with mild/moderate gestational hypertension. *British Journal of Obstetrics and Gynaecology* **93**, 260–263.

Groenendijk, R., Trimbos, J.B.M.J. & Wallenburg, H.C.S. (1984) Hemodynamic measurements in pre-eclampsia: preliminary observations. *American Journal of Obstetrics and Gynecology* **150**, 232–236.

Gupta, M., Shennan, A.H., Halligan, A., Taylor, D.J. & de Swiet, M. (1997) Accuracy of oscillometric blood pressure monitoring in pregnancy and pre-eclampsia. *British Journal of Obstetrics and Gynaecology* **104**, 350–355.

Haelterman, E., Breart, G., Paris, L.J., Dramaix, M. & Tchobroutsky, C. (1997) Effect of uncomplicated chronic hypertension on the risk of small-for-gestational age birth. *American Journal of Epidemiology* **145**, 689–695.

Hall, D.R., Odendaal, H.J., Steyn, D.W. & Smith, M. (2000) Nifedipine or prazosin as a second agent to control early severe hypertension in pregnancy: a randomised controlled trial. *British Journal of Obstetrics and Gynaecology* **107**, 759–765.

Hanretty, K.P., Whittle, M.J., Howie, C.A. & Rubin, P.C. (1989) Effect of nifedipine on Doppler flow velocity waveforms in severe pre-eclampsia. *British Medical Journal* **299**, 1205–1206.

Harper, M.A., Murnaghan, G.A., Kennedy, L., Hadden, D.R. & Atkinson, A.B. (1989) Phaeochromocytoma in pregnancy. Five cases and a review of the literature. *British Journal of Obstetrics and Gynaecology* **96**, 594–606.

Hayashi, M., Kiumi, F. & Mitsuya, K. (1999) Changes in platelet ATP secretion and aggregation during pregnancy and in preeclampsia. *American Journal of Medical Science* **318**, 115–121.

Heller, P.J., Scheider, E.P. & Marx, G.F. (1983) Pharolaryngeal edema as a presenting symptom in preeclampsia. *Obstetrics and Gynecology* **62**, 523–524.

Hennessy, T.G., MacDonald, D. *et al.* (1996) Serial changes in cardiac output during normal pregnancy: a Doppler ultrasound study. *European Journal of Obstetrics, Gynecology, and Reproductive Biology* **70**, 117–122.

Herpolsheimer, A., Brady, K., Yancey, M.K., Pandian, M. & Duff, P. (1991) Pulmonary function of preeclamptic women receiving intravenous magnesium sulfate seizure prophylaxis. *Obstetrics and Gynecology* **78**, 241–244.

Hibbard, L.T. (1973) Maternal mortality due to acute toxemia. *Obstetrics and Gynecology* **42**, 263–270.

Hiett, A.K., Devoe, L.D., Brown, H.L. & Watson, J. (1995) Effect of magnesium on fetal heart rate variability using computer analysis. *American Journal of Perinatology* **12**, 259–261.

Higgins, J.R., Walshe, J.J., Halligan, A., O'Brien, E., Conroy, R. & Darling, M.R. (1997) Can 24-hour ambulatory blood pressure measurement predict the development of hypertension in primigravidae? *British Journal of Obstetrics and Gynaecology* **104**, 356–362.

Hinchey, J., Chaves, C. *et al.* (1996) A reversible posterior leukoencephalopathy syndrome. *New England Journal of Medicine* **334**, 494–500.

Hodgkinson, R., Husain, P.J. & Hayashi, R.H. (1980) Systemic and pulmonary blood pressure during cesarean section in parturients with gestational hypertension. *Canadian Anaesthetists' Society Journal* **27**, 385–394.

Holmes, F. (1960) Incidence of the supine hypotensive syndrome in late pregnancy. *Journal of Obstetrics and Gynaecology of the British Empire* **67**, 254–258.

Horn, E.H., Filshie, M., Kerslake, R.W., Jaspan, T., Worthington, B.S. & Rubin, P.C. (1990) Widespread cerebral ischaemia treated with nimodipine in a patient with eclampsia. *British Medical Journal* **301**, 794.

Howard, W., Hunter, C. & Huber, C.P. (1961) Intervillous blood oxygen studies. *Surgery, Gynecology, and Obstetrics* **112**, 435–438.

Howie, P.W., Begg, C.B., Purdie, D.W. & Prentice, C.R.M. (1976) Use of coagulation tests to predict the clinical progress of pre-eclampsia. *Lancet* **2**, 323–325.

Hutton, J.D., James, D.K., Stirrat, G.M., Douglas, K.A. & Redman, C.W.G. (1992) Management of severe pre-eclampsia and eclampsia by UK consultants. *British Journal of Obstetrics and Gynaecology* **99**, 554–556.

Iseri, L.T. & French, J.H. (1984) Magnesium: nature's physiologic calcium blocker. *American Heart Journal* **108**, 188–194.

Isler, C.M., Rinehart, B.K., Terrone, D.A., Martin, R.W., Magann, E.F. & Martin, N.J. (1999) Maternal mortality associated with HELLP (hemolysis, elevated liver enzymes, and low platelets) syndrome. *American Journal of Obstetrics and Gynecology* **181**, 924–928.

Jacobs, M. (1984) Mechanism of action of hydralazine on vascular smooth muscle. *Biochemistry and Pharmacology* **33**, 2915–2919.

Janes, S.L. & Goodall, A.H. (1994) Flow cytometric detection of circulating activated platelets and platelet hyper-responsiveness in pre-eclampsia and pregnancy. *Clinical Science (Colchester, Essex)* **86**, 731–739.

Janes, S.L., Kyle, P.M., Redman, C. & Goodall, A.H. (1995) Flow cytometric detection of activated platelets in pregnant women prior to the development of pre-eclampsia. *Thrombosis and Haemostasis* **74**, 1059–1063.

Jeffcoate, T.N.A. & Scott, J.S. (1959) Some observations on the placental factor in pregnancy toxemia. *American Journal of Obstetrics and Gynecology* **77**, 475–489.

Jellinek, E.H., Painter, M., Prineas, J. & Russell, R.R. (1964) Hypertensive encephalopathy with cortical disorders of vision. *Quarterly Journal of Medicine* **33**, 239–256.

Johansson, B., Strandgaard, S. & Lassen, N.A. (1974) On the pathogenesis of hypertensive encephalopathy. *Circulation Research* **34** (Suppl. 1), 167–171.

Jones, H.M.R. & Cummings, A.J. (1978) A study of the transfer of alpha-methyldopa to the human fetus and newborn infant. *British Journal of Clinical Pharmacology* **6**, 432–434.

Jonsdottir, L.S., Arngrimsson, R., Geirsson, R.T., Sigvaldason, H. & Sigfusson, N. (1995) Death rates from ischemic heart disease in women with a history of hypertension in pregnancy. *Acta Obstetrica et Gynecologica Scandinavica* **74**, 772–776.

Jouppila, R., Jouppila, P. & Hollmen, A. (1980) Laryngeal oedema as an obstetric anaesthesia complication: case reports. *Acta Anaesthesiologica Scandinavica* **24**, 97–98.

Jouppila, P., Jouppila, R., Hollmen, A. & Koivula, A. (1982b) Lumbar epidural analgesia to improve intervillous blood flow during labour in severe preeclampsia. *Obstetrics and Gynecology* **59**, 158–161.

Jouppila, P., Jouppila, R. & Koivula, A. (1982a) Albumin infusion does not alter the intervillous blood flow in severe pre-eclampsia. *Acta Obstetrica et Gynecologica Scandinavica* **62**, 345–348.

Kaaja, R., Laivuori, H., Laakso, M., Tikkanen, M.J. & Ylikorkala, O. (1999) Evidence of a state of increased insulin resistance in preeclampsia. *Metabolism* **48**, 892–896.

Kaar, K., Jouppila, P., Kuikka, J., Luotala, H., Toivanen, J. & Rekonen, A. (1980) Intervillous blood flow in normal and complicated late pregnancy measured by means of an intravenous 133Xe method. *Acta Obstetrica et Gynecologica Scandinavica* **59**, 7–10.

Katz, V.L. & Cefalo, R.C. (1989) Maternal death from carotid artery thrombosis associated with the syndrome of hemolysis, elevated liver function, and low platelets. *American Journal of Perinatology* **6**, 360–362.

Kemp, P.A., Gardiner, S.M., March, J.E., Rubin, P.C. & Bennett, T. (1999) Assessment of the effects of endothelin-1 and magnesium sulphate on regional blood flows in conscious rats, by the coloured microsphere reference technique. *British Journal of Pharmacology* **126**, 621–626.

Killam, A.P., Dillard, S.H., Patton, R.C. & Pederson, P.R. (1975) Pregnancy-induced hypertension complicated by acute liver disease and disseminated intravascular coagulation. Five case reports. *American Journal of Obstetrics and Gynecology* **123**, 823–828.

Kirby, J.C. & Jaindl, J.J. (1984) Cerebral CT findings in toxemia of pregnancy. *Radiology* **151**, 114.

Kirkendall, W.M., Feinleib, M., Freis, E.D. & Mark, A.L. (1981) Recommendations for human blood pressure determination by sphygmomanometers. Sub-committee of the AHA post-graduate education committee. *Hypertension* **3**, 510A–519A.

Klarr, J.M., Bhatt, M.V. & Donn, S.M. (1994) Neonatal adrenergic blockade following single dose maternal labetalol administration. *American Journal of Perinatology* **11**, 91–93.

Klonoff Cohen, H., Cross, J.L. & Pieper, C.F. (1996) Job stress and preeclampsia. *Epidemiology* **7**, 245–249.

Knight, M., Duley, L., Henderson-Smart, D.J. & King, J.F. (2000) Antiplatelet agents for preventing and treating pre-eclampsia (Cochrane Review). In: *The Cochrane Library*, Issue 2, CD000492. Update Software, Oxford.

Kreft-Jais, C., Plouin, P.F., Tchobroutsky, C. & Boutry, M. (1988) Angiotensin converting enzyme inhibitors during pregnancy: a survey of 22 patients given captopril and nine given enalapril. *British Journal of Obstetrics and Gynaecology* **95**, 420–422.

Kreines, K. & Devaux, W.D. (1971) Neonatal adrenal insufficiency associated with maternal Cushing's syndrome. *Pediatrics* **47**, 516–519.

Kupferminc, M.J., Eldor, A. *et al.* (1999) Increased frequency of genetic thrombophilia in women with complications of pregnancy. *New England Journal of Medicine* **340**, 9–13.

Kyle, P.M., Buckley, D., Kissane, J., de Swiet, M. & Redman, C.W.G. (1995) The angiotensin sensitivity test and low-dose aspirin are ineffective methods to predict and prevent hypertensive disorders in nulliparous pregnancy. *American Journal of Obstetrics and Gynecology* **173**, 865–872.

Lafayette, R.A., Druzin, M. *et al.* (1998) Nature of glomerular dysfunction in pre-eclampsia. *Kidney International* **54**, 1240–1249.

Lamming, G.D., Symonds, E.M. & Rubin, P.C. (1990) Phaeochromocytoma in pregnancy: Still a cause of maternal death. *Clinical and Experimental Hypertension, Part B: Hypertension in Pregnancy* **9**, 57–68.

Lancet (1983) Acute fatty liver of pregnancy. *Lancet* **1**, 339.

Lang, R.M., Pridjian, G., Feldman, T., Neumann, A., Lindheimer, M.D. & Borow, K.M. (1991) Left ventricular mechanics in preeclampsia. *American Heart Journal* **121**, 1768–1775.

Lees, M.M., Scott, D.B., Kerr, M.G. & Taylor, S.H. (1967) The circulatory effects of recumbent postural change in late pregnancy. *Clinical Science* **32**, 453–465.

Levine, R.J., Hauth, J.C. *et al.* (1997) Trial of calcium to prevent preeclampsia. *New England Journal of Medicine* **337**, 69–76.

Liebowitz, H.A. (1984) Cortical blindness as a complication of eclampsia. *Annals of Emergency Medicine* **13**, 365–367.

Lin, M.-S., McNay, J.L., Shepherd, A.M.M., Musgrave, G.E. & Keeton, T.K. (1983) Increased plasma norepinephrine accompanies persistent tachycardia after hydralazine. *Hypertension* **5**, 257–263.

Lindheimer, M.D., Spargo, B.H. & Katz, A.I. (1974) Eclampsia during the 16th week of gestation. *Journal of the American Medical Association* **230**, 1006–1008.

Lipsitz, P.J. (1971) The clinical and biochemical effects of excess magnesium in the newborn. *Pediatrics* **47**, 501–509.

Little, W.A. (1960) Placental infarction. *Obstetrics and Gynecology* **15**, 109–130.

Longmire, S., Leduc, L., Jones, M.M., Hawkins, J.L., Joyce, T.H. & Cotton, D.B. (1991) The hemodynamic effects of intubation during nitroglycerin infusion in severe preeclampsia. *American Journal of Obstetrics and Gynecology* **164**, 551–556.

Lopez Espinoza, I., Dhar, H., Humphreys, S. & Redman, C.W.G. (1986) Urinary albumin excretion in pregnancy. *British Journal of Obstetrics and Gynaecology* **93**, 176–181.

Lopez Llera, M. (1993) Recurrent eclampsia. Clinical data, morbidity and pathogenic considerations. *European Journal of Obstetrics, Gynecology, and Reproductive Biology* **50**, 39–45.

Lopez Llera, M., Linares, G.R. & Horta, J.L.H. (1976) Maternal mortality rates in eclampsia. *American Journal of Obstetrics and Gynecology* **124**, 149–155.

Lorentzen, B., Drevon, C.A., Endresen, M.J. & Henriksen, T. (1995) Fatty acid pattern of esterified and free fatty acids in sera of women with normal and pre-eclamptic pregnancy. *British Journal of Obstetrics and Gynaecology* **102**, 530–537.

Lucas, M.J., Leveno, K.J. & Cunningham, F.G. (1995) A comparison of magnesium sulfate with phenytoin for the prevention of eclampsia. *New England Journal of Medicine* **333**, 201–205.

Luckas, M., Hawe, J., Meekins, J., Neilson, J. & Walkinshaw, S. (1998) Second trimester serum free beta human chorionic gonadotrophin levels as a predictor of pre-eclampsia. *Acta Obstetrica et Gynecologica Scandinavica* **77**, 381–384.

Lunell, N.O., Lewander, R., Nylund, L. Sarby, B. & Thornstrom, S. (1983) Acute effect of dihydralazine on uteroplacental blood flow in hypertension during pregnancy. *Gynecological Obstetrics and Investigations* **16**, 274–282.

Mabie, W.C., Ratts, T.E. & Sibai, B.M. (1989) The central hemodynamics of severe preeclampsia. *American Journal of Obstetrics and Gynecology* **161**, 1443–1448.

MacGillivray, I. (1959) Some observations on the incidence of preeclampsia. *Journal of Obstetrics and Gynaecology of the British Commonwealth* **65**, 536–539.

MacGillivray, I. (1961) Hypertension in pregnancy and its consequences. *Journal of Obstetrics and Gynaecology of the British Commonwealth* **68**, 557–569.

MacGillivray, I., Rose, G.A. & Rowe, B. (1969) Blood pressure survey in pregnancy. *Clinical Science (Colchester Essex)* **37**, 395–407.

Magee, L.A., Ornstein, M.P. & von Dadelszen, P. (1999) Fortnightly review: management of hypertension in pregnancy. *British Medical Journal* **318**, 1332–1336.

Marcoux, S., Berube, S., Brisson, J. & Fabia, J. (1992) History of migraine and risk of pregnancy-induced hypertension. *Epidemiology* **3**, 53–56.

Martin, J.N.J., Blake, P.G., Lowry, S.L., Perry, K.G.J., Files, J.C. & Morrison, J.C. (1990) Pregnancy complicated by preeclampsia–eclampsia with the syndrome of hemolysis, elevated liver enzymes, and low platelet count: how rapid is postpartum recovery? *Obstetrics and Gynecology* **76**, 737–741.

Maxwell, M.H., Waks, A.U., Schroth, P.C., Karam, M. & Dornfeld, L.P. (1982) Error in blood-pressure measurement due to incorrect cuff size in obese patients. *Lancet* **2**, 33–35.

McCarron, D.A. & Morris, C.D. (1985) Blood pressure response to oral calcium in persons with mild to moderate hypertension. A randomized, double-blind, placebo-controlled, crossover trial. *Annals of Internal Medicine* **103**, 825–831.

McCubbin, J.H., Sibai, B.M., Abdella, T.N. & Anderson, G.D. (1981) Cardiopulmonary arrest due to acute maternal hypermagnesaemia. *Lancet* l, 1058.

McFarlane, C.N. (1963) An evaluation of the serum uric acid level in pregnancy. *Journal of Obstetrics and Gynaecology of the British Commonwealth* **70**, 63–68.

McKay, D.G. (1972) Hematologic evidence of disseminated intravascular coagulation in eclampsia. *Obstetrical and Gynecological Survey* **27**, 399–417.

McKay, D.G., Merrill, S.J., Weiner, A.E., Hertig, A.T. & Reid, D.E. (1953) The pathologic anatomy of eclampsia, bilateral renal cortical necrosis, pituitary necrosis, and other acute fatal complications of pregnancy, and its possible relationship to the generalised Shwartzman phenomenon. *American Journal of Obstetrics and Gynecology* **66**, 507–539.

McKenna, P. & Shaw, R.W. (1979) Hyponatremic fits in oxytocin-augmented labours. *International Journal of Gynaecology and Obstetrics* **17**, 250–252.

Milliez, J., Dahoun, A. & Boudraa, M. (1990) Computed tomography of the brain in eclampsia. *Obstetrics and Gynecology* **75**, 975–980.

Ministry of Health (1957). *Report on Confidential Enquiries into Maternal Deaths in England and Wales 1952–54.* HMSO, London: 5–14.

Mires, G.J., Christie, A.D., Leslie, J., Lowe, E., Patel, N.B. & Howie, P.W. (1995) Are 'notched' uterine arterial waveforms of prognostic value for hypertensive and growth disorders of pregnancy? *Fetal Diagnosis and Therapy* **10**, 111–118.

Mires, G.J., Williams, F.L., Leslie, J. & Howie, P.W. (1998) Assessment of uterine arterial notching as a screening test for adverse pregnancy outcome. *American Journal of Obstetrics and Gynecology* **179**, 1317–1323.

Moller, B. & Lindmark, G. (1986) Eclampsia in Sweden 1976–1980. *Acta Obstetrica Gynecologica* **65**, 307–314.

Moore, M.P. & Redman, C.W.G. (1983) Case-control study of severe pre-eclampsia of early onset. *British Medical Journal (Clinical Research ed.)* **287**, 580–583.

Morris, J.A. & O'Grady, J.P. (1979) Volume expansion in severe edema-proteinuria-hypertension gestosis. *American Journal of Obstetrics and Gynecology* **135**, 276.

Muller, F., Savey, L. *et al.* (1996) Maternal serum human chorionic gonadotropin level at fifteen weeks is a predictor for pre-eclampsia. *American Journal of Obstetrics and Gynecology* **175**, 37–40.

Mutch, L.M.M., Moar, V.A., Ounsted, M.K. & Redman, C.W.G. (1977) Hypertension during pregnancy, with and without specific hypotensive treatment. II. The growth and development of the infant in the first year of life. *Early Human Development* **1**, 59–67.

Muttukrishna, S., Knight, P.G., Groome, N.P., Redman, C.W.G & Ledger, W.L. (1997) Activin A and inhibin A as possible endocrine markers for pre-eclampsia. *Lancet* **349**, **1285–1288.**

Naeye, R.L. & Friedman, E.A. (1979) Causes of perinatal death associated with gestational hypertension and proteinuria. *American Journal of Obstetrics and Gynecology* **133**, 8–10.

National High Blood Pressure Education Program (1990) National High Blood Pressure Education Program Working Group Report on High Blood Pressure in Pregnancy. *American Journal of Obstetrics and Gynecology* **163**, 1691–1712.

Nelson, T.R. (1955) A clinical study of pre-eclampsia. *Journal of Obstetrics and Gynaecology of the British Empire* **62**, 48–57.

Ness, R.B. & Roberts, J.M. (1996) Heterogeneous causes constituting the single syndrome of preeclampsia: a hypothesis and its implications. *American Journal of Obstetrics and Gynecology* **175**, 1365–1370.

Newsome, L.R., Bramwell, R.S. & Curling, P.E. (1986) Severe pre-eclampsia: hemodynamic effects of lumbar epidural anesthesia. *Anesthesia and Analgesia* **65**, 31–36.

Nezu, M., Miura, Y., Noshiro, T. & Inoue, M. (2000) Primary aldosteronism as a cause of severe postpartum hypertension in two women. *American Journal of Obstetrics and Gynecology* **182**, 745–746.

Nisell, H., Lintu, H., Lunell, N.O., Mollerstrom, G. & Pettersson, E. (1995) Blood pressure and renal function seven years after pregnancy complicated by hypertension. *British Journal of Obstetrics and Gynaecology* **102**, 876–881.

Odendaal, H.J., Pattinson, R.C., Bam, R., Grove, D. & Kotze, T.J. (1990) Aggressive or expectant management for patients with severe preeclampsia between 28 and 34 weeks' gestation: a randomized controlled trial. *Obstetrics and Gynecology* **76**, 1070–1075.

Olsen, K.S. & Beier Holgersen, R. (1992a) Fetal death following labetalol administration in pre-eclampsia. *Acta Obstetrica et Gynecologica Scandinavica* **71**, 145–147.

Olsen, K.S. & Beier Holgersen, R. (1992b) Hemodynamic collapse following labetalol administration in preeclampsia. *Acta Obstetrica et Gynecologica Scandinavica* **71**, 151–152.

van Oppen, A.C., Stigter, R.H. & Bruinse, H.W. (1996) Cardiac output in normal pregnancy: a critical review. *Obstetrics and Gynecology* **87**, 310–318.

Overgaard, J. & Skinhoj, E. (1975) A paradoxical cerebral hemodynamic effect of hydralazine. *Stroke* **6**, 402–404.

Paterson, M.E. (1979) The aetiology and outcome of abruptio placentae. *Acta Obstetrica et Gynecologica Scandinavica* **58**, 31–35.

Paterson, Brown. S., Robson, S.C., Redfern, N., Walkinshaw, S.A. & de Swiet, M. (1994) Hydralazine boluses for the treatment of severe hypertension in pre-eclampsia. *British Journal of Obstetrics and Gynaecology* **101**, 409–413.

Penny, J.A., Halligan, A.W. *et al.* (1998) Automated, ambulatory, or conventional blood pressure measurement in pregnancy: which is the better predictor of severe hypertension? *American Journal of Obstetrics and Gynecology* **178**, 521–526.

Perry, I.J., Stewart, B.A. *et al.* (1990) Recording diastolic blood pressure in pregnancy. *British Medical Journal* **301**, 1198.

Pickering, G. (1968) *High Blood Pressure.* J. and A. Churchill, London.

Pickering, T.G. (1996) White coat hypertension. *Current Opinions in Nephrology and Hypertension* **5**, 192–198.

Pickup, J.C., Mattock, M.B., Chusney, G.D. & Burt, D. (1997) NIDDM as a disease of the innate immune system: association of acute-phase reactants and interleukin–6 with metabolic syndrome X. *Diabetologia* **40**, 1286–1292.

Piering, W.F., Garancis, J.G., Becker, C.G., Beres, J.A. & Lemann, J. (1993) Preeclampsia related to a functioning extrauterine placenta: report of a case and 25–year follow-up. *American Journal of Kidney Disease* **21**, 310–313.

Pirani, B.B.K., Campbell, D.M. & MacGillivray I. (1973) Plasma volume in normal first pregnancy. *Journal of Obstetrics and Gynaecology of the British Commonwealth* **80**, 884–887.

Plouin, P.F., Breart, G. *et al.* (1990) A randomized comparison of early with conservative use of antihypertensive drugs in the management of pregnancy-induced hypertension. *British Journal of Obstetrics and Gynecology* **97**, 134–141.

Pollak, V.E. & Nettles, J.B. (1960) The kidney in toxemia of pregnancy: a clinical and pathologic study based on renal biopsies. *Medicine* **39**, 469–526.

Porapakkham, S. (1979) An epidemiologic study of eclampsia. *Obstetrics and Gynecology* **54**, 26–30.

Pouta, A.M., Hartikainen, A.L., Vuolteenaho, O.J., Ruokonen, A.O. & Laatikainen, T.J. (1998) Midtrimester N-terminal proatrial natriuretic peptide, free beta hCG, and alpha-fetoprotein in predicting preeclampsia. *Obstetrics and Gynecology* **91**, 940–944.

Pritchard, J.A. & Pritchard, S.A. (1977) Blood pressure response to estrogen-progestin oral contraceptive after pregnancy-induced hypertension. *American Journal of Obstetrics and Gynecology* **129**, 733–739.

Pritchard, J.A. & Stone, S.R. (1967) Clinical and laboratory observations on eclampsia. *American Journal of Obstetrics and Gynecology* **99**, 754–765.

Pritchard, J.A., Cunningham, F.G. & Mason, R.A. (1976) Coagulation changes in eclampsia: their frequency and pathogenesis. *American Journal of Obstetrics and Gynecology* **124**, 855–864.

Pritchard, J.A., Cunningham, F.G. & Pritchard, S.A. (1984) The Parkland Memorial Hospital protocol for treatment of eclampsia: evaluation of 245 cases. *American Journal of Obstetrics and Gynecology* **148**, 951–963.

Qureshi, A.I., Frankel, M.R., Ottenlips, J.R. & Stern, B.J. (1996) Cerebral hemodynamics in preeclampsia and eclampsia. *Archives of Neurology* **53**, 1226–1231.

Raftery, E.B. & Ward, A.P. (1968) The indirect method of recording blood pressure. *Cardiovascular Research* **2**, 210–218.

Ramanathan, J., Sibai, B.M., Mabie, W.C., Chauhan, D. & Ruiz, A.G. (1988) The use of labetalol for attenuation of the hypertensive response to endotracheal intubation in preeclampsia. *American Journal of Obstetrics and Gynecology* **159**, 650–654.

Ramsay, I.D. (1980) The adrenal gland. In: Hytten, F. & Chamberlain G., eds. *Clinical Physiology in Obstetrics.* Blackwell Scientific Publications, Oxford: 415–416.

Redman, C.W.G. (1980) Treatment of hypertension in pregnancy. *Kidney International* **18**, 267–278.

Redman, C.W.G. (1987) The definition of pre-eclampsia. In: Sharp, F. & Symonds, E.M., eds. *Hypertension in Pregnancy.* Perinatology Press, New York: 3–17.

Redman, C.W.G. (1991) Current topic: pre-eclampsia and the placenta. *Placenta* **12**, 301–308.

Redman, C.W.G., Beilin, L.J. & Bonnar, J. (1976a) Variability of blood pressure in normal and abnormal pregnancy . In: Lindheimer, M.D., Katz, A.I. & Zuspan, F.P., eds. *Hypertension in Pregnancy.* John Wiley, New York: 53–60.

Redman, C.W.G., Beilin, L.J. & Bonnar, J. (1976b) Renal function in pre-eclampsia. *Journal of Clinical Pathology* **10**, 91–94.

Redman, C.W.G., Beilin, L.J., Bonnar, J. & Ounsted, M.K. (1976c) Fetal outcome in trial of antihypertensive treatment in pregnancy. *Lancet* **2**, 753–756.

Redman, C.W.G., Beilin, L.J., Bonnar, J. & Wilkinson, R.H. (1976d) Plasma urate measurements in predicting fetal death in hypertensive pregnancy. *Lancet* **1**, 1370–1373.

Redman, C.W.G., Denson, K.W.E., Beilin, L.J., Bolton, F.G. & Stirrat, G.M. (1977) Factor VIII consumption in pre-eclampsia. *Lancet* **2**, 1249–1252.

Redman, C.W.G., Bonnar, J. & Beilin, L.J. (1978) Early platelet consumption in pre-eclampsia. *British Medical Journal* **1**, 467–469.

Redman, C.W.G. & Jefferies, M. (1988) Revised definition of pre-eclampsia. *Lancet* **1**, 809–812.

Redman. C.W.G., Sacks, G.P. & Sargent, I.L. (1999) Preeclampsia: an excessive maternal inflammatory response to pregnancy. *American Journal of Obstetrics and Gynecology* **180**, 499–506.

Reinthaller, A., Mursch-Edlmayr, G. & Tatra, G. (1990) Thrombin-antithrombin III complex levels in normal pregnancy with hypertensive disorders and after delivery. *British Journal of Obstetrics and Gynaecology* **97**, 506–510.

Riaz, M., Porat, R., Brodsky, N.L. & Hurt, H. (1998) The effects of maternal magnesium sulfate treatment on newborns: a prospective controlled study. *Journal of Perinatology* **18**, 449–454.

Rijhsinghani, A., Yankowitz, J., Strauss, R.A., Kuller, J.A., Patil, S. & Williamson, R.A. (1997) Risk of preeclampsia in second-trimester triploid pregnancies. *Obstetrics and Gynecology* **90**, 884–888.

Roberts, J.M., Taylor, R.N., Musci, T.J., Rodgers, G.M., Hubel, C.A. & McLaughlin, M.K. (1989) Preeclampsia: an endothelial cell disorder. *American Journal of Obstetrics and Gynecology* **161**, 1200–1204.

Robertson, E.G. (1971) The natural history of oedema during pregnancy. *Journal of Obstetrics and Gynaecology of the British Commonwealth* **78**, 520–529.

Robertson, W.B., Brosens, I. & Dixon, H.G. (1967) The pathological response of the vessels of the placental bed to hypertensive pregnancy. *Journal of Pathology Bacteriology* **93**, 581–592.

Robertson, W.B., Brosens, I. & Dixon, G. (1975) Uteroplacental vascular pathology. *European Journal of Obstetrics, Gynecology, and Reproductive Biology* **5**, 47–65.

Robillard, P.Y. & Hulsey, T.C. (1996) Association of pregnancy-induced-hypertension, pre-eclampsia, and eclampsia with duration of sexual cohabitation before conception. *Lancet* **347**, 619.

Rodriguez, M.H., Masaki, D.I., Mestman, J., Kumar, D. & Rude, R. (1988) Calcium/creatinine ratio and microalbuminuria in the prediction of preeclampsia. *American Journal of Obstetrics and Gynecology* **159**, 1452–1455.

Ros, H.S., Cnattingius, S. & Lipworth, L. (1998) Comparison of risk factors for preeclampsia and gestational hypertension in a population-based cohort study. *American Journal of Epidemiology* **47**, 1062–1070.

Rosa, F.W., Bosco, L.A., Graham, C.F., Milstien, J.B., Dreis, M. & Creamer, J. (1989) Neonatal anuria with maternal angiotensin-converting enzyme inhibition. *Obstetrics and Gynecology* **74**, 371–374.

Rotchell, Y.E., Cruickshank, J.K. *et al.* (1998) Barbados Low Dose Aspirin Study in Pregnancy (BLASP): a randomised trial for the prevention of pre-eclampsia and its complications. *British Journal of Obstetrics and Gynaecology* **105**, 286–292.

Rovinsky, J.J. & Jaffin, H. (1965) Cardiovascular hemodynamics in pregnancy. I. Blood and plasma volumes in multiple pregnancy. *American Journal of Obstetrics and Gynecology* **93**, 1–15.

Rubin, P.C., Butters, L. *et al.* (1983) Placebo-controlled trial of atenolol treatment of pregnancy-associated hypertension. *Lancet* **1**, 431–434.

Rubin, P.C., Butters, L. & McCabe, R. (1988) Nifedipine and platelets in preeclampsia. *American Journal of Hypertension* **1**, 175–177.

Ryding, E.L., Wijma, B. & Wijma, K. (1997) Post-traumatic stress reactions after emergency cesarean section. *Acta Obstetrica et Gynecologica Scandinavica* **76**, 856–861.

Sacks, G.P., Studena, K., Sargent, K & Redman, C.W.G. (1998) Normal pregnancy and preeclampsia both produce inflammatory changes in peripheral blood leukocytes akin to those of sepsis. *American Journal of Obstetrics and Gynecology* **179**, 80–86.

Saftlas, A.F., Olson, D.R., Franks, A.L., Atrash, H.K. & Pokras, R. (1990) Epidemiology of preeclampsia and eclampsia in the United States, 1979–1986 *American Journal of Obstetrics and Gynecology* **163**, 460–465.

Samuels, B. (1960) Postpartum eclampsia. *Obstetrics and Gynecology* **15**, 748–752.

Sanders, T.G., Clayman, D.A., Sanchez Ramos, L., Vines, F.S. & Russo, L. (1991) Brain in eclampsia: MR imaging with clinical correlation. *Radiology* **180**, 475–478.

Sawhney, H., Sawhney, I.M., Mandal, R., Subramanyam, B. & Vasishta, K. (1999) Efficacy of magnesium sulphate and phenytoin in the management of eclampsia. *Journal of Obstetric and Gynaecologic Research* **25**, 333–338.

Schatz, M., Zeiger, R.S., Harden, K., Hoffman, C.C., Chilingar, L. & Petitti, D. (1997) The safety of asthma and allergy medications during pregnancy. *Journal of Allergy and Clinical Immunology* **100**, 301–306.

Schenker, J.G. & Chowers, I. (1971) Pheochromocytoma and pregnancy. *Obstetrical and Gynecological Survey* **26**, 739–747.

Schimmel, M.S., Eidelman, A.I., Wilschanski, M.A., Shaw, D., Ogilvie, R.J. & Koren, G. (1989) Toxic effects of atenolol consumed during breast feeding. *Journal of Pediatrics* **114**, 476–478.

Schrocksnadel, H., Sitte, B., Steckel, B.G. & Dapunt, O. (1992) Hemolysis in hypertensive disorders of pregnancy. *Gynecologic and Obstetric Investigation* **34**, 211–216.

Seligman, S.A. (1971) Diurnal blood-pressure variation in pregnancy. *British Journal of Obstetrics and Gynaecology* **78**, 417–422.

Sengar, A.R., Gupta, R.K., Dhanuka, A.K., Roy, R. & Das, K. (1997) MR imaging, MR angiography, and MR spectroscopy of the brain in eclampsia. *American Journal of Neuroradiology* **18**, 1485–1490.

Shanklin, D.R. & Sibai, B.M. (1989) Ultrastructural aspects of pre-eclampsia. I. Placental bed and uterine boundary vessels. *American Journal of Obstetrics and Gynecology* **161**, 735–741.

Sheehan, H.L. & Lynch, J.P. (1973) *Pathology of Toxaemia of Pregnancy*. Churchill Livingstone, London.

Sheeler, L.R. (1994) Cushing's syndrome and pregnancy. *Endocrinology and Metabolism Clinics of North America* **23**, 619–627.

Shennan, A., Gupta, M., Halligan, A., Taylor, D.J. & de Swiet, M. (1996) Lack of reproducibility in pregnancy of Korotkoff phase IV as measured by mercury sphygmomanometry. *Lancet* **347**, 139–142.

Sheppard, B.L. & Bonnar, J. (1976) The ultrastructure of the arterial supply of the human placenta in pregnancy complicated by fetal growth retardation. *British Journal of Obstetrics and Gynaecology* **83**, 948–959.

Shoemaker, C.T. & Meyers, M. (1984) Sodium nitroprusside for control of severe hypertensive disease of pregnancy: a case report and discussion of potential toxicity. *American Journal of Obstetrics and Gynecology* **149**, 171–173.

Sibai, B.M. (1991) Diagnosis and management of chronic hypertension in pregnancy. *Obstetrics and Gynecology* **78**, 451–461.

Sibai, B.M. (1998) Prevention of preeclampsia: a big disappointment. *American Journal of Obstetrics and Gynecology* **179**, 1275–1278.

Sibai, B.M., el Nazer, A. & Gonzalez Ruiz, A. (1986) Severe preeclampsia-eclampsia in young primigravid women: subsequent pregnancy outcome and remote prognosis. *American Journal of Obstetrics and Gynecology* **155**, 1011–1016.

Sibai, B.M., Ewell, M. *et al.* (1997) Risk factors associated with preeclampsia in healthy nulliparous women The Calcium for Preeclampsia Prevention (CPEP) Study Group. *American Journal of Obstetrics and Gynecology* **177**, 1003–1010.

Sibai, B.M., Gonzalez, A.R., Mabie, W.C. & Moretti, M. (1987b) A comparison of labetalol plus hospitalization versus hospitalization alone in the management of preeclampsia remote from term. *Obstetrics and Gynecology* **70**, 323–327.

Sibai, B.M., Mabie, B.C., Harvey, C.J. & Gonzalez, A.R. (1987a) Pulmonary edema in severe preeclampsia-eclampsia: analysis of thirty-seven consecutive cases. *American Journal of Obstetrics and Gynecology* **156**, 1174–1179.

Sibai, B.M., Mabie, W.C., Shamsa, F., Villar, M.A. & Anderson, G.D. (1990) A comparison of no medication versus methyldopa or labetalol in chronic hypertension during pregnancy. *American Journal of Obstetrics and Gynecology* **162**, 960–966.

Sibai, B.M., McCubbin, J.H., Anderson, G.D., Lipshitz, J. & Dilts, P.V. (1981) Eclampsia I. Observations from 67 recent cases. *Obstetrics and Gynecology* **58**, 609–613.

Sibai, B.M., Mercer, B. & Sarinoglu, C. (1991) Severe preeclampsia in the second trimester: recurrence risk and long-term prognosis. *American Journal of Obstetrics and Gynecology* **165**, 1408–1412.

Sibai, B.M., Mercer, B.M., Schiff, E. & Friedman, S.A. (1994) Aggressive versus expectant management of severe preeclampsia at 28–32 weeks' gestation: a randomized controlled trial. *American Journal of Obstetrics and Gynecology* **171**, 818–822.

Sibai, B.M., Ramadan, M.K., Chari, R.S. & Friedman, S.A. (1995) Pregnancies complicated by HELLP syndrome (hemolysis, elevated liver enzymes, and low platelets). Subsequent pregnancy outcome and long-term prognosis. *American Journal of Obstetrics and Gynecology* **172**, 125–129.

Sibai, B.M., Ramadan, M.K. *et al.* (1993) Maternal morbidity and mortality in 442 pregnancies with hemolysis, elevated liver enzymes, and low platelets (HELLP syndrome). *American Journal of Obstetrics and Gynecology* **169**, 1000–1006.

Simanis, J., Amerson, J.R., Hendee, A.E. & Anton, A.H. (1972) Unresectable pheochromocytoma in pregnancy. *American Journal of Medicine* **53**, 381–385.

Sladek, S.M., Magness, R.R. & Conrad, K.P. (1997) Nitric oxide and pregnancy. *American Journal of Physiology* **272**, R441–R463.

Smith, K., Browne, J.C.Mc., Shackman, R. & Wrong, O.M. (1968) Renal failure of obstetric origin. *British Medical Bulletin* **24**, 49–58.

Solomon, C.G., Thiet, M., Moore, F. & Seely, E.W. (1996) Primary hyperaldosteronism in pregnancy. A case report. *Journal of Reproductive Medicine* **41**, 255–258.

Spargo, B., McCartney, C.P. & Winemiller, R. (1959) Glomerular capillary endotheliosis in toxemia of pregnancy. *Archives of Pathology* **68**, 593–599.

Spital, A. & Greenwell, R. (1991) Severe hyperkalemia during magnesium sulfate therapy in two pregnant drug abusers. *Southern Medical Journal* **84**, 919–921.

Stamilio, D.M., Sehdev, H.M., Morgan, M.A., Propert, K. & Macones, G.A. (2000) Can antenatal clinical and biochemical markers predict the development of severe preeclampsia? *American Journal of Obstetrics and Gynecology* **182**, 589–594.

Steyn, D.W. & Odendaal, H.J. (1997) Randomised controlled trial of ketanserin and aspirin in prevention of pre-eclampsia. *Lancet* **350**, 1267–1271.

Strandgaard, S., Olesen, J., Skinhoj, E. & Lassen, N.A. (1973) Autoregulation of brain circulation in severe arterial hypertension. *British Medical Journal* 1, 507–510.

Stubbs, T.M., Lazarchik, J., Van Dorsten, J.P., Cox, J. & Loadholt, C.B. (1986) Evidence of accelerated platelet production and consumption in nonthrombocytopenic preeclampsia. *American Journal of Obstetrics and Gynecology* **155**, 263–265.

Studd, J.W.W., Blainey, J.D. & Bailey, D.E. (1970) Serum protein changes in the pre-eclampsia–eclampsia syndrome. *Journal of Obstetrics and Gynaecology of the British Commonwealth* **77**, 796–801.

Suonio, S., Saarikoski, S., Tahvanainen, K., Paakkonen, A. & Olkkonen, H. (1986) Acute effects of dihydralazine mesylate, furosemide, and metoprolol on maternal hemodynamics in pregnancy-induced hypertension. *American Journal of Obstetrics and Gynecology* **155**, 122–125.

Swartjes, J.M., Schutte, M.F. & Bleker, O.P. (1992) Management of eclampsia: cardiopulmonary arrest resulting from magnesium sulfate overdose. *European Journal of Obstetrics, Gynecology, and Reproductive Biology* **47**, 73–75.

Taufield, P.A., Ales, K.L., Resnick, L.M., Druzin, M.L., Gertner, J.M. & Laragh, J.H. (1987) Hypocalciuria in preeclampsia. *New England Journal of Medicine* **316**, 715–718.

Taylor, R.N., Crombleholme, W.R., Friedman, S.A., Jones, L.A., Casal, D.C. & Roberts, J.M. (1991) High plasma cellular fibronectin levels correlate with biochemical and clinical features of preeclampsia but cannot be attributed to hypertension alone. *American Journal of Obstetrics and Gynecology* **165**, 895–901.

Tepperman, H.M., Beydoun, S.N. & Abdul-Karim, R.W. (1977) Drugs affecting myometrial contractility in pregnancy. *Clinical Obstetrics and Gynecology* **20**, 423–445.

Theron, G.B. & Thompson, M.L. (1993) The usefulness of weight gain in predicting pregnancy complications. *Journal of Tropical Pediatrics* **39**, 269–272.

Thomson, A.M., Hytten, R.E. & Billewicz, W.Z. (1967) The epidemiology of edema during pregnancy. *Journal of Obstetrics and Gynaecology of the British Commonwealth* **74**, 1–10.

Thorley, K.J. (1984) Randomised trial of atenolol and methyl dopa in pregnancy related hypertension. *Clinical and Experimental Hypertension* **B3**, 168.

Thornton, J.G. & Macdonald, A.M. (1999) Twin mothers, pregnancy hypertension and pre-eclampsia. *British Journal of Obstetrics and Gynaecology* **106**, 570–575.

Tillmann Hein, H.A. (1984) Cardiorespiratory arrest with laryngeal oedema in pregnancy-induced hypertension. *Canadian Anesthaesia Society Journal* **31**, 210–212.

Trofatter, K.F.J., Howell, M.L., Greenberg, C.S. & Hage, M.L. (1989) Use of the fibrin D-dimer in screening for coagulation abnormalities in preeclampsia. *Obstetrics and Gynecology* **73**, 435–440.

Trommer, B.L., Homer, D. & Mikhael, M.A. (1988) Cerebral vasospasm and eclampsia. *Stroke* **19**, 326–329.

Ulmsten, U. (1984) Treatment of normotensive and hypertensive patients with preterm labor using oral nifedipine, a calcium antagonist. *Archives of Gynecology* **236**, 69–72.

Villar, M.A. & Sibai, B.M. (1989) Clinical significance of elevated mean arterial blood pressure in second trimester and threshold increase in systolic or diastolic blood pressure during third trimester. *American Journal of Obstetrics and Gynecology* **160**, 419–423.

Vink, G.J. & Moodley, J. (1982) The effect of low-dose dihydralla-zine on the fetus in the emergency treatment of hypertension in pregnancy. *South African Medical Journal* **62**, 475–477.

Visser, M., Bouter, L.M., McQuillan, G.M., Wener, M.H. & Harris, T.B. (1999) Elevated C-reactive protein levels in overweight and obese adults. *Journal of the American Medical Association* **282**, 2131–2135.

Visser, W. & Wallenburg, H.C.S. (1991) Central hemodynamic observations in untreated preeclamptic patients. *Hypertension* **17**, 1072–1077.

Visser, W. & Wallenburg, H.C. (1995a) Temporising management of severe pre-eclampsia with and without the HELLP syndrome. *British Journal of Obstetrics and Gynaecology* **102**, 111–117.

Visser, W. & Wallenburg, H.C. (1995b) Maternal and perinatal outcome of temporizing management in 254 consecutive patients with severe pre-eclampsia remote from term. *European Journal of Obstetrics, Gynecology, and Reproductive Biology* **63**, 147–154.

Waisman, G.D., Mayorga, L.M., Camera, M.I., Vignolo, C.A. & Martinotti, A. (1988) Magnesium plus nifedipine: potentiation of hypotensive effect in preeclampsia? *American Journal of Obstetrics and Gynecology* **159**, 308–309.

Wallenburg, H.C.S. & Hutchinson, D.L. (1979) A radioangiographic study of the effects of catecholamines on uteroplacental blood flow in the rhesus monkey. *Journal of Medical Primatology* **8**, 57–65.

Walters, B.N.J., Thompson, M.E., Lee, A. & de Swiet, M. (1986) Blood pressure in the puerperium. *Clinical Science (Colchester Essex)* **71**, 589–594.

Wasserstrum, N., Kirshon, B., Willis, R.S., Moise, K.J.J. & Cotton, D.B. (1989) Quantitative hemodynamic effects of acute Volume expansion in severe preeclampsia. *Obstetrics and Gynecology* **73**, 546–550.

Watson, D.L., Sibai, B.M., Shaver, D.C., Dacus, J.V. & Anderson, G.D. (1983) Late postpartum eclampsia: an update. *Southern Medical Journal* **76**, 1487–1489.

Weiner, C.P., Kwaan, H.C., Chu, X.U.C., Paul, M., Burmeister, L. & Hauck, W. (1985) Antithrombin III activity in women with hypertension during pregnancy. *Obstetrics and Gynecology* **65**, 301–306.

Weinstein, L. (1982) Syndrome of hemolysis, elevated liver enzymes, low platelet count: a severe consequence of hypertension on pregnancy. *American Journal of Obstetrics and Gynecology* **142**, 159–167.

van Wersch, J. & Ubachs, J.M. (1991) Blood coagulation and fibrinolysis during normal pregnancy. *European Journal of Clinical Chemistry and Clinical Biochemistry* **29**, 45–50.

Whitelaw, A. (1981) Maternal methyldopa treatment and neonatal blood pressure. *British Medical Journal* **283**, 471.

Wiggers, C.J. (1956) Dynamic patterns induced by compression of an artery. *Circulation Research* **4**, 4–7.

Williams, M.A., Lieberman, E., Mittendorf, R., Monson, R.R. & Schoenbaum, S.C. (1991) Risk factors for abruptio placentae. *American Journal of Epidemiology* **134**, 965–972.

Witlin, A.G. & Sibai, B.M. (1998) Magnesium sulfate therapy in preeclampsia and eclampsia. *Obstetrics and Gynecology* **92**, 883–889.

World Health Organization (1988) Geographic variation in the incidence of hypertension in pregnancy. World Health Organization International Collaborative Study of Hypertensive Disorders of Pregnancy. *American Journal of Obstetrics and Gynecology* **158**, 80–83.

Yoneyama, Y., Suzuki, S., Sawa, R., Otsubo, Y., Power, G.G. & Araki, T. (2000) Plasma adenosine levels increase in women with normal pregnancies. *American Journal of Obstetrics and Gynecology* **182**, 1200–1203.

Zabriskie, J.R. (1963) Effect of cigarette smoking during pregnancy. Study of 2000 cases. *Obstetrics and Gynecology* **21**, 405–411.

Zech, P., Rifle, G., Lindner, A., Sassard, J., Blanc-Brunat, N. & Traeger, J. (1975) Malignant hypertension with irreversible renal failure due to oral contraceptives. *British Medical Journal* **4**, 326–327.

Zeek, P.M. & Assali, N.S. (1950) Vascular changes with eclamptogenic toxemia of pregnancy. *American Journal of Clinical Pathology* **20**, 1099–1109.

Zinaman, M., Rubin, J. & Lindheimer, M.D. (1985) Serial plasma oncotic pressure levels and echoencephalography during and after delivery in severe pre-eclampsia. *Lancet* **1**, 1245–1247.

Women with renal problems often consult the clinician on the advisability of becoming pregnant or continuing a pregnancy already in progress. When counselling such women, emotions must not be allowed to override objectivity and this requires knowledge of the physiological changes that occur during normal pregnancy and of the various pitfalls in the detection and diagnosis of obstetric renal problems. In some areas, accurate information is lacking from clinical practice and animal models have therefore been developed to examine rigorously the mechanisms controlling the altered renal function of normal pregnancy as well as the long-term consequences of pregnancy in health and disease [1].

Therefore, this chapter first summarizes the changes that occur in the urinary tract in pregnancy, including data derived from animal models, and then discusses the management of problems associated with chronic renal disease.

The kidney in normal pregnancy

Anatomical changes

The kidney increases approximately 1 cm in length during normal pregnancy. More striking, however, are the anatomical changes in the calyces, renal pelvis and ureters, which dilate markedly, often giving the erroneous impression of obstructive uropathy [2,3].

By the third trimester about 80% of women show evidence of stasis or hydronephrosis [4,5], with fetal pyelectasis more likely to occur in such women. Dilatation is more pronounced in the right than in the left urinary tract at all stages of pregnancy, perhaps related to the customary dextrorotation of the uterus. Ultrasound studies suggest that renal parenchymal volumes also increase during pregnancy, probably the result of increases in intrarenal fluid [6,7]. An increment of about 70% has occurred by the beginning of the third trimester with a slight reduction during the last weeks of pregnancy [8].

These anatomical changes have important clinical implications.

1 Dilatation of the urinary tract may lead to collection errors in tests based on timed urine volume (e.g. 24-h creatinine or protein excretion).

2 Urinary stasis within the ureters may predispose pregnant women with asymptomatic bacteriuria to develop acute symptomatic pyelonephritis.

3 Acceptable norms of kidney size should be increased by 1 cm if estimated during pregnancy or immediately after delivery. Since dilatation of the ureters persists into the puerperium, elective radiological examination of the urinary tract should be deferred until at least 16 weeks after delivery.

4 Rarely the changes may be extreme and precipitate the 'overdistension syndrome' (see p.226) and/or hypertension [9].

Functional changes

RENAL HAEMODYNAMIC CHANGES IN NORMAL PREGNANCY

When a woman becomes pregnant her glomerular filtration rate (GFR) increases by about 50% (Fig. 7.1), reaching the maximum at the end of the first trimester, and is maintained at this augmented level until at least the 36th gestational week [10–12]. Because GFR increases less than renal plasma flow (RPF) during early pregnancy, the ratio of GFR/RPF, the filtration fraction (FF) decreases. Late pregnancy is associated with an increase in FF to values similar to the non-pregnant norm.

Endogenous 24-h creatinine clearance is a convenient, non-invasive method that measures GFR when inulin infusion studies are impracticable. Studies performed at weekly intervals after conception have shown that 24-h creatinine clearance increases by 25% 4 weeks after the last menstrual period and by 45% at 9 weeks [13] (Fig. 7.2). During the third trimester a consistent and significant decrease towards non-pregnant values occurs

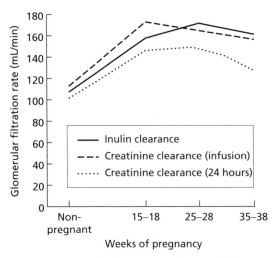

Fig 7.1 Mean glomerular filtration rate (GFR) in 10 healthy women during pregnancy and 8–12 weeks after delivery (non-pregnant). (Modified from [11].)

preceding delivery [14], and daily measurements postpartum have suggested a small transient increase during the first few days of the puerperium [10].

In the rat, pregnancy lasts 22 days and GFR increases early to a maximum (+30–40%), which is maintained throughout pregnancy, until near term when a return towards non-pregnant values is evident [15,16]. The rise in GFR is paralleled by an increase in RPF due to a fall in renal vascular resistance (RVR), which reaches a nadir by mid-pregnancy. The pressures and flows at the glomerulus that determine the GFR of a single nephron (SNGFR) are controlled by the tone of the preglomerular (afferent) and postglomerular (efferent) resistance vessels. The ratio of the tone of these resistances determines the glomerular blood pressure, P_{rmGC}, which directly controls SNGFR. The overall level of renal vascular tone controls glomerular plasma flow, which also controls SNGFR.

Micropuncture studies allow measurement of SNGFR and all its determinants, and in the pregnant rat show 30% increases in superficial cortical SNGFR by mid-pregnancy. This is the result exclusively of a proportional increase in glomerular plasma flow, because the oncotic pressure of systemic blood (π_A), the intraglomerular hydrostatic pressure, P_{GC}, the glomerular hydrostatic pressure gradient (ΔP) and the glomerular capillary ultrafiltration coefficient, K_f (the product of filtration surface area and water permeability), are unchanged by mid-pregnancy. Micropuncture studies show that P_{GC} does not increase at any stage in gestation in pregnant Munich–Wistar rats [15–18], despite the renal vasodilatation of pregnancy, due to close proportionality in the

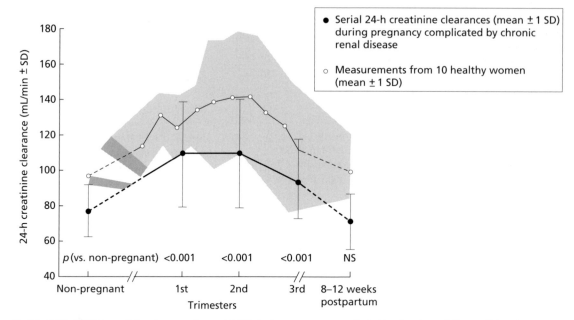

Fig 7.2 (●) Serial 24–h creatinine clearances (mean ± 1 SD) during pregnancy complicated by chronic renal disease. Thirty-three pregnancies of 26 women studied preconception, each trimester and 8–12 weeks after delivery. Measurements from 10 healthy women (mean ± 1 SD) shown by shaded area (○). (From [94].)

declines in preglomerular and efferent arteriolar resistances.

In normal human pregnancy, computer simulation of the glomerulus using theoretical models of hindered solute transport that represent the capillary wall as a heteroporous membrane suggests that P_{GC} is also unchanged [19,20] as in the rat (see above). Thus, all the evidence points to the increased GFR being due entirely to the increment in RPF with a contribution from decreased oncotic pressure, particularly in the third trimester.

Renal ultrasound assessment in the human, with colour flow mapping displays a real-time map of the mean Doppler shift within blood vessels on a colour overlay on the B-mode image. Analysis of waveforms from interlobar and interlobular arteries have failed to reveal any change in pregnancy, which is surprising as the large increments in renal blood flow are thought to be due to reduced RVRs [21]. It is likely, however, that waveform pulsatility reflects an interaction of several haemodynamic factors many of which are altered during pregnancy. It is not yet possible to access the individual effect on renal waveform variation of changes in maternal heart rate, stroke volume, blood pressure and blood flow because alterations in one variable affects the others. Haemodynamic modelling suggests that pulsatility (as indexed by pulsatility index and A : B ratio) correlates closely with vascular resistance [22], an effect that is independent of flow and

pressure, but the relationship has not been specifically tested for the unique conditions of the renal circulation in pregnancy.

Initiation of gestational renal changes

The causes of the renal and peripheral vasodilatation and of the plasma volume expansion of pregnancy remain unknown although it has been suggested that the primary change is a fall in total peripheral resistance, which creates an underfill signal, thus stimulating sodium retention and plasma volume expansion [23]. This is consistent with the increases that occur in renin–angiotensin–aldosterone levels in normal pregnancy in human and rodent pregnancy [23]. However, this view is not universally accepted because the changes that occur in plasma atrial natriuretic peptide (ANP), the sympathetic nervous system and the arginine vasopressin osmoregulatory system [24,25] are consistent with a continually integrated readjustments in volume regulatory and perception systems to sense the increasing plasma volume as *normal*. Furthermore, our studies in rats show that plasma volume expansion in early pregnancy can occur on a sodium-free diet, suggesting redistribution of fluids between body fluid compartments rather than sodium retention [26]. However, more recent work directly measuring fluid volumes in the rat shows that under normal dietary conditions, total body water, extracellular fluid volume and plasma volume all increase similarly in early pregnancy, suggesting that early renal sodium retention in pregnancy is the norm [27]. There is no question that a marked and demonstrable renal sodium retention occurs later in pregnancy [28,29]. Maternal factors initiate the renal vasodilatation and plasma volume expansion of pregnancy, since the pseudopregnant rat, in which the fetoplacental unit is absent, also undergoes a renal vasodilatation and plasma volume expansion [17].

FUNCTIONAL CHARACTERISTICS OF THE RENAL VASCULATURE IN PREGNANCY

Renal autoregulation and responsiveness of the renal vasculature in pregnancy

The kidney is able to maintain blood flow and GFR over a range of blood pressure (i.e. autoregulation) mainly by variations in preglomerular arteriolar tone [30,31].

In normal non-pregnant humans and animals, a protein meal or an amino acid infusion elicit substantial increases in GFR due to a selective renal vasodilatation with increased RPF [32–34]. In the human, observations have been conflicting. One group observed a substantial rise in creatinine clearance following a meat meal [35] while others report no increments in inulin and *para*-aminohippuric acid (PAH) clearances in pregnant women after a high-protein meal [36]. Healthy pregnant women, in response to intravenous amino acids, however, do show a marked renal vasodilatory response. Overall, therefore the kidneys in pregnancy do possess a significant reserve of vasodilatory capacity despite a state of chronic renal vasodilatation [20,37].

Responses to vasoactive hormones

The renin–angiotensin II (AII) system is greatly modified in normal pregnancy with increases in plasma renin activity and plasma AII and decreased responsivity to administered AII [38–39]. Some functional studies indicate that this loss of sensitivity to the vasoconstrictor actions of AII extends to the renal resistance vessels [40–42], although others indicate unchanged responsivity [43]. Although peripheral responsivity to administered noradrenaline (norepinephrine) and arginine vasopressin (AVP) is also reduced during pregnancy [39,40] these systems have not been extensively studied with regard to control of renal haemodynamics. Blockade of the vascular AVP (V_1) receptor has no renal haemodynamic or blood pressure effects in pregnancy [44]. Although thromboxane A_2 (TXA$_2$) is not involved in regulation of RVR in normals [45], this may become important in pre-eclamp-

sia, when TXA$_2$ production increases markedly (see Chapter 6). Overall, however, it is unlikely that withdrawal of active renal vasoconstrictor tone is the primary cause of the gestational renal vasodilatation.

ANP is a vasodilator and although vascular responsiveness is unchanged during pregnancy [46,47], normal women show moderate increases in plasma ANP during the second and third trimesters [48]. ANP is, however, unlikely to be involved in the renal vasodilatation of pregnancy because although pharmacological doses of ANP increase GFR, this is by a complex mechanism that includes increases in efferent resistance and P_{GC} [49], a pattern that differs from the glomerular haemodynamic alterations of normal pregnancy. There are potent endothelial factors that may participate in the renal vasodilatation of pregnancy. Increased urinary prostaglandin and prostacyclin levels have been reported in pregnant women and rats [40,50] but functional studies in the rat using cyclo-oxygenase inhibitors suggest that prostaglandins do not mediate the gestational rise in GFR [18,40].

In contrast, nitric oxide (NO) is a potent and physiologically active renal vasodilator in humans and non-pregnant animals [51,52], and there is now increasing evidence from the rat that NO plays a major role in the gestational rise in GFR [53,54]. Although oestrogen has been suggested as the hormone responsible for the pregnancy stimulus to NO production, animal data do not support this.

An elegant study has suggested a key role for the ovarian hormone relaxin [55], which may signal increased renal NO production in pregnancy via the endothelin (ET) B receptor [56].

As yet there is no clinical information on a role for renal NO in pregnancy. The lack of a rise in plasma NO$_X$ (the stable oxidation products of NO) and 24-h excretion of NO$_X$ in normal pregnant women [57], in contrast to the rise seen in pregnant rats [58] does not exclude a role for NO human pregnancy. There is because of increasing evidence [59] that NO$_X$ levels in body fluids cannot be used as indices of 'haemodynamically active' NO. The possible role of NO in the peripheral vasodilatation of pregnancy is still controversial and is discussed in detail elsewhere [60].

Physiological consequences of altered renal haemodynamics

Because GFR increases without substantial alterations in the production of creatinine and urea, plasma levels of these solutes decrease. Creatinine levels change from a non-pregnant value of 73 mmol/L to 60, 54 and 64 mmol/L in successive trimesters (Table 7.1).

Table 7.1 Changes in common indices of renal function during pregnancy (mean ± SD). (From [7,10,11,13,14,19,62,68].)

	Non-pregnant	First trimester	Second trimester	Third trimester
Effective renal plasma flow (mL/min)	480 ± 72	841 ± 144	891 ± 279	771 ± 175
Glomerular filtration rate (mL/min)				
Inulin clearance	105 ± 24	162 ± 19	174 ± 24	165 ± 22
24-h creatinine clearance	98 ± 8	151 ± 11	154 ± 15	129 ± 10
Plasma				
Creatinine (µmol/L)	73 ± 10	60 ± 8	54 -t 10	64 ± 9
Urea (mmol/L)	4.3 ± 0.8	3.5 ± 0.7	3.3 ± 0.8	3.1 ± 0.7
Urate (µmol/L)	246 ± 59	189 ± 48	214 ± 71	269 ± 56
Osmolality (mosmol/kg)	290 ± 2.2	280 ± 3.4	279 ± 2.9	279 ± 5.0

Average plasma urea levels are 3.5, 3.3 and 3.1 mmol/L in successive trimesters, rising to 4.3 mmol/L 6 weeks postpartum. Urea levels can be reported in a number of different ways; results may be given as either plasma (or serum) or whole blood levels, the latter being 10% below plasma levels. Some of the fall in plasma urea may be due to reduced protein degradation as well as increased clearance of this solute.

Normal pregnancy induces relative hypouricaemia. Plasma urate concentrations decrease by over 25% as early as week 8 of pregnancy, but increase again during the third trimester to attain levels close to the non-pregnant mean. The main reason for this is alteration in the renal handling of urate, which, although freely filtered, is subsequently so actively reabsorbed that only about 10% of the original filtered load appears in the urine. Later in pregnancy the kidney appears to excrete an even smaller proportion of the filtered urate load and it is this increase in net reabsorption that is associated with an increase in plasma urate concentration [61].

A number of other changes in normal pregnancy [62], including increased excretion of nutrients, calcium (along with an inhibitor of crystalluria) and protein, are due to alterations in tubular function as well as augmented renal haemodynamics [63,64]. Plasma osmolality is markedly reduced (by 8–10 mosmol/L) from the early weeks of pregnancy [65] but this is not associated with the water diuresis that would occur in the non-pregnant individual. Whilst the process of osmoregulation is effective during pregnancy, it is now clear that there are important changes in the osmotic thresholds that trigger control mechanisms such as the sensation of thirst and the release of the antidiuretic hormone AVP [65,66]. Other changes include a substantial increase in the metabolic clearance rate (MCR) of AVP, which rises fourfold after the first trimester, paralleling the appearance of, and marked increases in, circulating levels of a placental enzyme vasopressinase (also called oxytocinase), which is a cystine aminopeptidase capable of inactivating large quantities of AVP *in vitro*. The MCR of 1-deamino-8-D-AVP (desmopressin acetate, dDAVP), an analogue of vasopressin that is resistant to degradation by vasopressinase, is unaltered during pregnancy, suggesting that the aminopeptidase enzymes are also active *in vivo* [25,67].

Clinical consequences of functional changes

It is important to realize the extent to which the dramatic alterations in physiological norms may affect clinical interpretation in pregnancy (see Figs 7.1–7.3, Table 7.1).

1 Values considered normal in non-pregnant women may reflect decreased renal function during pregnancy. Plasma levels of creatinine and urea exceeding 75 mmol/L and 4.5 mmol/L, respectively, should alert the clinician to investigate renal function further.

2 Urate concentrations are significantly higher in pregnancies complicated by pre-eclampsia. Above a critical blood level of 350 mmol/L there is significant excess perinatal mortality in hypertensive patients, and serial measurements can be used to monitor progress in pre-eclampsia (see Chapter 6). It must be remembered, however, that physiological variability can be such that some healthy women have high blood levels without problems and that single random measurements are of no use clinically [68].

3 Glycosuria in pregnancy reflects an alteration in renal physiology and does not necessarily signify hyperglycaemia [10].

4 Increased urinary protein excretion should not be considered abnormal until it exceeds 500 mg in 24 h [64] and increasing proteinuria in women with chronic renal disease does not necessarily signify deterioration.

5 The osmoregulatory changes must be taken into account when managing women with known central diabetes insipidus (DI) (see Chapter 13) and when diagnosing the rare syndrome of 'transient DI of pregnancy', which usually presents during the second half of pregnancy and remits postpartum [1,69] (see Chapter 13).

Long-term significance of augmented renal haemodynamics

In animal models and in humans, sustained increments in GFR—whether induced by excessive protein intake, early diabetes, partial renal ablation or compensatory changes in the remaining glomeruli of kidneys with renal disease—can cause progressive glomerular injury [70]. The 'hyperfiltration' in these states is associated with sustained increases in glomerular blood pressure, and the glomerular hypertension is thought to play a primary role in initiation of kidney damage. Could the glomerular hyperperfusion of normal pregnancy lead to similar progressive nephropathy? The augmented GFR of pregnancy is due mainly to an increase in glomerular plasma flow, without coexistent glomerular hypertension, and the evidence so far argues against hyperfiltration-induced sclerosis in normal pregnancy both in humans and rats [1].

Data are somewhat limited for human pregnancy [71,72]. There is certainly an increase in total protein excretion [73] and a small increase in albumin excretion particularly during the third trimester and early puerperium [74]—changes related to altered tubular and probably not glomerular function. Although, unable to detect an overall increase in albumin excretion during normal pregnancy, Wright *et al.* [75,76] reported that ratios between clearances and urinary concentrations of albumin and creatinine increased progressively throughout pregnancy. The same group of workers have also suggested that these changes may indicate altered glomerular function and are more marked in women of high than of low parity, approximately matched for age. The results, however, were based upon urine collection during the afternoon, a protocol that must give rise to reservations about the validity of creatinine clearance estimations [10].

With the exception of the aforementioned report, the consensus is that there is no reversible deterioration in renal function during normal pregnancy or as a result of successive pregnancies, whether assessed by 24-h creatinine clearance, by inulin clearance or by total protein excretion [64,73,77]. Furthermore, women studied in consecutive pregnancies show similar GFR increments in the later compared with the first pregnancy and it is known that women do not show any tendency for GFR to decline during the reproductive years; overall they show far less of an age-dependent decline than men [78]. The clinical implications of the effect of pregnancy on glomerular physiology in the presence of chronic renal pathology are discussed later (page 219).

Volume homeostasis

Healthy women eating an unrestricted diet gain an average of 12.5 kg during their first pregnancy and 11.5 kg in subsequent pregnancies. Until fairly recently, clinicians regarded published averages as the upper limits of permissible weight gain, forgetting that there is a plus as well as a minus to deviations about a mean. Consequently many pregnant women were admonished for excessive weight gain, and their intakes of calories, sodium or both were needlessly restricted.

The increase in weight is largely fluid, total body water increasing by 6–8 L, 4–6 L of which are extracellular [12,79]. There is also cumulative retention of approximately 900 mmol of sodium distributed between the products of conception and the maternal extracellular space. This accumulation occurs gradually, and even in late pregnancy, the period of most rapid maternal weight gain, the amount retained is only 3–4 mmol/day, which is too small to be detected by conventional balance techniques.

Most of the maternally sequestered sodium is located in the extracellular space. Plasma volume increases by 40–50%, starting in the first trimester, accelerating to a peak in the second and remaining elevated until near term (see Chapter 2). However, increases in maternal interstitial volume (as well as fetal storage of sodium) are greatest in the third trimester. The increase in maternal plasma volume and interstitial space constitute a physiological hypervolaemia (Fig. 7.3). However, as discussed above, many of the mother's volume receptors sense these changes as normal; when salt restriction or diuretic therapy limits the expansion, the maternal response resembles that of salt-depleted non-pregnant subjects. Whether or not the increases in the fluid spaces are 'necessary' remains to be elucidated, but this seems to be likely, because failure of plasma volume to increase appropriately has been correlated with poor reproductive performance [79].

The factors that initiate and maintain the plasma volume expansion of normal pregnancy are the subject of debate. The 'underfill' theory [23], in which a primary peripheral vasodilatation drives renal sodium retention, is attractive but, as discussed above, many of the volume-sensing systems do not display 'underfill' responses in normal pregnancy [1,24,25]. There are many, and conflicting, changes during pregnancy in the systems that regulate renal sodium excretion [79,80].

Chronic renal disease and pregnancy

Pregnancy will usually end successfully if there is no significant hypertension or overt renal insufficiency

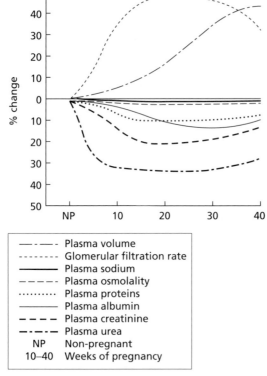

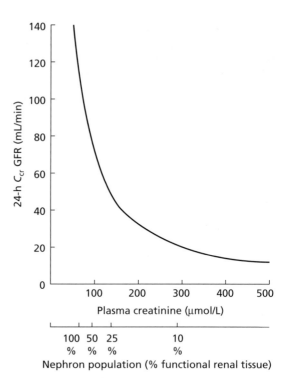

Fig 7.3 Physiological changes induced by pregnancy. Increments and decrements in various parameters are shown in percentage terms with reference to the non-pregnant baseline.

Fig 7.4 Relationship of clearance of creatinine (glomerular filtration rate, GFR) in mL/min to plasma creatinine concentration μmol/L) and nephron population (%) assuming a constant 24-h creatinine excretion of about 11.5 mmol. (Non-pregnant data: J. Davison, unpublished observations.)

prior to conception. If hypertension is present and it requires more than one drug for control, then obstetric success is substantially reduced.

Pathophysiology of renal dysfunction

To assess pregnancy and its altered renal physiology in the presence of chronic renal disease it is necessary to understand what happens when nephron mass has been lost. The relationship between plasma creatinine concentration, creatinine clearance (GFR) and nephron population shown in Fig. 7.4 reveals that an individual may lose about 50% of renal function and still have a plasma creatinine <130 mmol/L. However, if renal function is more severely compromised then a small further decrease in GFR causes a marked increase in plasma creatinine. Nevertheless, a patient who has lost 75% of her nephrons may have only lost 50% of function and may have a deceptively normal plasma creatinine. Thus, evaluation of renal function should ideally be based on the clearance of creatinine rather than on its plasma concentration.

Pre-pregnancy counselling (Box 7.1)

In patients with renal disease, pathology may be clinically silent and biochemically subtle because most individuals remain symptom free until their GFR falls to <25% of its original level. Many plasma constituents are frequently normal until a late stage of the disease.

As renal function declines so does the ability to conceive and to sustain a viable pregnancy. Degrees of impairment that do not cause symptoms or appear to disrupt homeo-

> **Box 7.1 Pre-pregnancy counselling**
> - Type of chronic renal disease under consideration
> - General health considerations
> - Diastolic BP <**80mmHg** or 'well-controlled hypertension'
> - Renal function:
>   Plasma creatinine <**250 μmol/L** but preferably
>   <180 μmol/L
>   Plasma urea <0 mmol/l
>   Presence or absence of proteinuria
> - Need to review pre-pregnancy drug therapy

stasis in non-pregnant individuals can jeopardize pregnancy. Normal pregnancy is rare when non-pregnant plasma creatinine and urea levels exceed 275 mmol/L and 10 mmol/L, respectively. These increments above normal non-pregnant levels appear trivial, but they represent decrements in function of approaching 80% (Fig. 7.4).

Assessment of a patient with chronic renal disease presents two basic and often conflicting issues: fetal prognosis and the maternal prognosis, both during pregnancy and in the long term. These issues must be carefully weighed and this delicate, 'balance' is illustrated in Fig. 7.5.

Renal function and the impact of pregnancy

Because of the different obstetric and remote prognoses in women with different degrees of renal insufficiency, the impact of pregnancy on maternal renal function is best predicted by the level of functional renal status prior to conception (Table 7.2).

PRESERVED/MILDLY IMPAIRED RENAL FUNCTION

Women with chronic renal disease, but normal or mildly decreased pre-pregnancy renal function (plasma creatinine <125 mmol/L), usually have a successful obstetric outcome and pregnancy does not adversely affect the course of their disease [81–101] (Table 7.3).

Although true for most patients, some authors suggest that this statement be tempered somewhat in lupus nephropathy, membranoproliferative glomerulonephritis (MPGN), focal glomerular sclerosis and perhaps IgA and reflux nephropathies, which appear more sensitive to intercurrent pregnancy [102]. For example, where there is a history of surgery in childhood for reflux, there may be an increased risk of ureteric obstruction, pre-eclampsia and/or possibly acute renal failure [103].

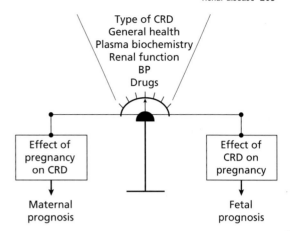

Fig 7.5 Pregnancy and chronic renal disease (CRD) depicting the balance between maternal and fetal prognosis and the role of factors such as the type of CRD, the degree of renal insufficiency, the presence or absence of hypertension and the type of drug therapy that is needed.

Many women with underlying renal disease show increments in GFR, but smaller in magnitude than those of normal pregnant women (Fig 7.2). Increased proteinuria is common, occurring in 50% of pregnancies (although rarely in women with chronic pyelonephritis), and it can be massive (often exceeding 3 g in 24 h), with nephrotic oedema. Two recent retrospective studies emphasize several important issues: Abe [81] analysed 240 pregnancies in 166 women and Jungers et al. [92] 254 pregnancies in 148 women, all with biopsy-proven disease. Perinatal outcome was poor in the presence of poorly controlled hypertension, nephrotic range proteinuria in early pregnancy and/or GFR ≤70 mL/min prior to pregnancy, or in the first trimester, whatever the type of renal

Table 7.2 Pre-pregnancy renal functional status.

Classification	Plasma creatinine (μmol/l)
Preserved/mildly impaired renal function	≤125
Moderate renal insufficiency	≥125
Severe renal insufficiency	≥250

Table 7.3 Pregnancy prospects for women with chronic renal disease.

Renal status	Plasma creatinine (μmol/L)	Problems in pregnancy (%)	Successful obstetric outcome (%)	Problems in long term (%)
Mild	≤125	26	96 (85)	<3 (9)
Moderate	≥125	47	90 (59)	25 (80)
Severe	≥250	86	71 (25)	53 (92)

Estimates based on 2370 women/3495 pregnancies (1973–95), which attained at least 28 weeks' gestation (J. Davison, unpublished data). Figures in brackets refer to prospects when complications developed prior to 28 weeks' gestation.

disease. Significant hypertension, renal functional abnormalities and proteinuria are rare between pregnancies and during long-term follow-up. When renal failure does supervene, it usually reflects the inexorable course of a particular renal disease.

MODERATE AND SEVERE RENAL INSUFFICIENCY

Prognosis is definitely more guarded where renal function is moderately impaired before pregnancy (plasma creatinine 125–250 mmol/L). In one series in the 1980s, a high incidence of renal morbidity occurred early in pregnancy; nearly half (five of 11) developed serious deterioration of renal function culminating in terminal renal failure several months postpartum [104]. An earlier study in the 1970s [86] revealed no immediate loss of renal function in 29 patients whose creatinine levels were <135 mmol/L, but in four of eight patients with initial creatinine levels >145 mmol/L there were significant further increases during pregnancy, which was complicated in every case. Four women were in end-stage renal failure within 18 months of delivery. Due to these experiences and the fact that apparent deterioration can occur unpredictably and unexpectedly in patients with stable renal function, most have adopted a rather cautious approach to pregnancy in women with both mild and moderate renal disease. Furthermore, it is now recognized that uncontrolled hypertension is an important factor in overall deterioration [105–112] (Tables 7.4 and 7.5).

The customary recommendation has been that pregnancy is best avoided in women who have lost 50% of their kidney function, but since the late 1980s and the 1990s the question has been reopened [87,113–116]. Hou et al. [114] recorded a successful obstetric outcome in 92% of the pregnancies in 22 women with creatinine levels of 150–240 mmol/L, whose pregnancies were allowed to go beyond the second trimester, but many had escalating hypertension and in 25% there was an accelerated decline in renal function. Cunningham et al. [87] also had significantly successful obstetric outcome (85%) in pregnancies in 26 women.

In a multicentre study by Jones and Hayslett [115] the infant survival rate was over 90% in 82 pregnancies in 67 women with moderate or severe disease but maternal complications were the rule (70%) and pregnancy-related loss of renal function occurred in almost 50%, of whom 10% progressed rapidly to end-stage renal failure. In another study [116] spanning 20 years and 43 pregnancies in 30 women, obstetric success was achieved in 82% (55% in 1976–85 and 84% in 1986–95) but acceleration towards end-stage renal failure was evident in seven women (23%) postpartum, all of whom had severe and poorly controlled hypertension and heavy proteinuria pre-pregnancy. The better obstetric success nowadays reflects specialist obstetric, nephrological and neonatal care in tertiary referral centres (Table 7.6).

The messages emerging from these experiences in the early 1990s continue to be reiterated. A recent single centre experience [117] documents short- and long-term outcomes in 38 patients in 46 pregnancies. Successful outcome was defined as a live healthy infant without handicap by age 2 years. This occurred in 96% of pregnancies from women with diabetic nephropathy and 89% from those with transplants. Again poorly controlled pre-existing hypertension was the best predictor of success. The influences of plasma creatinine and urate levels and of proteinuria were more variable but in general a worse outcome and poorer renal prognosis occurred in those with moderate and severe renal dysfunction.

	Intrauterine growth retardation (%)	Preterm delivery	Renal deterioration (%)
Normotension	2.3	11.4	3.0
Hypertension	15.6	20.0	15.0

Table 7.4 Effect of blood pressure on pregnancy complications in 123 pregnancies in 86 women with chronic renal disease [99].

	Hypertension	Renal deterioration	Both
Absent throughout pregnancy	18	12	10
Present at some time during pregnancy	34	27	40
Present from first trimester and controlled	20	–	–
Present from first trimester and uncontrolled	100	–	–
Present only during third trimester	12	–	–

Table 7.5 Effect of blood pressure and/or renal deterioration on fetal mortality (%) in 240 pregnancies in 122 women with chronic renal disease [110].

Table 7.6 Pregnancy prospects for women with moderate and severe chronic renal disease.

Problems in pregnancy (%)	Successful obstetric outcome (%)	Problems in long term (%)	End-stage renal failure within 1 year (%)
90 (81–97)	84 (65–93)	50 (30–57)	15 (10–23)

Data are from 107 women in 125 pregnancies; mean (range) from Jungers and Chauveau [112] & Jones and Hayslett [115].

Most women with severe renal insufficiency (plasma creatinine >250 mmol/L) are in fact amenorrhoeic and/or anovulatory [118]. The likelihood of conception, let alone having a normal pregnancy and delivery, is low but not, as some have been misled to believe, impossible. The risk of severe maternal complications is greater than the probability of a successful obstetric outcome (see Table 7.3). Realistically, these patients should not take additional health risks. Perhaps the aim should be to preserve what little renal function remains and/or to achieve renal rehabilitation via a dialysis and transplant programme, after which the question of pregnancy can be considered if appropriate. Some women, however, will be prepared to take a chance and even seek assisted conception in the face of their infertility. This obsessional pursuit of pregnancy and the issues surrounding the clinician's obligation to refuse (or accede to) care that poses a risk to the woman's health are admirably discussed by Stotland and Stotland [119].

Management of chronic renal disease in pregnancy (Box 7.2)

ANTENATAL CARE

Teamwork and good antenatal care are crucial for reducing maternal and perinatal morbidity and mortality. The value of such care is greatly enhanced by early and regular attendance so that trends may be detected and the significance of an abnormal observation assessed when taken in context with previous observations. Where patients have chronic renal disease the following factors are important:
1 careful monitoring of blood pressure; detection of hypertension and assessment of its severity and long-term effects;

Box 7.2 Management during pregnancy
- Type of chronic renal disease, if known
- General health considerations
- Effect of pregnancy on blood pressure
- Effect of pregnancy on renal function and plasma biochemistry
- Past obstetric history
- Use of medications and appropriateness for pregnancy

---

2 assessment of renal function (by 24-h creatinine clearance and protein excretion) and also nutritional status in heavily proteinuric patients;
3 assessment of the size, development and well-being of the fetus;
4 early detection of asymptomatic bacteriuria or confirmation of urinary tract infection.

CRITERIA FOR HOSPITAL ADMISSION

As long as the antenatal course is uncomplicated the patient should be seen at 2-weekly intervals until 32 weeks' gestation and then weekly thereafter. Immediate hospital admission is indicated in the following circumstances:
1 deterioration of renal function as evidenced by decrements in creatinine clearance to 20% and/or the onset of proteinuria or marked, *persistent* increases in proteinuria;
2 development of even moderate hypertension, i.e. blood pressure >140/90 mmHg on two or more occasions separated by an interval of at least 6 h;
3 signs of intrauterine growth restriction and/or deterioration of placental function;
4 change in rate of weight gain, either cessation or excess;
5 symptoms of impending eclampsia.

DIAGNOSIS DURING PREGNANCY

When the question of renal disease is raised for the first time during a pregnancy it is essential to try to establish a diagnosis and a course of management that will be helpful to both mother and fetus. When a patient presents with hypertension, proteinuria and/or abnormal renal function it is difficult to distinguish parenchymal renal disease from pre-eclampsia. A previous history of renal disorders, abnormal urine analysis, a family history of renal disease or a history of systemic illness known to involve the kidneys is obviously helpful, but even so parenchymal renal disease and pre-eclampsia may coexist. Also, think about the diagnosis of renal artery stenosis [120] (see Table 7.8, p.211).

The assessment of the patient and subsequent blood and urine testing are similar to those of non-pregnant patients but the definitive diagnosis usually has to wait until after delivery. Such patients should be hospitalized and their pregnancies allowed to continue if renal function and blood pressure remain stable. The use of interim or prophylactic haemodialysis to 'buy time' has been advocated but this is not established practice [121–126].

THE ROLE OF RENAL BIOPSY IN OBSTETRIC PRACTICE

Experience with renal biopsy in pregnancy is sparse, mainly because clinical circumstances rarely justify the minimal risks of biopsy at this time and the procedure is usually deferred to the postpartum period [80]. Reports of excessive bleeding and other complications in pregnant women have led some to consider pregnancy a relative contraindication to renal biopsy [127], although others have not observed any increased morbidity [128]. When the biopsy is performed in the immediate puerperium in subjects with well-controlled blood pressure and normal coagulation indices, the morbidity is certainly similar to that reported in non-pregnant patients [129].

Packham and Fairley [130] have reported on 111 biopsies in pregnant women, all preterm, confirming and extending the impression that risks of the procedure resemble those in the non-pregnant population. In fact, their incidence of transient gross haematuria was considerably lower than in non-pregnant patients, where it is 3–5%. Such excellent statistics no doubt reflect the experience and technical skills of the unit. Statistics have also been improved by refinement of the prebiopsy evaluation, which includes verifying that the patient is not significantly hypertensive and has not ingested drugs that interfere with clotting (i.e. aspirin) for at least 7–10 days prior to the procedure, as well as the usual tests to exclude bleeding diatheses.

There can be no doubt that given these data, it is in order to restate that pregnancy adds little or no risk to the procedure. However, because complications do occur, it is still important to have specific indications for renal biopsy in pregnancy. Packham and Fairley [130] suggest that closed (percutaneous) needle biopsy should be undertaken quite often, because they believe certain glomerular disorders to be adversely influenced by pregnancy, and that this effect might be blunted by specific therapy, such as antiplatelet agents. The consensus goes against such broad indications and reiterates that renal biopsy should be performed infrequently during gestation [131,132]. (Even in non-pregnant populations the reasons for renal biopsy are not clearly defined, and experts categorize indications as 'most useful', 'possibly useful' and of 'little or no use' [73].) The few widely agreed indications for ante-partum biopsy are as follows.

1 When there is a sudden deterioration of renal function prior to 32 weeks' gestation and with no obvious cause. This is because certain forms of rapidly progressive glomerulonephritis may respond to aggressive treatment with steroid 'pulses', chemotherapy and perhaps plasma exchange, when diagnosed early.

2 When there is symptomatic nephrotic syndrome occurring before the 32nd week of gestation. While some might consider a therapeutic trial of steroids in such cases, it is best to determine beforehand whether the lesion is likely to respond to steroids, because pregnancy is itself a hypercoagulable state prone to worsening by such treatment. On the other hand, proteinuria alone in a normotensive woman with well-preserved renal function, and who has neither marked hypoalbuminaemia nor intolerable oedema, would mean that the patient should be examined at more frequent intervals and biopsy deferred to the postpartum period. This is because the consensus amongst most investigators [84,85,94,99,102,110] is that prognosis is determined primarily by the level of renal function and the presence or absence of hypertension. A similar approach applies in the management of pregnancies with asymptomatic microscopic haematuria alone, when neither stone nor tumour is suggested by ultrasonography.

3 Where there is a presentation characterized by 'active urinary sediment' (red and white blood cells and casts) with proteinuria and 'borderline' renal function, in a patient who has not been evaluated in the past. This is a controversial area and it could be argued that diagnosis of some collagen disorders such as scleroderma or periarteritis would be grounds for termination of the pregnancy, or that classification of the type of lesion in a woman with systemic lupus erythematosus (SLE) would determine the type and intensity of therapy. The first two diseases are only infrequently diagnosed by renal biopsy. A normotensive woman with stable renal function and neither systemic involvement nor laboratory evidence of these collagen disorders is usually watched closely without intervention. Biopsy may be indicated, however, in the latter condition, i.e. in selected patients with SLE and lupus nephropathy of uncertain histopathology.

ASSESSMENT OF RENAL FUNCTION IN PREGNANCY

Serial data on renal function are needed to supplement routine antenatal observations. Tests that are available for use in routine clinical practice include the estimation of plasma creatinine, urea and electrolytes and determination of the clearances of creatinine and urea. A few words of caution are needed. Although plasma creatinine, its reciprocal or its logarithm are often used to estimate or even calculate GFR (in relation to age, height and weight), this approach should not be used in pregnancy, because bodyweight or size does not reflect kidney size. Ideally, evaluation of renal function in pregnancy should be based on the serial surveillance of clearance and not plasma concentration of creatinine, even though this is not the ideal measure of GFR. As creatinine levels may increase shortly after ingesting cooked meat (because cooking converts preformed creatine into creatinine), the timing of the blood sample during a clearance period must take meals and their content into account [133].

When reporting renal function values, it must be remembered that correcting data to a standard body surface area of $1.73\,m^2$ (and thus, by implication, to a standard kidney size) is not applicable in pregnancy [134]. Serial renal function tests should be performed and where possible compared to pre-pregnancy values.

The 'gold standard' for assessing proteinuria is still the 24-h urine collection [73,135] because dipstick testing can be deceptive. Urinary protein excretion rate above 500 mg/24 h should be regarded as significant in pregnancy. Some advocate near bedside automated urinalysis devices to quantify spot urine protein/creatinine ratios with 300 mg/mmol creatinine having a good predictive value for proteinuria >300 mg/24 h [136]. If renal function deteriorates during any stage of pregnancy, reversible causes should be sought such as urinary tract infection (UTI) or obstruction and dehydration or electrolyte imbalance, which may be subtle, perhaps secondary to diuretic therapy. (Near term, a 15% decrement in function that affects plasma creatinine minimally is normal [14].) Failure to detect a reversible cause for the decrease is an indication for ending the pregnancy by elective delivery. The use of dialysis to 'buy time', without really knowing the cause of the renal deterioration, is not generally accepted. If hypertension accompanies any observed decrease in renal function, the outlook is usually more serious and the fetus should be delivered.

Decisions regarding treatment of hypertension

This is perhaps the most controversial area in the management of renal disease during pregnancy and is also discussed in Chapter 6. Most current practices have not been validated by controlled trials in pregnant patients so that many clinicians, not cognizant of pregnancy pathophysiology, prescribe therapy that has been determined to be appropriate by careful studies in non-pregnant populations but that may be unwise in pregnant women [1]. Caution is certainly needed in treating pregnant women and, more important, there is a need for more concentrated and collaborative efforts in evaluating therapy in pregnancy especially with regard to possible effects of antihypertensive therapy on fetal growth [137].

Most of the specific risks of hypertension appear to be mediated through superimposed pre-eclampsia. There is

still controversy about the incidence of pre-eclampsia in women with pre-existing renal disease [89,138]. The diagnosis cannot be made with certainty on clinical grounds alone, because hypertension and proteinuria may be manifestations of the underlying renal disease.

In deciding what, if any, treatment is appropriate for hypertension several factors should be considered. These are thoroughly discussed in Chapter 6 and include the level of hypertension under consideration, the underlying cause of the hypertension, the effects on maternal complication rate and on perinatal morbidity and mortality, the detrimental effects of any treatment, and, lastly, the effect on long-term maternal prognosis.

CONTROL OF BLOOD PRESSURE IN SEVERE CHRONIC HYPERTENSION

This is invariably as a continuation of treatment started before conception. If a woman is stabilized effectively with drugs not specifically contraindicated in pregnancy, these drugs (with the exception of diuretics) should be continued during pregnancy. The most obvious contraindicated drugs are angiotensin-converting enzyme (ACE) inhibitors. Hospitalization is usually necessary for initiation or alteration of therapy.

PREVENTION OR AMELIORATION OF SUPERIMPOSED PRE-ECLAMPSIA IN SEVERE CHRONIC HYPERTENSION

The earlier the presentation, the more justified it is to attempt conservative management in order to allow fetal maturation, provided there are no other features necessitating delivery. If *de novo* treatment is indicated in pregnancy it must take place in hospital where the responses can be monitored. If the hypertension is not severe enough to require this, then it does not require treatment. If treatment is indicated for maternal reasons then hospital admission is mandatory. Antihypertensive therapy merely controls only one of the potentially dangerous problems but it allows further maturation before delivery becomes necessary for maternal and fetal reasons.

CONTROL OF ACUTE SEVERE HYPERTENSION

This is usually due to pre-eclampsia and includes hypertensive emergencies. Where such acute episodes occur early in the third trimester without marked deterioration in renal function, then some attempt might be made to control the blood pressure in the short term to enhance neonatal survival. Despite lowering the blood pressure to protect the mother against dangerous consequences, the other changes of pre-eclampsia will progress. Blood pressure may prove increasingly difficult to control and, if blood pressure 'escapes', this is then an indication to end the pregnancy by elective delivery.

The roles of volume expansion therapy and antiplatelet agents such as aspirin along with calcium and/or vitamin supplementation (all of which may also prevent pre-eclampsia) are discussed in Chapter 6.

Fetal surveillance

Serial assessment of fetal well-being is essential because renal disease can be associated with intrauterine growth restriction and, when complications do arise, the judicious moment for intervention is influenced by fetal status [139,140]. Current technology should minimize intrauterine fetal death as well as neonatal morbidity and mortality. Regardless of gestational age, most babies weighing 1500 g or more survive better in a special care nursery than in a hostile intrauterine environment. Increasingly, there is reliance on deliberate preterm delivery if there are signs of impending intrauterine fetal death, if renal function deteriorates substantially, if uncontrollable hypertension supervenes or if eclampsia occurs (Table 7.7). It must be realized, however, that 'buying time' for the immature fetus, for example by attempting to control escalating hypertension, is really only controlling a sign without necessarily modifying the underlying disorder.

Decisions regarding delivery

If pregnancy proceeds satisfactorily, it is probably advisable to induce labour at 38 weeks because prolonging the pregnancy beyond this time can be associated with greater risks of placental failure and intrauterine death. Moreover, at this gestation, the fetus should be relatively free of risk if the expected date of delivery is correct.

Delivery before 38 weeks may be necessary if renal function deteriorates markedly, if there are signs of impending intrauterine death, if uncontrollable hypertension supervenes or if eclampsia occurs. In addition the nephrotoxic effects of increased protein traffic in propagating injury in the glomerulus as well as the tubulointerstitium, leading to parenchymal damage may have been underestimated in the past. There is now good evidence in the non-pregnant setting that proteinuria has a predictive value regarding the rate of disease progression. More is known about the mechanisms underlying the gradual erosion of renal function and how medication can limit the deleterious effects of protein trafficking [141].

Patients should be delivered where full facilities and personnel are available for fetal monitoring, operative delivery and neonatal resuscitation. The use of regional analgesia in labour is discussed in Chapter 6.

BLOOD TRANSFUSION POLICY IN HYPERTENSIVE EMERGENCIES

A woman with a shrunken intravascular compartment is less tolerant of blood loss than is the normal pregnant woman [142]. Blood replacement must therefore be initiated sooner, although managed very carefully, to guard against the dangers of underfilling and overfilling. Close monitoring of the central venous pressure (CVP) is helpful, especially where there is oliguria (see Chapter 6).

Pregnancy and specific renal diseases

Table 7.8 summarizes the course of pregnancy in a number of specific diseases. In all types of disease plasma creatinine levels above $\sim 150\,\mu M$ carry an increased risk of accelerated loss of renal function due to pregnancy. Certain specific diseases are associated with risks of further long-term decrease in maternal renal function. Tables 7.9–7.11, from an in-depth review by Imbasciati and Ponticelli [91] describe outcomes in over 1000 women with a variety of specific renal lesions, usually documented by kidney biopsy. Therapeutic abortions were excluded when pregnancy success rates were calculated.

Renal status		1950s	1960s	1970s	1980s	1990s
Mild	Preterm delivery	9	10	19	25	28
	Perinatal mortality	18	15	7	<5	<3
Moderate	Preterm delivery	15	21	40	52	57
	Perinatal mortality	58	45	23	10	10
Severe	Preterm delivery	100	100	100	100	100
	Perinatal mortality	99	91	59	52	49

Table 7.7 Changing prospects and preterm delivery in women with chronic renal disease. (From J. Davison, unpublished data.)

Estimates based on 3010 women and 5270 pregnancies (1954–2000). All results expressed as a percentage.

Table 7.8 Pregnancy and specific renal diseases.

Renal disease	Effects
Chronic glomerulonephritis	Usually no adverse effect in the absence of hypertension. One view is that glomerulonephritis is adversely affected by the coagulation changes of pregnancy. Urinary tract infections may occur more frequently
Focal glomerulosclerosis	Risks of escalating hypertension and renal deterioration often not reversed postpartum. Increased fetal losses are likely
IgA nephropathy	Risks of uncontrolled and/or sudden escalating hypertension and worsening of renal function
Pyelonephritis	Bacteriuria in pregnancy can lead to exacerbation. Multiple organ system derangements may ensue including adult respiratory distress syndrome
Reflux nephropathy	Risks of sudden escalating hypertension and worsening of renal function
Urolithiasis	Infections can be more frequent, but ureteral dilatation and stasis do not seem to affect natural history. Data on lithotripsy in pregnancy are limited
Polycystic disease	Functional impairment and hypertension usually minimal in childbearing years
Diabetic nephropathy	Usually no adverse effect on the renal lesion, but there is increased frequency of infection, oedema and/or pre-eclampsia
Systemic lupus erythematosus	Controversial; prognosis most favourable if disease in remission >6 months prior to conception. Steroid dosage should be increased postpartum
Periarteritis nodosa	Fetal prognosis is dismal and maternal death often occurs
Scleroderma	If onset during pregnancy then can be rapid overall deterioration. Reactivation of quiescent scleroderma may occur postpartum
Previous urinary tract surgery	Might be associated with other malformations of the urogenital tract. Urinary tract infection common during pregnancy. Renal function may undergo reversible decrease. No significant obstructive problem but caesarean section often needed for abnormal presentation and/or to avoid disruption of the continence mechanism if artificial sphincter present
After nephrectomy, solitary kidney and pelvic kidney	Might be associated with other malformations of urogenital tract. Pregnancy well tolerated; dystocia rarely occurs with a pelvic kidney
Wegener's granulomatosis	Limited information. Proteinuria (± hypertension) is common from early in pregnancy. Immunosuppressives are safe but cytotoxic drugs are best avoided
Renal artery stenosis	May present as chronic hypertension or as recurrent isolated pre-eclampsia. If diagnosed then transluminal angioplasty can be undertaken in pregnancy if appropriate

ACUTE GLOMERULONEPHRITIS

Acute poststreptococcal glomerulonephritis complicating pregnancy is very rare but does occur [143–146], and has been mistaken for pre-eclampsia.

CHRONIC GLOMERULONEPHRITIS [84,99,110,111,114,147]

The prognosis of chronic glomerulonephritis during pregnancy is hard to evaluate primarily because most reports are poorly documented, often failing to list the degree of functional impairment, the blood pressure prior to conception and the histology of 'glomerulonephritis'. One suggestion is that most glomerular diseases are 'aggravated' because of the hypercoagulable state of pregnancy; thus patients are more prone to hypertensive crises early in pregnancy or later to superimposed pre-eclampsia [148]. The Melbourne group [104,149–151] have stated that pregnancy tends to aggravate most glomerular diseases

due to the hypercoagulable state that accompanies pregnancy; in particular they claim that crescentric glomerular lesions occur more readily. They also indicate that such patients are more prone to superimposed pre-eclampsia or hypertensive crises early in pregnancy. Other experience is that kidney function decreases most often in patients where hypertension is severe; nevertheless, most pregnancies are successful [94,152,153,154]. The subtypes of primary glomerulonephritis are all now regarded as distinct and separable disease entities, and with few exceptions can be specifically distinguished only by renal biopsy. Those subtypes present in women of childbearing age are given in Table 7.9.

FOCAL GLOMERULOSCLEROSIS

Increased proteinuria and hypertension during pregnancy are frequent but usually reversible. The renal lesion may be accelerated by pregnancy but this is rare if pre-

Name (abbreviation)	Synonyms
Focal glomerulosclerosis (FGS)	Focal and segmental glomerulosclerosis
	Focal and segmental hyalinosis
	Focal sclerosing GN
Membranous glomerulonephritis (MGN)	Membranous nephropathy
Diffuse proliferative GN (DPGN)	Mesangial proliferative GN
	Endocapillary proliferative GN
Membranoproliferative GN (MPCN)	Mesangiocapillary GN
	(Type II = dense deposit disease)
Mesangial IgA nephropathy (IgA-GN)	Berger's nephritis
	Focal proliferative GN
Minimal change nephrotic syndrome (MCNS)	Lipoid nephrosis
	Idiopathic nephrotic syndrome
	Minimal change glomerulonephritis

Table 7.9 Subtypes of primary glomerulonephritis (GN) in women of childbearing age.

pregnancy renal function is normal. Overall fetal loss rates are about 25%.

MEMBRANOUS GLOMERULONEPHRITIS

If renal function is satisfactory and stable and hypertension absent or under control then the outlook is good. Pregnancy does not damage the renal lesion.

DIFFUSE PROLIFERATIVE GLOMERULONEPHRITIS

This label covers a heterogeneous group of patients with prolonged proteinuria. Hypertension and proteinuria invariably worsen during pregnancy but the rate of subsequent progression into renal failure is not hastened. Fetal loss rates average 15%.

MEMBRANOPROLIFERATIVE GLOMERULONEPHRITIS

It is difficult to assess whether the course of MPGN, which is usually not good, is worsened by pregnancy. Certainly hypertension arising in pregnancy invariably persists afterwards and even when pre-pregnancy status is 'mild' (plasma creatinine <125 mmol/L) pregnancy can have an overall deleterious effect and fetal loss rates may be as high as 50%. Some women with persistent hypocomplementaemia have a circulating antibody 'C3 nephritic factor' and placental transmission and transient neonatal hypocomplementaemia (without long-term sequelae) have been described [155] (see Table 7.10).

MESANGIAL IGA NEPHROPATHY

Mesangial IgA nephropathy (IgA-GN) accounts for 15–20% of all glomerulonephritis in Europe and 30–40% in Japan but less than 10% in North America [156]. The risk of hypertension during pregnancy is probably higher than for other subtypes, and its persistence after delivery can be problematical. If pre-pregnancy status is 'moderate' (plasma creatinine 125–250 mmol/L) then progressive renal failure after delivery is highly likely, but of course this may have happened anyway because 1–2% of adult patients with IgA-GN enter renal failure each year. Fetal loss rates are around 15% except in the Melbourne series [150] where the figure is 30%, perhaps related to a selected referral pattern. IgA-GN is associated with human leucocyte antigen (HLA)-BW35 and in some cases may be an inheritable disease but as yet the genetic counselling implications are unclear. Abe [81–83] has examined the impact of IgA nephropathy and pregnancy on each other. Consistent findings were that: (i) pregnancy is well tolerated without effect on the course of the disease if blood pressure is normal and GFR is >70 mL/min before conception; (ii) the live birth rate is extremely low if hypertension exists before pregnancy and/or is not well controlled during pregnancy.

MINIMAL CHANGE NEPHROTIC SYNDROME

Most women of childbearing age are in stable remission with 'mild' status and pregnancy is well tolerated without risk of relapse. For women who are 'frequent relapsers' prednisone can be restarted or continued throughout pregnancy [157] but some decide to stop therapy and take a calculated risk of further relapse during pregnancy.

HEREDITARY NEPHRITIS

Most cases (85%) of this disorder are in males who have inherited the disease as an X-linked dominant disorder [158]. The majority of female carriers manifest mild abnormalities of renal function and urinary microscopy as dictated by the Lyon hypothesis. The remaining patients are examples of autosomal dominant or recessive inherit-

Table 7.10 Fetal and maternal outcome of pregnancies in women with primary glomerulonephritis. Data are the proportion (%) of all pregnancies. (From Imbasciati and Ponticelli [91]. See [91] for details of the six reports surveyed in this table.)

Histology	Pregnancies/patients	Spontaneous abortion (%)	Perinatal loss (%)	Preterm delivery (%)	Renal function decrease		Blood pressure increase	
					Reversible (%)	Progressive (%)	Reversible (%)	Permanent (%)
Focal glomerulosclerosis	85/61	3	23	32	13	5	32	10
Membranous nephropathy	110/70	12	4	35	3	2	22	3
Membranoproliferative	165/98	17	8	19	6	3	20	12
IgA nephritis	268/166	5	15	21	12	2	25	12
Mesangial proliferative	278/163	5	12	9	2	3	36	7
All types	906/558	8	13	19	8	3	27	9

ance. These diseases therefore may not become clinically manifest until pregnancy. Pregnancy in these women is usually successful from a renal viewpoint but can be complicated by bleeding problems usually due to disordered platelet morphology and function [159,160]. There is an interesting report of two sisters with this disorder who developed rapidly progressive crescentric glomerulonephritis associated with pregnancy [161].

This heterogeneous group, sometimes called familial glomerulonephritis, raises the question of renal disease transmission to the next generation, a problem not seen in any of the primary glomerulonephritis group, except possibly IgA-GN. The inheritance of Alport's syndrome (familial glomerulonephritis with deafness) is usually through less affected females and typically has greater expression in males. Benign familial haematuria syndrome is inheritable sometimes as an autosomal dominant disease [162].

COLLAGEN DISEASES OR DIFFUSE CONNECTIVE TISSUE DISEASES (see also Chapter 8)

Systemic lupus erythematosus

This relatively common disease with or without other diffuse connective tissue diseases (DCTDs) (overlap syndrome) has a predilection for the childbearing age group, and coincidence with pregnancy poses complex clinical problems due to the profound disturbance of the immunological system and multiple organ involvement in SLE and the complicated immunology of pregnancy itself [163,164]. The majority of pregnancies succeed, especially when the maternal disease is in complete clinical remission for 6 months prior to conception, even if there were severe pathological changes in the original renal biopsy and heavy proteinuria in the early stages of the disease [165,166]. Continued signs of disease activity or increasing renal dysfunction certainly reduce the likelihood of an uncomplicated pregnancy and the clinical course [167] (see Table 7.11). Obviously pre-pregnancy counselling must take account of the actual form of the lupus nephritis (mild vs. aggressive) as well as the medications that are currently being used either separately or in combination, for example glucocorticoids, cyclophosphamide, azathioprine and nowadays mycophendate mofetil, MMF (CellCept) [168].

SLE nephropathy may sometimes become manifest during pregnancy and when accompanied by hypertension, and renal dysfunction may be mistaken for pre-eclampsia. From recent reviews of the literature it appears that as many as 19% (progressive in 8%) and 42% experience decrements in GFR and hypertension, respectively. The figures are worse if renal insufficiency (plasma creatinine >125 mmol/L) antedates the pregnancy [91,169].

Some patients have a definite tendency to relapse, occasionally severely in the puerperium, and therefore it is prudent to prescribe or increase steroids at this time [170,171]. Rarely a particularly severe postpartum syndrome may develop consisting of pleural effusion, pulmonary infiltration, fever, electrocardiogram (ECG) abnormalities and even cardiomyopathy, with extensive IgG, IgM, Ig and C3 deposition in the myocardium [138]. The concept of the 'stormy puerperium' has been disputed [172]. Many now observe postpartum patients and do not institute or increase steroid therapy unless signs of increased disease activity are noted.

The fetal and thrombotic implications of the presence of maternal lupus anticoagulant, anticardiolipin antibodies and extractable nuclear antigen (ENA) antibodies (e.g. anti-Ro) are discussed in Chapter 8.

Systemic sclerosis

Scleroderma is a term that includes a heterogeneous group of limited and systemic conditions causing hardening of the skin. Systemic sclerosis implies involvement of both skin and other sites, particularly certain internal organs. Renal involvement is thought to occur in about 60% of patients with systemic sclerosis, usually within 3–4 years of diagnosis. The presentation may be the sudden onset of malignant hypertension, rapidly progressive renal failure or slowly worsening proteinuria and/or azotemia [173].

The combination of systemic sclerosis and pregnancy is unusual because systemic sclerosis occurs most often in the fourth and fifth decades, and patients with systemic sclerosis are usually infertile. When systemic sclerosis has its onset in pregnancy, there is a much greater tendency for deterioration. Patients with scleroderma and no evidence of renal involvement prior to conception can develop severe kidney disease in pregnancy. There are also

	Pregnancies	Spontaneous abortions (%)	Perinatal loss	Fetal loss
1952–70	587	20	9	29
1971–80	184	20	5	25
1981–88	224	13	13	26

Table 7.11 Systemic lupus erythematosus and pregnancy. (From Imbasciati and Ponticelli [91]. See [91] for details of literature surveyed in this table.)

instances when pregnancy has been uneventful and successful but many required the use of converting enzyme inhibitors, which are contraindicated from the fetal viewpoint. Most maternal deaths involve rapidly progressive scleroderma with severe pulmonary complications, multiple infections, hypertension and/or renal failure [174].

The extent of systemic involvement is probably more important than the duration of the disease, and limited mild disease carries a better prognosis. Sclerosis usually spares the abdominal wall skin but there is one report of hydronephrosis, presumed secondary to thickened skin and decreased abdominal wall compliance, in a twin pregnancy complicated by polyhydramnios [175].

WEGENER'S GRANULOMATOSIS

More information is accruing on pregnancy course and outcome in women with granulomatosis [176,177]. Proteinuria is common from early in pregnancy [178] and reports to date have described both complicated and uneventful pregnancies [179,180], including women taking either azathioprine or cyclophosphamide (see also Chapter 1). A significant flare of Wegener's granulomatosis (WG) in pregnancy remains a life-threatening condition and needs to be treated very aggressively. Whether the risk/benefit ratio for treatment is in favour of cyclophosphamide or an alternative such as plasma exchange and immunoglobulin remains a difficult clinical decision and a matter for debate [181].

PERIARTERITIS NODOSA

The outcome of pregnancy in women with renal involvement due to periarteritis nodosa is very poor, largely because of the associated hypertension, which is frequently malignant. Although a few successful pregnancies have been reported, in most cases fetal prognosis is dismal and many have ended with maternal death. This may merely reflect the nature of the disease itself, but it is an important consideration when making decisions about pregnancy. Early therapeutic termination has less maternal risk [182].

DIABETIC NEPHROPATHY (see Chapter 11)

Because many pregnant patients have been insulin-dependent diabetics since childhood, they probably already have microscopic changes in their kidneys [183,184]. Renal disease develops in 30% with a peak incidence 16 years after presentation [185]. Maternal hazards and perinatal loss are twice as common in diabetics with clinically overt renal disease as in those without (see Table 7.12).

During pregnancy, diabetic women have an increased prevalence and incidence of covert bacteriuria (and may be more susceptible to UTI), pre-eclampsia, peripheral oedema and occasionally severe, but transient, nephrotic syndrome [186]. Most women with diabetic nephropathy demonstrate the normal GFR increment, and pregnancy does not accelerate renal deterioration [187–189]. Perinatal survival averages about 90% with one in four women delivered before 34 weeks' gestation. Poor glycaemic control in early pregnancy and failure to improve immediately thereafter are significant risk factors for pre-eclampsia [190–192].

There is a report of diabetic women with moderate renal dysfunction (plasma creatinine >125 mmol/L) whose renal function permanently deteriorated in pregnancy in comparison to the changes before and afterwards—GFR decrements of 1.8 mL/min/month in pregnancy and 1.4 mL/min/month postpartum until the start of dialysis [193]. Such changes occurred despite good metabolic control and might have been related to hypertension, which often accelerates in late pregnancy, regardless of intensified treatment. It should be remembered, however, that these observations are uncontrolled and that non-pregnant diabetics with plasma creatinine >125 mmol/L also often progress rapidly to end-stage renal failure.

Some predictions of outcome can be based on initial renal studies in pregnancy. In an analysis of 45 women (46 pregnancies) those with proteinuria in excess of 3 g/24 h and/or plasma creatinine >130 mmol/L before 20 weeks' gestation had higher incidences of small babies, prematurity and pre-eclampsia. Until creatinine clearance was reduced markedly, the best predictor of pregnancy

Table 7.12 Outcome of pregnancy in women with diabetic nephropathy, polycystic kidney disease and reflux nephropathy. Data are the proportion (%) of all pregnancies. (From Imbasciati and Ponticelli [91]. See [91] for details of five reports surveyed in this table.)

Nephropathy	Pregnancies/ patients	Perinatal loss	Preterm delivery (%)	Renal function decrease	Blood pressure increase	Progressive course after delivery
Diabetic nephropathy	97/94	6	36	32	58	13
Polycystic disease	464/242	3	10	3	14	0.3
Reflux nephropathy	137/53	7	15	0.7	11	3

outcome was proteinuria <1 g/24 h having better outcomes in all categories and a significantly lower risk of long-term deterioration in renal function [194]. In this study there was a 100% perinatal survival but 53% developed pre-eclampsia, 58% had 1 g/24 h proteinuria by the third trimester and 35% demonstrated more than 15% fall in creatinine clearance.

Whether or not hypertension should be treated more aggressively, especially before conception, is open to question [187,195]. Diabetes already causes glomerular hyperfiltration, which theoretically may be further exacerbated by pregnancy if renal autoregulation fails to prevent excessive transmission of arterial pressure to the glomerular capillaries. Normalizing pressures may help to prevent (further) glomerular damage. Some of the antihypertensive agents used pre-pregnancy, in particular ACE inhibitors, may be contraindicated during pregnancy [158, 196] (see Chapter 6) but use right up to conception certainly reduces proteinuria and apparently could have a prolonged renoprotective effect during pregnancy [117,197] (Table 7.13).

PYELONEPHRITIS (TUBULOINTERSTITIAL DISEASE)

Acute pyelonephritis will be dealt with separately (see below). In chronic pyelonephritis (tubulointerstitial disease) the prognosis in pregnancy is similar to that of patients with glomerular disease, in that outcome is best in patients with adequate renal function and normal blood pressure. Compared to the non-pregnant state, there is an increased frequency of symptomatic infection in pregnant women, but overall, they have a more benign antenatal course than do women with glomerular disease [102].

Of interest is a report suggesting that women who develop frank pyelonephritis manifest greater degrees of pelvicalyceal dilatation in pregnancy, that may not regress after delivery, and which underscores the need for postpartum investigation of this population [198].

Table 7.13 Diabetic nephropathy in pregnancy and ACE inhibitors.

Prevalence 6–10% with 70% exacerbation rate (proteinuria + + ++)	
24-h protein excretion (g) in 8 women	
1.6 ± (SD) 0.67	Pre-pregnancy
0.3 ± 0.15	Pre-pregnancy + ACE inhibitor for 6 m
0.6 ± 0.52	1st trimester
0.8 ± 0.81	2nd trimester
1.0 ± 1.19	3rd trimester
0.6 ± 0.41	3 m postpartum
Prolonged protective effect on renal function during pregnancy?	

Reproduced with permission from [197].

REFLUX NEPHROPATHY

This term is used to describe renal morphological and functional changes that are the urodynamic consequence of vesicoureteric and intrarenal reflux, often complicated by recurrent infection. There are glomerular lesions (focal and segmental hyalinosis and sclerosis) and parenchymal atrophy and scarring. It is one of the most frequent renal diseases in women of childbearing age; one-third of cases are clinically unmasked by pregnancy; up to 30% of women developing end-stage renal failure have reflux nephropathy and this is usually present before 40 years [199].

It is frequently associated with hypertension and moderate to severe renal dysfunction, features that, as discussed earlier (see above), adversely affect pregnancy outcome [200,201]. Specific obstetric worries in these patients include severe fetal intrauterine growth restriction and the risk of sudden rapid worsening of hypertension and renal function with accelerated progression to renal failure.

As the disease may be inherited, children born to parents with vesicoureteric reflux or reflux nephropathy, or who have affected siblings, should be screened in infancy [202].

UROLITHIASIS

The prevalence of urolithiasis in pregnancy is 0.03–0.35% [152]. Most stones contain calcium salts and some are infectious in origin. Occasionally the more malicious struvite stones (e.g. staghorn) are seen. Uric acid and cystine stones are much more infrequent [203]. Renal and ureteric calculi are one of the most common causes of non-uterine abdominal pain severe enough to necessitate hospital admission during pregnancy [204]. Despite these dramatic complications, pregnancy has little influence on the course of stone disease, although there may be an increased incidence of both UTI and perhaps spontaneous abortion, as well as premature labour. The relatively benign prognosis is surprising, because pregnant women are normally hypercalciuric and their urinary supersaturation ratios for calcium oxalate and phosphate are substantially increased. This, in the face of urethral dilatation, stasis and perhaps obstruction, raises the question of why stone disease is not even more prevalent in pregnancy. The answer to this, however, may be that there is concomitant increase in the excretion of magnesium and citrate as well as several glycoproteins that inhibit stone formation (i.e. nephrocalcin) [67,205].

Management should be conservative initially, with adequate hydration, appropriate antibiotic therapy and pain relief with systemic analgesics [206]. The use of continuous segmental (T11–L2) epidural block has been advocated, as in non-pregnant patients with ureteric colic, and may even favourably influence spontaneous passage of stone(s). With good pain relief, the patient micturates without difficulty, moves without assistance and is less at risk from thromboembolic problems than if drowsy, nauseated and bedridden with pain.

When there are complications that might need surgical intervention, then pregnancy should not be a deterrent to intravenous urography (IVU), even though there is an understandable reluctance to consider radiological investigation and the absence of ureteric jets can be utilized if urolithiasis is suspected [207]. Specific clinical criteria should be met before undertaking an IVU: (i) microscopic haematuria; (ii) recurrent urinary tract symptoms; and (iii) sterile urine culture: the presence of two of these indicates a diagnosis of calculi in 60% of women [208]. Ultrasonography may be useful but it is less efficient at detecting very small stones (<5 mm in diameter) and in defining the degree or site of obstruction [204,209].

Alternative management involves the placement of an internal ureteral tube, or stent, between bladder and kidney, under local anaesthesia using cystoscopy or endoluminal ultrasound [210,211]. The stent retains its position because it has a pigtail or J-like curve at each end (double-J) and to prevent encrustation it can be changed every 8 weeks. Early empirical use for presumed stone obstruction in pregnant women with flank pain could be helpful especially when hydration, analgesia and antibiotics do not resolve pain or fever. When the pregnancy is over the usual radiographs should be obtained and standard management resumed.

Ultrasound-guided percutaneous nephrostomy is another effective and safe method of treating pregnant women with ureteric colic or symptomatic obstructive hydronephrosis [212]. The procedure is rapid, requires minimal anaesthesia and is perhaps a preferable alternative to retrograde stenting or more invasive approaches.

Information on lithotripsy during pregnancy is limited [213] and the procedure is best avoided.

In patients with cystinuria, assiduous maintenance of high fluid intake is the mainstay of management. Although D-penicillamine appears relatively safe it should only be used for severe cases, where urinary cystine excretion is known to be very high [214].

AUTOSOMAL DOMINANT POLYCYSTIC KIDNEY DISEASE (ADPKO)

This is an autosomal dominant disorder, spontaneous mutations occurring in fewer than 10% of cases [215]. It is the most common single-gene genetic disease of humans with an incidence of perhaps about one in 400–1000 [215–217]. Most cases do not have clinical manifestations until the fourth and fifth decade—only 17% are

diagnosed by the age of 25 [218]. It may therefore remain undetected during pregnancy, but careful questioning for a history of familial problems and the use of ultrasonography may lead to earlier detection. Patients do well when functional impairment is minimal and hypertension absent, as is often the case in childbearing years. Compared to the pregnancies of sisters unaffected by this autosomal dominant disease, they do have an increased incidence of hypertension late in pregnancy (20 vs. 2%) and a slightly higher perinatal mortality [219].

Women with advanced renal failure are best advised against pregnancy, although use of prophylactic dialysis has been advocated, despite lack of controlled studies, for just this type of patient [220].

Liver cysts are larger and more prevalent in women, especially those who have been pregnant, and enlargement of cysts, but not rupture, may occur during pregnancy [215].

It has been suggested that multiparity (three or more pregnancies) leads to an earlier onset of renal insufficiency [215], which might reflect the effects of pregnancy once moderate renal insufficiency was present. The consensus view, however, is that pregnancy has no long-term effect on renal prognosis [219].

If one or other parent has autosomal dominant polycystic kidney disease (ADPKD) they may seek genetic counselling. Patients from families where there is evidence of clustering of intracranial aneurysms or subarachnoid haemorrhage should be screened before considering pregnancy [221]. There will be a 50% chance of transmitting the disease to their offspring. DNA probe techniques are now being developed so that antenatal diagnosis is possible by chorionic villus sampling allowing women to undergo selective termination of pregnancy [222].

PERMANENT URINARY DIVERSION

Permanent urinary diversion is still used in the management of patients with congenital lower urinary tract defects but its use has declined for neurogenic bladders since the introduction of self-catheterization. The most common complication of pregnancy is urinary infection. Preterm labour occurs in 20% and the use of prophylactic antibiotics throughout pregnancy may reduce its incidence. Decline in renal function may occur, invariably related to infection and/or intermittent obstruction. With an ileal conduit, or augmentation cystoplasty, elevation and compression by the expanding uterus can cause outflow obstruction whereas with a ureterosigmoid anastomosis, actual ureteral obstruction may occur [223,224]. The changes usually reverse after delivery.

The mode of delivery is dictated by obstetric factors. Abnormal presentation accounts for a caesarean section rate of 25%, related no doubt to minor genital tract abnormalities. Vaginal delivery is safe but as the continence of a ureterosigmoid anastomosis depends on an intact anal sphincter, this must be protected with a mediolateral episiotomy.

INHERITED RENAL DISEASE

Inherited renal disorders are not rare, ADPKD affecting one in 400–1000 individuals [215] (see above). Some of the rarer hereditary diseases manifest during childhood and then progress to end-stage renal failure before or by adolescence (i.e. cystinosis and nephronophthisis). Thus pregnancy occurs when on dialysis or after transplantation [189]. In contrast, the most prevalent disorders, hereditary nephritis (see above) and polycystic disease (see below) have a later onset. Table 7.14 gives examples of inherited kidney disorders in which antenatal diagnosis is technically possible [225]. All such women contemplating pregnancy or in early pregnancy should be referred for genetic counselling [226].

Tuberous sclerosis is an autosomal dominant disease, comprising skin lesions, involvement of the central nervous system and visceral lesions, including renal angiomyolipoma [98,227].

Renal involvement in the von Hippel–Landau disease includes cysts and bilateral multifocal renal cell carcinoma. Twenty-five per cent of these women have phaeochromocytomata, often bilateral (which may cluster in families, and be the only manifestation of the disorder [228]). Therefore there is substantial risk of fatal outcome especially in pregnancy, and women with this condition should be screened to rule out phaeochromocytoma as well as for haemangioblastomata involving retina or central nervous system.

THE SOLITARY KIDNEY

Some patients have either a congenital absence of one kidney or marked unilateral hypoplasia. Most, however, have had a previous nephrectomy because of pyelonephritis (with abscess *or* hydronephrosis), unilateral tuberculosis, congenital abnormalities, trauma, tumour or donor nephrectomy [229]. Occasionally the woman may have been a living-related kidney donor [230]. It is important to know the indication for and the time since the nephrectomy [204]. In patients with an infectious and/or structural renal problem sequential pre-pregnancy investigation is needed for detection of any persistent infection.

There is no difference whether the right or left kidney remains as long as it is located in the normal anatomical position. If function is normal and stable, all women with this problem seem to tolerate pregnancy well despite the superimposition of GFR increments on already hyperfiltering nephrons.

Ectopic kidneys (usually pelvic) are more vulnerable to infection and are associated with impaired fetal outcome, probably because of associated malformations of the urogenital tract [204]. If infection occurs in a solitary kidney during pregnancy and does not quickly respond to antibiotics, then termination may have to be considered for preservation of renal function. Pregnancy in women who have survived childhood treatment for a nephroblastoma (Wilms' tumour) has a 30% perinatal loss, perhaps because of the late effects of radiotherapy on the uterus [231].

Table 7.14 Examples of inherited kidney diseases in which antenatal diagnosis may be technically possible.

			DNA study	
	Mode of inheritance	Biochemical diagnosis	Linkage analysis	Gene defect*
Polycystic kidney disease	AD		+	
Alport's syndrome	XD		+	+
	AR		+	+
Primary hyperoxaluria	AR	+		
Fabry's disease	XR	+	+	+
Finnish congenital nephrotic syndrome	AR	+ (raised amniotic fluid α-fetoprotein concentration)		
Congenital diabetes insipidus	XR		+	+
Oculocerebrorenal syndrome of Lowe	XR		+	+
von Hippel–Lindau disease	AD		+	

AD, autosomal dominant; AR, autosomal recessive; XD, X-linked dominant; XR, X-linked recessive.
*In certain families in which the gene defect has been identified.

NEPHROTIC SYNDROME AND PREGNANCY

The most common cause of nephrotic syndrome in late pregnancy is pre-eclampsia [89,232]. This form of pre-eclampsia has a poorer fetal prognosis than pre-eclampsia with less heavy proteinuria, but the maternal prognosis is similar.

Other causes of nephrotic syndrome in pregnancy include membranous nephropathy, proliferative glomerulonephritis or MPGN, lipid nephrosis, lupus nephropathy, hereditary nephritis, diabetic nephropathy, renal vein thrombosis, amyloidosis, sarcoidosis and secondary syphilis [80,233]. Some of these possibilities emphasize the importance of establishing a tissue diagnosis before initiating steroid therapy [157].

If renal function is adequate and hypertension is absent, there should be few complications during pregnancy; however, several of the physiological changes occurring during pregnancy may simulate aggravation or exacerbation of the disease. For example, increments in renal blood flow as well as increase in renal vein pressure may enhance protein excretion. Levels of serum albumin usually decrease by 5–10 g/L in normal pregnancy, and the further decreases that can occur in the nephrotic syndrome may enhance the tendency toward fluid retention. Despite oedema, diuretics should not be given as these patients have a decreased intravascular volume and this therapy could further compromise uteroplacental perfusion or aggravate the increased tendency to thrombotic episodes.

While the majority of these pregnancies succeed and are maintained near to term, there is evidence that the hypoalbuminaemia and the associated decreased intravascular volume may cause small-for-dates infants [234]. Furthermore, there is a report that infants of normotensive mothers who had heavy proteinuria during pregnancy manifested impaired neurological and mental development [235].

Long-term effects of pregnancy in renal disease

CLINICAL STUDIES

Pregnancy does not cause any deterioration or otherwise affect the rate of progression of the disease beyond what might be expected in the non-pregnant state, provided kidney dysfunction was minimal and hypertension was absent before pregnancy [91,112,132,148]. An important factor in remote prognosis could be the sclerotic effects that hyperfiltration might already have had in the residual (intact) glomeruli of kidneys of these patients. The situation may be worse in a single diseased kidney where presumably more sclerosis has occurred within the fewer

(intact) glomeruli. Theoretically, further progressive loss of renal function could ensue in pregnancy. Nevertheless, in some women with renal disease there can be unpredicted, accelerated and irreversible renal decline in pregnancy or immediately afterwards. The mechanisms, which are unknown, will be slow to emerge from human data, if they are ever available from this source, and therefore animal research must be considered [102,236].

STUDIES IN ANIMALS

Animal models have been developed to investigate the mechanisms involved in renal dysfunction when pregnancy and disease interact, as well as to assess long-term renal prognosis. In particular the role of glomerular blood pressure (P_{GC}) has been examined because of its importance in the development of glomerular injury.

Unilateral nephrectomy

Multiple pregnancies in rats with chronic underlying renal vasodilatation induced by uninephrectomy plus high dietary protein feeding do not cause worsening of proteinuria or structural damage [237]. GFR and SNGFR were lower in repetitively pregnant compared to non-pregnant rats [237], perhaps related to a decreased renal NO activity [238] but of interest, the vasodilatory response to intravenous amino acids was intact in repetitively pregnant rats whereas this renal reserve was absent in the non-pregnant [237]. P_{GC} was elevated by long-term uninephrectomy plus high dietary protein feeding but not worsened by pregnancy, which may explain the lack of exacerbation of the underlying glomerular impairment due to sequential pregnancies.

Infarction and reduction of renal mass

With five-sixths reduction of renal mass by combined ablation and infarction, systemic hypertension was evident together with high P_{GC} in virgin females. The remnant kidney was still capable of marked and prolonged renal vasodilatation during pregnancy with preglomerular and efferent arteriolar resistances decreasing in parallel [239]. Of note, this model of chronic renal disease is associated with a relative renal NO deficiency [240], without increased nitric oxide synthase (NOS) activity in these remnant kidneys in pregnancy [241], suggesting activation of an alternative renal vasodilatory system. Because blood pressure also fell, there was no change in P_{GC} and no worsening of proteinuria during pregnancy, thus no haemodynamic basis for pregnancy to exacerbate the glomerular injury [239]. Studies by others have shown no long-term histological damage by pregnancy in this model [242].

Spontaneously hypertensive rat

Glomerular injury develops with advancing age although its evolution is much slower in females than males [12,243]. Repetitive pregnancies have no long-term effect on glomerular function and structure or protein excretion in 1-year-old spontaneously hypertensive rats (SHRs) nor is the already high P_{GC} further elevated [244]. It had been anticipated that in the presence of severe systemic hypertension (as occurs in the SHR), superimposed pregnancy would expose the kidney to additional increases in P_{GC} and injury. However the normal gestational renal vasodilatation was not seen in the pregnant SHR. This lack of a renal vasodilatory response in the pregnant SHR, despite peripheral vasodilatation (blood pressure falls markedly in pregnancy) [245,246] may reflect a protective mechanism, guarding the maternal kidney.

Experimentally produced hypertension

Attempts to produce a model of 'pre-eclampsia' by superimposition of pregnancy on a range of experimentally induced or genetic hypertensive states in the rats have been unsuccessful, and pregnancy in hypertensive rodents is usually powerfully antihypertensive [239,245]. In fact, there are few viable models of pre-eclampsia in quadrupeds, as reviewed recently [247]. In the model of systemic hypertension with renal disease produced by chronic NOS inhibition (see above) renal and peripheral vasodilatation as well as plasma volume expansion were absent, blood pressure remained elevated and proteinuria developed at term. Our original observation has subsequently been confirmed by many researchers [248]. Thus, an intact NO system appears to be essential for expression of the antihypertensive response to pregnancy. Indeed, in the SHR the marked antihypertensive response to pregnancy is due to enhanced NO production [249].

Immune-mediated glomerular disease

In a rat model of antiglomerular basement membrane glomerulonephritis [250] characterized by significant proteinuria with high P_{GC}, pregnancy was not acutely harmful. Despite the underlying glomerulonephritis, moderate renal vasodilatation occurred in mid-pregnancy withincreases in RPF but without further increasing P_{GC} [250]. There was no difference in proteinuria and glomerular damage in non-pregnant and pregnant rats. The F × 1A1A antibody produces Heymann nephritis, a model of membranous glomerulonephritis, with sustained and very heavy proteinuria, mild impairment in glomerular function and high P_{GC} [251]. Pregnancy normalized P_{GC} due predominantly to increased preglomerular tone. Although proteinuria remained unchanged there were substantial decrements in GFR and SNGFR, with marked functional impairment by late pregnancy [252]. Thus, in this model of membranous glomerulonephritis, pregnancy and underlying renal disease interacted negatively.

Endotoxin administration in pregnancy

Administration of low-dose bacterial endotoxin was uneventful in virgin females but produced moderate hypertension, proteinuria, low platelet counts and glomerular thrombosis when administered to pregnant rats. This was later confirmed and a role for arginine deficiency, leading to inadequate antiaggregatory NO was suggested [253]. A role for superoxide anion, perhaps secondary to activation of the cyclo-oxygenase enzyme has also been reported [254, 255].

Adriamycin nephropathy

A dose of adriamycin that has minimal impact on blood pressure, renal function and renal histology in virgin rats, is associated with hypertension, heavy proteinuria and decrease in GFR when pregnancy is superimposed [256]. Widespread endothelial dysfunction has been implicated with disturbances in both cyclo-oxygenase products and in the NO system [256–259]. Of note, superimposed pregnancies also produced a long-term, significant and irreversible worsening of the renal disease, characterized by a marked mesangial expansion [260]. Considering adriamycin nephrosis is not associated with glomerular hypertension in male rats [261], and in view of the failure of the kidney to vasodilate in pregnant rats given adriamycin [256], it is unlikely that the adverse interaction with pregnancy in this model is haemodynamically mediated, although this remains to be tested.

Chronic hyperinsulinaemia/diabetes

Pre-eclamptic women have high insulin levels [262] and hyperinsulinaemia and insulin resistance are often seen in non-pregnant patients with essential hypertension [263]. In rats, experimentally induced chronic hyperinsulinaemia in pregnancy has been shown to cause hypertension close to term, possibly due to reduced NO production, although renal haemodynamics were not deranged [264]. In contrast, a recent report has shown that hypoinsulinaemic rats, with experimentally induced type I diabetes (with streptozotocin) show an augmented, NO-dependent renal vasodilatation when pregnancy is superimposed [265].

In summary, short- and long-term responses of pregnancy with underlying maternal renal disease are quite variable. In none of the models studied is there any evidence of a pregnancy-induced increment in glomerular blood pressure although alterations in endothelial factors, particularly NO, are a consistent feature.

Renal disease and pregnancy: some conclusions

1 A balance must be struck between pregnancy outcome and the impact pregnancy has in the long term [95,200]. Crucial determinants are pre-pregnancy renal functional status, the absence or presence of hypertension (and its management) and the kidney lesion itself, as well as better fetal surveillance, more timely delivery and improvements in neonatal care (see Tables 7.3 and 7.7).

2 Once a renal disease patient always a renal disease patient. If a woman with chronic renal disease wishes to have children, the sooner she sets about it the better, because renal function will in any case diminish with age.

3 Absence of severe hypertension or renal insufficiency before pregnancy is favourable. If dysfunction is moderate, there is still a fair chance that pregnancy will succeed, but the risks are much greater (see Table 7.3).

4 Type of renal disease will influence outcome. Pregnancy outcome in the presence of focal glomerulosclerosis, MPGN the collagen disorders and IgA and reflux nephropathies is controversial.

5 Review of medication is essential.

6 Proteinuria is common during pregnancy (up to 3 g/24 h) but little is known about the longer-term implications of the increased protein trafficking within the kidney [141].

7 Severe hypertension is a much greater adverse feature than low but stable renal function. Beware of controlling a sign without modifying the basic disorder.

8 Pre-eclampsia cannot be diagnosed clinically with certainty.

9 Deteriorating renal function, even without hypertension, is ominous.

Urinary tract disorders of pregnancy

Asymptomatic bacteriuria

In this condition, also labelled covert bacteriuria, true bacteriuria exists but there are no symptoms or signs of acute UTI (see also Chapter 16).

DIAGNOSTIC PITFALLS

Pregnant women often complain of or will admit to symptoms of urgency, frequency, dysuria and nocturia, occurring singly or in combination. These symptoms are not in themselves diagnostic of UTI and can be elicited from women with sterile urine.

Urine collection and examination

The growth of bacteria on qualitative culture of a urine specimen may represent either true bacteriuria (the multiplication of bacteria within the urinary tract) or contamination of the urine with urethral or perineal organisms at the time of collection. True bacteriuria can be separated from contamination on the basis of colony counts from a freshly obtained midstream urine specimen (MSU), with 100 000 colonies/mL of urine as the dividing line [266]. Two consecutive clean-voided specimens containing the same organism in numbers greater than 100 000 colonies/mL of urine represents true bacteriuria, as does a single suprapubic aspiration with any bacterial growth [267,268].

The use of the clean-catch or clean-void technique is satisfactory provided each clinic determines the number of cultures needed to achieve a 95% or greater level of confidence that bacteriuria exists [269,270]. The use of antiseptic solutions for vulval cleansing should be avoided as contamination of the urine may result in a false-negative culture [271]. A plain soap solution or distilled water is satisfactory.

A number of presumptive tests based on changes in chemical indicators are available but the dependability of these varies greatly [272].

Recent studies raise the possibility that women with more than usual glycosuria in pregnancy may have sustained renal tubular damage from earlier untreated UTI, even though the women may be no longer bacteriuric when pregnant [273]. Why infection might cause an alteration in the renal handling of glucose is not known. Certainly infection can impair distal tubular function, as evidenced by reduced urine concentrating ability, a manifestation of tubular dysfunction that is reversed once infection is eradicated. However, with regard to the renal handling of glucose, full recovery may not occur.

Site of infection

Asymptomatic bacteriuria is a heterogenous condition and several different approaches have attempted to differentiate between upper and lower UTI [79,274]. Ureteric catheterization, bladder washout techniques, renal biopsy, urinary concentration tests, determination of serum antibody titres and identification of antibody-coated bacteria in the urine have all been tried [149,262,275–278]. No single test is sufficiently precise, however, to give complete confidence in localizing the site of infection.

Source of infection

It is probable that bacteria originate from the large bowel and colonize the urinary tract transperineally. By far the most common infecting organism is *Escherichia coli*, which is responsible for 75–90% of bacteriuria during pregnancy. Other organisms frequently responsible for urinary tract infection include *Klebsiella*, *Proteus*, coagulase-negative staphylococci and *Pseudomonas*.

The stasis associated with ureteropelvic dilatation and/or partial ureteric obstruction, increased nutrient content of the urine and the presence of potential pathogens are present in most gravidas [279], yet only a small minority develop bacteriuria. Susceptible women may differ immunologically from those who resist infection: they are less likely to express antibody to the O antigen of *E. coli* on the vaginal epithelium and may display less effective leucocyte activity against the organism. Bacteria isolated from asymptomatic bacteriuria have certain characteristics (e.g. 58% have type 1 fimbria) that differentiate them from bacteria causing lower or upper UTI or from intestinal contaminants [280].

CLINICAL IMPLICATIONS

Incidence

The reservoir of young women with asymptomatic bacteriuria acquired during childhood has been estimated at 5% but only 1.2% are infected at any one time. The incidence increases after puberty coincident with sexual activity and varies from 2% to 10% depending on the techniques employed for testing and the socioeconomic status of the patients [268,281]. There is some evidence to suggest that prophylactic antibiotics given to schoolgirls with asymptomatic bacteriuria prevent subclinical renal damage [282], which would in any case only be unmasked by the physiological demands of pregnancy.

In pregnancy, true asymptomatic bacteriuria is invariably diagnosed at the first antenatal visit if tested for at that time and <1.5% subsequently acquire bacteriuria in late pregnancy. One antenatal study [283], in which 99% of women took part in at least one screening, indicated that the risk of onset of bacteriuria was highest between the ninth and 17th weeks of gestation. The 16th week was the optimal time for a single screen for bacteriuria, calculated on the numbers of bacteria-free gestational weeks gained by treatment.

It must be remembered that asymptomatic bacteriuria is more common in women with a renal transplant or with diabetes mellitus. In the former, 4–60% is the variable proportion of women who screen positive, more common in the first 3–4 months post-transplant but this is a time when women are advised against pregnancy anyway (see below). In diabetic women the incidence is three times higher than in the normal female population and is not influenced by the quality of diabetic control. Factors such as bladder dysfunction due to autonomic nerve dysfunction and defective polymorphonuclear leucocyte function are likely to contribute [284].

Importance of diagnosis

It is important to identify and treat the infected group because up to 40% develop acute symptomatic urinary tract infection [285]. Treating this group should prevent approximately 70% of all cases of acute UTI (Fig. 7.6).

The need for and cost-effectiveness of routine screening for bacteriuria in pregnancy, however, have been seriously questioned [269]. It is known that 2% of those with negative cultures will also develop acute infections. Thus, of the 90–98% that do not have asymptomatic bacteriuria at the booking visit (and therefore will not be treated) the number actually at risk of developing an acute UTI is quite significant and accounts for about 30% of all cases of acute UTI in pregnancy.

A positive history of previous UTI may be almost as effective as screening in predicting UTI in pregnancy [286]. Furthermore, the combination of bacteriuria with a history of urinary tract infection gives the most accurate prediction. Such women are at 10 times greater risk than those with neither feature, and four times greater risk than those with asymptomatic bacteriuria alone.

Any other postulated benefits of eradication of asymptomatic bacteriuria are unsubstantiated. The available data suggest that the association of asymptomatic bacteriuria and increased fetal loss, prematurity, pre-eclampsia and anaemia are unproved [79,272,287,288]. Several of these apparent correlations may have resulted from inaccuracies in matching cases and controls and none appears to be supported by recent studies [66,289]. However, when evidence of previous parenchymal damage is present there may be a great propensity to hypertension [290]. Also there is good evidence of an association between any type of UTI in pregnancy and sudden unexpected infant death [291].

Some 30–40% of pregnant women with asymptomatic bacteriuria may have upper (renal) UTI, and these women

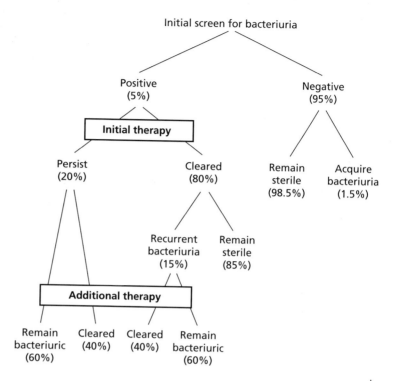

Fig 7.6 Natural history of asymptomatic bacteriuria and effects of treatment in pregnancy. Approximate percentages are given in parentheses

may be a special population at greatest risk of pregnancy problems as well as of acute UTI.

This assumption has been questioned by a study specifically designed to determine what adverse effects asymptomatic renal bacteriuria had on maternal and fetal well-being [292]. In a prospective study, pregnancy outcomes in women with treated asymptomatic bacteriuria of renal origin (diagnosed by the antibody-coated bacteria technique, with a 20% false-positive rate) were compared to outcomes in those with treated bladder bacteriuria as well as non-infected control subjects. Women with asymptomatic renal bacteriuria appeared to be at no greater risk than abacteriuric women of developing pregnancy problems, nor were their progeny at greater risk. Nevertheless, even though the impact of asymptomatic renal infection on ultimate pregnancy outcome is minimal, the need for screening for and eradication of asymptomatic bacteriuria in order to prevent pyelonephritis is still important. This study [292] also reconfirmed the fact that symptomatic infections may be implicated in delivery of low-birthweight infants when acute pyelonephritis complicates preterm labour, suggesting a causal role in its initiation.

Where underlying undiagnosed chronic pyelonephritis is present this could be responsible for the reported obstetric complications and increased perinatal losses.

Choice of drug

The choice of drug must be based on the sensitivity of the isolated organism(s). Short-acting sulphonamides or nitrofurantoin derivatives are often the initial therapy [272,293]. Other drugs are reserved for treatment of failures and for symptomatic infection. Ampicillin and the cephalosporins can be safely used in pregnancy. Tetracyclines are contraindicated because of staining of the teeth of infants by binding with orthophosphates, as well as the rare maternal complication of acute fatty liver of pregnancy if they are given parenterally (see Chapter 9). If sulphonamides are prescribed in late pregnancy they should be withheld during the last 2–3 weeks since they compete with bilirubin for albumin binding sites, increasing the risk of fetal hyperbilirubinaemia and kernicterus. Nitrofurantoin used during the last few weeks may precipitate haemolytic anaemia due to glucose-6-phosphate dehydrogenase deficiency in the newborn. Trimethoprim, a constituent of Bactrim and Septrin, is not recommended for use in pregnancy because it is a folic acid antagonist. Nevertheless, it is extensively used and probably safe, although not a drug of first choice.

Interestingly a prospective placebo-controlled trial has shown that in non-pregnant women, cranberry juice, an old folk medicine, effectively reduces pyuria and bacteriuria. Furthermore, substances in the juice of cranberries and other related species such as condensed tannins prevent the adhesion of *E. coli* to human uroepithelial cells. More specific agents interfering with bacterial adhesion may emerge in the future [294].

Duration of therapy

Opinions on optimal duration of therapy differ. Continuous antibiotic therapy from the time of diagnosis until after delivery has been recommended because of the belief that renal parenchymal involvement causes a high relapse rate. However, at least 60% of patients have bladder involvement alone and the administration of short-term therapy (2 weeks) should be satisfactory. Furthermore, if patient follow-up is meticulous, there is no advantage in using continuous long-term administration of antibiotics, and the possible hazards of such therapy to the fetus are avoided. Urine cultures should be obtained 1 week after therapy is discontinued and then at regular intervals throughout the pregnancy.

Relapses and reinfections

Relapse is the recurrence of bacteriuria caused by the same organism, usually within 6 weeks of the initial infection. Reinfection is the recurrence of bacteriuria involving a different strain of bacteria, after successful eradication of the initial infection [295]. Most patients with reinfections have infections limited to the bladder, usually occurring at least 6 weeks after therapy.

Approximately 15% of patients will have a recurrence during pregnancy and a second course of treatment should be given, based on a repeat culture with sensitivity testing. In the group of patients who relapse or who are resistant to the first course of therapy, only about 40% will have the asymptomatic bacteriuria cleared with subsequent therapy [296]. Since *E. coli* causes the majority of initial infections as well as recurrences, it may be necessary to employ an *E. coli* serotyping system to precisely distinguish different stains, although this does not help in clinical management.

Long-term considerations

As the interval between treatment of bacteriuria in pregnancy and postpartum follow-up becomes longer, the influence of the initial course of treatment on the incidence of bacteriuria becomes less noticeable [272]. Ten or more years after an initial episode of bacteriuria of pregnancy, the prevalence of bacteriuria in women not treated during pregnancy (25%) is virtually the same as in those women who were treated (29%). In contrast, women who have never been bacteriuric during pregnancy have rates of bacteriuria of about 5%. Thus, a single course of treatment during the index pregnancy does not appear to protect against persistent or recurrent bacteriuria years later. There are few prospective studies available, but there is no evidence that persistent asymptomatic bacteriuria in women with normal urinary tracts causes long-term renal damage or that treatment reduces the incidence of chronic renal disease [287].

Postpartum intravenous urography

There is no consensus of opinion regarding the need for postpartum IVU in patients who have had bacteriuria [297]. It is known that 20% of all patients with asymptomatic bacteriuria have IVU abnormalities [298] and this percentage is increased amongst patients with acute infections during pregnancy or with infections that have been difficult to eradicate [299].

The significance of an IVU abnormality is not so certain [300]. It may signify a predisposition to infection; it may result from infection or it may be unrelated to infection. Most abnormalities are minor and probably do not result from or cause renal infection. Furthermore, the role of infection in childhood, as indicated by scars on the IVU, is controversial [299].

In order to detect about 90% of the women with major urinary tract abnormalities or to document a non-obstructed urinary tract, an IVU should be performed in women who have asymptomatic bacteriuria during pregnancy who fulfil the following additional criteria:
1 difficulty in eradicating the bacteriuria during the pregnancy;
2 episode(s) of acute symptomatic UTI during the pregnancy;
3 history of acute infection(s) prior to the index pregnancy;
4 persistence/recurrence of asymptomatic bacteriuria or acute infection postpartum.
Those patients who do have major abnormalities demonstrated postpartum are more likely to require careful long-term follow-up for eradication of bacteriuria rather than surgery. However, a non-functioning kidney may be removed and major drainage anomalies may be corrected.

Acute symptomatic urinary tract infection

Where there is symptomatic UTI, two clinical syndromes are recognized: lower UTI or cystitis and upper UTI or acute pyelonephritis. The latter is the most common renal complication of pregnancy occurring in 1–2% of all pregnancies. It has been blamed as a cause of intrauterine growth restriction, congenital abnormalities, fetal death and can certainly cause premature labour [274,287,288, 292,301]. UTI may also occur in the puerperium, antecedent risk factors include placental abruptions, pre-eclampsia–eclampsia or renal disease, all of which are associated with catheterization, as are tocolysis and caesarean section which also predispose to postdelivery UTI [302].

ACUTE CYSTITIS

This occurs in about 1% of pregnant women of whom 60% have a negative initial screen. The symptoms are often difficult to distinguish from those due to pregnancy itself. Features indicating a true infection include haematuria, dysuria and suprapubic discomfort, as well as a positive urine culture. The spectrum of organisms found is the same as in women with asymptomatic bacteriuria (see above). Similar treatment is recommended with the aims of abolishing symptoms and preventing occurrence of acute pyelonephritis.

ACUTE PYELONEPHRITIS

The differential diagnosis includes other urinary tract pathology, other causes of pyrexia such as respiratory tract infection, viraemia, listeriosis (see Chapter 16) or toxoplasmosis (appropriate serological screening should be performed) and other causes of acute abdominal pain such as acute appendicitis, biliary colic, gastroenteritis, necrobiosis of a uterine fibroid or placental abruption. Always ask about a history of vesicoureteral reflux surgery in childhood because there is an increased risk of UTI in these women in pregnancy; to such an extent that some recommend the use of prophylactic antibiotics [303].

Pneumonia on the affected side should present no difficulties if attention is paid to the type of respiration, the respiratory rate and the physical signs in the chest. It should be noted, however, that so-called adult respiratory distress syndrome (ARDS), with accompanying liver and haematopoietic dysfunction, can be a significant complication of pyelonephritis [223,304]. These problems are all probably due to lipopolysaccharide-induced red cell membrane damage [305].

Acute appendicitis can be a difficult diagnosis to make, especially in the third trimester. Usually at the onset of appendicitis the pain is referred to the centre of the abdomen, vomiting is not a marked feature, the pyrexia is not as high as in acute pyelonephritis, and rigors rarely occur.

Once the diagnosis of pyelonephritis is considered, an MSU sample should be sent for culture and sensitivities.

Antibiotic treatment should be aggressive and must be undertaken in a hospital setting. It should be started once the diagnosis has been made and before the sensitivities are available. If the patient is dehydrated, due to vomiting and sweating, then intravenous fluids should be given. The use of tepid sponging and antipyretic drugs such as paracetamol may reduce the incidence of premature labour.

Regular assessment of renal function should be undertaken: although the infective attack is said to have little effect on renal function in non-pregnant patients, such attacks during pregnancy have been observed to cause transient but marked decrements in GFR [306]. Ultrasonographic examination of the renal tract of pregnant women with pyelonephritis has revealed significantly increased pelvicalyceal dilatation compared to normal physiological dilatation of pregnancy, but as treatment does not produce a consistent decrease, the anomaly may antedate the acute infection [198].

CHOICE AND DURATION OF THERAPY

Dogmatic statements cannot be justified regarding the type of antimicrobial therapy for acute UTI and the appropriate duration of regimens is also debatable [272]. Treatment should aim at giving the most effective drug to eradicate a particular infection without exposing the fetus to an unnecessarily harmful agent.

Antibiotics producing high blood levels and resultant high renal parenchymal concentrations are favoured, although the importance of these factors is still undetermined [307]. Two suitable groups of antibiotics are the broad-spectrum penicillins, for example ampicillin, and the cephalosporins; E. coli is the most common organism isolated in urinary infections and is usually sensitive to either of them. Trimethoprim/sulphonamide combinations, such as Septrin, are also used (see above). Aminoglycosides, such as kanamycin and gentamicin, can be given if there are problems with microbial resistance. Treatment should be monitored by blood levels. Whilst the patient is febrile, it is preferable to give intravenous antibiotics, which can be continued orally when the pyrexia has settled. Antibiotic sensitivities should be reviewed within 48 h.

The duration of treatment should be 2–3 weeks. In patients showing clinical deterioration or whose urine cultures reveal bacteria resistant to the selected antibiotic, repeat urine cultures are mandatory and alternative antibiotic therapy should be considered. In ill patients blood culture specimens should be taken. After the completion of the course of treatment urine cultures should be taken at every antenatal visit for the rest of the pregnancy.

Inpatient or outpatient treatment for acute pyelonephritis remains a vexed question tackled by a new study [308]. After ensuring that there was a prompt response to treatment in the first 24 h when hospitalized and that the women would be compliant if discharged, women were randomized to continuing inpatient or outpatient management. Of 246 women beyond 24 weeks' gestation with UTI, 151 were not eligible for randomization because of a variety of reasons including preterm delivery.

GRAM-NEGATIVE SEPSIS

This can occur in severely ill patients with acute pyelonephritis but the situation is commonly associated with instrumentation of an infected urinary tract. An aminoglycoside antibiotic is best because it is effective against nearly all of the Gram-negative urinary bacteria. Enterococci less commonly cause bacteraemia but because of resistance to aminoglycosides ampicillin can be used combined with an aminoglycoside until culture results are available. Patients who are sensitive to penicillin should receive a cephalosporin. Haematological aspects of the management of Gram-negative sepsis are considered in Chapter 3.

PERINATAL CONSIDERATIONS

Numerous studies in the last 30 years have reported links between urinary infections during pregnancy and adverse outcomes such as preterm birth. The difficulty of performing controlled studies in humans has promoted the development of animal models. In a murine model of UTI there was invariably histological evidence of metritis [309]. This is of importance in terms of uterine activity, which until now was thought to be associated with systemically mediated 'toxic' mechanisms.

Another possible association with UTI in pregnancy is the link with cognitive function in infancy. In a recent cohort study, 41 090 Medicaid-linked maternal and infant records were analysed together with collected and non-collected prescriptions. In the 23% of women without antibiotics there was a significant association between maternal UTI and mental retardation in childhood. Furthermore, the fetal death rate was 5.2% compared to no deaths in the group where antibiotics were taken [310].

Acute renal failure in pyelonephritis is discussed later.

Haematuria during pregnancy

The excretion of red blood cells increases (and one to two red cells per high-power field may be acceptable in the urine of pregnant women) but whether leucocyturia occurs is unclear [311]. Spontaneous gross or microscopic haematuria can be due to a variety of causes [312]. UTIs, particularly those associated with congenital anomalies, are difficult to eradicate and predispose to haematuria, especially if pyelonephritis is present. Rupture of small veins about the dilated renal pelvis may also cause bleeding. Spontaneous or traumatic rupture of the kidney can occur, usually where there are underlying anatomical abnormalities [313]. Spontaneous non-traumatic renal rupture, however, is very rare. Acute glomerulonephritis has been discussed earlier.

Haematuria may be secondary to any type of primary neoplasm, metastatic neoplasms, haemangiomata, calculi or fungal diseases involving the urinary system. Endometriosis, inflammatory bowel lesions, leukoplakia, amyloidosis and granulomata may involve the urinary tract and produce haematuria [314]. The ureteral stump after a nephrectomy (for either benign or malignant disease) may be involved by any of the aforementioned conditions and should be investigated.

An aggressive approach to evaluation is needed. This may be deferred until after delivery but the clinician should assess all the circumstances to decide whether or not it takes absolute priority. Until recently the general consensus was that in the absence of any demonstrable cause, haematuria can be classified as idiopathic with recurrences unlikely in the current or subsequent pregnancy [315,316]. However, it has been suggested that haematuria is associated with an increased likelihood of adverse maternal outcomes including preterm labour and pre-eclampsia [317]. From a retrospective case–controlled study, such women had an eightfold increased risk of pre-eclampsia and the mean duration from the dipstick detection of haematuria to diagnosis was 11.1 weeks.

Acute hydronephrosis and hydroureter

Very occasionally pregnancy can precipitate acute hydronephrosis or hydroureter. There is a broad spectrum of the so-called 'overdistension syndrome' [273,307]. Obstruction may occur at varying levels at or above the pelvic brim (Table 7.15). This condition is not to be confused with the massive ureteral and renal pelvic dilatations (as well as slight reduction in cortical width) that can occasionally occur in normal pregnancy without ill-effect [318]. Women who have had surgery for vesicoureteric reflux in childhood (especially bilaterally) can develop distal ureteral obstruction even in early pregnancy, which can masquerade as pre-eclampsia and/or renal failure [103].

Table 7.15 Clinical entities associated with pregnancy-induced urinary tract dilatation.

Clinical entity	Clinical features
Overdistension syndrome	Flank pain, renal colic
Pyelonephritis	Flank pain, fever, bacteriuria
Urinary tract rupture:	
Retroperitoneal	
parenchymal	Flank pain
	Mass: abscess, haematoma
	Anaemia/hypotension due to blood loss
	Haematuria
collecting system	Flank pain
	Mass: perinephric or subcapsular urinoma
	Haematuria (microscopic)
Intraperitoneal	
parenchymal	Peritonitis
collecting system	Flank pain
	Anaemia/hypotension due to blood loss
	Haematuria

The condition should be suspected when there are recurrent episodes of loin or low abdominal pain radiating to the groin and repeat MSU specimens are sterile. There may be small increments in plasma creatinine levels but urinalysis contains few or no red cells and repeat MSU specimens are negative. Diagnosis can be confirmed using excretory urography or ultrasound (no evidence of stone) and ureteral catheterization. If positioning the patient on the unaffected side (with antibiotic therapy if appropriate) fails to relieve the situation, then ureteral catheterization (stenting) or nephrostomy may be required. Typically, the pain is immediately relieved by ureteric catheterization or sonographically guided percutaneous nephrotomy so that corrective surgery can be delayed until the postpartum period [212,319,320].

Non-traumatic rupture of the urinary tract

The intrusion of unremitting pain and haematuria upon the course of pyelonephritis or the 'overdistension syndrome' suggests rupture of the urinary tract (Table 7.16). Furthermore, this complication can masquerade as other obstetric and surgical abdominal catastrophes, including appendicitis, pelvic abscess, cholecystitis, urolithiasis (see later) or abruptio placentae. Prompt recognition may prevent a small tear and urine leak, treatable by postural or tube drainage, from extending and/or expanding. Rupture of the renal parenchyma, with haemorrhagic shock, formation of a flank mass or dissection of urinary tract contents intraperitoneally compels prompt surgical intervention, usually with nephrectomy [307].

Pregnancy in renal transplant patients

The abnormal reproductive function and sexual disorders of haemodialysed women are usually reversed after renal transplantation. (The option of sterilization should not have been offered at this time.) The resumption of regular menstruation and ovulation correlate closely with the level of function achieved by the graft [118,321,322]. With the increase in the number of transplanted women of childbearing age and more recently those with pancreatic grafts [323], clinicians must now both counsel such patients as to whether or not they should conceive and also manage the pregnancies of those who do. It has been estimated that one of every 50 women of childbearing age who have a functional renal transplant will become pregnant [324]. There are now well over 14 000 pregnancies reported worldwide. Two new registries, one in the USA and the other in the UK are accruing data on complications and outcomes against the background of changing transplantation medical practice and immunosuppressive regimens [325–328].

Recent reviews of such pregnancies have emphasized the difficulty in assessing the exact incidence of the various management problems because some of the data in the literature are incomplete and many more pregnancies than those reported have occurred [77,112,325,326,329–343]. Excluding the large Denver series [344] where 75% of patients had received kidneys from living donors, only 20% of births occurred in recipients of living donor grafts. Transplants have been performed with surgeons unaware that the allograft recipient was in fact pregnant, and obstetric success in such cases does not negate the importance of contraception counselling for

Traumatic	Precipitating factor: trauma
Non-traumatic	
parenchymal	Congenital: tuberose sclerosis
	Tumour, especially hamartoma
	Pyelonephritis or abscess
	Vasculitis (polyarteritis nodosa)
	Cystic disease
non-parenchymal (obstructive)	Urolithiasis
	Reflux, stricture
	Infection

Table 7.16 Factors contributing to rupture of the urinary tract.

all renal failure patients including the exclusion of pregnancy prior to transplantation [345]. New data from established registries are very helpful to the clinician with regard to simple epidemiological queries (Table 7.17).

Pregnancy counselling

Management should start by counselling all couples who want a child, with a discussion of the implications of pregnancy as well as long-term prospects.

Pre-pregnancy assessment

Individual centres have their own specific guidelines. Most advise a wait of about 2 years post-transplant. This has turned out to be good advice because the patient will have recovered from the major surgical sequelae by then and renal function will have stabilized with a very high probability of allograft survival at 5 years [339]. Immunosuppression will also be at maintenance levels, which may account for higher birthweight babies in mothers becoming pregnant 2 years post-transplant as opposed

to in those conceiving earlier. In one series the mean birthweight was 2.9 kg in 18 pregnancies conceived on average 60 months after transplantation, compared to 1.7 kg in seven similar pregnancies conceived 16 months after transplantation [87].

Given is a list of suitability criteria [346], the absence of some of which is only a relative contraindication to pregnancy.

1 Good general health for 2 years after transplantation.

2 Stature compatible with good obstetric outcome.

3 No proteinuria.

4 No significant hypertension: due to the high incidence of hypertension in patients taking cyclosporine 'well-controlled hypertension' may be more appropriate. As well as drug effects, other causes of post-transplant hypertension include re-emergence of the original renal pathology, transplant renal artery stenosis and chronic rejection.

5 No evidence of graft rejection.

6 No evidence of pelvicalyceal distension on a recent excretory urogram.

7 Plasma creatinine of 180 µmol/L or less and preferably less than 125 µmol/L.

8 Drug therapy: prednisone 15 mg/day or less and

Table 7.17 UK National Transplantaion Pregnancy Registry (NTPR). Analysis of 261 recipients in 377 pregnancies (385 outcomes). Modified from Armenti *et al* 1998.

Maternal data	(%)	Outcomes	
Hypertension	62	Therapeutic abortion	9%
Pre-eclampsia	27	Spontaneous abortion	13%
Infection	22	Ectopic pregnancy	0.5%
Diabetes	12	Total first trimester loss ($n = 89$)	22.5%
Serum creatinine (mean) µmol/L		Pregnancies beyond 1st trimester ($n = 296$)	
Before	125	Live births	97%
During	115	Stillbirths	2%
After	142	Neonatal deaths	1%
		Caesarean section	51%
Graft dysfunction	12	Mean gestational age	35.8 w
Rejection	4	Mean birthweight	2.64 kg
Graft loss <2yr post delivery	7	Newborn complications	38%

azathioprine 2 mg/kg/day or less. A safe dose of cyclosporine is probably 2–4 mg/kg/day but with the introduction of new preparations with improved bioavailability and more predictable pharmacokinetics new appraisals are needed. There are only limited data for the most recent immunosuppressives (see below).

After full pre-pregnancy assessment, advice can be given, but it can only be advice, because patients must ultimately decide for themselves what degree of risk is acceptable. If the situation is tackled prospectively the final decision is more of an agreement than a judgement.

Long-term considerations and allograft survival

The ultimate measure of transplant success is the long-term survival of the patient and the graft. As it is only just over 35 years since this procedure became widely employed in the management of end-stage renal failure, there are few long-term data from sufficiently large series from which to draw conclusions. Furthermore, it must be emphasized that the long-term results for renal transplants relate to a period when several aspects of management would be unacceptable by present-day standards. Average survival figures of large numbers of patients worldwide indicate that 95% of recipients of kidneys from related living donors are alive 10 years after transplantation and with cadaver kidneys the figure is 60% [77,347–349]. Survival is increased if renal function is normal 2 years post-transplant, and this is probably the optimal time to contemplate pregnancy.

Even after transplantation and the joy of newfound health, everyday life still has a baseline of uncertainty. Nevertheless, many patients will choose parenthood in an effort to renew a normal life and possibly in defiance of the sometimes negative attitudes of the medical and nursing establishments. Psychologists are becoming more interested in why women in such circumstances get pregnant and what actually causes such overwhelming maternalism. The so-called 'burning building syndrome' [119] defines a maternal rashness and/or obsession, and attempts to distinguish between pathological and healthy levels of assumed risk. Couples should be aware of all implications including the harsh realities of maternal survival prospects. A major concern is that even in the medium term the mother may not survive or remain well enough to rear the child she bears.

Pregnancy does not necessarily cause irreversible decline in renal function or affect the natural history of the allograft [350,351]. The first proper study (in 1983), albeit on a very small scale, concluded that pregnancy had no effect on graft survival or function [352]. Data from the Registry of the European Dialysis and Transplant Association (EDTA) limited to approximately 3 years postpregnancy follow-up did not reveal any adverse influence of pregnancy on graft function [335]. Of interest is a survey that contained a considerable number of women in the 'poorer prognosis' category (hypertension, moderate renal insufficiency and long-standing diabetes mellitus): 18 women who underwent 34 pregnancies post-transplant were compared in case–controlled analysis with 18 allograft recipients who had never conceived. In a post-transplant follow-up in each group averaging 12 years (with a mean time from initial pregnancy of 5 years) there was no significant difference in GFR (inulin clearance or prevalence of hypertension) [353] (Fig. 7.7). These data are now contested by another study [354] based on plasma creatinine levels, which suggests that pregnancy could significantly jeopardize allografts.

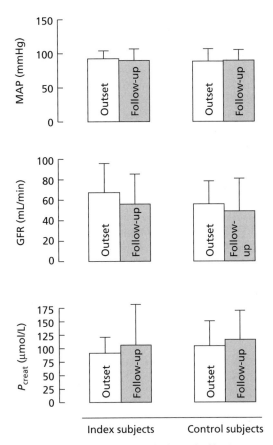

Fig 7.7 Mean arterial pressure (MAP), glomerular filtration rate (GFR) (inulin clearance) and P_{creat} (plasma creatinine) in renal transplant recipients ($n = 18$) who underwent pregnancy (index subjects) compared to control subjects ($n = 18$) who never conceived. Open bars ($\pm$ SEM) at onset just after transplantation and closed bars at end of follow-up, averaging 12 years. (Modified from [353].)

However, the significance of this study is derived from the very unusual feature that the control group suffered no graft failures in 10 years [351].

In a recent UK single-centre analysis of 33 pregnancies in 29 women the absence of chronic rejection and proteinuria (<1 g/day) pre-pregnancy were good prognosticators. Without exception all women with serum creatinine >200 fmol/L had progression of renal impairment and required dialysis within 2 years of delivery [355]. Analysis of 194 pregnancies from Japan revealed allograft deterioration in 20% after delivery [343]. Interestingly, women transplanted for renal failure secondary to lupus nephritis can successfully maintain a pregnancy with outcomes comparable to those of renal recipients who did not have SLE pathology and no differences in longer-term graft loss [356].

Reviews of the literature indicate that about 12% of women will have new long-term medical problems after pregnancy, although it is difficult to know whether such problems are merely time related or actually precipitated by pregnancy (Table 7.18) [77,331,347]. Interestingly, the incidence of later problems is doubled (25%) if pregnancy complications occur prior to the 28th week. Registry data indicate that 10% of mothers die within 1–7 years following childbirth. More long-term studies are needed to assess this (especially with the advent of the new immunosuppressive drugs), so that counselling is thorough and based on recorded experience and not clinical anecdote.

Management of renal transplant recipient in pregnancy (Box 7.3)

At the outset certain facts emerge from the literature [112,326,331]. About 25% of all conceptions do not go beyond the first trimester mainly because of therapeutic and spontaneous abortions. The overall complication rate in pregnancies going beyond the first trimester is 49% (Table 7.18). If complications (usually uncontrolled hypertension, renal deterioration or rejection) occur prior to the

---

Box 7.3 Renal transplants: pregnancy management

- Hospital-based antenatal care in conjunction with nephrologists
- Surveillance of renal function
- Graft rejection
- Hypertension/ pre-eclampsia
- Maternal infection
- Intrauterine growth restriction
- Preterm labour
- Effects of drug therapy on fetus and neonate
- Decision on timing and route of delivery

Table 7.18 Pregnancy prospects for renal allograft recipients. (From [331].)

Problems in pregnancy (%)	Successful obstetric outcome (%)	Problems in long term (%)
49	95 (75)	12 (25)

Estimates based on 5370 women in 7110 pregnancies, which attained at least 28 weeks' gestation (1961–2000). Figures in brackets refer to prospects when complications developed prior to 28 weeks' gestation.

28th gestational week then successful obstetric outcome occurs in 75% compared to 95% when pregnancy is trouble free prior to 28 weeks. Remote problems occur in 12% of women after delivery but where the pregnancy is complicated prior to 28 weeks remote problems occur in 25%, although it is difficult to know whether such problems are precipitated by pregnancy or are time dependent and would have occurred anyway. As to be expected those women with better graft function before pregnancy do much better overall (Table 7.19). This sets the scene.

Antenatal care

Patients must be monitored as high-risk cases. Management requires attention to serial assessment of renal function, diagnosis and treatment of rejection, blood pressure control, prevention or early diagnosis of anaemia, treatment of any infection as well as the meticulous assessment of fetal well-being.

Antenatal visits should be 2–weekly up to 32 weeks and weekly thereafter. At each visit, routine antenatal care should be supplemented with the following:
1 full blood count, including platelets (Coulter counter analysis);
2 blood urea, creatinine, electrolyte and urate levels;
3 24-h creatinine clearance and protein excretion;
4 MSU specimen for microscopy and culture;
5 plasma protein, calcium and phosphate levels [357] and liver function tests should be checked at 6-weekly intervals;
6 cytomegalovirus (CMV) and herpes homini virus (HHV) titres should be checked in each trimester if the initial screen is negative.
If the patient has diabetes mellitus then a very strict management protocol is needed. It is evident that the complication rate is at least double that in other pregnant renal allograft recipients [358,359]. This may relate to the cardiovascular changes that accompany diabetes. The outlook may be considerably better when women have received a pancreas as well as a kidney allograft, and successful preg-

Table 7.19 Pregnancy in renal allograft recipients: prospects and pre-pregnancy renal function.

Renal status	Problems in pregnancy (%)	Successful obstetric outcome (%)	Problems longterm (%)
$S_{cr} < 125$ μmol/L	30	97	7
$S_{cr} < 125$ μmol/L	82	75	27

Estimates (%) based in 5590 women and 7440 pregnancies from 1961–2001 which attained at least 28 weeks gestation. S_{cr} = non-pregnant serum creatinine. (From Davidson, unpublished data.)

nancies are increasing [48,358–361]. In one patient, however, the pancreatic graft was unexpectedly lost in acute rejection immediately after delivery, having functioned normally for 3 years prior to the pregnancy. For the future, the consensus generally is that simultaneous kidney/pancreas transplants are considered to be a treatment of choice for patients with diabetic nephropathy: inevitably such women will be potential mothers [362].

Screening all rhesus (Rh)-negative recipients for Rh antibodies is mandatory. In selecting donors for renal transplantation Rh antigens are usually disregarded because they are found only on red cells and not on leucocytes or other tissue cells. Nevertheless, several cases of Rh antibody response have occurred as a result of sensitization to the transplant and it is possible for these antibodies to contribute to transplant failures because they bind to the allograft. Rh isoimmunization and a rising antibody titre in a pregnant transplant patient could theoretically have serious renal as well as the better-known fetal consequences.

Immunosuppressive therapy is usually maintained at pre-pregnancy levels but adjustments may be needed if there are decreases in the maternal leucocyte and platelet counts, so as to at least ensure that the neonate is born with a normal blood count [363] (Table 7.20). Azathioprine liver toxicity and the rarer interstitial pneumonitis usually respond to dose reduction or changing to cyclosporine therapy, if necessary. Other controversies concerning immunosuppressives in pregnancy will be discussed later (see below).

Dietary counselling

Haematinics, vitamin D and calcium supplements should be prescribed if indicated [364–366]. (Metabolic bone disease in renal failure is mentioned in Chapter 14.) The role of dietary protein in augmenting glomerular function in pregnancy is controversial but it is important in these patients because their kidney is already hypertrophied. It has been suggested that graft failure may be hastened by hyperfiltration [367]. For safe dietary recommendations, more information is urgently needed about the intrarenal effects and the long-term renal sequelae of dietary protein manipulation as well as the effect restriction might have on fetal outcome, particularly central nervous system development.

Early pregnancy problems

Spontaneous abortion occurs in about 15%, the same as for the normal pregnant population. Between 0.2% and 0.5% of all conceptions are ectopic pregnancies. Hydatidiform mole has been reported in a transplant recipient and the potential for malignant transformation is possibly enhanced by immunosuppressive drugs [368]. Ovarian tumours in early pregnancy must be distinguished from pelvic blood vessel anomalies [369].

THERAPEUTIC TERMINATION

This procedure is an obvious option. In fact, 15% of pregnancies are terminated for various indications: psycho-

Table 7.20 Immunosuppressive dose adjustments during pregnancy in renal transplant recipients reported to NTPR.

	CsA 260 pregnancies (%)	Neoral® 59 pregnancies (%)	Tacro 23 pregnancies (%)
Increased	8.9	44	22
Varied	1.9	12	9
Decreased	5.4	0	4
No change	82	32	52
Switch	0	12	9
Discontinued	1	0	4

CsA, Sandoimmune® brand cyclosporine, Neoral®, Neoral® brand cyclosporine; Tacro, tacrolimus, FK506 or Prograf®. Modified from [326].

social problems associated with an unplanned pregnancy, uncertainty about long-term maternal prognosis, renal dysfunction before pregnancy and deteriorating renal function and/or severe hypertension during pregnancy [329].

ECTOPIC PREGNANCY

These patients may be at higher risk of ectopic pregnancy because of pelvic adhesions due to previous urological surgery, peritoneal dialysis or pelvic inflammatory disease. The diagnosis can be difficult because irregular bleeding and amenorrhoea accompany deteriorating renal function or even an intrauterine pregnancy [370]. The main clinical problem is that symptoms secondary to genuine pelvic pathology are erroneously attributed to the transplant.

Allograft function (Fig. 7.8)

Serial surveillance of creatinine clearance is essential. The following points are important.

1 The increase in GFR characteristic of early pregnancy and maintained thereafter is surprisingly also evident in transplant recipients even though the allograft is ectopic, denervated, possibly from an old donor, potentially damaged by previous ischaemia and immunologically different from both recipient and her fetus [346,371,372].

2 The better the renal function before pregnancy, the greater is the increment in GFR during pregnancy. For example in one series the stable problem-free group

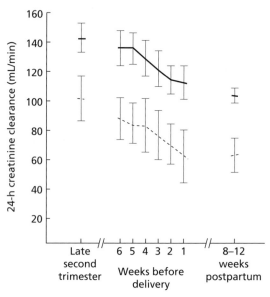

Fig 7.8 Changes in 24-h creatinine clearance in late pregnancy in 10 healthy women (upper) compared to 10 renal allograft recipients (lower) mean ± SEM. (Compiled from data of [579, 580, 14].)

had a mean pre-pregnancy serum creatinine of 80 μmol/L in contrast to 212 μmol/L in the group with problems in pregnancy [373]. Evidence from the US National Transplant Pregnancy Registry (NTPR) is that mean serum creatinine > 125 μmol/L (mean 132 μmol/L relative to a control group of 97 μmol/L) is associated with further decrements during pregnancy as well as more episodes of rejection and/or dysfunction or even graft loss within 2 years of delivery [374]. A report from the UK Registry (National Transplant Database Pregnancy Register) indicates that pregnancy success, defined as a live birth and survival after at least 24 weeks' gestation is above all significantly related to serum creatinine determined within 3 months before pregnancy [328].

3 There can be a transient reduction in GFR during the third trimester [322,375] just as occurs in normal pregnancy [14] and such a change does not necessarily represent a deteriorating situation with permanent impairment.

4 In 15% of patients significant impairment of renal function develops during pregnancy and may persist following delivery [322]. As a gradual decline in allograft function is a common occurrence in non-pregnant patients, it is difficult to delineate the specific role of pregnancy. Subclinical chronic rejection, with declining renal function, may occur as a late result of tissue damage after acute rejection or when immunosuppression has not been adequate.

5 There may be a non-immune contribution to chronic graft failure due to the damaging effect of hyperfiltration through remnant nephrons [367], perhaps even exacerbated during pregnancy (see above).

6 Proteinuria occurs near term in about 40% of patients but disappears postpartum, and in the absence of hypertension is not significant [64]. Pre-pregnancy proteinuria is a different matter as it is associated with a much higher incidence of graft deterioration during and/or after pregnancy [373,376]. The issue of the damaging effect of long-term renal protein trafficking is relevant here [141].

7 If renal function deteriorates by >15% at any stage of pregnancy, reversible causes should be sought such as UTI, subtle dehydration or electrolyte imbalance (occasionally precipitated by inadvertent diuretic therapy); allograft rejection must of course be considered. Inability to detect a treatable cause of a significant functional decrement is a reason to end the pregnancy by elective delivery. When proteinuria occurs and persists, but renal function is preserved and blood pressure is normal, the pregnancy can be allowed to continue.

Allograft rejection

Reviews in the 'azathioprine era' reported rejection episodes in pregnancy in pregnancy and immediately postpartum in 9% of women [377] whereas nowadays in women on cyclosporin regimens it is 4–5%. Tables 7.20 and 7.21 show comparison of pregnancy problems as well as disease-adjusted outcomes for female recipients reported to the NTPR including two of the newer immunosuppressive agents, Neoral (a cyclosporine preparation with improved bioavailability) and tacrolimus [326].

It has been reported that serious rejection episodes occur in 9% of women with pregnancies lasting into the third trimester [377]. Whilst the incidence of rejection is no greater than expected for non-pregnant transplant patients it might be considered unusual because it had always been assumed that the privileged immunological state of pregnancy would benefit the transplant. Furthermore, there are reports of reduction or cessation of immunosuppressive therapy during pregnancy without rejection episodes [378,379].

Chronic rejection may be a problem in all recipients and probably has a progressive subclinical course. If this is somehow influenced by pregnancy there do not appear to be any consistent factors serving to predict which patients will develop rejection episodes, as there is no relationship to prior rejection episodes, HLA types, the transplant–pregnancy time interval or problems in previous pregnancies [380]. The following points are important:

1 rejection at any time is difficult to diagnose;
2 if any of the clinical hallmarks such as fever, oliguria or deteriorating renal function associated with renal enlargement and tenderness are present, then the diagnosis must be considered;
3 ultrasonography can be helpful because alterations in the echogenicity of the renal parenchyma and the presence of an indistinct corticomedullary junction are indicative of rejection [381];
4 without renal biopsy, rejection cannot be distinguished from acute pyelonephritis, recurrent glomerulopathy, possible severe pre-eclampsia and even cyclosporine nephrotoxicity;

5 the diagnosis must be beyond doubt before embarking upon antirejection (rescue) therapy;
6 rejection occasionally occurs in the puerperium [364,379]; and this may be the result of the return to a normal immune state (despite immunosuppression) or possibly a rebound effect from the altered immunoresponsiveness associated with pregnancy.

Hypertension and pre-eclampsia

The appearance of hypertension and proteinuria in the third trimester and their relationship to deteriorating renal function, to the possibility of chronic underlying pathology and to pre-eclampsia are difficult diagnostic problems. Hypertension, particularly before 28 weeks' gestation, is associated with adverse perinatal outcome [382], which may be due to covert cardiovascular changes that accompany or are aggravated by chronic hypertension.

Pre-eclampsia is diagnosed clinically in about 30% of pregnancies and, interestingly, is not related to the chronological age of the donor organ [371]. Although many of the hypertensive syndromes are quite severe, there is only one report of a woman (a primigravida) where there was rapid progress to eclampsia, and interestingly, she subsequently had an uncomplicated successful pregnancy [75,383].

Unlike the situation in normal pregnant women, changes in urinary protein excretion, plasma urate levels, platelet count or liver-function tests do not appear to be useful markers for either the onset or the severity of pre-eclampsia, as all of these parameters can be substantially changed in otherwise uncomplicated pregnancies. The following points are important.
1 Many of the specific risks of hypertension are mediated through superimposed pre-eclampsia, a diagnosis that cannot be made with certainty on clinical grounds alone, because proteinuria, hypertension and renal deterioration may be manifestations of underlying transplant dysfunction or even rejection.

	CSA	Neoral®	Tacro
Livebirths (n)	350	57	17
Gestational age (weeks)	35.9	35	33
Birthweight (mean) (g)	2485	2449	2151
Premature (<37 weeks)	52	52	63
Low birthweight (<2500g)	46	54	63
Caesarean section	51	48	44
Newborn compications	40	49	53
Neonatal deaths (within 30 days of birth)	1	0	6

Table 7.21 424 Livebirth outcomes (% unless otherwise stated) in renal transplant recipients reported to NTPR.

2 It is not known whether systemic hypertension has any significant intrarenal effect in pregnancy, although in the single kidney situation, with or without pregnancy, it could theoretically contribute further to glomerular hyperfiltration and possibly glomerular hypertension and injury (reviewed in [237]).

3 Treatment of mild hypertension is not necessary during normal pregnancy but many would treat transplant patients more aggressively, believing this preserves renal function and regardless of its potential effect on birthweight [137,384].

Infections

Although some reports describe an increased incidence of all types of infection, this is controversial [385,386]. Nevertheless, there can be no doubt that immunosuppression, anaemia and debility make all recipients susceptible to infection. Infection with uncommon organisms is common, and cultures should always be obtained when infection is suspected. Fungal and related infections occur less frequently now that transplant teams have learnt more about the limits of the various immunosuppressive regimens. *Aspergillus*, *Mycobacterium tuberculosis*, *Listeria monocytogenes* and *Pneumocystis* have all been reported. The incidence of UTI may be as high as 40% and is said to occur in all women in whom chronic pyelonephritis was a primary cause of the renal failure. Viral infections, mainly CMV, herpes simplex (HSV) and hepatitis B, are always a potential hazard to mother and fetus [387–389].

Gastrointestinal disorders

Dyspepsia can cause considerable distress in any allograft recipient particularly in pregnancy. Although there is no correlation between dyspepsia and total steroid dosage, it does appear that problems are less common with low-dose immunosuppressive regimens.

Parathyroid dysfunction

(see also Chapter 14)

Up to 20% of women with successful renal transplants develop tertiary hyperparathyroidism. If maternal hyperparathyroidism is untreated (or undiagnosed) there is the risk of maternal hypercalcaemia followed by neonatal hypocalcaemia [390]. If parathyroidectomy is undertaken there is then the risk of hypoparathyroidism [365] with maternal hypocalcaemic seizures as well as congenital hypo- and hyperparathyroidism. Calcium and phosphate levels therefore need careful monitoring during pregnancy [112].

Immunosuppressive therapy during pregnancy

As mentioned above, routine clinical practice is to maintain therapy at pre-pregnancy levels but more research is needed in this area. Changes in therapy must not jeopardize overall suppression even though there are some reports where therapy was reduced or stopped during pregnancy without invoking rejection [378,379]. At no point after transplantation, barring serious drug toxicity, is it prudent to stop all immunosuppressive therapy [380].

The commonly used maintenance regimens are combinations of prednisone and azathioprine or cyclosporine. Evidence suggests that cyclosporine is more effective than the conventional drugs [391,392] and experience in pregnancy is still expanding [325,326,337,393–398].

PREDNISONE

This steroid decreases cell-mediated responses to the allograft with the disadvantages of increased risks of infection and/or malignancy and poor healing. Additional maternal side-effects include glucose intolerance, peptic ulcer development, osteoporosis and weakening of connective tissues, which may have predisposed to uterine rupture in one patient [379].

Prednisone crosses the placenta to a limited extent (see Chapter 1) and is converted to prednisolone, which, although not suppressing fetal adrenocorticotrophic hormone (ACTH), may have other adverse fetal effects (see later). Augmenting steroids postpartum to cover so-called 'rebound immunoresponsiveness' is controversial [399,400] and the consensus is that it is neither necessary nor beneficial.

AZATHIOPRINE

This purine analogue decreases delayed hypersensitivity and cellular cytoxicity while leaving antibody-mediated responses relatively intact. In the mother the primary hazards are increased risk of infection and/or neoplasia. Azathioprine crosses the placenta and the fetal and paediatric implications will be discussed later (see below). In theory, the fetus should be protected from the effects of azathioprine in early pregnancy, as it then lacks the enzyme inosinate pyrophosphorylase, which converts azathioprine to thioinosinic acid, the metabolite active on dividing cells [377,401].

The most sensitive method of monitoring azathioprine dosage and bioavailability is the measurement of red cell 6-thioguanine nucleotides (6-TGNs), which are metabolites of both azathioprine and 6-mercaptopurine and whose formation is catalysed by red cell thiopurine methyltransferase (TPMT). Low TPMT activity may be a risk factor for the development of thiopurine toxicity and there certainly are large individual variations in red cell 6-TGNs amongst patients receiving identical azathioprine dosage [402,403]. One in 300 patients inherits a lack of TPMT activity, and identification of such patients could be important, especially in pregnancy, if side-effects are to be avoided. A less sensitive, but nevertheless safe, approach involves adjustments in azathioprine dosage to maintain maternal leucocyte count within normal limits for pregnancy thus ensuring that the neonate is born with a normal blood count [363].

CYCLOSPORINE

This fungal metabolite's major inhibitory effect is on the T lymphocyte and other cells mediating allograft rejection. There is wide individual sensitivity and it is plasma rather than whole blood drug levels that correlate best with toxicity. The widely differing accumulation seen in various human tissues is related to variations in cyclophilin, the major intracellular cyclosporine-binding protein.

Although renal allograft survival data are better with cyclosporine [391,392], it actually reduces compensatory hyperfunction at the time of the transplant and has long-term nephrotoxic effects.

Consequently most patients have plasma creatinine levels of 100–260 μmol/L compared to 70–180 μmol/L in those on routine immunosuppression [404]. The relationship between higher creatinine and worse gestational outcome applies in cyclosporine-treated patients and > 175μmol/L is a cause for concern [405]. As well as nephrotoxicity, other adverse effects include neoplasia, hepatic dysfunction, tremor, convulsions, glucose intolerance, hypertension, haemolytic–uraemic syndrome (HUS) and predisposition to thromboembolic phenomena. The latter four are particularly significant and worrying in relation to pregnancy.

Little is known about either the maternal or fetal effects of this drug in pregnancy. Theoretically some of the maternal physiological adaptations could be blunted by cyclosporine, for example its depressive effects on extracellular volume and renal haemodynamics [404–407]. In the few cases in the literature, however, renal function was not adequately documented, and whether the kidney in pregnancy is more vulnerable to cyclosporine is not known [394,396,397,408]. Interestingly, the presence of *E. coli* kidney infection can increase susceptibility to nephrotoxicity and yet absence of renal innervation, as in a transplant, possibly affords some protection.

Pregnancy information has expanded enormously in the last 5 years and overall the pregnancy success rates with cyclosporine are comparable to those with azathioprine. Reports from NTPR are particularly enlightening [374,393] with over 1000 patients enrolled by 2000, about 50% of whom needed antihypertensive medication(s). Birthweights are reduced but this could also be related to graft dysfunction and/or to concomitant hypertension as well as to the immunosuppressive agent(s) [326, 398,409] (see Table 7.2). We suggest that if possible cyclosporine dosage be maintained at 2–4 mg/kg/day (see Table 7.20).

NEW IMMUNOSUPPRESSIVE AGENTS

It will be interesting to monitor the impact of the new cyclosporine preparation Neoral, which has improved bioavailability in non-pregnant transplant patients and where its use has enabled earlier maintenance of blood drug concentrations in the therapeutic range.

Reports are now appearing of successful pregnancies in liver and renal transplant recipients maintained on tacrolimus (FK506 or Prograf) (see Table 7.21). Twin pregnancies have been reported [410,411] in which one of both newborns developed respiratory and cardiac difficulties, one of whom died as a result of a thrombotic cardiomyopathy.

There is a paucity of pregnancy data for MMF (Cell-Cept), antithymocytic globulin, ATG (Atgam) and orthoclione, OKT3, although the latter has been used with steroids to treat acute rejection in pregnancy [325,326,345]. Some of these newer agents were originally considered to have a 'rescue role' only in kidney and kidney/pancreas transplantation but nowadays they are employed as primary immunosuppressive agents too [412].

Decisions regarding delivery

Preterm delivery is common (45–60%) because of intervention for obstetric reasons and the common occurrences of preterm rupture of membranes and preterm labour. Preterm labour is commonly associated with poor renal function and this may be a contributory factor in transplant patients [88,405]. In some, however, there is no obvious explanation and it has been postulated that long-term steroid therapy may weaken connective tissue and contribute to the increased incidence of preterm rupture of membranes [377].

MANAGEMENT DURING LABOUR

Vaginal delivery should be the aim and there is no evidence that there is any extra risk of mechanical injury to the transplanted kidney. Unless there are problems or unusual circumstances [413,414], the onset of labour should be spontaneous but of course induction should be undertaken if there are specific indications.

Careful monitoring of maternal fluid balance, cardiovascular status and temperature is essential. Aseptic technique is mandatory at all times [415]: any surgical procedure, however trivial, such as an episiotomy, should be covered with prophylactic antibiotics (ampicillin and metronidazole). Indeed, surgical induction of labour by amniotomy might be considered to warrant antibiotic cover.

Augmentation of steroids is necessary to cover the stress of delivery. A reasonable dose would be intramuscular hydrocortisone, 100 mg every 6 h during labour. Pain relief is conducted as for healthy women. If there are problems with acute hypertension then management should be as discussed in Chapter 6.

Fetal electronic monitoring should be undertaken. If fetal scalp blood samples are taken then a fetal platelet count would help to exclude fetal thrombocytopenia, which increases the risk of fetal intracerebral haemorrhage and is an indication for caesarean section [416] (but see also Chapter 3).

ROLE OF CAESAREAN SECTION

Although obstructed labour due to the position of the graft has been reported [417], the kidney does not usually obstruct the birth canal. Caesarean section is only necessary for purely obstetrical reasons [413,414]. However, from the literature, the 35–40% caesarean section rate is certainly much higher than might be expected, presumably reflecting fear of the unknown, rather than certainty that vaginal delivery would be hazardous for mother and/or child.

The following are important when making a final decision on the route of delivery.

1 Transplant patients may have pelvic osteodystrophy related to their previous renal failure (and dialysis) or prolonged steroid therapy, particularly if it occurred before puberty [418]. For instance, avascular necrosis, particularly of the femoral head, is a common problem, occurring in 20% of all transplant patients [419,420]. Patients with pelvic problems should be recognized antenatally and delivered by caesarean section if there is cephalopelvic disproportion.

2 Some authors have recommended that if there is any question of disproportion or kidney compression, then simultaneous IVU and radiographic pelvimetry should be performed at 36 weeks' gestation [379].

3 When a caesarean section is performed, a lower segment approach is usually feasible but previous urological surgery may make this difficult [421,422]. Care must be taken that the ureter and/or the graft blood supply are not damaged or compromised.

Paediatric management (Box 7.4)

PRETERM DELIVERY

Preterm delivery (<37 weeks' gestation) is common (45–60%) because of intervention for obstetric reasons and the tendency to preterm labour, which although commonly associated with renal impairment, is not always the obvious explanation. It has been suggested that long-term steroid therapy weakens connective tissue and contributes to the increased incidence of preterm rupture of membranes.

Average birthweights are low because most deliveries are preterm. Additionally, the incidence of fetal growth restriction is 30% (range 8–40% in the literature) and is not necessarily related to the severity of renal impairment, vascular disease or hypertension [423]. Certainly, immunogenetic disparity between conceptus and mother is advantageous, and placentae and fetuses are bigger when there is smaller maternofetal histocompatibility. Thus, in the renal transplant mother non-specific depression of the maternal immune system by immunosuppressives may contribute to fetal growth restriction. Congenital CMV infection may also be a contributory factor [387].

IMMEDIATE PROBLEMS

Over 50% of liveborns have no neonatal problems. As preterm delivery is common (45–60%) small-for-dates

---

Box 7.4 Factors causing neonatal problems in offspring of renal allograft patients
- Preterm delivery/small for gestational age
- Respiratory distress syndrome
- Depressed haemopoiesis
- Lymphoid/thymic hypoplasia
- Adrenocortical insufficiency
- Septicaemia
- Cytomegalovirus infection
- Hepatitis B surface antigen carrier state
- Congenital abnormalities
- Immunological problems
  Reduced lymphocyte phytohaemagglutinin (PHA) reactivity
  Reduced T lymphocytes
  Reduced immunoglobulin levels
- Chromosome aberrations in leucocytes

infants are delivered in at least 30% of cases and as occasionally the two problems occur together neonatal paediatric facilities must be available. There are also some special problems in these babies such as thymic atrophy, transient leucopenia, CMV and hepatitis B infection, bone-marrow hypoplasia, reduced blood levels of IgG and IgM, septicaemia, chromosome aberrations and polymorphism in lymphocytes, hypoglycaemia, hypocalcaemia and adrenocortical insufficiency [377,424–426].

Cord blood samples should be taken at delivery with the aim of excluding these problems. Adrenocortical insufficiency due to maternal steroid therapy increases the risk of overwhelming neonatal infection. Occasionally the neonate collapses shortly after delivery with overwhelming infection, and adrenocortical insufficiency should be suspected [427]. Once the diagnosis has been considered, the proper therapy consists of steroids, antibiotics, gammaglobulin and appropriate electrolyte solutions.

CONGENITAL ABNORMALITIES

No frequent or predominant developmental abnormalities have been reported. Azathioprine is teratogenic in animals but only with large doses, equivalent to >6 mg/kg bodyweight/day, much more than the modest ones (2 mg/kg/day or less) required by women with stable renal function [401,428]. In one series, however, where birth anomalies were present in seven out of 103 offspring, the mothers of abnormal babies had been taking a significantly higher daily dose of azathioprine than those who had normal babies: 2.64 mg/kg vs. 2.02 mg/kg [429]. (There was no significant difference in the daily dose of prednisone between the two groups.) This was based on a relatively small number of abnormal babies and could still be due to chance.

Very large doses of steroids in experimental animals can produce congenital abnormalities, but the risk to the fetus from doses used after transplantation is small. Cyclosporine is embryo- and fetotoxic in animals when given in doses 2–5 times greater than the human dose. There is still much to learn regarding potential toxicities of immunosuppressive agents. The effects of the improved regimens, which use newer and more potent (and possibly more toxic) medications, require further study in pregnancy [325].

VIRAL INFECTIONS

Infectious hepatitis (see Chapter 9)

It is likely that children born to renal transplant mothers who are carriers of HBsAg (during and after pregnancy) become antigen carriers themselves [425,430]. Of interest is the fact that any woman with acute hepatitis in late pregnancy or within 2 months after delivery transmits HBsAg to her offspring in at least 75% of cases, whereas in asymptomatic carriers the risk of the children becoming antigen positive is much less (see Chapter 9). Even if there is little effect on general health, however, serum aminotransferases may be elevated perhaps signifying chronic persistent hepatitis, which in some cases has been verified by biopsy [431].

The use of hyperimmunoglobulin against HBsAg given prophylactically to neonates has been investigated and it is known that the carrier state can be prevented in 75% if newborns are given hepatitis B immunoglobulin immediately after birth [323,432–434] (see also Chapter 9). Recently it has been shown that if hyperimmunoglobulin is given with hepatitis B virus vaccine within a few hours of birth this regimen is 90% effective in reducing the HBsAg carrier state in infants, but not if administration is delayed beyond 48 h or if either is given alone [435].

Cytomegalovirus (see Chapter 17)

CMV infection, a major cause of morbidity in transplant recipients, can present in a variety of ways in the mother including fever, leucopenia, thrombocytopenia and pneumonia as well as liver and renal dysfunction. CMV immunoglobulin can provide effective prophylaxis in women at risk for primary infection [436] and perhaps all potential mothers should be treated if appropriate.

Of most importance to the pregnant transplant recipient and her fetus are the implications of congenital CMV infection [437]. Therapeutic termination is not a practical approach because maternal infections are mostly symptomless, detectable only by serological monitoring, and many infants born to women with CMV infection are not seriously damaged but can be growth restricted. If primary maternal CMV infection is responsible for the majority of damaged CMV-infected infants, there may be a case for pre-pregnancy testing followed by CMV immunoglobulin or even CMV vaccination [438]. Live CMV vaccines are available but it is not known whether they can prevent congenital CMV infection.

Herpes simplex virus

Primary maternal infection prior to 20 weeks is associated with an increased rate of abortion. Caesarean section should be undertaken if a cervical culture is positive for HSV at term, because the risk of neonatal infection resulting from vaginal delivery is at least 50% (see Chapter 17).

Postnatal assessment and long-term maternal follow-up

A major concern is that the mother may or may not survive or remain well enough to rear the child she bears. It has been calculated that 10% will be dead within 7 years of pregnancy and 50% dead within 15 years [439], data that perhaps should be presented cautiously when undertaking pre-pregnancy assessment and long-term counselling (see above). Many women, however, will choose parenthood in an effort to re-establish a normal life and possibly in defiance of the sometimes negative attitudes of the medical establishment [440].

CONTRACEPTION

All women should be routinely counselled about contraception. The choice depends on balancing the desirability of pregnancy prevention against the potential risks of the contraceptive method. Contraceptive steroids can produce subtle changes in the immune system [441], but this is not necessarily a contraindication to their use. Low-dose oestrogen–progesterone preparations can be prescribed, although some have avoided them because of the possibility of causing or aggravating hypertension or further increasing the incidence of thromboembolism [442,443]. If the oral contraceptive is prescribed, careful and frequent surveillance is needed.

An intrauterine contraceptive device (IUCD) can aggravate any tendency towards menstrual problems and these in turn may confuse the signs and symptoms of abnormalities in early pregnancy, such as threatened abortion or ectopic pregnancy [370]. The risks of pelvic infection are increased and this could be disastrous in an immunosuppressed patient [444]. Insertion or replacement of an IUCD is normally associated with bacteraemia in at least one in every 10 women so in transplant patients antibiotic cover is essential at this time. Furthermore, there is a higher incidence of fungal infections with a plastic IUCD (42%) compared to a copper-containing device (2%). The efficacy of the IUCD may be reduced by immunosuppressive and anti-inflammatory agents, possibly due to modi-

fication of the leucocyte response [445,446]. Nevertheless, many request this method. Careful counselling and follow-up are essential.

GYNAECOLOGICAL PROBLEMS

These patients have the same problems that afflict the normal female population. There is a danger, however, that symptoms secondary to genuine gynaecological pathology may be erroneously attributed to the transplant due to its location near the pelvis. Transplant patients might be at slightly higher risk of ectopic pregnancy because of pelvic adhesions due to previous urological surgery, peritoneal dialysis, pelvic inflammatory disease or the use of an IUCD [446]. Diagnosis of ectopic pregnancy can be overlooked because irregular bleeding and amenorrhoea may be associated with deteriorating renal function as well as intrauterine pregnancy.

Transplant recipients receiving immunosuppressive therapy have a *de novo* malignancy rate estimated to be 100 times greater than normal, and the female genital tract is no exception [447–451]. For instance, there are reports of cervical changes ranging from cellular atypia through carcinoma *in situ* to invasive squamous cell carcinoma [452]. The malignancy association is probably related to factors such as loss of immune surveillance, chronic immunosuppression allowing tumour proliferation and/or prolonged antigenic stimulation of the reticuloendothelial system [453,454]. Regular gynaecological assessment is essential and any treatment should be conventional, with outcome unlikely to be influenced by stopping or reducing immunosuppression.

BREASTFEEDING

Steroids are secreted in breast milk but not in sufficient quantity to affect the infant at therapeutic doses. In theory, if the baby has been exposed to an immunosuppressive agent and its metabolites throughout pregnancy, it should be well accustomed to them, and if their concentrations in breast milk are minimal then breastfeeding

		Infant		
	Adult	Birth	6 months	>6 months
Mother 1	25	16	8	10
Mother 2	12	18	14	0
Renal transplant patients (non-pregnant)	26			
Normal	2.5	0.5–1	0.5–1	0.5–1

Table 7.22 Chromosome aberrations* (%) in cultured lymphocytes of two renal transplant mothers and their offspring compared to non-pregnant transplant patients and the normal population. (Modified from [458].)

*Caps, fragments, deletions, rings, etc. studied in metaphase.

would not be contraindicated. Despite the undoubted beneficial effects of breastfeeding, more specific information is needed about whether the amounts in breast are trivial or substantial from a biological point of view [371,455] and only then can sound advice be given. Cyclosporine is excreted in breast milk in amounts <2% of the maternal dose, and the blood concentration in infants is below the assay's sensitivity (i.e. $<30 \mu g/mL$) [394,456]. Despite the current weight of opinion that mothers should not breastfeed until more definitive data are available, some transplant recipients will choose to ignore this advice [457].

Potential long-term paediatric problems

If azathioprine causes chromosome aberrations in fetal lymphocytes (Table 7.22) [458], however transient, the fear is that these anomalies may not be temporary in other somatic cells not studied and in the germ cells. The sequelae could be future development of malignancies or impairment of reproduction in the affected offspring. There is some evidence concerning this from animal studies [459]. The ovaries of female offspring of mice treated with 6-mercaptopurine (the principal metabolite of azathioprine) equivalent to 3 mg/kg contained fewer oocytes and ovarian follicles compared to offspring of mothers that had not received the drug. Furthermore, these mice had fertility problems when they were bred. Despite normal bodyweight and general appearance, many proved to be sterile or if they became pregnant had smaller litters and more dead fetuses (Table 7.23).

This effect was probably initiated while the offspring were developing in the uteri of their mothers during treatment. It is unlikely that such damage would be eliminated or repaired, as seems to happen in somatic cells, because synthesis of DNA stops when the germ cells are arrested in the prophase of the first meiotic division *in utero*, and no new DNA is synthesized until after fertilization.

Thus, exposure of the fetus to low doses of potential mutagens may not cause immediate, obvious effects such as morbidity or birth defects, but may have severe consequences when otherwise normal female offspring reach puberty. As yet, there are no animal data on the reproductive performance of the male offspring.

Above all it is imperative that any child exposed to immunosuppressive therapy *in utero* has a careful evaluation of the immune system and long-term follow-up. To date, information about general progress in infancy and early childhood of the offspring of renal transplant mothers has been good [377,400,426,460]. The introduction of cyclosporine has prompted a study from the NTPR where 175 children of 133 women maintained on cyclosporine throughout pregnancy were examined at 4 months to 12 years (mean 4.4 years) [461]. At birth these children had a gestational age of mean 36 weeks and mean birthweight 2.49 kg. At follow-up 29 children (16%) had delays or needed educational support (Table 7.24). This study population had a high incidence of prematurity, more so in those identified with delays. Increased identification of delays, especially language, at older ages may have indicated difficulty in recognition at younger ages. The small size of this study precludes comparisons with the general US population, where incidentally 11% in state schools have special educational needs. Further study of associations between maternal and perinatal variables and developmental outcome is urgently needed.

Renal transplants and pregnancy: some conclusions

1 The reproductive endocrinology of uraemia is complex and has been reviewed elsewhere [118]; renal transplantation is usually quickly followed by improvements in reproductive function.

2 The possibility of conception in women of childbearing age emphasizes the need for compassionate and comprehensive counselling. Couples who want a child should be encouraged to discuss all the implications, including long-term maternal survival prospects.

3 Therapeutic abortion is an option taken up by 15% of women.

Table 7.23 Effect of 6-mercaptopurine (6-MP) in pregnancy in the mouse on subsequent reproduction of offspring. Mean ± SEM. (From [459].)

6-MP dose to mother (mg/kg/day)	Weight of ovaries of offspring (mg)	Number of offspring bred	Number of offspring achieving pregnancy	Number of fetuses per pregnancy	Percentage of dead fetuses
0	8.6 ± 0.4	33	33	13.0 ± 0.4	13
0.5	8.7 ± 0.3	46	44	12.8 ± 0.3	18
1.5	7.3 ± 0.6	33	26	10.6 ± 0.5	25
3.0	2.2 ± 0.6	9	2	6.5 ± 3.5	46

Table 7.24 Developmental delay or educational morbidity in 175 offspring of cyclosporine-treated renal transplant recipients reported to the National Transplantation Pregnancy Registry (NTPR) (data in parentheses are percentages of total). (Modified from [461].)

Age at assessment	Children with delay	Self-help delay	Social delay	Gross motor delay	Fine motor delay	Language delay
<1 year ($n = 20$)	1 (0.5)	0	0	1 (5)	1 (5)	0
1–5 years ($n = 84$)	11 (6.3)	3 (4)	1 (1)	2 (2)	4 (50)	7 (8)
5–12 years ($n = 71$)	Children with delay or educational morbidity 17 (9.7)	Early intervention 13 (18)	Grade failure 2 (30)	Tutoring or educational programming 10 (14)	ADD/HD 8 (11)	

ADD/HD, attention deficit/hyperactivity disorder. Modified from [461].

4 The spontaneous abortion rate is about 15% (the same as for the normal population) and of the conceptions that go beyond first trimester, 95% end successfully.

5 In most women, renal function is augmented during pregnancy, but permanent impairment occurs in 12% of pregnancies. In others there may be transient deterioration in late pregnancy (with or without proteinuria).

6 There is a 30% chance of developing hypertension, pre-eclampsia or both.

7 Preterm delivery occurs in 45–60%, and intrauterine growth restriction in at least 30% of pregnancies. The incidence is higher in women taking cyclosporine.

8 Despite its pelvic location, the transplanted kidney rarely obstructs labour and is not injured during vaginal delivery. Caesarean section should be reserved for obstetric reasons only but nowadays the rate is 35–40%.

9 Neonatal complications include respiratory distress syndrome, leucopenia, thrombocytopenia, adrenocortical insufficiency and infection. No predominant or frequent developmental abnormalities have been described. Better data on progress in infancy and childhood are urgently needed.

10 There is no room for complacency and further research is needed to improve understanding and management in the following areas: pre-pregnancy assessment criteria, the mechanisms of gestational renal dysfunction and proteinuria, the side-effects and implications of immunosuppression in pregnancy and the remote effects of pregnancy on both maternal renal prognosis and the offspring.

Pregnancy in haemodialysis patients

It has been several decades since the first documentation of conception and successful delivery in a patient undergoing chronic haemodialysis [462] and since then further case reports and registry data have been published [107,125,335,357,378,429,463–475]. In one of the cases reported [475] the renal function was so good that success might have been achieved without dialysis.

Any optimism must be tempered by remembering that clinicians are reluctant to publish their failures, and consequently the true incidence of unsuccessful pregnancies and their sequelae in women on haemodialysis cannot be determined. There is no doubt that the high surgical abortion rate (averaging 10–20% but decreasing in recent years) in these patients indicates that those who become pregnant do so accidentally, probably because they are unaware that pregnancy is a possibility. As the debate continues about the advisability or not of pregnancy, women are increasingly choosing to take the chance because childbearing and parenthood are important rehabilitation goals. This issue of considerable levels of assumed risk vs. admirable maternal self-sacrifice has already been discussed in relation to renal transplant patients (see above).

Pregnancy counselling

In spite of irregular or absent menstruation [476], decreased libido and potency, and impaired fertility, women undergoing haemodialysis should always use contraception if they wish to avoid pregnancy [118,321,477]. The introduction of recombinant human erythropoietin (rHuEpo) to the treatment of women with renal failure appears to be associated in some cases with return of normal menses (and ovulation), probably because of correction of hyperprolactinaemia and/or improved overall health [478]. The incidence of pregnancy in this group of women is about 1.5%.

There are substantial arguments against pregnancy and these should be pointed out, not least the risks to the patient and the greatly reduced likelihood of successful outcome [351]. Even when therapeutic terminations are excluded the live birth rate at very best has been only 40–50%. A 1998 literature survey (Tables 7.25 and 7.26) of 846 pregnancies [479] reviewed a 46% successful outcome in line with pre-1998 publications [107,330,357,480,481]. But more recent reports indicate that between 50 and 70% are 'successful' even though extreme prematurity and dis-

Table 7.25 Pregnancy in dialysis patients. Data (% unless otherwise stated) from an unpublished literature survey up to 1997 (J. Davison) and a questionnaire survey of 206 units (1281 women) in USA [236].

	1989	1992	1995	1997	[470]
Pregnancies (n)	182	287	327	384	60
Pregnancy rate	0.5	1.0	1.2	1.1	1.5
Therapeutic abortion	40	22	17	18	9
Spontaneous abortion	46	50	48	43	40
Perinatal loss	3	10	5	6	4
Successful outcome	11	18	30	33	47
Excluding therapeutic abortion	18	23	36	40	52

Table 7.26 Dialysis and pregnancy. From cumulative literature surveys to 1998: J. Davison (unpublished).

Literature skewed towards reporting success
Pregnancy rate of 1–2% in childbearing age group
846 pregnancies
   75% on dialysis pre-pregnancy
   Haemodialysis : Peritoneal dialysis = 3 : 1
   Dialysis time <1 year (37%), <2 years (60%), <5 years (78%), >10 years (9%)

turbing maternal problems are still commonplace [482] (Tables 7.27 and 7.28).

A great deal of information became available in 1998, specifically a report from the American Registry for Pregnancy in Dialysis Patients [126] analysing pregnancy data for 320 pregnancies in women on haemodialysis and peritoneal dialysis (Tables 7.29 and 7.30) plus a plethora of publications concerning single-centre and countrywide experiences. All have concluded that these risky and frequently disappointing pregnancies should only be handled in tertiary referral centres with continuous multidisciplinary management. Although the outcome is poor and needs to be constantly reappraised, this form of management is the best available at the moment [112,479,483,484].

The situation in Japan is given in a 1999 study of 74 pregnancies that revealed a 49% success rate compared to 9% in 1981 [343]. There were significant differences in mean gestational age and birthweight between surviving and non-surviving neonates: 33 weeks and 1.72 kg vs. 26 weeks and 0.70 kg; the extremely preterm babies that survived had severe long-term complications.

General management plan

EARLY PREGNANCY ASSESSMENT

Early diagnosis of pregnancy can be a problem. Irregular menstruation is common and a missed period will usually be ignored [118,485,486]. The big mistake the clinician may make is not even to consider the possibility of pregnancy. As urine pregnancy tests are unreliable [487], even if there is any urine available, early diagnosis and estimation of gestational age are best accomplished by ultra-

sound. Occasionally, rHuEpo requirements may increase without warning providing a diagnostic clue to the possibility of pregnancy [488].

Interestingly, in these patients there can be false-positive second-trimester Down's syndrome screening results because of extremely high maternal serum human chorionic gonadotrophin (hCG) levels (with normal α-fetoprotein (AFP) values) due to decreased renal clearance of hCG and possibly to cytotrophoblastic hyperplasia indicative of placental ischaemia. Follow-up management is difficult and at the very least ultrasound markers for fetal aneuploidy should be sought [489].

MANAGEMENT OBJECTIVES

For a successful outcome, scrupulous attention must be paid to blood pressure control, fluid balance, increased dialysis requirements and provision of good nutrition [263,465,470,471,490–492]. It should be emphasized that this will place many demands on the hospital team as well as the patient's family. It might even be considered to be a misuse of scarce resources and manpower.

Table 7.27 Dialysis and pregnancy. From cumulative literature surveys to 1998: J. Davison (unpublished).

846 pregnancies	
Therapeutic abortion	15%
Spontaneous abortion	20%
Perinatal loss	15%
Successful outcome	50%
Successful outcome excluding therapeutic abortion	62%

	[483]	[482]	[126]	[484]
Pregnancy rate (%)	0.3		2.2	(1.4)
Pregnancies (*n*)	15	110	320	17
Therapeutic abortions (%)	(30)	(20)	11	(15)
Spontaneous abortions (%)		11	32	17
Perinatal loss (%)	40	20	14	13
Successful outcome (%)	60	69	43	70
(excluding therapeutic abortions (%)			(49)	

Table 7.28 Pregnancy in dialysis patients (1998).

Data in parentheses are estimated from the information given. Where cells are blank, no accurate data were presented.

2299 centres with 930 replies (40%) for women aged 14–44 years
6230 women (48% of 12 992 women registered nationally)
Haemodialysis 4513; peritoneal dialysis 1699 (3 : 1)
344 pregnancies in 318 women (8 had 2 pregnancies and 9 had 3)
320 pregnancies analysed

Table 7.29 American Registry for Pregnancy in Dialysis Patients (1992–95).

Pregnancies (*n*)	Gestation (wks)	Mean birthweight (g)	Survival (%)
6	<24	520	0
4	24–25	647	0
4	26–27	705	25
8	28–29	807	50
10	30–31	1346	70
17	32–33	1570	82
19	34–35	1920	100
15	>36	2217	100

Table 7.30 Dialysis, birthweight and pregnancy outcome in 110 cases, 1971–96. (From [482].)

STRATEGY DURING PREGNANCY

Those women on dialysis for a shorter time (<5 years) and with residual renal function and satisfactory daily urine volumes (>50 mL/day), in whom biochemical control is easier, are more likely to become pregnant [112,126,493]. Some patients show increments in GFR even if the level of renal function is too poor to sustain life without haemodialysis. The dialysis strategy can vary from centre to centre [482,494,495] but should have the following aims.

1 Maintain plasma urea at <20 mmol/L. It has been suggested that intrauterine death is likely if levels are much in excess of 20 mmol/L [496] but in one case report [463] success was achieved despite levels of 25 mmol/L for many weeks.

2 Maintain pH and electrolyte levels near pregnancy norms. For instance, daily haemodialysis with dialysate bicarbonate reduced to 18–20 mmol/L may be needed in women who have no renal function.

3 Ensure good control of blood pressure.

4 Avoid hypotension during dialysis. In late pregnancy the gravid uterus and the supine posture may aggravate this by decreasing venous return. Doppler velocimetry of the umbilical artery reveals that haemodialysis induces significant alterations in fetal haemodynamics despite only small changes in maternal blood pressure and biochemistry and unchanged resistance to blood flow in the uteroplacental circulation [497].

5 Be on guard for dialysis-induced uterine contractions. Tocolytic agents can be used very carefully (when indicated) to good effect, and regular disinfection of the vagina has been advised by some to reduce the risk of preterm labour [493].

6 Ensure minimal fluctuations in fluid balance and limit volume changes.

7 Avoid maternal hypercalcaemia: the placenta produces 1,25-hydroxy vitamin D, and oral supplementation may have to be reduced.

8 Attempt to minimize heparin use, although this may be difficult as pregnancy is a hypercoaguable state.

9 Limit interdialysis weight gain to 0.5 kg until late pregnancy.

Inevitably this strategy means increased length and frequency of dialysis, in some instances by as much as 50% [357]. There is no doubt that frequent dialysis renders dietary management and control of weight gain much easier but the domestic problems caused might require that a combination of home and hospital dialysis is used [498].

In reports from Saudi Arabia and Belgium [499] comparing the pregnancies that ended before 28 weeks with those that went beyond, the authors found no significant differences in blood pressure, haemoglobin, creatinine levels, type of dialysate, postobstetric history or years on dialysis. Dialysis hours were, however, significantly longer in the successful groups—a fact now endorsed by data from the American Registry for Pregnancy in Dialysis Patients [126].

ANAEMIA

Increasing anaemia causes concern for maternal and fetal welfare. Patients are usually anaemic and blood transfusion may be needed, especially before delivery, for safe obstetric management [357,500]. Caution is needed because transfusion may exacerbate hypertension and might also impair the ability to control circulatory overload, even with extra dialysis. Fluctuations in blood volume can be minimized, however, if nitrogen-frozen packed red cells are transfused during dialysis. It should also be rembered that blood transfusion is associated with increased risk of transfusion-related reactions and infection. The risk of human immunodeficiency virus (HIV) transmission is 1 : 225 000 per unit of transfusion. The incidence of transfusion-related hepatitis B infection is 0.002% and that of hepatitis C virus is 0.1% [501] (see also Chapter 9). Additional risks of repeated transfusions include iron overload, reactions to leucocyte antigen and development of cytotoxic antibodies that may influence eventual renal transplantation. Hence, rHuEpo seems to be a safer approach and indeed has been used in pregnancy in situations other than dialysis patients, without ill-effect [33,465,502]. Specifically, the theoretical risks of anti-Epo antibody formation, hypertension and thrombotic complications have not been encountered so far [503]. No adverse effects have been noted in neonates in whom haematological indices and erythropoietin concentrations for gestational age suggest that rHuEpo does not have significant transplacental effects [504].

Unnecessary blood sampling should be avoided and, in any case, lack of venepuncture sites can be a problem. The protocol for the various routine tests performed in a particular unit should be followed meticulously, removing no more blood per venepuncture than is absolutely necessary. Screening for hepatitis B is mandatory.

HYPERTENSION

Blood pressure can fluctuate wildly. These patients have such abnormal lipid profiles and accelerated atherogenesis that it is difficult to predict the ability of the cardiovascular system to tolerate the stresses of pregnancy. Diabetic women on dialysis who have become pregnant are those in whom cardiovascular problems are most evident. Normal blood pressure is reassuring. Unfortunately, hypertension is a common problem, although it may be possible to control this by ultrafiltration to reduce circulating blood volume, provided exacerbation does not occur between dialyses. Any other measures must be carefully assessed in the light of possible side-effects.

DIETARY COUNSELLING

Despite more frequent dialysis, free dietary intake should be discouraged [366]. An oral intake of at least 70 g protein, 1500 mg calcium, 50 mmol potassium and 50 mmol sodium per day is advised and oral supplements of dialysable vitamins should be given. Vitamin D supplements can be difficult to judge in patients who have had a parathyroidectomy. It is not clear to what extent these dietary factors and maternal uraemia affect the fetus and its nutrition. The use of parenteral nutrition supplementation in pregnancy has been advocated [505].

DELIVERY

Caesarean section should only be necessary for obstetric reasons, although it could be argued that an elective caesarean section would always minimize potential problems of volume and blood pressure control during labour. In fact, preterm labour is generally the rule and the role of caesarean section under these circumstances needs to be carefully considered [126,506].

Pregnancy in patients on peritoneal dialysis

Since 1976 chronic ambulatory peritoneal dialysis (CAPD) and chronic cycling peritoneal dialysis (CCPD) have been utilized more frequently in the management of patients with all forms of renal insufficiency. Several features of peritoneal dialysis make it an attractive approach for the management of renal failure in pregnancy.

1 Maintenance of a more stable environment for the fetus in terms of fluid and electrolyte concentrations.

2 Avoidance of episodes of abrupt hypotension, a frequent occurrence during haemodialysis, which can cause fetal distress.

3 Continuous allowance for extracellular fluid volume control so that blood pressure control is augmented.

4 Lack of systemic heparinization.

5 Achievement of better maternal nutrition by allowing semirestricted diet.

6 Better blood sugar control in women with diabetes mellitus via intraperitoneal insulin.

7 Theoretically permitting safe use of intraperitoneal magnesium facilitating prevention and treatment of premature labour and possibly pre-eclampsia.

Young women can be managed with this approach and a few successful pregnancies have been reported [471,491,492,504,507–509]. Although anticoagulation and some of the fluid balance and volume problems of haemodialysis are avoided in these women, they nevertheless face the same problems: placental abruption, preterm labour, sudden intrauterine death and hypertension. Furthermore, it should be remembered that peritonitis can be a severe complication of CAPD, and accounts for the majority of therapy failures [510,511]. This, superimposed on a pregnancy, can present a confusing diagnostic picture with the potential for a whole series of treatment problems.

There are reports of gynaecological sequelae in these patients. Reflux of menstrual blood can occur through the intraperitoneal catheter under normal circumstances as well as due to possible endometriosis [512]. Severe pelvic peritonitis is always a possibility [513]. Psychosocial problems are common and can influence libido (and potency in males) [514].

Lastly, it has been argued that if dialysis is to be used in pregnancy then peritoneal dialysis is the method of choice and if a woman is already on haemodialysis then a change should be considered [471]. We, however, prefer that women continue on the mode of dialysis of the time of conception and this is certainly supported by analysis of results from the American Registry for Pregnancy in Dialysis Patients [126] and recent single-centre experiences [483,484,495,515,516].

Dialysis patients and pregnancy: some conclusions

See Boxes 7.5 and 7.6.

Acute renal failure

Acute renal failure is a clinical syndrome characterized by a sudden and marked decrease in glomerular filtration, rising plasma urea and creatinine levels, and usually by a

> **Box 7.5 Dialysis and pregnancy: worrying factors**
> - Age >35 years
> - Already on dialysis
> - Dialysis >5 years
> - Significant hypertension
> - Pregnancy diagnosed >16 weeks
> - Late increase in dialysis requirements
>
> **Box 7.6 Dialysis and pregnancy: clinical messages**
> - No preferred dialysis modality
> - Increased dialysis is essential
>   As soon as possible
>   >20 h/week
> - The shorter the previous time on dialysis, the better the outcome
> - Only 10% have haematocrit >30%
> - 75% require transfusion if not on rHuEpo
> - Hypertension, growth restriction and preterm delivery are inevitable

decrease in urine output to <400 mL in 24 h. As a clinical diagnosis the term only describes *the functional state of the kidneys* without distinguishing between the different forms of underlying pathology [517] (Table 7.30). For the most part, acute renal failure occurs in persons with previously healthy kidneys but it may also complicate the course of patients with pre-existing renal disease [517,518].

Before anuria or oliguria are ascribed to acute renal failure, obstruction to the renal outflow must be excluded, usually by infusion urography, if investigation is needed. This is particularly pertinent in obstetric practice, because it is all too easy to unwittingly damage the urinary tract when performing emergency surgery for obstetric disasters, such as postpartum haemorrhage, which are themselves causes of acute renal failure.

Rarely hydronephrosis leading to acute renal failure in late pregnancy can be due to obstruction from an enlarging uterus with or without polyhydramnios [403,519], a situation that resolves immediately after amniotomy [31], or if delivery is not appropriate then ultrasound-guided percutaneous nephrostomy is safe and reliable [212]. The effects of polyhydramnios are very occasionally added to by a fetal abdominal mass [520].

Perspective and trends

Forty years ago the incidence of acute renal failure in pregnancy was 0.02–0.05% [521] and represented about 2% of cases reported of renal failure of all causes. At that time acute renal failure was a substantial cause of maternal mortality, as at least 20% of women with this complication died [522].

There has been a marked decline in cases of acute renal failure related to obstetrics, largely attributable to liberalization of abortion laws and improvements in perinatal care which had reduced complications, such as sepsis, eclampsia, hypovolaemia and severe haemorrhage [518, 523–528] The current incidence is <0.005% [112], but complications with transient decrements in GFR of a mild to moderate degree probably occur in one in 8000 deliveries [529]. Acute renal failure still has a bimodal distribution corresponding to septic abortion in early pregnancy and pre-eclampsia and bleeding problems in the third trimester [90,530–532]. There are still parts of the world where the incidence of acute obstetric renal failure remains high (0.06%) [533] and in one unit in Northern India 10% of all renal failure cases are related to pregnancy [534].

Pathophysiology

There are three common patterns of altered renal function and anatomy, which are probably part of a spectrum of increasing severity of the same pathological process: preglomerular vasoconstriction causing renal hypoperfusion with preferential cortical ischaemia [208,535].

PRERENAL FAILURE OR VASOMOTOR NEPHROPATHY

This is a relatively mild form of acute renal failure and is caused by moderate degrees of renal ischaemia. It is partly a functional disorder, there are no changes in renal morphology and it is reversible if renal perfusion is improved.

ACUTE TUBULAR NECROSIS

This occurs if renal ischaemia is more severe or persistent. Damage is limited to the most metabolically active tubular cells. Blood vessels and glomeruli do not show significant alteration. It is also reversible after a variable period of renal shutdown.

ACUTE CORTICAL NECROSIS

This occurs if renal ischaemia is very severe or protracted or when there is intense intravascular coagulation. There is complete disintegration of glomeruli and tubules throughout the entire cortex of both kidneys, usually with an irreversible clinical course. In pregnancy, however, renal involvement may be patchy.

Phases of acute renal failure

Traditionally there are three consecutive phases and these have important management implications.

OLIGURIA

Urine volumes are <400 mL in 24 h. This phase may last from a few days to several weeks. Complete anuria is uncommon in acute tubular necrosis and is usually a manifestation of massive acute cortical necrosis or complete obstruction. Non-oliguric forms of acute cortical necrosis may be occasionally encountered in which urine volumes seem adequate but renal function is severely impaired [536] (Table 7.31).

POLYURIA

Urine volumes increase markedly and can be up to 10 L in 24 h. The polyuria may last from several days to 2 weeks. The urine is dilute and, despite the large volumes excreted, metabolic waste products are not efficiently eliminated. Consequently plasma urea and creatinine levels will continue to rise for several days in parallel with increased urine output. Profound fluid and electrolyte losses can endanger survival if not adequately replaced.

RECOVERY

Urine volumes decrease towards normal. Renal function gradually improves, nearing the level before the acute renal failure developed.

Diagnosis and investigation

A carefully taken history may reveal a background of abortion, severe hyperemesis gravidarum, haemorrhage, sensitization to drugs, incompatible blood transfusion pre-eclampsia and/or neglect of recent steroid intake (see Table 7.32). Once the diagnosis has been entertained, the possible causes must be pursued and, in conjunction with a nephrologist, a full initial assessment should be undertaken. The assessment should include the following.
1 Blood specimens: full blood count (Coulter counter analysis), urea, electrolytes and osmolality, glucose, liver-function tests, amylase, plasma proteins, in particular albumin, coagulation indices, acid–base status (arterial blood sample).
2 Urine specimens: specific gravity and osmolality, electrolyte concentrations, protein excretion.
3 Bacteriological assessment: blood cultures (aerobic and anaerobic), vaginal swabs, MSU.

Table 7.31 Differential diagnosis of oliguria.

	Prerenal failure (vasomotor nephropathy)	Acute tubular necrosis
History/background	Vomiting, diarrhoea, dehydration	Dehydration, ischaemic insult, ingestion of nephrotoxin (no specific history in 50%)
Physical examination	Decreased blood pressure, increased pulse, poor skin turgor	May have signs of dehydration, but physical examination often normal
Urinalysis	Concentrated urine; few formed elements on sediment, many hyaline casts	Isosthenuria; sediment contains renal tubular cells and pigmented casts, but may be normal
Urinary sodium	<20 mmol/L; most <10 mmol/L	$\geq$25, usually >60 mmol/L
$U:P$ ratios	High	Low
Osmolality	Often >1.5	<1.1
Urea	$\geq$20	$\leq$3
Creatinine	>40	<15
Fractional sodium excretion ($U:P_{Na}/U:P_{creatinine}$)	<1%	>1%
Renal failure index	<1	>1
($U:P_{Na}/U:P_{creatinine}$)	<1	>1

Modified from Lindheimer MD, Davison JM: *In Medical Disorders in Pregnancy*. Barron WM, Lindheimer MD (eds), Mosby-Yearbook, 1991. $U:P$, urine/plasma ratio.

Table 7.32 Some causes of obstetric acute renal failure.

Volume contraction/hypotension	Antepartum haemorrhage due to placenta praevia
	Post-partum haemorrhage: from uterus or extensive soft-tissue trauma
	Abortion
	Hyperemesis gravidarum
	Adrenocortical failure; usually failure to augment steroids to cover delivery in patient on long-term therapy
Volume contraction/hypotension and coagulopathy	Antepartum haemorrhage due to abruptio placentae
	Pre-eclampsia/eclampsia
	Amniotic fluid embolism
	Incompatible blood transfusion
	Drug reaction(s)
	Acute fatty liver
	Haemolytic-uraemic syndrome
Volume contraction/hypotension, coagulopathy and infection	Septic abortion
	Chorioamnionitis
	Pyelonephritis
	Puerperal sepsis
Urinary tract obstruction	Damage to ureters: during caesarean section and repair of cervical/vaginal lacerations
	Pelvic haematoma
	Broad ligament haematoma

4 ECG: abnormalities do not necessarily correlate with the degree of hyper- or hypokalaemia. Initially, in hyperkalaemia, there are peaked T waves with QRS prolongation and then disappearance of P waves with deformation of the QRS complex.

5 Assessment of fluid balance: the bladder should be catheterized and continuous drainage allowed so that hourly volumes can be recorded. A CVP line should be established, preferably via the antecubital vein. Where the patient is deeply shocked the subclavian vein may be used, but this route should be avoided when artificial ventilation is likely, because of the danger of pneumothorax. This complication is unlikely to arise using the right internal jugular vein, a route that has the added advantage that the catheter tip invariably enters the right atrium. The right atrial pressure (RAP) serves as an indicator of volume of blood returning to the right side of the heart and the response of the right ventricle to a volume load. A separate intravenous therapy line, preferably also in a central vein, should be established. Exact therapy will depend on the biochemical disturbance(s) and CVP or RAP readings. Administration of large amounts of fluid in acute tubular necrosis is both useless and fraught with danger. Blood loss must be taken into account; it is frequently underestimated especially if there has been an antepartum haemorrhage, which is often concealed.

6 Fetal salvage: if this has to be taken into consideration then a decision will have to be made regarding the timing and route of delivery.

Diagnostic pitfalls

It is difficult and often impossible to decide which of the three types of acute renal failure (acute tubular necrosis, acute cortical necrosis, prerenal failure) is present. Total anuria or alternating periods of anuria and polyuria strongly suggests obstruction, but normal urine volumes do not exclude obstruction. Complete anuria and/or evidence of disseminated intravascular coagulation (DIC) are suggestive of acute cortical necrosis but this diagnosis can only be firmly established by renal biopsy [531].

The differential diagnosis between functional renal insufficiency caused by dehydration or hypotension (prerenal failure or vasomotor nephropathy) and acute tubular or cortical necrosis is of practical importance as their therapy is diametrically different (see Table 7.31).

Urine/plasma (U:P) osmolality ratio. This ratio is the single most valuable indicator of early acute renal failure [537]. Pre-renal failure is suggested when the ratio is > 1.5, whereas in acute tubular or cortical necrosis it is closer to unity.

URINE-SPECIFIC GRAVITY

This is inadequate because misleadingly high values may be caused by sugar or protein admixture and comparison with plasma is not possible.

URINARY SODIUM CONCENTRATION

This index is only useful when oliguria is present because a low sodium concentration can be found in non-oliguric acute renal failure [267]. In prerenal failure the urine is concentrated with low sodium concentration (<20 mmol/L) and in acute tubular necrosis the urine is isotonic to

plasma with a relatively high sodium concentration (>60 mmol/L) [537].

TRIAL INTRAVENOUS INFUSION OF 100 ML 25% MANNITOL

Mannitol infusion is a relatively safe therapeutic test and may be helpful in distinguishing between reversible prerenal failure and established acute tubular necrosis provided the period of oliguria does not exceed 48 h and the $U:P$ osmolality ratio is >1.05 [537].

If a diuresis is established within 3 h (>50 mL/h or double the previous urine volume) then urine output should be replaced exactly with intravenous isotonic saline in an attempt to sustain adequate urine flow for at least 24–36 h, after which the danger of acute tubular necrosis has probably passed. By determining urinary electrolytes the losses can be replaced accordingly. If urine flow subsequently decreases to <30 mL then the mannitol infusion can be repeated 6–8-hourly.

If attempts to increase urine flow are unsuccessful, the objective is to support the functionally anephric patient until the kidneys recover.

USE OF DIURETICS

Increments in urine flow produced by 'loop diuretics' such as frusemide may represent conversion of oliguric renal failure to a polyuric form, rather than reversal of prerenal failure. Furthermore, there is no evidence of any beneficial effect of frusemide on the period of oliguria, immediate prognosis or mortality [538].

ROLE OF RENAL BIOPSY

Because acute cortical necrosis is usually irreversible, biopsy is indicated in patients with protracted oliguria or anuria who fail to improve, in order to allow an assessment of prognosis [131]. Diagnosing acute cortical necrosis early, however, is not mandatory, because the management of the acute stage is no different from that of acute tubular necrosis.

General management plan

PRERENAL FAILURE OR VASOMOTOR NEPHROPATHY

The basic principle is to replace blood and fluid losses adequately and maintain blood pressure at levels that will permit adequate renal perfusion. Evidence of continuing blood loss calls for localization and control of the bleeding. Volume correction should always precede the use of diuretics, with the exception of mannitol (both a volume expander and an osmotic diuretic), which may usefully reduce endothelial cell swelling and thereby help to restore renal blood flow.

VOLUME AND METABOLIC CONTROL

Fluid intake and output must be determined daily. Insensible fluid losses cannot be measured directly, but weighing the patient every day is helpful in assessing the state of hydration, and haematocrit and total protein determinations are additional evaluators.

Volume balance is achieved by allowing the adult, non-febrile patient an intake of 500 mL of fluid plus the total output of the preceding 24 h. If the patient is febrile, 200 mL of additional intake is needed for each 1°C increment. If fluid volume is in balance then bodyweight should decrease approximately 0.3–0.5 kg per 24 h because of tissue catabolism. Overhydration must be avoided and if present must be promptly corrected, if necessary by dialysis. Continuous careful supervision and replacement of urinary fluid electrolyte losses is even more important in the polyuric phase, as 50% of deaths occur at this time.

There is a need for oral or parenteral administration of at least 1500 calories of a protein-free fat/carbohydrate combination, which is low in potassium and sodium. Carbohydrate calories are important for decreasing gluconeogenesis from protein (protein-sparing effect), thus retarding the development of azotaemia/acidosis. Volume limitations dictate that glucose should be administered as a hypertonic (up to 50%) solution via a central vein.

Administration of essential L-amino acids improve wound healing, result in reductions of plasma potassium, magnesium and phosphate levels, and generally improve survival and hasten recovery [539].

In such circumstances dialysis should be started regardless of plasma biochemistry, but when creatinine and urea levels rise rapidly because of a hypercatabolic state, dialysis is indicated even if clinical symptoms have not yet appeared. Early 'prophylactic' dialysis, before the onset of uraemic symptoms, allows more liberal intake of protein, salt and water as well as preventing hyperkalaemic emergencies [530]. Furthermore, it decreases the incidence of infectious complications, improves wound healing, increases patient comfort and appears to improve patient survival.

PERITONEAL DIALYSIS

Peritoneal dialysis has many advantages and can be used in pregnant or recently delivered women [107,313]. It is easily available, simple, inexpensive and has a relatively low complication rate. There are no absolute contraindications and it can be used even in the presence of pelvic peritonitis. Relative contraindications are intraperitoneal adhesions, open wounds or drains in the abdomen and recent retroperitoneal operations [540]. Occasionally peritoneal dialysis may be complicated by peritonitis or trauma to the intra-abdominal viscera.

HAEMODIALYSIS

Haemodialysis depends on an adequate shunt blood flow and has limited usefulness in the presence of hypotension. It is contraindicated in the actively bleeding patient, because even well-controlled regional heparinization does not ensure the safety of the procedure.

Acute renal failure and septic shock (see also above)

Septicaemia associated with pregnancy is commonly due to septic abortion whereas pyelonephritis, chorioamnionitis and puerperal sepsis occur less frequently [524,532,534]. Only occasionally is the abortion spontaneous, although detailed questioning may be required to elicit evidence that abortifacients have been used. Although this life-threatening condition is now very rare, the clinician should not be lulled into a false sense of security given the ever-present potential of antibiotic-resistant bacterial strains.

PATHOLOGY

There are many reasons why acute renal failure should be associated with septic abortion. The patient is both dehydrated and hypotensive—a combination that leads to considerable renal ischaemia. Haemoglobinuria (due to haemolysis) and DIC are often present, and soap and lysol (common abortifacients) have specific nephrotoxic effects [541]. The severity of the renal dysfunction associated with clostridial infections suggest that clostridia produce a specific nephrotoxin [542]. However, most pregnancy sepsis is due to Gram-negative bacteria (clostridia is responsible for only 0.5%), so that marked haemolysis due to bacteria and/or abortifacients is sufficient by itself to provoke renal shutdown, although it is now apparent that antilipopolysaccharide antibodies may have a role [543].

DIAGNOSIS AND INVESTIGATION

The presentation can be quite dramatic, especially in cases of *E. coli* and clostridia infection. There is an abrupt rise in temperature (to 40°C) often associated with myalgias, vomiting and diarrhoea, the last occasionally bloody.

Once symptoms commence, hypotension, tachypnoea and progression to acute shock occur rapidly. The patients are usually jaundiced, with a particular bronze-like colour ascribed to the association of jaundice with cutaneous vasodilatation, cyanosis and pallor. Despite the presence of fever, the extremities are often cold, with purplish areas that may be precursors of small patches of necrosis on the toes, fingers or nose.

There is laboratory evidence of severe anaemia due to haemolysis with hyperbilirubinaemia of the direct type. There are also alterations in clotting factors that suggest DIC (see Chapter 3). Leucocytosis (25×10^9/L) with marked shifts to the left are the rule and thrombocytopenia of $<50 \times 10^9$/L is often observed. Hypocalcaemia, severe enough to provoke tetany, can occur [524].

Abdominal radiography may demonstrate air in the uterus or abdomen—the result of gas-forming organisms and/or perforation. Despite this toxic and septicaemic picture, bacterial identification may be difficult and the situation is further confused because clostridia are normally present in the female genital tract [544].

Full initial assessment should be conducted with an intensive care physician and a nephrologist [545] along the lines discussed for acute renal failure with the following additional important points.

Skin and core temperature differential

The relationship of skin temperature to central body temperature serves as an indicator of adequacy of peripheral perfusion. Peripheral temperature can be measured from the medial aspect of the big toe and central body temperature by a probe placed in the rectum, in the lumen of the oesophagus or over the sternum. A large difference between the two (>2°C) implies poor peripheral perfusion. This is commonly associated with lactic acidosis and occasionally with DIC.

Serum albumin

This should always be assessed in any patient with severe sepsis. Levels <25 g/L are commonly found, predisposing the patient to pulmonary oedema. Albumin replacement should be considered.

Blood sugar

Diabetes must be excluded. Blood from a finger prick should not be used if there is poor skin perfusion.

Acid–base status

The patient may be hypoxic, through ventilation/perfusion inequality. The $Paco_2$ is usually low in order to compensate for the increasing metabolic acidosis. An elevated $Paco_2$ is unusual: it may imply deterioration in the level of consciousness with loss of respiratory drive or, occasionally, may precede respiratory failure or depression due to sedative drugs.

Metabolic acidosis is generally related to inadequate peripheral oxygenation, anaerobic metabolism and the onset of lactic acidosis. An increasing and irreversible metabolic acidosis following initial resuscitation is a bad prognostic sign.

Coagulation indices (see Chapter 3)

Hypercoagulability may be seen early and can alternate with hypocoagulability. Haematological evidence of DIC correlates with the severity of the shock and poor peripheral oxygenation. The potential for blood loss in septic abortion increases the susceptibility to DIC. Thrombocytopenia alone can occur in the presence of significant sepsis.

Cardiovascular investigation

Routine cardiovascular assessment may be insufficient for haemodynamic evaluation [545]. More elaborate investigations may be needed such as right ventricular output assessment or pulmonary capillary wedge pressure (PCWP), and these require skilled personnel as well as specialized equipment. Therefore, should a patient fail to respond to volume replacement, metabolic correction and antibiotics or be severely shocked, treatment must be conducted in an appropriately equipped intensive care unit if the patient is not in one already.

DIAGNOSTIC PITFALLS

The clinician may be misled by an asymptomatic patient admitted with an incomplete abortion who rapidly becomes shocked within hours. The generalized muscular pains, often most intense in the thorax and abdomen, may lead to confusion with intra-abdominal inflammatory processes; this is especially true when a history of provoked abortion is denied or not sought, because heavy vaginal bleeding is often not a prominent feature.

Recent treatment with antibiotics or other drugs must be pursued, as it will give pointers to bacterial resistance, suppressed infection and drug-modified physiology.

GENERAL MANAGEMENT PLAN

The initial steps include vigorous supportive therapy and the use of antibiotics in high doses. The use of clostridia antitoxin, steroids and the role of surgical intervention are controversial.

The role of surgery

Three or four decades ago women with septicaemia due to septic abortion were usually considered too ill to undergo surgery. It was later suggested that in such patients the placenta served as a huge culture site for bacterial growth, from which bacteria and toxins could easily pass into the maternal circulation [546]. This led to the hypothesis that if this nidus could be contained by securing the ovarian and uterine vessels, the patient's blood pressure would respond favourably and rapidly. In a series of 77 women with soap-provoked septic abortion, 60% of patients who underwent surgery survived compared to 30% of those treated by supportive therapy alone [547]. Bartlett and Yahia [541] described five successive gravely ill women whose abortion had been induced by soap and/or phenol: each of them survived, and this success rate was attributed to the rapid performance of abdominal hysterectomy.

Such results led many to advocate a radical approach, where abdominal hysterectomy is performed in patients who are responding poorly to volume replacement and vasoactive agents [548,549]. However, this approach was questioned by Hawkins *et al.* [524] who described 20 patients managed with intensive antibiotic therapy, dialysis as required, and an absolute minimum of surgical intervention: 17 out of 19 of these patients survived while a 20th patient who had undergone hysterectomy died. These authors state that antibiotic therapy alone is usually capable of confining the infection to the pelvis and eventually eradicating it from the uterus. They further noted that many young women with septic abortion may want a pregnancy in the future, and in their series of 11 women who subsequently attempted to conceive, seven achieved normal pregnancies.

The debate concerning radical vs. conservative treatment continues [530]. Data supporting the surgical approach have not always been as favourable as the small series of Bartlett and Yahia [541], and none of the reported studies was controlled. On the other hand, the picture of a necrotic and grossly infected uterus that often accompanies these chemically produced abortions is sufficient to convince many that hysterectomy is necessary. Whilst the results of Hawkins *et al.* [524] are impressive, it should be noted that most of their patients were transferred from other hospitals, and constituted a group that had already survived for several days with a conservative approach.

Volume and metabolic control

It is essential to restore an adequate circulating volume as soon as possible, and the volume infused must be regulated according to CVP or RAP readings. When both the blood pressure and the CVP are low, fluid should be infused until the systolic pressure rises to 100 mmHg or higher and/or the CVP is up to 8 cmH$_2$O. An increase in urinary output to >40 mL/h is an excellent prognostic sign.

The fluid selected for volume replacement will depend upon whether there is an obvious electrolyte deficit, possible albumin depletion, or fluid is merely required to increase the circulating volume. Plasma protein fraction (PPF) is the solution of choice for volume replacement. Should the urinary output improve, potassium supplementation is generally necessary.

Sodium chloride (as normal saline) should only be given when there has been obvious sodium loss. A low serum sodium is common in the septic patient but does not necessarily reflect a fall in total body sodium. Blood should not be used for volume replacement, unless the haematocrit is 30% or less, because it increases viscosity and hence may encourage capillary sludging. Dextran 70 should not be used if there is evidence of a bleeding diathesis or a history of skin allergy or bronchospasm.

In an appreciable number of cases, anuria may persist for up to 3 or more weeks [550]. Often it is just when the patient is thought to have cortical rather than tubular necrosis that the diuretic phase commences. Some women with septic abortion do develop cortical necrosis, however, perhaps due to a severe ischaemic insult or massive DIC.

Drugs that may improve the haemodynamic state include dopamine, isoprenaline and phentolamine; their use must be based on expert assessment of the haemodynamic situation [551].

Bacteriological control

Appropriate antibiotic therapy is essential but in the shocked patient it is of secondary importance to restoration of adequate perfusion. Before antibiotics are given, the appropriate specimens for aerobic and anaerobic cultures must be taken. A bactericidal antibiotic may produce temporary clinical deterioration because of breakdown of bacteria and endotoxin release. This is an additional reason for performing basic resuscitation procedures before starting antibiotic therapy.

In patients without previous antibiotic therapy, it is reasonable to commence with a combination of a cephalosporin and metronidazole. Should the shock be severe and a *Pseudomonas* or *Proteus* infection be diagnosed or a resistant *Klebsiella* or coliform be suspected, then gentamicin should be included. The dosage of gentamicin must be regulated according to daily blood levels. Once the sensitivities are available, the antibiotic therapy may need to be modified. Antibiotics should be given intravenously at first, changing to the oral route once the shock phase is over.

Haematological control

Sequential assessment of the coagulation indices is essential. A steady deterioration may be seen consistent with a diagnosis of DIC, and is commonly associated with overall clinical deterioration. Active treatment is not required where there are minor changes in the coagulation indices without clinical evidence of bleeding and where shock is rapidly corrected.

Should the clotting factors continue to deteriorate, in spite of the preceding resuscitative measures, fresh frozen plasma (FFP) should be given. Heparin may be considered if there is a further fall in the fibrinogen titre, in spite of FFP. A persistent thrombocytopenia (platelet count $<40 \times 10^9/L$) and capillary oozing in spite of replacement of clotting factors is an indication for an infusion of platelets or platelet-enriched plasma.

Other measures

Hyperbaric oxygen and exchange transfusion have both been used to treat clostridial sepsis, but results are too fragmentary to recommend specific protocols [275].

Acute renal failure in pre-eclampsia/ eclampsia (see also Chapter 6)

The causes of renal failure in pre-eclampsia/eclampsia are considered in Chapter 6. Suffice to say that renal failure is usually due to acute tubular necrosis, but acute cortical necrosis may also occur. It is possible that acute tubular necrosis is the obligatory outcome of glomerular cell swelling and loss of anionic charge along with complete obliteration of the capillary lumen. The situation may be aggravated by haemorrhage or even inappropriate drug therapy [318]. If the renal failure is related solely to pre-eclampsia without chronic hypertension, renal disease or both (before pregnancy), then normal renal function resumes in about 80% of cases in the long term.

Underlying renal problems reduce this to 20%, with the remainder needing permanent renal replacement therapy.

HELLP syndrome (haemolysis, elevated liver enzymes and low platelets) was originally thought to be a rare complication of severe pre-eclampsia but as more attention is paid to liver and haematological functions it is now diagnosed more often [552]. It is not clear, however, whether acute renal failure is a specific component of the HELLP syndrome itself or a complication of a particularly severe multisystem condition. Certainly it may occur without haemolysis as in ELLP syndrome [553].

Treatment should follow the standard approach, although more specific therapies have been suggested such as prostacyclin infusion [554].

Acute renal failure and pyelonephritis

Acute pyelonephritis is the most common renal complication during pregnancy [274]. In the absence of complicating features such as obstruction, calculi, papillary necrosis and analgesic nephropathy, acute pyelonephritis is an extremely rare cause of acute renal failure in nonpregnant subjects, but this association appears to be more frequent in pregnant women [555]. The reason is obscure. It is known that, in pregnant women, acute pyelonephritis is accompanied by marked decrements in GFR as well as significant increments in plasma creatinine levels [306] and this contrasts with the situation in non-pregnant patients. The vasculature in pregnancy may be more sensitive to the vasoactive effect of bacterial endotoxins [556].

Acute renal failure and pre-existing chronic renal disease

In women with moderate and severe renal disease (serum creatinine $>180\mu mol/L$), gestational complications are inevitable (see above) and pregnancy-related loss of renal function occurs in almost 50% of pregnancies with 10% of women progressing rapidly to end-stage renal failure very soon after delivery but occasionally in pregnancy, when dialysis can be used to prolong pregnancy [112,115,135,557].

Haemolytic–uraemia syndrome

This rare and often lethal syndrome was first described 20 years ago [558] and named 'irreversible postpartum renal failure'. Several other labels have been used since then including 'idiopathic postpartum renal failure', 'postpartum malignant nephrosclerosis', 'idiopathic postpartum renal failure' and most commonly 'postpartum haemolytic–uraemia syndrome'. The haematological manifestations of HUS are considered in Chapter 3.

PATHOPHYSIOLOGY AND DIAGNOSIS

HUS is characterized by the onset of renal failure 3–10 weeks into the puerperium [90,559,560] after the patient has had an uneventful pregnancy and delivery. She develops marked azotemia and severe hypertension frequently associated with microangiopathic haemolytic anaemia and platelet aggregation with formation of microthrombi in the terminal portions of the renal vasculature. It should be remembered that renal failure, microangiopathic haemolytic anaemia and thrombocytopenia may be associated in pregnant women with severe preeclampsia, the HELLP syndrome [308], acute fatty liver of pregnancy and thrombotic thrombocytopenic purpura. Distinction between HUS and some of these disorders may be difficult because they may persist in the postpartum period. Although there is clinically a broad overlap between these conditions, correct identification is necessary because specific investigations or therapy are needed in some [561,562].

The pathophysiology is unknown and the controversies about management reflect this uncertainty [546,563,564]. HUS has a poor prognosis: in a review of 49 patients with HUS by Segonds *et al.* [564], death occurred in 61%, complete recovery of renal function in only 9.5%, and 12% of the patients had terminal renal failure requiring maintenance dialysis.

It has been suggested that endothelial damage is the key lesion in HUS. This may involve the Sanarelli–Schwartzman reaction [565], the action of an *E. coli*-produced vero-cell toxin (verotoxin) [566] and/or platelet aggregation and deposition. It has been demonstrated that endothelial production of NO may be critical to prevent endotoxin-induced glomerular thrombosis [567]. Genetic and environmental factors have been implicated as they have in postpill HUS, idiopathic HUS and thrombocytopenic purpura. Of interest are recent reports of two HLA-identical sisters, one of whom developed postpartum HUS and the other postpill HUS [234] and familial occurrence of thrombotic thrombocytopenic purpura during pregnancy. A pathogenic role for immunological factors has also been proposed as transient hypocomplementaemia can occur.

TREATMENT AND OUTCOME

Treatment has been with dialysis or plasmaphoresis, immunosuppression, heparin, streptokinase, dipyridamole, acetylsalicylic acid and corticosteroids in various combinations. Other forms of management have evolved in recent years and have been used with some success. A supposed lack of plasma prostacyclin (prostaglandin I_2, PGI_2)—a powerful vasodilator and potent endogenous inhibitor of platelet aggregation—can be counteracted by exchange transfusion or even plasma infusion alone [568] on the basis of its successful use in thrombotic thrombocytopenic purpura or in adult HUS [569]. Prolonged PGI_2 infusions have been tried with the aim of restoring the deficiency, thus controlling hypertension and reversing platelet consumption [570].

Because DIC may be of pathogenic significance, with placental thromboplastin release during labour, antithrombin III (ATIII) may have a protective effect. ATIII can be given as a concentrate and there have been reports of low plasma ATIII concentrations at the onset of the syndrome [571]. Interestingly, heparin increases the turnover rate of ATIII, and giving heparin to patients with potentially decreased plasma ATIII levels may therefore paradoxically increase an existing risk of thrombosis. Lastly, renal transplantation may be successful but there is a chance of recurrence of the HUS lesion in the allograft.

Bilateral renal cortical necrosis in pregnancy

Renal cortical necrosis is an extremely rare complication, which at one time seemed to be more common in pregnant compared to non-pregnant populations [532] but most recently its incidence during pregnancy has decreased to below one in 80 000. It is characterized by tissue death throughout the cortex with sparing of the medullary portions [160,572,573]. Although it may develop in patients with DIC or overwhelming septicaemia, most cases present in the third trimester or the puerperium when septic complications occur less often and when it is associated with specific obstetric complications such as placental abruption, unrecognized long-standing intrauterine death and occasionally pre-eclampsia [531]. Multigravidas beyond the age of 30 are more likely to develop this condition. It has been considered the clinical counterpart of the experimental Sanarelli–Schwartzman reaction [565].

While cortical necrosis may involve the entire renal cortex resulting in irreversible renal failure, it is the 'patchy' variety that occurs more often in pregnancy. This is characterized by an initial episode of severe oliguria, which lasts much longer than in uncomplicated acute tubular necrosis, followed by a variable return of function and stable period of moderate renal insufficiency. Years later, for reasons still obscure, renal function may decrease again, often leading to end-stage renal failure.

Miscellaneous causes of renal failure

Acute renal failure can occur during pregnancy in a variety of situations similar to those causing renal dysfunction in non-pregnant patients. These situations include primary renal diseases (acute nephritis, sarcoidosis, lymphoma, Goodpasture's syndrome), those related to systemic illnesses (endocarditis, ingestion of nephrotoxins, incompatible blood transfusions), structural infiltrations of the kidneys secondary to extrarenal disease [574] and non-surgical obstructive problems [103]. Acute renal failure in acute fatty liver of pregnancy is considered in Chapter 9.

Obstetric renal failure: some conclusions

1 Acute renal failure can occur during pregnancy in a variety of situations similar to those causing sudden renal dysfunction in non-pregnant patients [575]. Pathology peculiar to pregnancy, however, must always be considered. Acute fatty liver can be complicated by renal failure and its early recognition with prompt treatment could reduce fetal and maternal mortality rate. HUS is also associated with a high morbidity and mortality.

2 The need to actively treat acute renal failure cannot be questioned but the importance of reaching an early (histological) diagnosis of its cause must not be forgotten [576].

3 Treatment of sudden renal failure resembles that used in non-pregnant populations and aims at retarding the appearance of uraemic symptomatology, acid–base and electrolyte disturbances and volume problems. There must be constant awareness of the propensity of patients with acute renal failure to become infected, a complication that can be serious in pregnant women.

4 Some of the problems can be dealt with by judicious conservative management, but if such an approach is unsuccessful, dialysis will be necessary.

5 Dialysis in patients with acute renal failure is prescribed 'prophylactically'; that is prior to the appearance of electrolyte and acid–base disturbance imbalances or uraemic symptoms. Furthermore, as urea, creatinine and a presumed variety of metabolic waste products cross the placenta, 'prophylactic' dialysis could be more compelling in prepartum patients with immature fetuses and in whom temporization is desired. The policy of 'buying time' without modifying the underlying pathology should be continually reviewed.

6 The method of dialysis (peritoneal or haemodialysis) should be dictated by facilities available and by clinical circumstances. Peritoneal dialysis is effective and safe as long as the catheter is inserted high in the abdomen under direct vision through a small incision. It probably minimizes rapid metabolic pertubations.

7 Controlled anticoagulation with heparin (preferably including monitoring of activated clotting time to maintain it between 150 and 180 s) is desirable during haemodialysis. Volume shifts during haemodialysis must be minimized to avoid impairment of uteroplacental blood flow.

8 Increments in uterine activity or the onset of labour frequently occur during or immediately after dialysis. Therefore, when possible, early delivery (as dictated by fetal maturity) should be undertaken.

9 At or after delivery blood loss should be replaced quickly to the point of slight overtransfusion, because any haemorrhage may be underestimated.

10 The neonate can be subject to rapid dehydration because increased levels of urea and other solutes within the fetal circulation precipitate an osmotic diuresis in the neonate shortly after birth.

References

1 Lindheimer MD, Davison JM, Katz AI. The kidney and hypertension in pregnancy: twenty exciting years. *Sem Nephrol* 2001; 21: 173–89.

2 Peake SL, Roxburgh HB, Langlois S. Ultrasonic assessment of hydronephrosis of pregnancy. *Radiology* 1983; 128: 167–70.

3 Roberts J. Hydronephrosis of pregnancy. *Urology* 1976; 8: 1–5.

4 Cietak KA, Newton JR. Serial qualitative maternal nephrosonography in pregnancy. *Br J Radiol* 1985; 58: 399–404.

5 Graif M, Kessler A *et al.* Renal pyclectasis in pregnancy. Correlative evaluation of fetal and maternal collecting systems. *Am J Obstet Gynecol* 1992; 167: 1304–6.

6 Christensen T, Klebe JC *et al.* Changes in renal volume during normal pregnancy. *Acta Obstet Gynaecol Scand* 1989; 68: 541–3.

7 Dunlop W, Davison JM. Renal haemodynamics and tubular function in human pregnancy. *Clin Obstet Gynaecol* 1987; 1: 769–88.

8 Cietak KA, Newton JR. Serial quantitative nephrosonography in pregnancy. *Br J Radiol* 1985; 58: 405–13.

9 Satin AJ, Seikin GL, Cunningham FG. Reversible hypertension in pregnancy caused by obstructive uropathy. *Obstet Gynecol* 1993; 81: 823–5.

10 Baylis C, Davison JM. The urinary system. In: Chamberlain G, Broughton Pipkin F eds. *Clinical Physiology in Obstetrics*, 3rd edn. Blackwell Scientific Press, Oxford, 1998: 263–307.

11 Davison JM, Hytten FE. Glomerular filtration during and after pregnancy. *J Obstet Gynecol Br Commonwealth* 1974; 81: 588–95.

12 Conrad KP, Lindheimer MD. Renal and cardiovascular alterations. In: Lindheimer MD, Roberts JM, Cunningham FG, eds. *Chelsey's Hypertensive Disorders in Pregnancy*, 2nd edn. Appleton & Lange, Stanford, CN, 1999: 262–326.

13 Davison JM, Noble MCB. Serial changes in 24-hour creatinine clearance during normal menstrual cycles and the first trimester of pregnancy. *Br J Obstet Gynaecol* 1981; 88: 10–17.

14 Davison JM, Dunlop W, Ezimokhai M. Twenty-four hour creatinine clearance during the third trimester of normal pregnancy. *Br J Obstet Gynaecol* 1980; 87: 106–9.

15 Baylis C. The mechanism of the increase in glomerular filtration rate in the 12 day pregnant rat. *J Physiol* 1980; 305: 405–14.

16 Baylis C. Effect of early pregnancy on glomerular filtration rate and plasma volume in the rat. *Renal Physiol* 1980; 2: 333–9.

17 Baylis C. Glomerular ultrafiltration in the pseudopregnant rat. *Am J Physiol* 1982; 243: F300–5.

18 Baylis C. Renal effects of cyclooxygenase inhibition in the pregnant rat. *Am J Physiol* 1987; 253: F158–63.

19 Roberts M, Lindheimer MD, Davison JM. Altered glomerular permselectivity to neutral dextrans and heteroporous membrane modelling in human pregnancy. *Am J Physiol* 1996; 270: F338–F343.

20 Milne JEC, Lindheimer MD, Davison JM. Glomerular heteroporous membrane modeling in third trimester and postpartum before and during amino acid infusion. *AM J Physiol* 2002; 282: F170-F175.

21 Sturgiss SN, Martin K, Whittingham TA, Davison JM. Assessment of the renal circulation during pregnancy with colour Doppler ultrasonography. *Am J Obstet Gynecol* 1992; 167: 1250–4.

22 Legarth J, Thorup E. Characteristics of Doppler blood velocity waveforms in a cardiovascular *in-vitro* model. II. The influence of peripheral resistance, perfusion pressure and blood flow. *Scand J Clin Lab Invest* 1989; 49: 459–64.

23 Schrier RW. Body fluid volume regulation in health and disease: a unifying hypothesis. *Ann Intern Med* 1990; 113: 155.

24 Baylis C. Glomerular filtration and volume regulation in gravid animal models. *Clin Obstet Gynaecol* 1994; 8: 235–64.

25 Lindheimer MD, Barron WM, Davison JM. Osmoregulation and vasopressin release in pregnancy. *Am J Physiol* 1989; 257: F159–69.

26 Baylis C, Munger K. Persistence of maternal plasma volume expansion in midterm pregnant rats maintained on a zero sodium intake: evidence that early gestational volume expansion does not require renal sodium retention. *Clin Exp Hypertens* 1990; B9: 237–47.

27 Verkeste CM, Slagen BFM, Dubelaar ML, Van Kreel BK & Peeters LLH. 1998. Mechanism of volume adaption in the awake early pregnant rat. *American Journal of Physiology* 274, H1662–6.

28 Churchill SE, Bengele HH, Alexander EA. Sodium balance during pregnancy in the rat. *Am J Physiol* 1980; 239: R143–8.

29 Lichton IJ. Salt saving in the pregnant rat. *Am J Physiol* 1961; 201: 765–8.

30 Navar LG. Renal autoregulation: perspectives from whole kidney and single nephron studies. *Am J Physiol* 1978; 234: F357–70.

31 Baylis C. Acute blockade of alpha-1–adrenoceptors has similar effects in pregnant and nonpregnant rats. *Hypertens Preg* 1995; 14: 17–25.

32 Castellino P, Coda B, Defronzo RA. Effect of amino acid infusion on renal hemodynamics in humans. *Am J Physiol* 1986; 251: F132–40.

33 Hostetter TH. Human renal response to a meat meal. *Am J Physiol* 1984; 250: F613–8.

34 Meyer TM, Ichikawa I, Zatz R, Brenner BM. The renal hemodynamic response to amino acid infusion in the rat. *Trans Assoc Am Phys* 1983; 96: 76–83.

35 Brendolan A, Bragantini L *et al.* Renal functional reserve in pregnancy. *Kidney Int* 1985; 28: 232A.

36 Barron WM, Lindheimer MD. Effect of oral protein loading on renal hemodynamics in human pregnancy. *Am J Physiol* 1995; 269: R888–R895.

37 Sturgiss SN, Wilkinson R, Davison JM. Renal reserve during pregnancy. *Am J Physiol* 1996; 271: F16–F20.

38 Gant NF, Whalley PJ, Everett RB, Worley RJ, Macdonald PC. Control of vascular reactivity in pregnancy. *Am J Kidney Dis* 1987; 9: 303–7.

39 Paller MS. Mechanism of decreased pressor responsiveness to ANG II, NE and vasopressin in pregnant rats. *Am J Physiol* 1984; 247: H100–8.

40 Conrad KP, Colpoys MC. Evidence against the hypothesis that prostaglandins are the vasodepressor agents of pregnancy. *J Clin Invest* 1986; 77: 236–45.

41 Brown GP, Venuto RC . Renal blood flow response to angiotensin II infusions in conscious pregnant rabbits. *Am J Physiol* 1991; 261, F51–F59.

42 Novak J, Reckelhoff J, Bumgarner L, Cockrell K, Kassab S, Granger JP. Reduced sensitivity of the renal circulation to angiotensin II in pregnant rats. *Hypertension* 1997; 30: 580–84.

43 Masilamani S, Baylis C. The renal vasculature does not participate in the peripheral refractoriness to administered angiotensin II in the late pregnancy rat. *J Am Soc Nephrol* 1992; 3: 566.

44 Baylis C. Blood pressure and renal hemodynamic effects of acute blockade of the vascular actions of arginine vasopressin in normal pregnancy in the rat. *Hypertens Preg* 1993; 12: 93–102.

45 Kriston T, Engels K, Venuto R, Baylis C, Losonczy GY. Hemodynamic and renal effects of U46619, a TXA2/PGH2 analog, in late pregnant rats. *AM J Physiol* 1999; 276: R831–7.

46 Kristensen CG, Nakagawa Y, Coe FL, Lindheimer MD. Effect of atrial natriuretic factor in rat pregnancy. *Am J Physiol* 1986; 250: R589–94.

47 Nadel AS, Ballerman BJ, Anderson S, Brenner BM. Interrelationships among atrial peptides, renin and blood volume in pregnant rats. *Am J Physiol* 1988; 254: R793–800.

48 Irons DW, Baylis PH, Davison JM. Effects of atrial natriuretic peptide on renal hemodynamics and sodium excretion during human pregnancy. *Am J Physiol* 1996; 271: F239–F242.

49 Dunn BR, Ichikawa I, Pfeffer JM, Troy JL, Brenner BM. Renal and systemic hemodynamic effects of synthetic atrial natriuretic peptide in the anesthetized rat. *Circulation Res* 1986; 59: 237–46.

50 Ferris TF. Prostanoids in normal and hypertensive pregnancy. In: Rubin PC, ed. *Handbook of Hypertension*, Vol. 10: *Hypertension in Pregnancy*. Elsevier, Science Publishers, London, 1988: 102–17.

51 Moncada S, Palmer RMJ, Higgs EA. Biosynthesis and endogenous roles of nitric oxide. *Pharmacol Rev* 1991; 43: 109–42.

52 Kone BC, Baylis C. Biosynthesis and homeostatic roles of nitric oxide in the kidney. Editorial review. *Am J Physiol* 1997; 272, F561–F578.

53 Santmyire BR, Baylis C. The inducible nitric oxide synthase inhibitor aminoguanidine inhibits the pregnancy induced renal vasodilation and increase in kidney NOS activity in the rat. *J AM Soc Nephrol* (in press).

54 Deng A, Engels K, Baylis C. Increased nitric oxide production plays a critical role in the maternal blood pressure and glomerular hemodynamic adaptations to pregnancy in the rat. *Kidney Int* 1996; 50, 1132–8.

55 Davidson LA, sherwood OD, Conrad KP. Relaxin in a potent renal vasodilator in conscious rats. *J Clin Invest* 1999; 103: 525–533.

56 Conrad KR, Gandley RE, Ogawa T, Nakanishi S, Danielson LA. Endothelin mediates renal vasodilation and hyperfiltration during pregnancy in chronically instrumented concious rats. *Am J Physiol* 1999; 276(45), F767–F776.

57 Conrad KP, Kerchner LJ, Mosher MD. Plasma and 24-h NOX and cGMP during normal pregnancy and preeclampsia in women on a reduced NOX diet. *Am J Physiol* 1999; F48–F57.

58 Conrad KP, Joffe GM *et al.* Identification of increased nitric oxide biosynthesis during pregnancy in rats. *FASEB J* 1993; 7, 566–71.

59 Baylis C, Vallance P. Measurement of nitrite and nitrate (NOx) levels in plasma and urine; what does this measure tell us

about the activity of the endogenous nitric oxide. *Nephrol Hypert* 1998; 7, 1–4.

60 Baylis C, Beinder E, Suto T, August P. Recent insights into the roles of nitric oxide and renin-angiotensin in the pathophysiology of preeclampsia pregnancy. *Semin Nephrol* 1998; 18, 208–30.

61 Cano RI, Delman MR, Pitchumoni CS, Lev R, Fosenberg WS. Acute fatty liver of pregnancy. Complication of disseminated intravascular coagulation. *J Am Med Assoc* 1975; 231: 159–61.

62 Sturgiss SN, Dunlop W, Davison JM. Renal haemodynamics and tubular function in human pregnancy. *Bailliere's Clin Obstet Gynaecol* 1994; 8: 209–234.

63 Davison JM. Renal nutrient excretion. *Clin Obstet Gynaecol* 1987; 2: 365–80.

64 Davison JM. The effect of pregnancy on kidney function in renal allograft recipients. *Kidney Int* 1985; 27: 74–9.

65 Davison JM, Shiells EA, Philips PR, Lindheimer MD. Serial evaluation of vasopressin release and thirst in human pregnancy. the role of human chorionic gonadotrophin in the osmoregulatory changes of gestation. *J Clin Invest* 1988; 81: 798–806.

66 Davison JM, Gilmore EA, Durr J, Robertson GL, Lindheimer MD. Altered osmotic thresholds for vasopressin secretion and thirst in human pregnancy. *Am J Physiol* 1984; 246: F105–9.

67 Davison JM, Nakagawa Y, Coe FL, Lindheimer MD. Increases in urinary inhibiter activity and excretion of an inhibitor of crystalluria in pregnancy: a defense against the hypercalciuria of normal gestation. *Hypertens Preg* 1993; 12: 25–35.

68 Lind T, Godfrey KA, Otun H, Philips PR. Changes in serum uric acid concentrations during normal pregnancy. *Br J Obstet Gynaecol* 1984; 91: 128–32.

69 Barron WM. Water metabolism and vasopressin secretion during pregnancy. *Clin Obstet Gynaecol* 1987; 1: 853–71.

70 Brenner BM, Meyer TW, Hostetter TH. Dietary protein intake and the progressive nature of the kidney disease. The role of hemodynamically mediated glomerular injury in the pathogenesis of progressive glomerular sclerosis in ageing, renal ablation and intrinsic renal disease. *N Engl J Med* 1982; 307: 652–9.

71 Davison JM. The effect of pregnancy on long term renal function in women with chronic renal disease and single kidneys. *Clin Exp Hypertens* 1988; B8: 222A.

72 Davison JM, Hytten FE. Can normal pregnancy damage your health? *Br J Obstet Gynaecol* 1987; 94: 385–6.

73 Taylor AA, Davison JM. Albumin excretion in normal pregnancy. *Am J Obstet Gynaecol* 1997; 177: 1559–60.

74 Lopez-Espinoza I, Dhar H, Humphreys S, Redman CWG. Urinary albumin excretion in pregnancy. *Br J obstet Gynaecol* 1986; 93: 176–81.

75 Wright A, McIntoch C, Steele P, Bennet J, Polat A. Urinary albumin excretion during normal pregnancy in women of low and high parity: evidence of albumin leakage after prolonged hyperfiltration. *Proceedings of the Xth International Congress of Nephrology*, 1987, 513A.

76 Wright A, Steele P, Bennett JR, Watts C, Polak A. The urinary excretion of albumin in normal pregnancy. *Br J Obstet Gynaecol* 1987; 94: 408–12.

77 Davison JM. Pregnancy in renal allograft recipients: prognosis and management. *Clin Obstet Gynaecol* 1987; 1: 1027–45.

78 Brown WW, Davis BB, Spray LA, Wongsurawat N, Malone JD, Domoto DT. Aging and the kidney. *Arch Intern Med* 1986; 146: 1790–6.

79 Lindheimer MD, Katz AI. The renal response to pregnancy. In: Brenner BM, Rector FC Jr, eds. *The Kidney*. W.B. Saunders, Philadelphia, PA, 1981: 1762–815.

80 Lindheimer MD, Katz AI. *Kidney Function and Disease in Pregnancy*. Lea & Febiger, New York, 1977.

81 Abe S. An overview of pregnancy in women with underlying renal disease. *Am J Kidney Dis* 1991; 17: 112–15.

82 Abe S. Pregnancy in IgA nephropathy. *Kidney Int* 1991; 40: 1098–102.

83 Abe S. The influence of pregnancy on the long-term renal prognosis of IgA nephropathy. *Clin Nephrol* 1994; 41: 61–4.

84 Abe S, Amagasaki Y, Konishi K, Kato E, Sakaguchi H, Ilyori S. The influence of antecedent renal disease on pregnancy. *Am J Obstet Gynecol* 1985; 153: 508–14.

85 Barcelo P, Lopez-Lillo J, Caberto L, Del Rio G. Successful pregnancy in primary glomerular disease. *Kidney Int* 1986; 30: 914–19.

86 Bear RA. Pregnancy in patients with renal disease. A study of 44 cases. *Obstet Gynecol* 1976; 48: 13–18.

87 Cunningham FG, Cox SM, Harstad TW, Mason RA, Pritchard JA. Chronic renal disease and pregnancy outcome. *Am J Obstet Gynecol* 1990; 163: 453–9.

88 Felding CF. Obstetric aspects in women with histories of renal disease. *Acta Obstet Gynaecol Scand* 1969; 48: 2–43.

89 Fisher KA, Luger A, Spargo BH, Lindheimer MD. A biopsy study of hypertension in pregnancy. In: Bonnar J, Macgillivray I, Symonds EM, eds. *Pregnancy Hypertension*. MTP Press, Lancaster, 1980: 333–8.

90 Hayslett JP. Postpartum renal failure. *N Engl J Med* 1985; 312: 1556–9.

91 Imbasciati E, Ponticelli C. Pregnancy and renal disease: predictors for fetal and maternal outcome. *Am J Nephrol* 1991; 11: 353–62.

92 Jungers P, Houillier P, Forget D, Henry-Amar M. Specific controversies concerning the natural history of renal disease in pregnancy. *Am J Kidney Dis* 1991; 17: 166–71.

93 Kaplan AI, Smith JP, Tillman AJB. Healed acute and chronic nephritis in pregnancy. *Am J Obstet Gynecol* 1962; 83: 1519–25.

94 Katz AI, Davison JM, Hayslett JP, Singson E, Lindheimer MD. Pregnancy in women with kidney disease. *Kidney Int* 1980; 18: 192–206.

95 Katz AI, Lindheimer MD. Does pregnancy aggravate primary glomerular disease? *Am J Kidney Dis* 1985; 6: 261–5.

96 Klockars M, Saarikoski S, Ikonen E, Kuhlback P. Pregnancy in patients with renal disease. *Acta Med Scand* 1980; 207: 207–14.

97 Leppert P, Tisher CC, Shu-Chung SC, Harlan WR. Antecedent renal disease and the outcome of pregnancy. *Ann Intern Med* 1979; 90: 747–51.

98 Strauch BS, Hayslett JP. Kidney disease and pregnancy. *Br Med J* 1974; iv: 378–82.

99 Surian M, Imbasciati E *et al*. Glomerular disease and pregnancy: a study of 123 pregnancies in patients with primary and secondary glomerular disease. *Nephrology* 1984; 36: 101–5.

100 Werkö L, Bucht H. Glomerular filtration rate and renal blood flow in patients with chronic diffuse glomerulonephritis during pregnancy. *Acta Med Scand* 1956; 153: 177–86.

101 Williams DJ. Renal disease in pregnancy. *Curr Obstet Gynaecol* 1997; 7: 156–62.

102 Lindheimer MD, Katz AI. Gestation in women with kidney disease: prognosis and management. *Clin Obstet Gynaecol* 1987; 1: 921–38.

103 Thorp JA, Davis BE, Klingele C. Severe early onset preeclampsia secondary to bilateral ureteral obstruction reversed by stenting. *Obstet Gynecol* 1999; 94: 806–07.

104 Kincaid-Smith P, Whitworth JA, Fairley KF. Mesangial IgA nephropathy in pregnancy. *Clin Exp Hypertens* 1980; 2: 821–38.

105 Easterling TR, Brateng D, Coldman ML, Strandness DE, Zaccardi MJ. Renal vascular hypertension during pregnancy. *Obstet Gynecol* 1991; 78: 921–5.

106 Hou S. Pregnancy in women with chronic renal disease. *N Engl J Med* 1985, 312: 836–9.

107 Hou S. Peritoneal and hemodialysis in pregnancy. *Clin Obstet Gynaecol* 1987; 1: 1009–26.

108 Imbasciati E, Pardi C *et al*. Pregnancy in women with chronic renal failure. *Proceedings of the IVth World Congress of the International Society Study of Hypertension in Pregnancy*, 1984, 78A.

109 Imbasciati E, Pardi C *et al*. Pregnancy in women with chronic renal failure. *Am J Nephrol* 1986; 6: 193–8.

110 Jungers P, Forget D, Henry-Amar M, Grünfeld J-P. Chronic kidney disease and pregnancy. *Adv Nephrol* 1986; 15: 103–41.

111 Jungers P, Forget D, Houillier P, Henry-Amar M, Grünfeld J-P. Pregnancy in IgA nephropathy, reflux nephropathy and focal glomerular sclerosis. *Am J Kidney Dis* 1987; 9: 334–8.

112 Jungers P, Chauveau D. Pregnancy in renal disease. *Kidney Int* 1997; 52: 871–85.

113 Brem AS, Singer D, Anderson L, Lester B, Abuelo JG. Infants of azotemic mothers: a report of three live births. *Am J Kidney Dis* 1988; 12: 299–303.

114 Hou SH, Grossman SD, Madias NE. Pregnancy in women with renal disease and moderate renal insufficiency. *Am J Med* 1985; 78: 185–94.

115 Jones DC, Hayslett JP. Outcome of pregnancy in women with moderate or severe renal insufficiency. *N Engl J Med* 1996; 335: 226–32.

116 Jungers P, Chauveau D *et al*. Pregnancy in women with impaired renal function. *Clin Nephrol* 1997; 47: 281–8.

117 Bar J, Ben-Rafael Z *et al*. Predictions of pregnancy outcome in subgroups of women with renal disease. *Clin Nephrol* 2000; 53: 437–44.

118 Lim VS. Reproductive endocrinology in uremia. *Clin Obstet Gynaecol* 1994; 8: 469–80.

119 Stotland NL, Stotland NE. The mother and the burning building. *Obstet Gynecol Surv* 1997; 53: 1–2.

120 Heybourne KD, Schultz W, Goodlin RC, Durham JD. Renal artery stenosis during pregnancy: a review. *Obstet Gynecol Surv* 1991; 46: 509–14.

121 Coldsmith JH, Menzies DN, De Boer CH, Caplan W. Delivery of healthy infants after five week's dialysis treatment for fulminating toxaemia of pregnancy. *Lancet* 1971; ii: 738–40.

122 Mitra S, Vertes V, Roza O, Berman LB. Periodic haemodialysis in pregnancy. *Am J Med Sci* 1970; 259: 333–9.

123 Nalk RB, Clark AD, Warren DJ. Acute proliferative glomerulonephritis with crescents and renal failure in pregnancy successfully managed by intermittent haemodialysis. *Br J Obstet Gynaecol* 1979; 86: 819–22.

124 O'Donnell D, Sevitz H, Seggie JL, Meyers AM, Botha JR, Myburgh JA. Pregnancy after renal transplantation. *Aust NZ J Med* 1985; 15: 320–32.

125 Trebbin WM. Hemodialysis and pregnancy. *J Am Med Assoc* 1979; 241: 1811–12.

126 Okundaye IB, Abrinko P, Hou SH. Registry of pregnancy in dialysis patients. *Am J Kidney Dis* 1998; 31: 766–73.

127 Schewitz LJ, Friedman EA, Pollak VE. Bleeding after renal biopsy in pregnancy. *Obstet Gynecol* 1965; 26: 295–304.

128 Chenn HH, Lin HC, Yen JC, Chen CP. Renal biopsies is pregancies complicated by undertermined disease. *Acta Obstet Gynecol Scand* 2001; 80: 888–893.

129 Lindheimer MD, Fisher KA, Spargo BH, Katz AI. Hypertension in pregnancy: a biopsy study with long term follow-up. *Contrib Nephrol* 1981; 25: 71–7.

130 Packham D, Fairley KF. Renal biopsy; mdications and complications in pregnancy. *Br J Obstet Gynaecol* 1987; 94: 935–9.

131 Lindheimer MD, Davison JM. Renal biopsy during pregnancy: 'To b… or not to b…'. *Br J Obstet Gynaecol* 1987; 94: 932–4.

132 Kuller JA, D'Andrea N, McMahon MJ. Renal biospy and pregnancy *Am J Obstet Gynecol* 2001; 184: 1093–96.

133 Jacobsen FK, Christensen CK, Mogensen CE, Heilskow HCS. Evaluation of kidney function after meals. *Lancet* 1980; i: 319.

134 Chesley LC, Williams LO. Renal glomerular and tubular function in relation to the hyperuricaemia of pre-eclampsia and eclampsia. *Am J Obstet Gynecol* 1945; 50: 367–75.

135 Halligan AWF, Bell SC, Taylor DJ. Dipstick proteinuria: caveal eruptor. *Br J Obstet Gynaecol* 1999; 106: 1113–15.

136 Saudan PJ, Brown MA *et al*. Improved methods of assessing proteinuria in hypertensive pregnancy. *Br J Obstet Gynaecol* 1997; 104: 1159–64.

137 de Swiet M. Maternal blood pressure and birthweight. *Lancet* 2000; 355: 81–2.

138 Fisher K, Luger A, Spargo BH, Lindheimer MD. Hypertension in pregnancy: Clinical-pathological correlations and remote prognosis. *Medicine* 1981; 60: 267–74.

139 Thacker SB, Berkelman RL. Assessing the diagnostic accuracy and efficacy of selected antepartum fetal surveillance techniques. *Obstet Gynecol Surv* 1986; 41: 121–41.

140 Vintzileos AM, Campbell WA, Nochimson DJ, Weinbaum PJ. The use and misuse of the biophysical profile. *Am J Obstet Gynecol* 1987; 156: 527–33.

141 Abbate M, Beniqui A *et al*. Nephrotoxicity of increased glomerular protein traffic. *Nephrol Dial Transplant* 1999; 14: 304–12.

142 Tatum HJ, Mulé JG. Puerperal vasomotor tone in patients with toxemia of pregnancy. a new concept of the etiology and a rational plan of treatment. *Am J Obstet Gynecol* 1956; 71: 492–8.

143 Gabert HA, Miller JM. Renal disease in pregnancy. *Obstet Gynecol Surv* 1985; 40: 449–61.

144 Nadler N, Salinas-Madrigal L, Charles AG, Pollak VE. Acute glomerulonephritis during late pregnancy. *Obstet Gynecol* 1969; 34: 277–80.

145 Shepherd J, Shepard C. Poststreptococcal glomerulonephritis: a rare complication of pregnancy. *J Family Prac* 1992; 34: 630–2.

146 Feivenza F, Green A, Lafayette RA. Acute renal failure due to postinfection glomerulonephritis during pregnancy. *Am J Kidney Dis* 1997; 29: 273–6.

147 Cameron JS, Flicks J. Pregnancy in patients with pre-existing glomerular disease. *Contrib Nephrol* 1984; 37: 1459–5.

148 Epstein FH. Pregnancy and renal disease. *N Engl J Med* 1996; 335: 277–8.

149 Fairley KF, Whitworth JS, Kincaid-Smith P. Glomerulonephritis and pregnancy. In: Kincaid-Smith P, Mathew TH, Becker EL, eds. *Glomerulonephritis*, Part II. Wiley, New York, 1973: 997–1011.

150 Kincaid-Smith P, Fairley KF. Renal disease in pregnancy. Three controversial areas. Mesangial IgA nephropathy, focal glomerular sclerosis (focal and segmental hyalinosis and sclerosis) and reflux nephropathy. *Am J Kidney Dis* 1987; 9: 328–33.

151 Kincaid-Smith P, Fairley KF, Bullen M. Kidney disease and pregnancy. *Med J Aust* 1967; 2: 1155–9.

152 Katz AI, Davison JM, Hayslett JP, Lindheimer MD. Effect of pregnancy on the natural history of kidney disease. *Contrib Nephrol* 1981; 25: 53–60.

153 Jungers P, Houillier P, Forget D *et al*. Influence of pregnancy on the course of primary chronic glomerulonephritis. *Lancet* 1995; 346: 1122–1124.

154 Abe S. Pregnancy in glomerulonephritic patients with decreased renal function. *Hypertension in Pregnancy* 1996; 15: 305–12.

155 Kim Y, Shvil Y, Michael AF. Hypocomplementuria in a newborn infant caused by placental transfer of C3 nephritic factor. *J Pediatr* 1978; 92: 88–90.

156 Harper L, Savage COS. Treatment of IgA nephropathy. *Lancet* 1999; 353: 860–2.

157 Uribe LC, Thakur VD, Krane NK. Steroid-responsive nephrotic syndrome with renal insufficiency in the first trimester of pregnancy. *Am J Obstet Gynecol* 1991; 164: 568–9.

158 Grünfeld J-P. Alport's syndrome. In: Cameron JS, Davison AM, Grünfeld JP, Kerr D, Ritz E, eds. Oxford University Press, Oxford, 1992: 2197–205.

159 Grünfeld J-P, Boise EP, Hinglais N. Progressive and non-progressive hereditary chronic nephritis. *Kidney Int* 1973; 4: 216–20.

160 Grünfeld J-P, Noel LH, Hafez S, Droz D. Renal prognosis in women with hereditary nephritis. *Clin Nephrol* 1985; 23: 267–70.

161 Harris JP, Rakowski JA, Argy WP. Alport's syndrome presenting as crescentic glomerulonephritis. A report of two siblings. *Clin Nephrol* 1978; 10: 245–9.

162 Rogers PW, Kurtzman NA, Bunn SM. Familial benign essential hematuria. *Arch Intern Med* 1973; 131: 257–9.

163 Kuo VS, Koumantakis G, Gallery EDM. Proteinuria and its assessment in normal and hypertensive pregnancy. *Am J Obstet Gynecol* 1992; 167: 723–38.

164 Mor-Josef S, Navot D, Rabinowitz R, Sehenker JG. Collagen disease in pregnancy. *Obstet Gynecol Surv* 1984; 39: 67–83.

165 Hayslett JP, Lynn RI. Effect of pregnancy in patients with lupus nephropathy. *Kidney Int* 1980; 18: 207–20.

166 Jungers P, Dougados M, Pelissies C. Lupus nephropathy and pregnancy. *Arch Intern Med* 1982; 142: 771.

167 Hayslett JP. The effect of systemic lupus erythematosus on pregnancy and pregnancy outcome. *Am J Reprod Immunol* 1992; 28: 199–204.

168 Falk RJ. Treatment of lupus nephritis. *N Engl J Med* 2000; 343: 1182–3.

169 Nicklin JL. Systemic lupus erythematosus and pregnancy at the Royal Women's Hospital, Brisbane 1979–1989. *Aust NZ J Obstetrics Gynaecol* 1991; 31: 128–33.

170 Levy G. Pharmacokinetics in renal disease. *Am J Med* 1977; 62: 461–5.

171 Petri M, Howard D, Repke J. Frequency of lupus flare in pregnancy: The Hopkins Lupus Pregnancy Center experience. *Arthritis Rheum* 1991; 34: 1538–45.

172 Lockshin MD, Reinitz E, Druzin NL. Case control prospective study demonstrating absence of lupus exacerbation during and after pregnancy. *Am J Med* 1984; 77: 893–8.

173 Steen VD. Pregnancy in women with systemic sclerosis. *Obstet Gynecol* 1999; 94: 15–20.

174 Magmon R, Fejgin M. Scleroderma in pregnancy. *Obstet Gynecol Surv* 1989; 44: 530–4.

175 Moore M, Saffon JE, Barof HSB. Systemic sclerosis and pregnancy complicated by obstructive uropathy. *Am J Obstet Gynecol* 1985; 153: 893–5.

176 Luissiri P, Lance NJ, Curran JJ. Wegener's granulomatosis in pregnancy. *Arthritis Rheum* 1997; 40: 1354–60.

177 Dayoan ES, Diman LL, Boylen CT. successful treatment of Wegener's granulomatosis during pregnancy: a case report and review of the medical literature. *Chest* 1998; 113: 836–8.

178 Fields CL, Ossorio MA, Roy TM, Bunke CM. Wegener's granulomatosis complicated by pregnancy: a case report. *J Reprod Med* 1991; 36: 463–6.

179 Auzary C, Huong DLT *et al*. Pregnancy in patients with Wegener's granulomatosis: report of five cases in three women. *Ann Rheum Dis* 2000: 59: 800–04.

180 Murty GE, Davison JM, Cameron DS. Wegener's granulomatosis complicating pregnancy: first report of a case with a traceostomy. *J Obstet Gynecol* 1991; 10: 399–403.

181 Harber MA, Tso A *et al*. Wegener's granulomatosis in pregnancy—the therapeutic dilemma. *Nephrol Dial Transplant* 1999; 14: 1789–91.

182 Nagey DA, Fortier KJ, Linden J. Pregnancy complicated by periarteritis nodosa: Induced abortion as an alternative. *Am J Obstet Gynecol* 1983; 147: 103–95.

183 Cousins L. Pregnancy complications among diabetic women: Review 1965–85. *Obstet Gynecol Surv* 1987; 42: 140–9.

184 Hayslett JP, Reece EA. Managing diabetic patients with nephropathy and other vascular complications. *Clin Obstet Gynaecol* 1994; 8: 405–24.

185 Bojestig M, Arnqvist HJ *et al*. Declining incidence of nephropathy in insulin-dependent diabetes mellitus. *N Engl J Med* 1994; 330: 15–8.

186 Patterson KR, Lunan CB, MacCuish AC. Severe transient nephrotic syndrome in diabetic pregnancy. *Br Med J* 1985; 291: 1612.

187 Leguizaman G, Reece EA. Effect of medical therapy on progressive nephropathy: influence of pregnancy, diabetes and hypertension. *J Matern Fetal Med* 2000; 9: 70–78.

188 Schroder W, Heyl W, Hill-Grasshoff B, Rath W. Clinical value of detecting microalbuminuria as a risk factor for pregnancy-induced hypertension in insulin-treated diabetic pregnancies. *Europ J Obstet Gynecol Rep Biol* 2000; 91: 155–58.

189 Ekbom P, Damm P *et al*. Pregnancy out-come in Type 1 diabetic women with microalbuminia. *Diab Care* 2001; 24: 1739–44.

190 Gordon M, Landon MB *et al*. Perinatal outcome and long-term follow-up associated with modern management of diabetic nephropathy. *Obstet Gynecol* 1996; 87: 401–9.

191 Purdy LP, Hautsch CE *et al*. Effect of pregnancy on renal function in patients with moderate to severe renal insufficiency. *Diabetes Care* 1996; 19: 1067–74.

192 Hiilesmma V, Suhonen L, Teramo K. Glycaemic control is associated with pre-eclampsia but not with pregnancy induced hypertension in women with Type I diabetes mellitus. *Diabetalogia* 2000; 43: 1534–9.

193 Biesenbach G, Stöger H, Zaztgornik J. Influence of pregnancy on progression of diabetic nephropathy and subsequent requirements of renal replacement therapy in type 1 diabetic patients with impaired renal function. *Nephrol Dial Transplant* 1992; 7: 105–9.

194 Gordon M, Laudon MB *et al*. Perinatal outcome and long-term follow up associated with undermanagement of diabetic nephropathy. *Obstet Gynecol* 1996; 87: 401–9.

195 Parving H-H, Andersen AR, Smidt UM, Hommonel E, Mathiesen ER, Svendsen PA. Effect of antihypertensive treatment on kidney function in diabetic nephropathy. *Br Med J* 1987; 294: 1443–7.

196 Piper JM, Ray WA, Rosa FW. Pregnancy outcome following exposure to angiotensin converting enzyme inhibitors. *Obstet Gynecol* 1992; 80: 429–32.

197 Hod M, van Dijk DJ *et al*. Diabetic nephropathy and pregnancy: the effect of ACE inhibitors prior to pregnancy on fetomaternal outcome. *Nephrol Dial Transplant* 1995; 10: 2328–33.

198 Twickler D, Little BB, Satin AJ, Brown CE. Renal pelvicalyceal dilation in antepartum pyelonephritis: ultrasonographic findings. *Am J Obstet Gynecol* 1991; 165: 1115–19.

199 Jungers P, Houillier P, Chauveau D *et al*. Pregnancy in women with reflux nephropathy. *Kidney Int* 1996; 50: 593–9.

200 Becker GJ, Ihle BO, Fairley KF, Bastos M, Kincaid-Smith P. Effect of pregnancy on moderate renal failure in reflux nephropathy. *Br Med J* 1986; 292: 796–8.

201 Jungers P, Joillier P, Forget D. Reflux nephropathy and pregnancy. *Clin Obstet Gynaecol* 1987; 1: 955–70.

202 Bailey RR. Vesicoureteric reflux and reflux nephropathy. In: Cameron JS, Davison AM, Crunfeld JP, Kerr D, Ritz E, eds. *Oxford Textbook of Clinical Nephrology*. Oxford University Press, Oxford, 1992: 1983–2001.

203 Alexopoulos E, Tampakoudis P, Bili H, Mantalenakis S. Acute uric acid nephropathy in pregnancy. *Obstet Gynecol* 1992; 80: 488–9.

204 Shokeir AA, Mahran MR, Abdulmaaboud M. Renal colic in pregant women: role of renal resistive index. *Urol* 2000: 55: 344–47.

205 Maikrantz P, Holley JL, Parks JH. Gestational hypercalciuria causes pathological urine calcium oxalate supersaturation. *Kidney Int* 1989; 36: 108–13.

206 Evans H, Wollin TA. The management of urinary calculi in pregnancy. *Curr Opin Urol* 2001; 11: 379–84.

207 Asrat T, Roossin MC, Miller EI. Ultrasonographic detection of ureteral jets in normal pregnancy. *Am J Obstet Gynecol* 1998; 178: 1194–8.

208 Butler EL, Cox SM, Eberts EG, Cunningham FG. Symptomatic nephrolithiasis complicating pregnancy. *Obstet Gynecol* 2000: 96: 753–56.

209 Buchholz N-P, Biyabani MR *et al*. Urolithiasis in pregnancy—a clinical challenge. *Eur J Obstet Gynecol Reprod Biol* 1998; 80: 25–9.

210 Loughlin KR, Bailey RB. Internal ureteral stents for conservative management of ureteral calculi during pregnancy. *N Engl J Med* 1986; 315: 1647–9.

211 Wolf MC, Hollander JB, Salisz JA. A new technique of ureteral stent placement during pregnancy using endoluminal ultrasound. *Surg Gynecol Obstet* 1992; 175: 575–6.

212 Van Sonnenberg E, Casola G, Talner LB, Wittich GR, Varney RR, D'Agostino HB. Symptomatic renal obstruction or urosepsis during pregnancy: treatment by sonographically guided percutaneous nephrostomy. *Am J Roentgenol* 1992; 158: 91–4.

213 Algari MA, Sararinejad MR *et al*. Extracorporeal shock wave lithotripsy of renal calculi during early pregnancy. *Br J Urol* 1999; 84: 615–17.

214 Gregory MC, Mansell MA. Pregnancy and cystinuria. *Lancet* 1983; ii: 1158–60.

215 Gabow PA. Autosomal dominant polycystic kidney disease. *N Engl J Med* 1993; 329: 332–42.

216 Dalgaard OZ. Bilateral polycystic disease of the kidneys. a follow-up of 284 patients and their families. *Acta Med Scand* 1957; 328 (Suppl.): 1–10.

217 Pirson Y, Chauveau D, Grünfeld J-P. Autosomal dominant polycystic kidney disease. In: Davison AM, Cameron JS,

Grünfeld J-P *et al*., ed. *Oxford Textbook of Clinical Nephrology*, 2nd edn. Oxford University Press, Oxford, 1998: 2393–415.

218 Bear JC, McManamon P, Morgan P. Age at clinical onset and at ultrasonographic detection of adult polycystic kidney disease: data for genetic counselling. *Am J Med Genet* 1984; 18: 45–9.

219 Milutinovic J, Fialkow PJ, Agodoa LY. Fertility and pregnancy complications in women with autosomal dominant polycystic kidney disease. *Obstet Gynecol* 1983; 61: 566–70.

220 Alcaly M, Blau A, Barkai G. Successful pregnancy in a patient with polycystic disease and advanced renal failure: the use of prophylactic dialysis. *Am J Kidney Dis* 1992; 19: 382–4.

221 Wiebers DO, Torres VE. Screening for unruptured intracranial aneurysms in automsomal dominant polycystic kidney disease. *N Engl J Med* 1992; 327: 953–5.

222 Reeders ST, Zerres K *et al*. Prenatal diagnosis of autosomal dominant polycystic kidney disease with a DNA probe. *Lancet* 1986; ii: 6–7.

223 Barrett RJ, Peters WA. Pregnancy following urinary diversion. *Obstet Gynecol* 1983; 62: 582–56.

224 Hill DE, Chantigan PM, Kramer SA. Pregnancy after augmentation cystoplasty. *Surg Gynecol Obstet* 1990; 170: 485–7.

225 Knebelmann B, Antignac C, Gubler MC, Grünfeld JP. A molecular approach to inherited kidney disorders. *Kidney Int* 1993; 44: 1205–16.

226 Morgan SH, Grünfeld JP, eds. *Inherited Disorders of the Kidney*. Oxford University Press, Oxford: 1998.

227 Milliner DS, Torres VE. Renal manifestation of neurofibromatosis and tuberous sclerosis. In: Morgan SH, Grünfeld J-P, eds. *Inherited Disorders of the Kidney*. Oxford University Press, Oxford, 1998: 535–61.

228 Neumann HPH. von Hippel–Lindau syndrome. In: Morgan S, Grunfeld JP, eds. *The Investigation and Management of Inherited Disorders of the Kidney*. Oxford University Press, Oxford: 1994.

229 Wrenshall LE, McHugh L *et al*. Pregnancy after donor nephrectomy. *Transplantation* 1996; 62: 1934–6.

230 Buszta C, Steinmuller DR *et al*. Pregnancy after donor nephrectomy. *Transplantation* 1985; 40: 651–5.

231 Li FP, Gimbrere K, Gelber RD. Outcome of pregnancy in survivors of Wilm's tumor. *J Am Med Assoc* 1987; 257: 216–19.

232 First MR, Ooi BS, Wellington J, Pollak VE. Pre-eclampsia with the nephrotic syndrome. *Kidney Int* 1978; 13: 166–77.

233 Kublickas M, Bergström I, Randmaa I, Lunell N-O, Westgren M. Sarcoidosis in pregnancy: a review with reference to kidney involvement. *Curr Obstet Gynaecol* 1994; 4: 32–6.

234 Modesto A, Durand D, Orfila C, Suc JM. Syndrome hemolytique uremique chez deux germanius HLA identiques. *Nephrologie* 1984; 5: 47.

235 Rosenbaum AL, Churchill JA, Shakhasashiri ZA, Moody RL. Neuropsychologic outcome of children whose mothers had proteinuria during pregnancy. *Obstet Gynecol* 1969; 33: 118–23.

236 Baylis C. Renal disease in gravid animal models. *Am J Kidney Dis* 1987; 9: 350–3.

237 Baylis C, Wilson CB. Sex and the single kidney. *Am J Kidney Dis* 1989; 13: 290–8.

238 Reckelhoff JF. Age related changes in renal hemodynamics in female rats: role of multiple pregnancy and NO. *Am J Physiol* 1997; 272, R1985–R1989.

239 Deng A, Baylis C. Glomerular hemodynamic responses to pregnancy in the rat with severe reduction of renal mass. *Kidney Int* 1995; 48: 39–44.

240 Aiello S, Noris M *et al*. Renal and systemic nitric oxide synthesis in rats with renal mass reduction. *Kidney Int* 1997; 52, 171–81.

241 Santmyire BR, Zhang XZ, Baylis C. Changes in nitric oxide synthesis (NOS) during pregnancy (P) in the 5/6th nephrectomized (NX) rat. *J Am Soc Nephrol* 1998; 9, 347.

242 Leaker B, Becker GJ, El-Khatib M, Hewitson TD, Kincaid-Smith PS. Repeated pregnancy does not accelerate glomerulosclerosis in rats with subtotal renal ablation. *Hypertens Preg* 1992; B11: 1–23.

243 Feld LG, Brentjens JR, Van Liew JB. Renal injury and proteinuria in female spontaneously hypertensive rats. *Renal Physiol* 1981; 4: 46–56.

244 Baylis C. Immediate and long term effects of pregnancy on glomerular function in the SHR. *Am J Physiol* 1989; 257: F1140–5.

245 Aol W, Cable D, Cleary RE, Young PCM, Weinberger MH. The antihypertensive effect of pregnancy in spontaneously hypertensive rats. *Proc Soc Exp Biol Med* 1976; 153: 13–15.

246 Takeda T. Experimental study on the blood pressure of pregnant hypertensive rats. I. Effect of pregnancy on the course of experimentally and spontaneously hypertensive rats. *Jap Circ J* 1964; 28: 49–54.

247 Podjarny E, Baylis C, Losonczy G. Animal modes of preeclampsia. *Semin Perinatol* 1999; 23: 2–13.

248 Faas MM, Bakker WW, Poelman RT, Schuiling GA. Pregnancy aggravates proteinuria in subclinical glomerulonephritis in the rat. *J Lab Clin Med* 1999; 134: 267–74.

249 Ahokas RA, Mercer BM, Sibai BM. Enhanced endothelium-derived relaxing factor activity in pregnant, spontaneously hypertensive rats. *Am J Obstet Gynecol* 1991; 165: 801–7.

250 Baylis C, Reese K, Wilson CB. Glomerular effects of pregnancy in a model of glomerulonephritis in the rat. *Am J Kidney Dis* 1989; 14: 452–60.

251 Baylis C, Deng A, Couser WG. Glomerular hemodynamic effects of late pregnancy in rats with membranous glomerulonephritis produced by the anti Fx1A antibody. *J Am Soc Nephrol* 1995; 6: 1197–201.

252 Faas MM, Schuiling GA, Baller JFW, Visscher CA, Bakker WW. A new animal model for human preeclampsia: ultra-low-dose endotoxin infusion in pregnant rats. *Am J Obstet Gynecol* 1994; 171: 158–64.

253 Raij L. Glomerular thrombosis in pregnancy: role of the L-arginine-nitric oxide pathway. *Kidney Int* 1994; 45, 775–81.

254 Faas MM, Schuiling GA, Valkhof N, Baller JW, Bakker WW. Superoxide-mediated glomerulopathy in the endotoxin-treated pregnant rat. *Kidney Blood Press Res* 1998; 21(6), 432–7.

255 Faas MM, Schuiling GA, Baller JF, Valkhof N, Bakker WW. Aspirin treatment of the low-dose-endotoxin-treated pregnant rat: pathophysiologic and immunohistologic aspects. *J Lab Clin Med* 1997; 130(5), 496–508.

256 Podjarny E, Bernheim J et al. Adriamycin nephropathy: a model to study effects of pregnancy on renal disease in rats. *Am J Physiol* 1992; 263, F711–F715.

257 Rathaus M, Podjarny E et al. Adriamycin related hypertension in pregnant rats: response to a thromboxane receptor antagonist. *Clin Sci* 1992; 88: 623–7.

258 Podjarny E, Benchetrir S et al. Pregnancy induced hypertension in rats with adriamycin nephropathy is associated with an insufficient synthesis of nitric-oxide. *Hypertension* 1997; 4: 986–9.

259 Podjarny E, Pomeranz A et al. Effect of L-arginine treatment in pregnant rats with adriamycin nephropathy. *Clin Exp Hyper Pregnancy* 1993; 12: 517–24.

260 Pomeranz M, Podjarny E et al. Effect of recurrent pregnancies in the evolution of adriamycin nephropathy. *Nephrol Dial Transplant* 1995; 10: 2049–54.

261 Fogo A, Yoshida Y et al. Serial micropuncture analysis of glomerular function in two rat models of glomerular sclerosis. *J Clin Invest* 1988; 82: 322–30.

262 Clark H, Ronald AR, Cutler RE, Turck M. The correlation between site of infection and maximal concentrating ability in bacteriuria. *J Infect Dis* 1969; 120: 47–53.

263 Cohen D, Frenkley Y, Maschiach S, Eliahou HE. Dialysis during pregnancy in advanced chronic renal failure patients: outcome and progression. *Clin Nephrol* 1988; 29: 144–8.

264 Podjarny E, Bernheim J, Katz B, Green J, Mekler J, Bursztyn M. Chronic exogenous hyperinsulinemia in pregnancy: a rat model of pregnancy-induced hypertension. *J Am Soc Nephrol* 1998; 9: 9–13.

265 Omer S, Shan J, Varma DR, Mulay S. Augmentation of diabetes-associated renal hyperfiltration and nitric oxide production by pregnancy in rats. *J Endocrinol* 1999; 161: 15–23.

266 Kass EH. Asymptomatic infections of the urinary tract. *Trans Assoc Am Phys* 1956; 60: 56–63.

267 McFadyen IR, Eykryn SJ et al. Bacteriuria of pregnancy. *J Obstet Gynaecol Br Commonwealth* 1973; 80: 385–405.

268 Norden CW, Kass EH. Bacteriuria of pregnancy—a critical reappraisal. *Ann Rev Med* 1968; 19: 431–70.

269 Campbell-Brown M, McFadyen IR, Seal DV, Stephenson ML. Is screening for bacteriuria in pregnancy worthwhile? *Br Med J* 1987; 294: 1579–82.

270 Cohen SN, Kass EH. A simple method for quantitative urine culture. *N Engl J Med* 1967; 277: 176–80.

271 Roberts AP, Robinson RE, Beard RW. Some factors affecting bacterial colony counts in urinary infection. *Br Med J* 1967; i: 400–3.

272 Wing DA, Park AS et al. Limited clinical utility of blood and urine cultures in the treatment of acute pyelonephritis during pregnancy. *Am J Obstet Gynecol* 2000: 182: 1437–40.

273 Eckford SD, Gingell JC. Ureteric obstruction in pregnancy—diagnosis and management. *Br J Gynaecol* 1991; 98: 1337–40.

274 Cunningham FG, Lucas MJ. Urinary tract infections complicating pregnancy. *Clin Obstet Gynaecol* 1994; 8: 353–74.

275 Eaton CJ, Peterson EP. Diagnosis and acute management of patients with advanced clostridial sepsis complicating abortion. *Am J Obstet Gynecol* 1971; 109: 1162–5.

276 Heineman HS, Lee JH. Bacteriuria in pregnancy. *Obstet Gynecol* 1973; 41: 22–6.

277 Mundt KA, Polk BF. Identification of urinary tract infections by antibody-coated bacteria assay. *Lancet* 1979; ii: 1172–5.

278 Shelton SD, Boggess KA et al. Urinary interleukin-8 with asymptomatic bacteriuria in pregnancy. *Obstet Gynecol* 2001; 97: 583–6.

279 Lomberg H, Jodal U, Lefler H, DeMan P, Svanborg C. Blood group non-secretors have an increased inflammatory response to urinary tract infection. *Scand J Infect Dis* 1992; 24: 7.

280 Stein G, Fünfstück R. Asymptomatic bacteriuria—what to do. *Nephrol Dial Transplant* 1999; 14: 1618–21.

281 Savage WE, Hajj SN, Kass EH. Demographic and prognostic characteristics of bacteriuria in pregnancy. *Medicine (Baltimore)* 1967; 46: 385–407.

282 Davison JM, Sprott MS, Selkon JB. The effect of covert bacteriuria in schoolgirls on renal function at 18 years and during pregnancy. *Lancet* 1984; ii: 651–5.

283 Stenquist K, Dahlin-Nilsson I, Lidin-Janson G. Bacteriuria in pregnancy. Frequency and risk of acquisition. *Am J Epidemiol* 1989; 129: 372–9.

284 Geerlings SF, Erkeleus DW, Hoepelman IM. Urine weginfecties bij patienten met diabetes mellitus. *Nederlands Tijdschrift Voor Geneeskunde* 1997; 141: 372–5.

285 Whalley PJ. Bacteriuria of pregnancy. *Am J Obstet Gynecol* 1967; 97: 723–38.

286 Chng PK, Hall MH. Antenatal prediction of urinary tract infection in pregnancy. *Br J Obstet Gynaecol* 1982; 89: 8–11.

287 Brumfitt W. The significance of symptomatic and asymptomatic infection in pregnancy. *Contrib Nephrol* 1981; 25: 23–9.

288 Condie AP, Brumfitt W, Reeves DS, Williams JD. The effects of bacteriuria in pregnancy on fetal health. In: Brumfitt W, Asscher AW, eds. *Urinary Tract Infection*. Oxford University Press, London, 1973: 108–16.

289 Martinell J, Jodall U, Lipiu-Janson G. Pregnancies in women with and without renal seaming after urinary infections in childhood. *Br Med J* 1990; 300: 840–4.

290 McGladdery SL, Aparicio S, Verrier-Jones K. Outcome of pregnancy in an Oxford–Cardiff cohort of women with previous bacteriuria. *Q J Med* 1992; 303: 533–9.

291 Gardner A. Urinary tract infection during pregnancy and sudden unexpected infant death. *Lancet* 1985; ii: 495.

292 Gilstrap LS, Ramin SM. Urinary tract infections during pregnancy. *Obstet Gynecol Clin North AM* 2001; 28: 581–91.

293 Andriole VT. Bacterial infections. In: Burrow GN, Ferris TF, eds. *Medical Complications During Pregnancy*. W.B. Saunders, Philadelphia, PA, 1975: 382–95.

294 Baorto DN, Gao Z *et al.* Survival of FimH-expressing enterobacteria in macrophages relies of glycolipid traffic. *Nature* 1997; 389: 636–9.

295 Hart A, Nowicki BJ *et al.* Ampicillin-resistant Escherichia coli in gestational pyelonephritis: Increased occurrence and association with the Colonization Factor Dr Adhesion. *J Infect Dis* 2001; 183: 1526–29.

296 Leveno KJ, Harris RE, Gilstrap LC, Whalley PJ, Cunningham FG. Bladder versus renal bacteriuria during pregnancy: recurrence after treatment. *Am J Obstet Gynecol* 1981; 139: 403–6.

297 Andriole VT, Patterson TF. Epidemiology, natural history and management of urinary tract infection in pregnancy. *Med Clin North Am* 1991; 75: 359–73.

298 Powers RD. New directions in the diagnosis and therapy of urinary tract infections. *Am J Obstet Gynecol* 1991; 164: 1387–9.

299 Cower PE, Haswell B, Sidaway ME, de Wardener HE. Follow-up of 164 patients with bacteriuria of pregnancy. *Lancet* 1968; i: 990–4.

300 Briedahl P, Hurst PE, Martin JD, Vivian AB. The post-partum investigation of pregnancy bacteriuria. *Med J Aust* 1972; 2: 1174–7.

301 Gilstrap LC, Cunningham FG, Whalley PJ. Acute pyelonephritis in pregnancy: an anterospective study. *Obstet Gynecol* 1981; 57: 408–13.

302 Schwartz MA, Wang CC, Eckert L *et al.* Risk factors for urinary tract infection in the postpartum period. *Am J Obstet Gynecol* 1999; 181: 547–53.

303 Bukowski TP, Betrus GG *et al.* Urinary tract infections and pregnancy in women who underwent antireflux surgery in childhood. *J Urol* 1998; 159: 1286–9.

304 Pruett K, Faro S. Pyelonephritis associated with respiratory distress. *Obstet Gynecol* 1987; 69: 444–6.

305 Cox SM, Shelburne P, Mason RA, Cuss S, Cunningham FG. Mechanisms of hemolysis and anemia associated with acute antepartum pyelonephritis. *Am J Obstet Gynecol* 1991; 164: 587–90.

306 Whalley PJ, Cunningham FG, Martin FG. Transient renal dysfunction associated with acute pyelonephritis of pregnancy. *Obstet Gynecol* 1975; 46: 174–9.

307 Meyers SJ, Lee RV, Munschauer RW. Dilatation and nontraumatic rupture of the urinary tract during pregnancy: a review. *Obstet Gynecol* 1983; 66: 809–15.

308 Wing DA, Hendershott CM, Debuque L, Millar LK. Outpatient treatment of acute pyelonephritis in pregnancy after 24 weeks. *Obstet Gynecol* 1999; 94: 683–8.

309 Mussalli GM, Brunnert SR, Hirsch E. Preterm delivery in mice with renal abscess. *Obstet Gynecol* 2000; 95: 453–6.

310 McDermott S, Callaghan W *et al.* Urinary tract infections during pregnancy and mental retardation and developmental delay. *Obstet Gynecol* 2000; 96 (1): 113–19.

311 Gallery EDM, Ross M, Gyory AZ. Urinary red blood cell and cast excretion in normal and hypertensive human pregnancy. *Am J Obstet Gynecol* 1993; 168: 67–70.

312 Texter JH, Bellinger M, Kawamoto E, Koontz WE. Persistent haematuria during pregnancy. *J Urol* 1980; 123: 84–7.

313 Maresca L, Koucky CJ. Spontaneous rupture of the renal pelvis during pregnancy presenting as acute abdomen. *Obstet Gynecol* 1981; 58: 745–7.

314 Zanetta G, Webb MJ, Segura JW. Ureteral endometriosis diagnosed at ureteroscopy. *Obstet Gynecol* 1997; 91: 856–9.

315 Danielli L, Korchazak D, Beyar H, Lotan M. Recurrent hematuria during multiple pregnancies. *Obstet Gynecol* 1987; 69: 446–8.

316 Reid DE, Ryan KJ, Benirschke K. Medical and surgical diseases in pregnancy. In: *Principles and Management of Human Reproduction*. W.B. Saunders, Philadelphia, PA, 1972: 734–53.

317 Stehman-Breen C, Miller L *et al.* Pre-eclampsia and premature labour among pregnant women with haematuria. *Paediatr Perinatal Epidemiol* 2000; 14: 136–40.

318 Brown MA. Urinary tract dilatation in pregnancy. *Am J Obstet Gynecol* 1990; 164: 641–3.

319 Meares EM. Urologic surgery during pregnancy. *Clin Obstet Gynecol* 1978; 21: 907–15.

320 Schloss WA, Solomkin M. Acute hydronephrosis of pregnancy. *J Urol* 1952; 68: 885–8.

321 Editorial. Effect of transplantation on non-renal effects of renal failure. *Br Med J* 1981; 284: 221–2.

322 Merkatz IR, Schwartz GH, David DS, Stenzel KH, Riggio RR, Whitsell JC. Resumption of female reproductive function following renal transplantation. *J Am Med Assoc* 1971; 216: 1749–54.

323 Mulley AC, Silverstein MD, Dienstag JL. Indications for use of hepatitis B vaccine, based on cost-effectiveness analysis. *N Engl J Med* 1982; 307: 644–52.

324 Editorial. Pregnancy after renal transplantation. *Br Med J* 1976; i: 733–4.

325 Armenti VT, Moritz MJ, Davison JM. Medical management of the pregnant transplant recipient. *Adv Renal Reprod Ther* 1998; 5: 14–23.

326 Armenti VT, Moritz MJ *et al.* Pregnancy and transplantation. *Graft* 2000; 3: 49–63.

327 Davison JM, Redman CWG. Pregnancy post-transplant: the establishment of a UK Registry. *Br J Obstet Gynaecol* 1997; 104: 1106–7.

328 Briggs JD, Davison JM *et al.* National Transplant Database Register—First Report. *UKTSSA Users' Bull* 1999; 33: 8–9.

329 Davison JM. Renal transplantation and pregnancy. *Am J Kidney Dis* 1987; 9: 374–80.

330 Davison JM. Dialysis, transplantation and pregnancy. *Am J Kidney Dis*, 1991; 27: 127–32.

331 Davison JM. Pregnancy in renal allograft recipients: prognosis and management. *Clin Obstet Gynaecol* 1994; 8: 501–25.

332 Hadi HA. Pregnancy in renal transplant recipients: a review. *Obstet Gynecol Surv* 1986; 41: 264–71.

333 Kirk EP. Organ transplantation and pregnancy. *Am J Obstet Gynecol* 1991; 164: 1629–34.

334 Rizzoni G, Ehrich JHH *et al.* Combined report on regular dialysis and transplantation of children in Europe 1988. *Nephrol Dial Transplant* 1989; 4: 31–40.

335 Rizzoni G, Ehrich JHH *et al.* Successful pregnancies in women on renal replacement therapy: Report from the EDTA Registry. *Nephrol Dial Transplant* 1992; 7: 1–9.

336 Armenti VT, Ahlswede KM *et al.* Variables affecting birthweight and graft survival in 197 pregnancies in cyclosporine-treated female kidney transplant patients. *Transplantation* 1995; 59: 476–9.

337 Armenti VT, Moritz MJ, Davison JM. Drug safety issues in pregnancy following transplantation and immunosuppression. *Drug Saf Concepts* 1998; 19: 219–32.

338 Armenti VT, Jarrell BE *et al.* National Transplantation Pregnancy Registry (NTPR): cyclosporine dosing and pregnancy outcome in female renal transplant recipients. *Transplant Proc* 1996; 28: 2111–12.

339 Davison JM. Towards longterm graft survival in renal transplantation: pregnancy. *Nephrol Dial Transplant* 1995; 10 (Suppl. 1): 85–9.

340 Gaughan WJ, Moritz MJ *et al.* National Transplantation Pregnancy Registry: report on outcomes in cyclosporin-treated female kidney transplant recipients with an interval from transplant to pregnancy of greater than 5 years. *Am J Kidney Dis* 1996; 28: 266–9.

341 Ehrich JHH, Loirat C *et al.* Repeated successful pregnancies after kidney transplantation in 102 women. *Nephrol Dial Transplant* 1996; 11: 1314–17.

342 Bar J, Ben-Rafael Z *et al.* Prediction of pregnancy outcome in subgroups of women with renal disease. *Clin Nephrol* 1999; 53: 437–44.

343 Toma H, Tanabe K *et al.* Pregnancy in women receiving renal dialysis or transplantation in Japan: a nationwide survey. *Nephrol Dial Transplant* 1999; 14: 1511–16.

344 Penn I, Makowski EL, Harris P. Parenhood following renal transplantation. *Kidney Int* 1980; 18: 221–33.

345 Pergola PE, Kaucharla A, Riley DJ. Kidney transplantation during the first trimester of pregnancy: immunosppression with mycophenolate mofetil, tracolimus and prednisolone. *Transpl* 2001; 71: 994–97.

346 Davison JM, Lind T, Uldall PR. Planned pregnancy in a renal transplant recipient. *Br J Obstet Gynaecol* 1976; 83: 518–27.

347 Andrews PA. Renal transplantation. *Br Med J* 2002; 324: 530–34.

348 Renal Transplant Registry Advisory Committee. The 13th report of the human renal transplant registry. *Transplant Proc* 1977; 9: 9–26.

349 *UK Transplant Service Report*, 1986:4–30.

350 Lindheimer MD, Katz AI. Pregnancy in the renal transplant patient. *Am J Kidney Dis* 1992; 19: 173–6.

351 Lindheimer MD, Katz AI. Pregnancy in women receiving renal replacement therapy. *Kidney Curr Surv World Lit* 1994; 3: 135–7.

352 Whetam JCG, Cardelle C, Harding M. Effect of pregnancy on graft function and graft survival in renal cadaver transplant recipients. *Am J Obstet Gynecol* 1983; 145: 193–7.

353 Sturgiss SN, Davison JM. Effect of pregnancy on longterm function of renal allografts. *Am J Kidney Dis* 1992; 19: 167–72.

354 Salmela KT, Kyllonen LEJ, Homberg C, Grönhagen-Riska C. Impaired renal function after pregnancy in renal transplant recipients. *Transplantation* 1993; 56: 1372–5.

355 Crowe AV, Rustom R *et al.* Pregnancy does not adversely affect renal transplant function. *Q J Med* 1999; 92: 631–5.

356 McGrory CH, McCloskey LJ *et al.* Pregnancy outcomes in female renal recipients: a comparison of systemic lupus erythematosus to other diagnoses. *Transplantation* 2000; 69: S289.

357 Kobayashi H, Matsumoto Y, Otsubo O, Otsubo K, Naito T. Successful pregnancy in a patient undergoing chronic hemodialysis. *Obstet Gynecol* 1981; 57: 382–6.

358 McGrory, Groshek HW *et al.* Pregnancy outcomes in female pancreas-kidney recipients. *Transpl Proc* 1999; 31: 652–53.

359 Wilson GA, Coscia LA *et al.* National Transplantation Pregnancy Registry: Postpregnancy graft-loss among female pancreas-kidney recipients. *Transpl Proc* 2001; 31: 1667–9.

360 Endler M, Derfler K, Schaller A, Nowotny C. Schwangerschaft und Ceburt nach Nierentransplantation unter Cyclosporin A. Fallbericht und Literaturubersicht Geburtshilfe Frauenheilkd. 1987; 47: 660–3.

361 Tyden G, Brattstrom C *et al.* Pregnancy after combined pancreas–kidney transplantation. *Diabetes* 1989; 38 (Suppl. 1): 43–5.

362 Light JA. Experience with 50 kidney/pancreas transplants at the Washington Hospital Center. *Nephrol Dial Transplant* 1993; 22: 522–32.

363 Davison JM, Dellagrammatikas H, Parkin JM. Maternal azathioprine therapy and depressed haemopoiesis in the babies of renal allograft recipients. *Br J Obstet Gynaecol* 1985; 92: 233–9.

364 Parsons V, Bewick M, Elias J, Snowden SA, Weston MJ, Rodeck CH. Pregnancy following transplantation. *J R Soc Med* 1979; 72: 815–17.

365 Rabau-Friedman E, Maschiach S, Cantor E, Jacob ET. Association of hypoparathyroidism and successful pregnancy in kidney transplant recipient. *Obstet Gynecol* 1982; 59: 126–8.

366 Brookhyser J, Wiggens K. Medical nutrition therapy in pregnancy and kidney disease. *Adv Renal Replacement Ther* 1998; 5: 53–6.

367 Feehally J, Bennett SE, Harris KPG, Walls J. Is chronic renal transplant rejection a non-immunological phenomenon? *Lancet* 1986; ii: 486–8.

368 Manifold IH, Champsion AE, Goepel JR, Ramsewak S, Mayor PE. Pregnancy complicated by gestational trophoblastic disease in a renal transplant recipient. *Br Med J* 1983; 287: 1025–6.

369 Parer JT, Lichtenberg ES, Callen PW, Feduska N. Iliac venous aneurysm in a pregnant patient with a renal transplant. *J Reprod Med* 1987; 29: 869–71.

370 Scott JR, Cruikshank DP, Corry RJ. Ectopic pregnancy in kidney transplant patients. *Obstet Gynecol* 1978; 51: 565–85.

371 Coulam CB, Moyer TP, Jiang MS, Zincke H. Breastfeeding after renal transplantation. *Transplant Proc* 1985; 14: 605–9.

372 Coulam CB, Zincke H. Successful pregnancy in a renal transplant patient with a 75–year-old kidney. *Surg Forum* 1981; 32: 457–9.

373 Nojima M, Ihana H *et al.* Influence of pregnancy on graft function after renal transplantation. *Transplant Proc* 1996; 28: 1582–5.

374 Armenti VT, Ahlswede BA, Moritz MJ, Jarrell BE. National Transplantation Registry: Analysis of pregnancy outcomes of female kidney recipients with relation to time interval from transplantation to conception. *Transplant Proc* 1993; 25: 1036–7.

375 Warren SF, Mitas JA, Evertson LR. Pregnancy after renal transplantation: Reversible acidosis and renal dysfunction. *South Med J* 1981; 74: 1139–41.

376 Kozlowska-Boszko B, Lao M *et al.* Chronic rejection as a risk factor for deterioration of allograft function following pregnancy. *Transplant Proc* 1997; 29: 1522–3.

377 Rudolph JE, Shwihizir RT, Barius SA. Pregnancy in renal transplant patients: a review. *Transplantation* 1979; 27: 26–9.

378 Kaufmann JJ, Dignam W, Goodwin WE, Martin DC, Goldman R, Maxwell MH. Successful normal childbirth after kidney homotransplantation. *J Am Med Assoc* 1967; 200: 162–5.

379 Rifle G, Traeger J. Pregnancy after renal transplantation? An international review. *Transplant Proc* 1975; 7 (Suppl. 1): 723–8.

380 Guttman RD. Renal transplantation (I and II). *N Engl J Med* 1979; 301: 975–81 and 1038–48.

381 Editorial. Imaging the transplanted kidney. *Lancet* 1986; i: 781–3.

382 Sturgiss SN, Davison JM. Perinatal outcome in renal allograft recipients: prognostic significance of hypertension and renal function before and during pregnancy. *Obstet Gynecol* 1991; 78: 573–7.

383 Williams PF, Jelen J. Eclampsia in a patient who had had a renal transplant. *Br Med J* 1979; ii: 972.

384 Bakris GL. Is the level of arterial pressure reduction important for preservation of renal function? *Nephrol Dial Transplant* 1995; 11: 2382–9.

385 Horbach J, van Liebergen F, Mastboom J, Wijdeveld P. Pregnancy in a patient after cadaveric renal transplantation. *Acta Med Scand* 1973; 194: 237–40.

386 Sciarra JJ, Toledo-Pereyra LH, Bendel RP, Simmons RI. Pregnancy following renal transplantation. *Am J Obstet Gynecol* 1975; 123: 411–25.

387 Evans TJ, McCollum JPK, Valdimasson H. Congenital cytomegalovirus infection after maternal renal transplantation. *Lancet* 1975; i: 1359–60.

388 MacLean AB, Abbott CD, Aickin DR, Bailey RR, Bashford DH, Little PJ. Successful pregnancy after renal transplantation. *Aust NZ J Obstet Gynaecol* 1977; 17: 224–8.

389 Spencer ES, Anderson HK. Viral infections in renal allograft recipients treated with long-term immunosuppression. *Br Med J* 1979; i: 829–30.

390 Iqbal N, Steinberg H, Aldasouqi S, Edmonson JW. Nephrolithiasis during pregnancy secondary to primary hyperparathyroidism. *Urology* 2001; 57: 544iii–554v.

391 Calne RY. Cyclosporin in cadaveric renal transplantation: 5-year follow-up of a multi-centre trial. *Lancet* 1987; ii: 506–7.

392 European Multicentre Trial. Cyclosporin A as sole immunosuppressive agent in recipients of kidney allografts from cadaver donors. Preliminary results of a European multicentre trial. *Lancet* 1982; ii: 57–60.

393 Ahlswede KM, Armenti W, Mokritz MJ. Premature births in female transplant recipients: degree and effect of immunosuppressive regimen. *Surg Forum* 1992; 43: 524–5.

394 Flechner SM, Katz AR, Rogers AJ, van Buren C, Kahan BD. The presence of cyclosporine in body tissues and fluids during pregnancy. *Am J Kidney Dis* 1985; 5: 6–63.

395 Haugen G, Fauchald P, Sodal G, Halvorsen S, Oldereid N, Moe N. Pregnancy outcome in renal allograft recipients: influence of cyclosporin A. *Eur J Obstet Gynaecol Reprod Biol* 1991; 29: 25–9.

396 Khawar M, Pomrantz R, Tejani A. Two successful pregnancies in a cadaveric renal allograft recipient on cyclosporine (CsA) as the sole maintenance immunosuppressive. *Proceedings of the Xth International Congress of Nephrology*, Alden Press, Oxford, 1987, 620A.

397 Lewis GJ, Lamont CAR, Lee HA, Slapak M. Successful pregnancy in a renal transplant recipient taking cyclosporin A. *Br Med J* 1983; 286: 603.

398 Ghandour FZ, Krauss TC, Hricik DE. Immunosuppressive drugs in pregnancy. *Adv Renal Replace Ther* 1998; 5: 31–7.

399 Lau RJ, Scott JR. Pregnancy following renal transplantation. *Clin Obstet Gynecol* 1985; 28: 339–50.

400 Penn I. Pregnancy following renal transplantation. In: Andreucci VE, ed. *The Kidney in Pregnancy*. Martinus-Nijhoff, Boston, MA, 1985: 195–204.

401 Williamson RA, Karp LE. Azathioprine toxicity: review of the literature and case report. *Obstet Gynecol* 1981; 58: 247–50.

402 Lennard L, Brown CN, Fox M, Maddocks JL. Azathioprine metabolism in kidney transplant patients. *Br J Clin Pharmacol* 1984; 18: 693–700.

403 Lewis GJ, Chatterjee SP, Rowse AD. Acute renal failure presenting in pregnancy secondary to idiopathic hydronephrosis. *Br Med J* 1985; 290: 1250–1.

404 Oz BB, Hackman R *et al.* Pregnancy outcome after cyclosporine therapy during pregnancy: a meta analysis. *Transplant* 2001; 71: 1051–5.

405 Little MA, Abraham KA *et al.* Pregnancy in Irish renal transplant recipients in the cyclosporine era. *Ir J med Sci* 2000; 169: 19–21.

406 Kaskel TM, Devarajan P, Arbeit LA, Partin JS, Moore LC. Cyclosporine nephrotoxicity: sodium excretion, autoregulation and angiotensin II. *Am J Physiol* 1987; 252: F733–42.

407 Provoost AP. Cyclosporine nephrotoxicity in rats with an acute reduction of renal function. *Am J Kidney Dis* 1986; 8: 314–8.

408 Al-Khader A, Absy M, Al-Hasani MK, Joyce B, Sabbagh T. Successful pregnancy in renal transplant recipients treated with cyclosporine. *Transplantation* 1988; 45: 987–8.

409 Armenti VT, McGrory CH *et al.* Pregnancy outcomes in female renal transplant recipients. *Transpl Proc* 1998; 30: 1732–4.

410 Furman B, Wiznitzer A *et al.* Multiple pregnancies in women after renal transplantation: case report that raises a management dilemma. *Eur J Obstet Gynecol Reprod Med* 1999; 84: 107–10.

411 Vyar S, Kumar A *et al.* Outcome of twin pregnancy in a renal transplant recipient treated with tacrolimus. *Transplantation* 1999; 67: 490–2.

412 Shapiro R. Tacrolimus in renal transplantation—a review. *Graft* 2000; 3: 64–80.

413 MacLean AB, Sharp F, Briggs JD, MacPherson SC. Successful triplet pregnancy following renal transplantation. *Scott Med J* 1980; 25: 320–2.

414 Salant DJ, Marcus RG, Milne FJ. Pregnancy in renal transplant recipients. *S Afr Med J* 1976; 50: 1288–92.

415 Myerowitz RL, Medeiros AA, O'Brien TF. Bacterial infection in renal homotransplant recipients. a study of fifty-three bacteremic episodes. *Am J Med* 1972; 53: 308–14.

416 Scott JR, Cruikshank DP, Kochenour NK, Pitkin RM, Warenski JC. Fetal platelet counts in the obstetric management of immunologic thrombocytopenic purpura. *Am J Obstet Gynecol* 1980; 136: 459–9.

417 Nolan GH, Sweet RL, Laros RK, Roure CA. Renal cadaver transplantation followed by successful pregnancies. *Obstet Gynecol* 1974; 43: 732–9.

418 Huffer WF, Kuzela D, Popovtzer MM. Metabolic bone disease in chronic renal failure. II. Renal transplant patients. *Am J Pathol* 1975; 78: 385–98.

419 Elmstedt E. Avascular bone necrosis in the renal transplant patient. *Clin Orthop* 1981; 158: 149–57.

420 Ibels LS, Alfrey AC, Huffer WE. Aseptic necrosis of bone following renal transplantation: experience in 194 transplant recipients and review of the literature. *Medicine (Baltimore)* 1978; 57: 25–45.

421 Coyne SS, Walsh JW *et al.* Surgically correctable renal transplant complications: An integrated clinical and radiologic approach. *Am J Radiol* 1981; 136: 113–19.

422 Faber M, Kennison RD, Jackson HT, Sbarra AJ, Widnere B. Successful pregnancy after renal transplantation. *Obstet Gynecol* 1976; 48: 2–4.

423 Pirson Y, Van Lierde M, Chysen J, Squifflet JP, Alexandre GPJ, Van Ypersele de Strihou C. Retardation of fetal growth in patients receiving immunosuppressive therapy. *N Engl J Med* 1985; 313: 328.

424 Chahranmains N, Attaipour Y, Ghods AJ. Chromosomal aberrations among offspring of female renal transplant recipients. *Transplant Proc* 1993; 25: 2190.

425 Rasmussen P, Fasth A, Ahlmen J, Brynger H, Iwarson S, Kjellmer I. Children of female renal transplant recipients. *Acta Paediatr Scand* 1981; 70: 869–75.

426 Weil R, Barfield N, Schröter GPJ, Bauling PC. Children of mothers with kidney transplants. *Transplant Proc* 1985; 17: 1569–72.

427 Penn I, Makowski EL. Parenthood following renal and hepatic transplantation. *Transplantation* 1980; 30: 297–9.

428 Sarramon JP, Lhez JM *et al.* Crossesse chez les transplantes renales. *Ann Urol* 1985; 19: 57–9.

429 Registration Committee of the European Dialysis and Transplant Association. Successful pregnancies in women treated by dialysis and kidney transplantation. *Br J Obstet Gynaecol* 1980; 87: 839–45.

430 Skinhöj P, Cohn J, Bradburne AF. Transmission of hepatitis type B from healthy HBsAg-positive mothers. *Br Med J* 1976; i: 10–1.

431 Gerety RJ, Schweitzer IL. Viral hepatitis B during pregnancy, the neonatal period and infancy. *J Paediatr* 1977; 90: 368–74.

432 Flewett TH. Can we eradicate hepatitis B? *Br Med J* 1986; 293: 404–5.

433 Recommendations of the Immunization Practices Advisory Committee. Immune globulins for protection against viral hepatitis. *Ann Intern Med* 1982; 96: 193–7.

434 Zuckerman AJ. New hepatitis B vaccines. *Br Med J* 1985; 290: 492–6.

435 Beasley RP, Hwang L-U, Lee GY. Prevention of perinatally transmitted hepatitis B virus infections with hepatitis B immune globulin and hepatitis B vaccine. *Lancet* 1983; ii: 1099–102.

436 Syndman DR, Werner BG *et al.* Use of cytomegalovirus immune globulin to prevent cytomegalovirus disease in renal transplant recipients. *N Engl J Med* 1987; 317: 1049–54.

437 Jeffries DU. Cytomegalovirus infections in pregnancy. *Br J Obstet Gynaecol* 1984; 91: 305–96.

438 Best JM. Congenital cytomegalovirus infection. *Br Med J* 1987; 294: 1440–1.

439 Crespigny PCD, d'Apice AJF. Parenthood after renal transplantation. *Aust NZ J Med* 1986; 16: 245–9.

440 Stotland NL. Social change and women's reproductive health care. *Women's Hlth Iss* 1990:1: 4–11.

441 Keller AJ, Irvine WJ, Jordan JJ, London NB. Phytohemagglutin-induced lymphocyte transformation in oral contraceptive users. *Obstet Gynecol* 1976; 49: 83–91.

442 Rao VK, Smith EJ, Alexander JW. Thromboembolic disease in renal allograft recipients. *Arch Surg* 1976; 111: 1086–92.

443 Taylor ES. Editorial comments. *Obstet Gynaecol Surv* 1975; 30: 739.

444 Tatum HJ. Clinical aspects of intrauterine contraception: circumspection. *Fertil Steril* 1976; 28: 3–27.

445 Taylor ES, McMillan JH, Greer BE, Droegemueller W, Thompson HE. The intrauterine device and tuboovarian abscess. *Am J Obstet Gynecol* 1975; 123: 338–48.

446 Zerner D, Doil KL, Drewry J. Intrauterine contraceptive device failures in renal transplant patients. *J Reprod Med* 1981; 26: 99–101.

447 Caterson RJ, Furber J, Murray J, McCarthy W, Mahony JF, Shiels AGR. Carcinoma of the vulva in two young renal allograft recipients. *Transplant Proc* 1984; 16: 559–61.

448 Hoover R, Fraumeni JR. Risk of cancer in renal transplant recipients. *Lancet* 1973; ii: 55–7.

449 Sheil ACR. Cancer in organ transplant recipients: part of an induced immune deficiency syndrome. *Br Med J* 1984; 288: 659–61.

450 Dantal J, Hourmant M *et al.* Effect of longterm immunosuppression in kidney graft recipients on cancer incidence: randomised comparison of two cyclosporin regimens. *Lancet* 1998; 351: 623–8.

451 Newstead CG. Assessment of risk of cancer after renal transplantation. *Lancet* 1998; 351: 610–11.

452 Porreco R, Penn I, Droegemneller W, Greer B, Makowski EL. Gynecologic malignancies in immunosuppressed organ homograft recipients. *Obstet Gynecol* 1975; 45: 359–64.

453 Penn I. Cancers complicating organ transplantation. *N Engl J Med* 1990; 323: 1767–8.

454 London NJ, Farmery SM *et al.* Risk of neoplasia in transplant patients. *Lancet* 1995; 346: 403–6.

455 Fagerholm MI, Coularn CB, Moyer TP. Breast feeding after renal transplantation: 6–mercaptopurine content of human breast milk. *Surg Forum* 1980; 31: 447–9.

456 Nyberg G, Haljamee M *et al.* Breast feeding during treatment with cyclosporin. *Transplantation* 1998; 65: 253–5.

457 Thiru Y, Bateman AN, Coulthard MG. Successful breast feeding while mother was taking cyclosporin. *Br Med J* 1997; 345: 463.

458 Price HV, Salaman JR, Laurence KM, Langmaid H. Immunosuppressive drugs and the fetus. *Transplantation* 1976; 21: 294–8.

459 Reimers TJ, Sluss PM. 6–Mercaptopurine treatment of pregnant mice. Effects on second and third generations. *Science* 1978; 201: 65–7.

460 Willis FR, Findlay CA *et al.* Children of renal transplant recipient mothers. *J Paed Child Hlth* 2000; 36: 230–5.

461 Stanley CW, Gottlieb R *et al*. Developmental wellbeing in offspring of women receiving cyclosporine post-renal transplant. *Transplant Proc* 1999; 31: 241–2.

462 Confortini P, Galanti G, Ancona G, Giongo A, Bruschi E, Lorenzini E. Full term pregnancy and successful delivery in a patient on chronic haemodialysis. In: Cameron JS, eds. *Proceedings of the European Dialysis and Transplant Association*. Pitman Medical Limited, London, 1971: 74–8.

463 Ackrill P, Goodwin Fj Marsh FP, Stratton D, Wagman H. Successful pregnancy in patient on regular dialysis. *Br Med J* 1975; ii: 172–4.

464 Amoah E, Arab H. Pregnancy in a hemodialysis patient with no residual renal function. *Am J Kidney Dis* 1991; 17: 585–7.

465 Barri YM, Al-Furayh O, Qunibi WY, Rahman F. Pregnancy in women on regular hemodialysis. *Dial Transplant* 1991; 20: 652–7.

466 Challah S, Wing AW, Broyer M, Rizzoni G. Successful pregnancy in women or regular dialysis treatment and women with a functioning transplant. In: Andreucci VF, ed. *The Kidney in Pregnancy*. Martinus-Nijhoff, Boston, MA, 1986: 185–94.

467 Dominguez N, Cruz N, Ramos-Barroso A, Ramos-Umpierre E. Pregnancy in chronic hemodialysis. *Transplant Proc* 1991; 23: 1836–7.

468 Ehrich JHH, Rizzoni C *et al*. Combined report on regular dialysis and transplantation of children in Europe 1989. *Nephrol Dial Transplant* 1991; 6: 37–47.

469 Hou S. Pregnancy in organ transplant recipients. *Med Clin North Am* 1989; 73: 667–83.

470 Hou S. Peritoneal and haemodialysis in pregnancy. *Clin Obstet Gynaecol* 1994; 8: 481–500.

471 Redrow M, Cherem L *et al*. Dialysis in the management of pregnant patients with renal insufficiency. *Medicine* 1988; 67: 199–208.

472 Savdie E, Caterson RJ, Mahoney JF, Clifton-Bligh I, Birrell W, John E. Successful pregnancies in women treated by hemodialysis. *Med J Aust* 1982; 2: 9.

473 Sheriff MHR, Hardman M, Lamont CAR, Shepherd R, Warrent DJ. Successful pregnancy in a 44–year-old haemodialysis patient. *Br J Obstet Gynaecol* 1978; 85: 386–9.

474 Thomson NM, Rigby RJ, Atkins RC, Walters WAW. Successful pregnancy in a patient on recurrent haemodialysis. *Aust Soc Nephrol* 1978; 8: 243.

475 Unzelman RF, Alderfer GR, Chojnacki RE. Pregnancy and chronic hemodialysis. *Trans Am Soc Artificial Intern Organs* 1973; 19: 422–7.

476 Lim VS, Henriquez C, Sievertsen G, Frohman LA. Ovarian function in chronic renal failure: Evidence suggesting hypothalamic anovulation. *Ann Intern Med* 1980; 57: 7–12.

477 Soffer O. Sexual dysfunction in chronic renal failure. *South Med J* 1980; 73: 1599–601.

478 Schaefer RM, Kokot F, Werrize H. Improved sexual function in hemodialysis patients on recombinant erythropoietin: a possible role for prolactin. *Clin Nephrol* 1989; 31: 1–5.

479 Hou SH, Firanek C. Management of the pregnant dialysis patient. *Adv Renal Replace Ther* 1998; 5: 24–30.

480 Hou S. Incidence and outcome of pregnancy in endstage renal disease (ESRD). *J Am Soc Nephrol* 1992; 3: 77P.

481 Nageotte MP, Grundy HO. Pregnancy outcome in women requiring chronic hemodialysis. *Obstet Gynecol* 1988; 72: 456–9.

482 Giatras I, Levy DP, Malone F, Carlson J. Outcome of pregnancy during chronic dialysis. *Nephrol Dial Transplant* 1998; 13: A187.

483 Bagon JA, Vernaeve H, De Muylder X, Lafountaine JJ, Martens J, Van Roost G. Pregnancy and dialysis. *Am J Kidney Dis* 1998; 31: 756–65.

484 Romão JE, Luders C *et al*. Pregnancy in women on chronic dialysis. *Nephron* 1998; 78: 416–22.

485 Emmanouel DS, Lindheimer MD, Katz AI. Pathogenesis of endocrine abnormalities in uremia. *Endocrine Rev* 1980; 1: 28–44.

486 Schmidt RJ, Holley JL. Fertility and conception in end-stage renal disease. *Adv Renal Replacement Ther* 1998; 5: 38–44.

487 Hogan WJ, Price JW. Proteinuria as a cause of false positive results in pregnancy tests. *Obstet Gynecol* 1967; 29: 585–9.

488 Maruyama H, Akakawa M. Diagnostic clue in haemodialysis patients: progressive anemia resistant to eryropoietin. *J Am Soc Nephrol* 1997; 8: A1130.

489 Cheng P-J, Liu C-M *et al*. Elevated second trimester maternal serum hCG in patients undergoing haemodialysis. *Prenatal Diag* 1999; 19: 955–8.

490 Durant AQ. Treatment guidelines in a pregnant hemodialysis patient. *Dial Transplant* 1989; 18: 86–90.

491 Elliott JP, O'Keefe DF, Schon DA, Cherem LB. Dialysis in pregnancy: a critical review. *Obstet Gynecol Surv* 1991; 46: 319–24.

492 Yasin SY, Bey Doun SN. Hemodialysis in pregnancy. *Obstet Gynecol Surv* 1988; 43: 655–68.

493 Nakabayashi M, Adachi T *et al*. Perinatal and infant outcome of pregnant patients undergoing chronic hemodialysis. *Nephron* 1999; 82: 27–31.

494 Chan WS, Okun N, Kjellstrand CM. Pregnancy in chronic dialysis. A review of the literature. *Int J Artif Organs* 1998; 21: 259–68.

495 Levy DP, Giatris I, Jungers P. Pregnancy and end-stage renal disease—past experience and new insights. *Nephrol Dial Transplant* 1998; 13: Editorial comments.

496 Tenney B, Dandrow BV. Clinical study of hypertensive disease in pregnancy. *Am J Obstet Gynecol* 1961; 81: 8–15.

497 Oosterhof H, Navis CJ *et al*. Pregnancy in a patient on haemodialysis: fetal monitoring by Doppler velocimetry of the umbilical artery. *Br J Obstet Gynaecol* 1993; 100: 1140–1.

498 Hull AR. More dialysis appears beneficial for pregnant ESRD patients (at least in Belgium). *Am J Kidney Dis* 1998; 31: 863–4.

499 Souqiyyeh MZ, Huraffi SO, Mohd Salem AC, Aswad S. Pregnancy in chronic hemodialysis patients in the Kingdom of Saudia Arabia. *Am J Kidney Dis* 1991; 19: 235–8.

500 Rigenbach M, Renger B, Beavais P, Imbs JF, Eschbach J, Frey G. Crosesse et accouchment d'un enfant vivant chez une patiente traitde par haemodialyse interative. *J Urol Nephrol* 1978; 84: 360–6.

501 Naef RW, Morrison CJ. Infection and risk of blood transfusion: hematologic complication of pregnancy. *Clin Obstet Gynecol* 1995; 28: 547–57.

502 Vora M, Gruslim A. Erythropoietin in obstetrics. *Obstet Gynecol Surv* 1998; 53: 500–9.

503 Yankowitz J, Piraino B, Laifer SA. Erythropoietin in pregnancies complicated by severe anaemia of renal failure. *Obstet Gynecol* 1992; 80: 485–8.

504 Hou S, Orlowski J, Pahl M, Ambrose S, Hussey M, Wong D. Pregnancy in women with end-stage disease: treatment of anaemia and premature labor. *Am J Kidney Dis* 1993; 21: 16–22.

505 Brookhyser J. The use of percutanel nutrition supplementation in pregnancy complicated end-stage renal disease. *J Am Dietet Assoc* 1989; 89: 93–4.

506 Lim DTY, Fairweather DVI. The management of preterm labour. In: Elder MC, Hendricks CH, eds. *Preterm Labour.* Butterworths, London, 1981: 231–58.

507 Gadallah MF, Bashir A, Karubian F. Pregnancy in patients on chronic ambulatory peritoneal dialysis. *Am J Obstet Gynecol* 1992; 20: 407–10.

508 Jacobi P, Ohel G, Szylman P, Levit A, Lewin M, Paldi E. Continuous ambulatory peritoneal dialysis as the primary approach in the management of severe renal insufficiency in pregnancy. *Obstet Gynecol* 1992; 79: 808–10.

509 Kioko EM, Shaw KM, Clark AD, Warren DJ. Successful pregnancy in a diabetic patient treated with continuous ambulatory peritoneal dialysis. *Diabetes Care* 1983; 6: 298–300.

510 Goodship THJ, Heaton A, Rodger RSC, Ward MK, Wilkinson R, Kerr DNS. Factors affecting development of peritonitis in continuous ambulatory peritoneal dialysis. *Br Med J* 1984; 289: 1485–6.

511 Cotloib L, Shustak A, Varka I, Haas R, Mines M, Weiss Z. What is the acute incidence of peritonitis in maintenance peritoneal dialysis? A prospective study. *Artif Organs* 1985; 9: 160–3.

512 Blumenkrantz MJ, Gallagher N, Bashore RA, Teuckhoff MD. Retrogade menstruation in women undergoing chronic peritoneal dialysis. *Obstet Gynecol* 1981; 57: 667–70.

513 Rubin J, Rogers WA *et al.* Peritonitis during continuous ambulatory peritoneal dialysis. *Ann Intern Med* 1980; 92: 7–13.

514 Borgeson BD. Continuous ambulatory peritoneal dialysis (CAPD): some psychosocial observations. *Dial Transplant* 1982; 11: 54–6.

515 Hou SH, Firanek C. Management of the pregnant dialysis patient. *Adv Renal Repl Ther* 1998; 5: 24–30.

516 Nakabayashi M, Adachi T *et al.* Perinatal and infant outcome of pregnant patients undergoing chronic haemodialysis. *Nephron* 1999; 82: 27–31.

517 Kon V, Ichikawa I. Physiology of acute renal failure. *J Pediatr* 1984; 105: 351–7.

518 Turney JH, Ellis CM, Parson FM. Obstetric acute renal failure: 1956–87. *Br J Obstet Gynaecol* 1989; 96: 679–87.

519 Khauna N, Nguyen H. Reversible acute renal failure in association with bilateral ureteral obstruction and hydronephrosis in pregnancy. *Am J Obstet Gynecol* 2001; 184: 239–240.

520 Seeds JW, Cefato RC, Herbert WNP, Bowes WA. Hydramnios and maternal renal failure: Relief with fetal therapy. *Obstet Gynecol* 1984; 64: 268–95.

521 Kerr DNS, Elliott RW. Renal disease in pregnancy. *Practitioner* 1963; 190: 459–64.

522 Smith K, Browne JCM, Schackman R, Wrong OM. Renal failure of obstetric origin. *Br Med Bull* 1968; 24: 49–64.

523 Beaman M, Turney JH, Rodger RSC, McGonigle RSJ, Adu D, Michael J. Changing pattern of acute renal failure. *Q J Med* 1987; 62: 15–23.

524 Hawkins DF, Sevitt IH, Fairbrother PF, Tothil AU. Management of chemical septic abortion with renal failure: use of a conservative regimen. *N Engl J Med* 1975; 292: 722–5.

525 Stratta P, Canavese C, Dolgiani M. Pregnancy-related acute and renal failure. *Clin Nephrol* 1988; 32: 14–20.

526 Nzerue CM, Hewan-Lowe K, Nwawka C. Acute renal failure in pregnancy: a review of clinical outcomes at an inner city hospital from 1986–1996. *J Natl Med Assoc* 1998; 90: 486–90.

527 Krane K, Cuccazella A. Acute renal insufficiency in pregnancy. *J Maternal Fetal Med* 1995; 4: 12.

528 Nzerue CM, Hewan-Lowe K, Nwawka C. Acute renal failure in pregnancy: a review of clinical outcomes at an inner city hospital from 1986–1996. *J Natl Med Assoc* 1998; 90: 486–90.

529 Krane NK. Acute renal failure in pregnancy. *Arch Intern Med* 1988; 148: 2347–57.

530 Lindheimer MD, Katz AI, Ganeval D, Grünfeld. JP. Renal failure in pregnancy. In: Brenner BM, Lazarus JH, Myers BD, eds. *Acute Renal Failure.* 3; p. 510–526.

531 Pertuiset N, Grünfeld J-P. Acute renal failure in pregnancy. *Clin Obstet Gynaecol* 1987; 1: 873–90.

532 Pertiset N, Grünfeld JP. Acute renal failure in pregnancy. *Baillière's Clin Obstet Gynaecol* 1994; 8: 333–54.

533 Prakash J, Tripathi K, Malhotra V *et al.* Acute renal failure in Eastern India. *Nephrol Dial Transplant* 1995; 10: 2009–13.

534 Chugh KS, Singhal PC *et al.* Acute renal failure of obstetric origin. *Obstet Gynecol* 1976; 48: 642–6.

535 Myers BD, Moran SM. Hemodynamically mediated acute renal failure. *N Engl J Med* 1972; 314: 97–105.

536 Vertel RM, Knochel JP. Non-oliguric acute renal failure. *J Am Med Assoc* 1967; 200: 598–604.

537 Luke RG, Linton AI, Briggs JD, Kennedy AC. Mannitol therapy in acute renal failure. *Lancet* 1965; i: 980–1032.

538 Jorgensen KA. Acute renal failure: diuretic treatment. *Scand J Urol Suppl* 1981; 57: 31–5.

539 Abel RM, Abbott WM, Fischer JE. Intravenous essential L-amino acids and hypertonic dextrose in patients with acute renal failure. *Am J Surg* 1973; 123: 695–9.

540 Kleinknecht D, Grünfeld JP, Gomez PC, Moreau JF, Garcia-Torres R. Diagnostic procedures and long-term prognosis in bilateral renal necrosis. *Kidney Int* 1973; 4: 390–400.

541 Bartlett RH, Yahia C. Management of septic abortion with renal failure: Report of five consecutive cases with five survivors. *N Engl J Med* 1969; 281: 747–50.

542 Richet C, Alagille D. La proteolyse precose au course des anuries hemolytiques du postabortum. *Rev Fr Etudes Clin Biol* 1975; 2: 475–9.

543 Kniaz D, Eisenberg C, Elrad H. Postpartum hemolytic uremic syndrome associated with antiphospholipid antibodies. A case report and review of the literature. *Am J Nephrol* 1992; 12: 126–33.

544 Smith LP, MacLean APH, Maughan GB. *Clostridium welchii* septicaemia: a review and report of three cases. *Am J Gynecol* 1971; 110: 135–40.

545 Edwards JD. Management of septic shock. *Br Med J* 1993; 306: 1661–4.

546 Sun NCJ, Johnson WJ, Sung DTW, Woods JE. Idiopathic postpartum renal failure: Review and case report of a successful renal transplantation. *Mayo Clin Proc* 1975; 50: 395–401.

547 Janovski NS, Weimer LE, Ober WB. Soap intoxication following criminal abortion. *N Y Med J* 1963; 63: 1463–5.

548 Cavanaugh D, Singh KB. Endotoxin shock in abortion. In: Schurmer W, Nyhus LM, eds. *Corticosteroids in the Treatment of Shock.* University of Illinois Press, Illinois, 1970: 86–98.

549 Emmanouel DS, Katz AI. Acute renal failure in obstetric shock. Current views on pathogenesis and management. *Am J Obstet Gynecol* 1973; 117: 145–9.

550 Hamburger J, Richet G, Crosnier J, Funck-Brentano JL, Mery JP, Moutera HD. Acute tubular and interstitial nephritis ('acute tubular necrosis'). *Nephrology*, Vol. 1. W.B. Saunders, Philadelphia, PA, 1968: 501–12.

551 Hanson GC. Shock and infection. In: Hanson GC, Weight PL, eds. *The Medical Management of the Critically Ill.* Academic Press, London, 1978: 367–73.

552 Gaber LW, Lindheimer MD. Pathology of the kidney, liver and brain. In: Lindheimer MD, Roberts JM, Cunnignham FG, eds. *Chesley's Hypertensive Disorders in Pregnancy*, 2nd edn. Appleton & Lange, Stamford, Connecticut, 1999: 231–62.

553 Sibai BM, Ramadan MK. Acute renal failure in pregnancies complicated by hemolysis, elevated liver enzymes and low platelets. *Am J Obstet Gynecol* 1993; 168: 1682–7.

554 Fox JG, Sutcliffe NP, Walker JJ, Allison M. Postpartum eclampsia and acute renal failure: treatment with prostacyclin. Case report. *Br J Obstet Gynaecol* 1991; 98: 400–2.

555 Ober WE. Reid DE, Romney SL, Merrill JP. Renal lesions and acute renal failure in pregnancy. *Am J Med* 1956; 21: 781–810.

556 Cunningham FG, Lucas MJ, Hankins GDV. Pulmonary injury complicating ante-partum pyelonephritis. *Am J Obstet Gynecol* 1987; 156: 797–807.

557 Sibai BM, Kusterman L, Velasco J. Current understanding of severe pre-eclampsia, pregnancy-associated hemolytic ureteric syndrome, thrombotic thrombocytopenic purpura, hemolysis, elevated liver enzymes and low platelet syndrome and postpartum acute renal failure: different clinical syndromes or just different names? *Curr Opin Nephrol Hypertens* 1994; 3: 436–45.

558 Robson JS, Martin AM, Burkley VA. Irreversible postpartum renal failure: a new syndrome. *Q J Med* 1968; 37: 423–7.

559 Editorial. Haemolytic uraemic syndrome. *Lancet* 1984; ii: 1078–9.

560 Lazelmik N, Jaffa J, Peyeser MR. Hemolytic–uremic syndrome in pregnancy: Review of the literature and report of a case. *Obstet Gynecol Surv* 1985; 40: 618–21.

561 de Swiet M. Some rare medical complications of pregnancy. *Br Med J* 1985; 290: 2–3.

562 Saltiel C, Legendre C, Descamps JP, Hecht M, Grünfeld. J-P. Hemolytic and uremic syndrome in association with pregnancy. In: Kaplan BS, Thrompeter RS, Moake JL, eds. *Hemolytic Uremic Syndrome and Thrombocytopenic Purpura*. Marcel Dekker, New York, 1992: 241–54.

563 Drummond KN. Hemolytic uremic syndrome—then and now. *N Engl J Med* 1985; 312: 116–18.

564 Segonds A, Louradour N, Suc JM, Orfila C. Postpartum hemolytic uremic syndrome: a study of three cases with a review of the literature. *Clin Nephrol* 1979; 12: 229–42.

565 Conger JD, Falk SA, Guggenhheirn SJ. Glomerular dynamics and morphologic changes in the generalised Schwartzman reaction in postpartum rats. *J Clin Invest* 1981; 67: 1334–46.

566 Karmali MA, Petric M, Steele BT, Lim C. Sporadic cases of haemolytic uraemic syndrome associated with faecal cytotoxin and cytotoxin-producing *Escherichia coli* in stools. *Lancet* 1983; i: 619–29.

567 Schultz PJ, Raij L. Endogenously synthesized nitric oxide prevents indotoxin-induced glomerular thrombosis. *J Clin Invest* 1992; 90: 1718–25.

568 Remuzzi G, Misiani R *et al*. Treatment of hemolytic uremic syndrome with plasma. *Clin Nephrol* 1979; 12: 279–84.

569 Moake JL. An update on the therapy of the thrombotic thrombocytopenic purpura. In: Kaplan BS, Trompeter RS, Moake JL, eds. *Hemolytic Uremic Syndrome and Thrombotic Thrombocytopenic Purpura*. Marcel Dekker, New York, 1992: 541–6.

570 Webster J, Rees AJ, Lewis PJ, Hensby CN. Prostacylin deficiency in haemoytic uraemic syndrome. *Br Med J* 1980; 281: 271.

571 Brandt P, Jesperson J, Gregerson G. Post-partum haemolytic–uraemic syndrome successfully treated with antithrombin III. *Br Med J* 1980; i: 449.

572 Grünfeld J-P, Ganeval D, Bournerias F. Acute renal failure in pregnancy. *Kidney Int* 1980; 18: 179–91.

573 Grünfeld J-P, Pertuiset N. Acute renal failure in pregnancy. *Am J Kidney Dis* 1987; 9: 359–62.

574 Sheil O, Redman CWC, Pugh C. Renal failure in pregnancy due to primary lymphoma. Case report. *Br J Obstet Gynaecol* 1991; 98: 216–17.

575 Baylis C, Collins RC. Angiotensin II inhibition on blood pressure and renal hemodynamics in pregnant rats. *Am J Physiol* 1986; 250: F308–14.

576 Warren DJ. Acute renal failure: diagnosis of cause needed within hours. *Br Med J* 1987; 294: 1569.

8 Antiphospholipid syndrome, systemic lupus erythematosus and other connective tissue diseases

Michael de Swiet

The antiphospholipid syndrome

With regard to the outcome of pregnancy the presence of antiphospholipid antibodies has become so important that this must be considered first. The antiphospholipid syndrome (APS) [1–3] may be either primary if other features of connective tissue disease are absent or secondary to established connective tissue disease such as systemic lupus erythematosus (SLE). It is argued whether primary APS is a misnomer, i.e. whether primary APS is only a prodromal state before the patient develops other features of autoimmune disease—secondary APS [4].

It is now realized that the presence of lupus anticoagulant and cardiolipin antibodies is very closely related to the risk of abortion and later fetal loss [5–11].

The lupus anticoagulant is an inhibitor of the coagulation pathway found in 5–10% of patients with SLE [12], which causes prolongation of the kaolin clotting time. In contrast to the situation in coagulopathies, this prolongation is not corrected by mixing the patient's plasma with control plasma. There are increasingly complicated haematological tests to detect lupus anticoagulant [13–15] with little previous standardization between laboratories. Fortunately most laboratories are now coming to rely on the Dilute Russell Viper Venom Test (DRVVT) for the detection of lupus anticoagulant. Paradoxically the lupus anticoagulant is associated with an increased risk of thromboembolism, both arterial and venous [16] (see Chapter 4), and excessive bleeding is very rare [13,17].

Anticardiolipin antibodies are antibodies active against certain phospholipid components of cell walls. They are responsible for the 'false-positive Wasserman reaction', which has been known to occur in SLE. The higher the titre of anticardiolipin antibodies, the greater is the risk to the fetus [18]. Even in the absence of known lupus and without knowledge of cardiolipin antibody status, a retrospective study of patients with biologically false-positive tests for syphilis showed an increased fetal loss rate [19]. More recent studies suggest that the antibodies that really matter are those to β_2-glycoprotein, the cofactor by which anticardiolipin binds to phospholipid. These are usually present with cardiolipin antibodies. But sometimes the clinical features of APS may be apparent with no antibodies detectable in standard antiphospholipid assays [20]. Measurement of β_2-glycoprotein antibodies can be helpful in these circumstances; unfortunately this test is not yet generally available.

The features of the APS are summarized in Box 8.1 [21]. The possibility of pulmonary hypertension should be emphasized because this is so dangerous in pregnancy (see Chapter 5). In all patients who have APS or connective tissue disease without current evidence of APS, pulmonary hypertension should be excluded. This may be done clinically but if there is any doubt echocardiography should be performed (see Chapter 5).

In patients with SLE who have a bad obstetric history, both cardiolipin and lupus anticoagulant antibodies are often present in high titre. Patients who have cardiolipin antibodies in high titre usually have high levels of lupus anticoagulant [22,23]. If they do not, the level of cardiolipin antibodies is usually considered to be a better predictor of fetal outcome [7,24] probably because it is subject to less variability [6], although there is probably much variability between laboratories even with this test. Cardiolipin antibodies may belong to both IgG and IgM subtypes. The IgG antibodies seem to be better predictors of

Box 8.1 Clinical features of the antiphospholipid syndrome [21]

- Thrombosis

Venous

Recurrent deep vein thrombosis (also axillary, intravascular coagulation and retinal vein thromboses)

Arterial

    cerebrovascular accidents

    peripheral arterial gangrene

    coronary thrombosis

    retinal artery thrombosis

Other

    pulmonary hypertension

    ? avascular necrosis

- Abortion

recurrent IUD, placental thrombosis and infarction

- Thrombocytopenia

Intermittent, often acute

- Other occasional features

Coombs' positivity

Livedo reticularis

Migraine

Chorea

Epilepsy

Chronic leg ulcers

? Endocardial disease

? Progressive dementia due to repeated cerebrovascular thromboses

fetal outcome although the presence of IgM antibodies is not without risk to the fetus [24].

The risk to the fetus if the mother has lupus anticoagulant has been put at 85% [5] to 92% [10] mortality. However, the series of Lubbé and Liggins [9] was culled from the literature and represents patients where the lupus anticoagulant was often measured because of the patient's bad obstetric history. In a group of women attending a rheumatology clinic for SLE who have the lupus anticoagulant, or cardiolipin antibodies, the risk to the fetus may be much less, although Lockshin *et al.*'s retrospective study [7] of cardiolipin antibodies in patients with SLE does not support this concept. The problem is compounded by considerable methodological variation in assay procedures [22,25,26]. So what was thought to be a simple association between the presence of cardiolipin antibodies or lupus anticoagulant and high fetal risk has become rather blurred [27]. Furthermore, although the presence of these antibodies in the normal obstetric population is low, between 2% and 5% depending on the cut-off point used, the antibodies may be present in low titre in up

to 30% of patients with severe hypertension in pregnancy [28,29] or even in 10% of non-pregnant patients with endometriosis [29].

Studying patients with early fetal loss further confounds the problem. In patients presenting with unexplained recurrent abortion, the incidence of subclinical autoimmune disease varies between 1% and 29% [30]. The clearest association between cardiolipin antibodies and fetal loss is with second- and third-trimester losses. There is an increased risk of first-trimester loss, but first-trimester loss is so common that it is much more difficult to know whether the presence of cardiolipin antibodies relates to first-trimester loss in an individual patient. The prevalence of cardiolipin antibodies is 15% in patients with recurrent early abortion [31] (defined as three miscarriages or more) compared to 2% in women with low-risk obstetric histories [32]. These antibodies are therefore more likely to be relevant with patients who have had many miscarriages. Lupus anticoagulant is the most commonly detected antiphospholipid antibody in recurrent miscarriage followed by IgG and the IgM anticardiolipin antibodies [31]. In recurrent miscarriage with APS, miscarriage occurs in the first trimester after fetal heart activity has been established. In recurrent miscarriage without APS, the miscarriages are of anembryonic pregnancies [33].

The specificity of anticardiolipin antibodies for pregnancy complications is much increased by using an assay that is β_2-glycoprotein-1 dependent. In a study of 1600 unselected women with no previous history of pregnancy loss, the presence of such anticardiolipin antibodies was associated with a relative risk of 52.4 for adverse pregnancy outcome [34], whereas β_2-glycoprotein-1-independent anticardiolipin antibodies carried no significant increased risk. It is therefore clear that the fetus of the woman who has lupus anticoagulant or cardiolipin antibodies is at risk, but it is difficult to quantify that risk [11] and difficult to state what its excess risk is over that of the normal population [35–37]. This is of particular relevance to treatment options, some of which are not without maternal risk (see below). In addition, lupus anticoagulant and anticardiolipin antibody levels show spontaneous variation between non-pregnancy and pregnancy [35] and even within the same pregnancy. Because of this between-occasion variability a single abnormal antiphospholipid antibody test must be repeated after at least 8 weeks before it is considered clinically significant.

Box 8.2 gives the definition of APS that was arrived at by consensus following an international meeting in Sapporo in 1998. Note that the definition of APS in Box 8.2 gives the clinician responsibility to look for laboratory evidence of APS in unexplained fetal losses occurring after 10 weeks' gestation and in those requiring delivery before 34 weeks

Box 8.2 Definition of antiphospholipid syndrome (APS): consensus meeting, Sapporo, 1998, Criteria For the Classification of APS [38]

APS is present when one or more of the following clinical and one or more laboratory criteria are present

Clinical criteria

Vascular thrombosis: any confirmed thrombosis (arterial, venous or small vessel) in any organ or tissue

Pregnancy morbidity:

(a) any unexplained death of a morphologically normal fetus at or beyond the 10th week of gestation; normality documented by direct examination or ultrasound *or*

(b) any birth of a morphologically normal neonate before 34 weeks' gestation because of severe pre-eclampsia or severe placental insufficiency *or*

(c) at least three consecutive spontaneous abortions before the 10th week with maternal anatomic, hormonal and chromosomal (both parents) causes excluded

Laboratory criteria

1 Anticardiolipin (aCL) IgG and/or IgM in medium or high titre on two or more occasions at least 6 weeks apart measured by standardized ELISA for β_2-glycoprotein inhibitor-dependent aCL

2 Lupus anticoagulant on two or more occasions at least 8 weeks apart detected according to the guidelines of the standing subcommittee [181].

[45]. Inhibition of protein C [46,47] and of tissue plasminogen activator [48] have also been postulated as the mechanisms whereby lupus anticoagulant may cause thrombosis.

However, not all pregnancy loss in APS is associated with placental thrombosis, and it is likely that other mechanism are also operative particularly in first-trimester losses. Direct cellular injury caused by antiphospholipid antibodies binding to trophoblast [49] in a β_2-glycoprotein-1 dependant manner [50] and interference with the interleukin-3 cytokine pathway [51] are other possibilities. The possibility that the mechanism of first-trimester pregnancy loss in APS does not involve thrombosis, does of course question the use of heparin as an antithrombotic drug in this situation (see below).

Not surprisingly other causes of thrombophilia such as antithrombin, protein C and protein S deficiencies and hyperhomocysteinaemia are also being implicated in recurrent miscarriage [52].

Management of primary antiphospholipid syndrome

By definition primary APS presents without overt evidence of other connective tissue disease, i.e. either with thromboembolism or with previous fetal loss. Management is therefore directed towards the recurrence of these risks.

In secondary APS there may also have been previous thromboembolism or previous fetal loss and the management considerations discussed below also then apply. The separate management issues with regard to any underlying connective tissue disease are discussed later.

Treatment directed to improving fetal outcome in APS started with what we now realize was secondary APS in SLE. It was originally hoped that the use of corticosteroids would decrease the high abortion rate associated with SLE. In general, this has not been the case [53]. However, it was reported that aggressive treatment with aspirin 75–300 mg/day and prednisone in doses increasing to 60 mg/day could suppress lupus anticoagulant and anticardiolipin antibodies and consequently improve fetal outcome. Lubbé *et al.* [10] and Branch *et al.* [5] have reported series of 10 and eight patients, respectively, in which the outcome (50% and 62% survival, respectively) was much superior to that expected in untreated patients. In addition there have been several case reports of similar successes [54,55] but also larger studies indicating failure [56]. Furthermore, the high dose of prednisone often makes the patients Cushingoid [9] and induces diabetes, which requires further treatment. There is an increased risk of infection with *Listeria monocytogenes* [57] amongst other organisms. One patient has died of miliary tuberculosis

because of pre-eclampsia or growth restriction as well as those with recurrent miscarriage.

Measurement of anticardiolipin antibody has been proposed for screening the normal population [39] but in general it does not select a high-risk group [40] nor does it distinguish between normal pregnancy and all cases of fetal death including abortion [1]. Maternal thrombocytopenia in association with platelet antibodies appears to be an additional risk factor for fetal death in patients with the cardiolipin syndrome [41].

The mechanism(s) by which these agents might affect the fetus is unknown. The placenta is usually, but not invariably, severely infarcted [42], and the fetus is often growth restricted. Even in the pregnancies of those fetuses that survive, severe pre-eclampsia is very common. Current theories centre round the damage to placental vascular endothelium caused by cardiolipin antibodies, platelet deposition and imbalance in thromboxane/prostacyclin production tilted towards too much thromboxane and too little prostacyclin [43,44] all leading to inadequate maternal placental perfusion. A relative lack of Annexin V a naturally occurring anticoagulant on the intervillous surfaces of the placenta may be a contributing factor

[58]. Even with such treatment the pregnancies are usually complicated by hypertension and/or growth restriction and require very carefully monitoring [5].

In addition, suppression of anticardiolipin antibodies and lupus anticoagulant is not a guarantee of success [5,59], nor is failure to suppress the antibodies a guarantee of fetal death [15,36]. So a treatment strategy based on lowering antibody titres seems flawed. Furthermore, we still do not know the significance in fetal terms of these antibodies in an unselected population (see above). Therefore we need controlled clinical trials of this aggressive form of therapy, which are unfortunately very scanty [54,55].

For example one preliminary trial suggests that heparin and aspirin may be preferable to prednisone and aspirin in high-risk patients [60]. In another study, high-dose subcutaneous heparin (24 000 ± 7000 units/day) was associated with success in 14 of 15 high-risk lupus pregnancies [61]. Further support for heparin and aspirin came in two studies of pregnancies with APS [62,63]. Because of the Cowchock study referred to above [60], the high maternal morbidity from high-dose steroid therapy, and the success of heparin and aspirin in treating recurrent miscarriage (see below), it seems unlikely that further trials will be performed comparing steroids and aspirin with heparin and aspirin. Currently I prefer to use aspirin and heparin rather than aspirin and steroids, although I acknowledge that what is also needed is a trial to see whether heparin given in addition to aspirin in those who do not have a history of thromboembolism, improves fetal outcome other than in recurrent miscarriage. In patients where heparin, steroid and aspirin therapies have been unsuccessful, a variety of additional therapies have been tried including azathioprine [64,65], plasmapheresis, immunoglobulin and plasma exchange. Nevertheless, the place of these therapies is even less clear than the place of aspirin and heparin therapy.

Two trials have been performed supporting the use of heparin in addition to aspirin for recurrent miscarriage [66,67]. The study of Kutteh [66] suffered from alternate randomization and in neither the Kutteh nor the St Mary's trial [67] were placebo heparin injections used, so both had methodological problems. But both had a similar result: a take-home baby rate of more than 70% in the heparin and aspirin group compared to 40% in those treated with aspirin alone. Nevertheless, the lack of a placebo arm to the studies is important granted the potential for placebo effects in recurrent miscarriage. Where no pharmacological intervention was given the successful pregnancy rate is about 10% [33,52].

Interestingly all the benefit of additional heparin occurred in the first 14 weeks of pregnancy in the St Mary's study, even though the remainder of the pregnancies were stormy in both groups [68]; so there is currently indecision as to how long to continue heparin treatment. In practice most would continue until at least 34 weeks as in the original study 'to be on the safe side'. And most would adopt the original St Mary's scheme, i.e. start aspirin as soon as pregnancy is confirmed and then start heparin as soon as the fetal heart has been identified by ultrasound, usually at about 6 weeks. In the St Mary's trial unfractionated heparin was used, 5000 units given by subcutaneous injection 12 hourly. I prefer to use low molecular weight heparin (LMWH) and to give a higher dose, i.e. fragmin 5000 units or enoxaparin 40 mg because of the advantages of once daily treatment and because I believe that the lower dose of heparin would not be sufficiently effective for thromboprophylaxis. Granted the lack of teratogenicity of aspirin, it would also seem reasonable for patients to conceive taking aspirin rather than wait until they know that they are pregnant. The main concern about this form of treatment is osteopenia; this seems to less common with LMWH than with unfractionated heparin (see Chapter 4), which would be further reason for using LMWH rather than unfractionated heparin as in the original St Mary's study.

Patients who also have a past history of thromboembolism, arterial or venous, should be treated with subcutaneous heparin throughout pregnancy in addition to any aspirin or prednisone therapy that might be considered necessary. The heparin is given as described for patients with thromboembolism in pregnancy (see Chapter 4). Although this treatment will exacerbate any bone loss associated with steroid therapy, I believe it to be necessary in view of the dire consequences, particularly of cerebral arterial thrombosis [69]. Patients with lupus anticoagulant and/or cardiolipin antibodies and no history of thromboembolism are treated with low-dose aspirin alone (75 mg/day) unless it is judged that they also require heparin for fetal reasons.

Systemic lupus erythematosus (SLE)

SLE is a multisystem disease, which most frequently presents in young women. It is therefore relatively common in pregnancy, and it is certainly the connective tissue disease that has been studied most intensively. It is quite possible that SLE was the reason why Queen Anne lost 17 pregnancies and failed to produce an heir to the throne of England [70].

The apparent prevalence has increased as more mild forms of the disease are recognized. In 1974 Fessel [71] found the prevalence of SLE to be one in 700 women aged 15–64 years. In black women the prevalence was one in 245. Women in 'minority' races have a fivefold excess risk compared to white women [72]. The diagnosis may be

Box 8.3 Criteria for the diagnosis of systemic lupus (SLE) as suggested by the American Rheumatism Association [182]

To substantiate the diagnosis, the patient should have at least four features, either simultaneously, or following each other

- Facial butterfly rash
- Discoid lupus
- Photosensitivity—skin rash as a result of unusual reaction to sunlight
- Oral or nasopharyngeal ulceration
- Non-erosive arthritis involving two or more peripheral joints
- Pleurisy or pericarditis
- Proteinuria >0.5 g/day or cellular casts
- Psychosis or convulsions
- One of:
  haemolytic anaemia
  leucopenia, white blood cell count <4000/mm^3 on two or more occasions
  lymphopenia <1500/mm^3 on two or more occasions
  thrombocytopenia <100 000/mm^3
- Immunological disorder:
  positive LE cell preparation
  antibody to native DNA in abnormal titre
  antibody to smooth muscle nuclear antigen
  chronic false-positive syphilis serology for 6 months

based on the patient having at least four of the features noted by the American Rheumatism Association, either simultaneously or following each other (Box 8.3). However, the necessity to have four rather than three criteria has been challenged [73].

Since the publication of the American Rheumatism Association criteria, the measurement of antinuclear factor and of anti-DNA antibodies has replaced the lupus erythematosus (LE) cell test in the diagnosis of SLE. In pregnancy, proteinuria and thrombocytopenia can lead to confusion with pre-eclampsia. The clinical features of pre-eclampsia, which usually run a much more acute course, remit after delivery, and are not associated with other features summarized in Box 8.3. This enables the two conditions to be distinguished. However, proteinuria quite often appears early in pregnancy for a variety of reasons, the process may not be so acute, and in this situation, measurement of antinuclear factor and anti-DNA antibodies helps to distinguish SLE from other renal conditions and pre-eclampsia.

The disease runs a fluctuating course. In advanced forms, with severe nephritis or nervous system involvement, the overall prognosis is bad, but as less severe

forms are recognized, the prognosis has improved so that most centres would now report a >95% survival at 5 years. If treatment is required, the drugs most commonly used are aspirin, prednisone and antimalarials such as hydroxychloroquine and azathioprine. (For other reviews of connective tissue disease and SLE in pregnancy see [37,74,77].)

Overlap syndrome relates to diffuse connective tissue diseases overlapping in their clinical and immunological features. Olah and Redman [78] have described a single case where the fetus developed congenital heart block in association with anti-Ro antibodies (see below).

Effect of pregnancy on systemic lupus erythematosus

As is the case with most illnesses that run a fluctuating course, such as asthma or disseminated sclerosis, it is difficult to document any special effect of pregnancy on SLE. The general consensus is that pregnancy does not affect the long-term prognosis of SLE [79], but that pregnancy itself may be associated with more 'flare-ups', particularly in the puerperium [10,53]. Considering patients are usually observed more closely in pregnancy this is not surprising. Also, patients with SLE are normally advised against conceiving during an active phase of the disease and therefore conceive when they are well [80]. If the effect of pregnancy is judged by a comparison of the state of pregnancy with that before conception (see for example [81]), their condition can only either stay unchanged if they were well before pregnancy or deteriorate; this is a further cause of bias. In a comparison with the pre-pregnancy period, Garsenstein et al. [79] found that the exacerbation rate was three times greater in the first half of pregnancy, one and a half times greater in the second half, and at least six times greater in the puerperium— the time when maternal deaths have occurred [81]. These deaths have been due to pulmonary haemorrhage [82] or lupus pneumonitis [83] to which these women appear to be particularly susceptible [84].

In one case–control study from Toronto, there was no difference in the incidence of flares in 46 women during 79 pregnancies compared to well-matched controls who were not pregnant. Active disease at entry to the study did not predict flare in either pregnant or control group; however, inactive disease at the beginning of pregnancy did protect against flare during pregnancy [85]. Therefore, not surprisingly, the advice is that women with lupus should wait until their disease is quiescent before becoming pregnant. In another case–control study from London, flares occurred rather more frequently in the pregnant group (65%) than in the non-pregnant group (37%) [63,86].

Kincaid-Smith *et al.* [87] in Melbourne found specific renal biopsy changes in patients with renal 'flares' in pregnancy. These were similar to those found in haemolytic–uraemic syndrome (HUS) and were also associated with microhaemangiopathic haemolytic anaemia. Treatment directed toward HUS (aspirin, fresh frozen plasma, plasmapheresis) may be helpful for renal 'flares' in pregnancy; such flares may also be due to endothelial disease.

Chorea is a rare complication of SLE that may also be made worse by pregnancy (chorea gravidarum) [8,88]. It is interesting that successive pregnancies do not necessarily affect an individual in the same way [80].

The relationships of pregnancy to renal and skin diseases caused by SLE are also considered in Chapters 7 and 20, respectively.

Effect of systemic lupus erythematosus on pregnancy

There are three main ways in which SLE affects pregnancy and its outcome. First, SLE increases the risks of late pregnancy losses due to hypertension and renal failure; secondly, it is an important cause of heart block and other cardiac defects in the newborn. This effect may be part of a more general neonatal lupus syndrome. Thirdly, SLE increases the risk of fetal loss independently of hypertension or renal failure. This is usually in the presence of antiphospholipid antibodies, secondary APS considered separately above.

HYPERTENSION AND RENAL FAILURE

Patients are at risk of fetal morbidity if they have renal involvement and/or hypertension. For example, Houser *et al.* [89] studied 18 pregnancies in patients with SLE. Ten occurred in patients with no evidence of renal disease and were uncomplicated. The remaining eight occurred in patients with renal disease. There were four abortions (one elective), three premature deliveries, and only one normal term delivery. It is difficult to be precise as to what level of renal impairment is significant, but a creatinine clearance of $<65\,mL/min/m^3$ or proteinuria $>2.4\,g/24\,h$ would be ominous (see Chapter 7). Hayslett and Lynn [90] noted a 50% fetal loss rate in mothers with a serum creatinine in excess of $132\,mmol/L$ ($1.5\,mg/dL$).

THE NEONATAL LUPUS SYNDROME

This syndrome [91] includes haematological complications, cardiac abnormalities, babies in whom skin lesions are present [92] as the only abnormalities, and neonates who develop SLE in the absence of any involvement in the mother [93]. Maternal antibodies have been shown to cross the placenta [93] and it is likely that SLE is one of the conditions—such as rhesus disease, Graves' disease or myasthenia gravis—where transplacental passage of antibodies harms the fetus. However, in SLE, the precise antibody that affects the fetus has not been identified, and the fetal outcome cannot be correlated with fetal (or maternal) antibody levels apart from the relationship between congenital heart block and certain maternal antibodies (see below).

The haematological abnormalities are haemolytic anaemia, leucopoenia and thrombocytopenia. They are usually transient and not a major problem [94].

The cardiac abnormalities have been best defined by McCue *et al.* [95] and Esscher and Scott [96]. By far the most common abnormality is complete heart block which may be present and detected antenatally [97]. However, a variety of abnormalities have been described including endomyocardial fibrosis [96], pericarditis [98–100] and persistent sinus bradycardia [101]. Although the majority of infants born to mothers with SLE are normal, about one in three mothers (38%) who deliver babies with congenital heart block have, or will have, a connective tissue disease [96]. Most frequently, the disease is SLE, but in 16% of cases the mother had rheumatoid arthritis, and 25% have a less well-defined form of connective tissue disease. Reassuringly in a follow-up study 36 of 42 women who gave birth to a child with congenital heart block and who were asymptomatic at delivery, remained well on average 10 years later [102].

About 60% of mothers who deliver a child with congenital heart block have antibodies to soluble tissue ribonucleoprotein antigen (anti-Ro or SS-A and anti-La or SS-B antibodies). Because the production of anti-Ro and anti-La antibodies is correlated with the presence of HLA antigen DR3 which is more common in patients with Sjögren's syndrome [103], patients with Sjögren's syndrome are at particular risk of having an infant with congenital heart block [104–105]. The risk of congenital heart block is greater with anti-Ro than with anti-La but equally must not be overestimated. Anti-Ro antibodies are quite common so that the risk of congenital heart block in the presence of anti-Ro is at most one in 20, although this increases to one in three if the mother already has a child with congenital heart block [106]. In one prospective study there were no cases of heart block in 91 infants born to mothers with SLE despite 23% of the mothers being Ro positive [107]. In another series, these autoantibodies were invariably present in the mothers with SLE that delivered an affected child, but they were also present in some asymptomatic women who had a child with congenital heart block [108].

Antibody has been found in the site of the conducting tissue in the heart of a fetus that died with complete heart block. However, because it was both IgG and IgA antibody [109], some, the IgA antibody which does not cross the placenta, was presumably derived from the fetus. This is rather puzzling. In addition it is quite unclear why the anti-Ro antibody does not affect maternal cardiac conductive tissue.

It has also been shown that the mothers and their offspring may also have an IgG antibody that reacts with fetal cardiac tissue [110]. This antibody may also be involved in the pathogenesis of congenital heart block, and the presence of this and other autoantibodies may explain why the fetal prognosis is not invariably good even in the absence of well-established markers for fetal death such as antiphospholipid antibodies (see below). Thus, although the baby usually survives the perinatal period, and often does not require pacing, in a few cases with congenital heart block and without antiphospholipid antibodies the fetus dies antenatally or in labour [111]. Perhaps the antibodies directed against cardiac muscle are causing a fatal cardiomyopathy [112]. This would certainly be in keeping with findings of diffuse IgG antibody in all cardiac tissue of a fetus that died in association with high maternal titres of anti-Ro in early pregnancy [113] and with the clinical presentation before delivery as non-immune hydrops.

Of course fetuses may have congenital heart block because of a primary structural abnormality, frequently an atrioventricular canal defect [114]. Under these circumstances there is usually no association with maternal connective tissue disease.

McCuiston and Shock [115] first described discoid skin lesions in a neonate whose mother subsequently developed SLE. The lesions are usually on the face or the scalp and are present at birth or develop after birth possibly because fetal skin does not contain the anti-Ro antigen [116]. They have normally disappeared by 1 year of life, and only rarely are associated with other organ involvement [117]. Some skin lesions have been associated with maternal and fetal antibodies to U1RNP (nRNP) a protein found in normal human skin cells [118].

Secondary antiphospholipid syndrome

It is probable that those women with clinical lupus who do not have significant cardiolipin antibodies or lupus anticoagulant do not have excess fetal risk apart from the slight excess that may be present in association with anti-Ro or anti-La antibodies (see above) or because of hypertension or renal disease. For example Lockshin et al. [7] studied 21 patients with lupus. Twelve had normal pregnancies; their mean cardiolipin titre was only marginally raised to 27 units. Nine had abnormal pregnancies with fetal death or fetal distress. Their mean cardiolipin titre was 212 units. In the larger series of Loizou et al. [119] there were 129 pregnancies in women without cardiolipin antibodies; the abortion rate was 27%, whereas in 37 pregnancies with high levels of cardiolipin antibodies the abortion rate was 89%.

The incidence of abortion in patients with SLE may be as high as 40% [53]. On reviewing previous pregnancies, even those occurring before the onset of SLE, Fraga et al. [53] found that the incidence of abortion was 23%—about twice as high as in a group of control patients. Chesley [120] also analysed the outcome of 630 pregnancies in mothers with SLE and found that there was a 36% failure rate.

Baesnihan et al. [121] showed a high titre of lymphocytotoxic antibodies in three of four patients with SLE, whose pregnancies ended in abortion. These antibodies can be absorbed by trophoblast, which indicates a number of possible mechanisms for the cause of abortion in SLE [121] that are separate from APS. For example, Abramowsky et al. [122] have described necrotizing decidual vascular lesions with immunoglobulin deposition in placentas of women whose pregnancies were complicated by SLE.

Management of systemic lupus erythematosus in pregnancy

MATERNAL CONSIDERATIONS

The drugs most frequently used for the treatment of SLE [123] are simple analgesics such as paracetamol and non-steroidal anti-inflammatory drugs including aspirin. In more severe cases antimalarial drugs, corticosteroids, other immunosuppressives and cytotoxic agents are used.

Paracetamol has been used widely in pregnancy with no adverse effects in normal therapeutic doses. Aspirin has been extensively studied. Three large prospective studies [124–126], including the Perinatal Collaborative Project of over 14 000 women exposed to aspirin in the USA, have shown no teratogenic risk [125]. However, salicylates and other non-steroidal anti-inflammatory agents have been associated with neonatal haemorrhage because of their action in inhibiting platelet function [126,127]. The risk of bleeding from therapeutic doses of aspirin must be contrasted with the negligible risk from thromboprophylactic doses (75 mg daily) taken in pregnancy.

In addition there is the risk that prostaglandin synthetase inhibitors will cause premature closure of the ductus arteriosus and pulmonary hypertension [128]. This appears to be more of a theoretical than a practical risk

[129]. So far, only occasional cases have been reported following maternal indomethacin treatment [130]. There were no such complications in over 200 infants exposed to indomethacin in studies of its effect in preterm labour [131,132]. Chloroquine causes choroidoretinitis [133], although not usually in the doses employed for malaria prophylaxis or treatment [134]. However, withdrawal of chloroquine is associated with a high risk of SLE flare [135]. Therefore, it would seem sensible not to withdraw chloroquine in pregnancy but to treat exacerbations of SLE in pregnancy by an increase in steroid therapy rather than the *de novo* introduction of chloroquine.

Chloroquine has been contraindicated in pregnancy because of its potential to damage the retina. Also chloroquine has been reported to cause chromosome damage, but there is no evidence that this results in stable chromosome abnormalities, which might be of genetic or neoplastic significance [137]. Congenital deafness has also been reported [138]. However, in two series, one in the USA [138a] and one in the UK [139], there was no evidence of damage in the outcome of 42 pregnancies where the mothers were treated with 4-aminoquinolones including chloroquine. Also it is likely that the ocular risks from treatment with hydroxychloroquine have been exaggerated particularly in the first 5–7 years of treatment [140]. Because of the very definite risk of precipitating flare [135], it would seem prudent to continue chloroquine during pregnancy.

The safety of steroids is considered in Chapter 1.

Azathioprine is the cytotoxic agent that is most commonly used in rheumatic conditions and the only cytotoxic agent that can be considered for use in pregnancy. The possibility of induction of chromosome breaks and their long-term consequences for female fetuses is discussed in Chapter 7.

In summary, paracetamol is the best agent to use as an analgesic and an antirheumatic in pregnancy. Non-steroidal anti-inflammatory agents are best avoided in normal therapeutic doses in the last trimester and if a patient requires extra therapy for this relatively short time, corticosteroids should be used.

Since the erythrocyte sedimentation rate (ESR) is elevated in normal pregnancy, reduction of C3 complement can be used as an objective index of disease activity [142]; so too can the level of anti-DNA antibodies. C-reactive protein is not a marker for lupus activity. In patients taking long-term corticosteroids, parenteral steroid cover should be given in labour. Our practice is to use intramuscular hydrocortisone 100 mg 6-hourly, until the patient is taking oral medication. Because of the risk of dangerous exacerbation of SLE in the puerperium, steroid dosage should only be reduced with great care after delivery.

Some authors [143] have even arbitrarily increased steroid therapy in all patients from the 30th week of pregnancy until 4 weeks after delivery. The use of azathioprine should be reserved for cases where steroid therapy has failed or is contraindicated.

Plasmapheresis has been successfully used in pregnancy for maternal reasons in a patient with SLE, who developed severe proximal myopathy induced by steroids. The fetus was already growth restricted but did not appear to suffer further from the procedure [144]. A single successful case raises the possibility that plasmapheresis and steroid therapy may decrease the risk of the development of complete heart block in a patient who is anti-Ro positive [145] but there have also been failures.

In breastfeeding women, the non-steroidal anti-inflammatory drugs with short half-lives and rapidly elevated or inactive metabolites are best, i.e. ibuprofen, flurbiprofen and diclofenac [123]. Salicylates and antimalarial drugs should be avoided for the reasons given above. Minute quantities of prednisolone are secreted in breast milk and this drug and prednisone should therefore be considered safe.

FETAL CONSIDERATIONS

Aspects of management relating to APS have already been considered above.

The timing of delivery in patients with SLE and/or APS depends on the severity of the condition and whether the patients have renal involvement or hypertension. If there is none of these complications, the patient should be delivered at term. Increasing degrees of renal failure or hypertension will necessitate early delivery, either for these reasons alone or because of evidence of fetal compromise, as judged by poor growth, or cardiotocography or Doppler ultrasound measurement of fetal and maternal placental blood flow. With the advent of cardiotocography and widespread use of ultrasound to measure fetal growth, there is no longer any need for measurement of oestriol levels. But should oestriol levels be measured, note that they can be depressed purely by corticosteroid therapy, although usually only in dosages >75 mg cortisol per day [146].

Congenital heart block should be diagnosed before delivery from routine auscultation of the fetal heart and subsequent cardiotocography when bradycardia is discovered. If possible a detailed ultrasound examination of the fetal heart should then be performed. This will show atrioventricular dissociation confirming complete heart block and also demonstrate any structural heart disease which is present in 15–20% of cases [147]. If the fetus has complete heart block, it is difficult to assess its general condition *in utero* since accurate assessment usually depends on measurement of fetal heart rate and its variability. However, it is possible to measure the atrial rate and its variability by detailed ultrasound. Measurement of umbilical blood flow by Doppler ultrasound can be of value [148] and antenatal fetal blood sampling to measure fetal blood gases [149,150] is of real value in this situation. Labour can be monitored by repeated fetal blood gas estimation [104] but many such fetuses are understandably delivered by elective caesarean section.

The greatest problems occur in fetuses with heart block who are hydropic. They have low output intrauterine heart failure either due to the slow heart rate alone or to an additional cardiomyopathic process. The use of plasmapheresis and/or immunosuppressive or steroid therapy to prevent heart block occurring in high-risk cases (anti-Ro positive, previously affected fetus) has been mentioned above but there is no evidence that this form of treatment is of benefit once heart block has developed [151]. Nevertheless glucocorticoids that cross the placenta such as dexamethasone are frequently used [99,152] with the aim of achieving viability at which time the fetus should be delivered by caesarean section.

Rheumatoid arthritis

The finding by Hench [153] that rheumatoid arthritis improved in 24 of 30 pregnancies, coupled with a belief that cortisol levels were markedly elevated in pregnancy, was so important that it led to the successful use of steroids in patients with rheumatoid arthritis who were not pregnant. Kaplan and Diamond [154] have confirmed these observations, and difficulties in the management of rheumatoid arthritis are rare in pregnancy, although exacerbations may occur in the puerperium. The subject has been extensively reviewed by Thurnau [155]. There is no association between rheumatoid arthritis and infertility (expressed as nulliparity) [156]. Unger et al. [157] have correlated the improvement in rheumatoid arthritis with the level of pregnancy-associated α_2-glycoprotein, which has immunosuppressive action. However, pregnancy induces many other changes in the immune system and therefore there may be other reasons why rheumatoid arthritis improves. Nevertheless, a recent UK study of 140 pregnancies complicated by rheumatoid arthritis tends to weaken these comments, i.e. there was only a modest improvement in symptoms, with more than 25% of the women still having severe disability [158].

In contrast to SLE there is no increased risk of abortion in patients with rheumatoid arthritis [154] unless there is associated APS. This is uncommon. As indicated above, there is a small risk of congenital heart block in the newborn. Other potential problems are in abduction of the hip

during vaginal delivery, or extension of the neck and opening of the mouth for intubation in general anaesthesia.

The most common difficulty concerns drug administration. As indicated above, the dangers of steroid therapy have been exaggerated, and paracetamol is a better analgesic for use in pregnancy than aspirin. However, if paracetamol is inadequate it seems reasonable to use aspirin and other prostaglandin antagonists at least in the first two trimesters. However, there are case reports of convulsions in a breastfed infant, after the mother had taken indomethacin for analgesia [131,159], and therefore indomethacin should not be used in women who are breastfeeding. In any case other non-steroidal antagonists such as ibuprofen have a better safety profile and are preferred to indomethacin whether the patient is pregnant or not.

There is also little experience with the use of phenylbutazone in pregnancy. In non-pregnant patients, phenylbutazone can cause sodium retention and bone-marrow dyscrasias. It is not known whether these and other abnormalities occur in the fetus exposed to phenylbutazone before delivery but in any case phenylbutazone has also been replaced by safer non-steroidal anti-inflammatory drugs (NSAIDs) and should now be reserved for the inpatient treatment of (non-pregnant) patients with ankylosing spondylitis. The situation is similar concerning gold therapy. In the adult, gold causes blood dyscrasias, drug rashes and nephropathy. However, gold is very strongly protein bound and little appears to cross the placenta [160].

Antimalarial drugs such as chloroquine are also used in the treatment of rheumatoid arthritis and have been discussed in the section relating to SLE above. The risks of their use in pregnancy have been exaggerated and women should continue to take antimalarial drugs for the treatment of rheumatoid arthritis in pregnancy.

Sulphasalazine is increasingly used as second-line treatment for rheumatoid arthritis. Its safety in pregnancy is documented in Chapter 10.

With regard to immunosuppressive drugs, azathioprine is the drug that has been used most frequently. It appears to be relatively safe in the short term, although there are questions regarding the reproductive potential of female fetuses exposed to this drug in utero (see Chapter 7).

Penicillamine is also used in the treatment of rheumatoid arthritis. There are occasional reports of suspected teratogenesis [161] and neonatal abnormalities of connective tissue [162], which may be irreversible or reversible [163]. However, there are two series (totalling 56 pregnancies) in which the only abnormality (which could have occurred by chance) was one child with a small ventricular septal defect [164,165]. It would therefore seem that penicillamine is reasonably safe in pregnancy (see Chapter 9).

In summary, if a patient with rheumatoid arthritis requires treatment in pregnancy, she should be given paracetamol. If this does not give adequate relief in the first two trimesters, aspirin or other NSAIDs may be used. If these are inadequate and in the last trimester corticosteroids should be used despite the understandable concern that most rheumatologists have about corticosteroid therapy in rheumatoid arthritis [166]. Penicillamine treatment also appears to be safe.

Scleroderma and other connective tissue diseases

Scleroderma is a connective tissue disease affecting the skin, gastrointestinal tract (oesophagus), kidneys (see Chapter 7) and lungs. The cause is unknown and there is no known cure or disease modifying therapy. There have been several series of patients [167,168,169] and several case reports [170], describing the interaction of scleroderma and pregnancy (see also review in [86]).

The observation that nearly 30 times as many cells of fetal origin were found remote from pregnancy in women with scleroderma as in controls, caused much interest suggesting that microchimerism might be involved in the pathogenesis of the disease, a form of graft vs. host disease. The occurrence of the disease in men and in women who have not had children would make the explanation more complicated, i.e. these individuals would have had to have received cells from their mothers while *in utero* to develop microchimerism; but in any case explanations of this sort cannot be the whole answer, because the findings were not substantiated in a group of Japanese women with scleroderma [171].

Scleroderma has been divided into localized cutaneous and diffuse cutaneous forms. In the localized cutaneous form the scleroderma process is localized usually to the hands and arms distal to the elbow; it is associated with Raynaud's phenomenon and without organ involvement. The prognosis is good in general and in particular in pregnancy, although occasionally Raynaud's phenomenon may first appear as an aggressive manifestation of scleroderma in pregnancy [172]. Diffuse cutaneous scleroderma has more widespread cutaneous manifestations and is a much more aggressive illness. Raynaud's phenomenon is less common and the patient may have SCL-70 antibodies. Organ involvement is frequent, affecting heart, lungs and kidneys and is the cause of death. Not surprisingly the prognosis in general and in pregnancy in particular is worse. Because many patients deteriorate, they have been advised against pregnancy [170], particularly considering they may not be able to look after their children even if they survive pregnancy; but we still do not know whether pregnancy itself accelerates the deterioration that is inevitable in these patients. For example in a recent series of 91 pregnancies in 59 women with scleroderma there were only three episodes of renal crisis all with early diffuse disease. Four women took angiotensin-converting enzyme inhibitor drugs in five pregnancies with no ill effect in the fetus (see below) [173].

The fetal outcome is also impaired. In a review of 17 pregnancies reported in the literature, Karlen and Cook [170] documented five perinatal deaths, and five instances of premature delivery. Involvement of the cervix has been implicated as a cause of dystocia in labour [174]. These patients often have sclerotic skin and blood vessels, making venepuncture, venous access and blood pressure measurement difficult. Both regional and general anaesthesia are associated with technical problems particularly the difficulty of endotracheal intubation [175]. Such patients should see an anaesthetist early in their pregnancy so that anaesthetic management can be planned rather than guessed at in an emergency. Angiotensin-converting enzyme inhibitor drugs such as captopril have been advocated as treatment for crises in patients with scleroderma [176]. These drugs should be avoided in pregnancy because of concern about the fetus (see Chapter 6) unless there is no other treatment. In the case of a patient with scleroderma crisis, this is likely to be the case.

Other connective tissue diseases, which rarely complicate pregnancy, are polyarteritis nodosa [177,178], dermatomyositis [82] relapsing polychondritis [179], ankylosing spondylitis and Wegener's granulomatosis. Wegener's granulomatosis has already been considered in Chapter 1. In all these conditions there is insufficient experience to be confident of the effect of pregnancy. Because some patients have deteriorated in pregnancy, termination has been suggested for cases of polyarteritis nodosa [177] but this may not be justified [178].

Relapsing polychondritis is a condition where cartilage is inflamed and loses its structural integrity. Four cases have been described in pregnancy [179]. One deteriorated in pregnancy and required a tracheotomy [179]. In one case the neonate was also affected [180] suggesting transplacental passage of autoantibodies.

Finally, it has recently been suggested that patients are particularly at risk from developing polymyositis, an autoimmune disease of muscle, in the puerperium.

References

1 Infante-Rivard C, David M, Gauthier R, Rivard GE. Lupus anticoagulants, anticardiolipin antibodies, and fetal loss. A case-control study. *N Engl J Med* 1991; 325: 1063–6.

2 Rai R, Regan L. Antiphospholipid syndrome in pregnancy. *Curr Obstet Gynaecol* 1998; 8: 32–5.

3 Greaves M. Antiphospholipid antibodies and thrombosis. *Lancet* 1999; 353: 1348–53.

4 Gleicher N, Coulam C. Antiphospholipid antibodies and thrombosis. *Lancet* 1999; 354: 72–3.

5 Branch WD, Scott JR, Kochenour NK, Hershgold E. Obstetric complications associated with the lupus anticoagulant. *N Engl J Med* 1985; 313: 1322–6.

6 Derue GJ, Englert MJ *et al.* Fetal loss in systemic lupus: association with anticardiolipin antibodies. *J Obstet Gynaecol* 1985; 5: 207–9.

7 Lockshin NW, Gibofsky A, Peebles CL, Gigh I, Fotino M, Hurwitz S. Neonatal lupus erythematosus with heart block: family study of a patient with anti-SS-A and SS-B antibodies. *Arthritis Rheum* 1983; 26: 210–13.

8 Lubbé WE, Walker EB. Chorea gravidarum associated with lupus anticoagulant: successful outcome of pregnancy with prednisone therapy. *Br J Obstet Gynaecol* 1983; 90: 487–90.

9 Lubbé WE, Liggins GC. Lupus anticoagulant and pregnancy. *Am J Obstet Gynecol* 1985; 153: 322–7.

10 Lubbé WE, Butler WS, Palmer SJ, Liggins GC. Lupus anticoagulant in pregnancy. *Br J Obstet Gynaecol* 1984; 91: 357–63.

11 Ros JO, Tarres MV, Baucells MV, Maired JJ, Solano J. Prednisone and maternal lupus anticoagulant. *Lancet* 1983; ii: 576.

12 Schlieder MA, Nachman RL, Jaffe EA, Coleman MA. Clinical study of the lupus anticoagulant. *Blood* 1976; 48: 499–509.

13 Boxer M, Ellman L, Carvallho A. The lupus anticoagulant. *Arthritis Rheum* 1976; 19: 1244–8.

14 Exner T, Rickard KA, Kronenberg H. A sensitive test demonstrating lupus anticoagulant and its behavioural patterns. *Br J Haematol* 1978; 40: 143–51.

15 Reece EA, Romero R, Clyne LP, Kriz NS, Hobbins JC. Lupus like anticoagulant in pregnancy. *Lancet* 1984; i: 344–5.

16 Editorial. Anticardiolipin antibodies a risk factor for venous and arterial thrombosis. *Lancet* 1985; i: 912–13.

17 Ordi J, Vilardel M *et al.* Bleeding in patients with lupus anticoagulant. *Lancet* 1984; ii: 868–9.

18 Harris EN, Chan J, Asherson R, Charavi A, Hughes GRV. Predictive value of the anticardiolipin antibody for thrombosis, fetal loss and thrombocytopoenia. *Clin Sci* 1986; 70: 56P.

19 Thornton JR, Scott JS, Tovey LAD. Anticardiolipin antibodies in pregnancy. *Br Med J* 1984; 289: 697.

20 Cabral AR, Amigo MC, Cabiedes J, Alarcon-Segovia D. The antiphospholipid/co–factor syndromes: a primary variant with antibodies to β$_2$-glycoprotein-1 but no antibodies detectable in standard antiphospholipid assays. *Am J Med* 1996; 101: 472–81.

21 Hughes GRV, Harris EN, Gharavi AE. The anticardiolipin syndrome. *J Rheumatol* 1986; 13: 486–9.

22 Harris ENH, Gharavi AE *et al.* Anticardiolipin antibodies: detection by radioinummoassay and association with thrombosis in systemic lupus erythematosus. *Lancet* 1983; ii: 1211–14.

23 Harris EN, Louizou S *et al.* Anticardiolipin antibodies and lupus anticoagulant. *Lancet* 1984; ii: 1099.

24 Lockwood CJ, Reece EA, Romero R, Hobbins JC. Antiphospholipid antibody and pregnancy wastage. *Lancet* 1986; ii: 742–3.

25 Harris EN, Hughes GRV. Standardising the anticardiolipin antibody test. *Lancet* 1987; i: 277.

26 Lockshin MD, Druzin NIL. Antiphospholipid antibodies and pregnancy. *N Engl J Med* 1985; 313: 1351.

27 Walport MJ. Pregnancy and antibodies to phospholipids. *Ann Rheumatol Dis* 1989; 48: 795–7.

28 Branch WD, Rote NS, Scott RJ, Edwin S. The association of antiphospholipid antibodies with severe pre-eclampsia. *Clin Exp Rhuematol* 1988; 6: 198.

29 Taylor PV, Skerrow SM. Pre-eclampsia and antiphospholipid antibody. *Br J Obstet Gynaecol* 1991; 98: 604–6.

30 Cowchock S, Dehoratius RD, Wapner RJ, Jackson LG. Subclinical autoimmune disease and unexplained abortion. *Am J Obstet Gynecol* 1984; 150: 367–71.

31 Rai RS, Regan L *et al.* Antiphospholipid antibodies and beta 2–glycoprotein-1 in 500 women with recurrent miscarriage: Results of a comprehensive screening approach. *Human Reprod* 1995: 2001–5.

32 Pattison NS, Chamley LW, Mckay EJ, Liggins GC, Butler WS. Antiphospholipid antibodies in pregnancy: prevalence and clinical associations. *Br J Obstet Gynaecol* 1993; 100: 909–13.

33 Rai RS, Clifford K, Cohen H, Regan L. High prospective fetal loss rate in untreated pregnancies of women with recurrent miscarriage and antiphospholipid antibodies. *Human Reprod* 1995: 3301–4.

34 Katano K, Aoki A, Sasa H, Ogasawara M, Matsuura E, Yagami Y. β$_2$-glycoprotein-1 dependent anticardiolipin antibodies as a predictor of adverse pregnancy outcomes in healthy pregnant women. *Human Reprod* 1996; 11: 509–12.

35 Kilpatrick DC. Anti-phospholipid antibodies and pregnancy wastage. *Lancet* 1986; ii: 185–6.

36 Prentice RL, Gatenby PA, Loblay RM, Shearman RP, Kronenberg M, Basten A. Lupus anticoagulant in pregnancy. *Lancet* 1984; ii: 464.

37 Scott JS. Systemic lupus erythematosus and allied disorders in pregnancy. *Clin Obstet Gynaecol* 1979; 6: 461–71.

38 Wilson WA, Gharavi AE *et al.* International consensus statement on preliminary classification criteria for definite antiphospholipid syndrome. *Arthritis Rheum* 1999; 42: 1309–11.

39 Kilpatrick DC, Liston WA. Obstetric significance of cardiolipin antibodies in subjects without systemic lupus erythematosus. *J Obstet Gynaecol* 1992; 12: 82–6.

40 Bendon RW, Hayden LE *et al.* Perinatal screening for anticardiolipin antibody. *Am J Perinatol* 1990; 7: 245–50.

41 McCormack MJ, Adu D, Weaver J, Michael J, Kelley J. Antiplatelet antibodies: a prognostic marker in pregnancies associated with lupus nephritis. Case reports. *Br J Obstet Gynaecol* 1991; 98: 324–5.

42 Out HJ, Kooijman CD, Bruinse HW, Derksen RH. Histopathological findings in placentae from patients with intra-uterine death and anti-phospholipid antibodies. *Eur J Obstet Gynecol Reprod Biol* 1991; 41: 179–86.

43 Carreras LO, Defreyn G *et al.* Arterial thrombosis, intrauterine death and 'lupus' anticoagulant: detection of immunoglobulin interfering with prostacyclin formation. *Lancet* 1981; i: 244–6.

44 de Castellarnau C, Vila L, Sancho MJ, Borrell M, Fontcuberta J, Rutllant NIL. Lupus anticoagulant, recurrent abortion, and prostacyclin production by cultured smooth muscle cells. *Lancet* 1988; ii: 1137–8.

45 Rand JH, Wu XX *et al.* Pregnancy loss in the antiphospholipid antibody syndrome: a possible thrombogenic mechanism. *N Engl J Med* 1997; 337: 154–60.

46 Cariou T, Tobelem G, Soria C, Caen J. Inhibition of Protein C activation by endothelial cells in the presence of lupus anticoagulant. *N Engl J Med* 1986; 314: 1193–4.

47 Comp PC, De Bault LE, Esmon NL, Esmon CT. Human thrombomodulin is inhibited by IgG from two patients with non-specific anticoagulants. *Blood* 1983; 1 (Suppl.): 1099.

48 Violi F, Ferro D *et al.* Tissue plasminogen activator inhibitor in patients with systemic lupus erythematosus and thrombosis. *Br Med J* 1990; 300: 1099–102.

49 Rote NS, Walter A, Lyden TW. Antiphospholipid antibodies: lobsters or red herrings? *Am J Reprod Immunol* 1992; 28: 31–7.

50 Chamley LW, Duncalf AM, Mitchell MD, Johnson PM. Action of anticardiolipin and antibodies to β₂-glycoprotein-1 on trophoblast proliferation as a mechanism for fetal death. *Lancet* 1998; 352: 1037–8.

51 Fishman P, Falach *et al.* Prevention of fetal loss in experimental antiphospholipid syndrome by in vivo administration of recombinant interleukin-3. *J Clin Invest* 1993; 91: 1834–7.

52 Vincent T, Rai R, Regan L, Cohen H. Increased thrombin generation in women with recurrent miscarriage. *Lancet* 1998; 352: 116.

53 Fraga A, Mintz G, Orozco J, Orozco JH. Sterility and fertility rates, fetal wastage and maternal morbidity in systemic lupus erythematosus. *J Rheumatol* 1974; 1: 1293–8.

54 Freinstein DI. Lupus anticoagulant, thrombosis and fetal loss. *N Engl J Med* 1985; 313: 1348–50.

55 Spitz B, Van Assche FA, Vermylen J. Lupus anticoagulant and pregnancy. *Am J Obstet Gynecol* 1986; 154: 1169.

56 Laskin CA, Bombardier C *et al.* Prednisone and aspirin in women with autoantibodies and unexplained recurrent fetal loss. *N Engl J Med* 1997; 337: 148–53.

57 Ramsden CH, Johnson PM, Hart CA, Farquharson RG. Listeriosis in immunocompromised pregnancy. *Lancet* 1989; i: 794.

58 Englert MG, Derue GM, Loizous S, Hawkins DF, Elder MG, de Swiet M. Pregnancy and lupus: Prognostic indications and response to treatment. *Q J Med* 1988; 66: 125–36.

59 Lockshin MD, Druzin NIL *et al.* Antibody to cardiolipin as a predictor of fetal distress or death in pregnant patients with systemic lupus erythematosus. *N Engl J Med* 1985; 313: 152–6.

60 Cowchock FS, Recce EA, Balaban D, Ware Banch D, Plouffe L. Repeated fetal losses associated with antiphospholipid antibodies: a collaborative randomized trial comparing prednisone with low-dose heparin treatment. *Am J Obstet Gynecol* 1992; 166: 1318–23.

61 Rosove MH, Tabsh K, Wasserstrum N, Howard P, Hahn BH, Kalunian KC. Heparin therapy for pregnant women with lupus anticoagulant or anticardiolipin antibodies. *Obstet Gynecol* 1990; 75: 630–4.

62 Ware Branch D, Silver RM, Blackwell JL, Reading JC, Scott JR. Outcome of treated pregnancies in women with antiphospholipid syndrome: an update of the Utah experience. *Obstet Gynaecol* 1992; 80: 614–20.

63 Lima F, Kamashta MA, Buchanan NMM, Kerslake S, Hunt BJ, Hughes GRV. A study of sixty pregnancies in patients with the antiphospholipid syndrome. *Clin Exp Rheumatol* 1996; 14: 131–6.

64 Chan JKM, Marris EN, Hughes GRV. Successful pregnancy following suppression of cardiolipin antibodies and lupus anticoagulant with azathioprine in systemic lupus erythematosus. *J Obstet Gynaecol* 1986; 7: 16–17.

65 Gregorini G, Setti G, Remuzzi G. Recurrent abortion with lupus anticoagulant and preeclampsia: a common final pathway for two different diseases? Case report. *Br J Obstet Gynaecol* 1986; 93: 194–6.

66 Kutteh WH. Antiphospholipid antibody-associated recurrent pregnancy loss; treatment with heparin and low-dose aspirin is superior to low-dose aspirin alone. *Am J Obstet Gynecol* 1996; 174: 1584–9.

67 Rai R, Cohen H, Dave M, Regan L. Randomised controlled trial of aspirin and aspirin plus heparin in pregnant women with recurrent miscarriage associated with phospholipid (or antiphospholipid antibodies). *Br Med J* 1997; 314: 253–7.

68 Backos M, Rai R, Baxter N, Chilcott IT, Cohen H, Regan L. Pregnancy complications in women with recurrent miscarriage associated with antiphospholipid antibodies treated with low dose aspirin and heparin. *Br J Obstet Gynaecol* 1999; 102: 102–7.

69 Farquharson RG, Compston A, Bloom AL. Lupus anticoagulant: a place for pre-pregnancy treatment? *Lancet* 1985; ii: 842–3.

70 Emson HE. For the want of an heir: the obstetrical history of Queen Anne. *Br Med J* 1992; 304: 1365–6.

71 Fessel WJ. Systemic lupus erythematosus in the community. Incidence, prevalence, outcome and first symptoms; the high prevalence in black women. *Arch Intern Med* 1974; 134: 1027–35.

72 Grimes DA, Le Bolt SA, Grimes RR, Wingo PA. Systemic lupus erythematosus and reproductive function: a case-control study. *Am J Obstet Gynecol* 1985; 153: 179–86.

73 Manu P. Serial probability analysis of the 1982 revised criteria for the classification of systemic lupus erythematosus. *N Engl J Med* 1983: 1460.

74 Horowitz GM, Hankins GDV. Cutaneous manifestations of collagen vascular disease in pregnancy. *Clin Obstet Gynecol* 1990; 33: 759–76.

75 Boelaert J, Ryckaert R, Tser Kezoglou A, Daneels R. Systemic lupus erythematosus and pregnancy. *Acta Clin Belg* 1980; 35: 183–92.

76 Devoe LD, Taylor RL. Systemic lupus erythematosus in pregnancy. *Am J Obstet Gynecol* 1979; 135: 473–9.

77 Syrop CH, Varner MW. Systemic lupus erythematosus. *Clin Obstet Gynecol* 1983; 26: 547–57.

78 Olah KS, Redman CWG. Overlap syndrome and its implications in pregnancy. Case report. *Br J Obstet Gynaecol* 1991; 98: 728–30.

79 Garsenstein M, Pollak VE, Karik RM. Systemic lupus erythematosus and pregnancy. *N Engl J Med* 1962; 267: 165–9.

80 Estes D, Larson DL. Systemic lupus erythematosus and pregnancy. *Clin Obstet Gynecol* 1965; 8: 307–21.

81 Zulman JI, Talal N, Hoffman CS, Epstein WV. Problems associated with the management of pregnancies in patients with systemic lupus erythematosus. *J Rheumatol* 1980; 7: 37–49.

82 Speira IF. Connective tissue disease in pregnancy. *Mount Sinai J Med* 1980; 47: 438–41.

83 Ainslie WH, Britt K, Moshipur JA. Maternal death due to lupus pneumonitis in pregnancy. *Mount Sinai J Med* 1979; 46: 494–9.

84 Leung ACT, Bolton Jones M. Why do patients with lupus nephritis die? *Br Med J* 1985; 290: 937.

85 Urowitz MB, Gladman DD, Farewell VT, Stewart J, McDonald J. Lupus and pregnancy studies *Arthritis Rheum* 1993; 36: 1392–7.

86 Black CM, Stevens WM. Scleroderma. *Rheum Dis Clin North Am* 1989; 15: 193–212.

87 Kincaid-Smith P, Fairley KF, Kloss M. Lupus anticoagulant associated with renal thrombotic microangiopathy and pregnancy related renal failure. *Q J Med* 1988; 69: 795–815.

88 Donaldson LM, Espiner EA. Disseminated lupus erythematosus presenting as chorea gravidarum. *Arch Neurol* 1971; 25: 240–4.

89 Houser MT, Fish AJ, Tagatz GE, Williams PP, Michael AF. Pregnancy and systemic lupus erythematosus. *Am J Obstet Gynecol* 1980; 138: 409–13.

90 Hayslett JP, Lynn RI. Effect of pregnancy in patients with lupus nephropathy. *Kidney Int* 1980; 18: 207.

91 Lee LA, Bias WB *et al.* Immunogenetics of the neonatal lupus syndrome. *Ann Intern Med* 1983; 99: 592–6.

92 Lockshin NW. Anticardiolipin antibodies in pregnant patients with systemic lupus erythematosus. *N Eng J Med* 1986; 314: 1392–3.

93 Hardy JB, Solomon S, Banwell GS, Beach R, Wright V, Howard FM. Congenital complete heart block in the newborn associated with maternal systemic lupus erythematosus and other connective tissue disease. *Arch Dis Child* 1979; 54: 7–13.

94 Nathan DJ, Snapper I. Simultaneous placental transfer of factors responsible for LE cell formation and thrombocytopenia. *Am J Med* 1958; 25: 647.

95 McCue CM, Matakas ME, Tinglesrad JB, Ruddy S. Congenital heart block in newborns of mothers with connective tissue disease. *Circulation* 1977; 56: 82–90.

96 Esscher E, Scott JS. Congenital heart block and maternal systemic lupus erythematosus. *Br Med J* 1979; i: 1235–8.

97 Altenburger KM, Jeciziniak M, Roper WL, Hernandez J. Congenital complete heart block with hydrops fetalis. *J Pediatr* 1977; 91: 618–20.

98 Doshi N, Smith B, Klionsky B. Congenital pericarditis due to maternal lupus erythematosus. *J Pediatr* 1980; 96: 699–701.

99 Fox R, Hawkins DF. Fetal-pericardial effusion in association with congenital heart block and maternal systemic lupus erythematosus. Case report. *Br J Obstet Gynaecol* 1990; 97: 638–40.

100 Richards DS, Wagman AJ, Cabaniss ML. Ascites not due to congestive heart failure in a fetus with lupus-induced heart block. *Obstet Gynecol* 1990; 76: 957–9.

101 Fox R, Lumb MR, Hawkins DF. Persistent fetal sinus bradycardia associated with maternal anti-Ro antibodies. Case report. *Br J Obstet Gynecol* 1990; 97: 1151–3.

102 Press J, Uziel Y, Laxer RM, Luy L, Hamilton RM, Silverman ED. Long-term outcome of mothers of children with complete congenital heart block. *Am J Med* 1996; 100 (3): 328–32.

103 Hughes GRV. Autoantibodies in lupus and its variants: experience in 1000 patients. *Br Med J* 1984; 289: 339–42.

104 Paredes RA, Morgan H, Lachelin GCL. Congenital heart block associated with maternal Sjögren's syndrome. Case report. *Br J Obstet Gynaecol* 1983; 90: 870–1.

105 Veffle JC, Sunderland C, Bennett RM. Complete heart block in a fetus associated with maternal Sjogren's syndrome. *Am J Obstet Gynecol* 1985; 151: 660–1.

106 Olah KS, Gee H. Fetal heart block associated with maternal anti-Ro (SS-A) antibody—current management. A review. *Br J Obstet Gynaecol* 1991; 98: 751–5.

107 Lockshin MD, Bonfa E, Elkon K, Druzin ML. Neonatal lupus risk to newborns of mothers with systemic lupus erythematosus. *Arthritis Rheum* 1988; 31: 697–701.

108 Maddison PJ, Skinner RP, Esseher E, Taylor PV, Scott O, Scott JS. Serological studies in congenital heart block. *Ann Rheum Dis* 1983; 42: 218–19.

109 Litsey SE, Noonan JA, O'Connor WM, Cottrill CM, Mitchell B. Maternal connective tissue disease and congenital heart block. Demonstration of immunoglobulin in cardiac tissue. *N Engl J Med* 1985; 312: 98–100.

110 Taylor PV, Scott JS, Gerlis LM, Esseher E, Scott O. Maternal autoantibodies against fetal cardiac antigens in congenital complete heart block. *N Engl J Med* 1986; 315: 667–72.

111 Singsen BM, Akhter JE, Weinstein MW, Sharp GC. Congenital complete heart block and SSA antibodies: obstetric implications. *Am J Obstet Gynecol* 1985; 152: 655–8.

112 Herreman G, Galelowski N. Maternal connective tissue disease and congenital heart block. *N Engl J Med* 1985; 312: 1329.

113 Venning MC, Burn DJ, Ward RM, Henry JA, Davison JM. Neonatal lupus syndrome: Optimism justified? *Lancet* 1988; i: 640.

114 Shenker L, Reed KL, Anderson CF, Marx GR, Sobonya LE, Graham AR. Congenital heart block and cardiac anomalies in the absence of maternal connective tissue disease. *Am J Obstet Gynecol* 1987; 157: 248–53.

115 McCuiston CH, Shock EP. Possible discoid lupus erythematosus in a newborn infant, report of a case with subsequent development of acute systemic lupus erythematosus in the mother. *Arch Dermatol Syphilol* 1954; 70: 782–5.

116 Editorial. Neonatal lupus syndrome. *Lancet* 1987; ii: 489–90.

117 Vonderheid EC, Koblenzer PJ, Ming P, Ming L, Burgoon CF. Neonatal lupus erythematosus, report of four cases with a review of the literature. *Arch Dermatol* 1976; 112: 698–705.

118 Provost TT, Watson R, Gammon WR, Radowsky M, Harley JB, Riechlin M. The neonatal lupus syndrome associated with U 1 RNP (nRNP) antibodies. *N Engl J Med* 1987; 316: 1135–8.

119 Loizou S, Byron MA, Englert HJ, David J, Hughes GR, Walport MJ. Association of quantitative anticardiolipin antibody levels with fetal loss and time of loss in systemic lupus erythematosus. *Q J Med* 1988; 68: 525–31.

120 Chesley LC. *Hypertensive Disorders in Pregnancy*. Appleton-Century-Crofts, New York, 1978.

121 Baesnihan B, Grigor RR *et al.* Immunological mechanism for spontaneous abortion in systemic lupus erythematosus. *Lancet* 1977; ii: 1205–7.

122 Abramowsky CR, Vegas ME, Swinehart G, Gyves MT. Decidual vasculopathy of the placenta in lupus erythematosus. *N Engl J Med* 1980; 303: 668–72.

123 Byron MA. Treatment of rheumatic diseases. *Br Med J* 1987; 294: 236–8.

124 Buckfield P. Major congenital faults in newborn infants: a pilot study in New Zealand. *NZ Med J* 1973; 78: 159–204.

125 Slone D, Sisilind V, Hemonen OP, Monson RR, Kaufman DW, Shapiro S. Aspirin and congenital malformations. *Lancet* 1976; i: 1373–5.

126 Turner G, Collins E. Fetal effects of regular salicylate ingestion in pregnancy. *Lancet* 1975; ii: 338–9.

127 Stuart MJ, Gross SJ, Ellad H, Grateber JE. Effects of acetylsalicylic-acid ingestion on maternal and neonatal hemostasis. *N Engl J Med* 1982; 307: 909–12.

128 Editorial. PG-synthetase inhibition in obstetrics and after. *Lancet* 1980; ii: 185–6.

129 Heymann MA. Non steroidal anti-inflammatory agents. In: Eskes TKAB, Finster M, eds. *Drug Therapy During Pregnancy*. Butterworths, London, 1985: 85–99.

130 Goudie BM, Dossetor JFB. Effect on the fetus of indomethacin given to suppress labour. *Lancet* 1979; ii: 1187–5.

131 Eeg-Olofsson O, Malmros I, Elwin C, Steen B. Convulsions in a breast-fed infant after maternal indomethacin. *Lancet* 1978; ii: 215.

132 Niebyl JR, Witter FR. Neonatal outcome after indomethacin treatment for preterm labour. *Am J Obstet Gynecol* 1986; 155: 747–9.

133 Rees RB, Maubach MM. Chloroquine: a review of reactions and dermatologic indications. *Arch Dermatol* 1963; 88: 96–105.

134 Wolfe MS, Cordero JF. Safety of chloroquine in chemosuppression of malaria during pregnancy. *Br Med J* 1985; 290: 1466–7.

135 Canadian Hydroxychloroquine Study Group. A randomized study of the effect of withdrawing hydroxychloroquine sulfate in systemic lupus erythematosus. *N Engl J Med* 1991; 324: 150–4.

136 Leinwald I, Durgee AW. Scleroderma. *Ann Intern Med* 1954; 41: 1033–41.

137 Gifford RH. Rheumatic diseases. In: Burrow GN, Ferris TF, eds. *Medical Complications During Pregnancy*. W.B. Saunders, Philadelphia, 1975.

138 Hart CW, Nauton RF. The ototoxicity of chloroquine phosphate. *Arch Otolaryngol* 1964; 80: 407.

138a Parke A, West B. Hydroxychloroquine in pregnant patients with systemic lupus erythematosus. *J Rheumatol* 1996; 23: 1715–8.

139 Khamashta MA, Buchanan NM, Hughes GR. The use of hydroxychloroquine in lupus pregnancy: the British experience. *LUPUS* 1996; (Suppl 1): S 65–6.

140 Block JA. Hydroxychloroquine and retinal safety. *Lancet* 1998; 351: 771.

141 Lewis R, Lauersen NH, Birn Baum S. Malana associated with pregnancy. *Obstet Gynecol* 1973; 42: 696–700.

142 Zurier RB, Argyros TG, Urman JB, Warren J, Rothfield NF. Systemic lupus erythematosus. Management during pregnancy. *Obstet Gynecol* 1978; 51: 178–80.

143 Wong KL, Chan FY, Lee CP. Outcome of pregnancy in patients with systemic lupus erythematosus: a prospective study. *Arch Intern Med* 1991; 151: 269–73.

144 Thomson BJ, Watson ML, Liston WA, Lambie AT. Plasmaphaeresis in a pregnancy complicated by acute systemic lupus erythematosus. Case report. *Br J Obstet Gynaecol* 1985; 92: 532–4.

145 Barclay CS, French MAH, Ross LD, Sokol RJ. Successful pregnancy following steroid therapy and plasma exchange in a woman with anti-Ro (SS-A) antibodies. Case report. *Br J Obstet Gynaecol* 1987; 94: 369–71.

146 Oakey RE. The interpretation of urinary oestrogen and pregnanediol excretion in women receiving corticosteroids. *J Obstet Gynaecol Br Commonwealth* 1970; 77: 922–7.

147 Stephensen O, Cleland WP, Hallidie-Smith K. Congenital heart block and persistent ductus arteriosus associated with maternal systemic lupus erythematosus. *Br Heart J* 1981; 46: 101.

148 Kleinman CS, Copel JA, Hobbuns JL. Combined echocardiographic and Doppler assessment of fetal congenital atrioventricular block. *Br J Obstet Gynaecol* 1987; 94: 967–74.

149 Nicolaides KH, Soothill PW, Rodeck CH, Campbell S. Ultrasound-guided sampling of umbilical cord and placental blood to assess fetal wellbeing. *Lancet* 1986; i: 1065–7.

150 Soothill PW, Nicolaides KH, Rodeck CH, Campbell S. The effect of gestational age on blood gas and acid-base values in human pregnancy. *Fetal Ther* 1986; 7: 166–73.

151 Bunyon JP, Swersey SH, Fox HE, Bierman F, Winchester RJ. Intrauterine therapy for presumptive fetal myocarditis with acquired heart block due to systemic lupus crythematism. *Arthritis Rheum* 1987; 30: 44–9.

152 Bunyon JP, Roubey R *et al*. Complete congenital heart block: Risk of occurrence and therapeutic approach to prevention. *J Rheumatol* 1988; 15: 1104–8.

153 Hench AB. The ameliorating effect of pregnancy on chronic atrophic (infectious rheumatoid) arthritis; fibrositis and intermittent hydrothosis. *Proc Mayo Clinic* 1938; 13: 161.

154 Kaplan D, Diamond H. Rheumatoid arthritis and pregnancy. *Clin Obstet Gynecol* 1965; 8: 286–303.

155 Thurnau GR. Rheumatoid arthritis. *Clin Obstet Gynecol* 1983; 26: 558–78.

156 Pope JE, Bellamy N, Stevens A. The lack of associations between rheumatoid arthritis and both nulliparity and infertility. *Semin Arthritis Rheum* 1999; 28 (5): 342–50.

157 Unger A, Kay A, Griffin AJ, Panayi GS. Disease activity and pregnancy associated a2–glycoprotein in rheumatoid arthritis during pregnancy. *Br Med J* 1983; 286: 750–2.

158 Barrett JH, Brennan P, Fiddler M, Silman AJ. Does rheumatoid arthritis remit during pregnancy and relapse postpartum? Results from a nationwide study in the United Kingdom performed prospectively from late pregnancy. *Arthritis Rheum* 1999; 42 (6): 1219–27.

159 Fairhead FW. Convulsions in a breast-fed infant after maternal indomethacin. *Lancet* 1978; ii: 576.

160 Rocker I, Henderson WJ. Transfer of gold from mother to fetus. *Lancet* 1976; ii: 1246.

161 Solomon L, Abrams G, Dinner M, Berman L. Neonatal abnormalities associated with D-penicillamine, treatment during pregnancy. *N Engl J Med* 1977; 296: 54–5.

162 Mjolnerod JK, Rasmussen K, Dommerud SA, Gieruldsen ST. Congenital connective tissue defect probably due to D-penicillamine treatment in pregnancy. *Lancet* 1971; i: 673–5.

163 Linares A, Zarranz JJ, Rodriguez-Alarcon J, Diaz-Perez JL. Reversible cutis laxa due to maternal D-penicillamine treatment. *Lancet* 1979; ii: 43.

164 Lyle WH. Penicillamine in pregnancy. *Lancet* 1978; i: 606–7.

165 Scheinberg IH, Sternlieb I. Pregnancy in penicillamine-treated patients with Wilson's disease. *N Engl J Med* 1975; 293: 1300–2.

166 Dennison EM, Cooper C. Corticosteroids in rheumatoid arthritis. *Br Med J* 1998; 316: 789–90.

167 Haynes DM. Collagen diseases in pregnancy. In: Haynes BM, ed. *Medical Complications During Pregnancy*. McGraw Hill, New York, 1969.

168 Johnson TR, Banner EA, Winkelmann RK. Scleroderma and pregnancy. *Obstet Gynecol* 1964; 23: 467–9.

169 Slate WC, Graham AR. Scleroderma and pregnancy. *Am J Obstet Gynecol* 1968; 101: 335–41.

170 Karlen JG, Cook WA. Renal scleroderma and pregnancy. *Obstet Gynecol* 1974; 44: 349–54.

171 Murati H, Nakauchi H, Sumida T. Michrochimerism in Japanese women patients with systemic sclerosis. *Lancet* 1999; 354: 220.

172 Avrech OM. Raynaud's phenomenon and peripheral gangrene complicating scleroderma in pregnancy. *Br J Obstet Gynaecol* 1992; 99: 850–1.

173 Steen VD. Pregnancy in women with systemic sclerosis. *Obstet Gynecol* 1999; 94 (1): 15–20.

174 Bellucci MJ, Coustan DR, Plotz RD. Cervical scleroderma: a case of soft tissue dysbocia. *Am J Obstet Gynecol* 1984; 150: 891–2.

175 Thompson J, Conklin KA. Anesthetic management of a pregnant patient with scleroderma. *Anesthesiology* 1983; 59: 69–71.

176 McKenna F, Martin MFR, Bird HA, Wright V. Captopril. *Br Med J* 1983; 287: 1299.

177 Owen J, Hauth JC. Polyarteritis nodosa in pregnancy: a case report and brief literature review. *Am J Obstet Gynecol* 1989; 160: 606–7.

178 Debeukelaer MM, Travis LB, Roberts DK. Polyarteritis and pregnancy: report of a successful outcome. *South Med J* 1973; 66: 613–15.

179 Howard RJ, Tuck SM. Caesarean section in a pregnancy complicated by relapsing polychondritis. *J Obstet Gynaecol* 1992; 12: 120.

180 Arundell FD, Haserick JR. Familial chronic atrophic polychondritis. *Arch Dermatol* 1960; 82: 439.

181 Brandt JT, Triplett DA, Alving B, Scharrer I. Criteria for the diagnosis of lupus anticoagulants: an update. *Thrombosis Haemost* 1995; 74: 1185–90.

182 Tan EM, Cohan AS *et al.* The 1982 revised criteria for the classification of systemic lupus erythematosus. *Arthritis Rheum* 1982; 25: 1271–7.

9 Disorders of the liver, biliary system and pancreas

Elizabeth A. Fagan

Diseases of the liver remain rare in pregnancy (reviewed in [1]). Only 50 cases from 56 000 pregnancies were recorded in one non-specialized centre [2]. The majority are conditions unique to pregnancy. Most often these do not affect adversely maternal and fetal outcome. Early diagnosis of the exceptions is important because multidisciplinary management in a referral centre can improve outcome. In the triennial review of maternal mortalities for the UK between 1985 and 1987 the seven direct deaths from liver disease were as many as for each category associated with abortion, anaesthesia, genital sepsis and ruptured uterus [3]. In the latest review covering 1994–96, two of the 134 direct maternal deaths had primary hepatic dysfunction (one acute fatty liver of pregnancy, one alcoholic liver disease) and three of the deaths from hypertension were due to liver disease (two liver rupture, one liver failure) [4].

Liver disease can be difficult to diagnose. Jaundice is not invariable. Conversely, palmar erythema and spider naevae are commonly found in healthy pregnancy as well as in chronic liver disease and acute liver failure.

Anatomy and histopathology

In the third trimester, the liver occupies a more posterior–superior position with displacement to the right and sub-sequent reduction in dullness to percussion. A palpable liver is abnormal in pregnancy and usually indicates infiltration from fat as in acute fatty liver of pregnancy or alcoholic liver disease and malignancy or congestion as in congestive heart failure or Budd–Chiari syndrome. Liver size alone is not helpful in diagnosis and assessing severity of the liver disease except that a very small liver usually indicates massive necrosis or cirrhosis. Histopathological studies show no specific changes apart from mild steatosis. Percutaneous liver biopsy is safe in expert hands within the limitations of normal coagulation and ultrasonographic imaging.

Physiology and biochemistry

Table 9.1 summarizes the physiological changes observed in standard liver tests during pregnancy.

Abnormalities in liver tests suggest liver disease or a hepatic complication. In the non-pregnant individual, hepatic blood flow represents 25–35% of the cardiac output [5]. In pregnancy, absolute hepatic flow is not increased significantly. A smaller proportion of the increase in cardiac output (approximately 25%) passes through the liver. The total blood volume in pregnancy increases by up to 50% and is redistributed into the

Table 9.1 Liver tests in pregnancy [8].

Liver enzyme	Non-pregnant	1st trimester	2nd trimester	3rd trimester
AST (U/L)	7–40	10–27	10–28	11–29
ALT (U/L)	0–40	6–30	6–29	6–28
Bilirubin (μmol/L)	0–17	4–15	3–12	3–14
GGT (U/L)	11–50	5–37	5–43	3–41
ALP (U/L)	30–130	32–100	43–134	133–418

splanchnic circulation and great veins. Portal vein pressure is increased in late pregnancy. The additional pressure of the gravid uterus on the vena cava results in diversion of a portion of the venous return through the azygos system [6]. Venous pressure increases in the oesophagus leading to transient engorgement of oesophageal veins (varices) in up to 60% of healthy pregnant women [6] (see cirrhosis, below).

The liver in pregnancy shows no undue susceptibility to drugs and toxins. Clearance of drugs with high hepatic extraction ratios is unlikely to be altered significantly [5]. However, hepatic clearance may be reduced for drugs that rely on blood flow due to the larger volume of distribution [7].

Liver tests

The changes during pregnancy are summarized in Table 9.1. The most important changes are the falls in aspartate alanine transferase (ALT, serum glutamic pyruvic transaminase (SGPT)) and aspartate aminotransferase (AST, serum glutamic oxaloacetic transaminase (SGOT)) by about 25%, the maximum effect occurring in the third trimester [8,9]. The alkaline phosphatase is elevated because of the contribution from the placenta. Serum levels of alkaline phosphatase, AST and lactic acid dehydrogenase (LDH) also rise during labour and delivery. The alkaline phosphatase may remain elevated for up to 6 weeks postpartum but levels rarely exceed two times upper normal limits [10]. Levels of serum albumin fall through haemodilution by up to 25%. Serum α_1, α_2 and β globulins show a progressive rise by up to 50% but levels of gammaglobulin remain essentially unchanged [7].

Reliance on non-pregnant normal values for assessment of liver serum biochemistry to monitor liver disease activity and severity can be misleading [9]. Accordingly, over 50% of women with pre-eclampsia will have elevated liver enzymes by the adapted ranges compared with less than 20% by limits that are not adjusted for pregnancy [8]. Further, the increase in plasma volume from the first trimester leads to haemodilution with associated reductions in serum levels of albumin and other proteins. Also, increasing awareness of the widening spectrum of presentations for liver diseases during pregnancy reduces the specificity of tests once considered especially helpful in diagnosis. An elevated uric acid level commonly reported in acute fatty liver of pregnancy (AFLP) reflects typically the associated renal dysfunction with concurrent hypertension as well as massive hepatic cellular necrosis. A neutrophil leucocytosis is as likely to indicate sepsis as hepatocellular injury. The discordant finding of relatively low liver enzymes (AST and ALT <10× upper limit of normal) but persistently elevated prothrombin time typically indicates massive hepatocellular damage with few surviving hepatocytes.

Hypercholesterolaemia in pregnancy is well documented [10]. Plasma cholesterol rises by approximately 50% by the third trimester and triglycerides may rise two to three times upper normal limits. Serum levels of the bile acids chenodeoxycholic and cholic acids rise but remain within normal limits in most women.

Hyperbilirubinaemia and the fetus

Placental transfer of unconjugated bilirubin into the maternal system provides the major pathway for conjugation and subsequent elimination of fetal bilirubin and its degradation products. Only minor amounts are handled directly by the fetus or excreted into amniotic fluid [11]. Fetal exposure to high maternal levels of unconjugated and conjugated bilirubins may result in high circulating fetal levels because the unconjugated form can cross the placenta in both directions [11,12]. No simple relation links maternal with fetal levels of the bilirubins [12,13]. Prolonged exposure to elevated levels of unconjugated bilirubin and toxic metabolites, such as in maternal liver failure, does not result in neurological or developmental abnormalities [12,13]. Disruption of the fetal blood–brain barrier is as important as the level of unconjugated bilirubin for the development of kernicterus [14].

Certain maternal disorders are peculiar to pregnancy, others occurring coincidentally will be considered separately.

Liver disorders peculiar to pregnancy

Conditions as diverse as intrahepatic cholestasis of pregnancy (IHCP), hyperemesis gravidarum, AFLP, pre-eclampsia and HELLP (haemolysis, elevated liver enzymes, low platelets) syndrome are considered together because they arise only in association with pregnancy, resolve after delivery and have the propensity to recur in subsequent pregnancies.

Intrahepatic cholestasis of pregnancy

IHCP, also known as obstetric cholestasis (OC), is the most common condition peculiar to pregnancy and second only to viral hepatitis as a cause of jaundice in pregnancy [15] reviewed in [16,17]. However, most cases of IHCP diagnosed in recent years have not been associated with overt jaundice. Importantly, although IHCP affects adversely maternal well-being and fetal outcome, early diagnosis and careful interdisciplinary monitoring and prompt delivery at fetal maturity can improve outcomes in the mother and child.

EPIDEMIOLOGY

Geographic variation is wide. IHCP has been reported in up to 2% of deliveries [18–20] in Scandinavian [20,21] and Mediterranean countries [22], Poland [23], Chile [24,25], Canada [18], Australia [26] and China [19]. IHCP is also common in UK residents who originate from the Indian subcontinent.

CLINICAL FEATURES

The original description of generalized pruritus, mild jaundice and intrahepatic cholestasis occurring predominantly in the third trimester was attributed to Thorling [27] but was described by Ahlfeld in 1883 [28]. They noticed similar features in seven women and documented also fatigue, mild abdominal pain and subsidence after delivery, with recurrence in some in subsequent pregnancies. Today, the classical and predominant feature is generalized pruritus. Itching develops characteristically after the 30th week and becomes progressively severe but typically is relieved within 48 h following delivery [18–20]. More cases are being diagnosed with increasing awareness of the condition, and realization that overt jaundice is uncommon in all but the most severely affected mothers. Nocturnal itching of trunk, palms and soles can be intolerable with insomnia and fatigue. Anorexia, malaise, epigastric discomfort, steatorrhoea and dark urine are common. Rarely, pruritus can commence as early as the sixth week [18–20]. The frequency with which pruritus develops increases rapidly after the third month through to term [20]. For reasons that remain unclear, the onset of pruritus is distinctly uncommon in the seventh month

[20,27]. Occasionally, clearance of jaundice and resolution of abnormal liver tests have been delayed for up to 2 months postpartum [19,29].

Mild right upper quadrant pain is present in a minority. Any marked pain, hepatomegaly, splenomegaly or other findings should prompt exclusion of other causes of pruritus and jaundice, especially the cholestatic phase of viral hepatitis and gallstones. The increased risk of gallstones in IHCP probably relates to the combined presence of lithogenic factors such as the increased gallbladder volume, reduced ejection fraction of bile, and rise in serum bile acids [30].

Intrahepatic cholestasis has recurred with menstruation [31], oral contraceptive therapy and at the menopause [31–37]. Severe cases may be associated with multiple pregnancies [21].

LABORATORY FEATURES

The predominantly conjugated hyperbilirubinaemia (total serum bilirubin $<100\,\mu$mol/L; $n <17$) is mild and serum levels of AST, ALT and alkaline phosphatase [18–20] rarely exceed two times upper limits of normal for pregnancy [29]. The elevation in prothrombin time relates usually to vitamin K deficiency and is rapidly corrected by replacement therapy. Measurement of bile acids is available in many laboratories and is the most specific laboratory test.

Numerous other biochemical abnormalities have been reported in maternal serum including elevated levels of copper and markers of placental function [38] such as serum lipoprotein X (S-Lp X) [39] and plasma prolactin concentrations [40] but results are conflicting [18]. Serum levels of β_1-glycoprotein were reduced in some patients with IHCP [41] but the significance of these isolated findings requires further study.

PATHOGENESIS

The consensus holds that IHCP probably arises from a genetic predisposition for increased sensitivity and altered membrane composition of bile ducts and hepatocytes to normally produced oestrogens and progestagens and/or additionally as a response to the production of their abnormal metabolites. Abnormalities also occur in metabolism of bile acids and their transport at the canalicular level as well as across the placenta.

As a result, elevations in maternal levels of bile acids and their molar ratios seen in healthy pregnancy rise further in IHCP. Also, impairment of the normal fetal-to-maternal transfer of bile acids across the trophoblast results in accumulation of excess bile acids with abnormal profiles that are toxic to the fetus.

Genetic factors also play an important role, at least in high-prevalence regions [17]. A positive family history is found in up to half of the patients [18–20] in association with the histocompatibility antigen haplotypes human leucocyte antigen (HLA)-B8 and HLA-BW16. A genetic predisposition can explain the familial aggregation of cases over successive generations in high-prevalence regions such as Scandinavia and Chile and within certain ethnic groups such as the Araucanian-Indian population in Chile [25]. This genetic predisposition favours transmission as an autosomal dominant trait, and fathers also transmit the susceptibility to daughters [42]. In contrast, predisposing risk factors may be less apparent among affected women from low-prevalence regions. Out of 50 consecutive patients with IHCP in France, only one mother gave a family history of pruritus during pregnancy [43]. Also, pruritus was not noticed among any women who had taken oral contraceptives prior to the conception that evolved into IHCP [43]. Multiple pregnancies increase the severity of the disease [44] and may account for a significant proportion of cases of IHCP reported from low-prevalence regions.

Other familial disorders such as progressive familial intrahepatic cholestasis (PFIC: see below) and benign recurrent intrahepatic cholestasis (BRIC) may be linked to IHCP via alterations in the binding domains of liver cell receptors for DNA and oestrogens [45]. A higher than anticipated incidence of IHCP has been found in mothers of patients with PFIC and BRIC.

Oestrogens and progestagens have marked, and different, effects on the metabolism of bile salts, cholesterol and biliary lipids. Ethinyl oestradiol causes an increase in cholesterol content within the liver but decreases the secretion of bile salts. Also, high levels of circulating oestrogen in susceptible individuals may favour intrahepatic cholestasis [46] by impairing sulphation and transport of monohydroxy bile acids [45,47,48]. Normally, sulphation of oestrogens and bile acids such as lithocholic acid enhances their excretion in urine and bile. Impaired sulphation favours formation of glucuronide conjugates with cholestatic potential [47]. Also, impaired functioning of multidrug resistance protein 2 (Mrp 2), the canalicular isoform of the multidrug resistance protein that serves as an organic polyanion transporter, has been demonstrated in animal models of cholestasis including in rats treated with oestrogens [49].

The role for progesterone in the pathogenesis of IHCP is less clear although evidence is accumulating for this as an additional factor in some women with a predisposition to IHCP [43,50,51]. Progesterone increases the rate of esterification, but not synthesis, of cholesterol and causes an increase in bile salt-independent bile secretion. The net effect is to increase saturation of the bile with cholesterol. The most striking change in progesterone metabolism in IHCP is the increased concentration in maternal serum and urine and cord blood of sulphated metabolites, particularly those with a 3α-sulphoxy-5α (H) configuration [50,51]. Consequently, the ratio is increased of 3α- to 3β-hydroxylated steroids, and this effect is independent of the enterohepatic circulation [17,52]. In contrast, little change has been noted for the glucuronidated metabolites. One group [50,51] has suggested that progesterone and/or selected metabolites lead to a reduction in excretion of oestrogens by saturating the hepatic transport system especially of sulphated metabolites. Oral micronized progesterone seemed to exacerbate the disease in predisposed individuals in the study from France [43]. However, abnormalities of liver enzymes and serum total bile acids remained despite withdrawal of the tocolytic therapy, suggesting that the progesterone was acting as an additional factor rather than essential component in the pathogenesis of IHCP [43]. Whether the abnormal profile of sulphated progesterone metabolites in cholestasis is cause or effect, remains unclear. The limited evidence available favours a primary effect. This abnormal profile of sulphated steroids was detected in individual patients prior to the onset of IHCP [53] and was not found in cholestasis associated with viral hepatitis [54]. Reversal of the cholestasis and abolition of pruritus have been described after high-dose S-adenosyl-L-methionine pointing to an underlying metabolic defect and susceptibility [7,55]. External factors also contribute to IHCP. Seasonal variation, with more cases reported in the winter in some Scandinavian countries [20,25], as well as the general decline in the number of new cases, point to an additional environmental factor. Some authorities favour an inverse relation between selenium levels in plasma and expression of IHCP, at least in high-prevalence regions [25].

LIMITATIONS OF EXPERIMENTAL MODELS

Caution should be exercised when extrapolating to IHCP many of the results based on experimental models of cholestasis such as bile-duct ligation and endotoxin-related injury. Unlike in these models, in oestrogen-treated animals a post-translational mechanism has been implicated since levels of Mrp2 messenger RNA (mRNA) remained unaffected [54,56]. Further, levels of another transporter, C-CAM105 that is involved most likely in bile salt-dependent bile flow, also remained unchanged in oestrogen-treated rats. Feeding of deoxycholic acid to rats has been shown to exert a direct effect on post-translational regulation of steady-state mRNA levels in rodent hepatocytes [57]. However, normal levels of Mrp2 mRNA, despite decreased levels of the protein, support a defect in translation or defect in intracellular trafficking. Abnormalities in the movement of intracellular organelles have been described previously in IHCP and attributed to oestrogen [46].

Caution also should be noted on extrapolating data from other cholestatic disorders to IHCP. For example, oestradiol [58] and medroxyprogesterone [59] have been shown to reduce serum levels of liver enzymes in autoimmune chronic hepatitis and primary biliary cirrhosis (PBC). Whether this benefit reflected action on cholestatic mechanisms or an immunomodulating effect of medroxyprogesterone remains unproved.

BILE ACIDS AND TRANSPORTERS

In IHCP there is an increase in maternal serum levels of total bile acids compared with healthy pregnancy. Bile acids are the most abundant and important osmotic organic anions secreted into bile. In normal pregnancy by the end of the third trimester, the serum and plasma pool of cholic acid is raised whereas that for chenodeoxycholic acid is decreased [53]. Serum levels of cholic acid, chenodeoxycholic acid and total 3-α-hydroxy bile acids are elevated from 10- to 100-fold in patients with IHCP compared to healthy matched pregnant controls [18,20,21,38,60]. These elevations are a sensitive indicator of cholestasis. In general, serum levels of bile acids correlate with severity of maternal pruritus and increased risk of fetal distress [20,21]. Serum levels of total bile acids rise from early pregnancy and remain elevated throughout despite any clinical resolution that may occur prior to delivery [18,21,61–64]. Levels of cholic acid are raised further and especially relative to those of chenodeoxycholic acid, yielding an increase in the usual molar ratio of cholic/chenoxycholic acid. Glycine and taurine conjugates of chenodeoxycholic acid are the major bile acids found in the serum [64] and urine of patients with various causes of cholestasis [65,66]. IHCP, when compared to normal pregnancy, also is characterized by an elevation in the molar ratios of primary to secondary bile acids and of trihydroxylated to dihydroxylated bile acids. By contrast, a decrease occurs in the ratio for conjugated bile acids of glycine to taurine [63,64]. One explanation for the abnormally high ratio of cholic, to chenodeoxycholic, acid found in IHCP is the preference for excretion of the less polar bile acids as sulphates. The reduced enterohepatic circulation of cholic acid could explain the relatively low level of deoxycholic acid.

Although the exact causes of sudden fetal death remain unknown, any extrapolation to IHCP would implicate bile acids as toxic to the fetus. In rodent models of maternal cholestasis, excess concentration of bile acids, especially the secondary bile acids, was shown to endanger the fetus and compromise development of gestation [67].

Several transporters have been characterized that are located specifically to the canalicular membrane [17]. These transport substances such as organic anions (Mrp 2), phospholipid (multidrug resistance 3: Mdr 3) and bile acids (bile salt export pump: BSEP) actively into bile. Defects in these transporters account for several syndromes of familial intrahepatic cholestasis (see below). In IHCP, gene expression is altered at the level of canalicular, rather than sinusoidal, transporters, at least in experimental models of cholestasis [68]. The Na^+/taurocholic acid cotransporting polypeptide (ntcp) is responsible for 90% of the uptake of bile acids from sinusoidal (basolateral) blood via the basolateral membrane of hepatocytes. Another sinusoidal transporter, the organic anion transport polypeptide (Oatp1) is involved in the uptake of unconjugated bile acids as well as several organic anions including bromosulphthalein. Ntcp is down-regulated during normal pregnancy but up-regulated in the postpartum period. Secretion of prolactin facilitates binding of Stat5 to the *ntcp* promoter and transcriptional regulation of *ntcp* (reviewed in [69]).

Both sinusoidal transporters are down-regulated in various models of hepatocellular, as well as obstructive, cholestasis. However, no evidence was found for impaired excretion of bile acids in neonatal rats born of mothers with cholestasis caused by bile duct ligation [68]. Further, although *ntcp* is ontogenically regulated, no change in the pattern of expression of mRNA levels was detected during fetal and early life. This lack of effect of maternal cholestasis on expression of basolateral bile acid transporters in the rat fetus and neonate occurred despite higher levels of serum bile acids in, and lower body weights of, neonatal rats born of cholestatic mothers. The higher serum bile acid levels reflected transfer from mother to fetus by the placenta (see role of fetus and placenta, below).

Whether these observations are relevant to IHCP and studies in humans, remains to be determined. Fasting levels of total bile acids may be raised only modestly despite high levels of serum ALT [43]. There seems to be no correlation between serum levels of total bile acids and other liver tests such as AST and ALT, alkaline phosphatase, 5' nucleotidase and total bilirubin [43,70]. Further, some early studies report normal levels of bile acids in maternal serum in 42% of women with presumed IHCP; 20% of these had pruritus [62]. Whether IHCP includes pruritus despite normal bile salt levels, remains debatable.

One group from Portugal [63] was able to detect total bile acid levels in colostrum albeit at very low levels ($<1\,\mu$mol/L) compared with serum (mean $7.2\,\mu$mol/L) from nine healthy women. Values in colostrum varied significantly in women affected by IHCP but were elevated from two- up to 160-fold compared with women who had completed a healthy pregnancy [63].

Entrance of bile acids from fetal serum into trophoblast is impaired significantly in IHCP [70]. Importantly, impairment of efflux of glycocholate was corrected by treatment with ursodeoxychoic acid (UDCA). The fetus seems to lack the ability to excrete cholic acid because this remains elevated in meconium despite treatment with UDCA [71].

AETIOLOGY OF PRURITUS

The exact cause of such severe itching in IHCP is unknown. Pruritus is linked to cholestasis and abnormal bile salts regardless of most aetiologies. Although most women with high levels of total serum bile acids report itching, debilitating pruritus can occur despite low and declining levels, especially towards delivery.

A central hypothesis is that the pruritus associated with cholestasis reflects an increased availability of brain opiate receptors for binding their agonist ligands [72]. The possibility that the liver may act as a neuroendocrine organ was supported by the finding of raised concentrations in liver of three proenkephalin-derived opioid peptides following bile-duct resection in a rodent model of cholestasis [73].

MANAGEMENT PRINCIPLES

The treatment of IHCP is empirical as the exact aetiology remains unclear. The management of IHCP is dictated by the increased risks of fetal distress, spontaneous preterm delivery and sudden intrauterine death as well as by alleviating pruritus in the mother [16,43,74]. These risks to the fetus rise progressively through to delivery and remain regardless of serum levels of bile acids and liver enzymes (ALT). Close monitoring of these markers is essential but does not prevent sudden fetal distress and death. Provision should be made to deliver the fetus as soon as there is confidence about fetal lung maturity.

Fetal issues

All women with IHCP should be delivered no later than 37–38 weeks' gestation. Respiratory distress syndrome is extremely uncommon in fetuses born at this gestation. The only loss would be a greater incidence of failed induction and instrumental delivery. This outcome must be balanced against the risk of intrauterine death in the knowledge that at present there is no good way of detecting the fetus at risk. Delivery around 36 weeks or earlier should be considered for severe IHCP with jaundice, progressive elevations in serum bile acids and suspected fetal distress. Neonatal vitamin K_1 therapy should be given immediately postpartum to reduce the risk of intracranial bleeding particularly if the mother has taken cholestyramine or other resin sequestrants. However, extensive intracerebral hemorrhage in the fetus has been found at autopsy in one case in which the mother received no medication [75].

Close monitoring of fetal well-being is usual in all cases of IHCP, although it is not clear which parameters predict intrauterine death. Unfortunately, current prenatal testing does not prevent sudden intrauterine death. [43,74–76]. Abnormal patterns of intrapartum fetal heart rate have been reported in 22% of cases [77] but these are an unreliable indicator of fetal distress in IHCP [74,76]. Some authorities recommend regular amniocentesis to detect staining with meconium [77]. Passage of meconium in IHCP is common and has been recorded in 44% of cases [74].

Some authorities recommend regular non-stress, and contraction stress, tests but these also do not forewarn of intrauterine death [74–76]. Satisfactory detection of fetal movements and heart sounds have been reported only days before presentation with an intrauterine death [74–76]. Also, intrauterine death can present within days of the onset of pruritus [43,76].

There is no universally accepted monitoring programme for IHCP. At Queen Charlotte's Maternity Hospital, London, the usual practice is to monitor the fetus twice weekly from 30 weeks or from the diagnosis of IHCP if later. Monitoring consists of non-stressed cardiotocography. Weekly growth scans and estimations of liquor volume and Doppler umbilical blood flow also are performed. Maternal liver tests and blood clotting are tested at least weekly.

Limited studies have addressed haemostasis in IHCP. Elevated levels of plasma soluble fibrin [78] were found in women with cholestasis, including IHCP, but the anecdotal numbers precluded any correlation between elevated levels and outcome of pregnancy [18,19,79,80].

Maternal issues

The mother with IHCP should be reassured of her good outcome. Itching and jaundice will usually resolve immediately following delivery but almost certainly will recur in subsequent pregnancies. The diagnosis of IHCP in obstetric practice is based primarily on clinical features. Liver biopsy is unnecessary except in the untypical case when jaundice occurs without pruritus, symptoms commence before the 20th week, serum levels of bilirubin remains high 8 weeks or more after delivery [15,29] and to exclude other causes of intrahepatic cholestasis such as drug hepatotoxicity and the Dubin–Johnson syndrome (see below). Histological confirmation of IHCP reveals an acinar cholestasis with bile plugs in the canaliculi whereas hepatocellular necrosis and an inflammatory cell infiltrate, typical of hepatitis, are absent [15]. Percutaneous liver biopsy always should be carried out under ultrasonographic guidance, as clinical anatomical relationships may have altered, especially in the third trimester. Also, there is a risk of puncturing the exceptionally large gallbladder in IHCP [30].

All women with suspected IHCP should be screened for serological markers of viral hepatitis (see below) because presentation in the cholestatic phase is common. Autoimmune diseases should be sought by screening for autoantibodies, especially for antimitochondrial antibodies (see PBC, below). Hepatic ultrasonography should be carried out and repeated to exclude extrahepatic cholestasis including gallstones and cholangiocarcinoma.

Alleviation of pruritus

UDCA is the only therapy that has proven efficacy, albeit in small studies, in alleviating pruritus in IHCP. Clinical experience indicates that the majority of women will obtain total or partial relief of their symptoms between 1 day and 1 week after starting UDCA treatment. UDCA has no proven beneficial or adverse effects on the fetus but experience is insufficient to draw conclusions regarding teratogenicity and prevention of adverse outcomes. Reluctance to perform placebo-controlled trials follows the premature termination of the pivotal double-blind, controlled clinical trial in Chile after a baby was stillborn to a mother with IHCP; subsequently she was shown to have taken placebo [48]. Termination of this trial seems to have been premature because intrauterine death has also occurred in women taking UDCA.

UDCA, a minor naturally occurring hydrophilic bile salt, acts in IHCP to change towards normal the elevated and abnormal profiles of sulphated steroids in serum, urine, amniotic fluid and colostrum (but not in meconium) [50,63,71,81]. UDCA reduces concentrations in serum of sulphated metabolites of progesterone as well as bile acids [43,50]. UDCA stimulates biliary transport systems in-

volved in clearing steroid monosulphates and disulphates [48] and leads to reduced concentrations of bile acids within hepatocytes that are available for sulphation and hydroxylation, such as cholic acid. In particular, in IHCP, UDCA reduced significantly in serum and urine, levels and proportions of aminoacyl amidated cholic acid in positions 1β, 2β, 5β and 6β. UDCA caused a marked reduction in levels of monosulphated and disulphated $5\alpha/\beta$-pregnane-3α, 20α-diols and 5α-pregnane-3α, 20α and 21-triols, whereas changes were small or insignificant for levels of 5α-pregnane-3β and 20α-diol [50]. In the urine in pregnancy regardless of IHCP, the double conjugates of the major steroid 5α-pregnane-3α, 20α-diol were reduced by around 50% following introduction of UDCA [50,82].

Parallel changes in concentrations of bile acids between serum and urine and steroid sulphates are not invariable in IHCP. Furthermore, urinary excretion of these substances does not reflect faithfully their respective levels in serum [50]. In particular patients the level of cholestasis is reflected best in specific components such as elevated levels of sulphated steroids and increased ratio of 3α- to 3α-hydroxysteroids rather than total serum bile acids. The detectable levels of lithocholic acid in treated patients reflect the conversion of UDCA into lithocholic acid by bacteria in the intestine.

Guar gum was shown to improve pruritus in a double-blind study from Finland [83] by mechanisms which remain unclear. Treatment of pruritus with cholestyramine up to 20 g daily and phenobarbitone has been disappointing [18]. In general cholestyramine is safe in pregnancy [84]. This non-absorbable anion-exchange resin binds bile acids, anionic drugs and fat-soluble vitamins. Binding of vitamin K may result in elevations in prothrombin ratio. Postpartum haemorrhage has been reported in 8–22% of cases following delivery [18,19] and may be exacerbated by vitamin K deficiency. Vitamin K_1 (10 mg daily) should be administered regularly to women with IHCP throughout pregnancy, especially those receiving cholestyramine. Results from controlled trials of intravenous S-adenosyl-L-methionine (800 mg daily) have shown variable relief of pruritus with lessening of jaundice. A randomized placebo-controlled trial from Italy of 32 women with IHCP showed superiority of the combination of UDCA with S-adenosylmethionine over either drug alone or placebo for relieving pruritus and normalizing biochemical abnormalities, albeit for small numbers in each of four groups [85]. S-adenosylmethionine seems to be non-toxic to the fetus.

A single trial in Finland has shown that treatment with high-dose corticosteroids (dexamethasone 12 mg daily) is effective in improving the symptoms and biochemical changes of IHCP [37].

Recommendations regarding oral contraception

Although oestrogens have been linked to IHCP, pruritus and development of abnormal liver tests are not inevitable with their use in oral contraception. Accordingly, the combined oral contraceptive pill is not absolutely contraindicated in women with a prior history of IHCP [43]. Such women should be advised that oral contraceptives can result in pruritus and elevated liver enzyme tests (serum ALT and AST). Accordingly, these women may commence an oral contraceptive containing low-dose oestrogen [43] or a progesterone-only product once the liver tests have normalized from the index pregnancy, typically within 1 month postpartum. Women with a past history of IHCP taking oral contraceptive therapy should be followed with serial liver biochemistry and advised to report any pruritus or jaundice.

RECURRENCE OF INTRAHEPATIC CHOLESTASIS OF PREGNANCY

Women who have experienced IHCP should be advised that the chance of recurrence is high (45–70%) but not inevitable [43]. Further, IHCP may 'skip' consecutive pregnancies [43]. Also, the severity (or lack thereof) of any one pregnancy gives no indication of future severity or protection from future intrauterine death [43].

In one study of 27 multiparous women with IHCP, 15 experienced pruritus or jaundice in one subsequent pregnancy and three in more than one pregnancy. The remaining nine were not affected in later pregnancies [86]. The recurrence rate was 40% and 45%, respectively, in subsequent pregnancies in China [19] and Canada [18] and included two successive fetal losses for one patient [19].

Some authors recommend testing for genetic defects in MDR3 in women with IHCP [87] but this is not widely available and is unlikely to affect management.

PROGRESSIVE FAMILIAL INTRAHEPATIC CHOLESTASIS AND RELATION TO INTRAHEPATIC CHOLESTASIS OF PREGNANCY

PFIC describes a heterogeneous group of disorders of altered bile acid secretion and synthesis with autosomal recessive inheritance [88]. Recurrent prolonged cholestasis of pregnancy with pruritus related to oral oestrogen therapy, cholelithiasis and migraine headaches was described in four sisters from Puerto Rico [45]. Unlike IHCP, the liver disease continued to deteriorate after delivery and through successive pregnancies leading to fibrosis, cirrhosis and death. One sister received a liver graft

after the third pregnancy. Three of the 14 pregnancies led to stillbirth or preterm delivery. Interestingly, one variant of PFIC has been described in a boy of consanguinous parents whose mother had recurrent attacks of cholestasis during pregnancy that resembled IHCP. Mutations (1712delT) were detected in the *MDR3* gene as well as a high level of γ-glutamyl transpeptidase [88]. A detailed study from the same group in France [87] of another consanguinous family showed the coexistence of PFIC and IHCP in association with a gene defect (nonsense mutation) in *MDR3*. IHCP and other causes of cholestasis have been linked with adenosine triphosphate (ATP)-dependent aminophospholipid transport with discovery of mutations in a gene (*FIC1*), in PFIC that encodes for a subfamily of P-type ATPases that is important for the enterohepatic circulation of bile acids [87]. One hypothesis for the genetic basis of IHCP states that affected women are heterozygous for the gene defect/s in *MDR3* [87]. UDCA could alleviate IHCP by modulating nuclear transcription of transporter genes to effect delivery of more transporters to the canalicular membrane and/or by increasing the efficiency of transporter function within the membrane. Clinical presentation of IHCP depends on the interaction with non-genetic factors such as sex hormones and metabolites and their ability to regulate expression of the normal allele and/or bile transport systems [87].

Hyperemesis gravidarum (see also Chapter 10)

Nausea and vomiting sufficient to cause dehydration and acidosis occur in 0.2–1.6 women per 1000 deliveries [89]. Hepatic dysfunction from vomiting sufficient to require hospitalization is more common than thought previously [90]. Elevations in serum levels of AST to four times upper normal limits, and occasionally up to 22 times upper normal limits [91], have been found in 15–25% of women with hyperemesis gravidarum. The biochemical abnormalities do not correlate with severity of ketonuria [92]. Hepatic synthetic function, as measured by the prothrombin time, remains normal except with marked cholestasis and vitamin K deficiency. Reduced flow of bile and bile salts, as measured by impaired excretion of bromosulpthalein, has been demonstrated in the fasting rat, in kwashiorkor and in late pregnancy in women who experienced vomiting in the first trimester [93].

Pathogenetic mechanisms are unclear. Early reports included cases of viral hepatitis, drug-related hepatotoxicity and coincidental thyrotoxicosis. Current hypotheses favour a multifactorial origin for the liver injury including adverse effects of starvation and dehydration, high levels of oestrogens and a genetic predisposition. In hyperemesis, the elevated levels of serum cholesterol, triglycerides and phospholipids and alterations in low-density lipoproteins (LDL) and high-density lipoproteins (HDL) may reflect the effects of excess oestrogen on the liver. Severe hyperemesis gravidarum with accumulation of fat in the liver has been linked to deficiencies of mitochondrial β-oxidation pathways [94] (see AFLP, below). Successive pregnancies have been complicated by hyperemesis gravidarum and AFLP and HELLP syndrome [95].

The biochemical abnormalities reverse rapidly with restoration of fluid balance, improved nutrition and cessation of vomiting [91,92]. The main differential diagnoses are viral hepatitis and thyrotoxicosis. Liver biopsy usually is not required. The histopathology shows only non-specific changes.

Overlap syndromes with hepatic abnormalities (see also Chapter 6)

Pre-eclampsia and eclampsia, HELLP syndrome, AFLP, and hepatic rupture and infarction are the most common diseases involving the liver that arise in late pregnancy [10,96,97]. Their aetiologies and interrelations are being defined with discovery of genetic defects of fatty acid oxidation (see below). Nevertheless, dissent remains among authorities as to whether these disorders form a spectrum underwritten by pre-eclampsia as the common denominator or a series of distinct entities with a common pathway via the liver [98].

Characteristics will be described for each condition prior to discussing overlapping features.

THE LIVER IN PRE-ECLAMPSIA

Jaundice is uncommon but abnormal liver tests are evident in at least half of the cases of pre-eclampsia depending on how the condition is defined. The liver is not involved primarily in pre-eclampsia but becomes the target organ in severe cases. Liver disease occurs most often in advanced pre-eclampsia due to inadequate antenatal care. The associated constellation of signs and symptoms typically include marked hypertension (diastolic blood pressure >110 mmHg) and proteinuria with renal impairment (oliguria and raised serum creatinine), cerebral and visual disturbances and intrauterine growth restriction. Abnormalities of fatty acid oxidation seem to be common in pregnancies complicated by severe hypertension (see fatty acid oxidation, below).

Macroscopically, the liver in pre-eclampsia shows diffuse petechial haemorrhages over Glisson's capsule and the cut surface. Histopathological features are seen in over three-quarters of cases at postmortem [99]. Prominent features are hepatocellular necrosis with haemorrhage in the periportal regions and deposits of fibrin without any inflammatory infiltrate. Thrombi can be detected in capillaries in the portal tract and occasionally in branches of hepatic arteries and portal vein [15]. These features have been attributed to disseminated intravascular coagulation (DIC) [100] and resemble those of thrombotic thrombocytopenic purpura [101].

A vascular theory is now favoured [15,102]. Segmental vasospasm results in injury to endothelial cells and exposure of subendothelial collagen leading to platelet adherence and aggregation and precipitation of fibrin [15,102]. In dilated segments there is separation of endothelial cells and increased intraluminal pressure. Haemorrhage and rupture of anastomoses may occur between branches of the hepatic artery, portal vein and sinusoids [15]. Hepatic rupture may occur (see below). Rarely, hepatic infarction may result from gross ischaemia and obstruction to sinusoidal blood flow created by deposition of fibrin. Management is similar to that of acute liver failure (see below).

HELLP: SYNDROME

About 0.1–0.6% of women usually in the third trimester present principally with hepatic dysfunction and laboratory evidence of the HELLP syndrome: *H*aemolytic anaemia, *E*levated *L*iver transaminases and a *L*ow *P*latelet count [98,103,104]. Credit for discovery of thrombocytopenia and haemolysis, in association with severe pre-eclampsia, should go to Pritchard *et al.* [105], although Weinstein coined the term HELLP syndrome in 1982 [106].

HELLP syndrome should be considered a severe manifestation of pre-eclampsia. Occasionally HELLP presents before the 20th week. In 30%, HELLP is evident postpartum [103].

Hepatic dysfunction with the HELLP syndrome is reported to occur in around 10–15% of women with concurrent pre-eclampsia [107] and reviewed in [104]. Hypertension is obvious at presentation in over 80% of cases but is not invariable [104]. However, hypertension is not invariable in pre-eclampsia (see Chapter 6). Importantly, confusion over diagnostic criteria can delay appropriate management especially prompt delivery.

Most authorities will accept raised levels of AST (SGOT) above 50 IU/L (Normal range <30 in pregnancy, see Table 9.1) and lactate dehydrogenase above 180 IU/L with a platelet count below 100×10^9/L and haemolysis for the diagnosis of HELLP. The AST level usually is below 10 times upper normal limits but occasionally can exceed 1000 IU/L.

The HELLP syndrome probably represents a spectrum of disorders characterized by liver dysfunction with some haematological features of DIC. There is a microangiopathic haemolytic anaemia with the platelet count below 100×10^9/L (100 000 mm^{-3}) and abnormal forms of erythrocytes. Levels of antithrombin often are reduced below the usual fall that occurs in pregnancy [108]. The prothrombin time, a measure of synthetic function of the liver, and the partial thromboplastin time typically remain within, or near to, the normal range [106,109]. A mildly elevated prothrombin time usually indicates concurrent DIC whereas a grossly elevated prothrombin time can signify significant hepatic necrosis. Abnormal values occur for serum levels of unconjugated bilirubin, creatinine, LDH, and fibrinogen levels, fibrin degradation products, fibrin D-dimer, plasminogen activator inhibitor, protein C, anaphylatoxins (C3a, C5a) and creatinine.

The precise aetiology of HELLP syndrome within the spectrum of pre-eclampsia remains unclear. Injury to the vascular endothelium plays a pivotal role leading to abnormal vascular reactivity. Deposition of fibrin within the intravascular compartment ultimately leads to end-organ damage [98,110]. Further, genetic and biochemical links have been made with disorders of intramitochondrial β oxidation (see below).

Histopathological changes are not specific to HELLP. Deposition of fibrin in the periportal regions and, especially, the sinusoids is found early in the HELLP syndrome, including the milder cases. Fibrin is best demonstrated using immunofluorescence techniques [111,112]. Similar changes are found in pregnancy-associated hypertension with abnormal serum liver biochemistry but without evidence of HELLP, some cases of viral hepatitis and drug-related hepatotoxicity [112]. Fatty deposits are seen in HELLP as well as AFLP (see AFLP, below). Some authorities consider HELLP as a distinct histopathological entity from AFLP based on the different distribution of fat within the liver lobule [98] despite genetic links to disorders of fatty acid metabolism (see fatty acid oxidation, below).

Predictors of prognosis and maternal mortality

Elevation in levels of serum AST and unconjugated bilirubin reflect the severity of the haematological disturbances but do not correlate with trimester of presentation, clinical severity or propensity for complications and recovery. The serum level of AST usually returns to normal within 72 h after delivery, whereas the thrombocytopenia

may be protracted. Some authorities [98,113] further stratify HELLP syndrome according to maximum severity of the thrombocytopenia; class 1 with the nadir below 50×10^9/L; class 2 with nadirs between 51 and 100×10^9/L; and class 3 with nadirs between 101 and 150×10^9/L. The most severe thrombocytopenia (class 1 HELLP) is associated with the most complications. These stratifications require reappraisal with the finding that 11.6% of 6770 otherwise healthy women in Switzerland had platelet counts below 150×10^9/L at the time of delivery [114].

Elevated levels of circulating vascular, and endothelial, adhesion molecules may predict the development of pre-eclampsia and HELLP [115]. Unfortunately, many of these tests and values show too much variation for clinical use.

The spectrum of HELLP has widened to include milder cases with epigastric pain, elevated serum levels of AST and evidence of DIC but with normal or mild elevations in blood pressure, no significant proteinuria [112,116] and without haemolysis (HELLP syndrome).

Maternal mortality rates vary from 0% up to 25% [98,110,117,118]. In a retrospective analysis from the USA of the events surrounding death in 54 women with HELLP syndrome, maternal death was attributed to cerebral haemorrhage (45%), cardiopulmonary arrest (40%), DIC (39%), adult respiratory distress syndrome (28%), pulmonary oedema, renal failure (28%), sepsis (23%), hepatic haemorrhage (20%) and hypoxic ischaemic encephalopathy (16%) [118]. Apart from very low platelet counts (class 1 HELLP in 60% of maternal deaths), delay in diagnosis was considered contributary in 51% of the fatalities [118]. Less common complications include ascites, pleural and pericardial effusions, nephrogenic diabetes insipidus, hepatic haematoma and liver rupture (see liver rupture, below).

ACUTE FATTY LIVER OF PREGNANCY

The separate recognition of AFLP is usually attributed to Stander and Cadden in 1934 [119], although similar features were described by Rokitansky in 1843 and Tarnier in 1856 [120]. Differentiation from fulminant viral hepatitis is attributed to Sheehan in 1939 [90].

Estimates of occurrence are one in 6659 to 13 300 deliveries [121–123]. The greater awareness of AFLP and improvements in imaging have led to the recognition of milder cases and reporting of survivors [124,125]. Collected data from four series (Table 9.2) of biopsy-proven AFLP published from 1980 show a reduction in mortalities; the maternal to as low as 18% and fetal to 23% [121,126–128].

Such advances from specialized centres [117,123] have not been matched in general obstetric practice. AFLP

Table 9.2 Survival in biopsy-proven acute fatty liver of pregancy.

Author	Mothers		Infants	
	Number	Survival	Number	Survival
[126]	6	5	7*	4
[127]	12	8	15***	6**
[128]	5	4	6*	5*
[121]	10	9	12**	10**

Set of twins: * 1 set, ** 2 sets, *** 3 sets.

features consistently among the numbers of maternal deaths from direct causes surveyed for the UK [3,4]. These fatal cases illustrate the difficulties in diagnosing AFLP before death. Typical mistaken diagnoses were adult respiratory distress syndrome, DIC and cholecystitis requiring surgery. Jaundice may not be obvious and may be lacking. One presentation was in the second week postpartum after an uneventful pregnancy and delivery [3].

AFLP typically occurs in the obese woman in the third trimester. The predilection for primaparae is not emphasized in more recent series [121,129]. Multiparous women have presented as late as the eleventh gestation [129,130]. Common independent associations are pre-eclampsia in approximately 30–60% [117,127,130,131], twin pregnancy in 9–25% [117,127,130] and a male rather than female (ratio 3:1) fetus [124,130]. Distributions in age, parity and race do not differ significantly from normal obstetric practice [129,130]. The frequency of presentation rises after the 30th week but onset has been reported in the 20th week and postpartum [3,127,130,132].

Symptoms develop acutely but are non-specific such as abdominal pain (40–58%), nausea and vomiting (35–88%), headache (1–17%) and jaundice (50–90%) [3,121,127,130, 131]. Signs associated with pre-eclampsia such as hypertension, pedal oedema and proteinuria occur in over 50%.

More variable features are pruritus in 5–30% [121,130], fever in 40–53% [121,130], ascites in 40% [121], necrotizing enterocolitis [132] and clinical or postmortem evidence of pancreatitis in 16–100% [129,130,133,134]. The more severe cases may progress rapidly with impairment of conscious level, often related to profound hypoglycaemia, and development of acute liver failure, renal failure, bleeding diatheses, coma and death [117,121,124,127, 129,130] (see acute liver failure, below).

Laboratory findings include a marked neutrophil leucocytosis occasionally above $30\,000\,mm^{-3}$ with left shift. Other findings may be of a DIC with elevated levels of fibrin degradation products, very reduced levels of antithrombin [121,127,130,135–137] and/or overlap with HELLP syndrome (see above) with microangiopathic haemolytic anaemia and thrombocytopenia and abnormal red cell forms (burr cells, schistocytes, nucleated forms). Oliguria with elevated serum levels of creatinine and severe metabolic acidosis are common in severe cases [121,129,130].

Serum levels of bilirubin may be normal on presentation but rise with delayed delivery [124]. The AST is elevated between three and 10 times upper normal limits [121,129,130]. The association of a modest rise in serum AST and disproportionate elevations in serum alkaline phosphatase and uric acid no longer are considered discriminative for AFLP. Markedly elevated levels of serum AST ($>1000\,IU/L$) are found with shock, hepatic ischaemia and profound hypoglycaemia [129]. Some milder cases exhibited only minor elevations in serum alkaline phosphatase [121], which are comparable to levels seen in normal pregnancy (see Table 9.1). The serum level of uric acid often is elevated out of proportion to the impairment of renal function but this is considered a variable, and not distinguishing, finding [121]. Profound hypoglycaemia is common and, if unrecognized, contributes significantly to mortality of mother and child [121,129].

Morphological changes at postmortem in severe cases are widespread. Fatty infiltration and haemorrhages occur in many organs especially the gastrointestinal tract, pancreas, kidney, brain and bone marrow [15,129,138]. The liver is small and grossly yellow from steatosis [15]. The distribution characteristically is panlobular with sparing of periportal areas (Figs 9.1 & 9.2). Microvesicular steatosis commonly is accompanied by intrahepatic cholestasis with canalicular plugs of bile and an acute cholangiolitis. There may be extramedullary haematopoiesis and hyperplastic collections of Kupffer cells [15]. Microvesicular steatosis is the common denominator to several conditions other than AFLP that can be associated with deficiencies of congenital urea cycle enzymes and fatty acid oxidation. These include alcoholic hepatitis and hepatotoxicity due to tetracycline, sodium valproate and salicylates, vomiting disease of Jamaica, yellow fever, Reyes' syndrome and Wolman's disease. Importantly, fat may be overlooked with conventional histopathological stains and formalin-fixed liver tissue. Electron-microscopic examination is sensitive for detecting non-membrane bound fat in the hepatocytes and the abnormally large needle-shaped mitochondria containing large crystalline inclusions.

The risk of perinatal mortality rises with the quantity of fat, elevation in serum level of uric acid and reduction in platelet count.

CLINICAL OVERLAP BETWEEN PRE-ECLAMPSIA, HELLP AND ACUTE FATTY LIVER OF PREGNANCY

HELLP and AFLP present typically in the third trimester with non-specific symptoms and overlapping clinical, haematological and histological features [95,121,127, 139,140]. Epigastric pain from hepatic tenderness, nausea

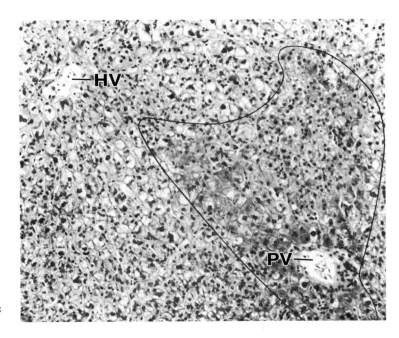

Fig 9.1 Acute fatty liver of pregnancy (H&E, × 150) showing typical sparing of periportal area (ringed). HV, hepatic vein; PV, portal vein.

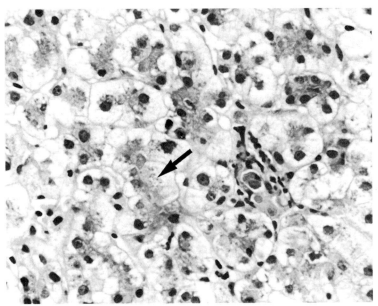

Fig 9.2 Acute fatty liver of pregnancy (H&E, × 600) showing perinuclear microvesicular steatosis (arrowed).

and vomiting, as well as elevated liver enzymes and a low platelet count are frequently found in these conditions as well as many others incidental to pregnancy (Box 9.1) [141].

Overall, evidence continues to accrue to suggest these form a spectrum of illnesses that correct with prompt delivery. Pre-eclampsia is present in 30–100% of AFLP [127,142]. Most of the evidence linking these conditions has relied on clinical correlates and individual case reports. Importantly, successive pregnancies may be complicated by pre-eclampsia, HELLP and/or AFLP [94,95,143]. Fatty liver has been suspected in some patients with the HELLP syndrome based on computed tomography (CT) imaging [110] and histopathological findings [98], albeit of a different distribution to AFLP. However, one exceptional study from Japan detailed the histopathological features using oil red O on frozen liver sections [144]. Microvesicular fat was detected in all 41 women presenting with pre-eclampsia, including those with normal liver tests [144].

Overlap with hyperemesis gravidarum

In a retrospective study of nine pregnant women with abnormal liver tests and variable presentations including hyperemesis gravidarum, pre-eclampsia and HELLP syndrome, all liver biopsy samples showed fatty liver with marked centrilobular microvesicular fat and cholestasis [142]. Hyperemesis gravidarum followed by AFLP in

---

Box 9.1 Differential diagnosis of hepatic disorders and hypertension

- HELLP
- Acute fatty liver
- Alcoholic hepatitis
- Biliary colic
- Budd–Chiari syndrome
- Cholecystitis
- Cocaine abuse
- Dissecting aortic aneurysm
- Disseminated intravascular coagulation
- Hepatic necrosis
- Hiatus hernia
- Pancreatitis
- Peptic ulcer
- Pyelonephritis
- Septicaemias
- SLE
- Thrombocytopenias
- Viral hepatitis

---

two successive pregnancies has been reported [145]. Interestingly, the common gene mutation (*G1528C*) associated with long-chain 3-hydroxyacyl-Co A dehydrogenase (LCHAD) deficiency was not detected in the mother and babies. Instead, both babies had undetectable activities for carnitine palmitoyl transferase (CPT-I) [145].

Fatty acid oxidation pathways

Our understanding of AFLP and related disorders has improved in parallel with recognition of disorders of intramitochondrial fatty acid oxidation especially in some babies born to mothers with AFLP, HELLP and pre-eclampsia [95]; reviewed in [146]. Early observations pointed indirectly to disorder/s of lipid metabolism, at least in the genesis of AFLP. Serum levels of cholinesterase fall in normal pregnancy. However, the rise in cholinesterase levels observed in a subsequent pregnancy in a survivor of AFLP 18 months previously suggested altered metabolism of lipids [147]. Subsequently, the discovery of defects in β oxidation in some patients with AFLP and their affected babies has linked objectively these conditions. Such defects have served as a marker to trace genetic defects across families and successive pregnancies [94,95,143].

Long-chain 3-hydroxyacyl-Co A dehydrogenase deficiency

In 1991, Schoeman *et al.* identified and characterized a defect in fatty acid oxidation in a mother with successive AFLP in two out of three pregnancies [148]. Both affected babies showed accumulation of lipid in multiple organs. Importantly, the third baby who remained healthy was born of the uncomplicated pregnancy. These observations linked the necessity for concurrence of an affected fetus and development of ALFP/HELLP syndrome in the mother likely to be heterozygous for LCHAD deficiency. In a study from Finland [95], pre-eclampsia, HELLP and/or AFLP occurred in pregnancies involving 31% of babies diagnosed with deficiency of LCHAD. Evidence suggests that the woman with AFLP and/or HELLP syndrome who carries an affected fetus has a low (but not undetectable) level of LCHAD consequent to being heterozygous for the mutant alleles. Stressful situations such as pregnancy especially in the third trimester can reveal latent deficiencies of fatty acid metabolism in the heterozygous mother. Fatty acid oxidation is inhibited in late pregnancy whereas substrates of long-chain fatty acids are liberated in pre-eclampsia. An affected fetus that is homozygous for mutant alleles relies on maternal pathways for fatty acid oxidation. Abnormal fatty acid metabolites produced by the affected fetus enter the maternal circulation and overwhelm the compromised mitochondrial oxidation pathways of the heterozygous mother.

Disorders of fatty acid oxidation including short-chain 3-hydroxyacyl-Co A dehydrogenase (SCHAD) and medium-chain 3-hydroxyacyl-Co A dehydrogenase (MCHAD) are reviewed by Treem [146]. The gene for LCHAD has been mapped to chromosome 2q34–q35. Different point mutations in the LCHAD portion of the α subunit of the mitochondrial trifunctional protein on exon 15 have been identified in children with LCHAD deficiency and their mothers affected by AFLP and/or HELLP syndrome [149]. The point mutation (*G1528C*) results in a change at the amino acid level from glutamic acid to glutamine at residue 474 of the mature α subunit. AFLP seems to segregate with specific mutant LCHAD alleles. This mutation seems to be responsible for around 50–87% of the mutant alleles in studies from Europe and the USA. Children with the *G1528C* mutation typically present with a Reyes-like syndrome characterized by microvesicular fat in the liver and death before 6 months of age [143]. Conversely, babies with defective enzyme activities relating to the trifunctional protein develop cardiac and neurological disorders without obvious liver disease.

Many of the clinical and laboratory features in AFLP and HELLP syndrome can be explained by defective energy production caused by failure of oxidation of long-chain fatty acids in tissues such as heart and skeletal muscle, and of synthesis of ketone bodies in the liver. The inability to oxidize fatty acids in the liver results in their diversion into triacylglycerol synthesis and marked hepatic steatosis. The predilection for the third (and fourth) trimesters, increased association of severe manifestations with multiple pregnancy and relief following delivery can be explained by the increasing stress on the normal physiological process of pregnancy. The rise in oestrogens accelerates near to term in normal pregnancy. Consequently, fatty acid oxidation is reduced and production of ketones altered leading to increased formation of triglycerides and secretion of very-low-density lipoproteins (VRDL) from the liver [148].

The rarity of AFLP and HELLP and uncommon recurrence in successive pregnancies can be explained by the likely heterozygous state in the mother and baby as well as the reluctance to risk further pregnancies. Only women carrying affected fetuses who are homozygous or compound heterozyous for the *G1528C* mutation responsible for isolated LCHAD deficiency have a history of severe AFLP and HELLP syndrome.

Additional predisposing factors for manifestation of AFLP have included protracted vomiting (see hyperemesis gravidarum, above) and fasting as well as toxins,

viruses and pre-eclampsia [124,146]. Pyelonephritis and urinary tract infection have been found in up to 25% of reports [130,150] and respiratory tract infection also is common [130]. Histopathological similarities are seen with jejuno-ileal bypass and protein malnutrition [151] but most cases recently have been well nourished [130]. Depression of protein synthesis by tetracyclines may have accounted for some of the early reports especially those presenting before the 28th week [130]. The chemical syndrome and liver histology of AFLP is very similar to that of Reyes' syndrome in children [15].

DIFFERENTIAL DIAGNOSIS OF OVERLAP SYNDROMES

No specific diagnostic features are found on clinical examination. The differential diagnosis from other causes of jaundice and encephalopathy, especially in the third trimester is wide (see Box 9.1 above, viral hepatitis, and acute liver failure, below). Diagnosis has become more difficult with inclusion of mild cases of AFLP with overlapping features.

AFLP should be considered in any pregnant woman presenting with one or more of the following: epigastric pain, symptoms suggestive of reflux oesophagitis, nausea, vomiting, jaundice and a bleeding diathesis regardless of hepatic encephalopathy [127]. Backache may indicate underlying pancreatitis. The main differential diagnosis is between other causes of acute liver failure such as viral hepatitis and drug hepatotoxicity, severe pre-eclampsia and alcoholic hepatitis [15,101]. Serological markers will distinguish viral causes such as hepatitis A, B (not C necessarily: see viral hepatitis), D, E and the herpes group. Clinical and histopathological distinction from hepatitis due to viruses and alcohol may be impossible, especially in mild AFLP. Several histological features overlap and cytoplasmic ballooning can mask the characteristic microvesicular steatosis [15].

Other confusing clinical conditions include a constellation of disorders such as haemolytic–uraemic syndrome, thrombocytopenic purpura, systemic lupus erythematosus (SLE), and disorders of the urea acid cycle, such as ornithine transcarbamylase (OTC) deficiency [152] and disorders of mitochondrial β oxidation. Thrombotic thrombocytopenic purpura and haemolytic–uraemic syndrome have been considered a spectrum of overlapping disorders with microangiopathic haemolytic anaemia, thrombocytopenia, renal failure and neurological disturbance [101], although recently specific features of thrombotic thrombocytopenic purpura have emerged (see Chapters 3 and 7). Common associations are with DIC and sepsis [101,135,153]. The degree of liver dysfunction is minor in these predominantly haematological conditions and elevations in levels of liver serum biochemistry such as the AST and bilirubin reflect haemolysis rather than abnormal liver function. Differential diagnosis of AFLP from the HELLP syndromes and pre-eclampsia may not be clinically relevant or only be possible using immuno-fluorescent techniques on liver histology [15]. The differential diagnosis of DIC in emergency obstetric practice is wide and considered in Chapter 3. In abruptio placentae, intrauterine death, amniotic fluid embolism, pre-eclampsia and sepsis, the haematological disorder usually is manifest before the onset of liver failure [135].

IMAGING

Ultrasonographic findings of increased reflectivity are consistent with fat. CT and magnetic resonance imaging (MRI) may show low attenuation [110]. Hepatic haemorrhage with haematoma and infarction can be found in some cases of HELLP and diagnosed by CT and MRI [110]. Hepatic infarction characteristically shows multiple non-enhancing lesions of low attenuation with mottled appearance and vessels coursing through [110,154].

These imaging tests are safe in pregnancy. A single 'slice' over the liver using modern CT equipment exposes the fetus to less irradiation than a conventional plain abdominal radiograph [155]. Overall, these tests are insensitive. A negative result does not exclude AFLP and related conditions. Liver histology may occasionally help to time delivery with mild disease and an immature fetus. Percutaneous sampling is often precluded by abnormal coagulation. The transjugular route can be successful in expert hands. Maternal and fetal outcome depend on clinical assessment of disease severity (see acute liver failure, below) and not the AST levels.

MANAGEMENT

Maternal outcome has improved significantly in recent years in HELLP syndrome and AFLP in parallel with earlier diagnosis. Nevertheless, prompt delivery is recommended because fetal mortality remains high especially from placental dysfunction in HELLP syndrome and from hypoglycaemia in AFLP.

Optimal management for hypertension and all but trivial liver dysfunction involves early discussion and transferral to a tertiary referral centre with intensive care facilities for managing hepatological, haematological and obstetric emergencies. Emphasis is on early diagnosis aided by improvements in radiological imaging techniques and intensive treatment of complications such as profound hypoglycaemia, gastrointestinal haemorrhage,

pancreatitis and sepsis [117,121,132] plus the ability to care for a preterm, and potentially sick, infant.

General measures include strict control and frequent monitoring of arterial blood pressure, correction of hypertension with hydralazine as well as abnormal levels of blood glucose, coagulation status and acid–base balance and instigation of prophylaxis against seizures in selected cases. Delivery should follow presentations beyond the 34th week. Milder cases may reach term. Spontaneous vaginal delivery is possible but close monitoring is essential to anticipate further impairment of liver function. Massive hepatic necrosis and a variety of neurological and cardiac abnormalities have been reported in these conditions. Bleeding complications are common in severe AFLP and HELLP syndrome. Major intra-abdominal bleeding may require laparotomy and evacuation of clot [117].

HELLP syndrome

The general consensus for HELLP syndrome is that correction of hypertension should be followed by delivery as soon as the fetus reaches a maturity that represents a reasonable chance of survival in the centre caring for the mother (reviewed in [98]). Some patients with mild HELLP syndrome may improve with conservative management and proceed to spontaneous vaginal delivery, but intrauterine growth restriction is common [112]. Prompt delivery may extend therapeutic manoeuvres considered unsafe for the fetus.

In contrast, there is no evidence that delivery improves outcome in other causes of thrombocytopenia such as haemolytic–uraemic syndrome, thrombocytopenic purpura and SLE. As with AFLP, postpartum recovery usually is rapid. Regardless, close monitoring should be extended into the first week postpartum and/or until normalization occurs of the platelet count. Large quantities of fresh blood and platelets may be required in severe (class 1) HELLP syndrome. Medical expertise should cover management of liver failure for the mother, including provision for liver transplantation [156], and for small-for-dates babies because intrauterine growth restriction is common.

Hepatic associations and complications include acute liver failure as well as hepatic haematoma and rupture. Budd–Chiari syndrome (see below) that developed postpartum in association with thrombotic thrombocytopenic purpura has been reported in a woman diagnosed as having HELLP syndrome during pregnancy [157].

Pulmonary oedema probably reflects adult respiratory distress syndrome and highlights the need for strict monitoring of fluid balance.

Individual case reports document some improvement with plasmapheresis [103,104,158] and antithrombotic

agents [159], including infusions of prostaglandin derivatives and inhibitors of thromboxane synthetase [113]. In
HELLP, individual reports showed that corticosteroids
and low-dose salicylates improved the level of AST and
platelets whereas heparin was without benefit. Accordingly, use of corticosteroids has been advocated for maternal as well as fetal reasons [98].

Acute fatty liver of pregnancy

In AFLP, the maternal hypoglycaemia may be profound
and protracted for many days following delivery, accounting for the continued deterioration in conscious level [126].
If there is significant hypoglycaemia a large centrally
placed venous catheter is essential for delivery of large
amounts of glucose. Monitoring and control of fluid balance will be helped by using a Swan–Ganz catheter. Low
levels of glucose and calcium may be aggravated by pancreatitis. Some authors have recommended reduction in
intake of dietary cholesterol as prophylaxis against the
development of AFLP, which is commonly associated with
hyperlipidaemia [160], but the benefit of this remains unproven. Correction of bleeding tendencies with fresh
frozen plasma, clotting factor concentrates and vitamin K_1
has improved the prognosis in severe cases of AFLP [121,
161]. Some authorities have advocated specific correction
of the deficiency of antithrombin which is common in AFLP
and other overlapping syndromes [108]. Others have cau-
tioned against the use of heparin and stressed correction of
hypovolaemia and oligohydramnios with plasma [137].

Anaesthesia

General anaesthesia should be carried out by an experienced anaesthetist. Epidural and other forms of nerve
block are contraindicated in patents with significant
thrombocytopenia and other abnormalities that compromise clotting. Regardless, platelet transfusions should
be given for counts below 30–50×10^9/L. If epidural anaesthesia has been used, the catheter should be removed
as soon as possible after delivery. The nadir in the platelet
count occurs typically 24–72h postpartum and may precipitate haemorrhage.

Timing and mode of delivery. The striking improvement in
liver function and conscious status achieved with rapid
delivery, and the absence of spontaneous recovery in a
proven case of AFLP and severe HELLP syndrome argue
strongly for induction of labour or delivery by caesarean
section (Table 9.6, p. 317).
Surprisingly, whether early delivery leads to improved
prognosis for mother and child [121,125,127], remains

unproved. In one series of 12 patients with AFLP, the
eight survivors had proceeded to immediate delivery via
induced labour or caesarean section [127]. However, two
of four maternal deaths occurred in the induced pregnancies [127]. Several survivors, albeit more recently, have
proceeded to term with spontaneous vaginal delivery of a
live fetus in up to 70% of cases [121]. Many of the cases
reported after 1980 have been mild based on clinical, but
not haematological, criteria [125,128].

Postpartum issues

As with pregnancy-induced hypertension, AFLP and
HELLP usually resolve within 1 week following delivery.
Nevertheless, intensive care facilities should be available.
The consumption coagulopathy may continue and be exacerbated following delivery [121]. Life-threatening postpartum haemorrhage is not uncommon [127] and fresh
plasma and platelets should be available.
In severe HELLP syndrome and AFLP the risks of liver
rupture, haemorrhage and infarction continue into the
postpartum period [121]. Other risks in AFLP include
hypoglycaemia, pancreatitis and pseudocyst formation.
Neurological complications such as cerebral oedema in
AFLP and intracranial haemorrhage in HELLP syndrome
also require monitoring. Rarely their onset is after delivery.
Postpartum eclampsia is especially common among
women with HELLP syndrome during pregnancy [162].
Liver transplantations for severe AFLP and for hepatic
rupture in relation to HELLP syndrome have been successful [110,163], including postpartum [164] (see liver transplantation below).
Liver metabolism returns to normal postpartum
according to magnetic resonance spectroscopy, except in
severe cases of HELLP [165]. However, one study from
the Netherlands found abnormalities in unconjugated (indirect) levels of bilirubin at a median of 31 months (range
3–101 months) in 54 women recovering postpartum from
HELLP syndrome [166].

NEONATAL FEATURES AND OUTCOMES FOR
THE OVERLAP SYNDROMES

Impaired hepatic synthetic function, neonatal thrombocytopenia, neutropenia and hypoprothrombinaemia unrelated to vitamin K and hypoalbuminaemia have been
reported in newborns when there was severe maternal
hypertension. Babies born to mothers with HELLP are at
especial risk for problems associated with prematurity and
intrauterine growth restriction [167]. In severe AFLP widespread fatty infiltration in the livers of the offspring has
been reported after several months of age [148]. Babies and

infants may present with a Reyes-like syndrome with refractory hypoglycaemia, fatty liver, coma and death, although this is rare [94,143]. Hypoglycaemia may be profound; fasting should be avoided. The occurrence of lethargy, hypotonia, hypoglycaemia, acidosis, hepatomegaly, cardiac dysfunction and elevated liver tests should prompt analysis of urine for accumulating organic acids and blood spots for abnormal acylcarnitine profiles. Meanwhile, suspected babies should be managed with frequent feeds, including through the night. Intravenous supplements of dextrose may be necessary, especially during intercurrent fevers and illnesses. Infants should be fed on a diet low in long-chain fat and high in carbohydrates for suspected metabolic illness [168].

Whether these families represent distinct recessive genetic errors of fatty metabolism, requires further study. Calcium supplements for the neonate may be necessary following maternal HELLP syndrome and pancreatitis. Additional vitamin K_1 may help prevent excess bleeding.

PREGNANCY OUTCOMES FOR SURVIVORS OF
ACUTE FATTY LIVER OF PREGNANCY AND
HELLP SYNDROME

Subsequent normal pregnancies have been reported for survivors of HELLP, AFLP and liver rupture. There are isolated reports of histologically proven recurrent AFLP and of HELLP in successive pregnancies [98,169]. A maternal defect in oxidation of long-chain fatty acids was demonstrated in one woman with AFLP occurring in successive pregnancies. Both infants died within the first year and autopsy revealed widespread fatty infiltration of their livers [148]. CPT-I deficiency was documented in babies born after successive hyperemesis gravidarum and AFLP without evidence of LCHAD deficiency [145].

Advice given to survivors of AFLP who desire a further pregnancy can be optimistic but recurrences may be more common than realized. Extrapolations from published data have limited meaning to the individual woman who desires another pregnancy. Some multiparous patients presenting with AFLP have documented hypertension in a preceding pregnancy.

In a review of women who became pregnant after documented HELLP syndrome in a previous pregnancy [169], the recurrence rate of HELLP syndrome was low (3% vs. 5%) in 13 hypertensive women compared with 139 normotensive women. However, ensuing maternal complications were much higher in the hypertensive group: pre-eclampsia (75% vs. 19%) and abruptio placentae (20% vs. 2%). Fetal complications also were higher and included

preterm delivery (80% vs. 21%), intrauterine growth restriction (45% vs. 12%) and perinatal death (40% vs. 4%).

GENETIC COUNSELLING

Survivors of AFLP and HELLP and related disorders who wish to consider further pregnancies should be counselled that the risks may be around 25% for recurrent AFLP and HELLP if the fetus is homozygous for LCHAD deficiency and both parents are heterozygous. Additional factors are likely to contribute to the manifestation of severe AFLP other than a maternal inborn error of metabolism. AFLP is not invariable in the heterozygous mother despite when carrying a fetus with LCHAD deficiency. Further, testing for LCHAD deficiency and mutations has low sensitivity and specificity especially for the individual patient. Mansouri *et al.* [170] reported no association between the LCHAD mutations and AFLP in 14 consecutive cases of French and North African origin. CPT-I should be sought in babies born to mothers with AFLP without genetic evidence for LCHAD deficiency. In a retrospective study from Finland, of 18 mothers with known LCHAD deficiency, the relative risk of developing pre-eclampsia, HELLP syndrome and AFLP was found to be 27% in pregnancies with an LCHAD-deficient fetus [95].

Nulliparity, twin gestation and male fetus have been associated with a slightly increased risk of AFLP. Again, these demographic data have limited application when counselling the individual patient.

There is a case for screening newborn babies born of women with AFLP and/or HELLP syndrome for disorders of fatty acid oxidation to allow early detection of treatable and potentially fatal metabolic disorders.

LCHAD and related enzymes can be detected from genomic DNA extracted from skin fibroblasts and their cultures and from a blood spot after amplification using the polymerase chain reaction (PCR) [94]. The point mutation (*G1528C* or *C1332T*) occurs in the active domain of LCHAD. The *G1528C* mutation results in a change at the amino acid level from glutamic acid to glutamine at residue 474 (Glu474Gln) of the mature α subunit. As this mutation creates a restriction site (Pst I), familial inheritance can be confirmed by gel electrophoresis of restriction digests of amplified genomic DNA. Testing can be carried out prenatally, including in the father and siblings; affected babies can be tested at autopsy. Fresh and frozen body fluids and tissues suitable for sampling include skin, muscle, kidney and many other organs. As fibroblast cultures take time, these should be sampled in anticipation, including at autopsy, and sent for appropriate biochemical, molecular and enzymic studies to document deficiencies in β-mitochondrial oxidation, carnitine and OTC [152].

Hepatic rupture and infarction

Spontaneous rupture of the liver was reported by Abercrombie in 1844 [171]. A recent survey gives its occurrence as one in every 45 000 live births [172]. The majority, although not all [173], of cases of hepatic rupture and infarction are associated with severe hypertension and the HELLP syndrome [98,117,154], especially in the older multiparous patient [110]. Rupture is most common in the third trimester but can occur at any time, including early in the puerperium [98,171,174–176]. For reasons that are obscure, hepatic rupture seems to be more common in black women resident in North America than in other population groups.

Vascular malformations, polyarteritis nodosa, mycotic aneurysms, fibromuscular dysplasia, Ehlers–Danlos syndrome type IV, cocaine use, amoebic abscess and tumours [177] account for a minority of cases in pregnancy [110,178]. As in the non-pregnant patient, liver rupture can be precipitated by blunt trauma [179], vomiting and convulsions.

Mechanisms surrounding spontaneous rupture remain obscure. Occlusion of the hepatic artery does not lead to widespread infarction because additional blood is supplied from the portal vein. Hepatic infarction and haemorrhage more likely result from several factors including gross ischaemia (as seen with cocaine abuse) and obstruction to sinusoidal blood flow by deposited fibrin and relative hypovolaemia.

Subcapsular haemorrhages in the liver are found in 80% of cases of pre-eclampsia and eclampsia [180] in association with a DIC. The altered haematological state may favour pathological deposition of fibrin thrombi in vessels and sinusoids leading to focal, and later confluent, subcapsular haemorrhagic necrosis [181–183] prior to rupture. This hypothesis has been challenged by the finding of a coagulopathy that developed after onset of rupture and following surgical repair [184]. The elevation in serum AST (SGOT) is usually accompanied by a rise in serum LDH and probably reflects red cell destruction [185]. Extensive necrosis of hepatocytes and a coagulopathy will result in high levels of AST (>1000 IU/L) [176, 186] and impaired synthetic function reflected in the elevated prothrombin ratio [184].

Differential diagnosis and management are similar to that of acute liver failure [117]. Rupture and infarction can occur at any time including in the puerperium. Onset is sudden with upper abdominal pain, nausea and vomiting. Usually the lower abdomen is soft and uterus not tender

[187]. Severe cases may be heralded by shock, hypotension, fever, vomiting, absent fetal heart sounds and vaginal bleeding from the haemorrhagic diathesis. Hepatic encephalopathy is compounded by severe hypoglycaemia. Levels of serum transaminases typically are grossly elevated (>10 times upper normal limits) and the prothrombin time is prolonged. Haemoperitoneum may be discovered at laparotomy for suspected perforated viscus, abruptio placenta and ruptured uterus. A subcapsular tear and haematoma may be seen with liver rupture. In over 90% these involve the anterior, superior aspect of the right lobe. Until recently, diagnosis was delayed and maternal mortality was as high as 75% [174,188]. Hepatic haemorrhage accounted for 20% of maternal deaths associated with HELLP syndrome in a retrospective analysis in the USA [118].

Hepatic rupture should be suspected with the triad of pre-eclampsia, right upper quadrant pain typically referred to the shoulder-tip, and shock. Occasionally pain is referred via the phrenic nerve to the region of the heart and oesophagus [98]. A chest radiograph may show elevation of the right hemidiaphragm. Urgent provision should be made for a general and/or vascular surgeon and obstetrician to proceed to theatre. In 10% of cases the left lobe of the liver is involved and a subcapsular haematoma may be overlooked at surgery [189]. Bleeding also may occur at intracerebral, intrathoracic and retroperitoneal sites [189].

The prognosis of liver rupture has improved with increased awareness of the complications of hypertension and advances in imaging techniques. Serial scanning for suspected haematoma, hepatic rupture and infarction is essential. In the acute phase, CT scanning with contrast, including spiral CT imaging and MRI are more sensitive than ultrasonography. CT imaging typically reveals a crescentic or oval lesion of low attenuation without distortion of the hepatic vasculature (absence of mass effect). In hepatic infarction (unlike acute liver failure with haemorrhage, infection and malignancy), enhancement after intravenous contrast medium is not seen. Diagnostic hepatic arteriography offers the option of transcatheter embolization in haemodynamically stable patients without intraperitoneal haemorrhage. Percutaneous diagnostic peritoneal lavage under aseptic technique has been carried out for suspected liver rupture. The presence of blood and haemodynamic instability should prompt urgent combined surgical and obstetrical intervention. Packing with subfascial drainage is preferred to radical hepatic resection [98,190]. Transcatheter embolotherapy should be considered especially when there is haemodynamic instability and when the risk of surgery is high. In expert hands, selective catheterization and embolization of the offending vessels can arrest bleeding abruptly but cessation may be temporary. Non-selective embolization may result in complications such as hepatic abscess, sepsis and ischaemia of the gallbladder [191]. Laparotomy is essential if arteriography fails. Hepatic resection is carried out only if the more conservative packing procedures fail.

Several authors favour immediate caesarean section, although the risks of stillbirth and perinatal death remain high [189,192–194]. Palpation, vomiting and straining should be minimized in women with severe HELLP syndrome and/or suspected hepatic haematoma. Early diagnosis may improve fetal and maternal outcome and obviate the need for surgery.

Later, uneventful pregnancies have been recorded in survivors of previous hepatic rupture [98,169,193–195]. One non-pregnant patient presented in shock and survived a 50% hepatic resection for rupture of a hepatic adenoma in the left lobe and excision of an unruptured adenoma in the right lobe. She conceived 5 months later and proceeded with an uneventful pregnancy to an elective caesarean section at term. Serial scans showed no recurrence [196] (see hepatic tumours below).

Liver transplantation for ruptured liver in association with HELLP syndrome has been successful but depends on the timely availability of a limited number of donor organs [117,163].

Liver disorders incidental to pregnancy

Areas of concern in obstetric practice are the adverse effects of any liver disease on the pregnant woman and her fetus as well as any adverse impact of the pregnancy on the liver disease.

Viral hepatitis A to E

General issues relating to viral hepatitis will be discussed before addressing specific concerns for the individual viral agents.

GENERAL ISSUES

Viral hepatitis remains the most common cause of jaundice in pregnancy [197]. The main hepatotropic agents likely to be seen in pregnancy are listed in Table 9.3. Clinical and epidemiological features of hepatitis A, B and D, C and E overlap. Specific diagnosis relies on detection of specific serological markers of acute and chronic infection. A viral infection, such as hepatitis B or C, or reactivation, such as with the herpes viruses, may be detected during pregnancy only as a result of screening. Presentation typically is delayed until the cholestatic phase with pruritus, jaundice and steatorrhoea. Discrimination from other viruses based on incubation periods and clinical features can be misleading. Presenting symptoms often are abrupt but non-specific with a flu-like illness, headache, fatigue, nausea, anorexia, vomiting and diarrhoea. Cholestatic jaundice with pale stools, dark urine and pruritus usually follow within days of the prodrome and is a common mode of presentation. Differentiation from other causes of jaundice may be difficult. Alcoholic hepatitis, biliary obstruction and intrahepatic cholestasis, and chronic liver diseases such as PBC may present in pregnancy. The main differential diagnosis is from other causes of cholestasis such as alcoholic hepatitis, biliary obstruction, IHCP (see above), drugs and autoimmune liver diseases (see below).

Name	Antibodies	Other markers
Hepatitis A	IgM antihepatitis A virus (HAV)	Nil
Hepatitis B	IgM antihepatitis B core antigen (HBc)	Hepatitis B virus DNA
Hepatitis C	Core region*	Hepatitis C virus RNA
Hepatitis D	IgM anti-HDV	Hepatitis B virus DNA (hepatitis D virus can interfere with B) Hepatitis D virus RNA
Hepatitis E	IgM antihepatitis E virus*	Hepatitis E virus RNA Ig G antibodies*
Herpes virus (simplex zoster, cytomegalovirus, Epstein–Barr)	IgM antibodies	Paired sera, cultures, liver inclusions and *in situ* hybridization
Exotic viruses	Panels of antibodies	Cytopathic effects in cell culture

Table 9.3 Serological diagnosis of acute viral hepatitis.

*Under evaluation.

MATERNAL ISSUES

Areas of particular concern in obstetric practice for the mother include the propensity for sexual transmission and issues relating to fertility as well as maternal outcome.

Sexual transmission

While sexual contact can result in transmission of all the hepatotropic agents, the risk of transmission varies greatly between the viruses. Hepatitis A and E virus (HAV, HEV) can be spread via the faeco-oral route during sexual contact particularly during the incubation phase of these infections. Hepatitis B virus (HBV) is easily and frequently spread via sexual contact. In contrast, sexual transmission is uncommon for hepatitis C virus (HCV) in the absence of confounding factors such as intravenous drug use between sexual partners and high levels of viraemia.

Fertility

This is not affected in acute, uncomplicated viral hepatitis. In fact, women can become pregnant subsequent to malabsorption of the contraceptive pill with significant diarrhoea, nausea and vomiting. Conversely, amenorrhoea and oligomenorrhoea are common with advanced liver disease, especially cirrhosis, and regardless of aetiology. Consequently, women with severe chronic viral hepatitis and advanced liver disease, especially cirrhosis, are often infertile or subfertile. Return of fertility is common in most young women following liver transplantation as it is following renal transplantation. In fact, persistent amenorrhoea may signify unsuspected pregnancy.

In vitro fertility

Seminal fluid should be considered a potential source of transmission for HBV. All donors of semen should be tested for hepatitis HBV markers. HBV DNA has been detected regularly in fractions of seminal fluid, including round cells, leucocytes and (rarely) spermatozoa. Heat-inactivated serum was identified as the source of contamination with HBV of culture medium used for *in vitro* fertilization [198]. An outbreak in the Netherlands identified 79 such women with serological evidence of HBV infection, including 24 who were pregnant, or became pregnant during their acute hepatitis infection. No adverse effects on mother and child were recorded for the 19 pregnancies that went to term [198].

The identification of HCV in semen remains controversial. HCV RNA was not detectable using PCR techniques in fractions of seminal fluid, round cells and spermatozoa from 56 viraemic men attending a tertiary referral centre in Italy with a particular expertise in processing seminal fluid from donors with human immunodeficiency virus (HIV) [199]. Thirty-four of the men had inhibitors to the PCR present in their fractions. Interestingly, hepatitis G virus (HGV, also known as GBV-C) was found in 50% of the fractions without PCR inhibitors, but the significance of these discordant findings remains unknown.

Contraception

Evidence from one large surveillance programme in Boston [200] indicated that viral hepatitis occurred more frequently in women using oral contraceptive therapy. Some authorities recommend discontinuation of combined therapy until normalization of liver serum biochemistry [201]. Others concluded that oral contraceptive therapy has no adverse effect on acute viral hepatitis [202] and chronic liver disease [203] but modern data relating to the individual viral agents are lacking.

Maternal outcome

Adverse maternal outcome relates to the propensity for developing severe viral hepatitis during pregnancy. In turn, reports on severity differ between developing, and developed, countries. Most data come from regions such as India and North Africa and report epidemics of hepatitis E that are severe among pregnant women. Acute viral hepatitis in an adult in a high prevalence country such as India is more likely to be due to HEV or HBV than HAV. There is widespread exposure to HAV in childhood and subsequent long-term immunity. In contrast, studies from Europe [27], the USA [204] and Zagreb [205] suggest no overall increase in severity but detail is lacking.

More research is needed to assess maternal and fetal outcomes in relation to influence of individual virus type. Variables to be considered are geographical region, socioeconomic status, nutrition, duration of immunity and temporal changes in prevalence of viral hepatitis within a given community. In developing countries malnutrition, poor socioeconomics and suboptimal obstetric care may combine significantly to contribute to the unusually severe outcome of hepatitis but information is conflicting. Data from Israel [206] support these conclusions. Studies before 1960 [207] coincide with poor socioeconomic conditions and report an increased severity of hepatitis in pregnant, compared with non-pregnant, women. In contrast, between 1967 and 1977, which marked rising socioeconomic progress, severities were similar [206]. A comparable study from Saudi Arabia [208] spanned more than 20 years and included a prospective period (1963–75) of rising socioeconomic growth. This showed a fall in mortality from 70.8% (1953–62) to 14.3% (1963–75) among pregnant women with viral hepatitis. The mortality among non-pregnant women fell similarly; 26.7% to 5.6% for the two respective time periods [208] indicating a high relative risk of death (approximately 4 : 1) for pregnancy. Maternal and fetal outcome may depend more on improvements in medical care than a reduction in severity of hepatitis in pregnancy. Whether malnutrition affects outcome, also remains controversial. Prospective studies from India for non-A, non-B hepatitis [209] and Libya for unspecified varieties of predominantly non-B viral hepatitis [210] have shown a persistence of high attack rate and mortality in pregnancy despite adequate nutrition and a similar outcome for non-A, non-B hepatitis despite malnutrition [211]. Other factors suggested as contributory to the adverse outcome of acute viral hepatitis in pregnancy have included hormonal changes [212], which may impair cellular immunity [213], but proof is lacking. Furthermore, evidence has accumulated that enhanced, rather than impaired, cellular immunity may play a role in the development of severe, including fulminant, hepatitis B (see acute liver failure, below). The suggestion that an enhanced coagulopathy may contribute to the excess mortality in pregnant women [208] does not take into account the common observation of the severely deranged coagulation status seen in all varieties of acute liver failure regardless of pregnancy [214,215]. Age and parity have no overriding effect on maternal and fetal outcome [204,206].

FETAL ISSUES

Areas of concern regarding the fetus are the risk of vertical transmission from the mother, including from amniocentesis and routes of delivery, and outcome especially the propensity to develop chronic infection and liver disease.

Amniocentesis

Amniocentesis in mothers who are HBV carriers does not seem to expose the infant to increased risk of HBV infection [216]. Data are insufficient to determine risks of transmission for HCV in relation to amniocentesis.

Caesarean section

There is no evidence that caesarean section protects against vertical transmission of HBV from mother to child. Data are insufficient to make a judgement on the other hepatotropic agents.

Breastfeeding

This is not contraindicated for viral hepatitis in pregnancy. The HAV and HBV vaccines are safe for breast-feeding mothers. Breastfeeding is not contraindicated with neonatal and maternal immunization.

Avoiding breastfeeding and immediate separation from the infectious mother do not prevent transmission of HBV infection within the first 6 months. The US Centers for Disease Control (CDC) and American College of Pediatrics do not recommend any precautions specific to hepatitis C for infected pregnant women and their babies. Breastfeeding is not contraindicated. HCV RNA and anti-HCV antibodies have been detected in colostrum and breast milk but show no correlation with levels in maternal serum.

Fetal outcome

The majority, although not all [27], of studies predating the 1980s have shown an increase in rate of intrauterine death and stillbirths [208,211,217,218] and prematurity [204,206,211,217,218]. A prospective study from Zagreb in 1986 [205], of 43 pregnant women with serologically defined acute uncomplicated viral hepatitis (A, 18%; B, 58%; non-A, non-B, 24%) showed an increase (27%) of preterm delivery. There do not seem to be any increased risks of spontaneous abortion, stillbirth, intrauterine growth restriction or congenital abnormalities following hepatitis A in pregnancy [204,205], although large specific surveys are lacking.

No excess in incidence of congenital abnormalities has been reported in retrospective [204,219], and prospective [220,221], studies.

No specific therapies are recommended for hepatitis A through E during pregnancy. Interferons, ribavirin, nucleoside analogues, ganciclovir and foscarnet are contraindicated in pregnancy (see herpes viruses, below for use of aciclovir).

Obstetric issues for specific major hepatotropic agents

HEPATITIS A VIRUS

HAV is endemic worldwide. HAV is an enteric RNA-containing virus spread predominantly by ingesting water contaminated with sewage (faecal–oral route) [222].

Transmission of HAV is almost exclusively horizontal via the faecal–oral route. In obstetric practice, vertical and perinatal transmission of HAV occur typically via contamination of maternal faeces in a mother presenting with hepatitis A in the third trimester or soon after delivery [197,223]. Faecal contamination during delivery is limited by the short interval of viral excretion.

Maternal issues

The prevalence of previous infection, determined by detecting IgG anti-HAV antibodies, relates inversely to standards of sanitation. Almost universal exposure occurs in infancy and childhood in the developing countries especially in Asia and the East, Africa, India, certain Mediterranean countries and South America. In contrast, infections among children and young adults in northern Europe, including the UK, and the USA have fallen in response to improved standards of hygiene [224]. Diagnosis of acute HAV infection relies on the detection of IgM anti-HAV antibodies in serum (Table 9.4). In pregnancy, testing is mandatory to make a diagnosis and exclude other causes. Testing for IgG anti-HAV is useful to demonstrate immunity in patients exposed to an index case and prior to travel abroad.

Fetal issues

Transmission of HAV from the mother to child is rare during the neonatal period [218,223,225–227]. Outbreaks of severe hepatitis A have been reported in paediatric intensive care units [228–233] and attributed to transfusion of contaminated blood [229,230] and to vertical transmission [231] with horizontal spread from attendant health-care personnel [228,230]. Severe infection, including acute liver failure, is rare but has been documented in this setting accompanied with sepsis and multiorgan failure.

Four recent case studies have documented vertical transmission following acute hepatitis A during pregnancy. In one case, the mother presented with jaundice immediately after delivery at 33 weeks' gestation [233]. In the second case, the mother contracted hepatitis A during the first trimester and remained unwell until after delivery [223]. In both cases, transmission occurred presumably from faecal contamination around delivery as HAV RNA was not detected in cord blood. HAV RNA was documented in serum in both cases and in faeces from the first baby at 32 (but not 101) days after birth [233]. In the first report [233], immunoglobulin was administered on day 5, IgM anti-HAV remained undetectable and the baby remained symptomless. In the second case [223], a naturally occurring (non-passaged) HAV variant originating in India was associated with severe, protracted hepatitis A in the pregnant mother and, subsequently in her baby born 4 months later. The third and fourth cases favour intrauterine transmission and document perforated ileum with meconium peritonitis and ascites in the fetus at 20 and 34 weeks' gestation, respectively, following maternal hepatitis A diagnosed during the first trimester [226,227].

Management

This is not affected by pregnancy. Hepatitis A and other causes of viral hepatitis occur more frequently as pregnancy progresses with a peak onset in the third trimester [204,205]. Whether symptoms in jaundiced cases are more likely than in anicteric cases, remains uncertain and may reflect the bias of reporting severe cases. In one prospective study [205] only 28.5% of cases were anicteric compared to 77.7% for non-A, non-B and 4.5% for hepatitis B.

Hepatitis A is a self-limiting illness noted for its complete recovery. A chronic carrier state is not recognized in humans. Occasionally, recovery may be delayed with protracted cholestasis and a biphasic course. Acute liver failure is rare [215] and not especially common in pregnancy (contrast hepatitis E and herpes hepatitis below).

Table 9.4 Serological diagnosis of acute and chronic viral hepatitis.

	A	B	C	D	E
Acute infection	IgM anti-HAV	IgM anti-HBc	IgM assays not commerically available	IgM anti-HDV	IgM-anti-HEV
Virus replication	HAV RNA	HBV DNA	HCV RNA	HDV RNA	HEV RNA
Chronic infection	N/A	HBV DNA HBsAg	HCV RNA HDAg (liver)	HDV RNA	N/A
Past infection	IgG anti-HAV	IgG anti-HBc	N/K	IgG anti-HDV	IgG anti-HEV
Past exposure	IgG anti-HAV	anti-HBs	N/K	IgG anti-HDV	IgG anti-HEV

N/A, not applicable; N/K, not known.

Protection and prophylaxis

Hepatitis A is most infectious in the presymptomatic phase prior to jaundice and early symptomatic phase when virus is excreted in stool. Poor personal hygiene and sanitation favour epidemics. Exposure to HAV is almost universal in promiscuous subjects, especially with oro-anal intercourse [234]. The risk of transmission rapidly wanes with development of symptoms and jaundice.

Normal immune globulin (NIG) contains antibodies to HAV (and also HBV; see below) and has been used as effective passive immunoprophylaxis for more than 40 years [235,236]. Intramuscular IG is safe if prepared to standards agreed by the World Health Organization and when given by the intramuscular route [237,238]. A single dose of 0.02 mL/kg given by deep, intramuscular injection immediately following an exposure, gives a protective efficacy rate of around 80% short term. IG can protect or attenuate the illness if given up to 2 weeks following exposure (contrast hepatitis B). This is surprising for a virus with an average incubation of 4 weeks. IG is recommended following close and sexual contacts with an index case and during an epidemic. Day-care centres for infants and institutions for custodial care are important settings for transmission. Immediate contacts of an index case should receive immunoprophylaxis (236–238).

Postexposure immunoprophylaxis may not prevent shedding of HAV in stool. Isolation of potentially infectious subjects is important in limiting spread in epidemics. No specific recommendations have been made for IG during pregnancy. IG should be given to symptomless women in contact with an index case during the third trimester in view of the increased rate of preterm deliveries [205]. Pregnant women about to travel to high-prevalence areas should be considered for prophylaxis with IG. Travellers should be prescreened for IgG anti-HAV antibodies to prevent unnecessary immunization because at least one-third will be found to be immune [239].

Neonatal hepatitis A should be considered if the mother develops features of infection in the puerperium or has been given IG, which may prolong the period of faecal excretion of HAV. Neonatal immunoprophylaxis is rarely necessary as most neonatal infections are mild and life-long immunity follows recovery.

NIG contains anti-HAV antibodies (and anti-HBs antibodies) and should be considered in the preterm neonate especially if exposed to HAV in the intensive care unit. Doses typically are between 0.06 and 0.12 mL/kg and offer some protection for around 2–3 months [197]. NIG may not be completely protective during outbreaks.

In 1992 in Europe at least one inactivated, whole-virus HAV vaccine was licensed for parenteral administration. No information is available for pregnancy but data show safety and high immunogenicity in the non-pregnant population.

The HAV vaccines are not licensed for children aged below 2 years. Similarly, the combined vaccines against HAV and HBV cannot be used as part of neonatal immunization against HBV. Whether universal active immunization against HAV of very young children is warranted requires assessment. The duration of protective immunity long term (>20 years) is unknown. The majority of infections are symptomless below the age of 5 years and this natural immunity is lifelong.

HEPATITIS E

HEV, like HAV, is spread by the faeco-oral route and causes acute self-limited hepatitis [197]. HEV infection is endemic in a zone stretching from Morocco to Hong Kong as well as in Central and South America.

Maternal issue

HEV and herpes simplex viruses (see below) have the propensity to cause severe disease in pregnancy in some regions of the world. In the study from Kashmir [209] acute liver failure was reported in 22.2% of pregnant, compared with less than 3% of non-pregnant, women. The hepatitis was more frequent and severe in late pregnancy; 9% developed hepatitis in the first trimester. This rose to approximately 19% in the second and third trimesters. Maternal deaths (44%) only occurred in late pregnancy [209]. In Rangoon, of 399 cases of hepatitis, the case-fatality rate among pregnant women was up to 12 times that for non-pregnant females and males for non-A, non-B, likely hepatitis E, but not hepatitis B [240].

Whether the severe outcome in pregnancy in developing countries reflects virus virulence, variants or host factors, especially malnutrition, remains inconclusive. For example, epidemic forms of non-A, non-B hepatitis from Japan [241] showed no especial adverse outcome in pregnancy.

Fetal issues

Transmission via faecal contamination during the perinatal period from a mother who contracts HEV during late pregnancy is feasible but not well documented due to the limited time for faecal excretion of virus. Intrauterine death is common with epidemics of severe hepatitis E that affect pregnant women in certain regions and due probably to the profound hypoglycaemia seen in the ensuing acute liver failure (see acute liver failure, below).

Management

Management does not differ from the non-pregnant counterpart. This is optimal in a centre with expertise in maternal and fetal intensive care, hepatology and infectious diseases (see acute liver failure, below).

Protection and immunoprophylaxis

Secondary spread to contacts is uncommon. Nevertheless, as with HAV, handling of faeces and bile should be minimized by washing hands thoroughly and disposing of contaminated clothes and fomites by autoclaving and incineration.

There are no forms of immunoprophylaxis against HEV. Pregnant personnel are best advised to avoid contact with cases of suspected HEV.

HEPATITIS B

Hepatitis B is a global public health problem. Worldwide, at least 280 million individuals are chronically infected with HBV. This is a major cause of liver disease worldwide, including chronic hepatitis, cirrhosis and primary liver cancer. In the West, the chronic carrier rate is between 0.5% and 5% of the general population.

In the USA, the reservoir of infectious carriers may be as high as one million [242]. More than 300 000 Americans become infected annually. Up to 30 000 of these can be expected to become hepatitis B surface antigen (HBsAg)-seropositive chronic carriers. Each year, more than 4000 Americans die from related cirrhosis and 800 from primary liver cancer [242,243].

HBV infection is spread predominantly via parenteral exposure, especially among intravenous drug users, and by sexual contact. Consecutive surveys from the CDC [244] between 1981 and 1988 showed that the number of reports of acute hepatitis B attributed to parenteral drug use rose by 80% and to heterosexual contact by 38%. The peak prevalence was in individuals aged 15–29 years, compared with less than 1% below 15 years and 26% for those aged 30–44 years.

Serological responses

The consensus view is that HBV is not cytopathic. Clearance of virus depends on the host's immune attack [197]. Serological responses remain the cornerstone of diagnosis of acute (see Table 9.4) and chronic infection. Acute infec-

tion typically leads to the detection of HBsAg in blood 2–8 weeks before development of abnormal serum liver biochemistry and onset of symptoms. Serum HBsAg usually remains detectable until the convalescent phase. Hepatitis B 'e' antigen (HBeAg) becomes detectable soon after HBsAg. HBeAg is a marker of high infectivity and closely associated with the inner core (HBcAg) and HBV DNA. IgG anti-HBc is present in the serum of HBsAg-positive chronic carrier mothers and may play an important role in immunomodulation of fetal serological responses to HBV infection.

In uncomplicated acute hepatitis B, recovery is associated with rapid clearance of serum HBV DNA and detection of anticore antibodies (IgM and, soon after, IgG), shortly followed by anti-HBe, with decline and disappearance of HBeAg and HBsAg antigenaemia within 3 months. The subsequent 'window' phase, defined by the serological presence of anti-HBc in the absence of HBeAg and anti-HBs, persists for 2–16 weeks. This phase terminates with detection of anti-HBs signalling recovery, viral clearance and immunity from future HBV infection. The window phase probably is an artefact. HBsAg can be detected using monoclonal antibodies and HBV DNA by PCR. Importantly, a pregnant woman who presents with acute hepatitis B, especially acute liver failure, may be misdiagnosed as having a non-B hepatitis if only HBsAg is sought using conventional polyclonal reagents. Serological testing for high-titre IgM anti-HBc is mandatory for the diagnosis of acute infection. Additional infection with delta virus can lead to an inhibition of the serological markers of HBV (see Table 9.4, and hepatitis D, below).

Acute hepatitis B

Infection may remain symptomless and anicteric. Any symptoms are non-specific such as a 'flu-like' illness, malaise, anorexia, nausea and vomiting and occasionally arthralgias and a skin rash. Clinically, hepatitis B cannot be distinguished easily from hepatitis due to other viruses, drugs, alcohol and autoimmune diseases.

While most adults clear the HBV (Fig. 9.3) within 1–3 months, clinical recovery from uncomplicated infection may take several months. A biphasic illness with resurgence of serum levels of transaminase and bilirubin is seen more commonly than with hepatitis A. At the other end of the spectrum is progression to acute liver failure with a mortality of more than 50%. Fortunately this is rare, especially in pregnancy [13,214], and accounts for fewer than 1% of hospitalized cases of acute viral hepatitis [197].

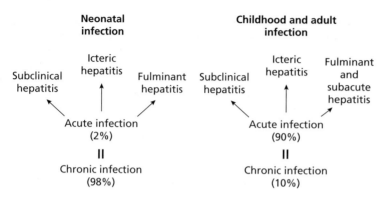

Fig 9.3 Contrasting presentations and outcomes between neonatal, childhood and adult HBV infection.

Chronic hepatitis B

The propensity for chronic infection depends on the age of acquisition (Fig. 9.3). Chronic infection is more likely with mild, anicteric illness. Conversely, chronic infection is uncommon following severe symptomatic hepatitis B, including fulminant hepatitis B.

The chronic carrier is defined as having seropositivity for HBsAg for a minimum of 6 months. At least half of long-term chronic carriers will die eventually from virus-related liver disease including chronic hepatitis, cirrhosis and its complications (see cirrhosis below). The lifetime risk of a chronic carrier from neonatal infection developing primary liver cancer may be as high as 40%, at least in high-prevalence areas [245]. In Taiwan and Korea, prevention of infection by instigation of a comprehensive neonatal immunization programme against HBV led to a reduction by more than 50% of primary liver cancer in children aged 6–14 years [246].

While the risk of developing primary liver cancer may be less in the West, HBV remains an important cause of chronic liver disease, cirrhosis and primary liver cancer. Spontaneous seroconversion from HBeAg to anti-HBe and from HBsAg to anti-HBs with clearance of virus following neonatal acquisition of virus is uncommon [247,248]. (See outcomes of neonatal infection (below) for further discussion of chronic hepatitis B.)

Maternal issues (see also amniocentesis and fertility, above). In prospective studies from Sydney [249] and Montreal [250] the prevalence of HBsAg seropositivity among blood donors and pregnant women was 0.07% and 1.9% respectively. HBsAg positivity among native Australian antenatal patients correlated with previous intravenous drug use, hepatitis, occupational exposure, blood transfusion, living in an institution and birth in Indo-China [249] or Africa [250]. The Montreal questionnaire was completed

by 30 315 pregnant women from nine hospitals between 1982 and 1984 [250]. Only around half of the seropositive Canadians declared a risk factor. Exposure to intravenous recreational drugs was sought only in the Australian study and found to be common.

For Senegal, there is no correlation between maternal HBsAg status and epidemiological factors such as parity, age, tribal origin, previous blood transfusion and caesarean section [251]. Other horizontally acting factors must explain the vast excess over anticipated numbers of chronic carriers. Direct evidence is lacking but scarification rituals, blood-sucking vectors and close person-to-person contact may account for some of the spread.

There is no evidence that a pregnant woman with acute or chronic hepatitis B pursues a more severe course than her non-pregnant counterpart. As with other types of viral hepatitis, the frequency of preterm delivery is increased when HBV is contracted in the third trimester [204].

Fetal issues. The impact of hepatitis B in obstetric practice is greatly underestimated. Transmission typically goes unnoticed. Symptoms are uncommon and non-specific, and disease becomes manifest only after many years. Serological responses remain the cornerstone of diagnosis of acute and chronic infection.

Three major, interrelated areas are of concern: (i) vertical transmission in neonates and horizontal transmission in early childhood; (ii) the propensity of the newborn of infected mothers to become a chronic carrier and its consequences; and (iii) the potential to irradicate HBV via immunoprophylaxis.

Vertical transmission. Acute hepatitis B infection occurring in late pregnancy and around delivery [204,252–254] favours vertical transmission from mother to child before or around birth. In one study from California [225] the risk of vertical transmission for mothers with acute hepatitis B manifest during the first (0%) and second trimesters (6%), respectively, was significantly less than that for the third trimester (67%) and within 5 weeks postpartum (100%).

Up to 40% of all chronic carriers of HBV arise following vertical transmission. Babies born of HBsAg-positive mothers with serological evidence of virus replication (seropositive for HBeAg and/or HBV DNA) have between a 20 and 95% chance of becoming infected, depending on the maternal ethnic origin [251,255–259].

Ethnic origin, especially coming from the Far East, is important even for mothers residing in low-prevalence countries [249,256,257,260,261]. As part of a large-scale, controlled prospective study on the efficacy of the hepatitis B vaccine among babies born of HBeAg-positive mothers in Taiwan, 95% without immunoprophylaxis became infected acutely and 93% became infected chronically by the sixth month of follow-up [262]. Studies from Hong Kong [263] showed a similar attack rate in unprotected infants.

It is not understood why vertical transmission from high-risk carrier mothers is much less frequent in certain regions, particularly in Senegal and Kenya (approximately 20%), than in the Far East [264]. Ethnic differences may reflect maternal levels of HBV DNA [251,265,266] but this has been disputed [261]. Standardization of assays for quantification of HBV DNA is required and comparisons made for general populations from different ethnic groups. Serum levels of HBV DNA in HBeAg-positive non-pregnant carriers seem to be much higher in Orientals than in Africans [266,267]. Furthermore, 58.3% of anti-HBe-seropositive Orientals had detectable levels of serum HBV DNA compared with only 13.3% of Africans and 5.5% of Northern Europeans [267].

Vertical transmission can occur in up to 25% of cases where the HBsAg-positive mother is HBeAg negative and in up to 12% of cases where the mother is anti-HBe positive [268]. There was no correlation with maternal seropositivity for IgM anti-HBc, an indirect measure of virus replication, in chronic carrier mothers and subsequent vertical transmission in Taiwan [259].

Most transmissions between mother and child occur at or around the time of birth. There is little serological evidence of infection in the newborn for acute hepatitis B before the third trimester [204,252,253,254,269]. In the infected neonate, serum HBsAg becomes detectable typically around 3 months implicating transmission around delivery. Specific high-titre IgM anti-HBc, an accurate predictor of recent infection, is absent in neonatal sera [270]. HBsAg, if present in cord blood, is often in low titre

and reflects contamination with maternal blood during delivery. The most persuasive argument against infection occurring *in utero* is the success of perinatal immunoprophylaxis [256,262,263,271] (see immunoprophylaxis, below).

Transmission postpartum can occur via mixing of maternal and fetal blood [272], contact with cervicovaginal epithelial cells shown to be positive for HBV DNA and ingestion of amniotic fluid [272] and breast milk that contains detectable HBsAg [273,274].

Although transmission usually occurs at or around the time of birth, evidence has accumulated in favour of infection *in utero* in some cases. Avoidance of breastfeeding, delivery by caesarean section and immediate separation from the infectious mother do not prevent subsequent infection within the first 6 months. Transplacental transmission seems to be common at least in the Far East. HBV DNA was detected in 44% of fetal livers from mothers following abortion [275]. This route may explain failure to protect up to 15% of neonates born of HBsAg-positive mothers despite optimum administration of immunoprophylaxis postpartum [256,275]. Also, following administration at birth of hepatitis B immune globulin (HBIG) containing high-titre anti-HBs and anti-HBc, levels of anti-HBs rise again after their initial predicted falls [271]. This pattern suggests passive–active immunity from exposure predating immunoprophylaxis.

In the HBsAg-seropositive mother, maternal anti-HBc antibody traverses the placenta leading to immunomodulation of fetal responses to the virus. Maternal anti-HBc antibody can suppress expression of viral antigens (HBsAg, HBcAg) and replication in the fetus that only responds to HBV-associated antigens when levels of maternal antibodies fall, typically around 3–6 months of age. HBIG may prevent neonatal infection by protracting the time period of effective inhibitory antibody on virus replication until maturation of the fetal immune system occurs after the first 2 months of life. Thereafter, the baby can mount an effective immune response, clear HBV and develop immunity (anti-HBs, anti-HBc) to future infection. In acute infection, HBcAg and HBsAg are expressed on the surface of infected hepatocytes. Maternal IgG anti-HBc may block recognition of virus-infected cells by cytotoxic T cells. Early exposure to soluble virus protein may induce a state of immune tolerance to virus antigen via induction of specific T-suppressor cells that serve also to inhibit the cytotoxic attack by the host. Also, maturation of the hepatocyte may be a prerequisite before virus replication can occur.

Horizontal transmission. Person-to-person contact [276], especially within communal living [277], is important in the West, the Mediterranean Littoral [278], the Middle East, Saudi Arabia and parts of Africa including Kenya [251], Senegal [264], Namibia [277], Nigeria [279], Zambia [280], Liberia [281], and New Zealand and Pacific Islands [282]. Up to 60% of neonates born of HBsAg-seropositive mothers who seem to escape vertical transmission become infected within 5 years [283]. The risk of spread from an infected neonate to susceptible members of an adopted, new household can be significant [278].

Outcome of neonatal infection. Retrospective [204] and prospective [220] studies have failed to demonstrate any increase in congenital abnormalities, in particular Down's syndrome [284,285], following maternal acute and chronic HBV infection.

The major concern is the propensity for developing chronic infection following infection with HBV within the first years of life (Fig. 9.3). Chronic carriage is uncommon in babies born following *acute* hepatitis B in the third trimester [286], and of carrier mothers with serological evidence of low levels of virus replication [287,288]. In the Californian study of acute hepatitis B in late pregnancy [225], HBsAg was detected in 12 of 18 babies at 1–3 months of age but none became a chronic carrier.

In contrast, over 90% of babies born to HBeAg-positive chronically infected mothers eventually show serological evidence of infection [245,262]. Furthermore, the vast majority will become chronic carriers—remain HBsAg seropositive for more than 6 months—into adult life [245,262]. This compares with only 1–10% of otherwise healthy adults becoming chronic carriers (Fig. 9.3) [289] following transmission in adulthood.

All neonates born to mothers seropositive for HBsAg and HBeAg are infected with HBV if HBeAg is detected in uncontaminated cord blood. Persistence of HBeAg beyond the second month is also predictive of chronic carriage. Conversely, a rapid reduction in titre of HBeAg after birth may predict subsequent clearance of virus and seroconversion to anti-HBs [258]. Genetic susceptibility to HBV infection via an autosomal recessive gene [290] remains unproven [291] and may be accounted for by differing levels of HBV DNA in the mothers.

Factors other than maternal anti-HBc influence the development of the chronic carrier state following neonatal infection. Development of a chronic carrier state correlates with the finding of high-titre [257,262] HBsAg found in cord blood that probably relates to the presence of maternal HBV DNA.

Chronic carriage is common among children born of HBsAg-positive carrier (HBeAg-negative/anti-HBe-negative) mothers if exposure to infection is delayed

beyond the first year [264]. In Senegal where horizontal transmission predominates, acquisition of HBV infection is typically delayed beyond the first 5 months of life [264]. Out of 34 such babies who showed no serological evidence of infection until the second year, four of six eventually became chronic carriers; none developed acute liver failure [264].

Chronic infection is uncommon in babies born to HBsAg-positive mothers with anti-HBe [287] and mothers also seronegative for HBeAg. Instead, these babies are at risk of severe acute neonatal hepatitis, including progression to acute liver failure [292–296]. Survivors show serological evidence of clearance of virus and subsequent immunity (anti-HBs) to future infection [294].

In adults as well as in babies, chronicity tends to follow a mild, anicteric illness [294]. The risk of developing the chronic carrier state in neonatal life and infancy is related to gender of the child and inversely to age at exposure (Fig. 9.3) [248]. In Senegal a gradation of risk of chronic carriage also was demonstrated within the first year; 82% of those infected before 6 months compared with 54% for infections between 6 and 12 months [248]. As in adults, males were more likely (87%) to become carriers than females (55%).

Management

Antenatal screening. All pregnant women should be screened for HBsAg and IgM anti-HBc antibodies. Seropositive mothers must be identified before delivery and in them screening for HBsAg should be extended to the family and close, especially sexual, contacts and children. Susceptible contacts should be offered immunization with vaccine and HBIG.

Neonatal immunoprophylaxis is most efficient if commenced at birth. Universal prenatal screening in the USA is estimated to identify 22 000 HBsAg-seropositive women. This strategy should prevent annually 3000 chronic infections and is cost saving [268,297,298]. Previous strategies from the National Center of Health Statistics in the USA until 1988 selected only high-risk women for screening. One-half or less of seropositive women are identified from demographic and epidemiological characteristics [268, 278].

Maternal immunization. Testing for HBsAg should be repeated in late pregnancy and postpartum in seronegative mothers with suspected acute infection or continued exposure to an HBsAg-positive subject via sexual, ocular and mucosal contact, needlestick, intravenous drug abuse, blood transfusion and parenteral exposures [237] (see indications for immunoprophylaxis, below).

Mothers with suspected *acute* infection should be tested also for IgM anti-HBc as a reliable marker of recent infection (Table 9.4). Seronegativity for HBsAg, anti-HBc and anti-HBs identifies susceptible individuals who require vaccination. A mother belonging to high-risk groups (Box 9.2). who presents in labour without prescreening, should be managed as high risk, until results become available. Her newborn must be considered high risk and immunoprophylaxis commenced immediately, and if necessary, before serological tests are confirmed. The decision to complete the immunization schedule should be assessed on the risk of future exposure via horizontal transmission (see above) [251,264,277,279–282], the serological results in the mother, and the cost of completion and follow-up. Babies born to mothers only identified as HBsAg positive more than 1 month after birth, such as at the postnatal visit, should be screened for HBsAg as evidence of recent infection and for anti-HBc and anti-HBs as markers of previous exposure with immunity. Seronegative babies should commence an immunization course without delay (see below).

Antiviral therapies. Following delivery, HBsAg-seropositive carrier mothers with serological evidence of virus

---

Box 9.2 High-risk women for hepatitis B presenting in pregnancy (after MMWR 1985 [238])
- Women from high-prevalence areas, whether immigrant or UK born:
  The Far East, SE Asia, Mediterranean, Middle East, United Arab Emirates, Sub-Saharan Africa, Haiti, Asian, Pacific Island or Alaskan Eskimo.
- Women with histories of:
  Acute or chronic liver disease
  Frequent occupational exposure to blood in medical or dental care:
  e.g. work or treat high-risk patients: in haemodialysis; work or residing in institutions for the mentally handicapped
  Rejection as a blood donor
  Multiple transfusions
  Tattoos from a high-risk area of the world or suspected contaminated needles
  Intravenous drug use
  Impaired immune responses
  Episodes of venereal disease
  Household and/or sexual contact with suspected HBV carrier:
  high-risk groups: with a bisexual partner, high-risk immigrant

---

replication (HBV DNA) should be considered for treatment with interferons. Clearance of HBsAg with seroconversion eventually to anti-HBs can be achieved in about half of adult females especially those with recent infection, elevated liver enzymes and chronic hepatitis. Long-standing viral persistence, impaired cell-mediated host defences and tolerance to the virus may explain the disappointing results of antiviral therapies for neonatally acquired infection. The long-term success of eradicating neonatally acquired HBV infection will depend on clearance of infected hepatocytes before integration of viral sequences and development of cirrhosis has occurred.

Prevention of transmission to the neonate. Caesarean section does not prevent transmission from an HBsAg-positive mother to her newborn. Provided immunization has commenced, the neonate need not be isolated from its mother and breastfeeding is not contraindicated [268]. Care should be taken to prevent the infant from direct contact with blood-soaked dressings and pads. Lactation is not a contraindication to receiving the hepatitis B vaccine.

Passive immunoprophylaxis. Specific HBIG contains high-titre anti-HBs and anti-HBc and offers good passive protection if given within 36 h of exposure to an HBsAg-positive subject or material [268,297]. Exposure includes babies born of infectious mothers and following needle-stick injury, sexual, ocular and mucosal contact [237,299]. IG, previously denoted as gammaglobulin, is used primarily as passive immunoprophylaxis against hepatitis A. IG contains moderate titres of anti-HBs (as well as anti-HAV antibodies) and should be used if HBIG is not available. The IGs offer only temporary protection. They are expensive, limited in supply and effective only if given immediately following a definite exposure. Many subjects requiring immediate protection remain at future risk from repeated exposure and should be assessed for vaccination. Examples include babies born of infectious mothers with acute [294] or chronic hepatitis B, the sexual partner of an HBsAg-positive carrier, an intravenous drug abuser and health-care personnel.

Passive immunoprophylaxis has been administered effectively and safely for more than 20 years. No specific adverse effects have been reported among many women later discovered to be pregnant. There is no evidence that preparations made to the specifications of the World Health Organization and administered intramuscularly transmit any blood-borne infections including HIV [237,238].

Active immunoprophylaxis. Hepatitis B immunization has been reviewed elsewhere [197,244,283,297,300]. Safe, efficacious vaccines have been licensed for clinical practice in the UK and USA since 1982. Several recombinant vaccines have been manufactured and licensed for clinical use since the late 1980s in the USA and Europe. In the West in clinical practice, these have superseded the plasma-derived vaccines. The HBsAg subunits (approximately 20 nm) are synthesized by molecular biology techniques rather than harvested from plasma of chronic carriers prior to rigorous inactivation. The recombinant and plasma vaccines share similar immunogenic properties including immunization schedules and numbers of suboptimal responses. Their safety has been endorsed by the World Health Organization [301] and the Immunization Practices Advisory Committee [268,297]. Serious adverse reactions are rare. Soreness at the site of injection and a low-grade fever occur in less than 5% of vaccinees.

Maternal immunization. Prudent practice dictates that no immunization be offered routinely in pregnancy or in cases of known allergy to the individual vaccine components (alum adsorbent and preservative). Manufacturers do not recommend immunization in pregnancy. However, in obstetric practice there are no specific contraindications to administering HBIG and a licensed hepatitis B vaccine. No specific adverse consequences have been reported among many women who received intramuscular IGs and vaccine and later were found to be pregnant. There is no possibility of transmission of viruses. The licensed vaccines are not made from whole virus, and inactivation procedures are exhaustive.

Immunization should not be withheld during pregnancy and lactation if a woman is perceived to be at high risk from HBV infection and provided she is assessed carefully and counselled. She should be pre-screened to avoid unnecessary immunization. Immunization with vaccine and HBIG should be offered only to susceptible women defined as seronegative for HBsAg, anti-HBc and anti-HBs and who remain at risk from repeated exposure from a regular HBsAg-seropositive sexual partner, occupation and intravenous drug use [237]. Immunization should be postponed with intercurrent infection to avoid exacerbation of fever.

All licensed vaccines require multiple, spaced doses administered as a deep intramuscular injection in the deltoid or anterior thigh. Anti-HBs levels are lower when administered into the fatty buttock or intradermally. Concern over the safety of multisite, automatic injectors for mass immunization and reduced efficacies of routes other than intramuscular have limited their appeal in mass vaccination.

The spacing of doses at times 0, 1, 2 and 12 months is superior to original recommendations for 0, 1 and 6 months in terms of speed of development and duration of detectable anti-HBs levels. The immunogenicity and protective efficacy rates exceed 90% in young adults. In adults, HBIG is usually given as a single dose (500 IU) by deep intramuscular injection at a contralateral site to the vaccine, and using a new disposable needle and syringe. There is no evidence of interaction when active and passive immunization are administered concurrently at separate sites [255]. Prior to the advent of effective vaccines, a second dose of HBIG was recommended 1 month later to complete postexposure passive prophylaxis [237]. This is unnecessary when a vaccine course has commenced unless there is uncertainty over the immune responsiveness of the vaccinee (see suboptimal responders, below). Proof of additional protective efficacy in the adult following a second dose of HBIG is lacking and doses should be conserved where supplies are limited. HBIG has limited protective efficacy if delayed 48 h or more after an exposure. In contrast, the hepatitis B vaccine can offer protection even if administered up to 2 weeks following an exposure [255]. HBV infection may be detected serologically but symptoms are uncommon and minor; seroconversion to anti-HBs is rapid and chronic carriage uncommon [255]. No information is available regarding transmission to the fetus following maternal immunization for acute HBV infection in pregnancy, but an optimistic outcome is likely in view of the rapid seroconversion in the mother.

Protection of health-care personnel. Immunization with hepatitis B vaccine is recommended for all clinical health-care personnel in direct and regular contact with patients [301,302].

Isolation and barrier nursing are unnecessary but direct contact with blood-soaked dressings and pads should be avoided. All attendants should wear protective clothing, cover exposed cuts and abrasions, and handle body fluids with care. Goggles and masks should be worn for anticipated splashes onto ocular and mucosal surfaces [303]. Five of 12 clusters involving transmitted HBV from health-care personnel to patients occurred in obstetricians and gynaecologists performing invasive procedures [303].

Neonatal immunization. Concurrent active and passive immunization is the prophylaxis of choice for preventing hepatitis B infection.

In 1992, the World Health Assembly endorsed the universal immunization targets for 1997 set by their Global Advisory Group to integrate hepatitis B vaccine into the Expanded Programme of Immunization (EPI). The strategy favouring universal immunization replaced selective targeting of high-risk groups that failed to make any epidemiological impact on hepatitis B infection. In the USA, the Immunization Practices Advisory Committee has recommended universal immunization of all babies regardless of maternal HBV status and teenagers and young adults where intravenous drug use and sexually transmitted diseases are common [268,297]. In countries with limited resources immunoprophylaxis should be given as priority to all infants born of HBsAg-positive mothers regardless of maternal ethnic origin and HBeAg and anti-HBe status.

Results with recombinant and plasma-derived vaccines are similar. In two important randomized controlled trials from Taiwan [262] and Hong Kong [263] the overall protective efficacy rate for dual immunoprophylaxis exceeded 93%. HBIG must be given in adequate dose as soon as possible after delivery (Table 9.5). Ideally, vaccine should be administered at the same time but at a different site and using a different disposable needle and syringe. There is no contraindication to the concurrent administration of other vaccines against polio, diptheria, tetanus or pertussis [268].

In the neonate, vaccination, but not HBIG, may be postponed up to 7 days after delivery with preservation of good (>90%) protective efficacy [237,238,262,304]. Whether any longer delay is justified in a high-risk neonate with an intercurrent bacterial infection is undecided.

Typical schedules are doses at 0, 1, 2 and 12 months and 0, 1 and 6 months. Doses vary according to the manufacturers' recommendations.

Side-effects of immunization. These are notably uncommon, apart from minor local reactions at the site of the injection and given the many million doses administered safely to newborn babies, children and adults.

Reports of neurological abnormalities following immunization include individual cases of Guillain–Barré syndrome, aseptic meningitis, transverse myelitis, seizures and later development of multiple sclerosis. These findings along with reports on an increase incidence of diabetes mellitus are considered to occur by random association.

Combination vaccines. Multivalent vaccines against hepatitis A and B have been licensed in Europe and the USA for children aged above 2 years and adults. A typical dose for the adult contains 720 ELISA Units HAAg and 20 µg HBsAg. These amounts are reduced 50% for the paediatric dose.

Immunization failures. The licensed hepatitis B vaccines are highly immunogenic and efficacious, especially in neonates. Approximately 5% of neonates and children and 10–20% of adults have a poor response (anti-HBs <100 IU/L). Failures are attributed to a genetically predetermined poor response, infection *in utero* (see vertical transmission, above), immunosuppression from intercurrent infection, in particular, HIV [305], drugs, other diseases (see vertical transmission, above) and the emergence of antibody escape variants of HBV.

The optimal policy for the poor responder groups has not been defined. The safest policy for poor responder adults continually exposed, such as health-care personnel, would be to ignore previous immunization. Instead, poor responders should be offered HBIG (and an additional dose of vaccine if some response is anticipated) following a definite exposure such as needlestick and await arrival of more immunogenic vaccines. Whether additional doses are justified in paediatric practice in the hope of some protection in poor- and non-responders has not been decided.

HEPATITIS D VIRUS

Patients with acute and chronic HBsAg-seropositive infection are at additional risk from hepatitis delta virus (HDV) [306,307]. Importantly, prevention of HBV via immunoprophylaxis protects against HDV infection. The decline in incidence of new HBV infections in certain areas, such as Italy, parallels the fall in HBV infection.

This highly pathogenic RNA-containing virus is very small and relies on HBV for helper functions. HDV has been found wherever HBV is endemic, is spread by the same routes and accounts for significant morbidity and mortality in patients with HBV infection. High-prevalence areas of the world for HDV and HBV include the Mediterranean Littoral, especially southern Italy and Israel, South America and the Middle East. In Northern

Table 9.5 HBV perinatal postexposure recommendations of the Advisory Committee on Immunization Practices, 1991.	HBIG		Vaccine*	
	Dose	Timing	Dose†	Timing
	0.5 mL (250 IU)	Within 12 h	5–10 (µg i.m.)	Within 12 h

*First dose given concurrently with HBIG, but at different intramuscular sites. Schedules for basic course: 0, 1 and 6 months or 0, 1, 2 and 12 months.
†Dose and schedule depend on manufacturers' recommendations.

Europe and the USA, dual infection is confined predominantly to high-risk groups specifically intravenous drug users, immigrants from high-prevalence areas and the multiply transfused.

Vertical transmission

Vertical transmission of HDV occurs but requires high levels of HBV replication. In one study from Italy [308], development of anti-delta positivity as evidence of vertical transmission of HDV infection was found in one of seven babies of HBsAg-positive mothers who were also antidelta positive. Vertical transmission is unlikely to play as significant a role as that for HBV. Subjects superinfected with HDV may have sufficient chronic liver disease to impair fertility and preclude pregnancy (see chronic hepatitis, below). More studies are required where the status of virus replication (HBV DNA) in the mother is confirmed.

Horizontal transmission

Evidence comes from Italy. Clustering of cases is seen within HBsAg-positive families without obvious risk factors [309]. The relative roles of intimate contact between sexual partners and spread between siblings are unclear. Why the spread of HDV via sexual contact among heterosexuals and homosexuals who are not intravenous drug users is uncommon, is not clearly understood. HDV can suppress replication of HBV, measured by falling titres of serum HBsAg, HBV DNA and IgM anti-HBc, leading to misdiagnosis. Testing must include HDVAg, HDV RNA and anti-HDV, as well as markers of HBV infection. Serial testing for seroconversion from IgM to IgG anti-HDV may be required in suspected cases (Table 9.4).

Immunoprophylaxis

Successful passive and active immunoprophylaxis against HBV infection protect against HDV regardless of route of transmission.

HEPATITIS C

Worldwide, HCV, an RNA-containing virus related to the pestiviruses and flaviviruses, is a major cause of sporadic (community-acquired) hepatitis. Parenteral exposure via injection of recreational drugs remains a major risk factor for acquiring HCV infection. Hepatitis C is common among intravenous drug users, multiply-transfused individuals and HIV-seropositive subjects.

Prior to the advent of screening blood donors for anti-HCV antibodies in the 1990s, HCV also was a major cause of post-transfusion non-A, non-B hepatitis. Vertical and sexual transmissions are much less common for HCV than for HBV.

In the USA, about 3–4 million individuals are infected with the HCV [197,310] with an estimated annual incidence of new infections in 1996 of 36 000 [310,311]. Chronic hepatitis commonly follows acute infection. Progression to cirrhosis occurs in about 20% of individuals infected beyond 10 years. Individuals with cirrhosis are at risk of developing primary liver cancer especially in certain countries such as Japan.

Serological diagnosis

Cloning of part of the virus genome was published in 1989 alongside development of an antibody test [312, 313]. Since 1990, all blood donors in Europe and the USA have been tested routinely for antibodies to HCV.

Unlike for HBV, conventional tests for detecting HCV antigens are not available. Instead, diagnosis relies on detecting antibodies in immunoassays and HCV RNA using PCR-based molecular techniques (Fig. 9.4).

Current serological markers do not discriminate acute from chronic infection. Patterns of seroconversion are difficult to define as most patients present with acute-on-chronic, rather than *de novo* acute, infection. The diagnosis of acute infection can be overlooked; seroconversion can be delayed many weeks and discrimination from chronic infection is difficult. Results correlate well with detection of HCV RNA using PCR. This detects viraemia by amplifying as little as one molecule of virus [197].

Maternal outcome

Anti-HCV antibodies were identified in about 1–2% of a total of 4680 consecutive pregnant women attending two antenatal clinics in Italy [81,314]; eight had concurrent HIV infection. Only two showed any elevation in liver enzyme tests during pregnancy and within a 6-month follow-up, and there were no adverse maternal and fetal outcomes. In Ireland, after 17 years' follow-up of a cohort of 232 young women infected with HCV after receiving contaminated anti-D globulin, only 2.4% had developed cirrhosis; the vast majority remain symptomless and 45% had liver enzymes remaining within the normal range [315].

In contrast, reports of non-pregnant patients from liver transplant centres tend to emphasize the severity of chronic liver disease with progression to cirrhosis and

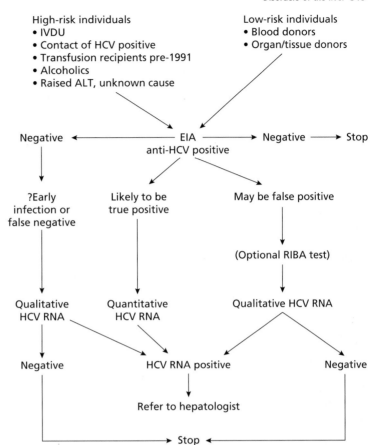

Fig 9.4 Algorithm for hepatitis C virus (HCV) screening. Notes: Recombinant immunoblot assay (RIBA) is optional to direct testing for HCV RNA; the qualitative polymerase chain reaction (PCR) is more sensitive ($\sim 100\,\text{geq/mL}$) (geq, genome equivalent) than the quantitative (bDNA) test (>200 000 geq/ mL); a positive qualitative HCV RNA indicates that virus is present in serum; a quantitative HCV RNA test gives an estimate of the level of viraemia (but is less sensitive than a qualitative test and may miss levels <1000 geq/mL); patients who are repeatedly reactive by Enzyme Immunoassay (EIA) should be tested for viraemia using reverse transcription (RT)- PCR regardless of supplemental testing using RIBA. A more cautious approach may be justified for 'low-risk' individuals [From Fagan & Harrison [197] with permission].

hepatoma especially in patients infected after 50 years of age.

Pregnant women with acute or chronic hepatitis C do not seem to be affected adversely by pregnancy (contrast hepatitis due to HEV and herpes viruses). Acute liver failure is an extremely rare consequence of acute HCV infection and no excess cases have been reported in pregnant women [197].

Sexual transmission

This is uncommon for HCV in the absence of confounding factors such as multiple sex partners, presence of genital herpes (as a surrogate marker of sexual exposure) and additional parenteral exposure through shared use of needles [310,311,316]. The average prevalence of HCV infection was 1.5% based on five studies in the USA involving long-term spouses of patients with chronic hepatitis C [311]. As with other blood-borne viruses, sexual transmission of HCV from males to females is more efficient than from females to males.

Fetal issues

Vertical transmission. This is less frequent than for HBV [317–320]; reviewed in [197], although individual case reports implicate successive vertical, and perinatal, transmission [317,321,322], including from an HCV-infected mother to her four sons [322].

As with HBV, the risk of transmission and the outcome relate to the level of viraemia and selection of quasispecies [197,317,322], as well as trimester of maximum exposure. Early data, based primarily on first-generation antibody tests and non-specific elevations in liver tests, probably overestimated the frequency of transmission. The consensus view is that vertical transmission is unlikely with chronic hepatitis C (0–18%) accompanied by low levels of viraemia (defined arbitrarily as $<1 \times 10^6$ genome equivalents per millilitre). Transmission is more common with concurrent HIV infection (6–36%) but this may reflect the propensity for high viraemias found in HIV-infected women, especially at delivery. In the study from Italy [314], of the 30 mothers with anti-HCV antibodies

(1.07%), none was seropositive for anti-HIV antibodies. Ten mothers had HCV RNA detected in serum around delivery. All cord bloods had undetectable HCV RNA but three of these 10 high-risk babies subsequently had HCV RNA detected at about 3 months of age. Postpartum transmission is implicated also in a prospective study from Japan.

Transmission also may occur with acute hepatitis C arising during pregnancy but data are limited [323].

Horizontal transmission. Horizontal transmission of HCV infection within the family is rare but can occur especially when the mother has a high level of HCV RNA. Early studies showed high rates of transmission from HIV-positive mothers but not all studies have confirmed these findings. In Asia and the Far East, anti-HCV seropositivity by second-generation enzyme immunoassay (EIA) is detectable in about 10–35% of children with a suspected viral aetiology (non-A, non-B hepatitis) for their chronic liver disease.

Management and follow-up testing

The CDC does not recommend routine screening of all pregnant women [311]. Instead, selective screening should focus on high-risk individuals [311]. These recommendations include pregnant women who are intravenous drug users, received blood transfusions, blood products or an organ tranplant before 1992, and those with selected medical conditions associated with abnormal liver tests and haemodialysis [311]. There are no specific recommendations for changing sexual practices for long-term steady sex partners of HCV-seropositive persons [311]. There are no recommendations against pregnancy for seropositive individuals [311]. Following delivery, women who are seropositive for HCV antibodies should be referred to a hepatologist for follow-up and consideration of antiviral therapy.

Perinatal transmission is sufficiently uncommon for the CDC and the American Academy of Paediatrics to consider unnecessary specific recommendations surrounding the mode of delivery and breastfeeding [311]. Whether caesarean section (vs. vaginal delivery) reduces transmission in highly viraemic mothers, requires further study.

Serial tests may be required to detect intermittent, low-level viraemia. Detection of anti-HCV antibodies in babies of less than 6 months of age may reflect maternal infection. Recommendations from the CDC are to delay testing for anti-HCV antibody to beyond 1 year (typically about 18 months) [311]. In obstetric practice, HCV RNA can be detected by 1–2 months of age in perinatally infected babies. An undetectable serum level of HCV RNA by

sensitive qualitative reverse transcription (RT)-PCR (detection limit above 100 copies/mL) at about 3 months of age makes vertical transmission unlikely.

Immunoprophylaxis. None is available for preventing hepatitis C infection.

Antiviral therapies (reviewed in [197]). IG and antiviral agents are not recommended by CDC as postexposure therapy for babies born of HCV-seropositive mothers [311].

Following delivery, HCV-RNA seropositive women should be referred to a hepatologist for evaluation of likely liver disease and chances of clearing HCV infection with antiviral therapy. The combination of interferon (category C) with ribavirin (category X) is the mainstay therapy for hepatitis C for adults and children with chronic hepatitis C. These drugs are contraindicated in pregnancy and in women practising unreliable contraceptive measures. Pregnancy tests are required regularly throughout antiviral therapy.

Ribavirin is a teratogen (category X) as shown in all animal studies. Accordingly, the manufacturers recommend a 'wash-out' period of a minimum of 6 months following discontinuation of ribavirin prior to discontinuing strict measures of birth control using the oral contraceptive pill with barrier methods. Safety data are insufficient to provide specific guidelines for women who have become pregnant during the time period in which ribavirin is retained in the body. Women who become pregnant within 6 months of discontinuing antiviral therapy should be referred for counselling as well as to a hepatologist.

HERPES VIRUSES (see also Chapter 17)

All members of the herpes group—herpes simplex, varicella zoster, cytomegalovirus (CMV) and Epstein–Barr virus (EBV)—can cause hepatitis.

Herpes simplex

Hepatitis is very uncommon in adults but well recognized in neonates. Fewer than 100 cases due to herpes simplex have been reported in the literature [324]. Types 1 and 2 are represented. More than half were associated with immunosuppression. Some were women in the third trimester [325–330]. Presenting features are non-specific and lead to delays in diagnosis. Mucocutaneous stigmata may be absent and jaundice is not invariable [327,329,331]. Herpes simplex hepatitis carries a grave prognosis without prompt antiviral therapy. Mortality exceeds 90% even with treatment [324].

Cytomegalovirus and Epstein–Barr virus

Both viruses are ubiquitous; more than 50% of adults have detectable antibodies. Reactivation of latent CMV infection is common in pregnancy and 3–5% of otherwise healthy women have viruria. CMV can be detected in 0.3–3% of babies screened routinely at delivery. Common transmission routes include sexual contact via body fluids such as saliva and blood especially from leucocyte fractions.

CMV hepatitis can have serious consequences in the pregnant and immunocompromised host, especially following organ transplantation and/or concurrent HIV infection (see HIV infection, below; [197]). Reactivation of latent infection or infection with new subtypes is more common than primary infection because most patients have pre-existing antibody. Reactivation of latent virus is favoured with an impaired T-cell response characteristically seen in the immunosuppressed. Acalculous cholecystitis and biliary strictures have been reported with CMV infection in the setting of immunosuppression, particularly HIV infection and AIDS (see below).

Transmission of EBV via blood is uncommon but outbreaks of hepatitis have been noted in haemodialysis units. Most primary infections occur in otherwise healthy children and young adults as infectious mononucleosis ('glandular fever'). Fewer than 5% of all cases develop hepatitis. This typically is symptomless but represents a significant number of cases. Acute liver failure is rare [197] and there is no predilection for pregnancy.

Maternal issues. Herpes simplex is the only virus in the West that seems to have a particular tendency to cause severe hepatitis in pregnancy. Early diagnosis and treatment with aciclovir can be successful. Herpes simplex type 2 commonly reactivates in pregnancy. Symptoms are three times as common in the pregnant, compared to non-pregnant, patient [332]. Herpes simplex type 2 is most common in the third trimester and most patients have cervical and genital lesions [330]. Genital herpes infection has been found in the non-pregnant patient with fulminant hepatitis [328,333]. Mechanisms predisposing towards dissemination of virus during pregnancy remain unclear. Impaired immune surveillance is implicated in the predisposition to disseminated EBV infection [334].

Fetal issues. Herpes simplex virus crosses the placenta but there seems to be no relation to congenital malformations [332] (cf. CMV, see below). In recurrent infection, high maternal levels of antibody offer some protection to the newborn. The risks of congenital dissemination are more common if primary infection occurs during pregnancy and increase to term.

Herpes simplex acquired at birth from cervical and vaginal contamination can lead to disseminated infection in over half the babies with 90% mortality from meningoencephalitis. Delivery by caesarean section should be considered in suspected cases of maternal primary infection [332]. Diagnosis depends on a battery of tests including serological markers and demonstration of inclusion bodies on histological examination of liver tissue. Viral DNA detected by *in situ* hybridization in liver tissue can provide a rapid diagnosis if sampling is feasible [324]. Antiviral therapy such as aciclovir can be successful if given early [335].

Vertical transmission of herpes viruses. Maternal transmission of herpes viruses may be blood borne via the placenta or from contamination with vaginal fluid and ulcers (herpetic) at delivery. Transmission from a symptomless mother may result in severe disseminated infection in the neonate. Individual cases of severe hepatitis, including acute liver failure, have been reported in neonates and babies for herpes simplex (especially HSV type 2), varicella zoster (including an illness resembling Reyes' syndrome), cytomegalovirus and human herpes virus 6 (HHV6).

Women who have received a graft and later become pregnant are at particular risk of transmitting CMV infection to their offspring. Transmission is common especially with primary infection resulting from a donor–recipient mismatch (organ donor is seropositive for CMV to seronegative recipient). Transmission following reactivation also can occur when a CMV-positive recipient receives a positive graft.

Fetal outcomes. CMV probably is the most common cause of post-transfusion hepatitis in seronegative neonates and children in the West [336] (cf. hepatitis C in adults). Over 30% of the population acquire CMV during the first few months of life. The newborn may acquire CMV from an infected mother during delivery or via breast milk and other body secretions. Most infections are mild, anicteric illnesses. After primary infection, the virus probably persists for life. Virus can be detected in 0.3–3% of babies screened routinely [337–339]. Up to 2% of neonates have signs of infection [340]. Following infection during pregnancy up to 10% will be severely handicapped [339]. This assessment is more optimistic than in previous reports [341] but, for England and Wales alone, CMV accounts for 180 children per annum with severe and permanent handicaps [339]. Various neonatal syndromes have been recorded following maternal reactivation with midbrain damage and cytomegalic inclusion disease [332]. Primary maternal infection in the first and second trimesters is associated with brain damage to the fetus. Five per cent of congenital infections include a neonatal hepatitis with hepatosplenomegaly, pneumonitis, chorioretinitis and a miriad of central nervous system disorders.

Severe hepatitis occurs most often in the preterm infant with interstitial pneumonitis. CMV infection should be considered especially in babies born to women who are immunosuppressed, including transplant recipients [177].

Diagnosis of herpes infections. Conventional tests rely on serological tests for antibodies (IgM anti-herpes antibodies); specifically, rising titres from paired sera, detection of early and late antigens, and detection of viruria. Analyses of amniotic fluid for viral DNA using PCR techniques is likely to supersede conventional virological tests especially for detection of vertical transmission in pregnancies with primary CMV infection [342]. The finding of CMV in cervical swabs in up to 28% of healthy women [343,344] does not always equate with congenital infection [332]. Instead, cultures of nasopharangeal secretions and urine from the newborn provide a ready and more reliable diagnosis.

Haemorrhage in the liver can be marked in herpes hepatitis. Viral DNA detected by *in situ* hybridization in liver tissue can provide a rapid diagnosis if sampling is feasible. Detection of virus in body fluids such as urine and in peripheral blood mononuclear cells using PCR techniques should be interpreted alongside results of serial serological tests.

Isolation of virus by culture of blood and tissues (e.g. the liver) on human fibroblasts along with a fourfold rise in titres of antibodies in paired samples is sufficient to diagnose acute CMV infection in most cases. Analysis of single samples often is insufficient for making the diagnosis. Monoclonal antibodies and DNA probes can detect CMV in tissues but, as with isolated findings in saliva and urine, a positive result does not differentiate acute from previous infection. CMV can be detected in about one-quarter of cervical swabs of healthy women and this does not correlate with risk and severity of congenital infection. Maternal CMV infection is symptomless despite transmission to the baby. Diagnosis relies on detection of virus in blood and rising titres of antibody.

CMV may persist in body fluids for months or years, especially following perinatal infection and CMV mononucleosis. Also, cultures may take weeks to show the characteristic cytopathic effects and rises in titres may be delayed.

Antiviral therapies. Ganciclovir and phosphonoformate (foscarnet) are useful in severe CMV infection but contraindicated in pregnancy. Mothers suspected of having herpes simplex hepatitis should be commenced without delay on aciclovir.

Passive immunization using specific, high-titre IG against CMV can offer some protection against primary infection after accidental exposure. This is very expensive and no information is available for use against primary infection during pregnancy. No vaccines are available. Studies to develop recombinant vaccines are in progress in Europe, the USA and Japan but fears remain over establishing long-term latency for viruses with oncogenic potential.

Human immunodeficiency virus infection, acquired immune deficiency syndrome and the liver (see Chapter 18 for a general review of HIV infection in pregnancy)

These topics are reviewed elsewhere [197].

MATERNAL ISSUES

Specific issues in obstetric practice for the mother include the diversity of liver diseases and practical implications of falsely negative serologies in the immunosuppressed patient as well as safety concerns that limit the use of certain antiretroviral therapies during pregnancy.

Concurrent liver disease is common in patients with HIV infection and AIDS (reviewed in [197]). Liver disease accounted for 4% of deaths in HIV-seropositive American women aged 15–44 years up until 1987 [345]. The high seroprevalence rates for concurrent HCV and HBV infection are consequent to sharing risk factors such as intravenous use of drugs and sexual practices.

The presenting features of HIV infection are protean with fever, hepatosplenomegaly and elevated serum levels of alkaline phosphatase and γ-glutamyl transpeptidase (GGT). Importantly, the immunosuppressed patient can remain seronegative for various antibodies used in the diagnosis of infectious diseases. Accordingly, diagnosis should focus instead on detection of nucleic acids (HBV DNA, HCV RNA) and antigens (HBsAg, HBeAg). Further, liver enzyme tests (AST, ALT levels) may remain low despite significant liver disease. Gross elevations of serum alkaline phosphatase and GGT are suggestive of infiltration of the liver with granulomata from opportunistic infections including *Mycobacterium avium* and various species of *Cryptosporidium*, *Histoplasmodium*, *Cryptococcus* and *Pneumocystis* as well as lymphomas and Kaposi's sarcoma of the liver. Other considerations include biliary disease such as cholecystitis, cholangitis and strictures from CMV (see above) as well as AIDS.

Differential diagnosis is correspondingly wide and includes all causes of cholestatic jaundice and biliary tract infections (see below).

Mothers with evidence of current or past HBV infection (see Table 9.4) who are immunosuppressed should be monitored for virus replication with levels of HBV DNA to assess the risks of vertical transmission.

FETAL ISSUES

Fetal issues include the increased risk of vertical transmission of infectious agents such as HCV, HBV and herpes viruses consequent to the high levels of viraemia seen in HIV-seropositive patients. Also, failure rates following immunization with the hepatitis B vaccine are high in the immunosuppressed host (see vertical transmission, above). Accordingly, babies born of mothers with detectable HBV DNA around the time of delivery, as well as HIV infections, should be immunized with HBIG as well as hepatitis B vaccine.

Acute liver failure

This rare and complex medical emergency requires early discussions and referral to a specialized centre with facilities for managing multiorgan failure and liver transplantation (reviewed in [197]). Early diagnosis and transfer are essential because prognosis without grafting depends on aetiology and speed of progression through the stages of hepatic coma.

Fulminant hepatic failure (FHF) is defined as the development of hepatic encephalopathy caused by severe liver dysfunction within 8 weeks of onset of symptoms in a patient with a previously normal liver [346]. Late-onset hepatic failure (LOHF; subacute hepatic necrosis) defines the development of encephalopathy between 8 and 26 weeks after onset of symptoms [347].

Clinical features of acute liver failure are non-specific and non-diagnostic (see acute fatty liver and HELLP syndromes, above). Systolic hypertension may be marked with cerebral oedema and may masquerade as pre-eclampsia and eclampsia. The liver usually is small in severe cases and end-stage illness regardless of aetiology. Conversely, hepatomegaly suggests fat and other infiltra-

tions but size is difficult to evaluate in pregnancy. Splenomegaly is uncommon but seen in Wilson's disease and other chronic liver diseases. A polymorphonuclear leucocytosis can be found in any liver failure complicated by microbial infection. Haematological features of DIC occur regardless of the aetiology. The presence of haemolytic anaemia should prompt exclusion of Wilson's disease. Levels of serum transaminase (AST or ALT) are often relatively low in acute fatty liver and the HELLP syndrome but can rise (>2000 IU/L) with hepatic necrosis from infarction and rupture. Relatively low serum levels of bilirubin and transaminase may indicate extensive hepatocellular necrosis with lack of regeneration of hepatocytes and, consequently, a poor prognosis.

Specific concerns in obstetric practice for the mother are the potential for certain liver diseases to pursue an especially adverse course in pregnancy and the possible benefits of early delivery in illnesses peculiar to pregnancy. The concerns for the fetus relate to whether it can survive to maturity and to the risks of vertical transmission with viral agents and other hepatotoxins.

DIFFERENTIAL DIAGNOSIS AND OBSTETRIC OUTCOME

The most common causes of acute liver failure likely to be encountered in pregnancy and the anticipated outcome following delivery are given in Table 9.6. Paracetamol (acetaminophen) overdose is the most common cause of fulminant hepatic failure in the UK and is prevalent in young women of childbearing age [348,349]. Serum levels should be sought in all patients. Hepatotoxicity of the fetal liver from metabolites of acetaminophen can lead to impaired coagulation and intraventricular haemorrhage [350]. N-acetylcysteine is a potent antioxidant and its use is being extended to all causes of acute liver failure. The very limited information suggests that this antidote is safe in pregnancy [349,350]. N-acetylcysteine, commenced as late as 36h following the overdose, can prevent the onset of hepatic encephalopathy.

In the West, acute liver failure of indeterminate aetiology (previously called non-A, non-B, non-C, non-E hepatitis) is the most common presumed viral cause of acute liver failure but data in pregnancy are lacking.

Table 9.6 Acute liver failure in pregnancy

Aetiology	Maternal outcome following delivery
Viral hepatitis	No effect
Drugs	No effect
Acute fatty liver	Improved
HELLP	Improved

Viral causes are rare in pregnancy but prevalent among series reported in Europe. Hepatitis E is prevalent in the developing countries and travellers returning from high-prevalence countries (see hepatitis E, above) [351]. Exotic agents such as Rift Valley fever, dengue and other arboviruses can cause the haemorrhagic fevers [197]. These should be considered in travellers bitten by insects in endemic areas such as the African countries. Other drugs and toxins include anticonvulsants and non-steroidal anti-inflammatory agents, carbon tetrachloride, halothane and poisonous mushrooms (*Amanita phalloides*).

SEROLOGICAL DIAGNOSIS

Rapid serological diagnosis is essential for the correct management of viral hepatitis. In expert hands, survival rates of 40–60% with medical management alone can be achieved for non-pregnant patients with acute liver failure due to excess acetaminophen or hepatitis A and B who are referred early but progress through to grades III–IV encephalopathy [197]. In contrast, the uniformly poor prognosis of most other causes of acute liver failure requires early assessment of the suitability for liver transplantation, which has revolutionized maternal outcome.

Serological markers remain the cornerstone for the diagnosis of viral hepatitis (see Table 9.4). While hepatitis C rarely is associated with acute liver failure, seronegativity for antibodies to HCV does not exclude the diagnosis because seroconversion can be delayed. Also, a negative test for HBsAg does not exclude HBV because this antigen is cleared unusually rapidly in acute liver failure [197]. Similarly, HBsAg, if present and persisting in high titre, may indicate a chronic carrier with an additional aetiology for the liver failure. Multiple viral aetiologies should be sought using panels of tests and repeated (see Table 9.4) in doubtful cases.

MANAGEMENT

This is similar regardless of pregnancy. Any of the following features should prompt early discussion and referral to a specialized centre [197]:
1 hepatic encephalopathy;
2 elevated prothrombin ratio (>2 times normal control);
3 renal impairment;
4 metabolic acidosis (blood pH <7.3 despite normovolaemia determined from the pulmonary capillary wedge pressure);
5 hypotension;
6 hyponatraemia;
7 thrombocytopenia.

The prothrombin time is the most sensitive indicator of severity of liver dysfunction, and hence prognosis (Table 9.7), and should be tested frequently. Administration of fresh frozen plasma is best avoided without overt bleeding because outcome is not affected and interpretation of the prothrombin time can be difficult. Blood and blood products should be available to support any surgical intervention and following delivery to help minimize blood loss. Parenteral vitamin K and folic acid should be given routinely. Blood glucose levels should be monitored closely and immediate provision made to administer large quantities of concentrated glucose (10–50%) via a central venous catheter. Hypoglycaemia remains a common cause of fetal and maternal death. Early manifestations of cerebral oedema include peaks of systolic hypertension and tachycardia and should be treated by mannitol-induced diuresis (100 mL of 20% as a bolus) with plasma osmolality maintained between 305 and 315 mosmol/kg. Mannitol is nephrotoxic and ineffective in renal failure. Ultrafiltration and haemodialysis may be required to remove excess fluid. Levels of blood urea may be misleadingly low. Renal function is best monitored by serial levels of serum creatinine and its clearance. Gastrointestinal bleeding from erosions is decreased by the prophylactic administration of an H_2 antagonist. All sedation should be withdrawn in the non-intubated patient. Elective endotracheal intubation and assisted ventilation may be required especially prior to travel and delivery and before the development of overt cerebral oedema. An experienced anaesthetist must carry out the intubation.

Corticosteroids are of no proven benefit in acute liver failure and may exacerbate complications such as infection. Microbial, including fungal, infection is common in liver failure. Detailed microbiological cultures and analyses should be carried out serially on all body fluids including blood, urine, sputum and ascites.

Data on management outcomes from controlled trials in fulminant viral hepatitis are lacking. In fulminant B, and D, virus replication is less than in uncomplicated acute infection and may have ceased before presentation. For continuing replication, the extent of liver damage may preclude regeneration. Interferons have been given to three pregnant women with fulminant viral hepatitis and two survived [352]. Lamivudine and other nucleoside analogues that inhibit virus replication have been shown to be safe in individual cases of fulminant hepatitis B but are not licensed for use in pregnancy. Aciclovir should be adminstered early for liver failure associated with herpes viruses (see above).

MATERNAL ISSUES

Accurate diagnosis is imperative because aetiology dictates management especially the requirement for early delivery to terminate diseases such as AFLP, HELLP and severe pre-eclampsia/eclampsia [117]. Conversely, delivery for viral hepatitis does not necessarily improve maternal outcome.

Differential diagnosis

In obstetric practice the major differential diagnoses include viral hepatitis, AFLP, severe pre-eclampsia and toxaemia of pregnancy, the HELLP syndrome and overlapping conditions such as thrombotic thrombocytopenic purpura and the haemolytic–uraemic syndrome (see above). Other confusing conditions include severe hyperemesis gravidarum, Budd–Chiari syndrome, alcoholic hepatitis, pancreatitis, septicaemias and other severe infections such as leptospirosis. In addition, chronic liver disease, especially Wilson's disease and autoimmune chronic hepatitis, and malignant infiltrations of the liver from lymphomas and metastases may present with a picture indistinguishable from acute liver failure [117].

FETAL ISSUES

Survival of the fetus in severe liver failure is exceptional. The fetus often is dead on presentation and this usually relates to profound fetal and maternal hypoglycaemia.

In maternal paracetamol overdose, metabolites can be hepatotoxic to the fetal liver and lead to impaired coagulation and intraventricular haemorrhage [350].

Liver transplantation

Medical and surgical issues of relevance in obstetric practice include the impact on mother and fetus when liver transplantation is carried out during pregnancy, adverse effects of the pregnancy in a transplant recipient, the safety and monitoring of immunosuppressive therapies, and the risk of recurrent disease in the graft. Further, the impact of transplantation on social, sexual, psychological and other personal needs cannot be overemphasized. Shared management is essential between transplant specialists, obstetricians and perinatologists.

Assessment for transplant candidacy includes the potential for recovery and suitability for grafting based on prognostic indicators (see Table 9.7). Knowledge of the patient's blood group is important for matching potential donors. HIV infection should be excluded and serological testing performed to document infection with HBV and HCV. Other microbial infections should be sought and treated aggressively. Patency of hepatic and portal venous anatomy should be confirmed by Doppler ultrasound with documentation of direction and velocity of blood flow. Tests should be commenced to exclude Wilson's disease (see below) and autoimmune chronic hepatitis as these have specific therapeutic options.

TRANSPLANTATION DURING PREGNANCY

Inevitably, transplantation during pregnancy is reserved for emergency cases of severe liver failure. Optimal timing of transplantation during pregnancy and the immediate postpartum period is restricted by the need to synchronize delivery and grafting. The narrow window of opportunity for survival of mother and baby is compromised further by the limited availability of donor organs. Nevertheless, successful maternal and fetal outcomes have been reported for grafting during pregnancy using cadaveric and living donor livers [353]. Individual cases relate to fulminant hepatitis B [13,214,354,355], acute fatty liver [164], the HELLP [156], and Budd–Chiari, syndromes [356,357], liver

Table 9.7 Poor prognostic indicators in acute liver failure.

Viral and other causes	Paracetamol
Any three of these: 0.96*	All three: 0.67*
• aetiology, e.g. non-ABC	• grade III encephalopathy
• age <10 or >40 years	• prothrombin time >100 s†
• prothrombin time >50 s†	• creatinine >300 μmol/L
• serum bilirubin >300 μmol/L	
• jaundice >7 days before encephalopathy	
or: 1.0*	*and/or:*
• prothrombin time >100 s 1.0†	• arterial pH <7.3 0.95*‡

*Positive predictive value.
†Based on UK thromboplastins. Prothrombin times are not comparable between USA and UK. These are for guidance only; other factors must be considered. Note that the prognosis is invariably poor (predictive value 1.0) if the prothrombin time is > 100s in viral causes.
‡With normovolaemia.

rupture relating to eclampsia as well as decompensated chronic hepatitis and sclerosing cholangitis. Maternal morbidity remains high mostly from haemorrhage surrounding delivery, especially caesarean section. Impaired haemostasis reflects the abnormal coagulopathy and thrombocytopenia. Common complications include infection, renal failure and respiratory distress syndrome.

The uniformly poor survival for acute liver failure, excluding hepatitis A and B or paracetamol hepatotoxicity, has emphasized the need for early liver grafting. Reinfection following transplantation in non-pregnant survivors has been documented for hepatitis B and D, and C with variable clinical outcomes. Data on the efficacy of immunoprophylaxis and antiviral therapies are sparse. Reinfection rates are below 5% for fulminant hepatitis B and B with D if HBIG is used during and after transplantation.

Liver 'assist' devices are being tested under clinical trial especially as a 'bridge' to transplantation but research studies exclude pregnant women.

IMPACT OF TRANSPLANTATION ON FERTILITY AND PREGNANCY

The menstrual cycle returns after successful grafting [358–360]. Amenorrhoea continuing after grafting may signify early pregnancy. Patients should be offered early advice on contraception. Deferral of pregnancy beyond the first year seems sensible because morbidity and mortality are greatest within this time. Oral contraceptive drugs can enhance the hepatotoxicity of cyclosporine [361] and are contraindicated in thrombogenic disorders such as Budd–Chiari syndrome.

Fetal outcome

Pregnancy in recipients of hepatic allografts is associated with good perinatal outcome [362], but there is an increased risk of preterm delivery [363]. Intrauterine growth restriction and poor postnatal infant growth have been reported [358] and denied [364]. All immunosuppressive drugs are known to cross the placenta and enter breast milk. Tacrolimus (FK506) and cyclosporine are concentrated also in the placenta but data are unavailable on OKT3 [365,366]. Significant amounts of drug are transmitted to the fetus and can result in transient impairment in renal function in the neonate. However, none of the conventional immunosuppressive drugs used in liver transplantation has been associated with marked excess of congenital birth defects [363–366] or protracted growth impairment. Azathioprine (category D) has been associated with growth restriction and immunosuppression in the neonate in some [355,365], but not all, studies [367].

Concern remains over possible effects of azathioprine on the subsequent reproductive performance of the female fetus (see Chapter 8).

Congenital CMV infection with hydrops fetalis, placental infection and preterm delivery has been reported in the offspring of graft recipients [177].

IMPACT OF PREGNANCY ON TRANSPLANTATION

Graft function and survival seem unaffected by pregnancy [355,362]. Wide fluctuations in levels of immunosuppressive drugs such as cyclosporine A during pregnancy and postpartum [364] are to be anticipated and may favour rejection [367] and explain some early cases of graft loss [368].

The National Cyclosporine Registry from Philadelphia, USA, recorded 37 pregnancies in 35 liver transplant recipients; all but two (FK506) were under cyclosporine [369]. Specific risks in the transplant recipient who becomes pregnant include the worsening of hypertension and increased risk of pre-eclampsia [335,362,363,370]. Rupture of a splenic artery aneurysm can occur [371]. Other complications include anaemia and infections [363] especially from CMV that can result in disseminated infection in the neonate [177] (see AIDS and the liver, above). Cervical dysplasia is not uncommon [369] and requires regular screening. Seven of 82 transplant recipients reported abnormal cervical cytology results following transplantation; four of the six who underwent colposcopy required ablative therapy.

Monitoring immunosuppressive agents

Confidence is increasing in line with experience and the safe use of immunosuppressive agents during pregnancy. Shared management is essential between transplant specialists and perinatologists.

Data remain sparse but most liver transplant centres use combinations that include corticosteroids and cyclosporine A, FK506 and azathioprine. Alterations in drug dosages of the conventional drugs and combinations are not usually neccessary in early pregnancy but likely as the changes in blood volume progress and resolve postpartum. Frequent monitoring of blood levels of cyclosporine A and FK506 is recommended [364,367,372]. Reduction in drug levels result from the elevation in blood volume of up to about 30% and reduced haematocrit. Cyclosporine is bound to erythrocytes. Conversely, clearance of some drugs is impaired following reduction in capacity of liver microsomal activity resulting from the sex steroids. Some authorities recommend measurements of serum, as well as blood (erythrocyte-bound), levels of cyclosporine during pregnancy and early postpartum. Divided daily doses may reduce maximum peaks. FK506 is often reserved for rejection resistant to corticosteroids and cyclosporine. The safety and efficacy of FK506 was supported in a prospective study of 21 pregnant transplant recipients [364]. These results, when compared with cyclosporine, showed better control of rejection, less arterial hypertension and reduced dependence on corticosteroids [364]. Strict control of blood levels reduces nephrotoxicity. Significant hyperkalaemia may require fluodrocortisone treatment. Elevated levels of serum creatinine and uric acid are notable in mother and neonate.

Chronic hepatitis, cirrhosis and portal hypertension

Amenorrhoea and infertility are common with untreated advanced liver disease regardless of aetiology. Accordingly, pregnancy is uncommon with advanced cirrhosis. Nevertheless, accurate diagnosis is essential especially to differentiate between such conditions as autoimmune chronic hepatitis, Wilson's disease and viral hepatitis. Treatment can reverse the infertility in some cases and improve significantly the long-term prognosis. Discussion will be limited to issues directly related to obstetric practice.

Chronic hepatitis

Chronic hepatitis is a histopathological diagnosis regardless of aetiology. The term chronic hepatitis embraces and replaces terms such as chronic persistent hepatitis and chronic active hepatitis as these are regarded within a spectrum, rather than discrete entities, that can lead to fibrosis and cirrhosis [197]. Chronic hepatitis is staged according to the amount of inflammatory cell infiltrate and destruction of liver cells (necroinflammatory activity) as well as the presence and extent of fibrosis, as these features have predictive value for development of cirrhosis.

Conversely, reliance on detection of clinical stigmata and liver serum biochemistry to monitor underlying disease activity may be misleading. Progression from chronic hepatitis to cirrhosis can occur despite a lack of symptoms and with serum liver enzymes maintained within the normal, or near-normal, ranges.

FETAL ALCOHOL SYNDROME

This is considered in Chapter 19.

AUTOIMMUNE CHRONIC HEPATITIS

In the West, the majority of cases occur in women who have autoimmune features with hypergammaglobulinae-

mia and autoantibodies to smooth muscle (SMA) and nuclear factor (ANF). The histological features include a chronic inflammatory cell infiltrate in the portal tracts extending beyond the limiting plate to surround islands of hepatocytes ('piecemeal necrosis'; syn. interface hepatitis). The inflammation and necrosis can extend towards the hepatic vein in the hepatic lobule ('bridging necrosis').

Untreated autoimmune chronic hepatitis is associated with amenorrhoea and infertility. Progression to cirrhosis and decompensated liver disease is not uncommon with untreated disease. Importantly, introduction of corticosteroids and azathioprine can reverse the infertility in early cases [373] and lead to a marked improvement in prognosis.

Liver function during pregnancy is preserved with well-controlled disease activity [374] but fetal prematurity and low birthweight have been recorded [373]. Obstetrical complications such as urinary infections and pre-eclampsia are common. In some series [373,375] fetal loss reached 55% but there was no increased incidence of congenital malformations.

Prednisolone therapy for autoimmune hepatitis should be continued throughout pregnancy in conventional doses (10–20 mg/day) and increased for suspected relapse [375], although this is unusual (10–15%) [373].

Regardless of pregnancy, azathioprine is considered an established therapy in the treatment of autoimmune chronic hepatitis (50–100 mg/day) with prednisolone [373]. The fetal risks of azathioprine are considered above. Maintenance of well-controlled disease is possible with azathioprine alone in certain patients, after cautious withdrawal of corticosteroids [376]. Whether monotherapy should be contemplated during pregnancy, is debatable. The risks to the fetus are high should relapse occur and evidence is lacking for adverse fetal effects of corticosteroids.

Uncontrolled disease and frequent relapses should prompt reappraisal of the diagnosis and exclusion of other conditions especially chronic hepatitis B and C (see above), Wilson's disease (see below), primary sclerosing cholangitis (PSC) (see below), alcoholic hepatitis and drugs including methyldopa and isoniazid. Histological and serological verification are important as immunosuppression is a long-term neccessity. Importantly, corticosteroids and other immunosuppressant drugs are contraindicated in viral hepatitis due to their adverse effects on enhancing virus replication (see above).

Cirrhosis and portal hypertension

Pregnancy remains uncommon in advanced cirrhosis, although there have been over 100 reports [377–383] following the first [384] in 1923. Cirrhosis is the main cause of intrahepatic portal hypertension. Non-cirrhotic causes of portal hypertension that may require different medical management include sarcoidosis, tuberculosis, schistosomiasis [385,386], metastatic malignancy, Gaucher's disease [387], polycystic liver disease and congenital hepatic fibrosis [388]. Information from two independent series [377,378] and a collective review of the literature [379] have identified the prognosis for the mother with cirrhosis and her fetus, the effects of pregnancy on coexisting liver disease and the role of surgical portal decompression [379].

EFFECTS ON FERTILITY

Infertility reflects the degree of hepatic dysfunction [378]. Irregular menses are common [389] and result from disturbances of the hypothalamic–pituitary axis rather than directly from the liver disease [390]. Malnutrition and altered hepatic metabolism of sex steroids may play a role but data are lacking. Fertility is normal or near-normal with well-compensated cirrhosis due to autoimmune hepatitis and Wilson's disease.

EFFECTS OF DISEASE ON PREGNANCY

Fetal loss is high in advanced cirrhosis. In early pregnancy there is an increased risk of spontaneous abortion [378,389,391]. In late pregnancy, only 45 babies from 69 pregnancies without surgical portal decompression [379] survived the neonatal period. Stillbirth was reported in 24% and there were 7% neonatal deaths. The prognosis for the fetus was better with previous portosystemic shunts prior to delivery. In this group 80% of pregnancies ended in live births although there were 13% stillbirths and 3% neonatal deaths [379].

EFFECTS OF PREGNANCY ON DISEASE

The once gloomy prognosis for mother and child has improved. Maternal prognosis depends more on the degree of hepatic dysfunction during pregnancy than aetiology, although well-compensated biliary, and postnecrotic, cirrhosis carry the best prognoses. Some early studies reported improved liver function during pregnancy in PBC [392] and Wilson's disease [393–395]. In Cheng's literature survey (1977), about half the women with documented advanced cirrhosis had successful term pregnancies without maternal complications.

Bleeding from oesophageal varices remains the most significant complication in pregnancy [382,396], especially in the second and third trimesters. The progressive increase in circulating blood volume, elevations in portal

pressure and added pressure from the gravid uterus on the inferior vena cava coincide to divert a greater proportion of the venous return through the azygos system [6]. The resultant increase in oesophageal pressure leads to transient oesophageal varices in at least half of healthy pregnant women [6,379]. Two early papers [378,379] reported divergent views on the outcomes of oesophageal varices in pregnancy. In the study by Britton [378], out of 160 pregnancies with documented coexisting oesophageal varices, bleeding occurred on 38 occasions. Associated maternal mortalities from variceal bleeds were 18% and 2% in cirrhotic and non-cirrhotic groups, respectively. In a literature review up until 1982 [379], gastrointestinal haemorrhage, from presumed oesophageal varices, occurred in eight of 60 (13%) cases without previous surgical portal decompression. Maternal mortality was high. Seven of 10 deaths in the non-shunted group were due to gastrointestinal bleeding. These figures, when compared with a 38% mortality in a non-pregnant cirrhotic control group [378], suggest there is no increased risk of fatal haemorrhage from oesophageal varices during pregnancy [378]. The literature survey [379] did not include a non-pregnant control group. However, a comparison was made with the maternal outcome for pregnant women who had previously undergone portosystemic shunting prior to pregnancy [379]. Only one of 23 pregnancies (21 mothers) resulted in a maternal death. This was due to hepatic coma on the eighth day postpartum and not to gastrointestinal bleeding. In a further seven cases, in which surgical portal decompression was performed during pregnancy (median 4 months prior to delivery), there were no maternal or fetal deaths [379]. The discordance between the two reports [378,379] can be partly explained. The literature review [379] highlighted the dangers of the postpartum period accounting for five of the seven deaths from gastrointestinal haemorrhage. This challenges the physiological explanation of haemodynamic alterations during pregnancy [6]. Other postpartum complications included early uterine haemorrhage (5.8% vs. 16.6%), hepatic coma (3.3% vs. 4.3%) and ascites (17.4% vs. 0%) in the shunted and non-shunted groups, respectively [379].

A later study from Hungary [382] with prospective data between 1980 and 1992, involved 11 pregnant women followed for anticipated complications of cirrhosis. Follow-up by a hepatologist included repeated upper endoscopies. Four of the six with documented oesophageal varices had gastrointestinal haemorrhage requiring endoscopic sclerotherapy. Bleeding was associated with rising levels of serum bilirubin and prothrombin time. Other complications included development of a haemorrhagic diathesis (five cases of excessive uterine bleeding and wound haematoma), puerperal sepsis (five cases) as well as ascites and hyperbilirubinaemia. Six of the 12 babies were small for dates, three were preterm and one died.

Other complications include rupture of splenic aneurysm [371] and portal vein thrombosis from protein C deficiency and thrombophilia.

Diagnosis of splenic artery aneurysm is best achieved with pulsed-wave Doppler ultrasound and CT imaging. A woman of childbearing age who has been diagnosed with splenic artery aneurysm should be considered for elective surgery via laparoscopic ligation [397]. Only 12 successful outcomes for mother and child were found in 100 cases of splenic artery aneurysm associated with pregnancy [371]. Two-thirds of the ruptures occurred in the third trimester of pregnancy.

MANAGEMENT

In advanced cirrhosis and following surgical portal decompression, attention should be paid to rest, vitamin supplementation and a diet high in carbohydrate and low in protein. A high-fibre diet should be encouraged to avoid constipation. Lactulose seems safe but specific data for human pregnancy are lacking. As with all drugs, laxatives should be used with caution in the first trimester.

The most significant complication likely to cause death is immediate blood loss from massive gastrointestinal bleeding due to ruptured oesophageal/and gastric varices. Further, complications include development of hepatic coma, postpartum haemorrhage, bacterial peritonitis and ruptured splenic artery aneurysm.

The death rate in pregnant women with cirrhosis has been reported to range from 10% to 18% (reviewed in [382,383]). Risks of bleeding peak in the third trimester and postpartum due to the impact on portal pressure of increased circulating volume. Women at particular risk of bleeding have preceding evidence of raised portal pressure, particularly a history of gastrointestinal haemorrhage prior to pregnancy.

General advice to the pregnant woman with cirrhosis and portal hypertension should include avoidance of situations that raise portal pressure such as straining, stooping and alcohol. Rebleeding and death are likely in non-compliant alcoholic patients with oesophageal varices. [396]. No specific measures to protect the oesophagus are of proven benefit in the absence of oesophageal reflux [396].

A woman presenting in pregnancy with suspected cirrhosis and portal hypertension requires a full medical investigation. Upper oesophagogastroduodenoscopy should be carried out for gastrointestinal haemorrhage. Liver biopsy may be required for diagnosis.

Survivors of a variceal bleed usually have end-stage irreversible disease. Additional medical therapy such as corticosteroids for autoimmune chronic hepatitis, D-penicillamine for Wilson's disease and abstinence from alcohol in alcoholic cirrhosis may induce a remission even in the presence of large varices [396].

Management of bleeding oesophageal varices has been simplified with the use of banding and sclerosing agents to obliterate venous channels [388,398] and also by the prophylactic use of β-blocking drugs. In non-pregnant patients, several controlled trials show the superiority of endoscopic techniques (banding vs. sclerotherapy) over surgical intervention such as portosystemic shunting and oesophageal transection, in reducing significantly rebleeding from varices for patients who present at the time of bleeding [388,396]. Portal pressure can be reduced by drugs such as β blockers and vasodilators. Venoconstriction and shunting of blood away from the oesophagus can be promoted using a combination of a vasoconstrictor and nitrate [388,396]. None of these measures has been shown to be superior to a course of sclerotherapy or to prevent rebleeding that recurs typically within 8 weeks [396]. Data are limited for pregnant women but reviews report the safety of banding [399] or sclerotherapy for bleeding varices in pregnancy [400]. These endoscopic techniques seem relatively safe and less traumatic than previously recommended surgical interventions [379–381]. Upper endoscopy should be repeated early on for each presentation of gastrointestinal bleeding as other non-variceal causes may be found. The fetal risks of β blockade are considered in Chapter 6 but are small compared to the risk of maternal death from bleeding varices.

Ascites should be managed with restriction of dietary sodium and, if severe, fluids. An ascitic tap carried out under ultrasonographic imaging should be analysed for a leucocytosis (>250 neutrophils/mm^3), microbial organisms and an acid pH (<7.35). Any one of these usually signifies peritonitis; fever and a peripheral blood leucocytosis may be absent. The prognosis with untreated spontaneous bacterial peritonitis or other sepsis is poor and frequently confounded by recurrent bleeding from the gastrointestinal tract, including from oesophageal varices. Appropriate antimicrobial therapy to cover gut-related organisms, such as *Escherichia coli*, should be instigated without delay. Tetracyclines are contraindicated in pregnancy (see Chapter 7).

In the non-pregnant patient with ascites, spironolactone remains the drug of choice. Spironolactone should not be used in pregnancy because of its antiandrogen activity. Triamterene, frusemide and bumetamide cross the placenta. Although their safety in pregnancy has not been established formally [84] these drugs have been used extensively and are probably safe with the proviso that the thiazide diuretics can precipitate hepatic coma in pregnant patients with cirrhosis [84,401]. Frusemide and a metabolite of spironolactone cross into breast milk, and breastfeeding is not recommended [84].

A pregnancy with well-compensated cirrhosis without jaundice and previously impaired liver function should be allowed to proceed to term. Vaginal delivery is safe in the majority of cases [378]. A protracted second stage should be avoided and interrupted by early forceps delivery to avoid excess straining with subsequent rise in portal pressure. The selection of forceps may explain the improved fetal outcome in shunted (26%) over non-shunted (13%) groups in the literature survey [379]. Excess blood loss should be anticipated especially in the puerperium [379].

Delivery should take place in a centre with expertise in handling bleeding oesophageal varices. Vitamin K_1, fresh frozen plasma and additional coagulation factors and platelets may be required. Sedatives, anaesthetics and diuretics should be used with caution because these can precipitate hepatic encephalopathy along with other factors such as excess blood loss, hypotension, occult infection, hypoglycaemia and constipation.

Caesarean section should be reserved for urgent situations to save the baby in the presence of rapidly deteriorating maternal liver function. The prognosis in these circumstances remains poor for mother and child [377]. Abdominal surgery may be technically difficult due to the large collateral circulation and adhesions from previous shunt surgery. Local anaesthesia with an epidural or pudendal block can be carried out safely [385] but advantages must be balanced against the increased risk of bleeding from the raised venous pressure and abnormal coagulation (cf. HELLP syndrome above). Elective termination of pregnancy should be considered only for decompensated cirrhosis in the first trimester.

Primary biliary cirrhosis

PBC is presumed to be an autoimmune disease of the liver but the exact aetiology is unknown (reviewed in [402]). PBC has a wide spectrum of disease severity and variable natural history [403] and is more common than was previously thought. Females outnumber males by a 10:1 ratio. There are no studies relating to the prognosis of PBC presenting in pregnancy.

The classical presentation is with jaundice, pruritus, fatigue and hepatosplenomegaly. Nevertheless, PBC may be symptomless and diagnosed on routine testing of liver function with elevated levels of serum alkaline phosphatase (liver isoenzyme) and GGT and hyperglobulinaemia

(IgM isotype). Diagnosis relies on detection of mitochondrial antibodies in almost all and characteristic liver histology in the absence of other biliary diseases.

Differential diagnosis includes other cholestatic diseases especially intrahepatic cholestasis of pregnancy (see above) that resolves in the puerperium and sclerosing cholangitis (see below) that may be associated with covert inflammatory bowel disease and cholelithiasis.

Maternal and fetal outcomes are variable but there is no evidence for a specific adverse effect during pregnancy. Prognosis is good for well-compensated disease. Features of relevance to obstetric practice are the pruritus that may be mistaken for IHCP (see above), high incidence (about 20%) of urinary tract infections, metabolic bone disease, in particular osteoporosis, and malabsorption of fat-soluble vitamins [402]. Other diseases that occur with PBC include thyroid disorders, sicca syndrome, Raynaud's syndrome, ulcerative colitis, coeliac disease and sarcoidosis [404].

Drug therapy is non-specific and aimed at relieving symptoms such as pruritus (see IHCP above). Cholestyramine resin binds fat-soluble vitamins (A, D, E, K) and vitamin K_1 supplements should be given especially before delivery. UDCA has become the mainstay of therapy in the non-pregnant patient. Controlled clinical trials indicate improved survival long term in PBC and a greater interval between diagnosis and need for liver transplantation (reviewed in [402]). Although no clinical trials have been conducted regarding the safety and efficacy for using UDCA for PBC during pregnancy, data from IHCP (see above) tend to favour its safety, albeit for use after the second trimester.

Wilson's disease

Wilson's disease should be considered in any young patient with liver disease including acute liver failure, especially with concomitant splenomegaly and Coombs-negative haemolysis [405]. The demonstration of Kayser–Fleischer rings by slit-lamp analysis assists the diagnosis. The rings may be absent especially when presenting with liver disease. Also, they can be found in PBC. Family members should be investigated. Detection of symptomless, but significant, liver disease is common in siblings. Specimens for analysis of urinary copper levels and diagnostic liver biopsy tissue must be handled in a copper-free environment to prevent contamination from skin, needles and containers. The prognosis is favourable if therapy with chelating agents is commenced before the development of cirrhosis. Liver grafting has been successful with clinical resolution of hepatic and neurological dysfunction but no data are available for pregnancy.

MATERNAL ASPECTS

Pregnancy is uncommon in untreated Wilson's disease [394,406,407], especially with advanced cirrhosis and portal hypertension. Subfertility and amenorrhoea are common, spontaneous abortions frequent, and there is high maternal morbidity and mortality in untreated disease [407]. Accumulated data from various sources and countries of 164 pregnancies in 111 women with Wilson's disease reported outcomes related to 153 live births [407]. Overall, maternal and fetal outcomes are good for women who continue treatment without interruption with either D-penicillamine (typically 0.75–1 g daily) or triethylene tetramine dihydrochloride (trientine) through the first and second trimesters. The dose of chelating agent required for successful cupriuresis probably is less in pregnancy than otherwise and can be cautiously reduced [408] by 25–50% (0.5 g daily dose) in the third trimester [407]. Toxicity is unusual and a full dose should be resumed immediately after delivery. D-penicillamine can be toxic in doses exceeding 1500 mg/day.

Treatment with the D-penicillamine (35 cases) or trientine (nine cases) up until 1986 resulted in good maternal and fetal outcomes [394,407]. Chelating agents can reduce serum levels of iron and zinc and should not be administered simultaneously with oral iron supplements. Pyridoxine (vitamin B_6) should be supplemented by a minimum of 50 mg/week to counteract the antipyridine effects of D-penicillamine [394,407].

Trientine is of equivalent cupriuretic value to D-penicillamine and possibly less toxic. Oral zinc has been used in 19 women during 26 pregnancies and resulted in 24 normal infants [409] but there are no data relating to trials in pregnancy, and experience is much less than with D-penicillamine and trientine [407]. The use of chelating agents in pregnancy generally is considered safe as long as therapy is not interrupted [407]. Therapy should be continued with the same agent; interruption of therapy and change of chelating agent can lead to relapse [407]. Rapid deterioration in liver function can occur after many years of successful therapy [407].

Reductions in maternal levels of serum copper have been attributed to an oestrogen effect of elevating the serum level of caeruloplasmin [410] but these changes are not invariable in pregnancy [408] or in patients taking oestrogen therapy [408].

Case reports document successful pregnancy in women grafted previously for end-stage Wilson's disease [405,411].

FETAL ASPECTS

Serum levels of copper and caeruloplasmin in cord blood and urinary levels of copper are normal in the heterozy-gote baby even if preterm and with poor maternal compliance of drug therapy [407,408,410]. Handling of copper by the fetus seems to be normal and there is no evidence of copper depletion [407]. Extraction of copper by the normal fetus may account for improvements in neurological status and liver function in some women during pregnancy [394,395].

D-penicillamine crosses the placenta and can affect the developing fetus [365]. The congenital abnormalities described are probably caused by the copper deficiency rather than direct effects of the chelating agent. Three babies with abnormalities of skin and connective tissue were born of mothers taking between 0.9 and 2.0 g/day of D-penicillamine during pregnancy for cystinuria [412] and rheumatoid arthritis [413,414] and two for Wilson's disease [394,415,416]. One further baby with reversible cutis laxa followed maternal D-penicillamine therapy (1.5 g/day) for Wilson's disease [417]. Cerebral palsy with blindness and arthrogryposis multiplex have been reported with maternal exposure to D-penicillamine for Wilson's disease [416] but the pregnancies were complicated by other factors that could have influenced outcome. These potentially adverse fetal effects should be discussed with the patient. However, as the maternal risks of discontinuing penicillamine are considerable, women with Wilson's disease should plan to take pencillamine throughout pregnancy.

In a study of 11 pregnancies in women with known Wilson's disease, trientine was given for a mean of 5 years before conception (reviewed in [407]). Seven of the 11 pregnancies were normal with up to 9 years of follow-up of the children [418]. One woman had a preterm delivery at 36 weeks and two had miscarriages unrelated to the Wilson's disease. One patient delivered a baby with the isochromosome X abnormality at 31 weeks (reviewed in [407]).

GENETIC TESTING

More than 100 mutations that result in Wilson's disease have been reported in the *ATP7B* gene that encodes a copper-transporting P-type ATPase (reviewed in [419,420]). DNA-based diagnosis is only feasible within selected families with an affected member to allow comparison of mutations against disease-carrying chromosomes in affected member/s [420]. Further, interpretation of genetic analyses is complicated since most patients will possess alleles with two different mutations of *ATP7B*. Nevertheless, prenatal exclusion of Wilson's disease was successful with DNA analysed from a chorionic villous biopsy at 9 weeks' gestation [421].

Budd–Chiari syndrome

The first description by Chiari in 1899 followed childbirth [422]. Over 50 cases have been described during pregnancy or, more commonly, postpartum [423–430].

This syndrome is defined as obstruction of the large hepatic veins that produces congestion and necrosis of the centrilobular areas of the liver [388]. Related disorders sharing clinical and haematological abnormalities include high inferior vena cava thrombosis, veno-occlusive disease with obstruction of centrilobular veins and peliosis hepatis with obstruction at the junction between hepatic sinusoids and centrilobular veins [388,430].

The aetiology of Budd–Chiari syndrome remains obscure. In the non-pregnant population in the West the most common associations are with polycythaemia rubra vera, paroxysmal nocturnal haemoglobinuria and other forms of altered coagulation. In some cases, thrombogenesis reflects resistance to activated protein C relating to the Leiden mutation in Factor V [431]. Pregnancy may lower further concentrations of antithrombin III, especially around delivery. Females predominate in more than three-quarters of cases regardless of pregnancy, oral contraceptive therapy and overt haematological disease [430]. This predilection may be enhanced further by alterations in hormonal status such as pregnancy and oral contraceptive use [7,427] taken from 20 days up to 10 years before presentation [432]. In the past, affected females were dissuaded from pregnancy for fear of an increased risk of hepatic venous thrombosis [432]. Activities of clotting factors are altered in pregnancy but no specific abnormality has been found in Budd–Chiari syndrome associated with pregnancy [427]. Out of 105 patients with Budd–Chiari syndrome, 15 presented between 4 days and 4 weeks postpartum and one further presented during pregnancy [427].

Clinical features include rapid abdominal distension due to accumulation of ascites that may be painless or associated with a vague discomfort. The liver typically is enlarged and occasionally tender. Serum liver biochemistry shows an elevation in level of alkaline phosphatase above that considered to reflect normal placental function (see Table 9.1). The serum levels of transaminase usually are modestly raised but can become markedly elevated causing diagnostic confusion with viral hepatitis. Rarely, the clinical presentation may be indistinguishable from acute liver failure (see above). The protein content of the ascitic fluid is usually characteristic of an exudate (albumin concentration above 40 g/L) but can be variable and not informative. Diagnosis in pregnancy is best achieved by ultrasonographic Doppler flow studies and percutaneous liver biopsy. Percutaneous hepatic venous catheterization is diagnostic should these techniques fail. Liver histology is not specific but typically shows outflow block with centrizonal venous congestion, haemorrhage, hepatocellular necrosis and dilatation of the sinusoids and central veins [423,425,433]. A search for abnormal haematological features should include a full thrombophilia screen making allowance for the normal changes of pregnancy (see Chapter 4). Haematological tests should be performed for paroxysmal nocturnal haemoglobinuria [434], haemolytic anaemia and thrombotic thrombocytopenic purpura [157].

Management of Budd–Chiari sydrome presenting in pregnancy has been disappointing. The fetus is not affected directly; outcome depends on maternal well-being. The ascites often is resistant to therapy with diuretics and salt restriction. (See above with regard to spironolactone and diuretic treatment in pregnancy.) In one series, only two of 16 patients gained relief of symptoms despite a variety of treatments including anticoagulation, reinfusion of ascites and surgery involving portocaval, splenorenal or mesocaval shunts. Maternal mortality with surgical intervention was 50% [427]. Transcatheter intrahepatic portosystemic shunting (TIPSS) in combination with heparin and plasminogen activator (tPA) have been used successfully to decompress the venous system in individual cases of Budd–Chiari syndrome.

Overall, the prognosis with pregnancy is poor [178]. Individual cases have been reported without maternal complications despite a mesocaval and cavoatrial shunt and intrauterine death in the sixth month [429]. Five successful pregnancies following Budd–Chiari syndrome had been reported up to 1984 [429,435,436]. One occurred 2 years after developing Budd–Chiari syndrome attributed to oral contraceptive therapy. Two consecutive pregnancies followed 3 and 4 years after developing the syndrome in association with polycythaemia rubra vera [436]. Successful pregnancies have been reported following grafting. Liver transplantation also has been successful during pregnancy [437,438] but the risk of recurrent thrombosis remains despite long-term anticoagulant therapy. Oral contraceptive drugs are contraindicated following grafting because the coagulation disorder remains.

Congenital disorders of metabolism of bilirubin

The hyperbilirubinaemias are relatively benign conditions characterized by persistent elevation in levels of serum bilirubin, which is predominantly unconjugated (Gilbert's disease) or conjugated (Dubin–Johnson and Rotor syndromes). The conjugated forms characteristically have bilirubinuria and deposition of dark, granular pigment in hepatocytes [439].

The patient is usually symptomless. Jaundice and dark urine may be noticed with excess alcohol, stress, fasting, exercise, oral contraceptive therapy and pregnancy [439–441].

The underlying mechanisms are not fully understood. The Dubin–Johnson syndrome is believed to relate to a functional inability to excrete organic ions including conjugated bilirubin, and certain dyes and porphyrins [442].

The only untoward effect in pregnancy is aggravation of jaundice [442] in up to half of the women [441]. Fetal outcome is good. An unconjugated hyperbilirubinaemia has been described in a neonate of a mother with Dubin–Johnson syndrome [443] but there is no specific risk of kernicterus [14]. The syndrome has been implicated as a cause of fetal death in some [444], but not all [442], cases of Dubin–Johnson syndrome. The main concern in obstetric practice is the differential diagnosis from other causes of cholestasis and jaundice in pregnancy, especially IHCP, biliary disease, gallstones and viral hepatitis that may alter management decisions for the fetus and mother [45]. Haemolytic anaemias, including that in Wilson's disease, and gallstones should be excluded. Dubin–Johnson syndrome, unlike IHCP and many other causes of cholestasis, is not associated with pruritus, and the serum alkaline phosphatase is within the normal range for pregnancy [440].

Inflammatory bowel disease and the liver

Abnormal liver tests and histological and radiological changes primarily affecting the biliary tract are common in ulcerative colitis and Crohn's disease. Surgical and postmortem liver specimens show histological abnormalities in 50–95%. The hepatic abnormalities do not seem to correlate with severity of inflammatory bowel disease. Symptomless patients may have significant sclerosing cholangitis and cholangiocarcinoma. Associations with HLA have been described but pathogenetic mechanisms remain obscure. There are no specific reports relating to outcome in pregnancy.

Sclerosing cholangitis

PSC is an uncommon form of progressive biliary disease; destruction of bile ducts and fibrosis that results in cirrhosis and cholangiocarcinoma [445]. The pathogenic mechanisms remain obscure. A significant number of patients have associated inflammatory bowel disease; 70 per cent, ulcerative colitis; and about 5 per cent, Crohn's disease. The clinical course is unpredictable. Hepatic abnormalities do not correlate with severity of inflammatory bowel disease. Elevation in serum alkaline phosphatase has been

shown to correlate with adverse prognosis but this marker is obscured by the placental component during pregnancy. Associations with HLA antigens B8 and DR3 have been described but do not correlate with prognosis [445].

Pruritus and abdominal pain are common presentations in pregnancy [446]. Itching may be sufficiently severe to prompt early delivery (see IHCP, above). No adverse outcome for mother or child was reported in a study of 13 pregnancies in 10 patients with a diagnosis of PSC preceding or presenting during pregnancy [446]. Individual reports of PSC warn of the potential for deterioration in liver function in the mother and accompanying severe elevations in fetal bile acids [447]. Transplantation has been carried out for PSC during pregnancy [448]. The differential diagnosis includes all presentations of cholestasis, especially PBC [449], IHCP (see above), including familial varieties [45], Caroli's disease and Dubin–Johnson syndrome.

Patients with PSC are at particular risk of developing cholangiocarcinoma as well as extrahepatic, and other hepatic, tumours [445]. Cholangiocarcinoma can be difficult to diagnose on endoscopic retrograde cholecystpancreatography (ERCP) and magnetic resonance cholecystpancreatography (MRCP), and cytology of brushings may be falsely negative. Prognosis remains abysmal and recurrence is almost invariable after liver transplantation.

Hepatic abscess

Amoebic abscess presenting in pregnancy is rare [450–454]. Outcome can be poor because the diagnosis is easily overlooked before catastrophic rupture. Presentation typically is in the third trimester or puerperium [451,452]. Clinical features are non-specific with abdominal discomfort, occasional fever or pulmonary features such as pain, pleural effusion and an elevated right diaphragm [454]. Rupture is common in late pregnancy and the puerperium [451]. Diagnosis often is late. Six of seven cases reviewed in one series [454] were diagnosed only at laparotomy for suspected appendicitis. Pregnancy, diabetes mellitus and immunosuppression are considered risk factors for amoebic colitis but no specific predilection has been linked to liver involvement.

Crohn's disease has been reported with intestinal fistula that was disclosed with septic shock and a liver abscess immediately postpartum [455] (see Crohn's disease, Chapter 10).

A strongly positive amoebic complement fixation test is diagnostic. For reasons that remain unclear, elevated serum levels of immunoglobulins are not invariable in pregnant patients with amoebiasis [456].

In pregnancy, liver abscess may be caused by unusual organisms such as *Listeria monocytogenes* [457], fungi especially in the immunocompromised patient, and *Echinococcus* spp. [458]. One-third of all reported cases of *L. monocytogenes* arise during pregnancy. For further details see Chapter 16.

Ultrasonographic analysis sometimes can differentiate between a pyogenic abscess and cyst due to *E. granulosus* (hydatid cyst) [459]. Hydatid disease must be excluded prior to surgical manipulation. Aspiration of a hydatid cyst has been carried out successfully in a primagravida during the 15th week of pregnancy [460] but is contraindicated in most cases, as dissemination of daughter scolices can prove fatal. Survival has improved significantly with earlier diagnosis using ultrasonographic techniques and effective antimicrobial agents such as metronidazole.

Polycystic liver disease

Polycystic liver disease shows an autosomal dominant inheritance and is found most often in multiparous women with concurrence of renal cysts [461]. Pregnant patients may present with abdominal pain due to enlargement of the cysts, infection and hepatomegaly [462]. Several factors, including age, female gender, pregnancy and the degree of renal involvement and functional impairment may modify the expression of hepatic cystic disease [463]. Differential diagnosis of an enlarged liver includes polycystic liver disease and congenital hepatic fibrosis. Serial transcutaneous aspirations through all trimesters were required for abdominal pain in one patient [462].

Hepatic tumours

ORAL CONTRACEPTIVE STEROIDS AND THE LIVER

A variety of benign and malignant hepatic lesions have been found more commonly in users than non-users of oral contraceptive steroids. Hepatic adenoma and follicular nodular hyperplasia are rare but recognized associations [464]. Development of hepatic adenomata was first linked to oral contraceptive use in 1973 [465]. This tumour has become more common since the dramatic rise in consumption of oral contraceptive steroids [466]. Overwhelming evidence for this association is available from case–control studies. The relative risk after 5 years of oral contraceptive therapy has been estimated at between 100 and 500 times that of non-users [467]. Importantly, regression of the lesion follows cessation of therapy.

In pregnancy, the main concern is rupture of this very vascular tumour [468]. Successful pregnancy has been reported following partial hepatectomy for removal of multiple adenomata [196]. Some adenomata show histological features of focal nodular hyperplasia and malignant change. This interrelation between hepatic adenoma, focal nodular hyperplasia and carcinoma [466,469] casts doubt on their benign classification.

PRIMARY LIVER CANCER (HEPATOCELLULAR CARCINOMA, HEPATOMA)

Primary liver cancer is linked with oral contraceptive use [467,470]. The number of cases in young women has risen since 1970 in line with rising use of oral contraceptive therapy [471]. One series from London reported that 18 of 26 white women aged less than 50 years with tumour arising in a non-cirrhotic liver had used oral contraceptive steroids for a median of 8 years [467]. Short-term use for less than 8 years was not associated with an increased risk of tumour development, although individual case reports attest to shorter intervals [470]. The risk increased 4.4-fold in users beyond 8 years and 7.2-fold when hepatitis B infection was excluded. These risks are significant but much less than those for development of hepatic adenoma [467]. Other confounding factors include HBV and smoking. High-dose oestrogen (e.g. mestranol >50 μg daily) had been implicated in earlier studies but seven of the 17 women in the London survey had taken low-dose (<30 μg daily) oestrogen [467]. Rarely, primary liver cancer may present in pregnancy. This can be associated with rapid growth of the tumour and an abysmal prognosis [472–474]. Although individual reports document survival of mother and child following extensive resection during pregnancy [470], few pregnancies result in a live infant [472].

The clinical findings are similar regardless of pregnancy. Most cases with cirrhosis show a marked elevation in serum level of α-fetoprotein. The main differential diagnosis is from treatable causes of a rapidly expanding mass such as benign hepatic tumours requiring resection and hepatic abscess (see above) and metastatic malignancy. Serological tests should include screening for HBV and HCV and an amoebic complement fixation test. Serum levels of carcinoembryonic antigen (CEA) and β-human choriogonadotropin (β-hCG) may be raised causing confusion with gestational trophoblastic disease (choriocarcinoma) [475] (see below).

Cholangiocarcinoma is rare (see PSC, above). Single case reports document presentation in pregnancy [476,477]. Prognosis remains poor. Clinically, the tumour presents with signs of extrahepatic cholestasis and pruritus. The main differential diagnosis is from the common causes of bile duct obstruction (see below), intrahepatic cholestasis, PBC and pancreatic abnormalities.

METASTATIC TROPHOBLASTIC DISEASE

Elevated or rising titres of serum and urinary β-hCG after evacuation of a hydatidiform mole or antecedent pregnancy indicate residual functional trophoblastic tissue and, possibly, malignant transformation to gestational trophoblastic disease (choriocarcinoma) [478–480]. In a retrospective study extending over 36 years, liver metastases were detected at presentation in 2.7% of 1676 women being treated for gestational trophoblastic disease at the national referral centre in the UK [481]. Liver metastases from gestational trophoblastic disease were found to be a significant independent variable carrying a poor prognosis; the additional finding of cerebral metastases worsened further the prognosis [481–484]. Overall survival in the poor prognosis category is 72% but falls to 33% with liver metastases [483]. In a study from North Carolina, USA, 15 of 126 women (12%) followed with gestational trophoblastic disease between 1966 and 1980 had liver metastases from a previous hydatidiform mole (seven cases), a previous full-term delivery (six cases) and presumed aborted pregnancy (two cases) [483]. Similar findings were reported from Texas [485] and Hong Kong [484]. Survival in the American studies [483,485] was less than 40% despite use of a modified Bagshawe regimen of multiagent chemotherapy and sublethal hepatic irradiation [480]. The majority with hepatic metastases had other risk factors associated with a poor prognosis such as a previous term pregnancy [485], multiple sites and high titres (>40 000 IU/L) of β-hCG in serum and urine [483]. More optimistic results were published from Hong Kong [484]. Complete remission was achieved in seven of 10 patients following vigorous multiagent chemotherapy. Partial remission was achieved in a further two who were changed to etoposide following resistance to the modified Bagshawe regimen. Improved results were attributed to aggressive and flexible chemotherapy regimes. Interestingly, these patients also had additional risk factors but in only two did their metastases arise from a previous full-term pregnancy [484].

Previous reports have stressed that hepatic, gastrointestinal and splenic haemorrhage [486] are the most significant complications of liver metastases in gestational trophoblastic disease [487]. Haemorrhage was not common in the above studies [483,484] and seemed amenable to embolization. Some authors recommended prophylactic irradiation to the liver [482]. The doses used were sublethal but not tumoricidal. No controlled trials have been carried out to prove the efficacy of sublethal irradiation in such patients [482]. Irradiation to the liver may result in enhanced hepatotoxicity in the presence of chemotherapeutic agents [483]. Other therapies tried for hepatic metastases have included embolization, surgical resection and regional perfusion with chemotherapeutic agents [483]. Future approaches aim to improve delineation of hepatic metastases because these place the patient into the high-risk category and affect the choice of chemotherapy [483,488]. The superiority of individual radiographic techniques for visualization of hepatic metastases remains undecided. Ultrasonography for tissue characterization is very useful [488], although some lesions are very diffuse and only visualized by hepatic arteriography [484] and CT scanning.

Gestational trophoblastic disease believed to arise from within the liver (primary choriocarcinoma) has been reported [489]. Differentiation from primary hepatocellular carcinoma is difficult due to overlapping histological features and elevated levels of β-hCG documented in up to 17% of cases of primary liver cancer [475].

The gallbladder and biliary tract

Anatomy and physiology

Fasting gallbladder volume increases through pregnancy [490,491] whereas residual volumes are increased in late pregnancy [491,492]. Results of dynamic studies remain controversial. Rates of contraction and emptying measured by ultrasonographic imaging were similar to non-pregnant controls [493]. No differences were found in patient characteristics between women with normal gallbladders and those with sludge or gallstones [491]. Gallbladder emptying was impaired in the luteal phase of the ovulatory cycle in one study [494] but was considered normal by others [495]. Oral contraceptive users may have normal gallbladder volumes and emptying [496] or increased fasting volumes on ultrasonographic imaging after a liquid meal [495]. In one study [497], although not another [498], the mean diameter of the common bile duct was increased through pregnancy compared to that in non-pregnant females. The relaxant action of progestagens on smooth muscle does not correlate with early dysfunction because serum progestagens rise significantly only after the first trimester. Oestrogens may impair water absorption by the gallbladder by inhibiting the sodium–potassium ATPase pump [496,498]. In primates, oestriol can effect a dose-dependent reduction in volume of bile [498].

The US Food and Drugs Administration (FDA) requires that information on the increased risks of gallbladder disease be included with instructions to users of oral contraceptive steroids [499]. In Australia, a large case–control study was conducted [500] on the interrelation between oral contraceptive steroids, pregnancy and gallbladder disease. Two hundred women with newly diagnosed gallstones based on ultrasonographic analysis were case-matched with women with suspected, but unproven, cholelithiasis and healthy controls. The risk of developing gallstones rose with parity only in young women and declined with rising age at first pregnancy. There was a dose–response relation between the relative risk of developing gallstones and exposure to pregnancy in the young patient [500].

A subpopulation of women seem susceptible to early development of gallstones after exposure to oral contraceptive steroids and pregnancy. The mean duration of oral contraceptive exposure for women with gallstones (<1 year) was lower than for healthy controls indicating that the increase in relative risk was of short duration. The rate of development of cholelithiasis fell with increasing duration of contraceptive use. These findings may explain the significant risk found only in short-term follow-up of pregnant women and oral contraceptive users. The authors [500] concluded that the degree, rather than period, of exposure to ovarian activity increased significantly the risk of developing gallstones. The increased risk seen in subsequent pregnancies may be related to 'oestrogenic shift'. Links with oestrogens include the finding of elevated levels of urinary oestrone in women with gallstones [500] and the statistical correlation between vomiting in pregnancy, gallbladder disease and a known intolerance to oral contraceptive steroids. The hormonal load on the liver in early pregnancy may be similar to that with oral contraceptive steroids [501] (see nausea and vomiting in pregnancy, Chapter 10).

Cholesterol cholelithiasis

Cholesterol gallstones are common in the West and found in women more often than men [502] and in users of oral contraceptive steroids. The sex difference commences at the menarche and remains throughout reproductive life. Other established risk factors include obesity, gastrointestinal disorders with malabsorption of bile salts such as Crohn's disease and small bowel resection, liver diseases and diabetes mellitus. The impact of pregnancy and parity remains unresolved due to the controversial interpretations of results of biliary physiology.

A prerequisite for stone formation includes the hepatic secretion of lithogenic bile [495]. In the non-pregnant female, when compared with the male, there is a reduction in total bile acid pool, in particular for chenodeoxycholic acid (CDCA). In users of oral contraceptive steroids the ratio of cholate to CDCA falls rendering the bile more saturated and therefore more lithogenic [7,503]. In the second and third trimesters there is a progressive decrease in the size of the pool of CDCA, but not of cholic acid. As the overall rate of cholesterol secretion is unchanged, its concentration is increased relative to the diminishing size of the bile acid pool, rendering the bile more lithogenic [7,504]. Oestrogens and progestagens have marked and different effects on metabolism of bile salts, cholesterol and biliary lipids, at least in the rat [505]. Ethinyl oestradiol causes an increase in cholesterol content within the liver but decreases the secretion of bile salts [506]. Progesterone increases the rate of esterification, but not synthesis, of cholesterol and causes an increase in bile salt-independent bile secretion. The net effect is to increase saturation of the bile with cholesterol [7,505].

CHOLELITHIASIS IN PREGNANCY

Gallbladder disease in pregnancy is the most common non-obstetric condition requiring surgery after acute appendicitis [507–510]. In a prospective study of 669 pregnant women in Greece, gallstones were detected in 1% at first screening and in an additional 2% at later follow-up [509]. Parity was found to be a significant factor for an increased risk of new gallstone formation as well as for the likelihood of cholelithiasis in the Greek [509], but not Chilean, study [508]. In Chile where cholelithiasis is common, gallstones were detected in 12% of 980 women in the immediate postpartum period compared with 1.3% of 150 age-matched nulliparous controls [508]. Biliary colic occurred in 70 women with stones in a contractile gallbladder. Pain was most common with stones above 10 mm in diameter. Stone formation correlated with saturation of bile with cholesterol during pregnancy [508]. Conversely, resolution of pain and disappearance of small stones occurred in those women after delivery that showed desaturation of their cholesterol with bile.

Acute cholecystitis requiring surgery and cholecystectomy has been reported in about one per 1000 deliveries [507,511–513]. Detection during pregnancy of symptomless gallstones by ultrasonography has varied between 2.5% (normal for non-pregnant young females) and 11% [514,515]. Echogenic bile—'biliary sludge'—was detected in 36% of pregnant women examined serially using ultrasonography [490]. Gallstones were seen to develop at 37 weeks following echogenic bile at 31 weeks [490]. The variable literature reflects biased reporting, variation in equipment and user expertise, and the prevalence of obesity and parity of the population sampled [492,515].

The classical presentation is with pain in the right upper quadrant that may radiate through to the back [507]. Nausea and vomiting are frequent but weight loss, intolerance to fatty food and fever are uncommon. The gallbladder usually is not palpable [507,511]. A past medical history may suggest gallbladder disease. Spontaneous perforation of the gallbladder has been reported in pregnancy [516].

The differential diagnosis of acute cholecystitis is wide and includes other causes of cholestatic jaundice and abdominal pain such as viral hepatitis, alcoholic hepatitis, acute pyelonephritis and other infections, including AIDS as well as HELLP syndrome.

Thickening of the gallbladder wall in severe pre-eclampsia probably reflects the marked hypoalbuminaemia and oedema and should not be mistaken for an attack of cholecystitis [517].

Cirrhosis and IHCP (see above) are associated with cholelithiasis.

MANAGEMENT

The role of routine screening for gallstones and management of the symptomless patient remain controversial [492,514]. Management of acute cholecystitis and biliary obstruction is the same as that in the non-pregnant patient. General measures are bed rest, withdrawal of oral feeding, rehydration with intravenous fluids and antibiotics that concentrate in bile. Detection of stones in the common bile duct is more difficult than for those in the gallbladder [518]. Ultrasonography is not helpful for determining the state of the papilla of Vater or the presence of a biliary stricture. Coexisting pancreatitis may be overlooked by obscuring gas from a small bowel ileus [519]. The biliary tree can be outlined using a technetium-99 (hepatobiliary iminodiacetic) HIDA scan with minimal irradiation to the fetus [519]. The use of ERCP and percutaneous transhepatic cholecystography (PTC) are not justified if the fetus cannot be shielded from the significant doses of irradiation given [520]. A film badge should be placed near the abdomen to monitor the exposure. Preference should be given to pre- and intraoperative ultrasonographic analysis. Fibre-optic endoscopic cannulation with retrieval of stones may be possible [520].

Laparoscopic cholecystectomy combined with caesarean section has been successful [513,521]. About 170 laparoscopic cholecystectomies during pregnancy have been reported up until 1999. A retrospective review of the literature up to 1997 indicated that when laparoscopic cholecystectomy is compared to open cholecystectomy, the risk of spontaneous abortion may be reduced in the first trimester, and preterm labour reduced in the third trimester [522]. Laparoscopic techniques should be reserved for the severely symptomatic patient [510,513]. Laparoscopic cholecystectomy seems safe throughout pregnancy when carried out by skilled surgeons. Guidelines have been formulated by the Society of American Gastrointestinal Endoscopic Surgeons that address laparo-

scopic surgery during pregnancy and issues such a pneumoperitoneum [523]. Risks include bleeding and in the third trimester the enlarged uterus imposes visual limitations. Some authors [519] recommend delaying cholecystectomy until after delivery but recurrent attacks are common [507,511].

Medical management may be less successful postpartum and there is an increase in postoperative complications such as deep venous thrombosis [507]. Fetal outcome [507,519] is optimal for surgery carried out in the second trimester. This timing coincides with less risk from spontaneous abortion and before the uterus is sufficiently large to displace significantly the liver [507,519]. Clinical and biochemical evidence of pancreatitis is common especially with stones in the common bile duct [519]. The risk of maternal and fetal mortality rises significantly when cholelithiasis is associated with pancreatitis complicated by pseudocyst [524] (see acute pancreatitis, below).

Stones in the common bile duct may be painless and jaundice in pregnancy is uncommon. The patient may develop a high fever, rigors and a polymorphonuclear leucocytosis due to cholangitis [507]. Surgical intervention is obligatory for large duct obstruction to avoid recurrent attacks and other complications including cholangitis, pancreatitis and empyema of the gallbladder. Rarely, biliary obstruction may be due to cholangiocarcinoma (see above) or *Clonorchis silensis* from the Far East. Management is the same as for non-pregnant individuals. HIV infection is associated with acalculous cholangitis and large duct dilatation.

Bile acid therapy with CDCA, ursocholic acid and their congeners that can dissolve cholesterol gallstones is contraindicated in pregnancy [525]. Bile acids cross the placenta. CDCA has been linked to liver toxicity and teratogenicity in animals [525]. Lithotrypsy is contraindicated in pregnancy.

The pancreas

The normal range for serum amylase is wide and its behaviour in normal pregnancy remains controversial [526–528]. Amylase is secreted by the pancreas, salivary, sweat and lactating mammary glands [528]. Production by the fallopian tube accounts for the very elevated serum levels found in a ruptured ectopic pregnancy [528].

A markedly elevated level of serum amylase remains the cornerstone for diagnosing pancreatitis. In pregnancy this may be difficult because the values in serum of amylase and its ratio to creatinine and lipases may be misleadingly low, even normal, in the first trimester despite severe pancreatitis. The high levels of serum triglycerides found in late pregnancy are associated with pancreatitis and can interfere with amylase levels. The renal clearances of amylase and creatinine are elevated in pregnancy. Whether the use of ratios is superior to a single elevated level of serum amylase, remains debatable. The level of serum lipase rises in parallel with amylase and may be of use in the diagnosis of acute pancreatitis in pregnancy but information is lacking.

Acute pancreatitis

This is an uncommon cause of abdominal pain in pregnancy and has been reported in 1:1100–11000 live births [529–533]. Reported series are biased towards the severe end of the spectrum. Pregnancy and the postpartum period do not precipitate or protect against severe pancreatitis. Fewer cases occurred postpartum than at any time during pregnancy [533].

The morbidity and mortality from acute pancreatitis remain high regardless of pregnancy. In early surveys, maternal deaths were as high as 20% [534–535] with neonatal losses in up to half [531,535]. Series after 1980 suggest that maternal mortalities are similar to the non-pregnant and fetal losses are about 10% [533].

There is no specific association between pancreatitis and pregnancy. The pathogenic mechanisms causing acute pancreatitis are poorly understood except for the link with gallstones. Other unproven mechanisms that predispose a pregnant patient to pancreatitis include the relaxant effect of progestagens leading to atony of the biliary tract, bile stasis in the duodenum and reflux [7,536]. Extreme elevations in abdominal pressure from vomiting in toxaemia could promote a rise in intrapancreatic pressure, rupture of the ducts and release of enzymes [537]. These suggestions lack scientific data and ignore the confounding influence of diuretic therapies in the treatment of hypertension, which may predispose to pancreatitis [84]. Pancreatitis can be associated with an underlying hypertriglyceridaemia, especially during pregnancy [532,538]. Alternatively, pregnancy and oral contraceptive steroids may unmask an underlying lipid disorder such as lipase-deficient familial hypertriglyceridemia [538] associated with high levels of VLDL and chylomicrons (type V hyperlipidaemia) or type I hyperlipidaemia [539]. A novel gene mutation (*Glutamine421Lysine*) in the gene for lipoprotein lipase was reported in a previously healthy primagravida who died from severe pancreatitis associated with reduced lipoprotein lipase and hypertriglyceridaemia during the third trimester of pregnancy [540].

Primary hyperparathyroidism remains a rare cause of pancreatitis during pregnancy, although over 50 cases have been reported (see Chapter 14) [541,542]. Other un-common associations are a hyperfunctioning parathyroid carcinoma [543], alcoholism [530,544], thiazides and corticosteroid treatment and infections such as mumps [537,545] and acute fatty liver [125]; see above).

CLINICAL PRESENTATION

Typically, this occurs in late pregnancy, possibly coinciding with the peak in serum levels of triglycerides. But acute pancreatitis can occur at any time and there seems to be no influence of maternal parity or age [533]. Abdominal pain is maximal in the epigastrum, often constant (not colicky) and may radiate through to the back. Pain is not invariable; up to one-quarter may present with only nausea and vomiting [530]. Physical examination may be unhelpful.

Severe haemorrhagic pancreatitis presents with profound shock, hypotension and marked hypovolaemia. Other features include ecchymoses, pleural effusions, hypoxia due to adult respiratory distress syndrome and milky ascites. A paralytic ileus and enlarged uterus may obscure ultrasonographic images. The detection of gallstones may point to underlying pancreatitis. A markedly elevated level of amylase in various body fluids, including a pleural effusion may persist after serum levels return to normal.

Pancreatitis associated with gallstones in the common bile duct is usually associated with an elevation in serum alkaline phosphatase beyond that attributed to placental growth and in GGT levels.

The differential diagnosis in pregnancy and the puerperium includes all other causes of abdominal pain, nausea and vomiting. This wide list includes acute appendicitis, peptic ulceration, hyperemesis gravidarum, pre-eclamptic toxaemia, renal infections and many liver disorders such as hepatitis, abscess, cholecystitis and AFLP. The differential diagnosis from a ruptured ectopic pregnancy or ruptured spleen may be difficult especially with bloody ascites.

MANAGEMENT

The aims are to induce a state of visceral rest and to prevent complications. Nasogastric suction is traditional and comforting but lacks evidence for efficacy and may promote elevations in serum amylase and delay the return of bowel sounds. There are no specific therapies. Various agents have been used as inhibitors of pancreatic secretion including anticholinergic agents, glucagon, corticosteroids, prostaglandins, vasopressin, trypsin inhibitors and ε-amino-caproic acid but results of trials are conflicting or absent. The H_2 antagonists inhibit the acid stimulus to pancreatic secretion but have no demonstrable effect on biliary or pancreatic secretion. Medium-chain triglycerides accompanied by a strict low-calorie diet with low fat have provided nutritional support in individual cases with good outcome [538].

Total parenteral nutrition has been used successfully in a malnourished pregnant woman with alcoholism [546]. Therapy was maintained for 83 days prior to elective caesarean section at 36 weeks' gestation with delivery of a 2.12-kg baby [546]. Total parenteral nutrition has also been used in the third trimester for acute pancreatitis complicated by a pseudocyst and marked hypoalbumi-naemia associated with intrauterine growth restriction [547] (see parenteral nutrition, Chapter 10).

A major consideration includes the prevention and management of other complications. Hypovolaemia may be marked. Strict attention should be paid to central monitoring of fluid balance and replacement with colloid and crystalloid solutions. Other problems include electro-lyte imbalance with hypocalcaemia and hypomagnesae-mia, carbohydrate intolerance, renal failure, fat necrosis, haemorrhage including DIC, venous thrombosis, ascites, peritonitis, intestinal damage, jaundice and hepatic and metabolic encephalopathies. Pulmonary oedema, pleural effusions and respiratory distress syndromes may pro-duce profound hypoxia requiring assisted respiratory support and oxygen therapy.

In the majority of uncomplicated cases in pregnancy, the disease settles with conservative management. Preg-nancy poses additional problems because the use of many of the therapeutic agents remains controversial. Termin-ation of pregnancy is rarely indicated and does not seem to improve maternal outcome [531]. Elective induction of labour in the third trimester has been recommended [531,536] but remains controversial and offers no guaran-tee of cessation of the pathological state after delivery. Fetal loss remains high [532].

The optimal timing for surgery for gallstones associated with pancreatitis is in the second trimester. Surgery is best performed during the same hospital admission but after the first attack has settled. Recurrent attacks of acute cholecystitis, biliary colic and pancreatitis are common.

Cystic fibrosis

This condition can affect the pancreas in pregnancy and is described in Chapter 1.

Pancreas transplantation

Pregnancy and outcome have been successful in recipi-ents of pancreas transplants with and without kidney grafts [548,549]. The National Transplantation Pregnancy

Registry recorded 15 pregnancies in recipients of com-bined pancreas and kidney allografts [366,549]. Prematur-ity and low birthweights were common among the 12 live births; two-thirds had been delivered by caesarean section. Complications were typical of those in the im-munosuppressed host with increased episodes of infec-tion especially of the urinary tract, also hypertension and eclampsia [366,549]. Two of the women experienced three subsequent graft losses within 2 years of giving birth, although retransplantations were successful [549]. False-negative pregnancy tests have been reported in a pan-creas transplant recipient in whom drainage was directed into the bladder rather than bowel [548].

Malignancies

In a 3-year survey from the CDC in the USA, 2.8% of patients with malignancies in the reproductive age group had carcinoma of the pancreas [550]. There are reports in pregnancy and the puerperium of pancreatic adenocarcinoma [551], mucin-secreting cystadenoma [552], adenocarcinoma [553], papillary cystic tumour [554] and insulinoma [555]. The outcome of these malig-nant tumours is poor regardless of pregnancy. The rapid growth of certain pancreatic tumours in pregnancy may reflect their dependency on sex hormones [552,554]. Isol-ated cases of adenocarcinoma and insulinoma have been reported in pregnancy and the puerperium [556]. In insu-linoma, early recognition of hypoglycemia, neurological features, and elevated levels of insulin and C peptide can lead to early diagnosis, surgery and successful outcome of pregnancy [556].

References

1 Craigo SD. Liver disease in pregnancy. *Semin Perinatol* 1998; 22: 97–182.

2 Klebanoff MA, Koslowe PA *et al.* Epidemiology of vomiting in early pregnancy. *Obstet Gynecol* 1985; 66: 612–16.

3 Department of Health and Social Security. *Report on Confidential Enquiries into Maternal Deaths in the United Kingdom 1985–87.* HMSO, London, 1991.

4 Department of Health and Social Security. *Report on Confidential Enquiries into Maternal Deaths in the United Kingdom 1994–96.* HMSO, London, 1998.

5 Robson SC, Mutch E *et al.* Apparent liver blood flow during pregnancy: a serial study using indocyanine green clearance. *Br J Obstet Gynaecol* 1990; 97: 720–4.

6 Kerr MG, Scott DB *et al.* Studies of the inferior vena cava in late pregnancy. *BMJ* 1964; 1: 532–3.

7 Van Thiel D. Effects of pregnancy and sex hormones on the liver. *Sem Liver Dis* 1987; 7: 1–66.

8 Girling JC, Dow E *et al.* Liver function tests in pre-eclampsia: importance of comparison with a reference range derived for normal pregnancy. *Br J Obstet Gynaecol* 1997; 104: 246–50.

9 Bacq Y, Zarka O *et al*. Liver function tests in normal pregnancy: a prospective study of 103 pregnant women and 103 matched controls. *Hepatology* 1996; 23: 1030–34.

10 Freund G, Arvan DA. Clinical biochemistry of pre-eclampsia and related liver diseases of pregnancy: a review. *Clin Chim Acta* 1990; 191: 123–51.

11 Bernstein RB, Novy MJ *et al*. Bilirubin metabolism in the fetus. *J Clin Invest* 1969; 48: 1678–88.

12 Waffarn F, Carlisle S *et al*. Fetal exposure to maternal hyperbilirubinaemia. *J Dis Child* 1982; 136: 416–17.

13 Baker VV, Cefalo RC. Fulminant hepatic failure in the third trimester of pregnancy. A case report. *J Reprod Med* 1985; 30: 229–31.

14 Levine RL, Fredricks WR *et al*. Entry of bilirubin into the brain due to opening of the blood-brain barrier. *Pediatrics* 1982; 69: 255–9.

15 Rolfes DB, Ishak KG. Liver disease in pregnancy. *Histopathology* 1986; 10: 555–70.

16 Fagan EA. Intrahepatic cholestasis of pregnancy. *Clin Liver Dis* 1999; 3: 603–32.

17 Lammert FL, Marschall H-U, *et al*. Intrahepatic cholestasis of pregnancy: molecular pathogenesis, diagnosis and management. *J Hepatol* 2000; 33: 1012–21.

18 Shaw D, Frohlich J *et al*. A prospective study of 18 patients with cholestasis of pregnancy. *Am J Obstet Gynecol* 1982; 142: 621–5.

19 Qui ZD, Wang QN *et al*. Intrahepatic cholestasis of pregnancy. Clinical analysis and follow-up study of 22 cases. *Chin Med J (Engl)* 1983; 96: 902–6.

20 Berg B, Helm G *et al*. Cholestasis of pregnancy. Clinical and laboratory studies. *Acta Obstet Gynecol Scand* 1986; 65: 107–13.

21 Laatikainen T, Tulenheiko A. Maternal serum bile acid levels and fetal distress in cholestasis of pregnancy. *Int J Gynaecol Obstet* 1984; 22: 91–4.

22 Bennett NMcK., Lehmann NI *et al*. Viral hepatitis and intrahepatic cholestasis of pregnancy. *Aust N Z J Med* 1979; 9: 54–7.

23 Roszkowski I, Wojcicka J. Jaundice in pregnancy. 1. Biochemical assays. *Am J Obstet Gynecol* 1968; 102: 839–46.

24 Reyes H, Ribalda J *et al*. Idiopathic cholestasis in a large kindred. *Gut* 1976; 17: 709–13.

25 Reyes H, Baez ME *et al*. Selenium, zinc and copper plasma levels in intrahepatic cholestasis of pregnancy, in normal pregnancies and in healthy individuals, in Chile. *J Hepatol* 2000; 32: 542–9.

26 Steel R, Parker ML. Jaundice in pregnancy. *Med J Aust* 1973; 1: 461.

27 Thorling L. Jaundice in pregnancy: clinical study. *Acta Med Scand* 1955; 302 (Suppl.): 1–123.

28 Svanborg A. A study of recurrent jaundice in pregnancy. *Acta Obstet Gynecol Scand* 1954; 33: 434–44.

29 Misra PS, Evanov FA *et al*. Idiopathic intrahepatic cholestasis of pregnancy. Report of an unusual case and review of the recent literature. *A J Gastroenterol* 1980; 73: 54–9.

30 Kirkinen P, Ylostalo P *et al*. Gallbladder function and maternal bile acids in intrahepatic cholestasis of pregnancy. *European J Obstet Gynecol Reprod Biol* 1984; 18: 29–34.

31 Kreek MJ, Sleisenger MH *et al*. Recurrent cholestatic jaundice of pregnancy with demonstrated estrogen sensitivity. *Am J Med* 1967; 43: 795–803.

32 Orellana-Alcalde JM, Dominguez JP. Jaundice and oral contraceptive drugs. *Lancet* 1966; 1: 1278–80.

33 Ockner RK, Davidson CS. Hepatic effects of oral contraceptives. *New Engl J Med* 1967; 276: 331–4.

34 Urban E, Frank BW *et al*. Liver dysfunction with mestranol but not with norethynodrel in a patient with Enovid-induced jaundice. *Ann Int Med* 1968; 68: 598–602.

35 Drill VA. Benign cholestatic jaundice of pregnancy and benign cholestatic jaundice from oral contraceptives. *Am J Obstet Gynecol* 1974; 119: 165–74.

36 Jeppsson S, Rannevik G. Effect of oral 17-beta-oestradiol on the liver in women with intrahepatic cholestasis (hepatosis) during previous pregnancy. *Br J Obstet Gynaecol* 1976; 83: 567–71.

37 Hirvioja ML, Tuimala, R, Vuori J. The treatment of intrahepatic cholestasis. Hirvioja ML, Tuimala R, Vuori J eds. The treatment of intrahepatic cholestasis of pregnancy with dexamethasone. *Br J Obstet Gynaecol* 1992; 99: 109–11.

38 Tiitinen A, Laatikainen T *et al*. Placental protein 10 (PP10) in normal pregnancy and cholestasis of pregnancy. *Br J Obstet Gynaecol* 1985; 92: 1137–40.

39 Johnson P. Studies in cholestasis of pregnancy with special reference to lipids and lipoproteins. *Acta Obstet Gynecol Scand* 1973; 27 (Suppl.): 1–80.

40 Ranta T, Vnnerus HA *et al*. Elevated plasma prolactin concentration in cholestasis of pregnancy. *Am J Obstet Gynecol* 1979; 134: 1–3.

41 Heikinheimo M, Aunnerus H *et al*. Pregnancy specific beta-1-glycoprotein levels in cholestasis of pregnancy. *Obstet Gynecol* 1978; 52: 276–8.

42 Holtzbach RT, Sivak DA *et al*. Familial recurrent interhepatic cholestasis of pregnancy: a genetic study providing evidence for transmission of a sex-linked dominant trait. *Gastroenterology* 1983; 85: 75–9.

43 Bacq Y, Sapey T *et al*. Intrahepatic cholestasis of pregnancy: a French prospective study. *Hepatology* 1997; 26: 358–64.

44 Gonzalez MC, Reyes H *et al*. Intrahepatic cholestasis of pregnancy in twin pregnancies. *J Hepatol* 1989; 9: 84–90.

45 Leevy CB, Koneru B *et al*. Recurrent familial prolonged intrahepatic cholestasis of pregnancy associated with chronic liver disease. *Gastroenterology* 1997; 113: 966–72.

46 Reyes H, Simon FR. Intrahepatic cholestasis of pregnancy: an estrogen-related disease. *Sem Liver Dis* 1993; 13: 289–301.

47 Davies MH, Ngong JM *et al*. The adverse influence of pregnancy upon sulphation: a clue to the pathogenesis of intrahepatic cholestasis of pregnancy? *J Hepatol* 1994; 21: 1127–34.

48 Palma J, Reyes H *et al*. Ursodeoxycholic acid in the treatment of cholestasis of pregnancy: a randomized, double-blind study controlled with placebo. *J Hepatol* 1997; 27: 1022–28.

49 Trauner M, Arrese M *et al*. The rat canalicular conjugate export pump (Mrp2) is down-regulated in intrahepatic and obstructive cholestasis. *Gastroenterology* 1997; 113: 255–64.

50 Meng L-J, Reyes H *et al*. Progesterone metabolites and bile acids in serum of patients with intrahepatic cholestasis of pregnancy: effect of ursodeoxycholic acid therapy. *Hepatology* 1997; 26: 1573–9.

51 Meng L-J, Reyes H *et al*. Effects of ursodeoxycholic acid on conjugated bile acids and progesterone metabolites in serum and urine of patients with intrahepatic cholestasis of pregnancy. *J Hepatol* 1997; 27: 1029–40.

52 Laatikainen T, Karjalainen O *et al*. Excretion of progesterone metabolites in urine and bile of pregnant women with intrahepatic cholestasis. *J Steroid Biochem* 1973; 4: 641–8.

53 Sjovall J, Sjovall K. Steroid sulphates in plasma from pregnant women with pruritus and elevated plasma bile acid levels. *Ann Clin Res* 1970; 2: 321–7.

54 Eriksson H, Gustafsson JA *et al.* Excretion of neutral steroids in urine and faeces of women with intrahepatic cholestasis of pregnancy. *Steroids Lipids Res* 1972; 3: 30–48.

55 Frezza M, Pozzato G *et al.* Reversal of intrahepatic cholestasis of pregnancy in women after high dose S-adenosyl-1-methionine. *Hepatology* 1984; 4: 274–8.

56 Trauner M, Arrese M *et al.* The rat canalicular conjugate export pump (M_{RP}2) is down-regulated in inter hepatic and obstructive cholestasis. *Gastroenterology* 1997; 113: 255–64.

57 Kren BT, Rodrigues CMP *et al.* Postranscriptional regulation of steady-state mRNA levels in rat liver associated with deoxycholic acid feeding. *A J Physiol* 1995; 269: G961.

58 Guattery JM, Faloon WW. Effect of estradiol upon serum enzymes in primary biliary cirrhosis. *Hepatology* 1987; 7: 737–42.

59 Sotaniemi EA, Hynnynen T *et al.* Effects of medroxyprogesterone on the liver function and drug metabolism of patients with primary biliary cirrhosis and chronic active hepatitis. *J Med* 1978; 9: 117–28.

60 Kiilholma P. Serum copper and zinc concentrations in intrahepatic cholestasis of pregnancy: a controlled study. *Eur J Obst, Gynecol Reprod Biol* 1986; 21: 207–12.

61 Heikkinen J, Maentausta O *et al.* Changes in serum bile acid concentrations during normal pregnancy, in women with intrahepatic cholestasis of pregnancy and in pregnant patients with itching. *Br J Obstet Gynaecol* 1981; 88: 240–5.

62 Lunzer M, Barnes P *et al.* Serum bile acid concentrations during pregnancy and their relationship to obstetric cholestasis. *Gastroenterology* 1986; 91: 825–9.

63 Brites D, Rodrigues CMP. Elevated levels of bile acids in colostrum of patients with cholestasis of pregnancy are decreased following ursodeoxycholic acid therapy. *J Hepatol* 1998; 29: 743–51.

64 Brites D, Rodrigues CMP *et al.* Correction of maternal serum bile acid profile during ursodeoxycholic acid therapy in cholestasis of pregnancy. *J Hepatol* 1998; 28: 91–8.

65 van Berge Henegouwen GP, Brandt KH *et al.* Sulfated and unsulfated bile acids in serum, bile and urine in patients with cholestasis. *Gut* 1976; 17: 861–9.

66 Setchell KDR, Kritchevsky D, Nair PP, Back P. Urinary bile acids. In: Setchell KDR Kritchevsky D, Nair PP, eds. *The Bile Acids: Chemistry, Physiology, and Metabolism,* 1988; Vol. 4. New York, Plenum Press: 404.

67 Monte MJ, Morales AI *et al.* Reversible impairment of neonatal hepatobiliary function by maternal cholestasis. *Hepatology* 1996; 23: 1208–17.

68 Arrese M, Trauner M *et al.* Maternal cholestasis does not affect the ontogenic pattern of expression of the Na^+/taurocholate cotransporting polypeptide (ntcp) in the fetal and neonatal rat liver. *Hepatology* 1998; 28: 789–95.

69 Muller M, Jansen PLM. The secretory function of the liver: new aspects of hepatobiliary transport. *J Hepatol* 1998; 28: 344–54.

70 Serrano MA, Brites D *et al.* Beneficial effect of ursodeoxycholic acid on alterations induced by cholestasis of pregnancy in bile acid transport across the human placenta. *J Hepatol* 1998; 28: 829–39.

71 Rodrigues CM, Marin JJ *et al.* Bile acid patterns in meconium are influenced by cholestasis of pregnancy and not altered by ursodeoxycholic acid treatment. *Gut* 1999; 45: 446–52.

72 Jones EA, Bergasa NU. The pruritus of cholestasis: from bile acids to opiate antagonists. *Hepatology* 1990; 11: 884–7.

73 Bergasa NV, Vergalla J *et al.* Hepatic concentrations of proenkephalin-derived opioids are increased in a rat model of cholestasis. *Liver* 1996; 16: 298–302.

74 Alsulyman OM, Ouzounian JG *et al.* Intrahepatic cholestasis of pregnancy: perinatal outcome associated with expectant management. *A J Obstet Gynecol* 1996; 175: 957–60.

75 Matos A, Bernardes J *et al.* Antepartum fetal cerebral hemorrhage not predicted by current methods in cholestasis of pregnancy. *Obstet Gynecol* 1997; 89: 803–4.

76 Londero F, San Marco L. Intrahepatic cholestasis of pregnancy. Are we really able to predict fetal outcome? (letter) *Am J Obstet Gynecol* 1997; 177: 1274.

77 Fisk NM, Storey GNB. Fetal outcome in obstetric cholestasis. *Br J Obstet Gynaecol* 1988; 95: 1137–43.

78 Ostlund E, Bremme K *et al.* Soluble fibrin in plasma as a sign of activated coagulation in patients with pregnancy complications. *Acta Obstet Gynecol Scand* 1998; 77: 165–9.

79 Reid R, Ivey KJ *et al.* Fetal complications of obstetric cholestasis. *B M J* 1976; 1: 870–2.

80 Wilson BR, Haverkamp AD. Cholestatic jaundice of pregnancy; new perspectives. *Obstet Gynecol* 1979; 54: 650–2.

81 Floreani A, Paternoster D *et al.* Hepatitis C infection in pregnancy. *Br J Obstet Gynaecol* 1996; 103: 325–9.

82 Crosignani A, Podda M *et al.* Changes in bile acid composition in patients with primary biliary cirrhosis induced by ursodeoxycholic acid administration. *Hepatology* 1991; 14: 1000–7.

83 Gylling H, Rjikonen S *et al.* Oral guar gum treatment of intrahepatic cholestasis and pruritus in pregnant women: effects on serum cholestanol and other non-cholesterol sterols. *Eur J Clin Invest* 1998; 28: 359–63.

84 Lewis JH, Weingold AB. The use of gastrointestinal drugs during pregnancy and lactation. *Am J Gastroenterol* 1985; 80: 912–23.

85 Nicastri PL, Diaferia A *et al.* A randomised placebo-controlled trial of ursodeoxycholic acid and S- adenosylmethionine in the treatment of intrahepatic cholestasis of pregnancy. *Br J Obstet Gynaecol* 1998; 105: 1205–7.

86 Furhoff AK, Hellstrom K. Jaundice in pregnancy. Follow-up study of the sera of women originally reported by L. Thorling. I: The pregnancies. *Acta Med Scand* 1973; 193: 259–66.

87 Jacquemin E, Cresteil D *et al.* Heterozygous non-sense mutation of the MDR3 gene in familial intrahepatic cholestasis of pregnancy. *Lancet* 1999; 353: 210–11.

88 de Vree JML, Jacquemin E *et al.* Mutations in the MDR3 gene cause progressive familial intrahepatic cholestasis. *Proc Acad Sci USA* 1998; 95: 282–7.

89 Abell TL, Riely CA. Hyperemesis gravidarum. *Gastroenterol Clin North Am* 1992; 21: 835–49.

90 Sheehan HL. The pathology of hyperemesis and vomiting of late pregnancy. *J Obstet Gynaecol Brit Emp* 1939; 46: 685–9.

91 Larrey D, Rueff B *et al.* Recurrent jaundice caused by recurrent hyperemesis gravidarum. *Gut* 1984; 25: 1414–15.

92 Morali GA, Braverman DZ. Abnormal liver enzymes and ketonuria in hyperemesis gravidarum. A retrospective review of 80 patients. *J Clin Gastroenterol* 1990; 12: 303–5.

93 Jarnfelt-Samsioe A, Eriksson B *et al.* Serum bile acids, gamma glutamyltransferase and routine liver function tests in emetic and nonemetic pregnancies. *Gynecol Obstet Invest* 1986; 21: 169–76.

94 Sims HF, Brackett JC *et al.* The molecular basis of pediatric long chain 3-hydroxyacyl-CoA dehydrogenase deficiency associated with maternal acute fatty liver of pregnancy. *Proc Nat Acad Sci USA* 1995; 92: 841–5.

95 Tyni T, Ekholm E *et al.* Pregnancy complications are frequent in long-chain 3-hydroxyacyl-coenzyme A dehydrogenase deficiency. *Am J Obst Gynecol* 1998; 178: 603–8.

96 Krueger KJ, Hoffman BJ *et al.* Hepatic infarction associated with eclampsia. *Am J Gastroenterol* 1990; 85: 588–92.

97 Schorr-Lesnick B, Lebovics E *et al.* Liver diseases unique to pregnancy. *Am J Gastroenterol* 1991; 86: 659–70.

98 Barton JR, Sibai BM. HELLP and the liver diseases of pre-eclampsia. *Clin Liver Dis* 1999; 3: 31–48.

99 McKay DG. Clinical significance of the pathology of toxemia of pregnancy. *Circulation* 1964; 30 (Suppl. 2): 66–75.

100 Hibbard LT. Spontaneous rupture of the liver in pregnancy: a report of eight cases. *Am J Obstet Gynecol* 1976; 126: 334–8.

101 de Swiet M. Some rare medical complications of pregnancy (editorial). *B M J* 1985; 290: 2–4.

102 Mattar F, Sibai BM. Pre-eclampsia clinical characteristics and pathogenesis. *Clin Liver Dis* 1999; 3: 15–29.

103 Sibai BM, Ramadan MK. Maternal morbidity and mortality in 442 pregnancies with hemolysis, elevated liver enzymes and low platelets (HELLP syndrome). *Am J Obstet Gynecol* 1993; 169: 1000–6.

104 Saphier CJ, Repke JT. Hemolysis, elevated liver enzymes, and low platelets (HELLP) syndrome, a review of diagnosis and management. *Semin Perinatol* 1998; 22: 118–33.

105 Pritchard JA, Weisman R *et al.* Intravascular hemolysis, thrombocytopenia and other hematologic abnormalities associated with severe toxemia of pregnancy. *N Engl J Med* 1954; 250: 89–98.

106 Weinstein L. Syndrome of hemolysis, elevated liver enzymes, and low platelet count; a consequence of hypertension in pregnancy. *Am J Obstet Gynecol* 1982; 142: 159–67.

107 Crosby ET. Obstetrical anaesthesia for patients with the syndrome of haemolysis, elevated liver enzymes and low platelets. *Can J Anaesth* 1991; 38: 227–33.

108 Minakami H, Watanabe T *et al.* Association of a decrease in antithrombin III activity with a perinatal elevation in aspartate aminotransferase in women with twin pregnancies: relevance to the HELLP syndrome. *J Hepatol* 1999; 30: 603–11.

109 Killam AP, Dillard SH *et al.* Pregnancy-induced hypertension complicated by acute liver disease and disseminated intravascular coagulation. *Am J Obstet Gynecol* 1975; 123: 823–28.

110 Sheikh RA, Yasmeen S *et al.* Spontaneous intrahepatic hemorrhage and hepatic rupture in the HELLP syndrome: four cases and a review. *J Clin Gastroenterol* 1999; 28: 323–8.

111 Goodlin RC, Holdt D. Impending gestosis. *Obstet Gynaecol* 1981; 58: 743–5.

112 Aarnoudse JG, Houthoff HJ *et al.* A syndrome of liver damage and intravascular coagulation in the last trimester of normotensive pregnancy. A clinical and histopathological study. *Br J Obstet Gynaecol* 1986; 93: 145–55.

113 Martin JN, Blake PG *et al.* Pregnancy complicated by pre-eclampsia–eclampsia with the syndrome of hemolysis, elevated liver enzymes and low platelet count. How rapid is post-partum recovery? *Obstet Gynecol* 1990; 76: 737–41.

114 Boehlen F, Hohlfeld P *et al.* Platelet count at term pregnancy: a reappraisal of the threshold. *Obstet Gynecol* 2000; 95: 29–33.

115 Krauss T, Kuhn W *et al.* Circulating endothelial adhesion molecules as diagnostic markers for the early identification of pregnant women at risk for the development of pre-eclampsia. *Am J Obstet Gynecol* 1997; 177: 443–9.

116 Goodlin RC, Anderson JC *et al.* Conservative treatment of liver hematoma in the postpartum period: a report of two cases. *J Reprod Med* 1985; 30: 368–70.

117 Pereira SP, O'Donohue J *et al.* Maternal and perinatal outcome in severe pregnancy-related liver disease. *Hepatology* 1997; 26: 1258–62.

118 Isler CM, Rinehart BK *et al.* Maternal mortality associated with HELLP (hemolysis, elevated liver enzymes, and low platelets) syndrome. *Am J Obstet Gynecol* 1999; 181: 924–8.

119 Stander HJ, Cadden JF. Acute yellow atrophy of the liver in pregnancy. *Am J Obstet Gynecol* 1934; 28: 61–9.

120 Tarnier M. Note sur L'etal grasseux du foie dans la fievire puerperale. 1856. *C R Seances Mem Soc Biol* 1857; III: 209–14.

121 Pockros PJ, Peters RI *et al.* Idiopathic fatty liver of pregnancy: findings in ten cases. *Medicine (Baltimore)* 1984; 63: 1–11.

122 Purdie JM, Walters BN. Acute fatty liver of pregnancy: clinical features and diagnosis. *Aust N Z J Obstet Gynaecol* 1988; 28: 62–7.

123 Castro MA, Fassett MJ *et al.* Reversible peripartum liver failure: a new perspective on the diagnosis, treatment, and cause of acute fatty liver of pregnancy, based on 28 consecutive cases. *A J Obstet Gynecol* 1999; 181: 389–95.

124 Kaplan MM. Acute fatty liver of pregnancy. *N Engl J Med* 1985; 313: 367–70.

125 Pockros PJ, Reynolds TB. Acute fatty liver of pregnancy (letter). *Dig Dis Sci* 1985; 30: 601–2.

126 Davies MH, Wilkinson SP *et al.* Acute liver disease with encephalopathy and renal failure in late pregnancy and early puerperium, a study of fourteen patients. *Br J Obstet Gynaecol* 1980; 87: 1005–14.

127 Burroughs AK, Seong NH *et al.* Idiopathic acute fatty liver of pregnancy in 12 patients. *Q J M* 1982; 204: 481–97.

128 Bernauau J, Degott C *et al.* Non-fatal acute fatty liver of pregnancy. *Gut* 1983; 24, 340–4.

129 Rolfes DB, Ishak KG. Acute fatty liver of pregnancy: a clinicopathologic study of 35 cases. *Hepatology* 1985; 5: 1149–58.

130 Hague WM, Fenton DW *et al.* Acute fatty liver of pregnancy. *J R Soc Med* 1983; 76: 652–61.

131 Bacq Y. Acute fatty liver of pregnancy. *Semin Perinatol* 1998; 22: 134–40.

132 Varner M, Rinderknecht NK. Acute fatty metamorphosis of pregnancy. A maternal mortality and literature review. *J Reprod Med* 1980; 24: 177–80.

133 Hatfield AK, Stein JH *et al.* Idiopathic acute fatty liver of pregnancy. Death from extrahepatic manifestations. *Am J Dig Dis* 1972; 17: 167–78.

134 Holzbach RT. Acute fatty liver of pregnancy with disseminated intravascular coagulation. *Obstet Gynecol* 1974; 43: 740–4.

135 Laursen B, Frost L *et al.* Acute fatty liver of pregnancy with complicating disseminated intravascular coagulation. *Acta Obstet Gynecol Scand* 1983; 62: 403–7.

136 Liebman HA, McGeehee WG *et al.* Severe depression of antithrombin III associated with disseminated intravascular coagulation in women with fatty liver of pregnancy. *Ann Intern Med* 1983; 98: 330–3.

137 Goodlin RC. Acute fatty liver of pregnancy (letter). *Acta Obstet Gynecol Scand* 1983; 63: 379.

138 Slater DN, Hague WM. Renal morphological changes in idiopathic acute fatty liver of pregnancy. *Histopathology* 1984; 8: 567–81.

139 Goodlin RC. Pre-eclampsia as the great impostor. *Am J Obstet Gynecol* 1991; 164: 1577–80.

140 Heilmann L, Hojnacki B *et al.* Hemostasis and pre-eclampsia (German). *Gerburt Frauenheilkd* 1991; 51: 223–7.

141 Egley CC, Gutliph J *et al.* Severe hypoglycaemia associated with HELLP syndrome. *Am J Obstet Gynecol* 1985; 152: 576–7.

142 Riely CA, Latham PS *et al.* Acute fatty liver of pregnancy. A reassessment based on observations in nine patients. *Ann Intern Med* 1987; 106: 703–6.

143 Ibdah JA, Bennett MJ *et al*. A fetal fatty-acid oxidation disorder as a cause of liver disease in pregnant women. *N Engl J Med* 1999; 340: 1723–31.

144 Minakami H, Oka N *et al*. Pre-eclampsia: a microvesicular fat disease of the liver. *Am J Obstet Gynecol* 1988; 159: 1043–7.

145 Innes AM, Seargeant LE *et al*. Hepatic carnitine palmitoyltransferase I deficiency presenting as maternal illness in pregnancy. *Pediatr Res* 2000; 47: 6–8.

146 Treem WR. Beta oxidation defects. *Clin Liver Dis* 1999; 3: 49–67.

147 Sakamoto S, Tsuji Y *et al*. Idiopathic fatty liver of pregnancy with a subsequent uncomplicated pregnancy and a progressive increase in serum cholesterase activity during the third trimester. A case report. *Hepatogastroenterology* 1986; 33: 9–10.

148 Schoeman MN, Batey RG *et al*. Recurrent acute fatty liver of pregnancy associated with a fatty-acid oxidation defect in the offspring. *Gastroenterology* 1991; 100: 544–8.

149 Isaacs JD, Sims HF *et al*. Maternal acute fatty liver of pregnancy associated with fetal trifunctional protein deficiency: molecular characterization of a novel mutant allele. *Pediatr Res* 1996; 40: 393–8.

150 Kunelis CT, Peters JL *et al*. Fatty liver of pregnancy and its relationship to tetracycline therapy. *Am J Med* 1965; 38: 359–77.

151 Harrison RA, Araujo JG. Aetiology of acute fatty liver of pregnancy (letter). *J R Soc Med* 1983; 76: 1079.

152 Schimanski U, Krieger D *et al*. A novel two-nucleotide deletion in the ornithine transcarbamylase gene causing fatal hyperammonia in early pregnancy. *Hepatology* 1996; 24: 1413–5.

153 Brandt P, Jespersen J *et al*. Post-partum haemolytic uraemic syndrome treated with antithrombin III. *Nephron* 1981; 27: 15–8.

154 Zissin R, Yaffe D *et al*. Hepatic infarction in pre-eclampsia as part of the HELLP syndrome: CT appearance. *Abdom Imaging* 1999; 24: 594–6.

155 McKee CM, Weir PE *et al*. Acute fatty liver of pregnancy and diagnosis by computed tomography. *B M J* 1986; 292: 291–2.

156 Gubernatis G, Pichlmayr R *et al*. Auxiliary partial orthotopic liver transplantation (APOLT) for fulminant hepatic failure: first successful case report. *World J Surg* 1991; 15: 660–5; discussion 665–6.

157 Hsu HW, Belfort MA *et al*. Postpartum thrombotic thrombocytopenic purpura complicated by Budd–Chiari syndrome. *Obstet Gynecol* 1995; 85: 839–43.

158 Martin JN, Files JC *et al*. Plasma exchange for pre-eclampsia–eclampsia with HELLP syndrome. *Am J Obstet Gynecol* 1990; 162: 126–37.

159 Sibai BM. The HELLP syndrome (Hemolysis, Elevated Liver enzymes, and Low Platelets): much ado about nothing? *Am J Obstet Gynecol* 1990; 162: 311–16.

160 Minakami H, Kimura K *et al*. Acute fatty liver of pregnancy with hyperlipidemia, acute hemorrhagic pancreatitis and disseminated intravascular coagulation. *Asia Oceania J Obstet Gynaecol* 1985; 11: 371–6.

161 Hou SH, Levin S *et al*. Acute fatty liver of pregnancy. Survival with early cesarian section. *Dig Dis Sci* 1984; 29: 449–52.

162 Miles JF, Martin JN *et al*. Post-partum eclampsia: a recurring perinatal dilemma. *Obstet Gynecol* 1990; 76: 328–31.

163 Hunter SK, Martin M *et al*. Liver transplant after massive spontaneous hepatic rupture in pregnancy complicated by pre-eclampsia. *Obstet Gynecol* 1995; 85: 819–22.

164 Amon E, Allen SR *et al*. Acute fatty liver of pregnancy associated with pre-eclampsia: management of hepatic failure with postpartum liver transplantation. *Am J Perinatol* 1991; 8: 278–9.

165 Magee LA, Dixon RM *et al*. ^{31}P magnetic resonance spectroscopy of the liver in HELLP syndrome. *B J Obstet Gynaecol* 1999; 106: 582–8.

166 Knapen MF, van Altena AM *et al*. Liver function following pregnancy complicated by HELLP syndrome. *Br J Obstet Gynaecol* 1998; 105: 1208–10.

167 Dotsch J, Hohmann M *et al*. Neonatal morbidity and mortality associated with maternal haemolysis, elevated liver enzymes, and low platelets syndrome. *Eur J Pediatrics* 1997; 156: 389–91.

168 Treem WR, Shoup M *et al*. Acute fatty liver of pregnancy, hemolysis, elevated liver enzymes, and low platelets syndrome, and long chain 3-hydroxyacyl-coenzyme A dehydrogenase deficiency. *Am J Gastroenterol* 1996; 91: 2293–300.

169 Sibai BM, Ramadan MK *et al*. Pregnancies complicated by HELLP syndrome (hemolysis, elevated liver enzymes, and low platelets): subsequent pregnancy outcome and long-term prognosis. *Am J Obstet Gynecol* 1995; 172: 125–9.

170 Mansouri A, Fromenty B *et al*. Assessment of the prevalence of genetic metabolic defects in acute fatty liver of pregnancy. *J Hepatol* 1996; 25: 781 (letter).

171 Abercrombie J. Case of haemorrhage of the liver. *London Med Gazette* 1844; 34, 792.

172 Smith LG, Moise KJ *et al*. Spontaneous rupture of the liver during pregnancy: current therapy. *Obstet Gynecol* 1991; 77: 171–5.

173 Schwartz ML, Lien JM. Spontaneous liver hematoma in pregnancy not clearly associated with pre-eclampsia: a case presentation and literature review. *Am J Obstet Gynecol* 1997; 176: 1328–32.

174 Bis KA, Waxman B. Rupture of the liver associated with pregnancy: a review of the literature and report of two cases. *Obstet Gynecol Surv* 1976; 31: 763–73.

175 Sloan DA, Schlegel DM. Spontaneous hepatic rupture associated with pregnancy. *Contemp Surg* 1984; 24: 39–42.

176 Manas KJ, Welsh JD *et al*. Hepatic hemorrhage without rupture in pre-eclampsia. *N Eng J Med* 1985; 312: 424–6.

177 Laifer SA, Ehrlich GD *et al*. Congenital cytomegalovirus infection in offspring of liver transplant recipients. *Clin Infect Dis* 1995; 20: 52–5.

178 Steven MM. Pregnancy and liver disease. *Gut* 1981; 22: 592–614.

179 Icely S, Chez RA. Traumatic liver rupture in pregnancy. *Am J Obstet Gynecol* 1999; 180: 1030–1.

180 Margolis K, Naidoo BN. Spontaneous postpartum subcapsular haematoma of the liver. *S Afr Med J* 1974; 48: 1997–8.

181 Castaneda H, Garcia-Romero H *et al*. Hepatic haemorrhage in toxaemia of pregnancy. *Am J Obstet Gynecol* 1970; 107: 578–84.

182 Aziz S, Merrell RC *et al*. Spontaneous hepatic hemorrhage during pregnancy. *Am J Surg* 1983; 146: 680–2.

183 Gonzalez GD, Rubel HR *et al*. Spontaneous hepatic rupture in pregnancy: management with hepatic artery ligation. *South Med J* 1984; 77: 242–5.

184 Heller TD, Goldfarb JP. Spontaneous rupture of the liver during pregnancy. A case report and review of the literature. *N Y State J Med* 1986; 86: 314–16.

185 Herbert WNP. Hepatic rupture and pregnancy. *N Y State J Med* 1986; 86: 286–8.

186 Loevinger EH, Vujic I *et al*. Hepatic rupture associated with pregnancy: treatment with transcatheter embolotherapy. *Obstet Gynecol* 1985; 65: 281–4.

187 Ibrahim N, Payne E *et al.* Spontaneous rupture of the liver in association with pregnancy. Case report. *Br J Obstet Gynaecol* 1985; 92: 539–40.

188 Henny CP, Lim AE *et al.* A review of the importance of acute multidisciplinary treatment following spontaneous rupture of the liver capsule during pregnancy. *Surg Gynecol Obstet* 1983; 156: 593–8.

189 Ekberg H, Leyon J *et al.* Hepatic rupture secondary to pre-eclampsia—a report of a case treated conservatively. *Ann Chir Gynaecol* 1984; 73: 350–3.

190 Feliciano DV, Mattox KL *et al.* Management of 1000 consecutive cases of hepatic trauma 1979–84. *Ann Surg* 1986; 204, 438–45.

191 Wagner WH, Lundell CJ *et al.* Percutaneous angiographic embolization for removal of hepatic arterial hemorrhage. *Arch Sur* 1985; 120: 1241–9.

192 Greca FH, Coelho JC *et al.* Ultrasonographic diagnosis of spontaneous rupture of the liver in pregnancy. *J Clin Ultrasound* 1984; 12: 515–16.

193 Winer Muram HT, Muram D *et al.* Hepatic rupture in pre eclampsia: the role of diagnostic imaging. *J Can Assoc Radiol* 1985; 36: 34–6.

194 Sakala EP, Moore WD. Successful term delivery after previous pregnancy with ruptured liver. *Obstet Gynecol* 1986; 68: 124–6.

195 Portnuff J, Ballon S. Hepatic rupture in pregnancy. *Am J Obstet Gynecol* 1972; 114: 1102–4.

196 Barnes AD, Harder E *et al.* Successful pregnancy following partial hepatectomy for removal of hepatocellular adenomas. *Am J Obstet Gynecol* 1984; 150: 998.

197 Fagan EA, Harrison TJ. *Viral Hepatitis: a Handbook for Clinicians and Scientists.* Bios Publications, 2000, Oxford Springer-Verlag, New York, 233–67.

198 Van Os HC, Drogendijk AC *et al.* The influence of contamination of culture medium with hepatitis B virus on the outcome of *vitro* fertilization pregnancies. *Am J Obstet Gynecol* 1991; 165: 152–9.

199 Semprini AE, Persico T *et al.* Absence of hepatitis C virus and detection of hepatitis G virus/GB virus C RNA sequences in the semen of infected men. *J Infect Dis* 1998; 177: 848–54.

200 Morrison AS, Jick H *et al.* Oral contraceptives and hepatitis: a report from the Boston Collaborative Drug Surveillance Program, Boston University Medical Center. *Lancet* 1977; 1: 1142–3.

201 Potts M, Diggory P, eds. *Textbook of Contraceptive Practice.* 1983; Cambridge University Press, Cambridge; 164.

202 Schweitzer IL, Weiner JM *et al.* Oral contraceptives in acute viral hepatitis. *J Am Med Assoc* 1975; 233: 979–80.

203 Jenny S, Markoff N. Oral contraceptives in liver disease. *Schweizer Med Wochenschr* 1967; 97: 1502–5.

204 Hieber JP, Dalton D *et al.* Hepatitis and pregnancy. *J Pediatr* 1977; 91: 545–9.

205 Palmovic D. Acute viral hepatitis in pregnancy. Results of a prospective study of 99 pregnant women. *Lijecnicki Vjesnik* 1986; 108: 296–300.

206 Shalev E, Bassan HM. Viral hepatitis during pregnancy in Israel. *Int J Obstet Gynaecol* 1982; 20: 73–8.

207 Peretz A, Paldi E *et al.* Infectious hepatitis in pregnancy. *Obstet Gynecol* 1959; 14: 435–441.

208 Gelpi AP. Viral hepatitis complicating pregnancy: mortality trends in Saudi Arabia. *Int J Gynaecol Obstetr* 1979; 17: 73–7.

209 Khuroo MS, Teli MR *et al.* Incidence and severity of viral hepatitis in pregnancy. *Am J Med* 1981; 70: 252–5.

210 Christie AB, Allam AA *et al.* Pregnancy hepatitis in Libya. *Lancet* 1976; 2: 827–9.

211 Singh DS, Balasubramaniam M *et al.* Viral hepatitis during pregnancy. *J Indian Med Res* 1979; 73: 90–2.

212 Borhanmanesh F, Haghighi P *et al.* Viral hepatitis during pregnancy: severity and effect on gestation. *Gastroenterology* 1973; 64: 304–8.

213 Tripathi BM, Misra NP. Viral hepatitis with pregnancy. *J Associ Physicians India* 1981; 29: 463–9.

214 Mallia CP, Nancekivell AF. Fulminant virus hepatitis in late pregnancy. *Ann Trop Med Parasitol* 1982; 76: 143–6.

215 O'Grady J, Williams R. Acute liver failure. In: Gilmore I, Shields R, eds. *Gastrointestinal Emergencies.* 1991; Bailliere Tindall, London: 104–22.

216 Ko TM, Tseng LH *et al.* Amniocentesis in mothers who are hepatitis B virus carriers does not expose the infant to increased risk of hepatitis B virus infection. *Arch Gynecol Obstet* 1994; 225: 25–30.

217 Akhtar KAK, Akhtar MA. Viral hepatitis in pregnancy. *J Pakistan Med Assoc (Karachi)* 1979; 29: 31–5.

218 Mehrotra R. Histopathological and immunohistochemical changes in placenta due to acute viral hepatitis during pregnancy. *Indian J Med Res* 1986; 83: 282–92.

219 Matsaniotis N, Kiossoglou K *et al.* Chromosomal aberrations in infectious hepatitis. *J Clin Pathol* 1970; 23: 553–7.

220 Dietzman DE, Madden DL *et al.* Lack of relationship between Down's syndrome and maternal exposure to Australia antigen. *Am J Dis Child* 1972; 124: 195–7.

221 Sever JL, Kapikian AZ *et al.* Hepatitis A in Down's syndrome: lack of an association. *J Infect Dis* 1976; 134: 198–200.

222 Lemon SM. Type A viral hepatitis. New developments in an old disease. *N Engl J Med* 1985; 313: 1059–69.

223 Fagan EA, Hadzic D *et al.* Vertical transmission from early pregnancy of a naturally occurring hepatitis A virus variant: evidence for persistent infection in man. *Pediatr Infect Dis J* 1999; 18: 389–91.

224 Frosner GG, Papaevangelou G *et al.* Antibody against hepatitis A in seven European countries. I. Comparison of prevalence data in different age groups. *Am J Epidemiol* 1979; 110: 63–9.

225 Tong MJ, Thursby M *et al.* Studies on the maternal-infant transmission of the viruses which cause acute hepatitis. *Gastroenterol* 1981; 80: 999–1004.

226 Leikin E, Lysikiewicz, A *et al.* Intrauterine transmission of hepatitis A virus. *Obstet Gynecol* 1996; 88: 690–1.

227 McDuffie RS, Bader T. Fetal meconium peritonitus after maternal hepatitis A. *Am J Obstet Gynecol* 1999; 180: 1031–2.

228 Klein BS, Michaels JA *et al.* Nosocomial hepatitis A. A multinursery outbreak in Wisconsin. *J Am Med Assoc* 1984; 252: 2716–21.

229 Noble RC, Kane MA *et al.* Posttransfusion hepatitis A in a neonatal intensive care unit. *J Am Med Associ* 1984; 252: 2711–15.

230 Rosenblum LS, Villarino ME *et al.* Hepatitis A outbreak in a neonatal intensive care unit: risk factors for transmission and evidence of prolonged viral excretion among preterm infants. *J Infect Dis* 1991; 164: 476–82.

231 Watson JC, Fleming DW *et al.* Vertical transmission of hepatitis A resulting in an outbreak in a neonatal intensive care unit. *J Infect Dis* 1993; 167: 567–71.

232 Linder N, Karetnyi YV *et al.* Symptomatic hepatitis A virus infection during the first year of life. *Pediatr Infect Dis J* 1995; 14: 628–29.

233 Tanaka I, Shima M *et al*. Vertical transmission of hepatitis A. *Lancet* 1995; 345: 397.

234 Fagan EA, Tolley P *et al*. Hepatitis B vaccine: immunogenicity and follow-up including two year booster doses in high-risk health care personnel in a London Teaching hospital. *J M Virol* 1987; 21: 49–56.

235 Morbidity Mortality Weekly Report (MMWR). Centers for Disease Control: Protection against viral hepatitis. Recommendations of the Advisory Committee on Immunization Practices (ACIP). *Morbid Mortal Weekly Rep* 1990; 39: 5–22.

236 Morbidity Mortality Weekly Report (MMWR). Prevention of hepatitis A through active or passive immunization. Recommendations of the Advisory Committee on Immunization Practices (ACIP). *Morbid Mortal Weekly Rep* R45 1997; 46: 588.

237 Morbidity Mortality Weekly Report (MMWR). Recommendations for protection against viral hepatitis. *Morbid Mortal Weekly Rep* 1985; 34: 313–24.

238 Morbidity Mortality Weekly Report (MMWR). Leads from the MMWR. Recommendations for the protection against viral hepatitis. *J Am Med Assoc* 1985; 254: 197–8.

239 Cossar JH, Reid D. Not all travellers need immunoglobulin for hepatitis A. *Br Med J* 1987; 294: 1503.

240 Myint Hla, Soe MM *et al*. A clinical and epidemiological study of an epidemic of non-A, non-B hepatitis in Rangoon. *Am J Trop Med Hyg* 1985; 34: 1183–9.

241 Yamauchi M, Nakajima H *et al*. An epidemic of non-A/non-B hepatitis in Japan. *Am J Gastroenterol* 1983; 78: 652–5.

242 Morbidity Mortality Weekly Report (MMWR). Public Health Service Interagency Guidelines for screening donors of blood, plasma, organs, tissues, and semen for evidence of hepatitis B and hepatitis C. *Morbid Mortal Weekly Rep* R4 40: 1991; 1–17.

243 Hoofnagle J, Shafritz DA *et al*. Chronic type B hepatitis and the 'healthy' HBsAg carrier state. *Hepatology* 1987; 7: 758–63.

244 Alter MJ, Hadler SC *et al*. The changing epidemiology of hepatitis B in the United States. Need for alternative vaccination strategies. *J Am Med Assoc* 1990; 263: 1218–22.

245 Beasley RP. Hepatitis B virus as the etiologic agent in hepatocellular carcinoma epidemiologic considerations. *Hepatology* 1982; 2 (Suppl.): 21–26S.

246 Chang M-H, Chen C-J *et al*. Universal hepatitis B vaccination in Taiwan and the incidence of hepatocellular carcinoma in children. *N Engl J Med* 1997; 336: 1855–9.

247 Lok ASF, Lai C-L *et al*. Interferon therapy of chronic hepatitis B virus infection in Chinese. *J Hepatol* 1986; 3 (Suppl. 2) S209–S215.

248 Coursaget P, Yvonnet B *et al*. Age and sex-related study of hepatitis B virus chronic carrier state in infants from an endemic area (Senegal). *J Med Virol* 1987; 22: 1–5.

249 Britton WJ, Parsons C *et al*. Risk factors associated with hepatitis B infection in antenatal patients. *Aust New Zeal J Med* 1985; 15: 641–4.

250 Delage G, Montplaisir S *et al*. Prevalence of hepatitis B virus infection in pregnant women in the Montreal area. *Canad Med Assoc J* 1986; 134: 897–901.

251 Greenfield C, Osidiana V *et al*. Perinatal transmission of hepatitis B virus in Kenya: its relation to the presence of serum HBV DNA and anti-HBe in the mother. *J Med Virol* 1986; 19: 135–42.

252 Schweitzer IL, Spears RL. Hepatitis-associated antigen (Australia antigen) in mother and infant. *N Engl J Med* 1970; 283: 570–2.

253 Cossart YE, Hargreaves FD *et al*. Australia antigen in the human fetus. *Am J Dis Child* 1972; 123: 376–8.

254 Merrill DA, Dubois RS. Neonatal onset of the hepatitis associated antigen carrier state. *N Engl J Med* 1972; 287: 1280–2.

255 Fagan EA, Eddleston AWLF. Hepatitis vaccination. *Clin Immunol Allergy* 1985; 5: 43–85.

256 Stevens CE, Toy PT *et al*. Perinatal hepatitis B virus transmission in the United States. Prevention by passive-active immunization. *J Am Med Assoc* 1985; 253: 1740–5.

257 Woo D, Cummings M *et al*. Vertical transmission of hepatitis B surface antigen in carrier mothers in two west London Hospitals. *Arch Dis Child* 1979; 54: 670–5.

258 Inaba N, Ijichi M *et al*. Placental transmission of hepatitis B e antigen and clinical significance of hepatitis B e antigen titers of children born to hepatitis B e antigen-positive carrier women. *Am J Obstet Gynecol* 1984; 149: 580–1.

259 Hwang L-Y, Roggendorf M *et al*. Perinatal transmission of hepatitis B virus: role of maternal HBeAg and anti-HBc IgM. *J Med Virol* 1985; 15: 265–9.

260 Derso A, Boxall EH *et al*. Transmission of HBsAg from mother to infant in four ethnic Groups. *Br Med J* 1978; 1: 949–52.

261 Boxall EH, Tarlow MJ. Hepatitis B vaccine in the prevention of perinatally transmitted hepatitis B virus infections: initial report of a study in the West Midlands of England. *J Med Virol* 1986; 18: 255–60.

262 Beasley RP, Hwang L-Y *et al*. Prevention of perinatally transmitted hepatitis B virus infections with hepatitis B immune globulin and hepatitis B vaccine. *Lancet* 1983; ii: 1099–02.

263 Wong VCV, Ip H *et al*. Prevention of the HBsAg carrier state in newborn infants of mothers who are chronic carriers of HBsAg and HBeAg by administration of hepatitis-B vaccine and hepatitis-B immunoglobulin. *Lancet* 1984; 1: 921–6.

264 Marinier E, Barrois V *et al*. Lack of perinatal transmission of hepatitis B virus infection in Senegal, West Africa. *J Pediatr* 1985; 106: 843–9.

265 Heijtink RA, Boender PJ *et al*. Hepatitis B virus DNA in serum of pregnant women with HBsAg and HBeAg or antibodies to HBe (letter). *J Infect Dis* 1984; 150: 462.

266 Lee S-D, Lo J-K *et al*. Prevention of maternal-infant hepatitis B virus transmission by immunization: the role of serum hepatitis B virus DNA. *Hepatology* 1986; 6: 369–73.

267 Karayiannis P, Fowler MJF *et al*. Detection of serum HBV-DNA by molecular hybridization-correlation with HBeAg/anti-HBe status, racial origin, liver histology and hepatocellular carcinoma. *J Hepatol* 1985; 1: 99–106.

268 Morbidity Mortality Weekly Report (MMWR). Update on adult immunization. Recommendations of the Advisory Committee on Immunization Practices (ACIP). *Morbid Mortal Weekly Rep* R12 1991; 40: 33–89.

269 Holzbach RT. Australia antigen hepatitis in pregnancy: evidence against transplacental transmission of Australia antigen in early and late pregnancy. *Arch Int Med* 1972; 130: 234–6.

270 Goudeau A, Yvonnet B *et al*. Lack of anti-HBc IgM in neonates with HBsAg carrier mothers argues against transplacental transmission of hepatitis B virus infection. *Lancet* 1983; 2: 1103–4.

271 Beasley RP, Hwang L-Y *et al*. Efficacy of hepatitis B immune globulin (HBIG) for prevention of perinatal transmission of the HBV carrier state: final report of a randomized, double-blind, placebo-controlled trial. *Hepatology* 1983; 3: 135–41.

272 Lee AKY, Ip HMH *et al*. Mechanisms of maternal-fetal transmission of hepatitis B virus. *J Infect Dis* 1978; 138: 668–71.

273 Boxall EH, Flewett TH *et al*. Hepatitis B surface antigen in breast milk. *Lancet* 1974; 2: 1007–8.

274 Linneman CC, Goldberg S. HBsAg in breast milk (letter). *Lancet* 1974; 2: 1550.

275 Tang S. (Chinese) Study on the HBV intrauterine infection and its rate. *Chung Hua Liu Hsing Ping Hsueh Tsa Chih* 1990; 11: 328–30.

276 Nordenfelt E, Dahlquist E. HBsAg positive adopted children as a cause of intrafamilial spread of hepatitis B. *Scand J Infect Dis* 1978; 10: 161–3.

277 Botha JF, Ritchie MJ *et al.* Hepatitis B virus carrier state in black children in Ovamboland: role of perinatal and horizontal transmission. *Lancet* 1984; 1: 1210–12.

278 Bogomolski-Yahalom V, Granot E *et al.* Prevalence of HBsAg carriers in native and immigrant pregnant female populations in Israel and passive/active vaccination against HBV of newborns at risk. *J Med Virol* 1991; 34: 217–22.

279 Tabor E, Gerety RJ. Hepatitis B virus infection in infants and toddlers in Nigeria: the need for early intervention. *J Pediatr* 1979; 95: 647–50.

280 Tabor E, Bayley AC *et al.* Horizontal transmission of hepatitis B virus among children and adults in five rural villages in Zambia. *J Med Virol* 1985; 15: 113–20.

281 Prince AM, White T *et al.* Epidemiology of hepatitis B infection in Liberian infants. *Infect Immun* 1981; 32: 675–80.

282 Moyes CD, Milne A *et al.* Very-low-dose hepatitis B vaccine in newborn infants: an economic option for control in endemic areas. *Lancet* 1987; i: 29–31.

283 Margolis HS, Alter MJ *et al.* Hepatitis B: evolving epidemiology and implications for control. *Sem Liver Dis* 1992; 11: 84–92.

284 Stoller A, Collmann RD. Incidence of infectious hepatitis followed by Down's syndrome nine months later. *Lancet* 1965; 2: 1221–3.

285 Kucera J. Down's syndrome and infectious hepatitis. *Lancet* 1970; 1: 569–70.

286 Gerety RJ, Schweitzer IL. Viral hepatitis, type B during pregnancy, the neonatal period and infancy. *J Pediat* 1977; 90: 368–74.

287 Shiraki K, Yoshihara N *et al.* Acute hepatitis B in infants born to carrier mothers with the antibody to hepatitis B e antigen. *J Pediatr* 1980; 97: 768–70.

288 Foschini M, De Toni A *et al.* prevention of perinatally transmitted hepatitis B virus infection by hepatitis B immunoglobulin immunoprophylaxis: an account of 201 newborn babies of hepatitis Bs antigen carrier mothers. *J Pediatr Gastroenterol Nutr* 1985; 4: 523–7.

289 Anderson MG, Murray-Lyon IM. Natural history of the chronic carrier. *Gut* 1985; 26: 848–60.

290 Blumberg BS, Fredlander JS *et al.* Hepatitis and Australia antigen: autosomal recessive inheritance of susceptibility to infection in humans. *Proc Nat Acad Sci USA* 1969; 62: 1108–15.

291 Stevens CE, Beasley RP, Lack of an autosomal recessive genetic influence in vertical transmission of hepatitis B antigen. *Nature* 1976; 260: 715–16.

292 Sinatra FR, Shah P *et al.* Perinatal transmitted acute icteric hepatits B in infants born to hepatitis B surface antigen-positive and anti hepatitis Bc-positive carrier mothers. *Pediatrics* 1982; 70: 557–9.

293 Delaphane D, Shulman ST. Immunoprophylaxis for infants born to HBsAg positive mothers. *Lancet* 1983; ii: 170–1.

294 Tong MJ, Sinatra FR *et al.* Need for immunoprophylaxis in infants born to HBsAg-positive carrier mothers who are HBeAg negative. *J Pediatr* 1984; 105: 945–7.

295 Ewing CI, Davidson DC. Fatal hepatitis B in infant born to an HBsAg carrier with HBeAb. *Arch Dis Child* 1985; 60: 265–7.

296 Beath SV, Boxall EH *et al.* Fulminant hepatitis B in infants born to anti-HBe hepatitis B carrier mothers. *Br Med J* 1992; 104: 1167–70.

297 Morbidity Mortality Weekly Report (MMWR). Centers for Disease Control: Protection against viral hepatitis. Recommendations of the Advisory Committee on Immunization Practices (ACIP). Recommended childhood immunisation schedule—United States 1999. *Morbid Mortal Weekly Rep* 1999; 48: 12–13.

298 Morbidity Mortality Weekly Report (MMWR). Centers for Disease Control: Notice to readers update: recommendations to prevent hepatitis B virus transmission—United States. *Morbid Mortal Weekly Rep* 1999; 48 (02): 33–4.

299 Winsnes R, Siebke JC. Efficacy of post-exposure prophylaxis with hepatitis B immunoglobulin in Norway. *J Infect* 1986; 12: 11–21.

300 Hollinger FB, Lemon SM, Margolis HS eds. *Viral Hepatitis and Liver Disease. Proceeding of the 1990 International Symposium*, 1991; Houston, Texas. Williams & Wilkins, Baltimore, MA.

301 Deinhardt F, Zuckerman AJ. Against hepatitis B: a report on a WHO meeting on viral hepatitis in Europe. *J Med Virol* 1985; 17: 209–17.

302 Department of Health and Social Security. *Report on Confidential Enquiries into Maternal Deaths in the United Kingdom 1979– 81.* HMSO, London, 1986.

303 Morbidity Mortality Weekly Report (MMWR). Recommendations for preventing transmission of human immunodeficiency virus and hepatitis B virus to patients during exposure-prone invasive procedures. *Morbid Mortal Weekly Rep* 1991; R8 40: 1–9.

304 Tabor E. Hepatitis B vaccine: different regimens for different geographic regions (Editor's column). *J Pediatr* 1985; 106: 777–8.

305 Carne CA, Weller IVD *et al.* Impaired responsiveness of homosexual men with HIV antibodies to plasma derived hepatitis B vaccine. *Br Med J* 1987; 294: 866–8.

306 Rizzetto M, Ponzetto A *et al.* Hepatitis delta virus as a global health problem. *Vaccine* 1990; 8: S10–S14.

307 Negro F, Rizzetto M. Pathobiology of delta virus. In: Hollinger FB Lemon SM, Margolis HS eds. *Viral Hepatitis and Liver Disease. Proceeding of the 1990 International Symposium*, Houston, 1991; Texas. Williams & Wilkins, Baltimore, MA: 477–80.

308 Zanetti AR, Ferron P *et al.* Perinatal transmission of the hepatitis B virus and of the HBV associated delta agent from mothers to offspring in Northern Italy. *J Med Virol* 1982; 9: 139–48.

309 Caporaso N, Del Vecchio-Blano, *et al.* Delta infection: intrafamily spreading. In: Verme G Bonino F, Rizzetto M eds. *Viral Hepatitis and Delta Infection.* 1983; Alan R Liss, New York: 139–43.

310 Alter MJ, Kruszon-Moran D *et al.* The prevalence of hepatitis C virus infection in the United States 1988–94. *N Engl J Med* 1999; 341: 556–62.

311 Morbidity Mortality Weekly Report (MMWR). Recommendations for prevention, control of hepatitis, C virus (HCV) infection and HCV-related chronic disease. *Morbid Mortal Weekly Rep* R-19 1998; 47: 1–39.

312 Kuo G, Choo Q-L *et al.* An assay for circulating antibodies to a major etiologic virus of human non-A, non-B hepatitis. *Science* 1989; 244: 362–4.

313 Choo Q-L, Kuo G *et al.* Isolation of a cDNA clone derived from a blood-borne non-A, non-B viral hepatitis genome. *Science* 1989; 244: 359–61.

314 Sabatino G, Ramenghi LA *et al*. Vertical transmission of hepatitis C: an epidemiological study on 2,980 pregnant women in Italy. *Eur J Epidemiol* 1996; 12: 443–7.

315 Kenny-Walsh E. Clinical outcomes after hepatitis C infection from contaminated anti-D immune globulin. Irish Hepatology Research Group. *N Engl J Med* 1999; 340: 1228–33.

316 Caporaso N, Ascione A *et al*. Spread of hepatitis C virus infection within families. Investigators of an Italian Multicenter Group. *J Viral Hep* 1998; 5: 67–72.

317 Weiner AJ, Thaler MM *et al*. A unique, predominant hepatitis C virus variant found in the infant born to a mother with multiple variants. *J Virol* 1993; 67: 4365–8.

318 Ohto H, Terazawa S. Transmission of hepatitis C virus from mother to infant. The vertical transmission of hepatitis C virus collaborative study Group. *N Engl J Med* 1994; 330: 744–50.

319 Zanetti AR, Tanzi, E *et al*. Mother-to-infant transmission of hepatitis C virus. *Lancet* 1995; 345: 289–91.

320 Hunt CM, Carson KL *et al*. Hepatitis C in pregnancy. *Obstet Gynecol* 1997; 89: 883–90.

321 Tahara T, Toyoda S *et al*. Vertical transmission of hepatitis C through three generations (letter). *Lancet* 1996; 347: 409.

322 Halfon P, Quentin Y *et al*. Mother-to-infant transmission of hepatitis C virus: molecular evidence of superinfection by homologous virus in children. *J Hepatol* 1999; 30: 970–8.

323 Lynch-Salamon DI, Combs CA. Hepatitis C in obstetrics and gynecology. *Obstet Gynecol* 1992; 79: 621–9.

324 Wolf H, Kuhler O *et al*. [Liver dystrophy in disseminated herpes simplex infection in pregnancy.] Leberdystrophie bei disseminierter Herpes-simplex-Infektion in der Schwangerschaft. *Geburts Frauenheil* 1992; 52: 123–5.

325 Hensleigh PA, Glover BD *et al*. Systemic herpesvirus hominis in pregnancy. *J Reprod Med* 1979; 22: 171–6.

326 Wertheim RA, Brooks BJ *et al*. Fatal herpetic hepatitis in pregnancy. *Obstet Gynecol* 1983; 62: 38S–42S.

327 Goyert GL, Bottoms SF *et al*. Anicteric presentation of fatal herpetic hepatitis in pregnancy. *Obstet Gynecol* 1985; 65: 585–8.

328 Rubin MH, Ward DM *et al*. Fulminant hepatic failure caused by genital herpes in a healthy person. *J Am Med Assoc* 1985; 253: 1299–301.

329 Jacques SM, Qureshi F. Herpes simplex virus hepatitis in pregnancy: a clinicopathologic study of three cases. *Hum Pathol* 1992; 23: 183–7.

330 Young EJ, Chafizadeh E *et al*. Disseminated herpesvirus infection during pregnancy. *Clin Infect Dis* 1996; 22: 51–8.

331 Shlien RD, Meyers S *et al*. Fulminant herpes simplex hepatitis in a patient with ulcerative colitis. *Gut* 1988; 29: 257–61.

332 Taina E, Hanninen P *et al*. Viral infections in pregnancy. *Acta Obstet Gynecol Scand* 1985; 64: 167–73.

333 Whorton CM, Thomas DM *et al*. Fatal herpes simplex virus type 2 infection in a healthy young woman. *South Med J* 1983; 76: 81–3.

334 Purtilo DT. Fulminant hepatic failure due to genital herpes in a healthy woman: was she healthy? (letter). *J Am Med Assoc* 1985; 254: 3421–2.

335 Klein NA, Mabie WC *et al*. Herpes simplex hepatitis in pregnancy. Two patients successfully treated with acyclovir. *Gastroenterology* 1991; 100: 239–44.

336 Adler SP, Chandrika T *et al*. Cytomegalovirus infections in the neonate acquired by blood transfusion. *Paediatr Infect Dis* 1982; 2: 114–18.

337 Starr JG, Bart RD *et al*. Inapparent congenital cytomegalovirus infection. Clinical and epidemiologic characteristics in early infancy. *N Engl J Med* 1970; 282: 1075–8.

338 Melish ME, Hanshaw JB. Congenital cytomegalovirus infection. Developmental progress of infants detected by routine screening. *Am J Dis Child* 1973; 126: 190–4.

339 Best JM. Congenital cytomegalovirus infection. *Br Med J* 1987; 294: 1440–1.

340 Leinikki P, Heinonen K *et al*. Incidence of cytomegalovirus infections in early childhood. *Scand J Infect Dis* 1972; 4: 1–5.

341 Marx JL. Cytomegalovirus: a major cause of birth defects. *Science* 1975; 190: 1184–6.

342 Antsakis AJ, Daskalakis GJ *et al*. Prenatal diagnosis of fetal primary cytomegalovirus infection. *Br J Obstet Gynaecol* 2000; 107: 84–8.

343 Numazaki Y, Yano N *et al*. Primary infection with human cytomegalovirus: virus isolation from healthy infants and pregnant women. *Am J Epidemiol* 1970; 9: 410–17.

344 Vesterinen E, Savolainen ER *et al*. Occurrence of herpes simplex and cytomegalovirus infections. *Acta Obstet Gynecol Scand* 1977; 56: 101–4.

345 Chu SY, Buehler JW *et al*. Impact of the human immunodeficiency virus epidemic on mortality in women of reproductive age, United States. *J Am Med Assoc* 1990; 264: 225–9.

346 Trey C, Davidson CS. The management of fulminant hepatic failure. *Progr Liver Dis* 1970; 3: 282–98.

347 Gimson AES, O'Grady J *et al*. Late-onset hepatic failure: clinical, serological and histological features. *Hepatology* 1986; 6: 288–94.

348 Czeizel AE, Timar L *et al*. Timing of suicide attempts by self-poisoning during pregnancy and pregnancy outcomes. *Int J Gynaecol Obstet* 1999; 65: 39–45.

349 Sancewicz-Pach K, Chmiest W *et al*. Suicidal paracetamol poisoning of a pregnant woman just before a delivery. *Przeglad Lekarski* 1999; 56: 459–62.

350 Kurzel RB. Can acetaminophen excess result in maternal and fetal toxicity? *South Med J* 1990; 83: 953–5.

351 Hussaini SH, Skidmore SJ *et al*. Severe hepatitis E infection during pregnancy. *J Viral Hep* 1997; 4: 51–4.

352 Levin S, Leibowitz E *et al*. Interferon treatment in acute progressive and fulminant hepatitis. *Isr J Med Sci* 1989; 25: 364–72.

353 Kato T, Nery JR *et al*. Successful living related liver transplantation in an adult with acute liver failure. *Transplantation* 1997; 64: 415–17.

354 Fair J, Klein AS *et al*. Intrapartum orthotopic liver transplantation with successful outcome of pregnancy. *Transplantation* 1990; 50: 534–5.

355 Laifer SA, Darby MJ *et al*. Pregnancy and liver transplantation. *Obstet Gynecol* 1990; 76: 1083–8.

356 Schmid R, Newton JJ. Childbirth after liver transplantation (letter). *Transplantation* 1980; 29: 432.

357 Kirk EP. Organ transplantation and pregnancy. A case report and review. *Am J Obstet Gynecol* 1991; 164: 1629–34.

358 Cundy TF, O'Grady JG *et al*. Recovery of menstruation and pregnancy after liver transplantation. *Gut* 1990; 31: 337–8.

359 de Koning ND, Haagsma EB. Normalization of menstrual pattern after liver transplantation: consequences for contraception. *Digestion* 1990; 46: 239–41.

360 Brown KA, Lucey MR. Liver transplantation restores female reproductive endocrine function. *Hepatology* 1991; 13: 1255–7.

361 Deray G, le Hoang P *et al*. Oral contraceptives interaction with cyclosporin (letter). *Lancet* 1987; 1: 158–9.

362 Wu A, Nashan B *et al*. Outcome of 22 successful pregnancies after liver transplantation. *Clin Transpl* 1998; 12: 454–64.

363 Rayes N, Neuhaus R *et al*. Pregnancies following liver transplantation—how safe are they? A report of 19 cases under cyclosporine A and tacrolimus. *Clin Transpl* 1998; 12: 396–400.

364 Jain A, Venkataramanan R *et al*. Pregnancy after liver transplantation under tacrolimus. *Transplantation* 1997; 64: 559–65.

365 Little BB. Immunosuppressant therapy during gestation (Review). *Semin Perinatol* 1997; 21: 143–8.

366 Armenti VT, Moritz MJ *et al*. Drug safety issues in pregnancy following transplantation and immunosuppression: effects and outcomes. *Drug Safety* 1998; 19: 219–32.

367 Patapis P, Irani S *et al*. Outcome of graft function and pregnancy following liver transplantation. *Transpl Proc* 1997; 29: 1565–6.

368 Radomski JS, Moritz MJ *et al*. National Transplantation Pregnancy Registry: analysis of pregnancy outcomes in female liver transplant recipients. *Liver Transpl Surg* 1995; 1: 281–4.

369 Mass K, Quint EH *et al*. Gynecological and reproductive function after liver transplantation. *Transplantation* 1996; 62: 476–9.

370 Scantlebury V, Gordon R *et al*. Childbearing after liver transplantation. *Transplantation* 1990; 49: 317–21.

371 Hillemanns P, Knitza R *et al*. Rupture of splenic artery aneurysm in a pregnant patient with portal hypertension. *Am J Obstet Gynecol* 1996; 174: 1665–6.

372 Laifer SA, Guido RS. Reproductive function and outcome of pregnancy after liver transplantation in women. *Mayo Clin Proc* 1995; 70: 388–94.

373 Steven MM, Buckley JB *et al*. Pregnancy in chronic active hepatitis. *Q J Med* 1979; 48: 519–33.

374 Colle I, Hautekeete M. Remission of autoimmune hepatitis during pregnancy: a report of two cases. *Liver* 1999; 19: 55–7.

375 Whelton MJ, Sherlock S. Pregnancy in patients with hepatic cirrhosis. Management and outcome. *Lancet* 1968; 2: 995–9.

376 Keating JJ, O'Brien CJ *et al*. Influence of aetiology, clinical and histological features on survival in chronic active hepatitis: an analysis of 204 patients. *Q J Med* 1987; 62: 59–66.

377 Cheng YS. Pregnancy in liver cirrhosis and/or portal hypertension. *Am J Obstet Gynecol* 1977; 128: 812–22.

378 Britton RC. Pregnancy and esophageal varices. *Am J Surg* 1982; 4: 421–5.

379 Schreyer P, Caspi E *et al*. Cirrhosis, pregnancy and delivery: a review. *Obstet Gynecol Surv* 1982; 37: 304–12.

380 Krol Van Straaten J, De Maat CE. Successful pregnancies in cirrhosis of the liver before and after portacaval anastomosis. *Neth Med J* 1984; 27: 14–15.

381 Teisala K, Tuimala R. Pregnancy and esophageal varices. *Ann Chirurg Gynaecol Suppl* 1985; 197: 65–6.

382 Pajor A, Lehoczky D. Pregnancy in liver cirrhosis. Assessment of maternal and fetal risk in eleven patients and review of the management. *Gynecol Obstet Invest* 1994; 38: 45–50.

383 Russell MA, Craigo SD. Cirrhosis and portal hypertension in pregnancy. *Sem Perinatol* 1998; 22: 156–65.

384 Scaglione S. Cirrosi di Laennec in gravidanza. *Riv Ital Ginecol* 1923; 1: 489.

385 Soto-Albors CE, Rayburn WF *et al*. Portal hypertension and hypersplenism in pregnancy secondary to chronic schistosomiasis. A case report. *J Reprod Med* 1984; 29: 345–8.

386 Obata NH, Kurauchi, O *et al*. Pre-eclampsia with fetal death in a patient with shistosomiasis japonica. *Arch Gynecol Obstet* 1998; 261: 101–4.

387 Mazor M, Wiznitzer A *et al*. Gaucher's disease in pregnancy associated with portal hypertension. *Am J Obstet Gynecol* 1986; 154: 1119–20.

388 Benhamou JP, Lebrec D. Non-cirrhotic intrahepatic portal hypertension in adults. *Clin Gastroenterol* 1985; 14: 21–31.

389 Varma RR, Michelsohn NH *et al*. Pregnancy in cirrhotic and non-cirrhotic portal hypertension. *Obstet Gynecol* 1976; 50: 217–22.

390 Cundy TF, Butler J *et al*. Amenorrhoea in women with non-alcoholic chronic liver disease. *Gut* 1991; 32: 202–6.

391 Huchzermeyer H. Schwangershaft bei Leberzirrhose und chronischer Hepatitis (Pregnancy in patients with liver cirrhosis and chronic hepatitis). *Acta Hepatogastroenterol (Stuttgart)* 1971; 18: 294–305.

392 Ahrens EH, Payne MA. Primary biliary cirrhosis. *Medicine (Baltimore)* 1950; 29: 299–364.

393 Bihl JH. Congenital cytomegalovirus infection. *Br Med J* 1959; 78: 1182–8.

394 Sherwin AL, Beck IT *et al*. The course of Wilson's diseases (hepatolenticular degeneration) during pregnancy and after delivery. *Canad Med Assoc J* 1960; 83: 160–3.

395 Dreifuss FE, McKinney WM. Wilson's disease (hepatolenticular degeneration) and pregnancy. *J Am Med Assoc* 1966; 195: 960–2.

396 Schalm SW, van Buuren HR. Prevention of recurrent variceal bleeding: non-surgical procedure. *Clin Gastroenterol* 1985; 14: 209–32.

397 Mattar SG, Lumsden AB. The management of splenic artery aneurysms: experience in 23 cases. *Am J Surg* 1995; 169: 580–4.

398 Kochlar R, Goenka MK *et al*. Endoscopic sclerotherapy during pregnancy. *Am J Gastroenterol* 1990; 85: 1132–5.

399 Starkel P, Horsmans Y *et al*. Endoscopic band ligation: a safe technique to control bleeding esophageal varices in pregnancy. *Gastrointest Endosc* 1998; 48: 212–14.

400 Dhiman RK, Biswas R *et al*. Management of variceal bleeding in pregnancy with endoscopic variceal ligation and N-butyl-2-cyanoacrylate: report of three cases. *Gastrointest Endosc* 2000; 51: 91–3.

401 Aneckstein AE, Weingold AD. Chlorthiazide-induced hepatic coma in pregnancy. *Am J Obstet Gynecol* 1966; 95: 136–7.

402 Heathcote EJ. Management of primary biliary cirrhosis. *Hepatology* 2000; 31: 1005–13.

403 Nir A, Sorokin Y *et al*. Pregnancy and primary biliary cirrhosis. *Int J Obstet Gynaecol* 1989; 28: 279–82.

404 Fagan EA, Moore-Gillon JC *et al*. Multiorgan granulomas and mitochondrial antibodies. *N Engl J Med* 1983; 308: 572–5.

405 Rath HC, Enger IM *et al*. Acute hemolytic crisis as the initial manifestation of Wilson's disease [German]. *Zeitschr Gastroenterol* 1997; 35: 199–203.

406 Toaff R, Toaff ME *et al*. Hepatolenticular degeneration (Wilson's disease) and pregnancy. A review and report of a case. *Obstet Gynecol Surv* 1977; 32: 497–507.

407 Sternlieb I. Wilson's disease and pregnancy. *Hepatology* 2000; 31: 531–2.

408 Morimoto I, Nonomiya H *et al*. Pregnancy and penicillamine treatment in a patient with Wilson's disease. *Jap J Med* 1986; 25: 59–62.

409 Brewer GJ, Dick RD *et al*. Treatment of Wilson's disease with zinc: XV long-term follow-up studies. *J Lab Clin Med* 1998; 132: 264–78.

410 Biller J, Swiontoniowski M *et al*. Successful pregnancy in Wilson's disease: a case report and review of the literature. *Eur Neurol* 1985; 24: 306–9.

411 Baruch Y, Weiner Z *et al*. Pregnancy after liver transplantation. *Int J Gynaecol Obstet* 1993; 41: 273–6.

412 Mjolnerod OK, Rasmunssen K *et al*. Congenital connective-tissue defect probably due to D-penicillamine in pregnancy. *Lancet* 1971; i: 673.

413 Marecek Z, Graf M. Pregnancy in penicillamine-treated patients with Wilson's disease. *N Engl J Med* 1976; 295: 841–2.

414 Solomon L, Abrams G *et al.* Neonatal abnormalities associated with D-penicillamine during pregnancy (letter). *N Engl J Med* 1977; 296: 54–5.

415 Harpey JP, Jaudon MC *et al.* Cutis laxa and low serum zinc antenatal exposure to penicillamine (letter). *Lancet* 1983; ii: 858.

416 Rosa FW. Teratogen Update: penicillamine. *Teratology* 1986; 33: 127–31.

417 Linares A, Zarranz JJ *et al.* Reversible cutis laxa due to maternal D-penicillamine treatment (letter). *Lancet* 1989; ii: 43.

418 Walshe JM. The management of pregnancy in Wilson's disease treated with trientine. *Q J Med* 1986; 58: 81–7.

419 Forbes JR, Cox DW. Functional characterization of missense mutations in ATP7B: Wilson disease mutation or normal variant? *Am J Hum Genet* 1998; 63: 1663–74.

420 Gollan JL, Gollan TJ. Wilson's disease in 1998: genetic, diagnostic and therapeutic aspects. *J Hepatol* 1998; 28: 28–36.

421 Cossu P, Pirastu M *et al.* Prenatal diagnosis of Wilson's disease by analysis of DNA polymorphism (letter). *N Engl J Med* 1992; 327: 57.

422 Chiari H. Uber die Selbstandige Endophlebitis Obiterans der Haupstamme der Venae Hepaticae als Todesurache. *Beitr Pathol Anatom* 1899; 26: 1–18.

423 Krass IM. Chiari's syndrome: report of a case following pregnancy. *J Obstet Gynaecol Br Emp* 1957; 64: 715–19.

424 Hancock KW. The Budd–Chiari syndrome in pregnancy. *J Obstet Gynaecol Br Commonw* 1968; 75: 746–8.

425 Datta DV, Chhuttani PN *et al.* Clinical spectrum of Budd–Chiari syndrome in Chandigarh with particular reference to obstruction of intrahepatic portion of the inferior vena cava. *Gut* 1972; 13: 372–8.

426 Dentsch V, Rosenthal T *et al.* Budd–Chiari syndrome study of angiographic findings and remarks on aetiology. *Am J Roentgenol* 1972; 116: 430–9.

427 Khuroo MS, Datta DV. Budd–Chiari syndrome following pregnancy. Report of 16 cases with roentgenologic, hemodynamic and histologic studies of the hepatic outflow tract. *Am J Med* 1980; 8: 113–21.

428 Covillo FV, Nyong AO *et al.* Budd–Chiari syndrome following pregnancy. *Missouri Med* 1984; 81: 356–8.

429 Huguet C, Deliere T *et al.* Budd–Chiari syndrome with thrombosis of the inferior vena cava: long-term patency of mesocaval and cavoatrial prosthetic bypass. *Surgery* 1984; 95: 108–11.

430 Dilawari JB, Bambery P *et al.* Hepatic outflow obstruction (Budd–Chiari syndrome). Experience with 177 patients and a review of the literature. *Medicine (Baltimore)* 1994; 73: 21–36.

431 Fickert P, Ramschak H *et al.* Acute Budd–Chiari syndrome with fulminant hepatic failure in a pregnant woman with factor V Leiden mutation. *Gastroenterology* 1996; 111: 1670–3.

432 Mitchell MC, Boitnott JM *et al.* Budd–Chiari syndrome: aetiology, diagnosis and management. *Medicine (Baltimore)* 1982; 61: 199–218.

433 Tavill AS, Wood EJ *et al.* The Budd–Chiari syndrome. Correlation between hepatic scintigraphy and clinical, radiological and pathological findings in 19 cases of hepatic venous outflow obstruction. *Gastroenterology* 1975; 68: 509–18.

434 Bais J, Pel M *et al.* Pregnancy and paroxysmal nocturnal hemoglobinuria. *Eur J Obstet Gynecol Reprod Biol* 1994; 53: 211–14.

435 Powell-Jackson PR, Melia W *et al.* Budd–Chiari syndrome: clinical patterns and therapy. *Q J Med* 1982; 201: 29–88.

436 Vons C, Smadja C *et al.* Successful pregnancy after Budd–Chiari syndrome (letter). *Lancet* 1984; 2: 975.

437 Valentine JM, Parkin G *et al.* Combined orthotopic liver transplantation and Cesarian section for the Budd–Chiari syndrome. *Br J Anaesth* 1995; 75: 105–8.

438 Salha O, Campbell DJ *et al.* Budd–Chiari syndrome in pregnancy treated by Caesarian section and liver transplant. *Br J Obstet Gynaecol* 1996; 103: 1254–6.

439 Dubin IM, Johnson FB. Chronic idiopathic jaundice with unidentified pigment in liver cells: new clinicopathologic entity with report of 12 cases. *Medicine (Baltimore)* 1954; 33: 155–97.

440 Cohen L, Lewis C *et al.* Pregnancy oral contraceptives and chronic familial jaundice with predominantly conjugated hyperbilirubinemia (Dubin–Johnson syndrome). *Gastroenterology* 1972; 62: 1182–90.

441 Seligsohn U, Shani M. The Dubin–Johnson syndrome and pregnancy. *Acta Hepatogastroenterol* 1977; 24: 167–9.

442 Arias IM. Inheritable and congenital hyperbilirubinemia. *N Engl J Med* 1971; 285: 1416–21.

443 Cotton DB. Infantile hepatic cholestasis with maternal Dubin–Johnson syndrome. *South Med J* 1984; 77: 1213–14.

444 Zoglio JDD, Cardillo E. The Dubin–Johnson syndrome and pregnancy. *Obstet Gynecol* 1973; 42: 560–3.

445 Farrant JM, Hayllar KM *et al.* Natural history and prognostic variables in primary sclerosing cholangitis. *Gastroenterology* 1991; 100: 1710–17.

446 Janczewska I, Olsson R *et al.* Pregnancy in patients with primary sclerosing cholangitis. *Liver* 1996; 16: 326–30.

447 Nolan DG, Martin LS *et al.* Fetal compromise associated with extreme fetal bile acidemia and maternal primary sclerosing cholangitis. *Obstet Gynecol* 1994; 84: 695–6.

448 Paternoster DM, Floreani A *et al.* Liver transplantation and pregnancy. *Int J Gynaecol Obstet* 1995; 50: 199–200.

449 Rabinovitz M, Appasamy R *et al.* Primary biliary cirrhosis diagnosed during pregnancy. Does it have a different outcome? *Dig Dis Sci* 1995; 40: 571–4.

450 De Silva K. Intraperitoneal rupture of an amoebic liver abscess in a pregnant woman at term. *Ceylon Med J* 1970; 15: 51–3.

451 Navaratne RA. Postpartum intraperitoneal rupture of an amoebic liver abscess. *Ceylon Med J* 1972; 17: 160–3.

452 Wagner VP, Smale LE *et al.* Amoebic abscess of the liver and spleen in pregnancy and the puerperium. *Obstet Gynecol* 1974; 45: 562–5.

453 Cowan DB, Houlton MC. Rupture of an amoebic liver abscess in pregnancy. A case report. *S Afr Med J* 1978; 53: 460–1.

454 Mitchell RW, Teare AJ. Amoebic liver abscess in pregnancy. Case report. *Br J Obstet Gynaecol* 1984; 91: 393–5.

455 Dominguez S, Boudghene F *et al.* Septic shock during the immediate post-partum period revealing a liver abscess in a woman with Crohn's disease [French]. *Gastroenterol Clin Biol* 1999; 23: 775–8.

456 Abioye AA, Edington GM. Prevalence of amoebiasis at autopsy in Ibadan. *Trans Roy Soc Trop Med Hyg* 1972; 66: 754–63.

457 Lindgren P, Pla JC *et al.* Listeria monocytogenes-induced liver abscess in pregnancy. *Acta Obstet Gynecol Scand* 1997; 76: 486–8.

458 Van Vliet W, Scheele F *et al.* Echinococcosis of the liver during pregnancy. *Int J Gynaecol Obstet* 1995; 49: 323–4.

459 Golaszewski T, Susani M *et al.* A large hydatid cyst of the liver in pregnancy. *Arch Gynecol Obstet* 1995; 256: 43–7.

460 Ustunsoz B, Alemdaroglu A *et al.* Percutaneous treatment of hepatic hydatid cyst in pregnancy. *Arch Gynecol Obstet* 1999; 262: 181–4.

461 Gabow PA, Johnson AM *et al*. Risk factors for the development of hepatic cysts in autosomal dominant polycystic kidney disease. *Hepatology* 1990; 11: 1033–7.

462 Kesby GJ. Pregnancy complicated by symptomatic adult polycystic liver disease. *Am J Obstet Gyneol* 1998; 179: 266–7.

463 Everson GT. Hepatic cysts in autosomal dominant polycystic kidney disease (comment). *Mayo Clin Proc* 1990; 65: 933–42.

464 Scott LD, Katz AR *et al*. Oral contraceptives, pregnancy, and focal nodular hyperplasia of the liver. *J Am Med Assoc* 1984; 251: 1461–3.

465 Baum JK, Holz F *et al*. Possible association between benign hepatomas and oral contraceptives. *Lancet* 1973; ii 926–9.

466 Davis M, Portmann B *et al*. Histological evidence of carcinoma in a hepatic tumour associated with oral contraceptives. *Br Med J* 1975; 4: 496–9.

467 Neuberger J, Forman D *et al*. Oral contraceptives and hepatocellular carcinoma. *Br Med J* 1986; 292: 1355–7.

468 Kent DR, Nissen ED *et al*. Effect of pregnancy on liver tumor associated with oral contraceptives. *Obstet Gynecol* 1978; 51: 148–51.

469 Klatskin G. Hepatic tumours: possible relationship to the use of oral contraceptives. *Gastroenterology* 1977; 73: 386–94.

470 Gisi P, Floyd R. Hepatocellular carcinoma in pregnancy. *J Reprod Med* 1999; 44: 65–7.

471 Khoo SK. Cancer risks and the contraceptive pill. What is the evidence after nearly 25 years of use? *Med J Aust* 1986; 144: 185–90.

472 Seaward PG, Koch MA *et al*. Primary hepatocellular carcinoma in pregnancy. A case report. *S Afr Med J* 1986; 69: 700–1.

473 Jeng LB, Lee WC *et al*. Hepatocellular carcinoma in a pregnant woman detected by routine screening of maternal alpha-fetoprotein. *Am J Obstet Gynecol* 1995; 172: 219–20.

474 Lau WY, Leung WT *et al*. Hepatocellular carcinoma during pregnancy and its comparison with other pregnancy-associated malignancies. *Cancer* 1995; 75: 2669–76.

475 Purtilo DJ, Clark JV *et al*. Hepatic malignancy in pregnant women. *Am J Obstet Gynecol* 1975; 121: 41–3.

476 Egwuatu VE. Primary hepatocarcinoma in pregnancy. *Trans Roy Soc Trop Med Hyg* 1980; 74: 793–4.

477 Nakamoto SK, Van Sonnenberg E. Cholangiocarcinoma in pregnancy: the contribution of ultrasound-guided interventional techniques. *J Ultrasound Med* 1985; 4: 557–9.

478 Grumbine FC, Rosenshein NB *et al*. Management of liver metastasis from gestational trophoblastic neoplasia. *Am J Obstet Gynecol* 1980; 137: 959–61.

479 Huggins GR. Neoplasia and hormonal contraception. *Clin Obstet Gynecol* 1981; 24: 903–25.

480 Newlands ES. Trophoblastic tumours. In: Studd J, ed. *Progress in Obstetrics and Gynaecology*. 1983; Churchill Livingstone, Edinburgh: 158 *et seq*.

481 Crawford RA, Newlands E *et al*. Gestational trophoblastic disease with liver metastases: the Charing Cross experience. *Br J Obstet Gynaecol* 1997; 104: 105–9.

482 Hammond CB, Berchert L *et al*. Treatment of metastatic trophoblastic disease. Good and poor prognosis. *Am J Obstet Gynecol* 1973; 115: 451–7.

483 Barnard DE, Woodward KT *et al*. Hepatic metastases of choriocarcinoma: a report of 15 patients. *Gynecol Oncol* 1986; 25: 73–3.

484 Wong LC, Choo YC *et al*. Hepatic metastases in gestational trophoblastic disease. *Obstet Gynecol* 1986; 67: 107–11.

485 Gordon AN, Gershenson DM *et al*. High risk metastatic gestational trophoblastic disease. *Obstet Gynecol* 1985; 65: 550–6.

486 Vujic I, Stanley JH *et al*. Embolic management of rare hemorrhagic gynecologic and obstetrical conditions. *Cardiovasc Int Radiol* 1986; 9: 69–74.

487 Kristoffersson A, Emdin S *et al*. Acute intestinal obstruction and splenic hemorrhage due to metastatic choriocarcinoma. A case report. *Acta Chirurg Scand* 1985; 151: 381–4.

488 Woo JS, Wong LC *et al*. Sonographic patterns of pelvic and hepatic lesions in persistent trophoblastic disease. *J Ultrasound Med* 1985; 44: 189–98.

489 Heaton GE, Matthews TH *et al*. Malignant trophoblastic tumors with massive hemorrhage presenting as liver primary. A report of two cases. *Am J Surg Pathol* 1986; 10: 342–7.

490 Bartoli E, Calonaci N *et al*. Ultrasonography of the gallbladder in pregnancy. *Gastrointest Radiol* 1984; 9: 35–8.

491 Van Bodegraven AA, Bohmer CJ *et al*. Gallbladder contents and fasting gallbladder volumes during and after pregnancy. *Scand J Gastroenterol* 1998; 33: 993–7.

492 Stauffer RA, Adams A *et al*. Gallbladder disease in pregnancy. *Am J Obstet Gynecol* 1982; 144: 661–4.

493 Radberg G, Asztely M *et al*. Gastric and gallbladder emptying in relation to the secretion of cholecystokinin after a meal in late pregnancy. *Digestion* 1989; 42: 174–80.

494 Nilsson S, Stattin S. Gallbladder emptying during the normal menstrual cycle. *Acta Chirurg Scand* 1967; 133: 648–52.

495 Everson GT, McKinley C *et al*. Gallbladder function in the human female: effect of the ovulatory cycle, pregnancy and contraceptive steroids. *Gastroenterology* 1982; 82: 11–19.

496 Braverman DZ, Johnson ML *et al*. Effects of pregnancy and contraceptive steroids on gallbladder function. *N Engl J Med* 1980; 302: 362–4.

497 Radberg G, Friman S *et al*. The influence of pregnancy and contraceptive steroids on the biliary tract and its reference to cholesterol gallstone formation. *Scand J Gastroenterol* 1990; 25: 97–102.

498 Mintz MC, Grumbach K *et al*. Sonographic evaluation of bile duct size during pregnancy. *Am J Roentgenol* 1985; 145: 575–8.

499 Food and Drug Administration (FDA). Department of Health, Education and Welfare. Oral contraceptive labelling. *Food Drug Admin Drug Bull* 1978; 8: 12–13.

500 Scragg RK, McMichael AJ *et al*. Oral contraceptives, pregnancy and endogenous oestrogen in gall stone disease—a case control study. *Br Med J* 1984; 288: 1795–99.

501 Jarnfelt-Samsioe A, Eriksson B *et al*. Gallbladder disease related to use of oral contraceptives and nausea in pregnancy. *South Med J* 1985; 78: 1040–3.

502 Bennion LJ, Grundy SM. Risk factors for the development of cholelithiasis in man (second of two parts). *N Engl J Med* 1978; 299: 1221–7.

503 Kern F, Everson GT *et al*. Biliary lipids, bile acids and gallbladder function in the human female: effects of contraceptive steroids. *J Clin Invest* 1982; 99: 798–805.

504 Kern F, Everson GT *et al*. Biliary lipids, bile acids and gallbladder function in the human female. Effects of pregnancy and the ovulatory cycle. *J Clin Invest* 1981; 68: 1229–42.

505 Stone B, Erickson SK *et al*. Regulation of rat biliary cholesterol secretion by agents which alter cholesterol metabolism. Evidence for a distinct biliary precursor pool. *J Clin Invest* 1985; 76: 1773–81.

506 Davis RA, Kern F. Effects of ethinyl estradiol and phenobarbital on bile acid synthesis and biliary bile acid and cholesterol excretion. *Gastroenterology* 1976; 70: 1130–35.

507 Woodhouse DR, Haylen B. Gallbladder disease complicating pregnancy. *Aust N Zeal J Obstet Gynaecol* 1985; 25: 233–7.

508 Valdivieso V, Covarrubias C et al. Pregnancy and cholelithiasis: pathogenesis and natural course of gallstones diagnosed in early pregnancy. *Hepatology* 1993; 17: 1–4.

509 Tsimoyiannis EC, Antoniou NC et al. Cholelithiasis during pregnancy and lactation. Prospective study. *Eur J Surg* 1994; 160: 627–31.

510 Yates MR, Baron TH. Biliary tract disease in pregnancy. *Clin Liver Dis* 1999; 3: 131–46.

511 Hill LM, Johnson CE et al. Cholecystectomy in pregnancy. *Obstet Gynecol* 1975; 9: 291–3.

512 Kammerer WS. Non-obstetric surgery during pregnancy. *Med Clin N Am* 1979; 6: 1157–63.

513 Glasgow RE, Visser BE et al. Changing management of gallstone disease during pregnancy. *Surg Endosc* 1998; 12: 241–6.

514 Chesson RR, Gallup DG et al. Ultrasonographic diagnosis of asymptomatic cholelithiasis in pregnancy. *J Reprod Med* 1985; 30: 920–2.

515 Williamson SL, Williamson MR. Cholecystosonography in pregnancy. *J Ultrasound Med* 1984; 3: 329–31.

516 Petrozza JC, Mastrobattista JM et al. Gallbladder perforation in pregnancy. *Am J Perinatol* 1995; 12: 339–41.

517 Gadwood KA, Reynes CJ et al. Gallbladder wall thickening in pre-eclampsia. *J Am Med Assoc* 1985; 253: 71–3.

518 Machi J, Sigel B et al. Operative ultrasonography in the biliary tract during pregnancy. *Surg Gynecol Obstet* 1985; 160: 119–23.

519 Hiatt JR, Hiatt JC et al. Biliary disease in pregnancy: strategy for surgical management. *Am J Surg* 1986; 151: 263–5.

520 Bar-Meir S, Rotmenesch S. Investigation of obstructive jaundice by ultra-thin-caliber endoscope: a new technique for potential use in pregnancy. *Am J Obstet Gynecol* 1984; 150: 1003–4.

521 Pelosi MA, Pelosi, MA et al. Laparoscopic cholecystectomy at Cesarian section. A new surgical option. *Surg Laparosc Endosc Percut Tech* 1997; 7: 369–72.

522 Graham G, Baxi L et al. Laparoscopic cholecystectomy during pregnancy: a case series and review of the literature. *Obstet Gynecol Surv* 1998; 53: 566–74.

523 Anonymous. Guidelines for laparoscopic surgery during pregnancy. Society of American Gastrointestinal Endoscopic Surgeons (SAGES). *Surg Endosc* 1998; 12: 189–90.

524 Printen KJ, Ott RA. Cholecystectomy during pregnancy. *Am J Surg* 1978; 44: 432–4.

525 Palmer AK, Heywood R. Pathological changes in the rhesus fetus associated with oral administration of chenodeoxycholic acid. *Toxicology* 1974; 2: 239–46.

526 Kaiser R, Berk JE et al. Serum amylase changes during pregnancy. *Am J Obstet Gynecol* 1975; 122: 283–6.

527 Strickland DM, Hauth JC et al. Amylase and isoamylase activities in serum of pregnant women. *Obstet Gynecol* 1984; 63: 389–91.

528 Garrison R. Amylase. *Emerg Med Clin N Am* 1986; 4: 315–27.

529 Chang CC, Hsieh YY et al. Acute pancreatitis in pregnancy. *Chung Hua I Hsueh Tsa Chih—Chin Med J* 1998; 61: 85–92.

530 Corlett RC, Mishell DR, Pancreatitis in pregnancy. *Am J Obstet Gynecol* 1972; 113: 281–90.

531 Wilinson EJ. Acute pancreatitis in pregnancy: a review of 98 cases and a report of 8 new cases. *Obstet Gynecol Surv* 1973; 28: 281–303.

532 Chang G, Wilkins-Haug L et al. Alcohol use and pregnancy: improving identification. *Obstet Gynecol* 1998; 91: 892–8.

533 Klein KB. Pancreatitis in pregnancy. In: Rustgi VK, Cooper JN, eds. *Gastrointestinal and Hepatic Complications in Pregnancy*. 1986; J. Wiley & Sons, New York: 138–61.

534 Langmade CF, Edmondson HA. Acute pancreatitis during pregnancy and the postpartum period: report of 9 cases. *Surg Gynecol Obstet* 1951; 92: 43–52.

535 Montgomery WH, Miller FC. Views and reviews. Pancreatitis and pregnancy. *Obstet Gynecol* 1970; 35: 658–65.

536 Jouppila P, Mokka R et al. Acute pancreatitis in pregnancy. *Surg Gynecol Obstetr* 1974; 139: 879–82.

537 Berk JE, Smith BH et al. Pregnancy pancreatitis. *Am J Gastroenterol* 1971; 56: 216–26.

538 Mizushima T, Ochi K et al. Prevention of hyperlipidemic acute pancreatitis during pregnancy with medium- chain triglyceride nutritional support. *Int J Pancreatol* 1998; 23: 187–92.

539 Stuyt PM, Demacker PN et al. Pancreatitis induced by oestrogen in a patient with type I hyperlipidaemia. *Br Med J* 1986; 293: 734.

540 Henderson H, Leisegang F et al. A novel Glu421Lys substitution in the lipoprotein lipase gene in pregnancy-induced hypertriglyceridemic pancreatitis. *Clin Chim Acta* 1998; 269: 1–12.

541 Thomason JL, Sampson MB et al. Pregnancy complicated by concurrent primary hyperparathyroidism and pancreatitis. *Obstet Gynecol* 1981; 57 (Suppl. 6) 34S–6S.

542 Kondo Y, Nagai H et al. Primary hyperparathyroidism and acute pancreatitis during pregnancy. Report of a case and review of the English and Japanese literature. *Int J Pancreatol* 1998; 24: 43–7.

543 Hess HM, Dickson J et al. Hyperfunctioning parathyroid carcinoma presenting as acute pancreatitis in pregnancy. *J Reprod Med* 1980; 25: 83–7.

544 McKay AJ, O'Neill J et al. Pancreatitis, pregnancy and gallstones. *Br J Obstet Gynaecol* 1980; 87: 47–50.

545 Trapnell JE, Duncan EHL. Patterns and incidence of acute pancreatitis. *Br Med J* 1975; ii: 179–83.

546 Gineston JL, Capron JP et al. Prolonged total parenteral nutrition in a pregnant woman with acute pancreatitis. *J Clin Gastroenterol* 1984; 6: 249–52.

547 Stowell JC, Bottsford JE et al. Pancreatitis with pseudocyst and cholelithiasis in third trimester of pregnancy: management with total parenteral nutrition. *South Med J* 1984; 77: 502–4.

548 Carmona F, Cararach V et al. Successful pregnancy after combined pancreas-kidney transplantation. *Eur J Obstet Gynecol Reprod Biol* 1993; 52: 143–5.

549 McGrory CH, Radomski JS et al. Pregnancy outcomes in 10 female pancreas-kidney recipients. *J Transpl Coordin* 1998; 8: 55–9.

550 Donegan WL. Cancer and pregnancy. *Cancer* 1983; 33: 194–214.

551 Gamberella FR. Pancreatic carcinoma in pregnancy: a case report. *Am J Obstet Gynecol* 1984; 149: 15–17.

552 Ganepola GA, Gritsman AY et al. Are pancreatic tumors hormone dependent? A case report of unusual, rapidly growing pancreatic tumor during pregnancy, its possible relationship to female sex hormones, and review of the literature. *Am Sur* 1999; 65: 105–11.

553 Smithers BM, Welch C et al. Cystadenocarcinoma of the pancreas presenting in pregnancy. *Br J Surg* 1986; 73: 591.

554 Morales A, Ruiz Molina JM et al. Papillary-cystic neoplasm of the pancreas. A sex-steroid dependent tumor. *Int J Pancreatol* 1998; 24: 219–25.

555 Galun E, Ben-Yehuda A et al. Insulinoma complicating pregnancy: a case report and review of the literature. *Am J Obstet Gynecol* 1986; 155: 64–5.

556 Bardet S, Mahot P et al. Discovery of an insulinoma during the first trimester of pregnancy (French). *Presse Med* 1994; 23: 285–7.

10 Disorders of the gastrointestinal tract

Elizabeth A. Fagan

Management problems in pregnancy

Disorders relating to the gastrointestinal tract, such as nausea and vomiting and infections including parasitic diseases are common in pregnancy and account for a significant proportion of hospitalizations during antenatal care [1]. Alterations in the neuroendocrinological axis and gut motility have been implicated but the underlying physiological changes remain controversial. Delayed gastric emptying has been implicated in the impaired absorption of glucose in some [2], but not all [3], studies. Most recent data show no significant delay for solids in gastric emptying [4] and intestinal transit in otherwise healthy pregnant women when compared with non-pregnant females (see constipation, below). These gestational problems are self-limiting and most do not affect maternal or fetal outcome. Their importance in obstetric practice is the need to differentiate them from the many diseases with similar presentations requiring a specific diagnosis and management.

Self-medication for gastrointestinal disorders is widespread. Proprietary antacids, antiemetics, laxatives and antidiarrhoeal agents may be taken before awareness of pregnancy. Warnings about drug ingestion also apply to these readily available preparations. Patients with pre-existing diseases, such as inflammatory bowel disease (IBD), on regular medication require close monitoring. The decision to alter treatment will depend on the relative risks of maternal relapse and perceived danger to the fetus.

Suggestions for therapy are given on the understanding that many drugs have not been subjected to extensive trials in pregnancy. A drug always should be prescribed with caution and only for disorders that are not self-limiting.

Safety of diagnostic imaging

Diagnostic ultrasonographic techniques, including duplex Doppler imaging, are not contraindicated during pregnancy and should be employed whenever necessary to improve the specificity of diagnosis, especially prior to surgery.

The advent of magnetic resonance imaging (MRI) with angiography (MRA), cholecyst-pancreatography (MRCP) and fast single-shot turbo spin–echo (HASTE) MR, as well as computed tomography (CT), including spiral CT, have revolutionized the diagnosis of many gastrointestinal disorders. The American College of Pediatrics and American College of Obstetricians and Gynecologists, published guidelines in 1992 for perinatal care. These stated that diagnostic radiological procedures should not be performed during pregnancy unless the information to be obtained from them is necessary for the care of the patient and cannot be obtained by other means (especially ultrasound).

The fetal brain is especially sensitive to radiation damage between weeks 8 and 15 after conception (weeks 10–17 of gestation). Exposure of below 200 mGy seems without harmful effect on the developing fetal brain and is well above that delivered by most modern, well-maintained diagnostic equipment [5].

While concern over the potential for adverse effects to the fetus has limited the use of diagnostic imaging modalities in pregnant patients, accumulating data attest to their safety, at least in the medium term.

The American College of Radiology stated in 1991 that no single diagnostic procedure results in a radiation dose that threatens the well being of the developing embryo and fetus [6].

Successful diagnosis using MRI has been reported in individual cases during pregnancy complicated by gastrointestinal disorders, particularly hyperemesis gravidarum complicated by vasospasm of the cerebral arteries [7], Wernicke's encephalopathy [8,9] and central pontine myelinolysis.

Fast MR techniques have improved significantly the resolution of maternal and fetal anatomies without the requirement for sedation [10]. MR techniques such as HASTE show promise in diagnosing conditions such as small bowel obstruction [11]. Although no adverse effects on the fetus have been reported, the National Radiological Protection Board and American College of Obstetricians and Gynecologists advise arbitrarily against the use of MRI during the first trimester.

Safety of endoscopic procedures

The reader is referred to the excellent review by Regan *et al.* [12]. Data from prospective, controlled studies are lacking. Nevertheless, the consensus view is that in expert hands, flexible fibre-optic upper endoscopy is safe and preferred to conventional barium studies for diagnosis of suspected gastro-oesophageal reflux, gastric lesions, peptic ulcer and coeliac disease. Duodenal biopsy is safe but jejunal biopsy should be avoided during pregnancy.

Flexible fibre-optic sigmoidoscopy also is safe if carried out carefully and by an experienced endoscopist [13]. Fibre-optic flexible sigmoidoscopy is essential for investigating persistent diarrhoea and blood in the stools [13] particularly in the management of colonic IBD. While maternal and fetal outcomes following eight colonoscopies were reported as favourable [13,12], much larger numbers are required before guidelines can be established regarding safety and efficacy.

Concerns in obstetric practice include the potential for adverse effects and consequences of sedation and other medications and intubation to cause hypotension, hypertension and hypoxia [12], bronchospasm and gastric aspiration. Vagal tone can increase during intubation, including colonic distension, causing bradycardia. Complications such as disruption of the placenta and trauma to the fetus are uncommon in expert hands.

The lack of evidence for teratogenic effects on the fetus should not promote complacency. Although a multicentre, case–controlled study of 83 upper endoscopies reported no excess adverse fetal outcomes, this study was retrospective and lacked sufficient statistical power to evaluate a negative correlation [13].

Attention to detail is essential for optimizing the safety of any diagnostic procedure during pregnancy. The pregnant woman should be given priority on the endoscopy list. Adequate venous access should be secured prior to intubation and sedation. Dehydration, hypotension and hypoglycaemia from fasting should be avoided by supplementation with intravenous fluids and glucose. A nasogastric tube should be used to aspirate gastric contents prior to sedation and intubation. Close monitoring of vital signs including oxygen saturations, blood pressure and fetal monitoring should be carried out in all cases. Facilities available should include ready access to ventilatory support, adequate suction aspiration equipment and availability of an experienced anaesthetist. The gravid patient should be placed in the left lateral position or right lateral decubitus position, including during colonoscopy, to limit compression by the uterus of the inferior vena cava. Recommendations for sedation during pregnancy, based on categorization of drug safety by the Food and Drug Administration (FDA), include use of meperidine (category B) in preference to benzodiazepines such as diazepam and midazolam (category D).

Water perfusion followed by endoscopic aspiration is preferred to use of simethicone for upper endoscopy and endoscopic retrograde cholecyst-pancreatography (ERCP) and to polyethylene glycol for preparation of the large bowel [12].

ERCP should only be carried out by an expert and in a hospital with all support facilities. It poses considerable risk to mother and unborn child due to complications such as pancreatitis, bleeding and exposure to irradiation. Nevertheless, ERCP has been carried out successfully and safely during pregnancy, albeit in small numbers of women. ERCP should be considered only in special circumstances such as obstruction of the common bile duct associated with jaundice and/or complications such as pancreatitis and cholangitis. The majority of indications for ERCP during pregnancy relate to cholelithiasis. Accordingly, diagnostic endoscopic ultrasonography is preferable to ERCP, especially if combined with endoscopic extraction of impacted stone. MRCP also would seem advantageous for diagnosis but data are lacking in pregnancy.

Contrast agents that contain iodine, such as diatrizoate (category D), have the potential to cause hypothyroidism in the baby. Risks during ERCP may be minimized by use of low concentrations of diatrizoate, especially of the water-soluble form, limiting the number of intraductal injections and avoiding unnecessary pancreatography [12].

Dietary habits in pregnancy

Changes in dietary selection are common. Aversion to coffee, alcohol, cigarettes, fried food, poultry and herbs are common and exacerbated by nausea, vomiting and gastro-oesophageal reflux. Dietary cravings also are common but their mechanisms are poorly understood [2]. In a study of 1772 women in the first trimester [14], dietary cravings were reported in 68% of urban black women and 84% of white women. Typical alterations in tastes and cravings included those for sour, savoury and sweet flavours and especially for fruit and milk. Aversions reported in above 45% were typically against meat, fish, fatty foods and coffee [14].

Pica also is common [15]. Cravings admitted are geophagy—for soil [16], clay and chalk as well as starch, baby powder, baking soda, coal, soap, toothpaste and disinfectants [14,15]. Ethnic factors may play a role [14–16]. In the studies by [14] and [16], pica, particularly for soil and ash, was reported in 38–73% of black women, compared with 5% of Indian and white women; the latter preferred chalk and ice. Underlying mechanisms are not understood. Pica is not necessarily related to gestational nausea and vomiting [14,16] or to parity. Some authors found a relation between geophagy, pica and iron-deficiency anaemia [15,17,18], especially resulting from blood loss in the gastrointestinal tract [19]. However, the reductions in haemoglobin were mild and seemed unrelated to pregnancy outcome. Geophagy usually resolves after delivery but typically recurs in later pregnancies. Pica usually is harmless but has been implicated in some cases of maternal and perinatal mortalities [15], chronic constipation, bowel obstruction, including from trichobezoar, and parasitosis such as toxoplasmosis [19], bilharzia (schistosomiasis) and congenital plumbism [20].

Malnutrition and vitamin deficiencies

Well-nourished women use various metabolic strategies to meet the energy demands of pregnancy. Alterations include reductions in diet-induced thermogenesis and activity-related energy expenditure, and deposition of less body fat than anticipated while increasing energy intake [21]. Overall, prospective studies of Western women show minimal effect of maternal diet in late pregnancy on placental weights, birthweights [22] or reduction of preterm birth [23,24]. Data on the impact of poor maternal nutrition during early pregnancy on these outcomes

also remain controversial. Other confounding factors, such as vomiting and smoking, interact to result in a baby of small-for-gestational age and low birthweight. Further, there is little evidence that nutritional counselling alters significantly the eating habits of pregnant women or fetal outcomes. Moreover, provision of protein supplementation has been associated with little beneficial, or even adverse, effects [23,24]. Supplementation of calories is associated with some increase in birthweights in developing regions and areas of famine but does not necessarily reduce the frequency of preterm birth [23,24].

Regardless, women with 'food fads' and strict vegetarians may be deficient in several essential dietary substances including, among others, certain vitamins, iron, polyunsaturated fatty acids and calcium. Cultural differences need to be addressed when assessing the impact of the environment and maternal diet on well-being and fetal outcome. In certain African countries and South-East Asia, night blindness due to vitamin A deficiency has been reported in up to 16% of pregnant women, and interferes significantly with domestic and social interactions. Night blindness typically is associated with suboptimal intake of preformed vitamin A in milk products, meat and fish and provitamin A from leafy green vegetables and fruits [25]. Individual studies report an association between maternal vitamin A deficiency and low male/female ratio in babies [26]. Other factors should be considered such as an increased risk of infections (especially urinary tract), diarrhoea and dysentery, as well as anorexia, nausea and vomiting, pre-eclampsia, obesity and short stature [26]. Caution should be exercised before recommending supplementation of vitamin A, as excess can lead to hepatotoxicity and teratogenic effects on the fetus.

Interest is emerging on the impact of maternal deficits of carotenoids, essential fatty acids and amino acids, such as total glutathione, on maternal hormones. In turn, studies are continuing to assess the impact of their deficits on fetal development, potential teratogenicity and future development of cancers in the offspring. Excess maternal intake of linoleic acid has been linked in some cases to neurological damage in the baby.

Unfortunately, most studies are of limited statistical power to separate individual dietary deficits (and sometimes excesses) from other confounding variables such the consequences of low socio-economic status (low education, poor housing, poor diet), smoking and excess exposure to alcohol and potential environmental toxins.

Iron deficiency remains common among fertile women in the West as well as in developing countries especially in women infected with intestinal parasites [27,28] (see

Chapter 2 where folic acid deficiency and the prevention of neural tube defects are also considered).

In all patients with gastrointestinal diseases, regardless of their compliance to diet, serial monitoring is essential through pregnancy and lactation. Supplements of folate may have to be increased considerably to achieve satisfactory levels in serum and red cells. Severe zinc deficiency may occur in acrodermatitis enteropathica and is an established cause of congenital malformation, particularly neural tube defects [29,30]. Breastfed babies and those born to mothers with low serum levels of vitamin B_{12} will have low serum and liver stores and the latter should receive supplements of B_{12} [31,32].

A trend towards statistical significance has been shown in certain randomized trials assessing the benefits to fetal outcome (reduction in preterm deliveries and low birthweights) of supplements of calcium as well as iron, zinc and fish oils [33], especially among undernourished women with low dietary intakes of these nutrients [24]. The question of prevention of pre-eclampsia by calcium supplementation is considered in Chapter 6. The efficacy of combined vitamin and mineral supplements, taken typically as over-the-counter medicines in many Western countries, has not been evaluated in randomized trials, which need to address confounding factors such as self-selection bias and lifestyle.

Disorders of the oral cavity

Apthous stomatitis

Benign ulceration has been reported in up to 20% of the general population [34]. Complaints among pregnant women are common in clinical practice although a survey of peer-reviewed literature between 1942 and 1991 concluded there was no evidence for associations between apthous stomatitis and the menstrual cycle, pregnancy or the menopause [35]. Objective, large studies are lacking. Most cases are idiopathic and a family history is common. The importance in obstetric practice is to recognize the exceptions that can herald many diseases such as coeliac disease, inflammatory bowel disease, Behçet's syndrome, pemphigus vulgaris, Reiter's syndrome, nutritional deficiencies, immunodeficiencies, particularly human immunodeficiency virus (HIV) infection, and various haematological disorders. In HIV-seropositive subjects the oral cavity can be infected with herpes simplex virus (typically type I) and *Candida albicans*. Hairy leukoplakia of the tongue also is well recognized [36].

The numerous and diverse medications used testify to their limited success and understanding of idiopathic apthous ulceration. Management generally is palliative, aimed at relieving pain, reducing the number of ulcer days, extending the periods of remission and identifying and treating any underlying disorders, especially deficiency of vitamins such as folic acid and B_{12} and iron, and fungal infection. Treatment should focus on good dental hygiene, antifungal lozenges for superinfections with *Candida* spp. and, if necessary, topical corticosteroids.

Hyperplastic gingivitis

Hyperplasia of gingival tissues can occur with puberty in association with elevated levels of gonadotropins and sex hormones [34] as well as with pregnancy [37,38]. In pregnancy, elevations in sex hormones and gonadotropins and selective growth of microbes such as *Prevotella intermedia* serve to intensify the inflammatory response in the gingiva [38]. In an extensive study of periodontal disease in pregnancy, [37] gingivitis was found in all women between the second and eight month, with regression at term and after delivery. Lobulated and nodulated gingival tissue (pregnancy tumour, pregnancy granuloma) have been reported in 2% of pregnancies [39]. In extreme cases, the gingival margin and interdental papillae may become deep purple and red with excessive bleeding on contact [34]. Histological features may be similar to pyogenic granuloma and include nodular inflammatory hyperplasia with endothelial proliferation and vascular dilatation. Gingival oedema seems to be the primary feature; debris and other irritants are not considered to be the major cause [2]. Management is difficult as these conditions may recur. Some improvement can occur with attention to oral hygiene, removal of dental plaque and use of soft toothbrushes.

Dental caries

Attention to dental health should continue throughout and beyond pregnancy [40]. The increase in frequency of dental caries during pregnancy by one to two times that of the non-pregnant population relates to the increase in incidence of acidophilic microorganisms in plaque and subgingiva associated with progressive periodontitis. Measurements of the pH of saliva have given conflicting results [2]. Predisposing factors include raised levels of sex hormones [41]. Deficiency of calcium plays only a secondary role. Although poor periodontal health is associated with delivery of a low birthweight infant [42], other factors such as suboptimal weight gain during pregnancy and socio-economic status linked to low education may contribute to the poor fetal outcome.

Gastro-oesophageal disorders

Gastro-oesophageal reflux

PATHOPHYSIOLOGY

Dyspepsia and heartburn due to gastro-oesophageal reflux are distressing symptoms that often commence in early pregnancy and occur in up to 80% of pregnant women [43–46]. Reflux is most common in the third trimester but can occur at any time during gestation. Various hypotheses have been postulated to explain the predisposition to reflux during pregnancy but the roles of oestrogen and progesterone in reducing the lower oesophageal sphincter pressure (LOSP) remain controversial [46]. Apart from reductions in LOSP [47–49], other contributing factors include increased intragastric pressure [50,51], reduced competence of the pyloric sphincter with backwash of alkaline bile [52], failure of acid clearance, diet and racial predisposition [53].

Gastro-oesophageal reflux is related to a reduced 'barrier' pressure—the difference between gastric, and LOSP, pressures—rather than an elevation in intragastric pressure alone [49,54,55], except in late pregnancy [49]. The lower oesophageal sphincter (LOS) is under control from a variety of humoral agents [54] including gut hormones, particularly motilin [56], acetylcholine, noradrenaline (norepinephrine), histamine, 5-hydroxytryptamine (5-HT) and prostaglandins [56]. In the non-pregnant individual, there is an adaptive response to any rise in intragastric pressure with an increase in LOSP [54,57]. This response prevents reflux by maintaining the barrier pressure. In pregnancy, in the luteal phase of the menstrual cycle, and in women taking combined progesterone and oestrogen oral contraceptive therapy [54], there is a failure of this adaptive response. The LOSP [49] is reduced under the combined influence of progesterone and oestrogen, rather than oestrogen [55], or progesterone [46], alone. Drugs can promote gastro-oesophageal reflux by lowering the LOSP especially those used in anaesthesia such as atropine, halothane, enflurane, opiates and thiopentone, and also tricyclic antidepressant agents [57]. Other factors in pregnancy include the impaired contractile response and alterations in the pattern of intermittent transient relaxations of the LOS, mechanisms of clearance of acid from the oesophagus and stimulation of sensory neuronal mechanisms. How these interact with exogenous stimuli such as a protein meal and pentagastrin [54,55], remains unclear because plasma levels of gastrin, gastric pH and gastric acid output are unchanged by pregnancy [58].

OESOPHAGITIS

Inflammation of the oesophageal mucosa results from contact with acid, or alkaline gastric contents. The most common cause is gastro-oesophageal reflux of acid peptic juice with or without a hiatus hernia [50]. Alkaline oesophagitis also may occur [59]. There is no direct correlation between severity of symptoms and the degree of gastro-oesophageal reflux [49], extent of oesophagitis seen at endoscopy and histopathology or the presence of a hiatus hernia. In a retrospective literature survey of the complications in pregnancy, Scott and Deutsch [60] collected 34 cases of severe, erosive and haemorrhagic oesophagitis most often associated with gestational vomiting.

HIATUS HERNIA

Hiatus hernia is common in the general population and can be demonstrated in around 10–20% of women in late pregnancy [61]. Controversy continues over the relation between the 'barrier' pressure, symptoms of gastro-oesophageal reflux and the presence of a hiatus hernia [50,53].

MANAGEMENT OF GASTRO-OESOPHAGEAL REFLUX

Gastro-oesophageal reflux and oesophagitis are distressing symptoms that often require treatment after exclusion of other disorders. Similar symptoms, especially dyspepsia, can herald many disorders ranging from infections and infestations, liver and biliary diseases, pancreatitis, and myocardial infarction. Reflux can present as bronchospasm simulating asthma.

In early pregnancy, ingestion of small carbohydrate-rich meals with avoidance of excess fat and alcohol [62] and avoiding bending, stooping and lying supine are sufficient to alleviate symptoms in over half the patients [45,63]. In late pregnancy, during labour and obstetrical anaesthesia there are additional concerns regarding the increased risk of vomiting and regurgitation. Tracheal aspiration of acid gastric contents can lead to a chemical pneumonitis, hypoxia and pulmonary oedema (Mendelson's syndrome; see below).

Antacids (see also peptic ulceration; antiulcer therapy, below)

A retrospective study showed that up to one-third of women take antacids at some time during pregnancy [64]. Studies on the teratogenicity of conventional, simple antacids containing aluminium, magnesium and calcium suggest that they are probably safe [64], although prospective data from controlled trials are lacking [65]. Aluminium and magnesium hydroxide do not cross into breast milk in appreciable amounts and probably are safe [66]. Aluminium products tend to cause constipation. Magnesium trisilicate in high dose over a protracted time can cause respiratory distress, hypotonia, silica nephrolithiasis and cardiovascular complications as well as diarrhoea [66]. First-line therapy is with single preparations of magnesium trisilicate, magnesium hydroxide and non-absorbable alginates in doses of 10–15 mL two to three times daily, between meals and at night. Preparations containing non-absorbed alginates, such as alginic acid (Gaviscon), are considered to be safe.

Proprietary antacids are best avoided. Many contain anticholinergic agents that are well absorbed, reduce the LOSP [51,57,67] and are excreted into breast milk [68]. Sodium bicarbonate should be avoided; metabolic alkalosis and fluid overload can occur in the fetus and mother. Misoprostol, an analogue of prostaglandin E_1, increases uterine tone and contractions and is contraindicated in pregnancy. In patients with coeliac disease, milk and lactose intolerance, Nulacin, should be avoided because this contains gluten, milk fats and lactose.

Acid suppressant agents (see peptic ulceration; antiulcer therapy, below)

Use of non-prescription drugs in early pregnancy, including H_2-receptor antagonists, continues to increase despite lack of controlled trials with sufficient statistical power to provide reliable safety data [45,63,69,70]. The H_2-receptor antagonists, such as cimetidine (category B), ranitidine (category B), famotidine (category B) and nizatidine (category C), and proton pump inhibitors, such as omeprazole (category C) and lansoprazole (category B), have not been approved by the FDA for use during pregnancy and lactation (see peptic ulcer, below). Nevertheless, small studies attest overall to their safety [71,72].

In a combined database from the UK and Italy between 1991 and 1996, the relative rate of non-genetic congenital malformations among live births from 2236 pregnancies with recorded exposure during the first trimester compared to non-exposed was 1.2 for cimetidine, 1.4 for ranitidine, and 0.9 for omeprazole [72]. Further, there was no relation between exposure to drug and excess risk of preterm delivery or growth restriction [72]. Cimetidine and ranitidine freely cross the placenta [73–75]. High levels have been achieved in breast milk compared to serum [73–76] but the effects on the suckling baby are unknown. Antiandrogenic effects of cimetidine, such as gynaecomastia and galactorrhoea, are recognized in humans. The significance of uterine H_2 receptors is unclear. In rabbits given H_1- and H_2-receptor blockers there was interference with the uterine vascular response at the time of implantation [77] but no adverse effects on fertility and gestation have been noted in humans.

Conflicting results from teratology studies [76,78] and anecdotal adverse effects [79] include hepatic dysfunction with severe jaundice in two newborn infants exposed to cimetidine 1 month prior to delivery [79]. One multicentre, prospective controlled study in Canada followed fetal outcome after maternal exposure to omeprazole during organogenesis [80]. Of 113 women, the 4% incidence of major congenital malformations was not statistically significant compared with 2% controls (non-exposed) and 2.8% paired for disease. Pregnancy complications such as low-birthweight, preterm delivery and small for gestational age were comparable for all groups. Similar (non-statistically significant) rates were found in a study of 51 pregnant women exposed to proton pump inhibitors [71]. The relative risk of congenital malformation was 1.6 and of preterm delivery, 2.3 compared to 13 327 controls [71]. Caution is required in interpreting such statistical data because even very large studies may not have sufficient power to exclude specific malformations. For example, 38 babies with cardiac malformations were born to women exposed to proton pump inhibitors from 30 days prior to conception through to the end of the first trimester [71].

In conclusion, the H_2-receptor antagonists should be reserved for use after the first trimester in women with severe peptic ulceration that has failed to show healing on effective antacid therapy and strict supervision of conservative measures. Proton pump inhibitors should be used with caution and only in late pregnancy until more data are available to attest to their safety in pregnancy [45,63,81].

The prokinetic agents, metoclopramide and domperidone raise LOSP [57] but experience in early pregnancy [82,83] is limited (see Antiemetics below). Metoclopramide interacts with anticholinergic agents. Individual publications have reported safety and efficacy of omeprazole in the treatment of hyperemesis gravidarum and in prevention of gastric aspiration prior to anaesthesia. Their safety in human pregnancy and lactation remains to be established.

Emergency anaesthesia (see also Chapter 1)

Gastric pressure and gastric volumes increase during labour and emergency caesarean section [84]. Concern that commonly used antacid suspension gels may be pulmonary irritants if inhaled has led to the preferential use of non-particulate antacid solutions such as sodium citrate. These seem to mix more effectively with gastric juice than their particulate counterparts and probably are safer at least in late pregnancy and prior to emergency anaesthesia [85].

Cimetidine and ranitidine continue to be used in preparation for obstetrical anaesthesia. Data are limited concerning their efficacy in rapidly neutralizing gastric contents and so preventing pulmonary complications following gastric aspiration. In a controlled trial in Italy of 75 women given ranitidine (50 mg intravenously) 30–60 min before caesarean section, there was a significant reduction in gastric acidity (pH above 2.5) and gastric fluid volume (below 25 mL) compared with no therapy [86]. Addition of metoclopramide was without extra benefit [86]. Gastric emptying can be delayed following extradural lumbar anaesthesia and fentanyl. The volume of gastric contents can be assessed using ultrasonography. Prior to anaesthesia, the pH of gastric contents should be raised with a non-particulate antacid such as sodium citrate and an H_2 antagonist. Parenteral antiemetics commonly used are promethazine and promazine.

Nausea and vomiting

These occur so frequently [1,14,87,88] as often to be considered diagnostic of pregnancy and its normal physiological consequences. Risk factors implicated in some studies are active and passive smoking, intolerance to oral contraceptive therapy, gallbladder disease and twin pregnancy. Ptyalism—excessive salivation and spitting—can be a distressing accompaniment of severe vomiting and probably results from the impaired ability of the nauseated woman to swallow normal quantities of saliva [2].

By contrast, hyperemesis gravidarum (see below) is defined as vomiting occurring before the 20th week and requiring admission to hospital [89]. Some definitions include a minimum loss of 5% bodyweight and/or the inability to maintain fluid and electrolyte balance without admission to hospital.

EPIDEMIOLOGY

Nausea and vomiting occur worldwide and cross cultural, genetic and environmental boundaries [45,90,91]. Symptoms occur most commonly between the sixth and 16th week [87] but in 20% of cases continue into the second and third trimesters [92]. In a large prospective epidemiological study carried out between 1959 and 1966 by the National Institutes of Health (NIH), USA, 9098 healthy women without any predisposing factors were followed

from the first trimester [87]. Vomiting (excluding hyperemesis gravidarum) was reported in 56% and associated more commonly with being a white primapara, young, of low education, non-smoker and obese [87]. Several factors considered not significant in the NIH study included the presence of a twin pregnancy (compared to singleton), primiparity in black women, smoking, degree of weight gain, known intolerance to oral contraceptive therapy and the presence of gallbladder disease [93], unplanned or planned pregnancy and a past obstetric history of fetal death, hypertension, diabetes or thyrotoxicosis [87]. A tendency to vomit in future pregnancies was significant, as an independent factor, despite adjustment for age and smoking history. In a prospective study in Sweden of 102 women followed through pregnancy, 61% complained of vomiting in the first trimester [93,94]. In contrast to the NIH study [87], vomiting was more common in multiparae. Other significant risk factors included a relatively short interpregnancy (< 4 years) interval, and a higher diastolic blood pressure in late pregnancy in those who had vomiting in the first trimester [94]. No correlation was found with previous intolerance to oral contraceptive therapy, motion sickness, alcohol intake and smoking and complications in late pregnancy such as oedema or eclampsia [94].

Factors associated with a reduced risk of gestational nausea and vomiting seem easier to identify than those associated with increased risk. A multivariate analysis of 825 women in California surveyed between 1983 and 1984 correlated a reduced risk of gestational nausea and vomiting with being white, aged over 35 years, previous infertility, of professional occupation, with a history of drinking alcohol that predated conception and no previous gestational nausea and vomiting if multiparous [90,91].

HYPEREMESIS GRAVIDARUM

Vomiting is a common indication for hospitalization during pregnancy [1]. Hyperemesis gravidarum occurs in around 0.5–1.5% of pregnancies and occurs regardless of race, marital status, age and gravidity [95]. Hyperemesis is associated with multiple pregnancy in most, but not all [96], studies, and occurs in up to 26% of patients with hydatidiform mole [89,97]. Other risk factors are similar to those for vomiting (see above).

Elevated levels of aspartate aminotransferases (AST, SGOT) have been reported in 15–25% of patients with hyperemesis gravidarum independently of ketonuria but return to normal with cessation of vomiting and rehydration [98]. Elevated levels of serum amylase originate from the salivary glands; elevated pancreatic amylase indicates vomiting complicating pancreatitis. Isolated studies have linked the presence of *Helicobacter pylori* with some cases of intractable hyperemesis gravidarum [99,100], but the prevalence of this organism in pregnant women remains unknown. These contradictions can be resolved only by large prospective studies that clearly define and separate hyperemesis gravidarum from uncomplicated gestational vomiting and from nausea alone.

FETAL OUTCOME

Statistical meta-analyses confirm a small reduction in risk of spontaneous abortion before 20 weeks with gestational vomiting. Birthweight is within the normal range following uncomplicated emesis. The incidences of miscarriage, stillbirth and preterm delivery are significantly less, including following hyperemesis gravidarum [101], compared with non-vomiting pregnancies [87,102]. Intrauterine growth restriction and small-for-dates babies can occur with severe hyperemesis gravidarum in association with maternal weight loss [96] and multiple hospital admissions [103]. In a retrospective study of 64 women, intrauterine growth restriction occurred in 32% of babies where mothers lost more than 5% of bodyweight through emesis compared with 6% born if vomiting mothers maintained their weight [96].

Vomiting *per se* is not considered to be teratogenic. No significant association has been found between gestational nausea and vomiting, perinatal mortality and fetal anomalies [101]. The Collaborative Perinatal Project group at the NIH conducted a prospective study on the epidemiology of vomiting in pregnancy in the 1960s that involved 16398 women registered before the 20th week and, subsequently the mothers of 2433 babies with abnormalities and minor anomalies [104]. No single category of congenital defects was found to be significantly different between vomiting pregnancies on no therapy and non-vomiting pregnancies [104]. In addition, there were no statistically significant differences for congenital defects or preterm delivery between cases of 'morning sickness' and those with hyperemesis gravidarum or non-vomiting pregnancies [103–105] except for macrosomia in severe hyperemesis reported in one study [96].

MECHANISMS OF NAUSEA AND VOMITING

These remain unclear. Pregnant women with nausea and vomiting have gastric slow-wave dysrhythmias (tachygastria and bradygastria), instability of fasting electrical activities and altered electrical responses to ingestion of food [106,107]. Such altered gastric electrical rhythms documented in early pregnancy using manometric and neuroelectrical techniques [106] reverse on recovery 2

months after voluntary termination [107] but their relation to gestational nausea and vomiting remains unproven. Higher levels of human chorionic gonadotropin (β-hCG) and a specific β_1-glycoprotein (schwangerschaftsprotein; SP1) have been found in vomiting, compared to non-vomiting, pregnancies and in hyperemesis gravidarum in some [108,109], although not all [89,101], studies. In turn, elevated levels of β-hCG correlate with elevations in serum levels of free thyroxine, C3 and C4 and IgG and IgM and lymphocyte counts [110].

A central role for oestrogens is favoured but unproven. Neuroregulatory hormones such as the β-lipotrophins (endorphins) are detectable in placenta and amniotic fluid. Their binding to opioid receptors in the vomiting centre in the hypothalamus that have been sensitized to β-hCG may promote nausea and vomiting [111]. Other neurotransmitters implicated in vomiting are dopamine, 5-HT, acetylcholine and histamine but their roles in gestational emesis remain unclear.

The roles of progesterone, cortisol and thyroxine in gestational vomiting also are controversial. Serum levels of progesterone and cortisol were reduced in vomiting, compared with non-vomiting, pregnancies in one study in the 14th week [112]. These differences were maintained through pregnancy even after resolution, but were not confirmed by others [109]. High levels of progesterone can inhibit the effects of gut hormones such as motilin [113] but such interactions require further investigation.

Hyperemesis gravidarum may represent the extreme end of the spectrum of gestational vomiting although the pathogenic mechanisms and relation to uncomplicated gestational emesis remain obscure. Whether there is an additional genetic predisposition for hyperemesis requires further study.

Lessening of symptoms with nasogastric feeding is a unique feature of hyperemesis gravidarum and contrasts with other causes of nausea and vomiting. This observation favours one hypothesis that hyperemesis gravidarum represents a severe, albeit masked, form of hunger [114]. Accordingly, symptoms are worse after fasting particularly overnight, and improve with short intervals between meals.

Mean levels of total oestradiol were elevated above those seen in uncomplicated gestational vomiting in one study [101]. In hyperemesis, the elevated levels of serum cholesterol, triglycerides and phospholipids and alterations in low-density lipoproteins (LDL) and high-density lipoproteins (HDL) may reflect the effects of excess oestrogen on the liver.

The relation of hyperemesis to elevated levels of free thyroxine is discussed in Chapter 12.

MANAGEMENT

Overall, pregnant women with protracted vomiting can be assured that there is no major risk of adverse fetal outcome [95,105].

Gestational vomiting

Morning sickness does not influence health. Symptoms generally improve with reassurance, small and dry, carbohydrate-rich meals and avoidance of large-volume drinks in the early morning [115]. Paradoxically, meals of high protein content can reduce nausea and slow-wave dysrhythmias in the stomach [116] despite a reduction in LOSP (see above). Alternative therapies such as acupuncture, ginger and vitamin B_6 may afford relief in some cases and seem safe [117]. Therapy with anti-emetics rarely is necessary (see below).

Persistent vomiting requires full investigation including screening for *Helicobacter pylori* (see below) and possibly upper endoscopy. Many disorders can masquerade as vomiting during pregnancy including pyelonephritis and other infections such as viral hepatitis, intestinal obstruction, appendicitis, raised intracranial pressure, thyrotoxicosis [118] and Addison's disease [115], porphyria, and ruptured tubal pregnancy and abdominal pregnancy [119]. Trophoblastic tumours, hydatidiform mole and chorioncarcinoma are often associated with clinical thyrotoxicosis because they secrete large amounts of hCG [118]. In the third trimester, vomiting may herald acute liver failure due to fatty liver, HELLP (haemolysis, elevated liver enzymes, low platelets syndrome) and other causes including cholecystitis, pancreatitis and, rarely, gastric cancer which may occur at any time in pregnancy [120].

Hyperemesis gravidarum

Management involves removal from a potentially stressful home environment, withdrawal of oral nutrition and fluids, rehydration with intravenous fluids, replacement of electrolytes and vitamins and antihistamine anti-emetics or metoclopramide [121,122]. Corticosteroids have been used in limited studies with some reported success [123,124].

Hyperemesis with protracted vomiting has been associated with various complications including the Mallory–Weiss oesophageal tear, Mendelson's syndrome [58,89], pneumomediastinum and jaundice. Neurological complications include psychosis that can be mistaken for a non-organic psychiatric disorder [125]. Three direct maternal deaths reported in the triennial review of maternal death

in the UK between 1991 and 1993 were due to the consequences of hyperemesis gravidarum (Wernicke's encephalopathy and/or aspiration) that went unrecognized [125]. Central pontine myelinolysis [126,127] and Wernicke's encephalopathy (over 20 cases reported since 1969) can occur in association with Korsakov's psychosis, rapid visual loss [128], central scotoma, retinal haemorrhage and rhabdomyolysis. The neurological disturbances may result from deficiency of vitamin B_1 as assessed by low levels of red cell transketolase and elevated levels of thiamine pyrophosphate. High carbohydrate loads, as with parenteral nutrition (see parenteral nutrition, below), without supplements of vitamins B and C may precipitate Wernicke's encephalopathy. MRI of the brain in Wernicke's encephalopathy may show characteristic changes in the thalamus and periaqueductal grey matter [8,9] and in the pons in central pontine myelinolysis.

The patient should be managed in a centre with special facilities. Symptoms should respond to the urgent replacement of thiamine (vitamin B_1 complex) and expert, judicious attention to restoration of fluids, electrolytes, specifically hyponatraemia and hypokalaemia, plasma osmolality and acid–base balance caused by the metabolic alkalosis and dehydration. The biochemical abnormalities reverse rapidly with restoration of fluid balance, improved nutrition and cessation of vomiting. An elevated prothrombin ratio indicates marked cholestasis and vitamin K deficiency. Thiamine should be given in high dose and intravenously (along with other vitamins and nutritional supplements) although the Committee on Safety of Medicines has advised caution when using the parenteral route due to the risk of allergic reactions.

Antiemetic drug therapy

Antiemetic therapy continues to be widely used and prescribed in pregnancy [129]. None is approved specifically for use in early pregnancy. The majority of cases of 'morning sickness' can be managed without recourse to drug therapy. Prescription should be reserved for exceptional cases and only after exclusion of intercurrent disease. Pyridoxine hydrochloride (vitamin B_6) is safe and has reduced gestational nausea and vomiting in randomized controlled trials although no relation was found between levels of pyridoxal 5′ phosphate and symptoms in 180 pregnant women with morning sickness in the first trimester [130]. Ginger significantly relieved symptoms in hyperemesis gravidarum compared with placebo in one study [131]. Drugs that block dopamine receptors such as metoclopramide, domperidone and phenothiazines seem safe but should be used with caution. Extrapyramidal side-effects can occur.

Drug safety

Concern over the teratogenic potential and consequent safety of many antiemetics in humans following the thalidomide tragedy has led to the reappraisal of the use of antiemetic drugs for human pregnancy and the unreliability of some animal studies [132,133]. This concern remains despite encouraging data from large retrospective [64], and prospective [104,134], studies, suggesting that a variety of antiemetics commonly used in early pregnancy, including meclozine, cyclizine and dimenhydrinate, probably do not cause a significant increase in congenital malformations [104]. In fact, these findings support earlier studies suggesting an inverse relation between nausea and vomiting (antiemetic therapy) and fetal abnormalities [64]. A smaller number of mothers of infants born with major abnormalities required antiemetics in the first trimester (7.4%) compared with mothers of normal infants (13.1%) [64].

The withdrawal of Bendectin/Debendox (doxylamine succinate and pyridoxine hydrochloride) from the market in June 1983 for suspected [135,136], but unproved, teratogenicity is an example of public pressure forcing a manufacturer (Merrell Dow: USA) to discontinue a product despite several carefully controlled studies that failed to support an association with congenital abnormalities [64,137–139].

There are isolated reports of cleft palate in babies born to mothers taking meclozine [140] and cyclizine [141]. Diphenhydramine has been linked to cleft palate [142] and trimethobenzamide, to other fetal anomalies [143]. Some phenothiazines are embryotoxic in animals. In addition, jaundice and extrapyramidal effects have occurred in neonates of mothers receiving chlorpromazine during pregnancy [144]. Promethazine is probably safe in early pregnancy despite anecdotal reports of congenital hip dislocation [134,145]. Dimenhydrinate has been associated with anecdotal reports of preterm labour [144].

Metoclopramide blocks central and peripheral dopamine D_2 receptors and, at high dose, 5-HT_3 receptors implicated in vomiting. Metoclopramide is a base that readily crosses the placenta and is excreted in breast milk [146]. Metoclopramide generally is considered safe, despite lack of data from controlled trials. Metoclopramide is being used increasingly in idiopathic vomiting of late pregnancy, labour [82,147] and during anaesthesia [83,148,149]. In the puerperium, metoclopramide causes hyperprolactinaemia and promotes lactation [146]. Other hormonal effects of unknown clinical significance include a reduction in levels of growth hormone, follicle-stimulating hormone and luteinizing hormone [148]. Droperidol, a major tranquillizer of the butyrophenone class, is being used increasingly to prevent vomiting in relation to spinal anaesthesia and caesarean section [150] as well as with diphenhydramine in hyperemesis gravidarum [151]. Any superiority over metoclopramide when used as a postoperative antiemetic is debatable [149] and information on its safety in early pregnancy is lacking. Prochlorperazine enjoyed popularity as a general antiemetic in pregnancy until the 1960s, particularly for hyperemesis gravidarum, but it has been superseded by metoclopramide, which causes fewer systemic side-effects. Possible links with cardiovascular and other abnormalities have limited its use [144]. Ondansetron and granisetron are potent and highly selective 5-HT_3 receptor antagonists. Ondansetron occasionally has been used when all other treatments of hyperemesis have failed but the safety and efficacy of these 5-HT_3 antagonists have not been evaluated sufficiently in large-scale trials in human pregnancy. Treatment with steroids (see above) and, if necessary, ondansetron should be considered before using parenteral nutrition.

Parenteral nutrition

This is recommended for severe cases of vomiting especially for suspected maternal protein–calorie malnutrition and when all other therapy has failed [152,153]. In a normal pregnancy, intake of adequate nutrition results in maternal changes directed at giving a healthy fetus and placenta [154]. A paradox arises in protein–calorie malnutrition and semistarvation whereby, on refeeding, there is preferential uptake by maternal, rather than fetal, tissues to replete maternal body stores [154]. Most studies have been limited to animal models although there is some evidence indicating this holds true for humans [154]. Guidelines for adequate replacement of nutrients in pregnancy are lacking. Apart from in hyperemesis gravidarum, successful outcomes using total parenteral nutrition (TPN) in pregnancy have been reported for severe IBD, massive gut resection, small bowel fistula, radiation enteritis, prolonged postoperative ileus and severe pancreatitis [155].

TPN is safe in expert hands with special care taken over insertion of the indwelling catheter, regular monitoring of maternal levels of nutrients, and provision for delivery of preterm, small-for-dates infants [153]. Lipid-containing solutions (emulsions) have been shown to damage the placenta in experimental animals [156] but seem safe from the limited data with human pregnancy [155]. Lipid emboli were not found in the placenta in single cases given solutions containing up to 50% lipid emulsions [155,157]. Concern remains over effects on the fetus of continual use of glucose-containing solutions from early in pregnancy. Whether this creates a state of continuous hypertonicity, akin to the situation in a poorly controlled diabetic pregnancy, is not known.

Nasogastric [114] and nasojejunal [158] feeding can maintain maternal and fetal bodyweights in some cases, although some weight loss should be anticipated. Individual reports attest to the safety of using percutaneous endoscopic gastrojejunostomy (PEG) as a safe and cost-effective alternative to TPN [159,160] especially if concern remains over the adverse effects of intravenous lipids on placental growth and risk of preterm birth.

Maternal monitoring (see coeliac disease, below)

Monitoring of serial blood levels of glucose, electrolytes, trace elements and minerals, vitamins and amino acids is essential throughout pregnancy (and lactation when TPN is used for indications other than hyperemesis) [161]. The optimal daily nutritional requirements such as for calories, nitrogen and trace elements and vitamins in a pregnant woman receiving TPN are not known.

More information on maternal: fetal ratios of nutrients is urgently needed. Deficiencies of fat-soluble vitamins, pyridoxine (vitamin B_6) and other group B vitamins, calcium, iron and free fatty acids among many other essential nutrients are common despite supplementation. Wernicke–Korsakoff syndrome due to thiamine deficiency developed in one patient with a twin pregnancy receiving TPN with B vitamins for a previous jejuno-ileal bypass [161] (see jejuno-ileal bypass, below).

Fetal outcome

The expected weight can be maintained provided TPN is commenced early and is adequate for fetal and maternal needs. Frequent serial monitoring of fetal growth using ultrasonography is essential. Preterm labour is a recognized complication of maternal nutritional deprivation and may occur despite fetal growth [157,162]. Neural tube defects have been related to deficiency of folic acid [163] around the time of conception and supplements should be given prior to, and through, pregnancy and lactation [164] (see coeliac disease, below).

Gastrointestinal disorders

Gastric acid secretion

Studies on gastric physiology during pregnancy are limited. The consensus from early papers is that basal and maximal acid outputs are not altered significantly [43,58]. Variation between, and within, individuals is wide, yielding conflicting results [2]. Any reduction in

outputs is limited to the second trimester [2,165]. Serum pepsinogen, an indirect marker of acid output, does not change significantly through pregnancy or the puerperium [166]. Serum levels of gastrin rise significantly only as term approaches and peak soon after birth [167]. The hypothesis that histaminase from the placenta might inactivate or block the effects of histamine at the level of the parietal cell, remains unproven [168].

Any reduction in acid output during pregnancy is insufficient to explain the reported reduction in peptic ulcer symptoms [166,169]. However, the rise in level of serum gastrin that peaks postpartum corresponds with the resurgence of ulcer symptoms. Oestrogens may play a role in cytoprotection independently of effects on acid output, because clinical trials have shown improved healing in men taking stilboestrol [170]. Effects on prostaglandins or similar pathways have not been studied in pregnancy.

Peptic ulceration

PREVALENCE

Peptic ulceration arising *de novo* in pregnancy is remarkably uncommon [81]. In nearly 23 000 deliveries, only six women had documented active ulceration [171] but this study predated endoscopic evaluation. In a study of 118 women with peptic ulceration documented prior to pregnancy, 89% improved clinically or became symptom free [172]. The reduction in symptoms of peptic ulceration seen during pregnancy also has been attributed to a healthier diet, increased intake of foods such as milk, emotional tranquillity and medical supervision [173].

Despite these encouraging reports from the early literature, peptic ulceration is probably under-recognized. Symptoms do not correlate with disease severity. There remains a reluctance to use diagnostic fibre-optic endoscopic techniques despite their safety in expert hands (see safety of endoscopic procedures, above). Furthermore, there are other reports of increased severity of peptic ulcer symptoms and complications during pregnancy [174,175], especially in association with pre-eclampsia [174,176]. In addition, quiescent ulcers may erupt [173], especially in the puerperium [172,177]. Presentation may be acute with massive haemorrhage [177] and perforation [178].

Zollinger–Ellison syndrome

Zollinger–Ellison syndrome is a rare condition associated with hypersecretion of gastric acid caused by excess secretion of gastrin by a gastrinoma. Although rare, this syndrome represents the most common of the symptomatic malignant pancreatic endocrine tumours. The challenge in obstetric practice is to diagnose the condition because presentation may be only with intractable gastro-oesophageal reflux and/or peptic ulceration. Further, there is the need to control the large volume of gastric acid with antisecretory drug therapies at high doses that have not been validated for safety in pregnancy. Also, some cases are associated with multiple endocrine neoplasia (MEN-I), especially tumours of the parathyroid glands, causing hypercalcaemia. Therapy is essential during pregnancy to prevent, or at least control, severe peptic ulceration, severe gastro-oesophageal reflux and malabsorption. Antacids typically fail to control symptoms. Treatment with ranitidine in high dose seems preferable to cimetidine or omeprazole, although these may have to be used in individual cases.

Helicobacter pylori

Infection with *H. pylori* is common among the general population and, overall, does not show gender bias. While almost 100% of infected cases have gastritis, only around 15% have peptic ulceration. Importantly, evidence of recent infection (IgM antibody isotype) is twice as common during pregnancy (26.6% vs. 11%) as in healthy non-pregnant controls [179]. Acquisition of *H. pylori* in early infancy has been linked to vertical transmission following decline of maternal immunity [180]. Whether *H. pylori* plays a pathogenic role (see hyperemesis gravidarum, above) in mother or infant, remains unclear.

Diagnosis of peptic ulcer relies on a high index of suspicion. Prodromal symptoms of pain exacerbated after meals may be absent or confused with simple dyspepsia. Physical examination may be normal or reveal minimal abdominal tenderness despite severe peptic ulceration, perforation and peritonitis. Upper oesophago-gastroduodenoscopy (endoscopy) is safe in pregnancy and, in experienced hands, can be carried out in many instances with only topical anaesthesia to the nasopharynx. Unfortunately, experience in pregnancy is limited (see safety of endoscopic procedures, above).

Haemorrhage and perforation of peptic ulcer are uncommon in late pregnancy and the puerperium but under-recognized in fatal cases [177,178]. The associated high maternal and fetal losses emphasize the need for a high index of suspicion in any mother with abdominal pain especially in the third trimester or puerperium.

MANAGEMENT

General principles are unaffected by pregnancy [176]. There are no clinical trials relating to treatment regimes

to eradicate *H. pylori* during pregnancy. Eradication of *H. pylori* has been reported to resolve hyperemesis gravidarum in individual patients (see hyperemesis gravidarum, above).

Conservative measures such as prohibition of smoking, rest and regular antacids should be used until after delivery [181]. Indications for surgery and outcome, including mortality, are similar to those out with pregnancy [176]. Following perforation, prompt resuscitation of the mother may be followed by surgery and, if appropriate, delivery by caesarean section [176].

Antiulcer therapy

Antacids (see management of gastro-oesophageal reflux, above) remain the treatment of choice for peptic ulceration in pregnancy despite some obvious disadvantages to the mother. There is sufficient evidence from studies in the non-pregnant population that adequate dosage can achieve the same rates of healing of duodenal ulcers as does cimetidine [181]. Relapse rates for duodenal ulcer also are not significantly faster or greater in patients receiving cimetidine therapy compared with antacids [181]. Diarrhoea (from magnesium-containing preparations) and constipation (from aluminium) can occur especially with the large, frequent amounts required. There is also the theoretical risk of phosphate depletion with aluminium-containing antacids. The H_2-receptor antagonists, cimetidine and ranitidine [182,183], and proton pump inhibitors have been used extensively in the management of peptic ulceration in the non-pregnant patient. They have not been approved for use in pregnancy or during lactation through lack of sufficient data on their safety [45,63,66,70] (see gastro-oesophageal reflux; management and acid suppressant agents, above). Sucralfate, carbenoxolone and tri-potassium di-citrato bismuthate (De-Nol) [184,185] each have healing efficacies equal to cimetidine in controlled clinical trials in the non-pregnant patient. De-Nol is efficacious in eradicating *H. pylori* [186], especially in combination with tetracycline and metronidazole but De-Nol and tetracycline are contraindicated in pregnancy. Sucralfate (category B), a basic aluminium salt of sucrose octa sulphate, is minimally absorbed and probably safe for use in pregnancy and during lactation. It acts by adsorption onto the exudative surface of ulcers and may act as a barrier against acid, pepsin and bile salts.

Side-effects of carbenoxolone such as fluid retention and electrolyte imbalance preclude its use in pregnancy. Misoprostol, a synthetic analogue of prostaglandin E_1, is contraindicated in pregnancy because it causes uterine contractions [187].

Gastric bypass for morbid obesity

Infertility remains common among women with morbid obesity. Data on outcomes are limited [188,189] (see jejuno-ileal bypass, below). Good maternal and fetal outcomes were documented via a patient-based questionnaire in 41 women who became pregnant subsequent to gastric bypass surgery for morbid obesity [189]. Individual complications include Wernicke's encephalopathy [190], Landry–Guillain–Barré syndrome, and other neurological sequelae.

Gastric cancer

Over 100 individual case reports document gastric cancer presenting during pregnancy [120,191–193]. Delays in diagnosis and high-grade malignancy contribute to the poor prognosis with only about 20% survival at 3 years.

Coeliac disease

Gluten-sensitive enteropathy is an abnormality of the small intestinal mucosa caused by the ingestion of gluten-containing substances in susceptible individuals. In most cases, histology from a jejunal and duodenal biopsy shows subtotal villous atrophy. Withdrawal of gluten from the diet results in marked clinical and histological improvement. The histopathological appearances, which may remain abnormal for months, are often incomplete in affected adults despite adherence to approved diets.

The onset of coeliac disease may be prevented, or delayed for months, by extended breastfeeding in infants with a strong family history, independent of their concurrent ingestion of gluten [194].

EPIDEMIOLOGY

The prevalence of coeliac disease in the West has been estimated at 0.03% [195]. The incidence varies considerably from one in 6500 of the general population in Sweden [196] to one in 890 in Switzerland and to between one in 2000 and one in 8000 in the UK [197]. The highest recorded incidence is one in 300 for western Ireland [198]. The true incidence may be higher because reports tend to reflect early studies with the classical, more florid presentations (see below). Coeliac disease probably occurs worldwide but histological documentation in developing countries is limited. The preponderance of females [199] in some reports has been matched by an equal sex ratio in others [200].

Up to 80% of patients are positive for the histocompatibility antigen human leucocyte antigen (HLA) B8 [201]

and there is a familial link [202]. Symptomless relatives may have biochemical abnormalities suggesting malabsorption such as a low serum folate, low xylose excretion and elevated faecal fats, making coeliac disease a likely diagnosis [203].

CLINICAL FEATURES

Coeliac disease can present at any age [197]. The classical features are diarrhoea, malabsorption, anorexia and weight loss. Importantly, many patients, especially adults [202,204], present with only mild and non-specific gastrointestinal symptoms. Presentation to departments other than gastroenterology is frequent, especially during pregnancy for haematological disorders such as megaloblastic and iron-deficiency anaemias [203]. Diarrhoea and steatorrhoea may be absent. Other presentations include bone pain from osteoporosis and osteomalacia and, rarely, tetany [205] secondary to malabsorption of calcium and vitamin D [206]. Neurological manifestations range from generalized muscle weakness to peripheral neuropathies, encephalopathy, syndromes associated with deficiencies of vitamins B_6 and B_{12} and psychoses. Changes in the skin and mucous membranes are common. Coeliac disease may present with glossitis, cheilosis, stomatitis, apthous ulceration, skin pigmentation, dermatitis herpetiformis and oedema [200,205].

EFFECTS ON FERTILITY

Female

Coeliac disease was detected in 4.1% of women referred for unexplained infertility in Finland [207]. Untreated disease is associated with delayed menarche of around 1 year, oligomenorrhoea, amenorrhoea and involuntary infertility [208,209]. Pathogenic mechanisms remain unclear. Infertility also has been reported in patients with pernicious anaemia [210]. Outcome improves with restoration of normal gut histology following withdrawal of gluten and correction of nutritional deficiencies.

Male

Infertility has been reported with untreated disease; impotence in 18 per cent, with sperm motility impaired in 75% [211]. Abnormal sperm forms, recorded in 46%, improved after gluten withdrawal [211]. In the untreated male, dysfunction of the hypothalamic–pituitary axis has been implicated in causing the elevations in plasma levels of testosterone and luteinizing hormone [211] and serum prolactin [212] found in some cases. Infertility was reversed on treatment in one study [213].

EFFECTS IN PREGNANCY

Maternal outcome

In known coeliacs, exacerbation of symptoms can occur during pregnancy and the puerperium [214]. Further, in a case–controlled study from Argentina of 130 coeliac women and age-matched female controls, first presentation during pregnancy or the puerperium was recorded in 11 patients; nine of these had underestimated features suggestive of coeliac disease [215]. Data relating to histological relapse, intercurrent infection and dietary factors are lacking. However, clinical deterioration during pregnancy [215] and the puerperium [204,216] is not infrequent among untreated cases.

Recall of gastrointestinal symptoms in childhood is common for women who present in pregnancy. Symptoms can remit around puberty despite persistently abnormal histology [217] and recur during pregnancy [200], surgery [218], stress and intercurrent infection [219].

A case–controlled study from the UK [209] paired 68 women with untreated disease and controls matched for age. Significantly larger numbers of pregnancies with untreated disease when compared with controls ended in spontaneous miscarriage (15 vs. 6%) and stillbirth (5.8 vs. 0.6%). Importantly, fetal outcomes improved toward control values with diagnosis and treatment [209].

Fetal outcome

In the Italian [208], and British [209], studies spontaneous abortions were two to three times more common in untreated coeliacs compared with controls. This finding agrees with early reports [220,214]. In the Italian study, recurrent spontaneous abortion among untreated coeliacs occurred independently of severity and duration of clinical disease or of biochemical abnormalities [208].

Spontaneous abortion has been linked with megaloblastic anaemia [200] secondary to folic acid deficiency [221] and iron-deficiency anaemia [207,209]. Deficiencies of folic acid and vitamin B_{12} are common in untreated coeliacs [214].

In Sweden between 1952 and 1961, five of 39 women with coeliac disease had megaloblastic anaemia documented in a previous pregnancy [218]. In a later study of 32 women with megaloblastic anaemia documented during pregnancy more than 10 years previously, 41% had low levels of serum folate compared with 10% of healthy matched controls [203,218]. Also, 27% of patients had elevated levels of faecal fat suggesting malabsorption.

Data are accumulating to show that strict adherence to a gluten-free diet can reduce poor fetal outcomes to levels comparable to controls including reduction in frequency of spontaneous abortion [214], stillbirths and low birth-weight [222,223]. Further, nursing mothers with treated coeliac disease breastfeed for 2.5 times as long as untreated mothers [222]. Overall, study samples have been too small to assess the impact of treated and untreated coeliac disease and related vitamin deficiencies on fetal outcomes, including congenital abnormalities. While deficiency of folic acid is common, there is no evidence for increased incidence of neural tube defect in babies born to mothers with coeliac disease [224].

DIAGNOSIS

This requires a high index of suspicion in clinical practice as signs and symptoms of malabsorption may be lacking. Women should be screened for suspected coeliac disease with presentations of unexplained iron-deficiency anaemia, diarrhoea and weight loss during pregnancy and the puerperium [215,216] and for associated concurrent conditions such as refractory IBD and collagenous colitis. Investigation of suspected iron and vitamin deficiencies (see management, below) should be carried out before indiscriminate prescription of supplements. Pregnant women with suspected coeliac disease require a full investigation. Duodenal biopsy via fibre-optic gastroduodenoscopy is safe in expert hands. Jejunal biopsy with a capsule and radiological imaging is not recommended in pregnancy (see safety of endoscopic procedures, above). In the West, less common causes of total villous atrophy of a jejunal biopsy include Crohn's disease, tropical sprue and intolerance to cows' milk protein [225] and soy protein [226]. The main differential diagnoses from other small bowel disorders are Crohn's disease and infestations and infections such as those with *Campylobacter* spp. and *Giardia* spp., and acquired immune deficiency syndrome (AIDS).

MANAGEMENT

A known coeliac should be encouraged to adhere strictly to a gluten-free diet if pregnancy is planned [214,227]. Careful attention should be paid to deficiencies of vitamin B_{12} [32], folic acid [228], iron and trace metals such as zinc [30] with supplementation through pregnancy and lactation.

Failure to respond to a gluten-free diet and clinical relapse should be investigated as in the non-pregnant with attention to dietary indiscretion, inadvertent ingestion of gluten-containing drugs [229], intercurrent infection and infestations such as giardiasis, IBD and associated disorders including autoimmune diseases, collagenous colitis [230] and malignancy.

Follow-up of coeliac disease should be life long. In the majority of non-compliant adults [231] there is histological evidence of relapse. Symptoms do not correlate necessarily with histological severity [231]. Haematological and nutritional abnormalities are common even in those who deny symptoms [232]. All coeliacs, including those who adhere strictly to a gluten-free diet, remain at significant risk of gastrointestinal malignancies, particularly intestinal lymphoma (>50% of malignancies) and oesophageal carcinoma [233]. Dyspepsia and dysphagia occurring in coeliac disease should be taken seriously. Upper endoscopy should be carried out in view of the association between oesophageal malignancy and coeliac disease.

Collagenous colitis

Lindstrom first described this condition in 1976. Clinical presentation is with watery stools, including nocturnal diarrhoea, malaise and weight loss [230,234]. Characteristic histopathological features include a thickened layer of collagen beneath the epithelial layer of the colon adjacent to the basement membrane [234]. Onset can be abrupt and mistaken for an infectious gastroenteritis. Although the aetiology is unknown, collagenous colitis is much more common in women than men (F/M ratio >6:1) and can present during childbearing years. In a large retrospective survey from Sweden between 1989 and 1995 [230], 142 of the 163 patients diagnosed were women; 25% were under 45 years of age. All five women who became pregnant after diagnosis experienced remission of symptoms. Interestingly, 40% of cases had associated diseases especially autoimmune disorders, rheumatoid arthritis, coeliac disease and diabetes mellitus [230]. The finding of concomitant IBD in four patients was considered coincidental.

Treatment with sulphasalazine prompted adverse reactions in 40%. Although corticosteroid therapy improved symptoms, relapse was common on cessation of therapy. Recommendations for therapy in the non-pregnant patient include loperamide, cholestyramine and corticosteroids. As remission is common during pregnancy, treatment can be delayed until after delivery, although these drugs are considered safe in pregnancy. Patients taking cholestyramine should be supplemented with vitamin K_1 as cholestyramine binds vitamins as well as bile salts (see Chapter 9).

Infections and infestations

Infections and infestations of the gastrointestinal tract cause significant morbidity worldwide (Box 10.1). Few studies address the detection of gastrointestinal patho-

---

Box 10.1 Gastrointestinal infections and infestations

Bacterial	**Protozoa**
Escherichia coli	*Giardia lamblia*
Salmonella spp.	*Entamoeba histolytica*
Shigella spp.	*Isospora belli*
Staphylococcus sp.	
Campylobacter spp.	**Nematodes (round worms)**
Cholera	*Trichinella spiralis*
Listeria spp.	*Enterobius vermicularis*
Aeromonas hydrophilia	*Trichuris trichiura*
Plesiomonas shigelloides	*Ascaris lumbricoides*
Balantidium coli	*Strongyloides stercoralis*
Cryptosporidium spp.	*Ancylostoma duodenale*
Clostridium difficile	
Necator americanus	**Cestodes (tapeworms)**
	Taenia sp.
Viral infections	*Echinococcus* spp.
Rotaviruses	*Hymenolepis nana*
Norwalk-like viruses	

---

gens and the safety and efficacy of therapies during pregnancy. In developed countries in the West, intestinal pathogens are an uncommon cause of gastroenteritis [235]; a viral aetiology is suspected in most cases [236]. These data contrast with the common finding of pathogenic parasites in developing countries, including in symptomless women.

BACTERIAL INFECTIONS

Travellers' diarrhoea and food poisoning

Acute diarrhoea associated with abdominal cramps, bloating, nausea, fever and malaise is well known to travellers. Symptoms typically begin abruptly, occur during travel or shortly after return, usually are self-limiting and require no specific therapy [237], including in pregnancy [238]. Infection occurs through ingestion of food and water contaminated with organisms and their toxins. Enterotoxigenic *Escherichia coli* accounts for 40–70% of cases. Other organisms such as the genus *Shigella* may be isolated from the stools in 5–20% of cases. Occasional causes of travellers' diarrhoea include viruses such as rotaviruses, Norwalk-like viruses and parasites such as *Giardia lamblia*.

Management principles. Acute diarrhoea lasting less than 72 h often can be managed conservatively with attention to rehydration with clear fluids and without recourse to drugs. Common remedies such as kaolin, pectin and hydrated aluminium silicate act to reduce stool frequency by absorbing water. There is no evidence to show a reduction in water loss by the gut [239]. Controlled prospective trials in non-pregnant subjects using charcoal, preparations containing kaolin and pectin and diphenoxylate showed no influence on outcome or speed of resolution of symptoms (typically within 72 h) compared with controls receiving simple fluid replacement [240]. Occasionally, these preparations may exacerbate symptoms and delay the excretion and clearance of organisms such as *Shigella* spp. [239].

Diarrhoea lasting longer than 72 h should be investigated. Fresh stools should be sent directly for microscopic examination for ova, cysts and parasites and microbial culture (Box 10.1). Flexible fibre-optic endoscopy and sigmoidoscopy with biopsy are safe in pregnancy in careful expert hands (see safety of endoscopic procedures, above). These should be carried out to exclude coeliac disease, IBD and collagenous colitis among other intestinal disorders.

Antimicrobial therapy. Controlled studies have indicated that doxycycline, trimethoprim–sulfamethoxazole or trimethoprim alone when taken prophylactically are consistently effective in reducing the incidence of travellers' diarrhoea in certain areas by up to 90% [237]. None, however, is recommended for use in pregnancy. Trimethoprim is a folate antagonist [241] and may be teratogenic [242]. There is no information on the safety of doxycycline in pregnancy. The injudicious use of antibiotics has led to problems such as increasing microbial resistance that may limit their efficacy. Furthermore, the widespread use of antimicrobial agents has led to an increase in incidence of pseudomembranous colitis [243].

Clostridium difficile

The diagnosis of antibiotic-associated colitis, in association with *Clostridium difficile*, should be considered in any pregnant patient with diarrhoea complicating recent or previous antimicrobial therapy, even after a single dose [244,245], as well as in recently hospitalized patients. Severity is independent of dose, duration of treatment and route of administration. Nosocomial spread has been reported in which three women from the same ward treated with cefoxitin as prophylaxis prior to caesarean section developed diarrhoea [246].

Fresh specimens of stool should be sent for detection of the enterotoxin [243,246]. Therapy includes withdrawal of all antimicrobial agents and oral administration of vancomycin, as the treatment of choice [246,247]. Vancomycin is poorly absorbed but serum levels should be monitored to prevent damage to the fetal eighth cranial nerve [248]. Metronidazole can be used as an alternative agent and seems safe during pregnancy [249].

Campylobacter

This is a common, under-recognized cause of acute diarrhoea. In a general survey of acute diarrhoea in adults and children in west Scotland between 1986 and 1987, *Campylobacter* spp. were the second most common identified cause after *Salmonella* spp. [250]. *Campylobacter fetus* is divided into subspecies *C. jejuni* (*C. coli*) and the more severe *C. fetus* (*C. intestinalis*).

In a review of the literature between 1977 and 1986 there were 97 (19 *C. fetus*) documented cases associated with pregnancy [251]. The 78 cases of *C. jejuni* resulted in 13 babies with meningitis; eight also had documented septicaemia [251]. Stillbirth occurred in eight cases [251]. In a retrospective study of enteric infections in pregnancy in Canada between 1984 and 1988, *Campylobacter* spp. were the most commonly identified pathogenic organisms being detected in 10 out of 24 000 pregnancies [252]; most (eight cases) occurred in the third trimester. Nine proceeded to full-term normal delivery; one baby of a well mother developed *C. jejuni* enterocolitis 3 days later. The 10th pregnancy was complicated by preterm labour at 28 weeks, neonatal sepsis and death [252].

Infection with *C. fetus* is more serious. In a retrospective review of seven women, there were three cases of preterm labour and stillbirth and a further baby died of neonatal sepsis [253]. The mothers had a febrile illness with respiratory symptoms. Although one woman pursued a fulminating course, two others were symptomless [253]. *Campylobacter fetus* was isolated from cultures of blood, fetal spleen, brain and placenta. The placenta can show necrosis, infarction and abscess and the sources of infection may remain unidentified [253,254]. In neonatal meningitis and enteritis the source probably is faecal–oral from mothers with diarrhoea at delivery [255,256].

Diagnosis. Gastrointestinal infection in pregnancy with the genus *Campylobacter* can cause abdominal pain, fever and often bloody diarrhoea [253]. *Campylobacter* spp. can cause diarrhoea in HIV-seropositive subjects [36]. The typical presentation in a woman without HIV infection is with a respiratory tract infection and fever [252,257]. Neonatal infection, including septicaemia, has been reported despite seemingly well mothers [252,253]. These Gram-negative bacilli can be grown from cultures of blood, stool and placenta but may require prolonged incubation under microaerophilic conditions with selective media

[253,255,258–260]. Blood cultures are preferred to stool cultures that often yield false-negative results [251].

Analysis and culture of multiple samples of blood, fresh stool and cervical swabs are essential for suspected *Campylobacter* enteritis especially near delivery [253,256, 261]. Appropriate cultures, especially of blood, should be taken also from the fetus in cases of septic abortion [253,262], intrauterine death [263] and neonatal gastroenteritis [261]. Samples should be delivered directly to the laboratory without refrigeration. *Campylobacter* infection should be considered in the differential diagnosis of toxic megacolon [264]. *Campylobacter* can be identified and sequenced for epidemiological tracking using RNA extracted and amplified from archival tissue (formaldehyde-fixed, paraffin-embedded tissue blocks).

Management. The advice to avoid unpasteurized milk and to cook poultry thoroughly should be reinforced in pregnancy. Prompt instigation of antimicrobial therapy should be considered because cultures may require extended time for growth. Treatment of maternal gastroenteritis consists of 4 weeks of oral erythromycin base or stearate. Erythromycin estolate is contraindicated because of potential hepatotoxicity. Addition of gentamicin and chloramphenicol should be considered for suspected systemic infection [251,253]. Susceptibility to the β-lactam antibiotics such as ampicillins and cephalosporins varies [251]. Relapses are common with short courses. Erythromycin is used extensively in pregnancy, especially for genital mycoplasma infections. Erythromycin crosses the placenta but fetal blood levels remain low [265]. Abnormal levels of serum (AST SGOT) can occur.

Outbreaks from cross-infection are rare [266] but high standards of hygiene are important, especially the thorough washing of hands and disposal of faeces and contaminated fomites. In suspected maternal gastroenteritis, delivery is best carried out under conditions of nursing isolation [236].

Microbial surveillance, particularly blood cultures, is essential in seemingly healthy neonates born to mothers who excrete *Campylobacter* spp. at delivery [236]. Breastfeeding can be assumed with adherence to strict hygiene to prevent cross-infection. Erythromycin is first-line therapy for suspected neonatal infection. CT and MRI scanning of the brain and, possibly, lumbar puncture should be considered in neonates with suspected meningitis, intracerebral haemorrhage and infarction [251].

Listeriosis

This is considered in Chapter 16.

Typhoid and paratyphoid fever, shigellosis and their carriers

Historically, typhoid fever was implicated in up to 3% of cases of spontaneous abortion and preterm labour [236] but this is rare in the West. These infections are common in the HIV-seropositive subject [36]. The acute infections run a similar course to those in the non-pregnant; transplacental infection has been recorded [267–269]. Amoxicillin remains the first-line antibiotic in pregnancy [270], although resistance of *Salmonella* spp. and *Shigella* spp. is increasing, especially in developing countries [271]. Nosocomial outbreaks are uncommon but reported more frequently for *Salmonella* than for *Shigella* spp. [236,272]. Breastfeeding can continue if mothers comply with strict standards of hygiene.

Delivery of symptomless carriers of *Salmonella* spp. and *Shigella* spp. should be carried out under conditions of isolation. Antibiotic therapy should be instigated in the newborn for symptoms and positive stool cultures. The choice of antibiotic should be anticipated in advance and will depend on expert advice and local microbiological surveillance. Ciprofloxacin and other synthetic quinolones pass into breast milk. They have been shown to cause damage to joints and cartilage in growing animals and are not recommended in pregnancy or with breastfeeding.

Immunization with typhoid vaccine is contraindicated in pregnancy. There are insufficient data regarding the safety of the parenteral vaccines of *Salmonella typhi* containing either purified Vi polysaccharide antigen Ty2 or the conventional heat-killed, whole organism.

Intestinal tuberculosis

This infection is uncommon in pregnancy in the West but should be considered in women returning from the developing countries, especially the Indian subcontinent. Intestinal tuberculosis is considered further in Chapter 1.

Miscellaneous

The treatments of bacterial overgrowth, tropical sprue and Whipple's disease (*Tropheryma whippelii*) traditionally involve tetracyclines but these are contraindicated in pregnancy. There are no specific guidelines for their management in pregnancy. HIV-seropositive patients can present with clinical features indistinguishable from Whipple's disease [36] (see below).

INTESTINAL PARASITES AND INFESTATIONS

Intestinal parasites were found in 44–93% of pregnant women from South-East Asia and South America

[27,273–276]. Most (93%) antenatal patients were infected with more than one intestinal parasite in a prospective cohort study of 91 pregnant women in Ecuador [27]. Importantly, although many women deny symptoms, impaired fetal growth and stillbirth are common among babies born of infected women with severe iron-deficiency anaemia related to high parasite burdens due to *Entamoeba histolytica* [27] and hookworm [28].

Multiple infestations are common with poor sanitation and faecal contamination [277]. The prevalence increases with congenital and acquired immunodeficiency syndromes [36]. Common species are hookworm (*Ancylostoma duodenale, Necator americanus*), whipworm (*Trichuris trichiura*), dwarf tapeworm (*Hymenolepis nana*), roundworm (*Ascaris lumbricoides*), threadworm (*Enterobius vermicularis*), tapeworm (*Taenia saginata* and *Taenia solium*) and *Entamoeba histolytica* [27,276–278].

Maternal aspects

The main consequence of helminthic infections is iron-deficiency anaemia in the mother. Severe iron deficiency is associated with increased perinatal morbidity and mortality. Maternal malnutrition should be corrected and the diet supplemented with iron, folic acid and other vitamins.

Fetal outcome

Outcomes are favourable for the well-nourished mother and child. Multiple infestations may account for around 10% of intrauterine growth restriction and reduced birthweight in developing countries in association with malnutrition and heavy parasite burden [27,28,275,279,280].

Congenital and neonatal infections are uncommon. Faecal contamination at birth is responsible for most cases. Neonatal parasitic infection must be suspected for babies with malaise, anaemia and gastrointestinal symptoms.

Treatments

Most infestations can be managed conservatively. Purgation using laxatives such as senna and liquid paraffin should be avoided in pregnancy (see below).

Treatment for most intestinal protozoan parasites is rarely required during pregnancy except in the presence of malnutrition and multiple infestations [275]. In most cases, specific therapies can be delayed until after delivery [279,280].

Treatments, such as with albendazole, mebendazole, ivermectin and praziquantel, all have embryotoxic, muta-

genic and teratogenic potential. Accordingly, specific therapies should only be considered for intractable symptoms and, if possible, deferred until after delivery or until the third trimester [279,280]. Important exceptions that require treatment before delivery are symptomatic infections with *Entamoeba histolytica, Giardia lamblia*, ascariasis and malaria (see below).

Helminthic infestations

Reinfection with hookworm is high in crowded circumstances such as refugee camps. Therapy with mebendazole [280,281], pyrantel pamoate or a single dose (5 g) of bephenium is reserved for very heavy worm burdens and preferably only after delivery or in late pregnancy. Relapses are common in the puerperium. Eradication of sporadic cases of hookworm in an urban society is usually successful after delivery since there is no intermediate host to sustain the reservoir of infection. Anaemia from hookworm may require supplementation with iron. Piperazine for roundworm and threadworm should be reserved for large worm burdens in pregnancy and not used concurrently with pyrantel that antagonizes its action. Abdominal discomfort, dyspepsia and diarrhoea from taenia are usually tolerated in pregnancy. Quinacrine (for *Taenia solium*) and niclosamide (for *Taenia saginata*) should only be given after delivery. Whipworm and mixed helminth infestations can be treated with mebendazole or albendazole. Treatment with mebendazole was not associated with a major increase in congenital abnormalities in a study from Sri Lanka between 1996 and 1997 of 1737 pregnant women, including 407 exposed inadvertently to the drug during the first trimester. Concern remains over the safety of mebendazole and albendazole during pregnancy.

Maternal ascariasis should be treated with pyrantel pamoate prior to delivery. Treatment reduces the risk of the parasite migrating into the trachea that has been the cause of several obstetric deaths in the USA [274]. Therapy should be continued immediately after delivery even for mild symptoms to prevent neonatal acquisition of worms.

Breastfeeding is permitted with quinacrine and pyrantel pamoate but should be avoided when the mother is being treated with mebendazole, thiabendazole, albendazole or niclosamide [274,278].

Trematodes

Schistosomiasis affects over 200 million individuals worldwide with an especially high prevalence in Africa, Egypt and South America. *Shistosoma mansoni* and *S. japonicum* affect predominantly the gastrointestinal tract (acute phase) and liver (chronic phase), whereas *S. haematobium* affects the urogenital system. *Chlonorchis sinensis*, a common liver fluke in the East, was found in 20% of pregnant refugees from South-East Asia [274] and can present with cholecystitis, obstructive jaundice and biliary problems. Schistosomiasis should be considered in the differential diagnosis of bloody diarrhoea, hepatospleno-megaly and portal hypertension. Severe pre-eclampsia with possible infestation of the placenta (as well as the liver) has been reported with chronic, otherwise symptom-less, *S. japonicum* infection [282]. One report from Niger documented 26 cases of schistosomiasis of the female genital tract in association with sterility (six cases), tubal pregnancy (one case) and various gynaecological tumours [283]. Diagnosis of schistosomiasis is by microscopic exam-ination of stools and rectal biopsy material for eggs. Sig-moidoscopy should be carried out to exclude the possible association of carcinoma of the colon. The course of the disease with these parasites is not affected adversely by pregnancy. In sporadic cases in urban populations in the West, spread of infection is uncommon because there is no intermediate host.

Therapy often can be withheld until the puerperium. All drugs used in the treatment of schistosomiasis, such as oxamniquine, praziquantel, niridazole and hycanthone, are effective but very toxic. Facilities for caesarian section should be available since vaginal delivery may be impos-sible because of scarring of the cervix in chronic disease. Cholecystitis due to *Chlonorchis* should be treated with praziquantel but therapy delayed, if possible, until after delivery. Breastfeeding is contraindicated in mothers re-ceiving drug therapy.

Entamoeba histolytica

Amoebiasis is the third leading cause of death worldwide due to parasites [284]. Amoebic infection of the gastro-intestinal tract may cause dysenteric, or non-dysenteric, colitis, appendicitis, amoeboma and hepatic abscess [277]. *Entamoeba histolytica* is endemic in the tropics and sub-tropics but also occurs in the UK, Europe and North America, especially among immigrants from developing countries. Amoebiasis can mimic and coexist with other diarrhoeal illnesses such as bacillary dysentery, hook-worm, schistosomiasis, giardiasis [273] and colonic IBD. These should be considered in the differential diag-nosis by regular examination of fresh stools and careful flexible sigmoidoscopy in all patients with a dysenteric illness.

Immunohaemagglutination (IHA) assays aimed at detecting antibodies to *E. histolytica* are only positive (>1:32 titre) in about 50–60% of cases of suspected liver

abscess [277] (see hepatic abscess, Chapter 9). The enzyme-linked immunosorbent assay (ELISA) assay is more sensitive (86% with titres above 1:64) than IHA [288] but a positive result does not correlate with parasite burden or the presence of cysts in stool. The ELISA may be falsely negative in 20% of cases of liver abscess [277] and in infected neonates [285]. Molecular techniques can be applied to tissue samples to detect *E. histolytica* [286].

Amoebiasis in pregnancy is reported to follow a severe course [287,288]. The neonate may acquire the infection from faecal contamination at birth [274], although clinical sequelae are uncommon in breastfed babies because anti-bodies to amoeba are present in breast milk [289]. In the general population, metronidazole has been used to treat intestinal and hepatic amoebiasis. Most studies on metro-nidazole have shown it to be free from teratogenic effects. Metronidazole crosses the placenta and is excreted into breast milk [66]. Earlier reports of infants born with cra-niofacial abnormalities to mothers who were treated in the first trimester for amoebiasis [290] have not been con-firmed. A recent case–controlled study involved a total of over 1000 women who received metronidazole during the first trimester [249]. Overall, there was no statistical evi-dence for excess incidence of major congenital abnormal-ities [249]. Tinidazole may be more effective than metronidazole in the treatment of amoebiasis [291] but has not been evaluated extensively in pregnancy. Paromo-mycin is an alternative drug that has been used in preg-nancy and postpartum; breastfeeding is permitted [274]. Diloxanide has been used to increase elimination of para-sites from the bowel [292] but should be reserved for use postpartum; breastfeeding is permitted [274]. Sur-gical drainage and percutaneous drainage of abscesses and empyema should be reserved for severe cases not controlled by medical therapy [284].

Giardiasis

Giardia lamblia (*G. intestinalis*) is one of the most common causes of travellers' diarrhoea and malabsorption and is endemic in Europe, the UK and the USA. Infestation is especially common in developing countries [275,285] and among immigrants resident in the West. In two studies of intestinal infestations in South-East Asian [273] and Mex-ican [275] women during pregnancy, 44% had intestinal parasites. Giardia (17–25%) was second only to hook-worm (47%) [273] and tapeworm (35.2%) [275]. *Giardia* cysts are common in children of infected mothers (con-trast *E. histolytica*).

This infestation may occur *de novo* but susceptibility to infection is increased with achlorhydria, hypogammaglobulinaemia, coeliac disease, chronic pancreatitis and protein malnutrition. Clinical features include nausea, headache, abdominal discomfort and diarrhoea with steatorrhoea and malabsorption. Unlike amoebic and bacillary dysentery, bloody diarrhoea and fever are uncommon. *Giardia lamblia* infests a variety of mammals including cattle, horses, rabbits and domestic pets, including cats and dogs. Transmission between hosts is by the faeco-oral route. One common route is ingestion of water contaminated by introduction of animal excreta and untreated sewage into the drinking water supply, as in streams. *Giardia* also can spread directly from person to person. Faecooral spread is particularly common in day-care centres and nursing homes [293,294]. Diagnosis is confirmed by isolation of parasites and/or cysts from stool but duodenal aspirates may improve diagnostic yields. Jejunal biopsy is contraindicated during pregnancy (see safety of endoscopic procedures, above). Metronidazole or paromomycin remain the treatment of choice for symptomatic infections in pregnancy and the puerperium and breastfeeding is permitted. Quinacrine is a cheap alternative for developing countries [294] but should be reserved for postpartum therapy. Tinidazole and furazolidone may also be used [294], although their safety in pregnancy has not been established. Neonates are especially prone to giardiasis particularly via faecal contamination during delivery. Mothers suspected of having giardiasis should be screened and treated before delivery [274]. Normal human milk rapidly kills *Giardia lamblia*, independent of its concentration of secretory IgA. Giardiasis is rare in breastfed babies (see amoebiasis, above) [289]. Poor hygiene plays a major role in the spread of giardiasis. Improvements in personal hygiene, such as the washing thoroughly of hands can greatly reduce spread [294].

VIRAL INFECTIONS AND THE GASTROINTESTINAL TRACT

Acquired immune deficiency syndrome (see also Chapter 19, human immunodeficiency virus infection)

The impact of HIV infection in the gut relates to the propensity to develop persistent opportunistic infections [36] as well as to the side-effects of antiretroviral therapy [295]. Studies specific to pregnancy are lacking. The spectrum of infection in HIV-seropositive subjects does not differ significantly from that seen out with pregnancy. HIV infection must be considered in all cases of unexplained bowel dysfunction and in the differential diagnosis of IBD, coeliac disease and Whipple's disease.

Oral manifestations include ulcers from herpes simplex virus and *Candida albicans*. Dysphagia can arise from *Candida albicans*, cytomegalovirus and Kaposi's sarcoma. Small-bowel watery diarrhoea typically is associated with infection from various species of *Cryptosporidium*, *Salmonella*, *Strongyloides*, *Isospora*, *Listeria* and *Mycobacterium* (*avium–intracellulare* and *tuberculosis*) [36]. Infections of the large bowel typically occur with cytomegalovirus and species of *Shigella* and *Campylobacter*.

Most of the drug therapies [36] recommended are contraindicated in pregnancy (reviewed in [296]). Conversely, diarrhoea is a common side-effect of many antiretroviral drugs [295]. Oral aciclovir has been used safely in pregnant women with severe genital ulcers due to herpes simplex and helps prevent transmission to the neonate. Close consultation with the microbiologist and virologist is essential.

HIV infection predisposes to several malignancies affecting the gastrointestinal tract, including Kaposi's sarcoma, non-Hodgkin's lymphoma and rectal carcinoma [36].

Viral gastroenteritis (see also Chapter 17, enteroviruses)

Acute diarrhoea and vomiting attributed to a virus is a common diagnosis in pregnancy but successful identification of the offending pathogen is rare [236,272]. Rotavirus has been detected in stool and by serology (ELISA) in individual women with diarrhoea at delivery [272] but is more common in children, especially in the West. Occasional reports have implicated adenovirus, Norwalk-like virus and the astroviruses and coronaviruses. The concern with regard to pregnancy is the potential to cause outbreaks of infection, including gastroenteritis, among neonates in nurseries. Attention to hygiene, especially washing hands thoroughly between handling babies, is important in limiting spread. Attendants with suspected gastroenteritis should be excluded from obstetrical wards and nurseries.

Polio

Polio in pregnancy is considered in Chapter 17.

Inflammatory bowel disease

The incidence and prevalence of IBD, i.e. ulcerative colitis, Crohn's disease and non-specific colitis and proctitis, have risen in the last 40 years (reviewed in [297]). IBD is common in North America, the UK and Scandinavia with annual prevalence rates per 100 000 population reported as high as 40–100 for ulcerative colitis and 4–6 for Crohn's disease [298]. IBD is reported as uncommon in areas such as Morocco and Saudi Arabia [298] and among black people rather than white people [299]. IBD is more common among Jews than non-Jews [300,301]. Family members with a history of unexplained diarrhoea should be investigated for IBD. Clusterings within families and close contacts suggests an environmental factor [301,302].

EFFECTS OF DISEASE ON PREGNANCY

The prevalence and incidence of IBD during reproductive years has focused awareness on the impact of the diseases and therapies in pregnancy.

Female fertility

Early studies suggested a higher than normal rate of involuntary infertility. However, data were weakened by insufficient numbers [303] and omission of relevant factors such as fertility of the partner, voluntary infertility of the couple, nutritional status [304–307] and psychological problems with sexual dysfunction, particularly after resective surgery [308] and with chronic disease [309,310].

Ulcerative colitis. Several studies suggest that fertility is not affected adversely with quiescent disease and little altered for all but severely active disease [311]. Crohn *et al.* [312] and Korelitz [313] found no impairment in fertility for well-controlled disease. In later studies with variable disease activity [314], the number of involuntarily infertilities was comparable (around 10–15%) to that for the general population [311]. Voluntary infertility can be high (21–45%), especially in patients with previous surgery [311] (see surgical therapy, below).

Crohn's disease. Amenorrhoea and involuntary infertility correlate with disease activity. Normal fertility can be anticipated in well-controlled disease including after surgical resection [305,311,313]. Data from Oxford [315] and northeast Scotland [311] show similar rates of involuntary infertility (11–14%) to those for the general population [316]. As with ulcerative colitis, voluntary infertility was high, especially among those with previous surgery (23–36%) [311] (see surgical therapy, below).

The impact of anatomical extent of disease is not clearly defined and to do so would require large studies. Two groups found that conception was less frequent in women with Crohn's colitis (67%) compared to those with small bowel disease alone [304], ileitis or ileocolitis [305]. In contrast, in another study [306], only women with small

intestinal disease had lower than normal fertility rates. In a case–controlled study of infertility in Crohn's disease by the European Collaborative Group [317] subfertility (46% vs. 29% control group) and number of children (0.4 vs. 0.7 per family) were independent of disease site.

Drug therapy. No direct data are available for salazopyrine (sulphasalazine) and female fertility. By contrast salazopyrine is an important, reversible cause of male infertility [318]. This is due probably to the sulphapyridine component. Infertility can be reversed by stopping therapy or transferring to 5-aminosalicylic acid (5-ASA) alone [318–320]. There were no statistically significant differences between treated and untreated men for levels of luteinizing hormone, follicle-stimulating hormone, testosterone, prolactin and levels in semen of acid phosphatase, fructose and prostaglandins (PGE_2) [318].

There is no evidence that corticosteroids cause infertility. The safety of azathioprine, used occasionally for severe IBD [311], is discussed in Chapter 8.

Deficiencies of trace metals also may contribute to infertility. Low serum levels of zinc and chromium have been reported in Crohn's disease associated with hypogonadism [321].

Fetal outcomes

Spontaneous abortion. Several early reports before the 1980s stressed the detrimental effect of IBD (reviewed in [297]. More recent data from a large retrospective community survey of 409 women with IBD extending over 20 years in north-east Scotland [311], showed that the rates of spontaneous abortion with pre-existing ulcerative colitis (7–16%) and Crohn's disease (6–18%) were not significantly different from those in the normal population.

Despite the consensus view that IBD has no gross adverse effect on fetal outcomes, recent studies from the USA, Canada, France and Denmark concur in demonstrating an increased risk of excess preterm birth, low birthweight, small-for-gestational age and caesarean section [322–326]. Odds ratios above 1.5 were demonstrated for each of these outcomes in a population-based cohort study in Sweden between 1991 and 1992 of 756 women identified with IBD [322]. Similar findings of low birthweight and increased risk of preterm birth were reported in a Danish study conducted between 1982 and 1992, which studied fetal outcomes in 510 babies born to women with Crohn's disease [324]. Whether these adverse outcomes relate to therapy [323,325,327], active disease requiring therapy or disease activity alone, requires further study.

Activity of inflammatory bowel disease at conception. The consensus view remains that a normal delivery and good fetal outcome can be anticipated in more than 80% of cases for quiescent disease around conception. This optimistic outcome persists despite subsequent relapse during pregnancy and for first presentations during pregnancy and the puerperium [297,311].

Severely active disease, particularly at conception, seems detrimental to mother and fetus. Such women may avoid conception [311]. Nevertheless, in the Scottish study, the IBD became clinically quiescent in more than half the patients with active disease at conception [311].

Presentation in pregnancy and the puerperium. Poor outcomes are not invariable [297,311,328] reported on 11 pregnancies in 10 women with Crohn's disease presenting during pregnancy. There was a 55% fetal loss; four fetal deaths occurred in the six women requiring surgery during pregnancy. In contrast, Crohn *et al.* [312] reported only one fetal death among 19 pregnancies for ulcerative colitis presenting during pregnancy. In the Scottish study, one of three first presentations for Crohn's disease in pregnancy was particularly severe [311] and associated with spontaneous preterm labour at 30 weeks. The 10 presentations in pregnancy with ulcerative colitis were uneventful as were all eight presentations in the puerperium [311].

Previous surgery for inflammatory bowel disease

In the Scottish study [311], involuntary infertility was higher (20–30%) than normal following surgery, especially for ulcerative colitis. Voluntary infertility also was high (see above).

Fetal outcome is less good for previous surgery and currently severely active disease [311] and for severe IBD requiring surgical resection during pregnancy (see emergency surgery, below). The rates for spontaneous abortion and stillbirth (36%) were higher for women with previous surgery and active disease compared with 23% for those with inactive disease [311].

EFFECTS OF PREGNANCY ON DISEASE (Box 10.2)

The conflicting and controversial results can be explained in part by the changes in management and follow-up that span 70 years since 1931. Improved outcomes of more recent cases reflect in part the benefits of earlier diagnosis, stricter control of inflammatory activity with drug therapies and resective surgery. In 1931, Barnes and Hayes [329] reported two maternal, and two fetal, deaths among three women who developed ulcerative colitis

postpartum. This report led to the initial pessimistic conclusion that women with pre-existing ulcerative colitis should avoid pregnancy. During 1950–56 there were several reports of pregnant women with pre-existing ulcerative colitis who experienced an increase in the number of relapses during pregnancy and, particularly, postpartum [312,330,331]. Several maternal deaths were recorded for first presentations of ulcerative colitis in pregnancy and postpartum. A more recent study reviewed and confirmed the high relapse rate (between 30 and 40% per annum) regardless of pregnancy for ulcerative colitis and Crohn's disease [311]. Clinical relapse may occur at any time during pregnancy but tends to be particularly common in the first trimester [304,311,332,333]. These findings are consistent with a report of changes in bowel habit in IBD in relation to the menstrual cycle [334].

Although results remain conflicting, there is general agreement that patients with Crohn's disease seemingly limited to the terminal ileum fare better in pregnancy and postpartum than those with colonic Crohn's disease or ulcerative colitis. More precise data are needed on disease site, extent and inflammatory activity.

PERIANAL AND PERINEAL DISEASE

Caesarean section is preferred in severe perianal and perineal disease as episiotomy can exacerbate the IBD and cause fistula formation in Crohn's disease [297].

PYODERMA GANGRENOSUM

This has been reported at the surgical wound site following caesarean section for ulcerative colitis [335]. Relapse

---

Box 10.2 Effects of inflammatory bowel disease (IBD) on pregnancy and management plan

Effects
- Overall, no deleterious effect
- Fertility is normal in well-controlled IBD
- Full-term, normal delivery and fetal outcome if IBD:
  is quiescent at conception
  preceded pregnancy and quiescent
- No deleterious effect on subsequent pregnancies
- Increased fetal loss if IBD:
  is first manifest in pregnancy and severe
  is colonic rather than small bowel alone
  required previous surgery
  requires surgery for severe IBD

Plan
- Postpone pregnancy if disease active

of pyoderma gangrenosum during the puerperium also has been reported [336].

SUMMARY

Most women with pre-existing IBD can anticipate normal fertility and a full-term normal delivery, especially for quiescent, rather than active, IBD at conception. Follow-up has shown no additional risk to the fetus. The risk of congenital defects is not increased significantly.

Rates of involuntary infertility and spontaneous abortion with IBD are similar to those for the general population. Fertility is impaired and fetal outcome less good for patients with IBD who have undergone previous surgery and have active disease. Relapses are frequent during pregnancy, especially in the first trimester for ulcerative colitis and in the puerperium for Crohn's disease. The impact on the mother who first presents in pregnancy and the puerperium remains unclear.

Overall, there seems to be no increase in the rates of elective termination of pregnancy or caesarean section.

Recent studies suggest that pregnancy does not seem to have a specific adverse impact on the course of IBD. The more optimistic outcome for mother and fetus can be attributed to better medical management and early therapeutic intervention with salazopyrine and corticosteroids (see below).

MANAGEMENT

Women with known IBD should be encouraged to embark on a pregnancy when the disease is quiescent [297,311] and while they are taking minimum medication. Overall, medical management is the same as for the non-pregnant patient [297,337,338]. The reports of a higher incidence of fetal complications when a pregnant woman requires active treatment are likely to reflect severe disease activity rather than the direct effect of drugs.

Vaginal delivery is feasible for most women with IBD except in those with severe perineal disease. Episiotomy also is contraindicated with perineal disease because of concern about fistula formation; caesarean section is preferable in such cases.

As always, breastfeeding should be encouraged.

Depression is very common in IBD, particularly in Crohn's disease [339] and may be exacerbated during pregnancy through fears regarding safety of drug therapy, fetal outcome and the added stress of uncontrolled disease.

Acute severe disease

The pregnant patient with active IBD should be admitted to hospital. Fresh stools should be taken for culture for pathogenic microorganisms and detection and analysis of their toxins (see infections and infestations, above). Stools should be screened for parasites, especially *E. histolytica* and *S. stercoralis* prior to treatment, particularly with corticosteroids, because the latter may cause disseminated parasitosis. HIV infection can cause problems in the differential diagnosis (see AIDS and the gastrointestinal tract, above). In general, treatment consists of rest, nil by mouth, oral corticosteroids such as prednisolone, rectal corticosteroids, oral sulphasalazine (salazopyrine) or related products containing 5-ASA and intravenous fluids.

In a moderately severe attack of colonic IBD, initial treatment is with topical corticosteroid enemas, oral sulphasalazine and oral prednisolone. In colitis predominantly confined to the left side, therapy with 5-ASA [340,341] seems to be effective (see drug safety, below).

Drug therapies

The mainstay maintenance therapies in IBD are 5-ASA and related products (mesalazine) and sulphasalazine. Corticosteroids are reserved for inducing remission in active disease. Drugs reserved for active disease refractory to corticosteroids include azathioprine, 6-mercaptopurine [342] and cyclosporine and pose only a small risk to the developing fetus. While no major excess of congenital abnormalities has been reported, use of such drugs (as well as refractory inflammation) has been associated with intrauterine growth restriction, and preterm birth [297,338].

Most gastroenterologists prescribe 5-ASA and related products as mainstay therapy. The component 5-ASA is unstable but believed to be the major active principle in the treatment of IBD. Some trials of the coated preparation (mesalazine) have shown an increase in premature birth and reduction in birthweight [323,325,327].

Most of the safety data in pregnancy relate to sulphasalazine (salazopyrine). This drug has been studied extensively in randomized, controlled, double-blind clinical trials. Sulphasalazine, a prodrug, is split (azo-reduction) by colonic bacteria into the components sulphapyridine and 5-ASA. Clinical efficacy is related to the 5-ASA component whereas general toxicity reflects the sulphapyridine and acetylator status of the mother (drug clearance). In general, sulphasalazine is considered safe for use throughout pregnancy and the puerperium and also during breastfeeding. Sulphasalazine and its components cross the placenta. Sulphasalazine and sulphapyridine reach a concentration in cord blood and breast milk of approximately half that of maternal serum [343] but levels are not considered detrimental to the fetus [344].

The ability of sulphapyridine to displace bilirubin from albumin binding sites [345] has been overemphasized. Salazopyrine impairs absorption, transport and metabolism of dietary folic acid [341] necessitating additional supplementation (see coeliac disease, above).

Before 1980 there were no reports of pregnant women given steroids for IBD. Current information is reassuring regarding their safety in pregnancy and IBD [314,346] [307,333,347]. The overall safety of corticosteroids in pregnancy is discussed in Chapter 1. The indications for their use in acute, active IBD are the same as in the non-pregnant patient [314] but doses should be kept below 20 mg/day whenever possible, particularly in early pregnancy. Breastfeeding probably is safe even with nursing mothers who may take up to 30 mg/day prednisolone for asthma; at these dose levels adrenal suppression has not been significant in the fetus.

The safety of azathioprine in pregnancy is considered in Chapter 8.

Pregnancy should be avoided in women taking methotrexate, a recognized abortifactant, as this is associated also with birth defects.

Metronidazole [249] and ciprofloxacin do not seem to cause adverse fetal outcome in the short term. However, individual studies maintain concerns regarding the safety of metronidazole [249], especially as long-term courses of these and other antimicrobial drugs have not been evaluated adequately in pregnancy.

No safety data are available for use of other immunomodulatory therapies such as monoclonal antibodies and levamisole for IBD during pregnancy.

Limited data are available for the treatment of IBD in pregnancy with elemental diets. Other treatments for acute IBD found to be safe during pregnancy have included total parenteral nutrition (see above) for small bowel Crohn's disease and use of the penicillin family of antibiotics.

Chronic disease

Sulphasalazine and 5-ASA are superior to placebo for the maintenance of remission of chronic ulcerative colitis. Results for chronic Crohn's disease are less convincing. There is no evidence that corticosteroids are useful in maintaining a remission in IBD.

Assessment of nutritional status is important (see coeliac disease and parenteral nutrition, above). Supplementation with folic acid 5 mg daily is advisable in all pregnant patients with IBD. Vitamin B_{12} is essential for ileal Crohn's disease and following ileal resection (see ileostomy and colostomy, below). Ideally, measurement and assessment of trace elements including chromium,

zinc and copper as well as vitamins should be carried out regularly during pregnancy and through lactation. Osteomalacia and vitamin D deficiency syndromes are well-recognized in Crohn's disease and require early therapeutic intervention (see Chapter 14). Additional supplementation with iron (see Chapter 2) may be required for chronic blood loss. Many oral preparations containing iron cause diarrhoea, especially in the ileostomy patient (see below). Colonic function often improves in the pregnant patient with IBD.

The use of antimotility agents and stool thickeners such as codeine phosphate and diphenoxylate with atropine (Lomotil) should be kept to a minimum. Many of the antimotility and antispasmodic compounds contain anticholinergic agents such as atropine, hyoscine and barbiturates. These have been associated with congenital abnormalities [66,348]. Their use is contraindicated during pregnancy and lactation. The severity of diarrhoea can be better assessed when such preparations are withheld. Emphasis should focus on treating the underlying inflammatory activity and any infection rather than treating symptoms alone. Constipation should be avoided in IBD, especially in patients with strictures. Constipation may impair the efficiency of action of oral sulphasalazine on the left colon ('constipated colitis'). All patients should be encouraged to take adequate fluids and a high-fibre diet if strictures are excluded (see constipation, below), and, if necessary, poorly absorbed processed hydrophilic agents [349]. Magnesium hydroxide and lactulose are preferred to many complex commercial laxatives (see below).

Colorectal carcinoma (see below) is an uncommon but well-known association with colonic IBD [297]. Colorectal carcinoma presenting in pregnancy is rare but should be considered in patients with long-standing (more than 10 years duration) and extensive IBD.

Emergency surgery

Resective surgery may be required for up to 25% of patients with fulminating ulcerative colitis [350,351] and up to 50% with Crohn's disease affecting the small bowel or ileocolitis when complicated by obstruction, fistulae and abdominal suppuration [350]. Prior to surgery, parenteral nutrition (see above) should be considered, including provision for a long-term, indwelling venous line for postoperative feeding. Surgery for severe colonic IBD involves a single-stage colectomy and ileostomy preferably with preservation of the rectal stump (see colectomy and ileostomy, below). In late pregnancy, a total colectomy may prove difficult. A partial colectomy with ileostomy may suffice until after delivery. In Crohn's disease, limited gut resection with end-to-end anastomosis is preferred to bypass procedures and extensive resections. Clinical relapse and disease recurrence around the site of previous resective surgery for Crohn's disease occur in over 90% regardless of disease site, severity of inflammation and extent of resection. Bypass procedures are discouraged today because the problems remain of the residual inflammation, potential blind-loop and bacterial overgrowth and increased risk of carcinoma.

Publications before the 1980s, often of individual cases, reported a poor outcome for mother and fetus for fulminating IBD requiring resective surgery [297]. In a later series, Mogadam *et al.* [346] followed 178 women with ulcerative colitis and 146 with Crohn's disease through pregnancy. Although there were no maternal deaths, only four of the nine fetuses survived where the mother had a resection during pregnancy [346]. Fulminating IBD during pregnancy is uncommon in more recent studies, probably reflecting earlier diagnosis and successful medical intervention.

Fetal outcome

As discussed above, the rates of spontaneous abortion and stillbirth for emergency resective surgery during pregnancy may exceed 50% [297].

Maternal outcome

A normal delivery and fetal outcome are possible after total proctocolectomy for fulminating ulcerative colitis during pregnancy. In Crohn's disease, in a review of 33 cases of free perforation [352], one woman in her third month of pregnancy was treated with resection and diversion and subsequently had a full-term, normal delivery. Fetal and maternal mortalities following surgery for Crohn's disease and ulcerative colitis that first present in pregnancy with very severe disease probably remain high as indicated in early studies [328,353].

Ileostomy and colostomy

Involuntary infertility following resective surgery has not been considered in most studies.

Pregnancy is not contraindicated in patients with an ileostomy or colostomy carried out for urinary or alimentary diversion.

In general, loss of up to 50% of small bowel and/or colon is well tolerated in the non-pregnant patient. Adaptation in the ileostomy occurs with time. More extensive small and large bowel resection can result in complex metabolic and neuroendocrine dysfunction [354,355]. The pregnant woman with an ileostomy or massive gut

resection may develop malabsorption of fat, fat-soluble vitamins, vitamin B_{12}, water and electrolyte imbalance, hyperoxaluria and cholelithiasis. Complications to be anticipated include obstruction of ureters and Fallopian tubes (pyosalpinx), and effects of surgery on subsequent fertility and sexual function. Adhesions, fistulae and infections add to the general morbidity [304,306,311, 356,357]. Less serious, but more common problems include cracking of the skin and bleeding around the peristomal area.

Pregnancy may interfere with function of the ileostomy, especially after the first trimester with mechanical displacement of the bowel. Intestinal obstruction is a serious complication in pregnancy (see intestinal obstruction, below). The diagnosis can be mistaken for hyperemesis gravidarum or abruptio placentae with a tender uterus, shock and absent fetal heart sounds [358].

INFLAMMATORY BOWEL DISEASE

Women with an ileostomy from a previous colectomy and quiescent IBD have a fair chance of a full-term normal vaginal delivery and healthy infant [353,356,357,359]. In one large review [356] using questionnaires from the Ileostomy Society, 75 women were followed through 89 pregnancies. All had had an ileostomy carried out at some time prior to pregnancy for vesicovaginal fistula following previous obstetric trauma or colectomy for IBD. Pregnancy was uneventful to term in 84 instances and a normal vaginal delivery was achieved in 71%. The increase in use of forceps occurred from impaired ability to push. Caesarean section was carried out in 16 cases for obstetrical reasons and in one case only for ileal prolapse. One maternal death in the UK reported between 1985 and 1987 occurred at 33 weeks in a patient with a previous total colectomy for ulcerative colitis [119]. She died from a massive haemorrhage through the ileostomy resulting from erosion of bowel by the placenta in an abdominal pregnancy that was not suspected despite 3 months of amenorrhoea [119].

Intestinal obstruction was reported in 10% of pregnant women with ileostomies with one maternal death following a caesarean section and one spontaneous abortion [356]. Details of disease activity and anatomical site were not given.

The ileal pouch–anal anastomosis aims to provide continence. Experience in pregnancy is limited but encouraging [355,360]. Out of 92 women who underwent proctocolectomy and fashioning of a 'J'-shaped anastomosis for IBD between 1981 and 1983 at the Mayo Clinic, four of six conceptions ended in normal vaginal deliveries [360]. Anal function returned to baseline postpartum.

Caesarean section was considered unnecessary except for cephalopelvic disproportion and any marginal anal continence before conception [360]. In a retrospective survey by questionnaire in Canada, of 16 pregnancies in 12 women with ileal pouch anal anastomosis for IBD, no pouch-related complications were reported during the 16 pregnancies and deliveries (10 vaginal, six caesarean sections), although complications may occur postpartum [361].

Appendicitis

This is the most common non-obstetric condition requiring surgery during pregnancy. The incidence in pregnancy (around one in 500–1500 pregnancies) is similar to that in the non-pregnant population [362].

In pregnancy, the appendix undergoes progressive upward displacement and reaches the level of the iliac crest around the fifth or sixth month. Accordingly, classical signs (see below) such as pain in the right lower quadrant may be lacking.

Maternal and fetal morbidities and mortalities relate mostly to delays in diagnosis.

MATERNAL OUTCOME

Maternal morbidity and mortality are increased with perforation [362]. In a retrospective review of the literature, of 713 maternal cases of confirmed appendicitis since 1960, rupture had occurred in one quarter in which there were five maternal deaths [363]. Abdominal complications, especially perforation, wall abscess and adynamic ileum are common with delayed diagnosis.

FETAL OUTCOME

Adverse fetal outcome remains significant in some [362,364], although not all [365], studies. In the survey from Sweden [362], spontaneous abortion occurred in 30% of cases arising in the first trimester. Preterm labour occurred in 11% of cases arising in the second trimester. There were no adverse outcomes for cases presenting in the third trimester [362]. Overall, perinatal death has been reported in about 20% of cases with perforation [363,364]. The risk of preterm delivery is much lower after the first week following appendectomy [364].

CLINICAL COURSE AND MANAGEMENT

Appendicitis during pregnancy can show an aggressive evolution. Whether this reflects a delay in diagnosis and the bias of reporting severe cases, remains unclear. Emphasis is on early diagnosis to avoid perforation. Pain may be colicky and confused with cholecystitis due to referral to the right upper quadrant and epigastrium. Vomiting may the sole symptom and be confused with hyperemesis gravidarum or pyelonephritis. Pyuria and leucocytosis are common in pregnancy regardless of appendicitis. Abdominal pain with rebound tenderness accompanied by nausea and vomiting are the most common features. A fever and/or extreme peripheral blood leucocytosis with neutrophilia are risk factors for perforation and should be considered late signs. The differential diagnosis is wide and includes cholecystitis, urinary tract infection, deep vein thrombosis, pulmonary embolism, acute pancreatitis and pneumonia. Obstetric conditions to be excluded include abruptio placentae, pre-eclampsia and adnexal torsion. Other conditions may coexist with appendicitis such as ruptured ectopic pregnancy [366,367], spontaneous rupture of the gallbladder from concurrent acute cholecystitis [368] and amoebic abscess [277].

Routine use of high-resolution ultrasonography has improved the diagnostic accuracy in suspected appendicitis and reduced the rates of negative laparotomy. In a prospective study of 121 German women of childbearing age with suspected appendicitis [369], the criteria for diagnosis included visualization of a non-compressible aperistaltic appendix, with a target-like appearance in transverse view and a diameter ≥ 7 mm. The overall accuracy was 96.7%; 82.6% sensitivity and 100% specificity. Twenty-four (89%) of 27 patients with appendiceal rupture (incidence 20.8%) were diagnosed correctly with ultrasound. Some authorities recommend routine use of antibiotics with coverage against Gram-negative organisms and anaerobic organisms [370] aimed at lessening the risk of perforation. Results are conflicting [362,370] with regard to the clinical efficacy of tocolytic agents for preventing or treating preterm labour.

A McBurney's incision and spinal anaesthesia should be considered for appendectomy during pregnancy, especially after 20 weeks' gestation [364].

LAPAROSCOPIC TECHNIQUES

Advances in laparoscopic techniques have made laparoscopic appendectomy [364,371] an option for selected patients during the first 20 weeks of gestation. Only a skilled surgeon and anaesthetist (to protect the airway), in the presence of an experienced obstetrician, should carry out any laparoscopic approach during pregnancy. Important additional considerations include avoiding a direct supine position to avoid compression of the inferior vena cava by the gravid uterus. Also, the initial site of insertion of the trocar should be carried out under direct vision within clear view of the uterus. A low pressure (<12 mmHg) should be used for abdominal insufflation to avoid reduction in perfusion of the placenta. Minimal CO_2 should be used and the woman monitored for levels of end-tidal CO_2 and oxygen saturation. Full operating facilities should be available including anaesthesia and ventilatory support. The patient should be prepared beforehand for the possibility of conventional surgery with anaesthesia.

Caesarean section is not necessary except for intercurrent obstetrical indications [364].

Intestinal obstruction

This is a serious complication in pregnancy [370,372] and, after appendicitis, is the second most common indication for non-obstetric surgery during pregnancy. The incidence in healthy pregnant women seems to be rising and can be similar to that seen for acute appendicitis. This increase relates to the rising number of laparotomies in young women carried out for appendicitis and gynaecological disorders and is independent of age and parity.

Volvulus of the sigmoid (right) colon [373] and caecum [374] account for around one-quarter of cases of intestinal obstruction in pregnancy compared to 3–5% in the non-pregnant population [375]. Volvulus during pregnancy carries a maternal mortality rate of 20–43% [372]. Predisposing factors include adhesions and appendiceal abscesses. Bowel obstruction accounted for two of the 100 indirect causes of maternal death reported between 1991 and 1993 in the UK [376]. Other causes of obstruction include gastric outlet obstruction [158], intussusception from congenital malrotation [375,377], diaphragmatic hernia, IBD including from ileal pouch—anal anastomosis (see inflammatory bowel disease, above), pseudo-obstruction of the colon (Ogilvie's syndrome), abdominal malignancies (see colon cancer, below), endometriosis and multiple pregnancy.

Presentation typically is in the third trimester when the uterus enlarges sufficiently to displace the viscera. Constipation and previous abdominal surgery may play a role. Caecal volvulus and pseudo-obstruction of the colon are recognized complications of caesarean section.

Management is similar to that in the non-pregnant patient with nasogastric suction and attention to correction of deficits in fluid balance and electrolytes. Endoscopic decompression may be successful in colonic pseudo-obstruction. In Ogilvie's syndrome, a plain abdominal radiograph shows dilatation of the caecum with or without dilatation in the ascending and transverse colon and no distal air. Imaging is essential for the diagnosis. Serial abdominal radiography is essential and requires close

monitoring for continued caecal distension and possible perforation. Parenteral nutrition may be necessary for protracted vomiting. Careful insertion of venous catheters is necessary to prevent sepsis and thrombosis [153]. In addition, the pregnant patient and fetus should be monitored closely in an intensive care setting. Although colonoscopy can reduce certain gut rotations extra caution is required in obstetric practice. The risk of perforation rises when the diameter of the caecum exceeds 9 cm. Successful outcomes have been reported with puncture decompression and/or caecostomy. Many patients with bowel obstruction require bowel resection and colostomy due to underlying infarction that may not be obvious clinically or by MRI [11] and CT imaging prior to surgery [375,376]. Broad-spectrum antibiotics are recommended preoperatively and before endoscopic intervention in view of the high morbidity and mortality associated with bowel ischaemia and infarction. Recommendations include combinations of ampicillin, cephalosporins, clindamycin and aminoglycosides. Mortality remains high for obstruction due to diaphragmatic hernia, and surgical correction is advised especially in symptomatic patients presenting before the third trimester [378]. Vaginal delivery is associated with increased intra-abdominal pressure and should not be attempted with diaphragmatic hernia presenting in the third trimester [378].

Bowel obstruction and perforation should be sought in all cases in which free fluid is found in the peritoneal cavity at caesarean section.

Abdominal complications of tubal pregnancy

Four of 16 maternal deaths in the UK from ruptured tubal pregnancy between 1985 and 1987 had significant involvement of the bowel [119]. Gastrointestinal complications included spontaneous perforation of the bowel, suspected gastroenteritis and abdominal pregnancy with erosion of the placenta into the bowel. Death has also been associated with bowel perforation following laparoscopy for ectopic pregnancy [125]. Typically tubal pregnancy is not suspected until late. Presentations can be with non-specific abdominal pain and vomiting [125]. One patient with a previous total colectomy for ulcerative colitis died from a massive haemorrhage through the ileostomy resulting from erosion of bowel by the placenta [119]. Pregnancy was not suspected despite 3 months of amenorrhoea [119]. The differential diagnosis in pregnancy of abdominal pain, nausea and vomiting is wide. Apart from intestinal obstruction, appendicitis and ruptured tubal and abdominal pregnancy, the list includes peptic ulceration, renal infections, many liver disorders such as hepatitis and hepatic abscess and cholecystitis, pancreatitis (see Chapter 9) and gastro-intestinal infestations. In obstetric practice presentation with a tender uterus, shock and absent fetal heart sounds can be mistaken for hyperemesis gravidarum, pre-eclamptic toxaemia and abruptio placentae. Ruptured ectopic pregnancy or ruptured spleen may be difficult to exclude especially with bloody ascites.

Jejuno-ileal bypass and biliopancreatic diversion

Individual case reports attest to the possibility of a success-ful outcome to pregnancy following these diversion pro-cedures carried out for morbid obesity [188], including after total parenteral nutrition [161]. One study reported normal frequency (no diarrhoea) of bowel function during preg-nancy in four women with a jejuno-ileal bypass, and normal fetal outcomes [379]. This study supports delayed small bowel transit in pregnancy. However, in a retrospective review of the literature of 113 pregnancies after jejuno-ileal bypass and 153 after biliopancreatic diversion (BPD), the authors concluded that pregnancy in the obese woman represents an increased risk to mother and child and en-dorsed poor fetal outcome relating to stillbirth, congenital defects and growth restricted babies. Parenteral nutrition should be considered early in these situations.

Constipation

Constipation is often considered a common consequence of the physiological effects of pregnancy, although difficulties in definition and lack of objective data are misleading.

Constipation is difficult to define. Most authorities agree to a definition of fewer than three stools in 1 week [380–382]. Drossman proposed three criteria to standard-ize the definition of constipation: straining at defecation and hard stools during more than 75% of bowel move-ments and two or less movements each week [383]. Re-duced stool frequency is usually accompanied by stool weights below 35 g daily and more than 25% of the time in defecation spent as straining [381].

Women, especially of childbearing age, have been shown to have a more constipated bowel habit than men [382,384]. Further, women with IBD and irritable bowel syndrome have a cyclical pattern to their symptoms of diarrhoea, constipation and abdominal pain in relation to their men-strual cycle [333], suggesting an interrelation between bowel motility and sex hormones.

The few studies on constipation in pregnancy have yielded conflicting results. Evaluation of patterns of bowel habit in one series of 1000 healthy Israeli women during pregnancy showed a reduction in stool frequency in only

11%; 1.5% required laxatives. In over half, there was no change in bowel habit and around one-third showed an increase in stool frequency [385]. Common complications are backache, faecal impaction and haemorrhoids (see below). The incidence of constipation (as well as urinary incontinence) during pregnancy is increased with parity as demonstrated in a questionnaire survey from Dublin of 7771 women who delivered live babies [386]. These and other data [387] suggest mechanical problems in the lower gastrointestinal tract, and especially at the anal sphincter [387]. However, studies are few, especially in humans, and mostly confined to transit times in the small bowel [388,389]. Parry et al. [388] assessed transit time from stom-ach to caecum using mercury-loaded capsules in 22 healthy pregnant women between the 12th and 20th week and in 12 non-pregnant female controls. Mean stomach-to-caecum transit times were 57.9 h compared to 51.7 h in the non-pregnant group. Transit times exceeded 60 h in over one-third of the pregnant women. In the small bowel of non-pregnant women, mouth-to-caecum transit time is in-creased during the luteal (days 18–20), compared with fol-licular, phases of the menstrual cycle [390]. This delay has been attributed to elevated serum levels of progesterone [390], and, possibly, to its inhibitory action on motilin, among other gut hormones (see nausea and vomiting, above) [113].

Direct studies on colonic motility have not been carried out in pregnant women. Absorption of water and sodium in the colon during pregnancy was increased in one study [389] and attributed to reduced colonic activity. Effects of hormones were not assessed directly.

Slow colonic transit may favour increased absorption of deoxycholic acid to account for the increase in lithogenic bile and predisposition to form biliary sludge and gall-stones in pregnancy [391] (see cholelithiasis, Chapter 9). Delays in whole-gut transit times have been found in non-pregnant women of normal bodyweight with gallstones [382,391].

The influence of diet was not considered directly but plays an important role in patterns of bowel habit. In a survey by Anderson et al. [392,393] in Cambridge, Eng-land, a detailed dietary questionnaire was taken of 18 women in the third trimester, nine of whom complained of severe constipation. No significant differences were found between the two matched groups for diet, includ-ing fibre content (around 18 g daily). Dietary intake of fibre of women who claimed to have increased their intake was similar to that of the general British population (20 g daily) [392,393]. Other factors that contribute to con-stipation include decrease in physical activity, oral iron supplementation, volitional suppression of the reflex to defecate, and use of tocolytic drugs such as magnesium and nifedipine that alter calcium homeostasis in smooth-muscle cells in the intestine [384].

IDIOPATHIC SLOW-TRANSIT CONSTIPATION

Severe constipation resistant to therapeutic manoeuvres such as high-fibre diets is recognized especially in young women [382]. In one study, this condition was diagnosed in 64 non-pregnant young women on the basis of delayed elimination of barium markers on radiographic imaging in the presence of a structurally normal radiograph [394]. The aetiology is unknown. Evidence cited in favour of a hormonal basis includes the occurrence around puberty in young women with dysmenorrhoea and previous gynaecological surgery but not previous pregnancy. Galactorrhoea was found in some cases but levels of prolactin and other hormones were not recorded [394]. Interestingly, one study found delayed gastric emptying for solids, but not liquids, in idiopathic slow transit constipation; half also had slow transit times through the small bowel and proximal colon [395]. In contrast, no delays were found in women with constipation following childbirth [395].

MANAGEMENT

Every patient with constipation requires detailed consideration and examination, in particular of the anal, and perineal, regions to exclude anal fissure [387], IBD and, rarely, malignancy. Occasionally manometric studies may be necessary. If negative, a full investigation should be carried out to exclude other disorders especially hypothyroidism, which may predispose to altered bowel habit. A thorough inquiry should include details of the patient's definition and their dietary and laxative habits and drug therapy.

General measures include education about the normal, variable pattern of bowel regulation. Emphasis should focus on the importance of an adequate fluid intake and, in the absence of bowel strictures, inclusion of a high intake of dietary fibre. Other behavioural modifications involve encouragement of exercise, including Kegel exercises, and scheduled defaecation after meals. Constipation was reduced significantly by supplementing the daily fibre intake (average 20 g daily in the UK at that time) by only an additional 7 g/day [392,393]. This amounted to an increase in wholemeal bread eaten daily from an average of 2.5 slices to 6 slices. The equivalent number of calories was maintained by reducing intake of fat [393].

Stool-bulking agents and laxatives

The choices in pregnancy include processed hydrophilic stool-bulking agents such as methyl cellulose, ispaghula, sterculia and unprocessed (Miller's) bran with a high fluid intake [349,396], magnesium hydroxide tablets (4–6 tablets daily) lactulose or Senokot. Magnesium hydroxide causes increased osmotic retention of fluid in the colon. Although up to 20% of magnesium salts are absorbed, no adverse effects have been reported in pregnancy. Lactulose, a synthetic disaccharide (fructose and galactose), is widely prescribed in pregnancy and seems to be safe. Lactulose in a dose of 30 ml daily for 15 days resulted in normalization of stool habit in 87% of pregnant women with prior constipation and was well tolerated. Direct information is lacking regarding any passage across the placenta and also into breast milk [66]. Lactulose is contraindicated in lactose intolerance and galactosaemia.

Senokot, an anthraquinone, is widely used in pregnancy and the puerperium [348,397,398]. Senna glycosides, the active principles, are released into the colon after bacterial breakdown and following enterohepatic circulation. Senna metabolites can pass into breast milk. Controlled studies have shown no adverse effect on infants [398–400]. Senokot is of particular value in the prevention of constipation in the puerperium. In one study, two Senokot tablets given daily during the first 4 days postpartum reduced the requirement for an enema from 83% to 1% without any adverse effects [398]. Senna can colour urine leading to the erroneous estimation of urinary oestrogens.

Senokot is safe in pregnancy and the puerperium but other anthraquinone laxatives such as aloe and danthron have been associated with congenital malformations [64]. Liquid paraffin, lubricants such as mineral oil, caster oil and soap are contraindicated in pregnancy. These impair absorption of fat-soluble vitamins, namely vitamins D and K, and may lead to neonatal coagulation defects with haemorrhage. There is also the risk of maternal aspiration with lipoid pneumonia during vomiting. Seepage through the anal sphincter may cause pruritus. The polyphenolic laxatives include phenolphthalein, oxyphenacetin and bisacodyl (Dulcolax). Phenolphthalein is excreted in breast milk and should not be used in pregnancy or during lactation. Bisacodyl has been safely used in pregnancy [401] in enema form and suppositories but has been superseded by oral lactulose. Faecal impaction may require tap-water enemata and emollient laxatives as well as manual disimpaction.

Irritable bowel syndrome

This includes a heterogeneous group of conditions characterized by intermittent abdominal pain—'spastic colon', altered bowel habit, incomplete evacuation of stool, and passage of clear mucus per rectum. [402]. The causes are unknown. Physiological changes in non-pregnant patients show abnormal myoelectrical activity throughout the gastrointestinal tract [403]. Studies in pregnancy are lacking.

MANAGEMENT

Diagnosis is by exclusion of many other causes of altered bowel habit. Patients require a full inquiry and investigation. IBD, laxative abuse, gut infections and infestations, bile-salt malabsorption, coeliac disease, lactose intolerance and hormone-secreting tumours (those secreting vasoactive inhibitory polypeptide (VIP) and calcitonin, among others) should be excluded especially for presentations with diarrhoea. Hypothyroidism is an important exclusion for constipation.

Therapies are empirical and depend on the predominant symptoms. Bulking agents are preferred to unprocessed bran, which may exacerbate symptoms and cause bloating [402]. Fluid intake should be encouraged. Antispasmodic agents such as hyoscine and dicyclomine (anticholinergic) and mebeverine, alverine and peppermint oil (smooth-muscle relaxant) are used widely in the non-pregnant patient with abdominal pain. Such antispasmodic agents and antidiarrhoeal agents such as loperamide are contraindicated in pregnancy.

Anorectal and perineal disorders

Anorectal disorders including haemorrhoids, tears of the anal sphincter resulting from obstetric injury and fissure-in-ano, anal incontinence, rectovaginal fistula and rectal prolapse cause significant discomfort and embarrassment [404]. Perianal fistulae in Crohn's disease and vaginal discharge following proctocolectomy in ulcerative colitis [405] can add to the morbidity in IBD. Dyspareunia is common in patients with IBD involving the perineal area, and its frequency is more than doubled (12–27%) following proctocolectomy [405].

Although these disorders are common, every case requires a careful history and examination to exclude the myriad of other disorders such as IBD and rectal and colonic malignancies (see below) that can masquerade as 'haemorrhoids' with pain, bleeding and rectal discharge.

ANAL FISSURE

Anal fissure is common after delivery despite low anal canal pressure. In a prospective study of 209 primigravidae, anal manometric pressures were measured 6 weeks before and after birth. Prepartum resting and squeeze pressures were similar in women regardless of development of anal fissure [387]. Anal canal pressures fell postpartum in both groups. Constipation postpartum was

common especially in women who had developed an anal fissure. The mode of delivery and use of epidural anaesthesia did not impact on the incidence of anal fissure [387]. The authors recommend caution with surgical interference of the anal sphincter in view of the reduced pressures in the anal canal [387].

HAEMORRHOIDS

These are extremely common in pregnancy and postpartum. Haemorrhoids can be exacerbated by constipation and straining during labour and infection following episiotomy resulting in thrombosis, strangulation and rectal prolapse. In a study of 40 patients studied in the puerperium with anorectal disorders, 95% had external haemorrhoids and, in 37.5%, these were accompanied by internal haemorrhoids [406]. Prolapse and thrombosis was found in 20% and *fissure-in-ano* in 5% [406]. Women prone to develop haemorrhoids commonly present during pregnancy and there is an increased incidence in multiparous patients [406].

Common presentations of anorectal disorders include pruritus, rectal bleeding and perineal pain. Mucoid and purulent discharge may occur with secondary inflammation and infection. Uncomplicated haemorrhoids are said not to cause pruritus [407]; their presence warrants investigation for underlying causes (see below). Haemorrhoidectomy has been carried out for severe symptoms during pregnancy [408].

Pathogenic mechanisms remain unclear. Suggestions include high pressure in the pelvic veins and undefined hormonal factors acting on the unique haemorrhoidal plexus [409,410].

SPHINCTER INJURIES

In one survey of 20 500 women with episiotomies, 1040 (5%) had third- and fourth-degree extensions, including some with a perianal tear [411]. In 101 (10%) of these severe injuries, the episiotomy wound had disrupted. Complications included anal ulcer and abscess, disruption of the sphincter, and rectovaginal fistula [411]. Surgical intervention was successful in most cases. In a retrospective cohort study of primigravid women from the USA between 1996 and 1997, anal continence was compared in 209 women who had received an episiotomy, 206 who had suffered second- to fourth-degree spontaneous lacerations and 211 who had no significant perineal injury [412]. Episiotomy was shown to increase by threefold the risk of faecal incontinence at 3 and 6 months postpartum compared to women who had a spontaneous laceration. The effect of episiotomy was independent of age, birthweight, duration of second-stage of labour, use of instrumentation during delivery, and complications of labour [412].

Patients with faecal incontinence resulting from obstetric injury may benefit from manometric and endosonographic techniques. Quantitative assessment of the degree of sphincter dysfunction may help to predict those who should benefit from surgery [413,414]. Use of ultrasound and pulsed electromagnetic energy therapies for perineal trauma following delivery showed no benefit in a randomised, placebo-controlled trial [415].

HERPES SIMPLEX VIRUS

Rectal and perianal ulcers can occur with herpes simplex virus (HSV), typically type II. Some success has been reported following oral aciclovir and this should be considered in late pregnancy to prevent transmission to the newborn (see Chapter 17).

PAPILLOMA VIRUSES AND WARTS

Flat condylomata of the cervix and anogenital area are common and occur in up to 2% of women of childbearing age [416]. Many result from transmission of human papilloma viruses (HPV) and are as common a sexually transmitted disease as herpes genitalis and gonorrhoea [416]. Some of the human papilloma viruses, such as HPV-6 and HPV-11, are considered of low oncogenic potential and are associated with condylomata acuminata [417]. By contrast, HPV-16 and HPV-18 carry high risk and are associated with squamous cell carcinoma of the vulva and cervical intraepithelial neoplasia [417,418].

Condylomata acuminata are associated with promiscuity and other sexually transmitted diseases, diabetes mellitus, corticosteroid therapy and depression of cell-mediated immunity [418]. At least half of vestibular warts will be accompanied by warts detectable on the cervix, and 70% of those with perianal warts also will have rectal warts [418]. Condylomata acuminata may grow rapidly during pregnancy. Caesarean section may have to be considered because anal warts have been associated with development of laryngeal papillomata in the infant [418]. Treatment is with podophyllin as a 25% solution in tincture of benzoic acid. However, this is contraindicated in pregnancy and therefore cryosurgery is preferable in pregnancy.

Gastrointestinal malignancies

Malignancy discovered during a normal pregnancy poses a considerable problem for the patient and her healthcare attendants [419]. The true incidence of gastrointestinal malignancy complicating pregnancy is unknown. Gastric cancer has been considered above.

References

1 Bennett TA, Korelchuck M *et al*. Pregnancy-associated hospitalizations in the United States in 1991 and 1992: a comprehensive view of maternal morbidity. *Am J Obstet Gynecol* 1998; 178: 346–54.

2 Hytten FE. The alimentary system. In: Hytten F, Chamberlain G, eds. *Clinical Physiology in Obstetrics*. 1991; Blackwell Scientific Publications, Oxford: 137–49.

3 Philipson EH, Rossi KQ *et al*. Glucose, insulin, gastric inhibitory polypeptide, and pancreatic polypeptide responses to polycose during pregnancy. *Obstet Gynecol* 1992; 79: 592–6.

4 Maes BD, Spitz B *et al*. Gastric emptying in hyperemesis gravidarum and non-dyspeptic pregnancy. *Aliment Pharmacol Ther* 1999; 13: 237–43.

5 Toppenberg KS, Ashley-Hill D, Miller DP. Safety of radiographic imaging during pregnancy. *Am Fam Phys* 1999; 59: 1813–18.

6 Hall EJ. Scientific view of low-level radiation risks. *Radiographics* 1991; 11: 509–18.

7 Kanayama N, Khatun S *et al*. Vasospasms of cerebral arteries in hyperemesis gravidarum. *Gynecol Obstet Invest* 1998; 46: 139–41.

8 Gardian G, Voros E *et al*. Wernicke's encephalopathy induced by hyperemesis gravidarum. *Acta Neurol Scand* 1999; 99: 196–8.

9 Hillborn M, Pyhtinen J *et al*. Pregnant, vomiting and coma. *Lancet* 1999; 353: 1584.

10 Levine D, Barnes PD *et al*. Obstetric MR imaging. *Radiology* 1999; 211: 609–17.

11 Regan F, Beall DP *et al*. Fast MR imaging and the detection of small-bowel obstruction. *Am J Roentgenol* 1998; 170: 1465–9.

12 Cappell MS. The safety and efficacy of gastrointestinal endoscopy during pregnancy. *Gastroenterol Clin N Am* 1998; 27: 37–71.

13 Cappell MS, Colon V *et al*. A study of eight medical centers of the safety and clinical efficacy of esophagogastroduodenoscopy in 83 pregnant females with follow-up of fetal outcome and with comparison to control groups. *Am J Gastroenterol* 1996; 91: 348–54.

14 Walker AR, Walker BF *et al*. Nausea and vomiting and dietary craving and aversions during pregnancy in South African women. *Br J Obstet Gynaecol* 1985; 92: 484–9.

15 Horner RD, Lackey CJ *et al*. Pica practices of pregnant women. *J Am Diet Assoc* 1991; 91: 34–8.

16 Geissler PW, Prince RJ *et al*. Perceptions of soil-eating and anaemia among pregnant women on the Kenyan coast. *Soc Sci Med* 1999; 48: 1069–79.

17 Rainville AJ. Pica practices of pregnant women are associated with lower maternal hemoglobin at delivery. *J Am Diet Assoc* 1998; 98: 293–6.

18 Crosby WH. Clay ingestion and iron deficiency. *Ann Int Med* 1982; 97: 456.

19 Feldman MD. Pica: current perspectives. *Psychosomatics* 1986; 27: 519–23.

20 Pearl M, Boxt LM. Radiographic findings in congenital lead poisoning. *Radiology* 1980; 136: 83–4.

21 Kopp-Hoolihan LE, van Loan MD *et al*. Longitudinal assessment of energy balance in well-nourished pregnant women. *Am J Clin Nutr* 1999; 69: 697–704.

22 Mathews F, Yudkin P *et al*. Influence of maternal nutrition on outcome of pregnancy: prospective cohort study. *Br Med J* 1999; 319: 339–43.

23 Kramer MS. Effects of energy and protein intakes on pregnancy outcome: an overview of the research evidence from controlled clinical trials. *Am J Clin Nutr* 1993; 58: 627–35.

24 Goldenberg RL, Rouse DJ. Medical progress: prevention of premature birth. *N Engl J Med* 1998; 339: 313–20.

25 Christian P, West KP *et al*. Night blindness of pregnancy in rural Nepal—nutritional and health risks. *Int J Epidemiol* 1998; 27: 231–7.

26 Andersson R, Bergstrom S. Is maternal malnutrition associated with low sex ratio at birth? *Hum Biol* 1998; 70: 1101–06.

27 Weigel MM, Calle A *et al*. The effect of chronic intestinal parasitic infection on maternal and perinatal outcome. *Int J Gynaecol Obstet* 1996; 52: 9–17.

28 Santiso R. effects of chronic parasitosis on women's health. *Int J Gynaecol Obstet* 1997; 58: 129–36.

29 Prasad AS. Zinc deficiency in human subjects. *Progr Clin Biol Res* 1983; 129: 1–33.

30 Prasad AS. Clinical manifestations of zinc deficiency. *Ann Rev Nutr* 1985; 5: 341–63.

31 Srikantia SG, Reddy V. Megaloblastic anaemia of infancy and vitamin B12. *Br J Haematol* 1967; 13: 949–53.

32 Davis RE. Clinical chemistry of vitamin B_{12}. *Adv Clin Chem* 1985; 24: 163–216.

33 Villar J, Gulmezoglu AM *et al*. Nutritional and antimicrobial interventions to prevent preterm birth: an overview of randomized controlled trials. *Obstet Gynecol Surv* 1998; 53: 575–85.

34 Antoon JW, Miller RL. Apthous ulcers—a review of the literature on etiology, pathogenesis, diagnosis and treatment. *J Am Den Assoc* 1980; 101: 803–8.

35 McCartan BE, Sullivan A. The association of menstrual cycle, pregnancy and menopause with recurrent oral apthous stomatitis. a review and critique. *Obstet Gynecol* 1992; 80: 455–8.

36 Weller IVD. AIDs and the gut. *Scand J Gastroenterol* 1985; 20 (Suppl. 114): 77–81.

37 Loe H, Silness J. Periodontal disease in pregnancy. *Acta Odont Scand* 1963; 21: 533–51.

38 Di Placido G, Tumini V *et al*. Gingival hyperplasia in pregnancy. II. Etiopathogenic factors and mechanisms [Italian]. *Min Stomatol* 1998; 47: 223–9.

39 Zegarelli EV, Kutscher AH, Hyman GA. *Diagnosis of the Mouth and Jaws*. 1978; Lea & Febiger, Philadelphia, 73.

40 Lee A, McWilliams M *et al*. Care of the pregnant patient in the dental office. *Dent Clin N Am* 1999; 43: 485–94.

41 Kornman KS, Loesche WJ. The subgingival microbial flora during pregnancy. *J Periodont Res* 1980; 15: 111–22.

42 Dasanayake AP. Poor periodontal health of the pregnant woman as a risk factor for low birth weight. *Ann Periodont* 1998; 3: 206–12.

43 Van Thiel DH, Gavaler JS *et al*. Heartburn of pregnancy. *Gastroenterology* 1977; 72: 666–8.

44 Feeney JG. Leading article. Heartburn in pregnancy. *Br Med J* 1982; 284: 1138–9.

45 Broussard CN, Richter JE. Treating gastro-oesophageal reflux disease during pregnancy and lactation: what are the safest therapy options? *Drug Safety* 1998; 19: 325–37.

46 Alvarez-Sanchez A, Rey E *et al*. Does progesterone fluctuation across the menstrual cycle predispose to gastroesophageal reflux? *Am J Gastroenterol* 1999; 94: 1468–71.

47 Byrne JJ. Diagnostic evaluation of patients with intestinal problems. *Clin Obstetr Gynecol* 1972; 15: 473–83.

48 Dodds WJ, Dent J *et al*. Pregnancy and the lower esophageal sphincter. *Gastroenterology* 1978; 74: 1334–6.

49 Baimbridge ET, Nicholas SD *et al*. Gastro-oesophageal reflux in pregnancy. Altered function of the barrier to reflux in asymptomatic women during early pregnancy. *Scand J Gastroenterol* 1984; 19: 85–9.

50 Cohen S, Harris LD. Does hiatus hernia effect competence of the gastro-esophageal sphincter? *N Engl J Med* 1971; 284: 1053–6.

51 Brock-Utne JG, Dow TGB *et al*. Gastric and lower oesophageal sphincter (LOS) pressures in early pregnancy. *Br J Anaesth* 1981; 53: 381–4.

52 Atlay RD, Gillison EW *et al*. A fresh look at pregnancy heartburn. *J Obstet Gynaecol Br Commonw* 1973; 80: 63–6.

53 Bassey OO. Pregnancy heartburn in Nigerians and Caucasians with theories about aetiology based on manometric recordings from the oesophagus and stomach. *Br J Obstet Gynaecol* 1977; 84: 439–43.

54 Van Thiel DH, Wald A. Evidence refuting a role for increased abdominal pressure in the pathogenesis of the heartburn associated with pregnancy. *Am J Obstet Gynecol* 1981; 140: 420–22.

55 Ogorek CP, Cohen S. Gastroesophageal reflux disease: new concepts in pathophysiology. *Gastroenterol Clin N Am* 1989; 18: 275–92.

56 Goyal RK, Rattan S. Neurohumeral, hormonal and drug receptors for the lower esophageal sphincter. *Gastroenterology* 1978; 74: 598–619.

57 Cotton BR, Smith G. The lower oesophageal sphincter and anaesthesia. *Br J Anaesth* 1984; 56: 37–46.

58 Singer AJ, Brandt LJ. Pathophysiology of the gastrointestinal tract during pregnancy. *Am J Gastroenterol* 1991; 86: 1695–712.

59 Kaye MD, Showalter JP. Pyloric incompetence in patients with symptomatic gastroesophageal reflux. *J Lab Clin Med* 1974; 83: 198–206.

60 Scott NM, Deutsch DL. The esophagus during pregnancy. *Am J Gastroenterol* 1955; 24: 305–13.

61 Burrow GN, Ferris TF, eds. *Medical Complications During Pregnancy*. 1975; WB Saunders, Philadelphia.

62 Hogan WJ, de Andrade SRV *et al*. Ethanol-induced acute esophageal motor function. *J Appl Physiol* 1972; 32: 755–60.

63 Katz PO, Castell DO. Gastroesophageal reflux during pregnancy. *Gastroenterology Clin N Am* 1998; 27: 153–67.

64 Nelson MM, Forfar JO. Associations between drugs administered during pregnancy and congenital abnormalities of the foetus. *Br Med J* 1971; i: 523–7.

65 Atlay RD, Weekes AR. The treatment of gastrointestinal disease in pregnancy. *Clin Obstet Gynaecol* 1986; 13: 335–47.

66 Lewis JH, Weingold AB. The use of gastrointestinal drugs during pregnancy and lactation. *Am J Gastroenterol* 1985; 80: 912–23.

67 Fisher RS, Roberts GS *et al*. Altered lower esophageal sphincter function during early pregnancy. *Gastroenterology* 1978; 74: 1233–7.

68 Wilson JT, Brown RD *et al*. Drug excretion in human breast milk: principles, pharmacokinetics and projected consequences. *Clin Pharmacokinet* 1980; 5: 1–66.

69 Larson JD, Patatanian E *et al*. Double-blind, placebo-controlled study of ranitidine for gastroesophageal reflux symptoms during pregnancy. *Obstet Gynecol* 1997; 90: 83–7.

70 Rayburn W, Liles E *et al*. Antacids vs antacids plus non-prescription ranitidine for heartburn during pregnancy. *Int J Gynaecol Obstet* 1999; 66: 35–7.

71 Nielsen GL, Sorensen HT *et al*. The safety of proton pump inhibitors in pregnancy. *Aliment Pharmacol Thera* 1999; 13: 1085–9.

72 Ruigomez A, Garcia Rodriguez LA *et al*. Use of cimetidine, omeprazole, and ranitidine in pregnant women and pregnancy outcomes. *Am J Epidemiol* 1999; 150: 476–81.

73 Riley AJ, Crowley P *et al*. Transfer of ranitidine to biological fluids; milk and serum. In: Misiewicz JJ, Wormsley KG, eds. *The Clinical Use of Ranitidine: the Second International Symposium on Ranitidine*. 1982; The Medicine Publishing Foundation, Oxford: 78–81.

74 Mihaly GW, Jones DB *et al*. Placental transfer and renal elimination of cimetidine in maternal and fetal sheep. *J Pharmacol Exp Ther* 1983; 227: 441–5.

75 Gillet GB, Watson JD *et al*. Ranitidine and single-dose antacid therapy as prophylaxis against acid aspiration syndrome in obstetric practice. *Anaesthesia* 1984; 39: 638–44.

76 Anand S, Van Thiel DH. Prenatal and neonatal exposure to cimetidine. results in gonadal and sexual dysfunction in adult males. *Science* 1982; 218: 493–4.

77 Hoos PC, Hoffman LH. Effective histamine receptor antagonists and indomethacin on implantation in the rabbit. *Biol Reprod* 1983; 29: 833–40.

78 Parker S, Schade RR *et al*. Prenatal and neonatal exposure of male rat pups to cimetidine but not ranitidine adversely affects subsequent adult sexual functioning. *Gastroenterology* 1984; 86: 675–80.

79 Glade G, Saccar CL *et al*. Cimetidine in pregnancy: apparent transient liver impairment in the newborn. *Am J Dis Child* 1980; 134: 87–8.

80 Lalkin A, Loebstein R *et al*. The safety of omeprazole during pregnancy: a multicenter prospective controlled study. *Am J Obstet Gynecol* 1998; 179: 727–30.

81 Cappell MS, Garcia A. Gastric and duodenal ulcers during pregnancy. *Gastroenterol Clin N Am* 1998; 27: 169–95.

82 Harrington RA, Hamilton CW *et al*. Metoclopramide: an updated review of its pharmacological properties and clinical use. *Drugs* 1983; 25: 451–94.

83 Desmond PV, Watson KJ. Metoclopramide—a review. *Med J Aust* 1986; 144: 366–9.

84 Hartsilver EL, Vanner RG *et al*. Gastric pressure during emergency caesarian section under general anaesthesia. *Br J Anaesth* 1999; 82: 752–4.

85 Moir DD. Cimetidine, antacids and pulmonary aspiration. *Anesthesiology* 1983; 59: 81–3.

86 Bifarini G, Favetta P *et al*. [Pharmacologic prevention of Mendelson syndrome. A controlled clinical trial.] Prevenzione farmacologica della sindrome di Mendelson. Studio clinico controllato. *Min Anestesiol* 1992; 58: 95–9.

87 Klebanoff MA, Koslowe PA *et al*. Epidemiology of vomiting in early pregnancy. *Obstet Gynecol* 1985; 66: 612–16.

88 Einarson A, Koren G *et al*. Nausea and vomiting in pregnancy: a comparative European Study. *Eur J Obstet Gynecol Reprod Biol* 1998; 76: 1–3.

89 Fairweather DV. Nausea and vomiting during pregnancy. *Am J Obstet Gynecol* 1968; 102: 135–175.

90 Weigel MM, Weigel RM. The association of reproductive history, demographic factors, and alcohol and tobacco consumption with the risk of developing nausea and vomiting in early pregnancy. *Am J Epidemiol* 1988; 127: 562–70.

91 Weigel RM, Weigel MM. Nausea and vomiting of early pregnancy and pregnancy outcome. A meta-analytical review. *Br J Obstet Gynaecol* 1989; 96: 1312–18.

92 Midwinter A. Causes of vomiting in pregnancy. *Practitioner* 1971; 206: 743–50.

93 Jarnfelt-Samsioe A, Samsioe G *et al*. Nausea and vomiting in pregnancy—a contribution to its epidemiology. *Gynecol Obstet Invest* 1983; 16: 221–9.

94 Jarnfelt-Samsioe A, Eriksson B *et al*. Some new aspects in emesis gravidarum. Relations to clinical data, serum electrolytes, total protein and creatinine. *Gynecol Obstet Invest* 1985; 19: 174–86.

95 Tsang IS, Katz VL *et al*. Maternal and fetal outcomes in hyperemesis gravidarum. *Int J Gynaecol Obstet* 1996; 55: 231–5.

96 Gross S, Librach, C *et al*. Maternal weight loss associated with hyperemesis gravidarum: a predictor of fetal outcome. *Am J Obstet Gynecol* 1989; 160: 906–9. Comment in: *Am J Obstet Gynecol* 1990; 162: 1349.

97 Glick MM, Dick EL. Molar pregnancy presenting with hyperemesis gravidarum. *J Am Osteopath Assoc* 1999; 99: 162–4.

98 Morali GA, Braverman DZ. Abnormal liver enzymes and ketonuria in hyperemesis gravidarum. A retrospective review of 80 patients. *J Clin Gastroenterol* 1990; 12: 303–5.

99 Frigo P, Lang C *et al*. Hyperemesis gravidarum associated with *Helicobacter pylori* seropositivity. *Obstet Gynecol* 1998; 91: 615–17.

100 Jacoby EB, Porter KB. *Helicobacter pylori* infection and persistent hyperemesis gravidarum. *Am J Perinatol* 1999; 16: 85–8.

101 Depue RH, Bernstein L *et al*. Hyperemesis gravidarum in relation to estradiol levels, pregnancy outcome and other maternal factors: a seroepidemiologic study. *Am J Obstet Gynaecol* 1987; 156: 1137–41.

102 Medalie JH. Relationship between nausea and / or vomiting in early pregnancy and abortion. *Lancet* 1957; 2: 117–19.

103 Godsey RK, Newman RB. Hyperemesis gravidarum. A comparison of single and multiple admissions. *J Reprod Med* 1991; 36: 287–90.

104 Klebanoff MA, Mills JL. Is vomiting during pregnancy teratogenic? *Br Med J* 1986; 292: 724–6.

105 Hallak M, Tsalamandris K *et al*. Hyperemesis gravidarum. Effects on fetal outcome. *J Reprod Med* 1996; 41: 871–4.

106 Koch KL, Stern RM *et al*. Gastric dyarhythmias and nausea of pregnancy. *Dig Dis Sci* 1990; 35: 961–9.

107 Riezzo G, Pezzolla F *et al*. Gastric myoelectric activity in the first trimester of pregnancy: a cutaneous electromyographic study. *Am J Gastroenterol* 1992; 87: 702–7.

108 Kauppila A, Heikinheimo M *et al*. Human chorionic gonadotrophin and pregnancy-specific beta-1-glycoprotein in predicting pregnancy outcome and in association with early pregnancy vomiting. *Gynecol Obstet Invest* 1984; 18: 49–53.

109 Masson GM, Antony F *et al*. Serum choriogonadotrophin (hCG), schwangerschaftsprotein 1 (SP1), progesterone and oestradiol levels in patients with nausea and vomiting in early pregnancy. *Br J Obstet Gynaecol* 1985; 92: 211–15.

110 Leylek OA, Toyaksi M *et al*. Immunologic and biochemical factors in hyperemesis gravidarum with and without hyperthyroxinemia. *Gynecol Obstet Invest* 1999; 47: 229–34.

111 Starks GC. Pregnancy-induced hyperemesis (hyperemesis gravidarum). A reassessment of therapy and proposal of a new etiologic theory. *Missouri Med* 1984; 81: 253–6.

112 Jarnfelt-Samsoie A, Bremme K *et al*. Steroid hormones in emetic and non-emetic pregnancy. *Eur J Obstet Gynecol Reprod Biol* 1986; 21: 87–99.

113 Christofides ND, Ghalei MA *et al*. Decreased plasma motilin concentrations in pregnancy. *Br Med J* 1982; 285: 1453–4.

114 Hsu JJ, Clark-Glena R *et al*. Nasogastric enteral feeding in the management of hyperemesis gravidarum. *Obstet Gynecol* 1996; 88: 343–6.

115 Biggs JSG, Vesey EJ. Treatment of gastrointestinal disorders of pregnancy. *Drugs* 1980; 19: 70–6.

116 Jednak MA, Shadigian EM *et al*. Protein meals reduce nausea and gastric slow wave dysrhythmic activity in first trimester pregnancy. *Am J Physiol* 1999; 277: G855–G861.

117 Aikins Murphy P. Alternative therapies for nausea and vomiting of pregnancy. *Obstet Gynecol* 1998; 91: 149–55.

118 Hershman JM. Human chorionic gonadotrophin and the thyroid: hyperemesis gravidarum and trophoblastic tumors. *Thyroid* 1999; 9: 653–7.

119 Department of Health. *Report on Confidential Enquiries into Maternal Deaths in the United Kingdom 1985–7*. HMSO, London, 1991: 54–8.

120 Hagen A, Becker C *et al*. Hyperemesis in late pregnancy should we think of cancer? A case report. *Eur J Obstet Gynecol Reproduct Biol* 1998; 80: 273–4.

121 Winship DH. Gastrointestinal diseases. In: Burrow GN, Ferris TF, eds. *Medical Complications During Pregnancy*. 1975; WB Saunders, Philadelphia: 275–350.

122 Sullivan CA, Johnson CA *et al*. A pilot study of intravenous ondansetron for hyperemesis gravidarum. *Am J Obstet Gynecol* 1996; 174: 1565–8.

123 Wells CN. Treatment of hyperemesis gravidarum with cortisone. *Am J Obstet Gynecol* 1953; 66: 598–601.

124 Safari HR, Alsulyman OM *et al*. Experience with oral methylprednisolone in the treatment of refractory hyperemesis gravidarum. *Am J Obstet Gynecol* 1998; 178: 1054–8.

125 Department of Health. *Report on Confidential Enquiries into Maternal Deaths in the United Kingdom 1991–93*. HMSO, London, 1996: 1–202.

126 Bergin PS, Harvey P. Wernicke's encephalopathy and central pontine myelinolysis associated with hyperemesis gravidarum. *Br Med J* 1992; 305: 517–18.

127 Tonelli J, Zurru MC *et al*. Central pontine myelinolysis induced by hyperemesis gravidarum [Spanish]. *Medicina* 1999; 59: 176–8.

128 Tesfaye S, Achari V *et al*. Pregnant, vomiting and going blind. *Lancet* 1998; 352: 1594.

129 Multicenter Study. Multicenter study of the use of drugs during pregnancy in Spain (III). Drugs used during the first pregnancy trimester. [DUP workshop of Spain.] Estudio multicentrico sobre el uso de medicamentos durante el embarazo en Espana (III). Los farmacos utilizados durante el primer trimestre de la gestacion. Grupo de Trabajo DUP Espana. *Med Clin Barcelona* 1991; 96: 52–7.

130 Schuster K, Bailey LB *et al*. Morning sickness and vitamin B6 status of pregnant women. *Hum Nutr Clin Nutri* 1985; 39C: 75–9.

131 Fischer-Rassmussen W, Kjaer SK *et al*. Ginger treatment of hyperemesis gravidarum. *Eur J Obstet Gynecol Reprod Biol* 1990; 38: 19–24.

132 McBride WG. Thalidomide and congenital abnormalities. *Lancet* 1961; ii: 1358.

133 Lenz W, Knapp K. Thalidomide embryopathy. *Deutsche Med Wochenschr* 1962; 87: 1232–42.

134 Kullander S, Kallen B. A prospective study of drugs and pregnancy. *Acta Obstetr Gynecol Scand Suppl* 1976; 55: 105–11.

135 Aselton P, Jick H *et al*. Pyloric stenosis and maternal Bendectin exposure. *Am J Epidemiol* 1984; 120: 251–6.

136 Zierler S, Rothman KJ. Congenital heart disease in relation to maternal use of Bendectin and other drugs in early pregnancy. *N Engl J Med* 1985; 313: 347–52.

137 Shapiro S, Heinonen OP *et al*. Antenatal exposure to doxylamine succinate and dicyclomine hydrochloride (Bendectin) in relation to congenital malformations, perinatal mortality rate, birthweight and intelligence quotient score. *Am J Obstet Gynecol* 1977; 128: 480–5.

138 Smithells RW, Sheppard S. Fetal malformation after Debendox in early pregnancy. *Br Med J* 1978; 1: 1055–6.

139 Federal Register Food and Safety Administration (on Bendectin). *Fed Reg* 1979; 44: 41068.

140 Lenz W. Malformations caused by drugs in pregnancy. *Am Dis Child* 1966; 112: 99–106.

141 McBride WG. An aetiological study of drug ingestion by women who gave birth to babies with cleft palate. *Aust N Zeal J Obstet Gynaecol* 1969; 9: 103–4.

142 Hill RM, Tennyson LM. Drug-induced malformations in humans. In: Stern L, ed. *Drug Use in Pregnancy*. 1984; ADIS Health Science Press, Sydney: 99–133.

143 Witter FR, King TM. Drugs and the management of chronic diseases in the pregnant patient. In: Stern L, ed. *Drug Use in Pregnancy*. 1984; ADIS Health Science Press, Sydney, 190–211.

144 Briggs GG, Bodendorfer TW *et al*., eds. *Drugs in Pregnancy and Lactation: a Reference Guide to Fetal and Neonatal Risk*. 1983; Williams & Wilkins, Baltimore, ML.

145 Huff PS. Safety of drug therapy for nausea and vomiting of pregnancy. *J Fam Pract* 1980; ii: 969–70.

146 Schulze-Delrieu K. Drug therapy: metoclopramide. *N Engl J Med* 1981; 305: 28–33.

147 Vella L, Francis D *et al*. Comparison of the antiemetics metoclopramide and promethazine in labour. *Br Med J* 1985; 290: 1173–5.

148 Solanki DR, Suresh M *et al*. The effects of intravenous cimetidine and metoclopramide on gastric volume and pH. *Anaesth Analg* 1984; 63: 599–602.

149 Waldmann CS, Verghese C *et al*. the evaluation of domperidone and metoclopramide as antiemetics in day care abortion patients. *Br J Clin Pharmacol* 1985; 19: 307–10.

150 Santos A, Datta S. Prophylactic use of droperidol for control of nausea and vomiting during spinal anaesthesia for Cesarean section. *Anaesth Analg* 1984; 63: 85–7.

151 Nageotte MP, Briggs GG *et al*. Droperidol and diphenhydramine in the management of hyperemesis gravidarum. *Am J Obstet Gynecol* 1996; 174: 1801–5.

152 Hamaoui E, Hamaoui M. Nutritional assessment and support during pregnancy. *Gastroenterol Clin N Am* 1998; 27: 89–121.

153 Russo-Stieglitz KE, Levine AB *et al*. Pregnancy outcome in patients requiring parenteral nutrition. *J Mat Fet Med* 1999; 8: 164–7.

154 Rosso P. Nutrition and maternal-fetal exchange. *Am J Clin Nutr* 1981; 34: 744.

155 Zibell-Frisk D, Jen KL *et al*. Use of parenteral nutrition to maintain adequate nutritional status in hyperemesis gravidarum. *J Perinatol* 1990; 10: 390–5.

156 Heller L. Parenteral nutrition in obstetrics and gynaecology. In. Greep JM, Soeters PB, Wesdorp RIC *et al*., eds. *Current Concepts in Parenteral Nutrition*. 1977; Nyhoff Medical Division, The Hague: 179–86.

157 Martin R, Trubow M *et al*. Hyperalimentation during pregnancy: a case report. *J Parent Ent Nutr* 1985; 9: 212–15.

158 Uchide K, Suzuki N *et al*. Pregnant women with transient gastric obstruction managed by naso-jejunal nutrition. *Nutrition* 1998; 14: 458–61.

159 Godil A, Chen YK. Percutaneous endoscopic gastrostomy for nutrition support in pregnancy associated with hyperemesis

gravidarum and anorexia nervosa. *J Parent Ent Nutr* 1998; 22: 238–41.

160 Serrano P, Velloso A *et al.* Enteral nutrition by percutaneous endoscopic gastrojejunostomy in severe hyperemesis gravidarum: a report of two cases. *Clin Nutr* 1998; 17: 135–9.

161 Rivera-Alsina ME, Saldana LR *et al.* Fetal growth sustained by parenteral nutrition in pregnancy. *Obstet Gynecol* 1984; 64: 138–41.

162 Tresadern JC, Falconer GF *et al.* Maintenance of pregnancy in a home parenteral nutrition patient. *J Parent Ent Nutr* 1984; 8: 199–202.

163 Hibbard ED, Smithells RW. Folic acid metabolism and human embryopathy. *Lancet* 1965; i: 1254.

164 Holmes-Siedle M, Lindenbaum RH *et al.* Vitamin supplementation and neural tube deffects (letter). *Lancet* 1982; i: 276.

165 Hunt JN, Murray FA. Gastric function in pregnancy. *J Obstet Gynaecol Br Emp* 1958; 65: 78–83.

166 Waldum HL, Straume BK *et al.* Serum Group I pepsinogens (PG1) during pregnancy. *Scand J Gastroenterol* 1980; 15: 61–3.

167 Rooney PJ, Dow TGB *et al.* Immunoreactive gastrin and gestation. *Am J Obstet Gynecol* 1975; 122: 834–6.

168 Clark DH, Tankel HI. Gastric acid and plasma histaminase during pregnancy. *Lancet* 1954; 2: 886.

169 Parbhoo SP, Johnston IDA. Effect of oestrogens and progestagens on gastric secretion in patients with duodenal ulcer. *Gut* 1966; 7: 612–18.

170 Truelove SC. Stilboestrol, phenobarbitone and diet in chronic duodenal ulcer. *Br Med J* 1960; ii: 559–66.

171 Baird RM. Peptic ulceration in pregnancy. Report of a case with perforation. *Can Med Assoc J* 1966; 94: 861–2.

172 Clark DH. Pregnancy and peptic ulcer in women. *Br Med J* 1953; i: 1254–7.

173 Crisp WE. Pregnancy complicating peptic ulcer. *Postgrad Med* 1960; 27: 445–7.

174 Langmade CF. Epigastric pain in pregnancy toxaemias. *West J Surg* 1956; 64: 540–4.

175 Peden NR, Boyd EJS *et al.* Women and duodenal ulcer. *Br Med J* 1981; 282: 866.

176 Jones PF, McEwan AB *et al.* Haemorrhage and perforation complicating peptic ulcer in pregnancy. *Lancet* 1969; iii: 350–1.

177 Aston NO, Kalaichandran S *et al.* Duodenal ulcer hemorrhage in the puerperium. *Can J Surg* 1991; 34: 482–3.

178 Parry GK. Perforated duodenal ulcer in the puerperium. *N Zeal Med J* 1974; 80: 448–9.

179 Lanciers S, Despinasse B *et al.* Increased susceptibility to *Helicobacter pylori* infection in pregnancy. *Inf Dis Obstet Gynecol* 1999; 7: 195–8.

180 Gold BD, Khanna B *et al.* *Helicobacter pylori* acquisition in infancy after decline of maternal passive immunity. *Pediatr Res* 1997; 41: 641–6.

181 Ippoliti AF, Elashoff J *et al.* Recurrent ulcer after successful treatment with cimetidine or antacid. *Gastroenterology* 1983; 85: 875–8.

182 Finkelstein W, Isselbacher KJ. Medical intelligence: drug therapy cimetidine. *N Engl J Med* 1978; 299: 992–6.

183 Langman MJ, Henry DA *et al.* Cimetidine and ranitidine in duodenal ulcer. *Br Med J* 1980; 281: 473–4.

184 Connon JJ. De Nol, an effective drug in the therapy of duodenal ulceration. *J Irish Med Assoc* 1977; 70: 206–7.

185 Poulantzas J, Polymeropoulos PS *et al.* Double- blind evaluation of the effect of tri-potassium di-citratobismuthate in peptic ulcer. *Br J Clin Pract* 1978; 32: 147–8.

186 *Drug and Therapeutics Bulletin. Helicobacter pylori* infection—when and how to treat. *Drug Ther Bull* 1993; 31: 13–15.

187 Monk JP, Clissold SP. Misoprostol. A preliminary review of its pharmacodynamic and pharmacokinetic properties, and therapeutic efficacy in the treatment of peptic ulcer disease. *Drugs* 1987; 33: 1–30.

188 Friedman D, Cuneo S *et al.* Pregnancy after surgical therapy for obesity. Bibliographic review and our experience with biliopancreatic diversion [Italian]. *Min Ginecol* 1996; 48: 333–44.

189 Wittgrove AC, Jester L *et al.* Pregnancy following gastric bypass for morbid obesity. *Obes Surg* 1998; 8: 461–4.

190 Seehra H, MacDermott N *et al.* Wernicke's encephalopathy after vertical banded gastroplasty for morbid obesity. *Br Med J* 1996; 312: 434.

191 Fazeny B, Marosi C. Gastric cancer as an essential differential diagnosis of minor epigastric discomfort during pregnancy. *Acta Obstet Gynecol Scand* 1998; 77: 469–71.

192 Ferrara R, Zago A *et al.* Gastric neoplasia in pregnancy: report of a case [Italian]. *Ann Ital Chir* 1998; 69: 665–7.

193 Tewari K, Asrat T *et al.* The evolution of linitis plastica as a consequence of advanced gastric carcinoma in pregnancy. *Am J Obstet Gynecol* 1999; 181: 757–8.

194 Auricchio S, Follo D *et al.* Does breast feeding protect against the development of clinical symptoms of celiac disease in children? *J Pediatr Gastroenterol* 1983; 2: 428–33.

195 Carter CO, Sheldon W *et al.* Coeliac disease. *Ann Hum Genet* 1959; 23: 266.

196 Borgfors N, Selander P. The incidence of coeliac disease in Sweden. *Acta Paediatr Scand* 1968; 57: 260.

197 Editorial. Coeliac disease. *Br Med J* 1970; 4: 1–2.

198 McCarthy CF, Mylotte M *et al.* Family studies on coeliac disease in Ireland. In: *Proceedings of the Second International Coeliac Symposium, Coeliac Disease.* 1974; Stenfert Kroese, Leiden.

199 Visakorpi JK, Immonen P *et al.* Malabsorption syndrome in childhood. The occurrence of absorption defects and their clinical significance. *Acta Pediatr Scand* 1967; 56: 1–9.

200 Mann JG, Brown WR *et al.* The subtle and variable clinical expressions of gluten-induced enteropathy (adult coeliac disease, nontropical sprue). An analysis of twenty-one consecutive cases. *Am J Med* 1970; 48: 357–66.

201 Falchuk ZM, Rogentine GN *et al.* Predominance of histocompatibility antigen HLA B8 in patients with gluten- sensitive enteropathy. *J Clin Invest* 1972; 51: 16025.

202 Mylotte MJ, Egan-Mitchell B *et al.* Familial coeliac disease. *Q J Med* 1972; 41: 527–8.

203 Ek B. Studies on idiopathic sprue. Familial incidence and relation to pregnancy and partial gastrectomy. *Acta Med Scand* 1969; 185: 463–4.

204 Anonymous. Case records of the Massachusetts General Hospital. Weekly clinicopathological excercises. Case 34–1999: a 37-year-old woman with liver disease and recurrent diarrhea. *N Eng J Med* 1999; 341: 1530–7.

205 Green PA, Wollaeger EE. The clinical behavior of sprue in the United States. *Gastroenterology* 1960; 38: 399–418.

206 Juergens JL, Scholz DA *et al.* Severe osteomalacia associated with occult steatorrhoea due to nontropical sprue. *Arch Int Med* 1956; 98: 774–82.

207 Collin P, Vilska S *et al.* Infertility and coeliac disease. *Gut* 1996; 39: 382–4.

208 Molteni N, Bardella MT *et al.* Obstetric and gynecological problems in women with untreated celiac sprue. *J Clin Gastroenterol* 1990; 12: 37–9.

209 Sher KS, Mayberry JF. Female fertility, obstetric and gynaecological history in coeliac disease: a case control study. *Acta Paediatr Supple* 1996; 412: 76–7.

210 Hall M, Davidson RJL. Prophylactic folic acid in women with pernicious anaemia pregnant after periods of infertility. *J Clin Pathol* 1968; 21: 599–602.

211 Farthing MJC, Rees LH *et al.* Male gonadal function in coeliac disease. II. Sex hormones. *Gut* 1983; 24: 127–35.

212 Stevens FM, Craig A. Prolactin and coeliac disease. *Irish J Med Sci* 1981; 150: 329–31.

213 Baker PG, Read AE. Reversible infertility in male coeliac patients. *Br Med J* 1975; ii: 316–17.

214 Ogborn ADR. Pregnancy in patients with coeliac disease. *Br J Obstet Gynaecol* 1975; 82: 293–6.

215 Smecuol E, Maurino E *et al.* Gynaecological and obstetric disorders in coeliac disease: frequent clinical onset during pregnancy or the puerperium. *Eur J Gastroenterol Hepatol* 1996; 8: 63–89.

216 Malnick SD, Atali M *et al.* Celiac sprue presenting during the puerperium: a report of three cases and a review of the literature. *J Clin Gastroenterol* 1998; 26: 164–6.

217 Mortimer PE, Stewart JS *et al.* Follow-up study of coeliac disease. *Br Med J* 1968; III: 7–9.

218 Ek B. Studies on idiopathic sprue. On the familiar incidence of idiopathic sprue and the significance of pregnancy and partial gastrectomy for the manifestation of the symptoms. *Acta Med Scand* 1967; 181: 125–6.

219 Brooks FP, Powell KC *et al.* Variable clinical course of adult celiac disease. *Arch Int Med* 1966; 117: 789–94.

220 Joske RA, Martin JD. Coeliac disease presenting as recurrent abortion. *J Obstet Gynaecol Br Commonw* 1971; 78: 754–8.

221 Martin JD, Davis RE. Serum folic acid activity and vaginal bleeding in early pregnancy. *J Obstet Gynaecol Br Commonw* 1964; 71: 400–3.

222 Ciacci C, Cirillo M *et al.* Celiac disease and pregnancy outcome. *Am J Gastroenterol* 1996; 91: 718–22.

223 Norgard B, Fonager K *et al.* Birth outcomes of women with celiac disease: a nationwide historical cohort study. *Am J Gastroenterol* 1999; 94: 2435–40.

224 Dickey W, Stewart F *et al.* Screening for coeliac disease as a possible maternal factor for neural tube defect. *Clin Genet* 1996; 49: 107–8.

225 Walker-Smith JA, Harrison M *et al.* Cow's milk-sensitive enteropathy. *Arch Dis Child* 1978; 53: 375–80.

226 Ament ME, Rubin CE. Soy protein—another cause of a flat intestinal lesion. *Gastroenterology* 1972; 62: 227–34.

227 Morris JS, Ajdukiewicz AB *et al.* Coeliac infertility: an indication for dietary gluten restriction? *Lancet* 1970; 1: 213–14.

228 Davis RE. Clinical chemistry of folic acid. *Adv Clin Chem* 1986; 25: 233–94.

229 Booth CC. The enterocyte in coeliac disease. *Br Med J* 1970; 4: 14–17.

230 Bohr J, Tysk C *et al.* Collagenous colitis: a retrospective study of clinical presentation and treatment in 163 patients. *Gut* 1996; 39: 846–51.

231 Kumar PJ. Reintroduction of gluten in adults and children with treated coeliac disease. *Gut* 1979; 20: 743–9.

232 Croese J. Coeliac disease. Haematological features and delay in diagnosis. *Med J Aust* 1979; 2: 335–8.

233 Swinson CM, Lavin GS *et al.* Coeliac disease and malignancy. *Lancet* 1983; i: 111–15.

234 Lindstrom CG. Collagenous colitis with watery diarrhea. New Entity? *Pathol Eur* 1976; 11: 87–9.

235 Sanghi A, Morgan-Capner P *et al.* Zoonotic and viral infection in fetal loss after 12 weeks. *Br J Obstet Gynaecol* 1997; 104: 942–5.

236 Grandien M, Sterner G *et al.* Management of pregnant women with diarrhoea at term and of healthy carriers of infectious agents in stools at delivery. *Scand J Infect Dis Supple* 1990; 71: 9–18.

237 Consensus Conference. Travelers diarrhea. NIH Consensus Conference. *J Am Med Assoc* 1985; 253: 2700–4.

238 Samuel BU, Barry M. The pregnant traveler. *Infect Dis Clin N Am* 1998; 12: 325–54.

239 Gorbach SL. Travelers' diarrhea. *N Engl J Med* 1982; 307: 881–3.

240 Alestig K, Trollfors B *et al.* Acute non-specific diarrhoea: studies on the use of charcoal, kaolin-pectin and diphenoxylate. *Practitioner* 1979; 222: 859–62.

241 Kahn SB, Fein SA *et al.* Effects of trimethoprim on folate metabolism in man. *Clin Pharmacol Ther* 1968; 9: 550–60.

242 Bushby SRM, Hitchings GH. Trimethoprim, a sulphonomide potentiator. *Br J Pharmacol* 1968; 33: 72–90.

243 Larson HE, Price AB. Pseudomembranous colitis: presence of clostridial toxin. *Lancet* 1977; 2: 1312–14.

244 McNeeley SG, Anderson GD *et al.* *Clostridium difficile* colitis associated with single-dose cefazolin prophylaxis. *Obstet Gynecol* 1985; 66: 737–8.

245 James AH, Katz VL *et al.* *Clostridium difficile* infection in obstetric and gynecologic patients. *S Med J* 1997; 90: 889–92.

246 Arsura EL, Fazio RA *et al.* Pseudomembranous colitis following prophylactic antibiotic use in Caesarian section. *Am J Obstet Gynecol* 1985; 151: 87–9.

247 Keighley MRB, Burdon DW *et al.* Randomised controlled trial of vancomycin for pseudomembranous colitis and post operative diarrhoea. *Br Med J* 1978; 2: 1667.

248 Stirrat GM, Beard RW. Drugs to be avoided or given with caution in the second or third trimesters of pregnancy. *Prescrib J* 1973; 13: 135–40.

249 Czeizel AE, Rockenbauer M. A population based case–control teratologic study of oral metronidazole treatment during pregnancy. *Br J Obstet Gynecol* 1998; 105: 322–7.

250 Shepherd RC, Sinha GP. Cryptosporidiosis in the West of Scotland. *Scot Med J* 1988; 33: 365–8.

251 Wong SN, Tam AY *et al.* *Campylobacter* infection in the neonate: a case report and review of the literature. *Pediatr Infect Dis J* 1990; 9: 665–9.

252 Simor AE, Ferro S. *Campylobacter jejuni* infection occurring during pregnancy. *Eur J Clin Microbiol Infect Dis* 1990; 9: 142–4.

253 Gribble MJ, Salit IE *et al.* *Campylobacter* infections in pregnancy. Case report and literature review. *Am J Obstet Gynecol* 1981; 140: 423–6.

254 Meyer A, Stallmach T *et al.* Lethal maternal sepsis caused by *Campylobacter jejuni*: pathogen preserved in placenta and identified by molecular methods. *Mod Pathol* 1997; 10: 1253–6.

255 Karmali MA, Tan YC. Neonatal *Campylobacter* enteritis. *Canad Med Assoc J* 1980; 122: 192–7.

256 Tabak MA, Hart MD *et al.* *Campylobacter* enteritis: prenatal and perinatal implications. *Am J Obstet Gynecol* 1983; 147: 845–6.

257 Vinzent R, Dumas J *et al.* Septicemie grave au couride la grossesse due a un vibrion avortement consecutif. *Bull Acad Nat Med (Paris)* 1947; 131: 90.

258 Blaser MJ, Berkowitz ID *et al.* *Campylobacter* enteritis: clinical and epidemiologic features. *Ann Int Med* 1979; 91: 179–85.

259 Gilbert GL, Davoren RA *et al.* Midtrimester abortion associated with septicaemia caused by *Campylobacter jejuni*. *Med J Aust* 1981; 1: 585–6.

260 Vesikari T, Huffunen L *et al*. Perinatal *Campylobacter fetus* ss. *jejuni* enteritis. *Acta Pediatr Scand* 1981; 70: 261–3.

261 Anders BJ, Lauer BA *et al*. *Campylobacter* gastroenteritis in neonates. *Am J Dis Child* 1981; 135: 900–2.

262 Jost PM, Galvin MC *et al*. *Campylobacter* septic abortion. *S Med J (Birmingham, Alabama)* 1984; 77: 924.

263 Farrell DJ, Harris MJ. A case of intrauterine fetal death associated with maternal *Campylobacter coli* bacteraemia. *Aust N Zeal J Obstet Gynaecol* 1992; 32: 172–7.

264 Pockros PJ, Weiss JB *et al*. Toxic megacolon complicating *Campylobacter* enterocolitis (letter). *J Clin Gastroenterol* 1986; 8: 318–19.

265 McCormack WM, George H *et al*. Hepatotoxicity of erythromycin estolate during pregnancy. *Antimicrob Ag Chemother* 1977; 12: 630–5.

266 Butzler JP, Skirrow MB. *Campylobacter* enteritis. *Clin Gastroenterol* 1979; 8: 737–65.

267 Diddle AW, Stephens RL. Typhoid fever in pregnancy. Probable intrauterine transmission of the disease. *Am J Obstet Gynecol* 1939; 38: 300–5.

268 Freedman ML, Christopher P *et al*. Typhoid carriage in pregnancy with infection of neonate. *Lancet* 1970; i: 310–11.

269 Ruderman JW, Stroller KP *et al*. Bloodstream invasion with *Shigella sonnei* in an asymptomatic newborn infant. *Pediatr Infect Dis* 1986; 5: 379–80.

270 Pillay N, Adams EB *et al*. Comparative trial of amoxycillin and chloramphenicol in treatment of typhoid fever in adults. *Lancet* 1975; 2: 333–4.

271 Mandal BK Modern treatment of typhoid fever (Editorial). *J Infect* 1991; 22: 1–4.

272 Sterner G, Granstrom G *et al*. Management of pregnant women with contagious infections at delivery. *Scand J Infect Dis* 1988; 20: 463–73.

273 D'Alauro F, Lee RV *et al*. Intestinal parasites and pregnancy. *Obstet Gynecol* 1985; 66: 639–43.

274 Roberts NS, Copel JA *et al*. Intestinal parasites and other infections during pregnancy in Southeast Asian refugees. *J Reprod Med* 1985; 30: 720–5.

275 Villar J, Klebanoff M *et al*. The effect on fetal growth of protozoan and helminthic infection during pregnancy. *Obstet Gynecol* 1989; 74: 915–20.

276 Navitsky RC, Dreyfuss ML *et al*. *Ancylostoma duodenale* is responsible for hookworm infections among pregnant women in the rural plains of Nepal. *J Parasitol* 1998; 84: 647–51.

277 Roche J, Benito A. Prevalence of intestinal parasite infections with special reference to *Entamoeba histolytica* on the island of Bioko (Equatorial Guinea). *Am J Trop Med Hyg* 1999; 60: 257–62.

278 Pawlowski ZS. Intestinal helminthiases. *Med Int* 1992; 108: 4535–42.

279 Bialek R, Knobloch J. Parasitic infections in pregnancy and congenital protozoan infections. Part I. Protozoan infections. *Zeitschr Geburt Neonatol* 1999; 203: 55–62.

280 Bialek R, Knobloch J. Parasitic infections in pregnancy and congenital parasitoses. Part II. Helminth infections. *Zeitschr Geburt Neonatol* 1999; 203: 128–33.

281 de Silva NR, Sirisena JL *et al*. Effect of mebendazole therapy during pregnancy on birth. *Lancet* 1999; 353: 1145–9.

282 Obata NH, Kurauchi O *et al*. Preeclampsia with fetal death in a patient with schistosomiasis japonica. *Arch Gynecol Obstet* 1998; 261: 101–4.

283 Nouhou H, Seve B *et al*. Schistosomiasis of the female genital tract: anatomoclinical and histopathological aspects. Apropos of 26 cases [French]. *Bull Soc Pathol Exot* 1998; 91: 221–3.

284 Lyche KD, Jensen WA. Pleuropulmonary amebiasis. *Sem Respir Infect* 1997; 12: 106–12.

285 Islam A, Stoll BJ *et al*. The prevalence of *Entamoeba histolytica* in lactating women and in their infants in Bangladesh. *Trans Roy Soc Trop Med Hyg* 1988; 82: 99–103.

286 Li E, Stanley SL. Protozoa. Amebiasis. *Gastroenterol Clin N Am* 1996; 25: 471–92.

287 Lawson JB, Stewart DB, eds. *Obstetrics and Gynaecology in the Tropics*. 1967; Edward Arnold, London, 52–9.

288 Wig JD, Bushnurmath SR *et al*. Complications of amoebiasis in pregnancy and puerperium. *Ind J Gastroenterol* 1984; 3: 37–8.

289 Gillon FD, Reiner DS *et al*. Human milk kills intestinal protozoa. *Science* 1983; 221: 1290–2.

290 Cantu JM, Garcia-Cruz D. Midline facial defect as a teratogenic effect of metronidazole. *Birth Defects* 1982; 18: 85–8.

291 Prakash C, Bansal BC *et al*. A comparative study of tinidazole and metronidazole in symptomatic intestinal amoebiasis. *J Assoc Phys India* 1974; 22: 527–9.

292 Beeley L. Adverse effects of drugs in later pregnancy. In: Wood SM, Beeley L, eds. *Prescribing in Pregnancy. Clin Obstet Gynaecol* 1981; WB Saunders, London: 281–90.

293 Sealy DP, Shuman SH. Endemic giardiasis and day-care. *Pediatrics* 1983; 72: 154–8.

294 Stevens DP. Selective primary health care: strategies for control of disease in the developing world. XIX. Giardiasis. *Rev Infect Dis* 1985; 7: 530–5.

295 Cameron DW, Japour AJ *et al*. Ritonavir and saquinavir combination therapy for the treatment of HIV infection. *AIDS* 1999; 13: 213–24.

296 Kotler DP. HIV in pregnancy. *Gastroenterol Clin N Am* 1998; 27: 269–80.

297 Korelitz BI. Inflammatory bowel disease and pregnancy. *Gastroenterol Clin N Am* 1998; 27: 213–24.

298 Kirsner JB, Shorter RG. Recent developments in nonspecific inflammatory bowel disease (second of two parts). *N Engl J Med* 1982; 306: 837–48.

299 Segal I, Tim LO *et al*. The rarity of ulcerative colitis in South African blacks. *Am J Gastroenterol* 1980; 74: 332–36.

300 Brahme F, Lindstrom C *et al*. Crohn's disease in a defined population. An epidemiological study of incidence, prevalence, mortality and secular trends in the city of Molmo, Sweden. *Gastroenterology* 1975; 69: 342–51.

301 Niv Y, Abukasis G. Prevalence of ulcerative colitis in the Israeli kibbutz population. *J Clin Gastroenterol* 1991; 13: 98–101.

302 Van Kruiningen HJ, Colubel JF *et al*. An in depth study of Crohn's disease in two French families. *Gastroenterology* 1993; 104: 351–60.

303 De Dombal FT, Watts JM *et al*. Ulcerative colitis and pregnancy. *Lancet* 1965; 2: 599–602.

304 Fielding JF, Cooke WT. Pregnancy and Crohn's disease. *Br Med J* 1970; 2: 76–7.

305 De Dombal FT, Burton IL *et al*. Crohn's disease and pregnancy. *Br Med J* 1972; 3: 550–3.

306 Homan WP, Thorbjarnarson NB. Crohn's disease and pregnancy. *Arch Surg* 1976; 111: 545–7.

307 Miller JP. Inflammatory bowel disease in pregnancy: a review. *J Roy Soc Med* 1986; 79: 221–5.

308 Gruner O-PN, Naas R *et al*. Marital status and sexual adjustment after colectomy. *Scand J Gastroenterol* 1977; 12: 193–7.

309 Gazzard BG, Price HL *et al*. The social toll of Crohn's disease. *Br Med J* 1978; 2: 1117–19.

310 Meyers S, Walfish JS *et al*. Quality of life after surgery for Crohn's disease: a psychosocial survey. *Gastroenterology* 1980; 78: 1–6.

311 Hudson M, Flett G *et al*. Fertility and pregnancy in inflammatory bowel disease. *Int J Gynaecol Obstet* 1997; 58: 229–37.

312 Crohn BB, Yarnis H *et al*. Ulcerative colitis and pregnancy. *Gastroenterology* 1956; 30: 391–403.

313 Korelitz BI. Pregnancy, fertility and inflammatory bowel disease. *Am J Gastroenterol* 1985; 80: 365–70.

314 Willoughby CP, Truelove SC. Ulcerative colitis and pregnancy. *Gut* 1980; 21: 469–74.

315 Khosla R, Willoughby CP. Crohn's disease and pregnancy. *Gut* 1984; 25: 52–6.

316 Templeton A, Fraser C *et al*. The epidemiology of infertility in Aberdeen. *Br Med J* 1990; 301: 148–52.

317 Mayberry JF, Weterman IT. European survey of fertility and pregnancy in women with Crohn's disease: a case control study by the European Collaborative Group. *Gut* 1986; 27: 821–25.

318 O'Morain C, Smethurst P *et al*. Reversible male infertility due to sulphasalazine: studies in man and rat. *Gut* 1984; 25: 1078–84.

319 Cann PA, Holdsworth CD. Reversal of male infertility on changing treatment from sulphasalazine to 5 aminosalicylic acid. *Lancet* 1984; i: 1119.

320 Shaffer JL, Kershaw A *et al*. Sulphasalazine- induced infertility reversed on transfer to 5 aminosalcylic acid. *Lancet* 1984; 1: 1240.

321 McClain C, Soutor C *et al*. Zinc deficiency: a complication of Crohn's disease. *Gastroenterology* 1980; 78: 272–9.

322 Kornfeld D, Cnattingius S *et al*. Pregnancy outcomes in women with inflammatory bowel disease—a population-based cohort study. *Am J Obstet Gynecol* 1997; 177: 942–6.

323 Diav-Citrin O, Park YH *et al*. The safety of mesalamine in human pregnancy: a prospective controlled cohort study. *Gastroenterology* 1998; 114: 23–8.

324 Fonager K, Sorensen HT *et al*. Pregnancy outcome for women with Crohn's disease: a follow-up study based on linkage between national registries. *Am J Gastroenterol* 1998; 93: 2426–30.

325 Marteau P, Tennenbaum R *et al*. Foetal outcome in women with inflammatory bowel disease treated during pregnancy with oral mesalazine microgranules. *Aliment Pharmacol Ther* 1998; 12: 1101–8.

326 Tennenbaum R, Marteau P *et al*. Pregnancy outcome in inflammatory bowel diseases [French]. *Gastroenterol Clin Biol* 1999; 23: 464–9.

327 Sachar D. Exposure to mesalamine during pregnancy increased preterm deliveries (but not birth defects) and decreased birth weight. *Gut* 1998; 43: 316.

328 Martinbeau PN, Welch JS *et al*. Crohn's disease and pregnancy. *Am J Obstet Gynecol* 1975; 122: 746–9.

329 Barnes CS, Hayes HM. Ulcerative colitis complicating pregnancy and the puerperium. *Am J Obstet Gynecol* 1931; 22: 907–12.

330 Tumen HJ, Cohn EM. Pregnancy and chronic ulcerative colitis. *Gastroenterology* 1950; 16: 1–11.

331 Abramson D, Jankelson IR *et al*. Pregnancy in idiopathic ulcerative colitis. *Am J Obstet Gynecol* 1951; 61: 121–9.

332 Crohn BB, Yarnis H *et al*. Regional ileitis complicating pregnancy. *Gastroenterology* 1956; 31: 615–28.

333 Nielsen OH, Andreasson B *et al*. Pregnancy in ulcerative colitis. *Scand J Gastroenterol* 1983; 18: 735–42.

334 Kane SV, Sable K *et al*. The menstrual cycle and its effect on inflammatory bowel disease and irritable bowel syndrome: a prevalence study. *Am J Gastroenterol* 1998; 93: 1867–72.

335 Steadman UA, Brennan TE *et al*. Pyoderma gangrenosum following cesarian section. *Obstet Gynecol* 1998; 91: 834–6.

336 Futami H, Kodaira M *et al*. Pyoderma gangrenosum complicating ulcerative colitis: successful treatment with methylprednisolone and cyclosporine. *J Gastroenterol* 1998; 33: 408–11.

337 Subhani JM, Hamilton MI. Review article: the management of inflammatory bowel disease during pregnancy. *Aliment Pharmacol Ther* 1998; 12: 1039–53.

338 Connell W, Miller A. Treating inflammatory bowel disease during pregnancy: risks and safety of drug therapy. *Drug Saf* 1999; 21: 311–23.

339 Helzer JE, Chammas S *et al*. A study of the association between Crohn's disease and psychiatric illness. *Gastroenterology* 1984; 86: 324–30.

340 Campieri M, Lanfranchi GA *et al*. Treatment of ulcerative colitis with high-dose 5 aminosalicylic acid enemas. *Lancet* 1981; 2: 270–1.

341 Peppercorn MA. Sulphasalazine. Pharmacology, clinical use, toxicity and related new drug development. *Ann Int Med* 1984; 101: 377–86.

342 Marion JF. Toxicity of 6-mercaptopurine/azathioprine in patients with inflammatory bowel disease. *Inflamm Bowel Dis* 1998; 4: 116–7.

343 Azad Khan AK, Truelove SC. Placental and mammary transfer of sulphasalazine. *Br Med J* 1979; 2: 1553.

344 Baiocco PJ, Korelitz BI. The influence of inflammatory bowel disease and its treatment on pregnancy and fetal outcome. *J Clin Gastroenterol* 1984; 6: 211–16.

345 Hensleigh PA, Kauffman RE. Maternal absorption and placental transfer of sulphasalazine. *Am J Obstet Gynecol* 1977; 127: 443–4.

346 Mogadam M, Dobbins WO *et al*. Pregnancy in inflammatory bowel disease: effect of sulphasalazine and corticosteroids on fetal outcome. *Gastroenterology* 1981; 80: 72–6.

347 Vender RJ, Spiro HM. Inflammatory bowel disease and pregnancy. *J Clin Gastroenterol* 1982; 4: 231–49.

348 Fagan EA, Chadwick VS. Drug treatment of gastrointestinal disorders in pregnancy. In: Lewis P, ed. *Clinical Pharmacology in Obstetrics*. 1983; Wright PSG, Bristol: 114–37.

349 Godding EW. Constipation and allied disorders. *Pharm J* 1976; 5: 17.

350 Kirsner JB, Shorter RG. Recent developments in 'non-specific' inflammatory bowel disease (first of two parts). *N Eng J Med* 1982; 306: 775–85.

351 Cooksey G, Gunn A *et al*. Case report. Surgery for acute ulcerative colitis and toxic megacolon during pregnancy. *Br J Surg* 1985; 72: 547.

352 Katz S, Schulman N *et al*. Free perforation in Crohn's disease: a report of 33 cases and review of literature. *Am J Gastroenterol* 1986; 81: 38–43.

353 McEwen HP. Ulcerative colitis in pregnancy. *Proc Roy Soc Med* 1972; 65: 279–81.

354 Cosnes J, Hecketsweiler P *et al*. Consequences of extensive bowel resections in Crohn's disease: a study of 53 cases. *Gastroenterol Clin Biol (Paris)* 1981; 5: 198–206.

355 Griffin GE, Fagan EA *et al*. Enteral therapy in the management of massive gut resection complicated by chronic fluid and electrolyte depletion. *Dig Dis Sci* 1982; 27: 902–8.

356 Hudson CN. Ileostomy in pregnancy. *Proc Roy Soc Med* 1972; 62: 281–3.

357 Barwin BN, Hartley JMG. Ileostomy and pregnancy. *Br J Clin Prac* 1974; 28: 256–8.

358 Davis MR, Bohon CJ. Intestinal obstruction in pregnancy. *Clin Obstet Gynecol* 1983; 26: 832–42.

359 Morowitz DA, Kirsner JB. Ileostomy in ulcerative colitis: a questionnaire study of 1803 patients. *Am J Sur* 1981; 141: 370–5.

360 Metcalf A, Dozois RR *et al.* Pregnancy following ileal pouchanal anastomosis. *Dis Col Rectum* 1985; 28: 859–61.

361 Scott HJ, McLeod RS *et al.* Ileal pouch-anal anastomosis: pregnancy, delivery and pouch function. *Int J Colorectal Dis* 1996; 11: 57–60.

362 Andersen B, Nielsen TF. Appendicitis in pregnancy: diagnosis, management and complications. *Acta Obstet Gynecol Scand* 1999; 78: 758–62.

363 Mahmoodian S. Appendicitis complicating pregnancy. *S Med J* 1992; 85: 19–24.

364 Retzke U, Graf H *et al.* Appendicitis in pregnancy [German]. *Zentr Chir* 1998; 123 (Suppl. 4): 61–5.

365 Hee P, Viktrup L. The diagnosis of appendicitis during pregnancy and maternal and fetal outcome after appendectomy. *Int J Obstet Gynaecol* 1999; 65: 129–35.

366 Bozoklu S, Bozoklu E *et al.* Ruptured ectopic pregnancy with undetectable beta-hCG levels coexisting with acute appendicitis. *Acta Obstet Gynecol Scand* 1997; 76: 181–2.

367 Barnett A, Chipchase J *et al.* Simultaneous rupturing heterotopic pregnancy and acute appendicitis in an in-vitro fertilization twin pregnancy. *Hum Reprod* 1999; 14: 850–1.

368 Grimes DA. Spontaneous perforation of the gallbladder from cholecystitis with acute appendicitis in pregnancy. A case report. *J Reprod Med* 1996; 41: 450–2.

369 Schwerk WB, Wichtrup B *et al.* Ultrasonography in the diagnosis of acute appendicitis: a prospective study. *Gastroenterology* 1989; 97: 630–9.

370 Coleman MT, Trianfo VA *et al.* Nonobstetric emergencies in pregnancy: trauma and surgical conditions. *Am J Obstet Gynecol* 1997; 177: 497–502.

371 Thomas SJ, Brisson P. Laparoscopic appendectomy and cholecystectomy during pregnancy: six case reports. *J Soc Laparoendosc Surg* 1998; 2: 41–6.

372 Firstenberg MS, Malangoni MA. Gastrointestinal surgery during pregnancy. *Gastroenterol Clin N Am* 1998; 27: 73–88.

373 Lopez Carral JM, Esen UI *et al.* Volvulus of the right colon in pregnancy. *Int J Clin Pract* 1998; 52: 270–1.

374 Montes H, Wolf J. Cecal volvulus in pregnancy. *Am J Gastroenterol* 1999; 94: 2554–6.

375 Ventura–Braswell AM, Satin AJ, Higby K. Delayed diagnosis of bowel infarction secondary to maternal midgut volvulus at term. *Obstet Gynecol* 1998; 91: 808–10.

376 Report on Confidential Enquiries. *Report on Confidential Enquiries into Maternal Deaths in the United Kingdom 1991–1993.* HMSO, London, 1996: 1–205.

377 Damore LJ, Damore TH *et al.* Congenital intestinal malrotation causing gestational intestinal obstruction. A case report. *J Reprod Med* 1997; 42: 805–8.

378 Kurzel RB, Naunheim KS *et al.* Repair of symptomatic diaphragmatic hernia during pregnancy. *Obstet Gynecol* 1988; 71: 869–71.

379 Olow B, Akesson BA *et al.* Pregnancy after jejuno-ileostomy because of obesity. *Acta Chir Scand* 1976; 142: 82–6.

380 Martelli H, Duguay C *et al.* Some parameters of large bowel motility in normal man. *Gastroenterology* 1978; 75: 612–18.

381 Sarna SK. Physiology and pathophysiology of colonic motor activity (Part 2 of 2). *Dig Dis Sci* 1991; 36: 998–1018.

382 Heaton KW, Radvan J *et al.* Defecation frequency and timing, and stool form in the general population: a prospective study. *Gut* 1992; 33: 818–24.

383 Drossman DA. Characterization of intestinal function and diagnosis of irritable bowel syndrome by surveys and questionnaires [French]. *Gastroenterol Clin Biol* 1990; 14: 37C–41C.

384 Bonapace ES, Fisher RS. Constipation and diarrhea in pregnancy. *Gastroenterol Clin N Am* 1998; 27: 197–211.

385 Levy N, Lemberg E *et al.* Bowel habit in pregnancy. *Digestion* 1971; 4: 216–22.

386 Marshall K, Thompson KA *et al.* Incidence of urinary incontinence and constipation during pregnancy and postpartum: a survey of current findings at the Rotunda Lying-In Hospital. *Br J Obstet Gynaecol* 1998; 105: 400–2.

387 Corby H, Donnelly VS *et al.* Anal canal pressures are low in women with postpartum anal fissure. *Br J Surg* 1997; 84: 86–8.

388 Parry E, Shields R *et al.* Transit time in the small intestine in pregnancy. *J Obstet Gynaecol Br Commonw* 1970; 77: 900–1.

389 Parry E, Shields R *et al.* The effect of pregnancy on the colonic absorption of sodium, potassium and water. *J Obstet Gynaecol Br Commonw* 1970; 77: 616–19.

390 Wald A, Van Thiel DH *et al.* Gastrointestinal transit: the effect of the menstrual cycle. *Gastroenterology* 1981; 80: 1497–500.

391 Heaton KW, Emmett PM *et al.* An explanation for gallstones in normal-weight women: slow intestinal transit. *Lancet* 1993; 341: 8–10.

392 Anderson AS, Whichelow M. Constipation during pregnancy: dietary fibre intakes and the effect of fibre supplementation. *Hum Nutr Appl Nutr* 1985; 39A: 202–7.

393 Anderson AS. Dietary factors in the aetiology and treatment of constipation during pregnancy. *Br J Obstet Gynaecol* 1986; 93: 245–9.

394 Preston DM, Lennard-Jones JE. Severe chronic constipation of young women: 'idiopathic slow-transit constipation'. *Gut* 1986; 27: 41–8.

395 MacDonald A, Baxter JN *et al.* Gastric emptying in patients with constipation following childbirth is due to idiopathic slow transit. *Br J Surg* 1997; 84: 1141–3.

396 Godding EW. Constipation and allied disorders. *Pharm J* 1976; 2: 8.

397 Sichel MS. Postpartum and postoperative bowel function. *Northwest Med* 1961; 60: 708–9.

398 Shelton MG. Standardized senna in the management of constipation in the puerperium: a clinical trial. *S Afr Med J* 1980; 57: 78–80.

399 Baldwin WF. Drugs in pregnancy. Senna—clinical study of senna administered to nursing mothers: assessment of effects on infant bowel habits. *Canad Med Assoc J* 1963; 89: 566–8.

400 Werthmann MW, Krees SV. Quantitative excretion of Senokot in human breast milk. *Med Ann Distr Columbia* 1973; 42: 4–5.

401 Sweeney WJ. Use of bisacodyl suppositories as a routine laxative in post partum patients. *Am J Obstet Gynecol* 1963; 85: 908–11.

402 Whorwell PJ. Irritable bowel syndrome. *Prescrib J* 1992; 32: 152–6.

403 Snape WJ, Carlson GM *et al.* Colonic myometric activity in the irritable bowel syndrome. *Gastroenterology* 1976; 70: 326–30.

404 Toglia MR. Pathophysiology of anorectal dysfunction. *Obstet Gynecol Clin N Am* 1998; 25: 771–81.

405 Wikland M, Jansson I *et al.* Gynaecological problems related to anatomical changes after conventional proctocolectomy and ileostomy. *Int J Colorect Dis* 1990; 5: 49–52.

406 Atkinson RE, Hudson CH. Ano-rectal and perineal disorders of pregnancy and the puerperium. *Practitioner* 1970; 205: 789–90.

407 Gallagher DM. Pruritus ani. *Mod Treat* 1971; 8: 963–70.

408 Saleeby RG, Rosen L *et al.* Hemorrhoidectomy during pregnancy: risk or relief? *Dis Colon Rectum* 1991; 34: 260–1.

409 Thomson H. Piles: their nature and management. *Lancet* 1975; 2: 494–5.

410 Thulesius O, Gjores JE. Arterio-venous anastomoses in the anal region with reference to the pathogenesis and treatment of haemorrhoids. *Acta Chir Scand* 1973; 139: 476–8.

411 Venkatesh KS, Ramanujam PS *et al.* Anorectal complications of vaginal delivery. *Dis Colon Rectum* 1989; 32: 1039–41.

412 Signorello LB, Harlow BL *et al.* Midline episiotomy and anal incontinence: retrospective cohort study. *Br Med J* 2000; 320: 86–90.

413 Fleshman JW, Dreznik Z *et al.* Anal sphincter repair for obstetric injury: manometric evaluation of functional results. *Dis Colon Rectum* 1991; 34: 1061–7.

414 Nielsen MB, Hauge C *et al.* Anal endosonographic findings in the follow-up of primarily sutured sphincteric ruptures. *Br J Surg* 1992; 79: 104–6.

415 Grant A, Sleep J *et al.* Ultrasound and pulsed electromagnetic energy treatment for perineal trauma. A randomized placebo-controlled trial. *Br J Obstet Gynaecol* 1989; 96: 434–9.

416 Meisels A, Morin C. Human papillomavirus and cancer of the uterine cervix. *Gynecol Oncol* 1981; 12: 5111.

417 Munger K, Scheffner M *et al.* Interactions of HPV E6 and E7 oncoproteins with tumour suppressor gene products. *Cancer Surv* 1992; 12: 197–217.

418 Lynch PJ. Condylomata acuminata (anogenital warts). *Clin Obstet Gynecol* 1985; 28: 142–51.

419 Walsh C, Fazio VW. Cancer of the colon, rectum and anus during pregnancy. The surgeon's perspective. *Gastroenterol Clin N Am* 1998; 27: 257–67.

11 Diabetes

Michael Maresh

Management of the pregnant woman with diabetes continues to present a challenge to the physician, obstetrician and other specialists involved in their care. Before insulin was available, those women with type I diabetes that survived to the age of reproduction and were able to become pregnant had less than a 50% chance of having a living child. Today, maternal mortality is rare with only about one woman a year in the UK dying in pregnancy in association with diabetes [1,2]. However, fetal and neonatal morbidity and mortality remains much higher than in the general population. This is unacceptable and at St Vincent in 1989 the World Health Organization (WHO) and the International Diabetes Federation listed a number of targets for Europe. One was 'to achieve pregnancy outcomes in women with diabetes that approximate to those in women without diabetes' [3]. This has been endorsed by successive governments in the UK [4].

It is widely accepted that if a diabetic woman can achieve normoglycaemia then the resulting normal metabolic environment in which the fetus develops should result in a near normal pregnancy outcome and reduce the current excess of congenital malformations and unexplained fetal death *in utero* [5,6]. But there is still a high degree of morbidity in the neonate, including macrosomia, and the long-term significance of some of these unfavourable outcomes is uncertain. Now that the evidence base is much clearer, all who care for women with diabetes who want children should be informed of how good outcomes can be achieved and should be striving to introduce these practices.

While the evidence is relatively clear for pregnant women with type I (insulin-dependent) diabetes mellitus there are much fewer data for women with type II (non-insulin-dependent) diabetes mellitus, but similarly poor outcomes do appear to be common in the latter group. With regard to gestational diabetes and impaired glucose tolerance much has been written, but the subject remains controversial. It is important to clarify the sometimes confusing terminology that is used.

Terminology and definitions

Diabetes

There is even confusion with regard to the definition of diabetes itself. The WHO definition, agreed in 1980 [7] is based on the 75-g oral glucose tolerance test (GTT). Diabetes is defined if the fasting blood glucose concentration is ≥7.8 mmol/L and 2-h value is ≥11.1 mmol/L. However, it is recognized that these two thresholds are not equivalent in terms of the risk of complications. Recent proposals by the American Diabetes Association [8], which are similar to those proposed in a WHO consultative document [9], recommend lowering the fasting threshold to ≥7.0 mmol/L. This lowering of the threshold will be welcomed by those caring for pregnant women as fasting glucose values in pregnancy of >7.0 mmol/L cause concern.

Women who are known to have diabetes prior to pregnancy are often referred to in the pregnancy literature as having established diabetes or pregestational diabetes. The former term is preferable because of the confusion surrounding the term gestational (see below). The vast majority of these women will have type I (insulin-dependent) diabetes, the remainder having type II (non-insulin-dependent) diabetes. There is also a subclassification into the various 'White' groups, where diabetes is graded from A to F/R according to the severity. This is judged by the age of onset, duration and the presence or absence of complications of the disease [10,11]. In pregnancy women are usually classified as either having vascular complications (group F and R) or not having them (group B, C and D).

Gestational diabetes mellitus and impaired glucose tolerance

Gestational diabetes is a term which is widely used, but not in a consistent manner. It should describe women who are found during pregnancy to have a GTT that meets the thresholds for diagnosing diabetes (see above). The same criteria should be used as in the non-pregnant state. A number of these women will have had undiagnosed diabetes before pregnancy.

The confusion has arisen around the term impaired glucose tolerance. This is defined using WHO criteria [7] as occurring in those having a 2-h GTT glucose concentration of between 8 and 11 mmol/L with a normal fasting value. Whether women with glucose tolerance in this range are at increased risk for perinatal problems is controversial (see below). If the GTT shows only impaired glucose tolerance then the term gestational impaired glucose tolerance [12] should be used and *not* gestational diabetes as is often done. Unfortunately, in the USA the term gestational diabetes is used to include both women with gestational diabetes and those with impaired glucose tolerance [13].

Physiology and pathophysiology

Pregnancy by itself induces profound metabolic alterations in all women, regardless of whether or not they have diabetes. These tend to become more marked with advancing gestational age. It seems likely that the changes are adaptive, ensuring an optimal environment for fetal growth and development. Knowledge of these changes is essential if an understanding of the principles of care of the diabetic mother and her baby is to be achieved.

Maternal glucose homeostasis

Figure 11.1 shows the remarkably stable concentration of plasma glucose that is maintained by the normal mother over a 24-h period. Both in early and late pregnancy the glucose concentration stays constant between 4.0 and 4.5 mmol/L, except after meals. This degree of homeostasis can only maintained by doubling the secretion of insulin from the end of the first to the third trimester of pregnancy. In general, the relative normality or otherwise of a diurnal profile is reflected by the GTT. It is generally agreed that glucose tolerance worsens as normal pregnancy advances. Longitudinal studies have shown glucose concentrations to be increased postprandially and decreased with fasting with increasing gestation. Insulin resistance increases in pregnancy, although the aetiology remains uncertain. Studies of insulin receptor binding in normal pregnancy have been conflicting, but Kuhl [14] reviewing the data, concluded that the pregnancy induced insulin resistance was likely to be a postreceptor defect.

The effect is likely to be mediated by the increased production of one or more of the pregnancy-associated hormones or of free cortisol which is also elevated in pregnancy. Changes in insulin activity result in other effects on intermediary metabolism. Withholding food from pregnant women results in a much earlier recourse to breakdown of triglyceride, leading to increased concentration of circulatory free fatty acids and ketone bodies, originally described by Freinkel [15] as 'accelerated starvation'.

Abnormalities of maternal glucose homeostasis

Both β-cell insufficiency and an increase in insulin resistance may contribute to the development of gestational

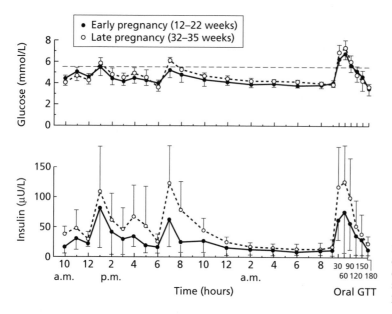

Fig 11.1 Plasma glucose and insulin concentrations over a 24-h period and during an oral glucose tolerance test (GTT) in nine women studied in early and late pregnancy [16]. Figures are mean ± SD.

impaired glucose tolerance and gestational diabetes. Those with severe β-cell insufficiency will not be able to increase their insulin secretion adequately, and will tend to show hyperglycaemia and hypo- or normo-insulinaemia [16]. Other studies of abnormal glucose tolerance [17,18] have shown women to have a more heterogeneous picture ranging from hypo- to hyperinsulinaemia. Those with a normal or increased plasma insulin concentration are likely to have a marked increase in peripheral resistance to insulin, which results in hyperglycaemia.

A further cause of abnormal glucose homeostasis in pregnancy occurs when pregnancy intervenes in the prodromal stage of insulin-dependent diabetes. This has been estimated to occur about once in 8000 deliveries [19]. The decrease in insulin activity in gestational diabetes and impaired glucose tolerance is associated with changes in more than just glucose levels. The concentrations of glycerol, free fatty acids, ketone bodies, and branched chain amino acids have all been found to be elevated in untreated women [17,18,20].

The established diabetic woman who has had the disease for some years before becoming pregnant usually has complete loss of endogenous insulin secretion as determined by plasma C-peptide concentration. The use of measurable C peptide could be used as an additional subclassification in insulin-dependent diabetes.

Fetal glucose homeostasis

The plasma glucose concentration of the fetus follows that of the mother closely, with the normal maternal–fetal difference in glucose concentration being about 0.5 mmol/L in favour of the mother. Oakley *et al.* [21] showed that, with an increase in glucose concentration in the mother, the maternal–fetal difference increases until the system of 'facilitated diffusion' by which glucose crosses the placenta, appears to be saturated at a maternal value of about 11–13 mmol/L. After this, despite a considerable increase in maternal hyperglycaemia, it is not possible to increase the concentration in the fetus further. This phenomenon is present in diabetic as well as nondiabetic mothers and can be viewed as a protective mechanism for the fetus to avoid the damaging effects of severe hyperglycaemia. Subsequent data obtained by cordocentesis at term has confirmed this close relationship [22].

Insulin appears in the fetal circulation as early as 10–12 weeks' gestational age. Fetal insulin concentrations in diabetic pregnancy have been shown to be elevated by the second trimester in samples obtained through cordocentesis but no relationship was demonstrated between fetal glucose and C-peptide concentrations. However, in the third trimester there is a relationship [22]. There is agreement that insulin does not cross the placenta at physiological concentrations. The β-cell pancreatic response of the fetus to a maternal glucose infusion is sluggish [21,23], and in the fetus of the non-diabetic mother it plays no part in the regulation of glucose homeostasis, its role being more likely as a growth-promoting hormone. Figure 11.2 compares the difference between the maternal and fetal glucose and insulin responses to a glucose load in a non-diabetic and a diabetic woman. The difference in the maternal fetal glucose concentration increases as the

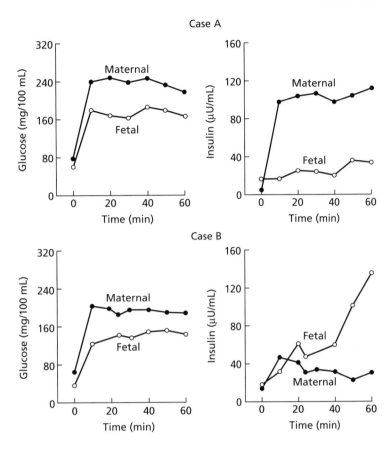

Fig 11.2 Examples of glucose and insulin response following 60 min of glucose infusion in a non-diabetic (case A) and a gestational diabetic (case B) (for conversion of glucose to mmol/L divide by 18) [21].

mother becomes more hyperglycaemic. This effect is the same for the diabetic as for the non-diabetic woman. The brisk fetal insulin response in the diabetic woman is in marked contrast to the sluggish response in the fetus of the non-diabetic mother. The fetus can also secrete insulin from the pancreas in response to amino acids [24].

Observations such as these have led to the acceptance of the 'hyperglycaemic–hyperinsulinism' theory of Pedersen [25]. Stated simply, this proposes that the fetal hyperglycaemia resulting from maternal hyperglycaemia stimulates fetal pancreatic β-cell hypertrophy resulting in an inappropriate release of insulin. This theory is accepted as it convincingly explains the aetiology of much of the fetal and neonatal pathology found in diabetic pregnancy. An expanded hypothesis is shown in Fig. 11.3. These observations are of particular clinical significance because they point to the possibility that normalization of the glucose environment of the fetus of the diabetic mother will diminish the tendency to hyperinsulinaemia and hence lead to a diminution of many perinatal problems.

Van Assche and Aerts [26] demonstrated that if growth is restricted *in utero* as indicated by being born light for gestational age, then the fetus will have fewer β cells. In later life other studies have shown that if adults who were light at birth then become overweight, they will have increased insulin resistance and are more likely to develop impaired glucose tolerance or type II diabetes than their counterparts who were of average birthweight [27]. Other subsequent research, for example the Dutch famine study, has supported these findings [28]. Thus, *in utero* effects on the fetal pancreas may have profound long-term effects.

Fetal haematology

Studies of cord blood at delivery have reported increased erythropoietin and haemoglobin concentrations in infants born to mothers with diabetes [29] with a suggested relationship to maternal glucose control [30]. Antenatal cordocentesis data have confirmed that the incidence of fetal polycythaemia is increased and that this relates to maternal diabetic control [31]. However, the cordocentesis data did not show that the concentrations of erythropoietin in the fetus related to maternal

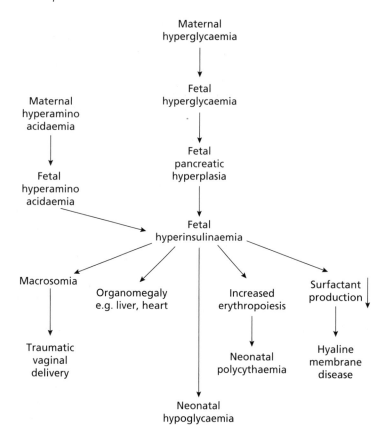

Fig 11.3 An expanded modification of the Pedersen hypothesis [25].

glucose control [32], but concentrations can change acutely. The erythropoietin concentration could be raised because of the effects of insulin on erythropoietin production or alternatively through poor tissue oxygenation. Fetal thrombocytopenia has also been demonstrated in association with maternal diabetes; the most likely cause is increased platelet consumption through aggregation [31].

Glycosylated haemoglobin and other glycated proteins

Glycosylated haemoglobin (HbA$_{1c}$) is a normally occurring moiety of haemoglobin which in non-pregnant normoglycaemic women is fairly constant at 5–6% of the total haemoglobin mass. The glucose is bound irreversibly to the red cell, and measurement of the percentage of HbA$_1$ that has been glycosylated gives an indication of the plasma glucose concentrations to which the current red cells have been exposed. Accordingly, the HbA$_{1c}$ percentage gives a retrospective estimate of average plasma glucose concentration over the preceding 2 months. Gly-

cosylated haemoglobin concentrations tend to decline in the second trimester of normal pregnancy because of the increased erythropoiesis of early pregnancy: the increased proportion of young erythrocytes have less chance to be glycosylated. Other compounds are also glycosylated and measurement of glycosylated serum proteins can be used as an alternative to measurement of HbA$_{1c}$.

Effect of diabetes on the fetus
Congenital malformations

There is an increased incidence of congenital malformations amongst the offspring of mothers with established diabetes. While the consensus view had been that there is about a threefold increase over the rate for non-diabetic pregnancy, two recent reports that comprehensively studied all diabetic women in two regions in the UK, suggested a four- to 10-fold increase [5,6]. However, some centres report a decrease in malformation rate with time. For example the 2.7% rate from Copenhagen [33], shows a significant decrease from earlier reports and is less than twice as much as the rate in their normal population.

Both minor and major malformations are increased. Specific abnormalities such as cardiac and neural tube defects are associated with diabetes. In addition, the incidence of caudal regression syndrome (an absence or hypoplasia of caudal structures), which is normally very rare, is increased in diabetic pregnancy [34].

The Copenhagen group [35] reported an association between malformations and maternal diabetic vascular disease. However, subsequently they showed [36] that this was an effect of poor diabetic control rather than the severity of the vascular disease. Leslie *et al.* [37] suggested that the malformation rate was higher amongst the offspring of mothers with established diabetes who had a higher than normal HbA_1 in early pregnancy. This has subsequently been confirmed by others [38–40]. One study investigating glycaemic control and congenital malformations in women seen by 21 days postconception [41] was unable to demonstrate such a relationship, but the women were moderately well controlled and few had the degree of elevation of HbA_{1c} found in the other studies. Their finding of a decreased malformation rate in those women seen early, in contrast to those seen later in pregnancy (4.9% vs. 9.0%) is in accord with studies that have shown that women seen in pre-pregnancy clinics are less likely to have babies with congenital malformations than those not seen before conception [42,43] (see pre-pregnancy care, below).

In the Diabetes Control and Complications Trial [44] in the USA there were a number of women who conceived during the study. Even though all the women had either well-controlled or moderately well-controlled diabetes, there was still a trend towards fewer malformations in the group who were intensively treated.

In conclusion, while there does appear to be a relationship between poor diabetes control during embryogenesis and subsequent malformations, there is a considerable overlap between diabetes control in those women who have babies with abnormalities compared to those who do not.

With regard to pathogenesis, it has long been known that malformations can be induced in animals by exposing the fetus to high concentrations of glucose at the time of organogenesis [45]. It has also been suggested [46] that ketonaemia potentiates this effect. Work in rats [47,48] has shown that lumbosacral defects in the fetus could only be induced if the mother was hyperglycaemic in the first days of pregnancy, i.e. the period when organogenesis is occurring in the rat. If diabetes was induced in rats after the first week of pregnancy or insulin treatment was given, the defects did not appear.

Hypoglycaemia has also been investigated in rats *in vivo*, and a slight increase in congenital malformations has been reported [49,50]. To date no clinical evidence supports such a relationship in the human [41,51]. Thus, an abnormal metabolic environment appears responsible for the increased congenital malformations found with maternal diabetes, the Fuel-Mediated Teratogenesis theory, proposed by Freinkel [52]. The exact mechanism is uncertain, but Eriksson and Borg [53] suggested that free oxygen radicals generated by embryonic mitochondria may be responsible, and clinical studies to investigate this are being undertaken.

There is no evidence of an increased incidence of malformations in the offspring of gestational diabetic women [54] presumably because the metabolic disturbance of diabetes does not appear in the mother until later in pregnancy when organogenesis is complete.

Malformations that are not obvious at birth or shortly thereafter may not be reported and therefore the total number may be underestimated. In addition, little is known about the 'malformation' rate in organ systems such as the brain where a relatively minor disruption of organogenesis might cause significant behavioural abnormalities in later life. A study by Yssing [55] from Denmark of 740 children of diabetic mothers showed that 36% had some form of cerebral dysfunction. Although this study was uncontrolled, it serves as a reminder of how seriously one should regard the damaging effects of uncontrolled diabetes throughout pregnancy. A number of studies have looked at the development of the child and attempted to correlate this with maternal metabolic control, particularly in relation to circulating ketone bodies. Earlier studies [56,57] caused controversy [58], but further studies have again suggested that maternal ketone body concentrations may be of relevance to subsequent intellectual development [59]. The relevance of this to management is discussed later.

Spontaneous miscarriage

As congenital malformations are a major cause of miscarriage it would be expected that the rate of miscarriage would be increased in women with established diabetes. Uncontrolled studies have suggested an increase [60], and that this is related to poor diabetic control during embryogenesis [61]. In contrast, no difference was found in a large controlled prospective study in women seen by 21 days postconception [62]. However, those with diabetes who did miscarry had higher fasting and postprandial glucose concentration and HbA_{1c} than those with continuing pregnancies. The Diabetes Control and Complications Trial Research Group [44] compared women with diabetes being managed conventionally or intensively prior to pregnancy and did not show a difference in miscarriage rates, but even the conventionally managed group had relatively well-controlled diabetes. Women who attend for pre-pregnancy counselling have also been shown to have no increased miscarriage rate compared to the general population [63].

In conclusion, it appears that poorly controlled diabetes is associated with an increased risk of miscarriage, but that the woman with moderately well-controlled diabetes has minimal increased risk.

Perinatal mortality in established diabetes

The perinatal mortality rate amongst women with established diabetes has always been higher than for the population as a whole. Almost all the published data relate to type I, insulin-dependent diabetes, but what data are available for women with type II, non-insulin-dependent diabetes suggest that the risks are similar. However, rates have been falling consistently as can be seen from the data from one large English hospital (Table 11.1). When considering perinatal mortality care must also be taken to ensure that a correction has not been made for fatal malformations. Another factor that has to be taken into account when considering perinatal mortality figures such as those in Table 11.1 is that most reports come from centres with a special interest in diabetic pregnancy. Two regional studies in England showed that the perinatal mortality rate was about five times higher for women with diabetes than for the general population [5,6]. It seems likely that the variations in perinatal mortality rates between hospitals can be attributed to the quality of medical and obstetric care. Series of cases looked after by individual clinicians have shown lower rates [64]. Data from Northern Ireland [65] suggest a trend towards decreased perinatal mortality in a central referral unit compared to national figures, despite the likelihood that more complex cases are cared for in such a centre.

Similar trends have been shown in pooled data from a number of large centres throughout the UK [66].

Table 11.1 also shows the changes in perinatal mortality rates relative to the cause of death. It can be seen that deaths due to obstetric problems, complications of diabetes, respiratory distress and 'unknown' have all fallen, whereas death rates due to congenital malformation remained unaltered until they too started falling in the 1980s. In this large central hospital, if malformations are removed from the figures, perinatal mortality rates would be essentially the same as for a non-diabetic population. This must point towards the effect of improved obstetric and diabetic care on outcome.

Unexplained fetal death *in utero*

Despite improvement in diabetic care, death *in utero* of a normally formed fetus accounted for over half of perinatal deaths in a recent English regional study [5]. Occasional perinatal deaths are also still reported from major centres using careful fetal monitoring programmes [67]. The aetiology is almost certainly multifactorial, but acidaemia is likely to be a key aspect. Initially, much of the evidence had to be obtained from post-mortem samples, amniotic fluid, cord blood at delivery and from animal studies. Data obtained by direct blood sampling from the fetus is now giving more insight. A number of factors are now considered.

PLACENTAL BLOOD SUPPLY

Doppler umbilical artery waveform studies initially produced some confusing results, but subsequent studies have suggested that values are within the normal range unless growth restriction or pre-eclampsia is present [68,69]. In addition the data available on women with diabetic vascular disease (diabetic nephropathy) does not suggest a specific impairment of umbilical artery velocity waveforms [70]. No relationship has been found between diabetic control and Doppler waveforms [68].

Table 11.1 Perinatal mortality rates and causes of death amongst 1449 diabetic babies born to diabetic mothers over a 40-year period at King's College Hospital, London. (J.M. Brudenell, personal communication.)

Years	*n*	Perinatal deaths (/1000)	Causes of death				
			Obstetric	Diabetic	Congenital malformations	Respiratory distress	Unknown
1951–60	318	72(226)	26	5	6	17	18
1961–70	389	39(100)	9	2	5	8	15
1971–80	352	13 (37)	3	1	6	1	2
1981–90	390	7 (18)	0	0	4	0	3

PLACENTAL ABNORMALITIES

Fox [71] reviewed this aspect and concluded that placental changes were not specific to diabetes and did not relate to the severity of the diabetes or its control and that rapid repair of any damage occurred. In addition, the evidence suggests that the area available for maternofetal exchange is increased. Accordingly, it seems unlikely that the placenta is a relevant factor in the unexplained fetal death.

PLACENTAL OXYGEN TRANSFER

This has been comprehensively reviewed by Madsen [72] and is likely to be a relevant factor. Although there is an increase in red blood cell 2,3-diphosphoglycerate (DPG) content in diabetic pregnancy throughout all trimesters, 2,3-DPG-induced changes in oxygen affinity are impaired. Increasing concentrations of maternal HbA_{1c} were found to be associated with a small, but significant decrease in arterial oxygen saturation. The women studied did not have poorly controlled diabetes (HbA_{1c} median 7.8% and maximum 9.9%) and with worse control the red cell oxygen release is likely to be further impaired. Women who smoke have a smaller increase in red cell 2,3-DPG and are therefore likely to have further impairment of oxygen release. In addition, when recovering from ketoacidosis there is a marked reduction in red cell oxygen release, which may account for the poor fetal prognosis in this situation.

FETAL ACID–BASE BALANCE

In the sheep, hyperglycaemia was not found to be of significance to a well-oxygenated fetus, unless there was mild hypoxia, when there was a rapid fall in pH [73]. Cord blood samples taken antenatally from fetuses of diabetic women in the third trimester have demonstrated relatively normal blood Po_2 concentrations, but a tendency to mild acidaemia with increased lactate concentrations [22]. In addition, the inverse relationship between fetal pH and glucose concentration was again demonstrated (Fig. 11.4). These findings suggest that the fetus of the diabetic mother has a tendency towards a metabolic acidosis. Increasing glucose concentrations worsen it and this can occur in the absence of hypoxaemia. As there is a correlation between fetal pH and Po_2 one can speculate that sudden rises in maternal glucose could be enough to cause fetal acidaemia and mild hypoxaemia to develop. Extrapolating from the animal work of Shelley et al. [73] it is suggested that this mild hypoxaemia might be sufficient to cause an irreversible pH decline and fetal demise.

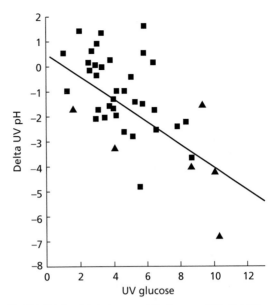

Fig 11.4 Relationship between umbilical venous (UV) cord pH and UV cord blood glucose obtained from antenatal cordocentesis in diabetic pregnancy. Six women had nephropathy and hypertension ▲. Value of ■ pH is in SD from normal mean for gestational age. $r = 0.603$, $p < 0.0001$ [22].

FETAL METABOLIC DEMAND

The organomegaly induced by hyperinsulinaemia [74] in the fetus of the diabetic mother will result in an increased oxygen demand as has been shown in animal studies [75].

FETAL THROMBOSIS

As mentioned in the section on fetal haematology, in diabetic pregnancy there is a tendency towards fetal polycythaemia and thrombocytopenia [31], the latter probably due to platelet aggregation. The fetus is likely to be at increased risk of thrombotic episodes and this has been documented in post-mortem studies [76]. This could also be a factor in fetal death occurring *in utero*.

In conclusion, it can be seen that a number of factors are likely to be relevant in the pathogenesis of intrauterine fetal demise, but the common factor, is that of less than ideal diabetic control.

Perinatal mortality in gestational diabetes and impaired glucose tolerance

In a group of women with gestational diabetes mellitus there will be a significant number (perhaps 20–30%) who had undiagnosed diabetes prior to pregnancy. Women with type II diabetes have increased perinatal mortality.

Accordingly a study of a large enough group of women with gestational diabetes is likely to demonstrate an increase in perinatal mortality. Most of the studies published have included a wide spectrum of glucose intolerance including both those with gestational impaired glucose tolerance and gestational diabetes. The randomized trial of O'Sullivan [77], which compared treating women to just giving routine antenatal care, demonstrated a non-significant increase in perinatal mortality in the untreated group (8.5% vs. 3.6%). Other controlled studies have demonstrated a fourfold increase in perinatal mortality in women with untreated gestational diabetes compared to controls [78], although this increase was confined to older more obese women. Similar results were reported from a study in Pima Indian women where those with impaired glucose tolerance had an increased perinatal mortality rate in contrast to controls with normal glucose tolerance [79].

Whether women with just impaired glucose tolerance have higher perinatal mortality rates is unknown [80,81]. The Toronto study [82] assessed the outcomes in women with varying degrees of glucose tolerance who did not have gestational diabetes. There were no interventions, but the study did not attempt to assess perinatal mortality. A similar larger international study is currently being undertaken which also will not have the power to address this issue granted the low perinatal mortality rates that exist today.

In conclusion it is probable that perinatal mortality is increased when there is gestational diabetes and possibly also at the more severe end of impaired glucose tolerance.

Effects of diabetes on the neonate

Because of the overwhelming concern about perinatal mortality, little attention had been paid until recently to reducing the neonatal morbidity commonly associated with maternal diabetes. The expanded Pedersen hypothesis, shown in Fig. 11.3, can be used to explain much of the neonatal morbidity that follows a diabetic pregnancy. Rates of morbidity remain high both in gestational and established diabetes and results of selected surveys are shown in Table 11.2.

Birthweight

Insulin-dependent diabetes is associated with an increased incidence of both large and small for gestational age infants, both conditions being associated with increased perinatal morbidity. The distribution of birthweight from a typical population with established diabetes is shown in Fig. 11.5. Typically, 25–40% of infants of mothers with established diabetes have birthweights over the 90th centile; the Northern Regional study [6] reported that 35% were more than the 95th centile. The term macrosomia is widely used to describe babies who are overweight, but it is variably defined in terms of either actual birthweight or centile weight. Excessive fetal growth rarely becomes apparent before 28 weeks' gestation, although longitudinal ultrasound studies of fetal abdominal circumference have suggested that increased growth rate may be present between 20 and 24 weeks [83,84]. Typically, the macrosomic baby of the diabetic mother is fat and plethoric, with all organs, with the exception of the brain, being enlarged due to an increase in cytoplasmic mass. There is much evidence to support the Pedersen hypothesis illustrated in Fig. 11.3 that birthweight is increased because of fetal pancreatic hyperplasia and hyperinsulinism. Using the hyperinsulinaemic, normoglycaemic monkey model, Susa and Schwartz [74] showed that it is hyperinsulinaemia that is responsible for these changes. In the human fetus, subcutaneous fat is markedly increased, the amount being directly related to the maternal plasma glucose concentration in the third trimester of pregnancy [85] and to the HbA_{1c} [86]. In addition, analysis of amniotic fluid C-peptide concentrations has shown a correlation with large for gestational age babies [87] A similar correlation was shown between the insulin/glucose ratio in fetal plasma obtained by cordocentesis and large babies [22]. Furthermore, morphological studies of the fetus of the diabetic mother have shown that the greater percentage area of

Table 11.2 Comparison of perinatal morbidity and mortality amongst women with diabetic pregnancy.

Location	Author	Year	No. of women	Respiratory distress (%)	Jaundice (%)	Hypoglycaemia (%)	Macrosomia (%)	Perinatal mortality 1/1000
UK	Beard & Lowy	1982	664	12	20	15	29	61
Dublin	Drury	1986	285	3	15	11	–	45
New York	Jovanovic	1981	55	0	0	1	0	0
Israel	Hod	1991	132	2	17	8	25	0

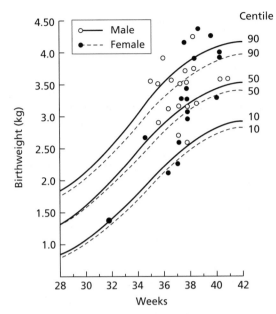

Fig 11.5 Birthweight and gestation distribution for infants of insulin-dependent diabetic mothers at St Mary's Hospital, Manchester. (Percentile charts [192].) (M. Maresh, unpublished observations).

total pancreatic tissue occupied by the insulin-secreting islet cells, the bigger the baby [88].

Whilst fetal hyperinsulinaemia is clearly associated with excessive fetal growth, the exact mechanism is uncertain. It could be mediated through insulin-like growth factors (IGFs) and their binding proteins (IGFBPs) [89]. However, a longitudinal study in normal and diabetic pregnancy has not shown a relationship between IGF-1 or IGFBP-1 with ultrasound-determined fetal growth or birthweight [90]. Further clarification is required which may come from molecular biology and other techniques that are now being used to study this issue.

The clinical importance of fetal macrosomia, which is often associated with hydramnios, is that it may indicate poor diabetic control and accordingly an increased risk of perinatal mortality. Whilst more common in the established diabetic woman, macrosomia may also occur with gestational diabetes. In addition, excessive fetal growth increases the risk of trauma during vaginal delivery and particularly of shoulder dystocia with its risk of Erb's palsy and asphyxial brain damage.

In gestational diabetes and impaired glucose tolerance, the increased birthweight of babies may be accounted for by the tendency for these women to be older and fatter than normal. The effect of maternal weight on birthweight has been demonstrated both when women have been

treated for their glucose intolerance [79,91] and when they have not been treated [82]. However, the lowering of birthweight by treatment has been shown in many studies including those of O'Sullivan et al. [92] and Roversi et al. [93]. Regardless of the cause of the increase in birthweight, the baby of the woman with abnormal glucose tolerance is still at increased risk of disproportion and operative delivery with its increased risk of trauma. Intensified treatment has been shown to reduce these risks [94,95].

Respiratory dysfunction

Respiratory distress syndrome of the newborn is a known complication of maternal diabetes. It is suggested that fetal hyperinsulinism reduces pulmonary phospholipid production, particularly phosphatidylglycerol, leading to surfactant deficiency [96]. There is evidence to associate poor diabetic control with an inadequate amniotic fluid phospholipid profile [97]. Although it was shown that prediction of subsequent neonatal respiratory distress syndrome could be improved by the measurement of the phospholipid profile in addition to the lecithin/sphingomyelin ratio [98], this test is now rarely used.

Respiratory distress syndrome is becoming less common no doubt due to less preterm elective delivery and to better diabetic control. It is being replaced by transient tachypnoea of the newborn, which is thought to be due to delayed removal of fetal lung liquid and is quite common especially after caesarean delivery. It is characterized by a rapid respiratory rate and transient cyanosis, usually disappearing within 24–36 h of birth.

Hypoglycaemia

This is usually asymptomatic in the newborn of the diabetic woman, and plasma glucose concentrations of <2.0 mmol/L without evidence of systemic disturbance are quite common. The hypoglycaemia is caused by endogenous hyperinsulinism developing in fetal life that becomes clinically apparent only when the fetus is separated from its supply of glucose from the mother. In addition, the combination of reduced hepatic phosphorylase activity and diminished glucagon and catecholamine release results in decreased output of glucose from the liver of these babies [99]. The concentration of plasma glucose in the newborn correlates inversely with the degree of carbohydrate intolerance of the mother in the third trimester of pregnancy [100] and also with maternal HbA_{1c} [101]. By encouraging early feeding and by performing regular glucose estimations on the newborn after birth, the condition can be detected and treated before symptomatic hypoglycaemia can occur. A value below 1.0 mmol/L is an indication for the intravenous administration of glucose because of the risk of cerebral damage.

Polycythaemia and jaundice

Polycythaemia is more common in infants of diabetic mothers. A venous haematocrit more than 65% is considered abnormal and has been shown to be present in 29% of infants of diabetic mothers in contrast to 6% in controls [102]. With impaired glucose tolerance the frequency increases in proportion to the greater degree of abnormality [91]. Cordocentesis has also demonstrated a relationship between maternal diabetic control and fetal polycythaemia [31]. Animal work suggests that fetal hyperinsulinism results in elevated levels of erythropoietin, leading to increased haematopoiesis. The erythropoietin concentration in the umbilical vein has been found to be higher in women with established diabetes than in those with gestational diabetes or in controls [29]. The clinical consequence of the polycythaemia is an increase in blood viscosity leading to increased cardiac work and microcirculatory disturbances. Hyperviscosity within the pulmonary bed may be a contributory factor to respiratory distress. It might also explain the increased incidence of renal vein thrombosis and necrotizing enterocolitis. The destruction of many cells and the relative immaturity of the liver enzyme systems of the newborn that handle bilirubin predispose to the high prevalence of jaundice in these babies. This varies between series, but a typical rate appears to be about 19% having bilirubin values exceeding 15 mg/dL [103]. These complications led to the recommendation of early clamping of the umbilical cord and exchange transfusion if the haematocrit exceeded 70% [104].

Hypocalcaemia and hypomagnesaemia

Hypocalcaemia is more common in infants of diabetic mothers and is reported to occur in between 5% and 22% [103,105]. In addition, hypomagnesaemia is also more frequent [106]. Reduced parathyroid hormone concentrations have been noted in pregnancy associated with normal calcium concentrations. The exact mechanism of these changes is uncertain, but again there appears to be a relationship with diabetic control. In view of the possibility of neonatal fits associated with these metabolic changes careful surveillance is required in neonates.

Hypertrophic cardiomyopathy

It has been suggested that about 30% of infants of mothers with insulin-dependent diabetes have cardiomegaly and

10% have evidence of cardiac dysfunction [107]. The characteristic abnormality, which is best demonstrated by echocardiography [108], is asymmetrical septal hypertrophy. This is similar to that seen in familial obstructive cardiomyopathy or hypertrophic obstructive cardiomyopathy, except that it is reversible over a period of weeks [109] and fibre disarray is not a prominent feature [107,109]. The animal work of Susa and Schwartz [74] suggests that the cardiomegaly is caused by hyperinsulinism and the clinical data of Gutgesell *et al.* [110] suggested a link with the degree of maternal diabetic control.

Summary of causes of neonatal morbidity

As mentioned in the individual sections it seems likely that fetal hyperinsulinism is an important factor underlying some if not all of these complications and that anything that can reduce this is likely to diminish the neonatal complication rate in diabetic pregnancy. In addition there is much clinical evidence to support the hypothesis that normalization of maternal plasma glucose in the latter part of pregnancy is likely to reduce neonatal morbidity. This is perhaps best shown when results of single specialist centres [64,111] are compared with those of national surveys [112] (Table 11.2). In the report of Jovanovic *et al.* [111] normoglycaemia in the mother was maintained for the greater part of pregnancy with the result that neonatal morbidity virtually disappeared. Hopefully, current large-scale studies will give further and up-to-date information.

Diagnosis and screening for diabetes and impaired glucose tolerance in pregnancy

Diagnosis

The diagnostic test is the oral GTT. Until recently there have been no agreed criteria for defining abnormality because of such variables as whether an oral or intravenous test is performed, the amount of glucose that is given and the variety of methods used for glucose assay. The criteria of O'Sullivan *et al.* [113] were generally regarded as being most acceptable because of the careful long-term follow-up of the women following the pregnancy during which they had their initial GTT. They used a 100-g load of glucose administered orally following prior dietary preparation and collected venous blood half-hourly over 3 h. They defined an abnormal result as two or more venous whole blood glucose values exceeding the following limits: fasting 5.0 mmol/L, 1 h 9.2 mmol/L, 2 h 8.1 mmol/L and 3 h 6.9 mmol/L. Subsequently these have been modified and venous plasma values of 5.8, 10.6, 9.2 and 8.1 mmol/L, respectively, are recommended in the USA [13].

The WHO [7], in an attempt to standardize the GTT, recommended a 75-g oral load. A diagnosis of impaired glucose tolerance is made if the glucose fasting plasma glucose is <7.8 mmol/L and the 2-h is ≤11.0 mmol/L and >7.8 mmol/L. These criteria were based on studies outwith pregnancy. A large multicentre pregnancy study was conducted by Lind [12], which confirmed earlier suggestions that a 2-h value ≥7.8 mmol/L was common after a 75-g GTT, being found in about 10% of pregnant women in the third trimester. It was recommended that the cut-off for the 2-h value should be raised to 9 mmol/L and that this should be combined with the 95th percentile value for the 1-h value which was 10.5 mmol/L. While there are some methodological problems with the data, until more are published these criteria are recommended for the diagnosis of impaired glucose intolerance in pregnancy. Lind [12] also recommended the use of the term gestational impaired glucose tolerance for this group, gestational diabetes being reserved for those with a diabetic GTT, i.e. a 2-h value greater than 11.0 mmol/L.

An alternative set of criteria for defining an abnormal GTT was developed by Gillmer *et al.* [100] using the neonatal end point of hypoglycaemia which has more clinical credibility than using statistical cut-offs. By defining neonatal hypoglycaemia 2 h after birth as a plasma glucose concentration of ≤1.7 mmol/L, they determined the upper limit of normal glucose tolerance in the mother. They found that their critical values differed little from those of O'Sullivan *et al.* [113].

Screening

A condition should not be screened for unless it can be clearly defined. If the condition is diagnosed, treatment should also improve health. While this applies to the detection of diabetes it is more controversial with regard to impaired glucose tolerance. Attempts to detect unrecognized diabetes in pregnancy are a routine part of established antenatal practice. The success of these efforts varies widely because of the generalized lack of any consistent and systematic approach to the problem. If screening is to be effective it must be comprehensive. Interpretation of the literature is made difficult by different definitions and methodologies used and the differences in the ethnic mix of the populations studied. The following screening techniques are widely used (see Table 11.3).

POTENTIAL DIABETIC FEATURES

There are certain features that a woman may have in her family or medical or obstetric history that predispose her to an increased possibility of developing diabetes in pregnancy. These are:

- diabetes in a first-degree relative;
- maternal obesity (>120% ideal bodyweight);
- previous large baby (>4 kg);
- previous unexplained stillbirth;
- previous abnormal glucose tolerance.

To these features identified at booking can be added glycosuria (more than one occasion) (see below) and hydramnios. Although the practice of only performing a glucose tolerance test on women with potential diabetic features remains widespread it is not an efficient screening method. The prevalence of potential diabetes depends considerably on the population served and has been reported to be 8.5% in Belfast [114] and 35% in inner London [115]. Screening studies of entire obstetric populations have shown that only about 45% of women found to have carbohydrate intolerance have defined features of potential diabetes [113].

Table 11.3 Comparison of screening methods for impaired glucose tolerance. Values approximated from articles referred to in text.

Method	Sensitivity percentage	Specificity percentage	% of population requiring GTT
Potential diabetic features*	50	65	10–30
Random glucose†	40	90	
Fasting glucose†	75	70	30
Glucose load*	75	80	10–15
Glycated Hb*	40	90	

*Positive outcome being an abnormal glucose tolerance test (GTT) as defined by O'Sullivan & Mahan, 1964 [193].

†Positive outcome being an impaired GTT as defined by WHO [7].

GLYCOSURIA

The traditional method of waiting for glycosuria to appear has a low pickup rate and, as such, is of limited value. Sutherland *et al.* [116] found that 11% of an unselected obstetric population of 1418 women had glycosuria at some time, but fewer than 1% of those with glycosuria had an abnormal GTT. Most women have glycosuria if all urine samples are tested throughout pregnancy while, in contrast, many women with impaired glucose tolerance never have glycosuria detected when they visit the antenatal clinic.

GLUCOSE CHALLENGE TEST

This test is advocated in the USA [117], but is only used in about 6% of hospitals in the UK [118]. The woman is given a 50-g glucose drink when she attends the antenatal clinic with no prior fasting or other special preparation. One hour later blood is taken for glucose assay. If the value is $\geq 7.8\,mmol/L$ (>2SD of the mean for an unselected obstetric population), a full GTT is done [113]. Originally it was proposed that this test was done early in pregnancy and then repeated later (e.g. at 28 weeks) in women who had a negative GTT or if they had one of the features of potential diabetes. However, currently where it is used it tends to be done only at about 28 weeks. The numbers of tests can be halved by confining the screening test to women aged 25 or over, with only a slight reduction in sensitivity. This is the approach recommended in the USA apart from advocating screening women under 25 who have potential diabetic features [117]. Support for this approach also comes from the Toronto Study [119]. In this population using thresholds of >30 years old or a prepregnancy body mass index (BMI) >22.0, would result in 35% of women not requiring screening tests with 82% of women with gestational diabetes being detected. Originally an overall sensitivity of 79% and a specificity of 83% were reported by O'Sullivan *et al.* [113]. A more recent study [120], using different criteria and methods, has reported a lower sensitivity (59%) with the 7.8 mmol/L threshold, but a high specificity (91%). Reducing the threshold to 7.0 mmol/L gave sensitivities of 68% for a specificity of 82%, with full glucose tests being required in 14% of women. In conclusion, studies of this method have been able to demonstrate relatively high sensitivities and specificities.

FASTING GLUCOSE

The use of fasting glucose as a screening test was proposed by Mortensen *et al.* [121] although they used it in a preselected group with potential diabetic features. A fasting blood glucose cut-off of 4.1 mmol/L produced a sensitivity of over 90%. Applying this criterion, Jowett *et al.* [122] also found a sensitivity of 92% with a specificity of 49%. Subsequently a European study on an unselected population, using the American Diabetes Association criteria, reported a sensitivity of 81% and a specificity of 76% [120]. However, with a threshold of 4.8 mmol/L, 30% of the population required a full GTT. A Brazilian study [123] using the WHO criteria, but with a similar 4.8-mmol/L threshold, differentiated between screening for diabetes and impaired glucose tolerance, and reported 69% sensitivity and specificity for impaired glucose tolerance with 35% requiring a full GTT.

RANDOM GLUCOSE

Random glucose measurement has been encouraged as a simple way to screen for abnormal glucose tolerance [124]. A positive cut-off was taken as 6.4 mmol/L if the women were tested less than 2 h after a meal and 5.8 mmol/L if more than 2 h after a meal. Data on sensitivity and specificity of this method of screening was subsequently obtained [122,125], which showed this to be a poor method of screening (see Table 11.3). Random glucose testing was reported to be used in 26% of hospitals in the UK in 1994 [118], but there appears to be a variety of cut-offs used. It has been suggested that combining random blood glucose with glycosuria may be an effective method [118], but there are no data to support this.

GLYCOSYLATED HAEMOGLOBIN

The use of HbA_{1c} and glycosylated proteins has been extensively investigated as a simple one sample screening test with no preparation required. Unfortunately after initial enthusiastic reports, multiple studies have, perhaps not surprisingly, shown that the tests have poor specificity and sensitivity.

CONCLUSIONS

The justification for any screening system is that it should be cost effective and also acceptable to the patient. A full GTT, apart from being expensive, is time consuming and unpleasant for pregnant women. Equally, limiting the test to women with potential diabetic features is not justified because of the relatively low pick-up rate (see Table 11.3). Accordingly the only tests that appear to have reasonable sensitivity and specificity are the fasting glucose and the glucose challenge test. However, until the relevance of impaired glucose tolerance is defined, major efforts to implement effective screening practice would not appear to be justified.

Medical management

Pre-pregnancy care

To be effective, medical management of established diabetes must start well before pregnancy. All affected teenage girls should be warned of the risks of poor diabetic control at the beginning of pregnancy to them and their babies. Attention to general health, contraception and good metabolic control are subjects that must be discussed by physicians, general practitioners, diabetes specialist nurses, health visitors, youth workers and indeed by all who have contact with women with diabetes in a caring capacity. The trend towards managing diabetes in special centres and the increasing use of diabetes specialist nurses will enable advice to be given more readily to some of the younger women who need it most. The decentralization of some care to general practice should also be beneficial when the care is concentrated and given by one member of the practice team who has a particular interest.

Whether a specific pre-pregnancy clinic is necessary remains controversial. Although some clinics have achieved very high attendance rates, with about 60% of pregnant women having been seen prior to conception [43], this is the exception. What is required is easy access to someone knowledgeable in the field; whether that person is a physician or obstetrician, specialist nurse or midwife is irrelevant. Similarly, whether a formal clinic is established or whether there is an alternative method of access to care, is irrelevant.

The establishment of a pre-pregnancy counselling service in centres with a large diabetic clinic population is advisable. The major objective is to ensure that good diabetic control prevails at the time of conception and embryogenesis. Studies have shown that women who were counselled before pregnancy were found to have lower HbA$_{1c}$ values [43] and lower glucose values [42] in the first trimester and had fewer babies with congenital malformations [42,43], compared to those women who did not have counselling.

Preconception care also gives the opportunity for a change to insulin for all diabetic women on oral hypoglycaemic drugs. Apart from the possible problems subsequent to transplacental drug passage, the major reason for changing to insulin is the tighter diabetic control that can be achieved.

The complications of diabetes and its interrelations with pregnancy also need discussing before pregnancy. Retinopathy should be treated prior to pregnancy if indicated. In cases of severe nephropathy it may be necessary to discourage pregnancy for the sake of the woman's health. In addition to improving diabetic control, the opportunity should be taken to give general advice regarding the importance of being as healthy as possible at the start of the pregnancy—stopping smoking, reducing alcohol intake and achieving an ideal bodyweight being obvious examples. Furthermore, contraceptive or fertility advice may be required and rubella immunity status can be checked. Folic acid supplementation should be started. Finally, pre-pregnancy discussions can raise the issue of how the pregnancy is likely to be managed and what effects it might have on lifestyle such as work and family commitments.

The joint pregnancy–diabetic clinic

The pregnant diabetic woman is best managed in a special antenatal clinic where all those with the necessary expertise can work together. Few obstetricians and diabetic physicians in the UK are likely to care for more than two pregnant women with insulin-dependent diabetes per year, unless these patients' care is centred on one obstetrician and physician within each maternity unit. Despite repeated recommendations that centralization should occur, in 1994 only 57% of hospitals in the UK had special diabetic antenatal clinics [118]. There is also a need for a referral unit that will take some of the more difficult cases within a region. The midwife should not be relegated solely to helping in the clinic organization, but can use her skills to complement those of the other members of the multidisciplinary team [126]. With outpatient care throughout pregnancy being the routine, the diabetes specialist midwife or nurse has a major role in teaching women blood glucose home monitoring, the administration of insulin and the alteration of insulin regimens. The presence of a dietitian is essential for initiating the treatment of gestational diabetes and fine tuning the diet in women with type I and particularly type II diabetes as they aim for tighter diabetic control. Medical and obstetric problems in diabetic pregnancy are often interdependent and need to be managed by an obstetrician and physician working together.

Principles of treatment

The major objective of medical management is to attain normoglycaemia. The non-diabetic woman maintains a plasma glucose in pregnancy within the range of 3.5–4.5 mmol/L [16] rarely exceeding 5.5 mmol/L except immediately after meals (see Fig. 11.1). However, this is a blood glucose concentration that is considerably lower than most with established diabetes are used to in the non-pregnant state and initially may lead to symptoms of hypoglycaemia. While this is clearly worrying and distressing initially, with close support and encourage-ment blood glucose levels near those of normoglycaemia usually can be achieved. Reasonable targets for the capil-lary blood glucose are <5.5 mmol/L fasting and before meals and < 7.5 mmol/L 1 h after meals.

All women should be given a glucagon kit and they should ensure that their partners are familiar with giving them glucagon injections. In a survey in the UK in 1994 the range of preprandial blood glucose concentrations being aimed at was 4.0–9.0 mmol/L with a worrying 20% of physicians being happy with a preprandial blood glucose concentration of more than 7.0 mmol/L [118]. Since then audit of management of diabetes in pregnancy has been introduced in a number of Regions in the UK and clear guidelines have been developed [127]. It is hoped that appropriate targets are now being used.

As pregnancy advances insulin requirements increase, eventually reaching a plateau and sometimes decreasing near term. The insulin-dependent diabetic woman there-fore requires considerable attention to the dosage regime. Women with established non-insulin-dependent diabetes usually require insulin to achieve normoglycaemia. Some with gestational diabetes may need to transfer from diet to insulin at some time during pregnancy for adequate control, although many can achieve acceptable normogly-caemia by following restrictive dietary advice alone.

The objective of diabetic control in pregnancy is to maintain normoglycaemia at all times. The usual practice in the UK is to perform glucose measurements four times a day with measurements before meals and a measure-ment at bedtime [118]. Measurements after meals are not widely used in the UK, whereas in the USA they are, as it has been suggested that these measurements correlate better with birthweight and therefore excessive fetal growth *in utero* [128,129]. Night-time measurements may be helpful as high prebreakfast levels can occasionally result from a rebound phenomenon after nocturnal hypo-glycaemia. Many insulin-dependent diabetic women are able to adjust their insulin dosages according to their results without the need for hospital advice. The use of blood glucose measurement strips with or without reflectance meters has made this easier to achieve, and pregnant women now routinely practise home monitor-ing of blood glucose. It is wise to obtain other estimations of blood glucose control such as measuring HbA$_{1c}$ on a monthly basis. Studies of how patients record their meter glucose values in their diaries have shown that there is a trend towards omitting or lowering high values [130].

Checking blood glucose levels when women attend the clinic is of limited value as that day is unlikely to be typical and the knowledge that they will be tested may be counterproductive to their overall care. However, it is important that their meters are checked on a regular basis.

Dietary advice is an essential part of the management of all diabetic women whether insulin dependent or not. Dietary compliance can be monitored by regular weighing of the woman as well as by observation of blood glucose concentrations. The major problems tend to be in women with non-insulin-dependent diabetes. A diet that is designed to achieve normoglycaemia should also produce a static bodyweight; any increase in weight suggests that the diet is not being adhered to.

If blood glucose concentration is to be well regulated, thought must be given to the effect of daily events on insulin requirements. Emotional lability is a potent factor in inducing hyperglycaemia and marked diurnal fluctu-ations in blood glucose. Many diabetic women do not alter their lifestyle when they become pregnant and may continue to do stressful jobs or expect to be able to cope with their other young children. When this occurs, con-siderable difficulty may be experienced in obtaining ideal diabetic control. Realistic discussions need to take place between the woman, her partner and the team looking after her. Ideally these should have taken place prior to pregnancy.

With the increasing realization in the 1960s that im-proved control of blood glucose in the third trimester led to better results, the philosophy of full inpatient care of pregnant diabetics from 32 weeks was advocated [131]. However, with the advent of home monitoring of blood glucose, admission to hospital should now only be neces-sary if significant complications are present or as a last resort if adequate control cannot be achieved by any other way. Clearly outpatient care is easier for the rest of the family. The actual number of outpatient visits will vary, but in general fortnightly is recommended with more or less frequent visits as indicated [132].

Insulin regimens

To achieve normoglycaemia throughout the 24 h, short- and longer-acting insulins are required. Since the intro-duction of pen-type syringes, these have become increas-ingly used, and now are almost the routine. Typically three doses of short-acting insulin are given preprandially combined with one dose of a long-acting insulin at night. However, a woman who is well controlled and happy on a biphasic insulin regimen should not be made to change unless she is unable to obtain normoglycaemia. The newer insulin analogues are being used in pregnancy and appear totally suitable for pregnancy. Continuous subcutaneous insulin infusion (CSII) has been used in pregnancy, but appears to offer no advantage to most diabetic pregnant women and should only be used if there is a well supported CSII service already established for the non-pregnant. In view of the state of 'accelerated starvation' found in pregnancy, ketoacidosis will develop more rapidly than in the non-pregnant state, should there be pump failure and an intrauterine death has been reported [133].

A method of giving insulin known as 'the maximum tolerated dose' was pioneered by Roversi *et al.* [93]. Short-acting insulin dosages were increased daily until symptomatic hypoglycaemia resulted and the dosage was then reduced to that of the previous day. Although the results

were good, women found the regimen distressing and there was a higher than expected rate of fetal growth restriction. This method is now rarely used.

Management of impaired glucose tolerance and gestational diabetes

Although there is no consensus view, in the UK most women with impaired glucose tolerance and gestational diabetes are initially managed with dietary advice. This can be a most effective way of reducing blood glucose as can be seen in Fig. 11.6. Dieting has not only decreased postprandial hyperglycaemia, but also fasting blood glucose concentrations. The effect of diet is to make insulin more efficient, as demonstrated by a decrease in the insulin/glucose ratio [18]. The general recommendations of

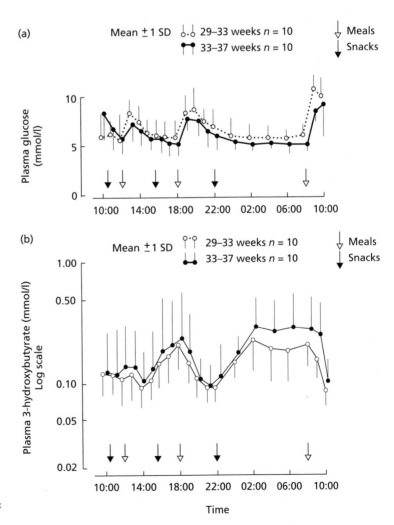

Fig 11.6 Twenty-four-hour metabolic profiles (mean ± 1 SD) in 10 women with abnormal glucose tolerance studied between 29 and 33 weeks and again between 33 and 37 weeks [18]. ○ Before dietary restriction; ● after dietary restriction for 4 weeks. (a) Plasma glucose; (b) plasma 3-hydroxybutyrate.

the British Diabetic Association [134] are that 50% of energy should be obtained from carbohydrate and this should also apply to pregnancy. The total calories in the diet should be between 1800 and 2000 daily. In the obese this should be restricted further so that in practice these women will put on little or no weight. While such an approach is less popular in the USA, current American Diabetes Association recommendations [8] are that women should restrict their calorie intake by about one-third if they are overweight (BMI >30 kg/m²).

As much fibre as possible is beneficial in pregnancy as it reduces the degree of postprandial hyperglycaemia [135]. Persuading the diabetic mother to keep to her diet is usually easier in pregnancy because of the incentive the mother has regarding her baby's well-being. However, cultural factors play a part, which are sometimes difficult to resolve, for example some Indian women believe that it is important to keep the baby well fed and their mothers-in-law will insist on a high calorie intake, regardless of the advice of the doctor! Restrictive dietary advice leads to an increase in ketonaemia. Although there is wide individual variation, ketonaemia in pregnancy tends to increase with gestation [18,136]. Figure 11.6 shows that treatment of women with gestational diabetes does not increase significantly the 24-h concentration of β-hydroxybutyrate, which could be reduced further by the use of high-fibre diets [137].

Oral hypoglycaemic agents have never been widely used and should not be used if compliance with insulin injections can be achieved. Drugs such as chlorpropamide cross the placenta and induce fetal hyperinsulinism. However, although neonatal hypoglycaemia was more prevalent when chlorpropamide was used compared to when insulin was used, hypoglycaemia was still uncommon [138]. Coetzee and Jackson [139] from South Africa have reported similarly good results using metformin.

Although there have been advocates for the routine use of insulin [140], the usual view is to only add insulin in those who, despite keeping to their diet, have fasting hyperglycaemia. The current UK recommendations are that if preprandial blood glucose measurements consistently are more than 6.0 mmol/L, insulin therapy should be commenced [118]. Studies have certainly shown that insulin therapy will decrease birthweight [93,94,141,142]. As with established diabetes, women can use pen syringes to give themselves short-acting insulin three times per day before each main meal starting at 6 units per dose. Alternatively, they can use an insulin regimen of twice-daily biphasic insulin, i.e. a fixed combination of short- and medium-acting insulins, with a starting dose of 20 units per day that can be altered to obtain control. Whilst insulin therapy has not been associated with clinical or

biochemical evidence of hypoglycaemia in reported series, the management should be conducted by the same team who look after those with insulin-dependent diabetes. Insulin therapy must be combined with restrictive dietary advice, for if it is not, the insulin will lead to excessive deposition of fat. This will increase the peripheral resistance to insulin, with the result that, despite increasing doses of insulin, hyperglycaemia will persist.

Control of blood glucose during labour

The key to a successful outcome to labour is also good diabetic control. Insulin requirements in labour tend to be low [143], but fluctuations in blood glucose concentrations due to the stresses of labour can be considerable if glucose levels are not well monitored and controlled. Normoglycaemia will reduce the risk of neonatal hypoglycaemia.

For women having a planned induction of labour or an elective caesarean section and who are taking long-acting insulin in the evening, consideration should be given to reducing their evening dose the night before delivery. For women with an unfavourable cervix being induced with vaginal prostaglandins, short-acting insulin and light snacks may be used until labour commences. Normoglycaemia is best achieved in both the established diabetic and the insulin-requiring gestational diabetic woman by the intravenous administration of both glucose and insulin, and this is the current practice in almost all hospitals in the UK [118]. However, with increasing desire for mobilization in labour, in a well-organized unit and with highly motivated women with well-controlled diabetes, multiple subcutaneous injections of insulin might be considered.

The following regimen is outlined as a guide to the practical management of the diabetic mother during labour. When the mother is admitted in spontaneous labour or prior to induction of labour, an intravenous infusion of 10% dextrose solution should be commenced. The infusion rate should be adjusted to provide 1 L of fluid every 8 h. Twenty units of soluble insulin (0.2 mL of 100 units/mL) should be mixed in 19.8 mL of normal saline BP in a 20-mL syringe which is then administered intravenously by infusion pump at a final concentration of 1 unit/mL. The plasma glucose concentration should be estimated prior to deciding whether to start an insulin infusion. It is useful to have a glucose reflectance meter on the delivery unit for this purpose provided there are staff who are familiar with its use. Alternatively, if the woman has her own then she or her partner can use that. Blood glucose concentrations are normally controlled by altering the insulin infusion rate. If the initial blood glucose is less than 7 mmol/L then the insulin infusion should be given at a rate of 1 unit/h; if it exceeds 7 mmol/L, then the infusion should commence at 2 units/h. Glucose estimations should initially be repeated at hourly intervals and the insulin infusion rate increased or decreased by 1 unit/h until a stable blood glucose concentration of between 4.5 and 5.5 mmol/L has been achieved. If the concentration falls below 3.5 mmol/L the glucose infusion rate should be increased. After a rise in early labour, the glucose concentration tends to fall as labour progresses so that eventually it may be necessary to stop insulin administration and even to give extra glucose intravenously. Women with impaired glucose tolerance may require intravenous insulin if glucose concentrations (which should be checked 2-hourly) are persistently above 7 mmol/L.

Should any additional intravenous fluids be necessary during labour such as for giving oxytocin, then isotonic saline or Hartman's solution should be used. Additional potassium is only advisable if labour is prolonged (e.g. >12 h) and then potassium chloride should be added to the infusate (e.g. at a concentration of 20 mmol/L). Prior to any operative procedure requiring an anaesthetic, the obstetrician should discuss blood glucose control with the anaesthetist to avoid hypoglycaemia and also the inadvertent use of glucose-containing fluids intravenously. Should problems arise with glucose control with this regimen, the usual causes are staff unfamiliarity with glucose measurements, the infusion pump being accidentally turned off or disconnected, or oxytocin being infused in a glucose solution.

Postnatal management

Immediately after delivery, insulin and glucose infusions should be discontinued. If this is not done, hypoglycaemia is likely to occur as a consequence of the increase in insulin sensitivity following the delivery of the placenta. For the insulin-dependent woman it is simplest to revert to the insulin regimen she was taking before pregnancy and to wait until breastfeeding is established before attempting more precise diabetic control. Women with gestational diabetes or impaired glucose tolerance who have been treated with insulin during pregnancy usually do not require any form of treatment, but should have blood glucose measurements made before leaving hospital to check that hyperglycaemia has not persisted.

Breastfeeding should be encouraged, but because of increased nutritional demands, an extra 50 g carbohydrate a day in the dietary intake is recommended [144]. An alternative philosophy is to reduce the insulin dosage [145]. If oral hypoglycaemic agents are used, breastfeeding is not advised because of their possible transfer to the

fetus in breast milk. Women who have had impaired glucose tolerance or gestational diabetes should have a GTT performed about 6–12 weeks after delivery. If this is normal they should be warned that the condition is likely to reoccur in a subsequent pregnancy unless they lose weight. Thus, all women who have had impaired glucose tolerance or gestational diabetes particularly those who are overweight (>120% of ideal bodyweight) should be encouraged to either reduce their weight or maintain it if they are within the range of their ideal bodyweight. This may be achieved by help from the dietitian who advised them during pregnancy. There is now good evidence to show that more than 50% of women who have had gestational diabetes will develop type II, non-insulin-dependent diabetes. The data are summarized in Table 11.4.

The longest follow-up is by O'Sullivan [146] who has shown that in women whose glucose tolerance reverts to normal after pregnancy there was a 50% risk of developing diabetes after 22–28 years of follow-up. O'Sullivan also demonstrated the importance of avoiding obesity, as in his study 47% of the obese, but only 28% of the non-obese showed abnormality at follow-up. In conclusion, the predictive power of impaired glucose tolerance in pregnancy for subsequent diabetes is such that one can argue strongly for routine screening of all pregnant women in order to detect those at risk. It seems likely that women with gestational impaired glucose tolerance and gestational diabetes can diminish this risk of developing type II diabetes in the long term by attention to diet and taking regular exercise.

Pregnancy in diabetic women with renal and/or vascular complications

About 20% of pregnant diabetic women have evidence of significant vascular complications. They deserve separate mention because their problems require special consideration, and may well be best cared for in tertiary centres.

DIABETIC NEPHROPATHY (see also Chapter 7)

The condition is manifested by increasing proteinuria, hypertension and fluid retention—all with or without evidence of diminishing renal function. It may worsen in pregnancy, and management must be determined according to the risk to the mother and fetus. If renal function is seriously impaired before pregnancy then termination must be considered in early pregnancy, particularly if hypertension is an associated complication. In the series of Steel et al. [51] a good outcome was achieved in ongoing pregnancies when creatinine clearance was more than 40 mL/min in the first trimester.

Table 11.4 Follow-up studies of the incidence of impaired glucose tolerance following a previous gestational diabetic pregnancy. Modified from O'Sullivan [179].

Location	Author	Year	Diagnostic criteria GDM	Follow-up period (years)	% diabetic or IGT
Sweden	Hagbard & Svanborg	1960	FBG > 11.2 mmol/L	1–7	62.0
Los Angeles, USA	Mestman *et al.*	1972	2 FBG > 5 mmol/L	0.5	55.6
Leningrad, Russia	Konradi & Matveeva	1974	Abnormal OGTT	0–6	44.2
Belfast, UK	Hadden	1979	Local criteria	10	2.0
			2 h >7.2 mmol/L	10	87.5
Phoenix, USA	Pettitt *et al.*	1980	Abnormal OGTT	4–8	45.5
Aberdeen, UK	Stowers *et al.*	1985	Abnormal IVGTT	<22	35.0
Chicago, USA	Metzger *et al.*	1985	Abnormal OGTT &		
			FBG <5.9 mmol/L	1	38.0
			FBG 5.9–7.3 mmol/L	1	67.0
			FBG >7.3 mmol/L	1	95.0
Melbourne, Australia	Grant *et al.*	1986	Abnormal OGTT	1–12	18.8
Stockholm, Sweden	Efendic *et al.*	1987	Abnormal OGTT	<3	65.0
Copenhagen, Denmark	Damm *et al.*	1989	Abnormal OGTT	2–10	34.0
Boston, USA	O'Sullivan	1989	Abnormal OGTT	<28	49.9
Trinidad, West Indies	Ali & Alexis	1990	Abnormal OGTT	3–7	78.3
Los Angeles, USA	Kjos *et al.*	1990	Abnormal OGTT	<2	40.0
London, UK	Dorhorst *et al.*	1990	Abnormal OGTT	6–12	64.0

FBG, fasting blood glucose; GDM, gestational diabetesmellitus; IGT, Impaired glucose tolerance; IVGTT, intraveneous glucose tolerance test.

Renal function must be closely monitored throughout pregnancy as it may deteriorate at any time and this may require interruption of the pregnancy. Fortunately, renal function does not deteriorate in the majority of cases [147]. Occasionally a severe diabetic nephrotic syndrome may develop [148–150]. Distinguishing this from pre-eclampsia may be difficult and in theory requires a renal biopsy but this is best avoided in pregnancy. However, admission to hospital for close monitoring of maternal and fetal condition is mandatory. Fortunately, with advances in neonatal care, fetal viability can nearly always be obtained without jeopardizing long-term maternal renal function. Fetal growth restriction is more commonly found with diabetic nephropathy. Antenatal fetal blood sampling in six women with diabetic nephropathy and hypertension showed the fetal pH to be below the 5th centile in all cases, but the umbilical artery Doppler flow measurements were relatively normal [70]. Antenatal fetal surveillance in the third trimester must therefore be very close (see below). Birthweight, as expected, is inversely related to maternal blood pressure and directly to creatinine clearance in the third trimester [147].

DIABETIC RETINOPATHY

Retinopathy should not be regarded as a contraindication to pregnancy, but one that needs assessing prior to pregnancy and treating as necessary. Almost all women will have features of background diabetic retinopathy after about 15 years of diabetes. Proliferative retinopathy may develop during pregnancy, and most series report a few cases ranging up to a maximum of about 20% [151–155]. Provided proliferative retinopathy (whether new or pre-existing) is actively treated there appears to be no deterioration in visual acuity after pregnancy. In addition background retinopathy may appear to deteriorate during pregnancy through improved diabetic control leading to an ischaemic retinopathy [155]. These changes usually resolve spontaneously. In view of this, all women with type I or type II diabetes should have fundoscopy performed at least twice during pregnancy and treatment given as necessary.

AUTONOMIC NEUROPATHY

Neuropathy can be demonstrated in diabetic women in pregnancy, but it is uncommon for it to be a clinical problem. It occasionally presents with gastric symptoms of severe and continued vomiting leading to metabolic disturbance. This can then be associated with fetal loss [156].

Obstetric management

There is a certain artificiality in attempting to distinguish between obstetric and medical management of diabetic pregnancy when there are so many problems that require a joint approach. Although, as has been repeatedly emphasized in this chapter, the most important contribution to management is good control of maternal blood glucose, there are numerous issues that really only the obstetrician can decide upon. The obstetrician has the responsibility of ensuring that fetal development is proceeding satisfactorily from the time of conception until delivery. For instance, in early pregnancy congenital malformations should be excluded, whilst in later pregnancy, detection of excessive fetal growth and/or hydramnios is often evidence that diabetic control needs to be improved. The management decisions with which the obstetrician is faced can be considered sequentially according to the stage of pregnancy.

First trimester

As soon as she thinks she may be pregnant, the diabetic woman should attend the hospital and preferably the joint clinic for initial assessment by the whole team. An ultrasound examination at this time is essential for dating the pregnancy and confirming a viable pregnancy. In the past, Pedersen and Molsted-Pedersen [157,158] suggested that the finding of a smaller than expected crown–rump length on ultrasound was peculiar to diabetic pregnancy and that it was evidence of future fetal growth restriction and likely congenital malformations. However, others have been unable to substantiate this observation [159]. If there is concern about the quality of diabetic control, which may particularly occur with hyperemesis, admission to hospital is advised. This provides a good opportunity to provide updating education. The patient may need to be advised on nutrition and to be convinced of the importance of achieving good control in the interests of her baby. It will also facilitate the institution of daily blood glucose monitoring.

The mother who is found to have gestational diabetes needs particularly careful counselling so that she understands that, although the diabetes may disappear after pregnancy, attention to diabetic control is essential if the risk to the fetus is to be minimized. All these women will be treated by some dietary restriction whether or not they have additional insulin and will need to be motivated to accept the discipline this requires in the interests of their babies. Effective counselling takes time and the diabetes specialist midwife or nurse and the dietician should be prepared to spend plenty of time with her at the first one to two visits or ideally to perform a home visit.

Second trimester

From the little that is known of intrauterine life in diabetic pregnancy, it appears that the second trimester is a time of relative security for the fetus. Organogenesis is virtually complete and the fetus does not appear to be at an increased risk of dying *in utero*. However, whether the fetus has subsequent growth acceleration is likely to be determined from early in the second trimester [84] so that strict diabetic control needs to be maintained.

Ultrasound screening for congenital malformations should be discussed with all women and is best done at 19–20 weeks' gestation. Offering fetal echocardiography at 20–22 weeks is ideal management in view of the increased risk of cardiac abnormalities associated with diabetes. However, most cannot offer this service as a routine in which case it should be reserved for those with poor diabetic control during embryogenesis. Scanning should also aim to exclude a neural tube defect and sacral agenesis, which are known to occur more frequently in diabetic pregnancy [160]. If maternal serum α-fetoprotein screening is performed, care is needed with interpretation due to the values being lower in diabetic pregnancy [161]. The incidence of Down's syndrome is not increased, but if serum marker screening is being used, again care is needed with interpretation. When compared to controls, in maternal diabetes the multiples of the median (MoM) were found to be 0.77 MoM for α-fetoprotein, 0.92 MoM for serum unconjugated oestriol and 0.95 MoM for human chorionic gonadotrophin [162].

The frequency of antenatal visits can be determined in general by the degree of blood glucose control that has been achieved. Should proteinuria occur, protein and creatinine excretion should be measured over 24 h together with plasma urea, urate and creatinine. Many obstetricians and physicians like to have baseline renal function tests done as early as possible in pregnancy in all diabetic mothers whether or not they have proteinuria. Ultrasound measurements of the fetal head and abdominal circumference should ideally start by 24 weeks' gestation, as even then an increase in growth rate may be seen [83,84].

The mother who is found to have gestational diabetes needs particularly careful counselling so that she understands that, although the diabetes may disappear after pregnancy, attention to diabetic control is essential if the risk to the fetus is to be minimized. All these women will be treated by some dietary restriction whether or not they have additional insulin, and will need to be motivated to accept the discipline this requires in the interests of their babies. Effective counselling takes time and the diabetes specialist midwife or nurse and the dietitian should be prepared to spend plenty of time with her at the first one to two visits or ideally to perform a home visit.

Third trimester

The last 12 weeks of pregnancy is the period when the combination of good medical and obstetric care is likely to have the greatest impact on fetal health. Complications such as pregnancy-induced hypertension, hydramnios and fetal macrosomia, preterm labour and perinatal death are all increased in the poorly controlled diabetic woman. Good control achieved in the earlier months of pregnancy has to be maintained in the face of increasing insulin requirements. The obstetrician must be constantly on the lookout for any deterioration in fetal well-being, in particular the development of hypertension, hydramnios or excessive fetal growth. A number of additional methods of fetal surveillance are used.

ULTRASOUND

Most studies have shown that the head size in diabetic pregnancy remains within normal limits [163]. Abdominal circumference measurements of the fetus are as good a indicator of fetal weight in diabetic pregnancy as in non-diabetic pregnancy and therefore have the same limitations. Fetal abdominal circumference measurements of >36 cm are a good predictor of the birthweight being more than 4 kg [164]. Measurements should ideally be performed every 2 weeks in the third trimester along with an assessment of amniotic fluid volume. Examples of two abnormal growth patterns are shown in Fig. 11.7.

Umbilical artery Doppler flow velocity waveforms have been studied widely in diabetic pregnancy. The current view is that abnormal results tend only to be found in cases where growth restriction has been already detected [68,69]. There is therefore no point in their routine use in all diabetic pregnancies, but the method should just be reserved for helping in the management of the growth restricted fetus, as in normal pregnancy.

ANTENATAL CARDIOTOCOGRAPHY

Antenatal cardiotocography is a useful means of assessing fetal health irrespective of whether maternal diabetes is present. In the uncomplicated diabetic pregnancy if the test is performed two or three times per week from 36 weeks' gestation onwards, many women who would have otherwise have been delivered before 38 weeks' gestation because of the obstetrician's anxiety about the possibility of intrauterine death, can be allowed to progress to nearer term. This is now the most widely accepted practice. Teramo *et al.* [165] found a significant correlation between abnormal tests and poor metabolic control. This is in agreement with the findings by Salvesen *et al.* [166] that fetal heart rate variation correlates well with the degree of fetal acidaemia in diabetic pregnancy. However, six of 12 fetuses in this study with a pH below the 5th centile had normal heart rate variability.

Great care must be taken in deciding how frequently cardiotocography should be performed and also in the interpretation of the results. This can only be conducted by experienced staff that are aware of the details of the case, and are either a part of or have good liaison with the obstetric/diabetic team. In the woman with well-controlled diabetes who has permanent normoglycaemia, it is probably unnecessary [153]. In the woman with

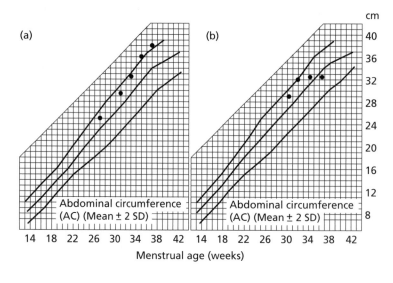

Fig 11.7 Abnormal fetal abdominal circumference growth patterns in diabetic pregnancy. (a) Excessive fetal growth. Diabetes not optimally controlled, induced at 38 weeks, shoulder dystocia. 4340-g female infant. (b) Excessive fetal growth with superimposed growth retardation. Spontaneous labour at 37 weeks, late decelerations, fetal acidosis, emergency caesarean section. 2580-g female infant. (M. Maresh, unpublished observations.)

hypertension and vascular disease it may be necessary to start earlier, and with any suggestion of growth restriction daily recordings may be advisable.

BIOPHYSICAL PROFILE

The biophysical profile has been proposed as part of routine care [118,167,168], although the Scottish Intercollegiate Guidelines Network [127] had reservations about advising routine usage. There is no evidence presented to support the addition of ultrasound detection of fetal breathing, movement and tone to a surveillance programme of serial ultrasound assessments and cardiotocography. Salvesen *et al.* [166] noted a correlation between fetal acidaemia and the biophysical profile score, but nine out of 12 fetuses with a pH <5th centile had normal scores.

In conclusion the biophysical profile does not appear to have a role in routine care and in the high-risk case a normal result should be interpreted with care.

Pregnancy complications

In the past, it was thought that the incidence of complications such as pregnancy-induced hypertension, antepartum haemorrhage and urinary tract infection was thought to be increased in diabetic pregnancy. A review by Cousins [169] showed little current evidence to support this. In the 1980 UK Survey of Diabetic Pregnancy the incidence of pregnancy-induced hypertension—at 12% amongst the established diabetic mothers—was the same as that for those with gestational diabetes [112]. However, what is of significance is the increased risk to the fetus from any one of these complications of pregnancy in association with diabetes. The appearance of a complication of pregnancy which is potentially life threatening to the fetus is an indication for hospital admission and possible delivery.

PRETERM LABOUR

In diabetic pregnancies the incidence of preterm delivery (less than 37 completed weeks of gestation) is increased. Molsted-Pedersen [170] reported a threefold increase in women with mild diabetes. In the UK Survey of Diabetic Pregnancy [112], 50% of women with established diabetes were delivered before 38 weeks of gestation. Approximately two-thirds of these women were induced or had an elective caesarean delivery, either because of suspected fetal compromise or because of established routine management. The remaining third went into spontaneous labour for reasons that are unknown, but some early

deliveries were likely to have been associated with hydramnios. The effect of preterm delivery on the baby of the diabetic mother is likely to be more serious than on that of the non-diabetic because of the known predisposition of the former to complications such as respiratory distress.

If a decision is made to try to prevent delivery by suppressing uterine activity, β-sympathomimetic drugs should be used with considerable caution as they have a gluconeogenic effect and can cause loss of diabetic control and diabetic ketoacidosis. Calcium-channel blockers, such as nifedipine, are equally effective and do not effect diabetic control. However, the corticosteroids administered to the mother to accelerate fetal lungs maturity also induce hyperglycaemia through antagonizing insulin, and can on their own cause loss of diabetic control and ketoacidosis. Accordingly once corticosteroids have been given, 2-hourly blood glucose monitoring should be instituted whilst awaiting the rise in blood glucose. This is likely to start within 6–12 h. Intravenous insulin should be given with a glucose infusion. However, if the woman is eating then glucose is unnecessary, and normal saline should be used. A standard sliding scale relating insulin infusion rate to blood glucose is unlikely to be adequate and usually about twice as much insulin is necessary for each level of blood glucose. If β-sympathomimetic drugs are given then the blood glucose increases more rapidly and blood glucose should be checked every 15 min following the start of the infusion until the clinical picture is stable. Even larger doses of insulin are required and additional potassium may be necessary to counteract the drug-induced hypokalaemia.

As there is no evidence that weekly courses of corticosteroids are of additional benefit, corticosteroid therapy should only be given once, when premature delivery is considered by experienced staff to be likely, as treatment is potentially dangerous to the mother and fetus. Worsening hyperglycaemia, despite intravenous insulin, is usually caused by underestimating the insulin requirement or by failing to realize that the insulin infusion pump is not working.

Timing and route of delivery

In the past, unexpected stillbirth was a relatively common event near term in the pregnant diabetic woman. This led in the 1930s to a policy of delivery at a gestational age when the fetus was considered to have a reasonable chance of extrauterine survival [171] usually between 36 and 38 weeks. As a result, the incidence of hyaline membrane disease and caesarean section rose [172]. Delayed pulmonary maturation of the fetus is a feature of diabetic pregnancy [96]. This is thought to be primarily due to a deficiency of one of the important constituents of pulmonary surfactant—phosphatidylglycerol. Measurement of phosphatidylglycerol in the amniotic fluid is a useful index of whether the baby is likely to develop respiratory distress, but it involves an amniocentesis near term. Fortunately, improved diabetic control and the recent tendency to allow an increasing number of women to go into spontaneous labour have diminished the need for amniocentesis for phosphatidylglycerol measurement. Ideally it should be measured prior to elective caesarean section if there is any doubt about the fetal maturity, and in cases of preterm labour if there is any doubt about whether or not to suppress labour. Unfortunately, because the test is rarely used it may be difficult to find a laboratory prepared to make the measurements. A policy of delivery between 36 and 38 weeks' gestation for women with established diabetes was common in the UK and was often applied as well to those with gestational diabetes. There is increasing evidence of the safety of waiting for the onset of spontaneous labour, providing that the diabetes is well controlled and the pregnancy is uncomplicated. Drury [64] in a personal series of women with established diabetes in Dublin allowed diabetic women to go into spontaneous labour unless complications supervened. His results showing only 18% being delivered under 38 weeks' gestation were in marked contrast with those of the Survey of Diabetic Pregnancy in the UK [112], where 50% delivered before 38 weeks. More recently a figure of 35% of women being delivered before 37 weeks has been reported [66]. No obvious adverse fetal or neonatal outcomes have been demonstrated from less interventionist obstetric management.

Maternal diabetes is commonly associated with high caesarean section rates. Drury [64] also had a low caesarean section rate of 26%, which contrasted to the UK survey rate of 58% [112]. As the general caesarean section rate in the UK has increased in the 1990s, attempts to be less interventional, particularly in women with well-controlled diabetes, have not surprisingly had minimal effects on the caesarean section rate in diabetic women. Recent reports suggest rates of 60–65% [6,66].

These results underline one of the basic tenets of modern obstetric practice. 'Across the board' policies on such an important issue as the route and timing of delivery are no longer acceptable—each case should be assessed on its merits, which in the case of maternal diabetes include diabetic control and fetal well-being. If the fetus is in good condition and normally grown, the mother's pregnancy is uncomplicated with her diabetes well controlled, there is no cause for invention. Nor is there any obvious reason to repeat a caesarean section if

the indications for the operation in a previous pregnancy were non-recurrent. However, elective caesarean section may be indicated for a number of valid reasons, such as demonstrable fetal compromise or a baby that, on clinical and ultrasound assessment, is so large that traumatic vaginal delivery appears a distinct possibility. It needs to be stressed that while a much more liberal view about allowing vaginal delivery can be taken nowadays, this approach must be accompanied by careful antenatal assessment by an experienced obstetrician, good control of the blood glucose of the mother, and the use of cardiotocography and fetal pH estimation if required, throughout labour.

Intrapartum care

The fetus of the gestational and of the established diabetic woman should always be regarded as being at particular risk during labour no matter how well controlled the diabetes. Fetal asphyxia and disproportion are particular hazards. Good control of blood glucose (see above) is required to assist in maintaining fetal normoglycaemia and preventing fetal acidaemia. Continuous cardiotocography is advised, and the traces should be interpreted in the normal ways. The most common cause of an abnormal pattern in labour is secondary to maternal hyperglycaemia so the first step in the management of an abnormal trace is to obtain normoglycaemia if it is not present. However, if there is no rapid improvement, fetal pH measurement should be undertaken in the normal way. Delay in the active phase of labour should usually be managed by active recourse to caesarean section rather than by using oxytocin. An experienced obstetrician should be available for the delivery with all staff well drilled in the management of shoulder dystocia. Similarly, seemingly simple forceps or ventouse deliveries should not be commenced by inexperienced staff because of the increased risk of problems with the shoulders. Prophylactic antibiotics should be given for both emergency and elective caesarean sections and also consideration should be given to thromboprophylaxis.

Contraception

Advice on contraception before and after pregnancy is an important part of the present day care of diabetic women during their reproductive years. The subject is a difficult one because of the adverse effects of some methods of contraception on metabolic and circulatory systems. Equally, diabetes may interfere with the effectiveness of contraceptives. For a further review the reader is referred to Skouby *et al.* [173].

Oral contraceptives

The combined oral contraceptive alters metabolism with a trend towards worsening glucose tolerance and rising triglyceride levels. The current consensus is that in combined preparations, it is the progestogenic component that is mainly responsible for the diabetogenic effect of oral contraceptives.

Steel [174] observed an increase in insulin requirements in only 17 out of 88 diabetic women who had started oral contraceptives and there was no difference between 30-mg and 50-mg oestrogen preparations. If, as seems likely, deterioration of glucose tolerance in diabetes is the product of increasing insulin resistance, then those women who have presented with gestational diabetes during pregnancy are more liable to remain diabetic if they take oral contraceptives after pregnancy. However, in general women with previous gestational diabetes mellitus were shown by Skouby et al. [175] not to have had a worsening of their glucose tolerance when contrasted to controls when given low-dose combined oral contraceptives even though the insulin response to glucose increased significantly. Similar results have been reported by Kjos et al. [176]. However, in contrast Kjos et al. [176] showed that progesterone-only contraception significantly increased the risk of developing type II diabetes in women who had had an abnormal glucose tolerance test in pregnancy.

Effects on lipid profile have been investigated and reviewed [173]; in general, current preparations do not appear to have effects with the possible exceptions of the monophasic ethinyloestradiol/norethisterone preparations. Few data have been published on the metabolic effects of the newer progestogens such as gestodene, but what is available suggests no change in glycaemic control [173].

An increased risk of thrombotic or thromboembolic lesions in diabetic women on oral contraceptives has long been postulated. The combination of proliferative intimal vascular lesions that are known to occur as a complication of diabetes, and an increase in platelet aggregation induced by oral contraceptives, sets the scene for thrombus formation. Steel and Duncan [174] reported an alarming incidence of near fatal lesions in insulin-requiring diabetic women aged less than 30 years taking oral contraceptives compared with a similar group not taking oral contraceptives. These ranged from cerebral ischaemia to myocardial infarction. These authors have argued that because it is the oestrogen component of the oral contraceptive that induces the abnormal clotting, it is logical to use a 'progestogen-only' oral contraceptive. The disadvantages of this method of contraception are an increased failure rate (six per 100 woman years) and a 50% rate of menstrual irregularity.

Intrauterine contraceptive device

This should be an ideal method of contraception for women with diabetes. Although it was suggested that copper-bearing devices are rendered ineffective more frequently in diabetic women as compared with non-diabetic women, by the tendency for the copper to become encrusted with sulphur and chloride, a large series found no increase in the failure rate for copper devices in diabetic women [177]. The corrosive process was no different from that found in controls and was purely time dependent.

Mechanical methods

While mechanical methods (male and female condom and diaphragm) are currently unfashionable they remain effective alternatives without the disadvantages of the oral contraceptive pill in particular.

Sterilization

Sterilization is particularly indicated when there is evidence of progressive vascular degeneration and/or nephropathy, but as usual should only be performed after full consultation with the woman and her partner. All diabetic women should consider some limitation of their family. Laparoscopic sterilization, as a day case, is the method of choice because it involves minimal disturbance of diabetic control and care of the baby.

Pregnancy may have such disastrous consequences for the diabetic woman with severe nephropathy or progressive retinopathy that occasionally it is necessary to advise termination of pregnancy. In such cases sterilization should obviously be discussed with the diabetic woman and her partner.

In conclusion the oral contraceptives may be used, particularly in the younger woman without vascular disease, to ensure effective contraception. Progestogen-only contraception is probably best avoided particularly in women who have had impaired glucose tolerance or gestational diabetes. Between children and until the woman is sure that her family is complete, barrier methods or intrauterine contraceptive devices may be a better alternative. The safety and efficacy of sterilization make this the preferred option once the family is complete.

References

1 Department of Health. *Report on Confidential Enquiries into Maternal Deaths in the United Kingdom 1991–93.* HMSO, London, 1996.

2 Department of Health. *Report on Confidential Enquiries into Maternal Deaths in the United Kingdom 1994–96*. HMSO, London, 1998.

3 Diabetes Care and Research in Europe: the St Vincent Declaration. *Diabet Med* 1990; 34: 655–61.

4 NHS Executive. Health Service Guidelines. Key features of a good diabetes service. *NHS Executive HSG* 1997; 97: 45.

5 Casson I, Clarke C *et al*. Outcomes of pregnancy in insulin dependent diabetic women: results of a five year population cohort study. *Br Med J* 1997; 315: 275–8.

6 Hawthorne G, Robson S *et al*. Prospective population based survey of outcome of pregnancy in diabetic women: results of the Northern Diabetic Pregnancy Audit 1994. *Br Med J* 1997; 315: 279–81.

7 World Health Organization. Expert Committee. *Diabetes Mellitus Technical Report Series*, 1980: 646

8 American Diabetes Association. Gestational diabetes mellitus. *Diabetes Care* 1999; 22 (Suppl. 1): S74–S76.

9 Alberti K, Zimmett P, for the WHO Consultation Group. Definition, diagnosis and classification of diabetes mellitus and its complications. Part 1: Diagnosis and classification of diabetes mellitus. Provisional report of a WHO consultation. *Diabet Med* 1998; 15: 539–53.

10 White P. Pregnancy and diabetes. Medical aspects. *Med Clin North Am* 1965; 49: 1015–24.

11 Hare J, White P. Gestational diabetes and White Classification. *Diabetes Care* 1980; 3: 394.

12 Lind T. A prospective multicentre study to determine the influence of pregnancy upon the 75g oral glucose tolerance test. In: Sutherland HW, Stowers JM, Pearson DWM, eds. *Carbohydrate Metabolism in Pregnancy and the Newborn IV*. Springer-Verlag, Berlin, 1989: 209–26.

13 Metzger B, Coustan D, eds. Proceedings of the Fourth International Workshop Conference on Gestational Diabetes Mellitus. *Diabetes Care* 1998; 21 (Suppl. 2): B1–167.

14 Kuhl C. Aetiology of gestational diabetes. In: Oats JN, ed. *Diabetes in Pregnancy. Bailliere's Clinical Obstetrics and Gynaecology*. W.B. Saunders, London, 1991: 5; 279–92.

15 Freinkel N. Effects of the conceptus on maternal metabolism during pregnancy. In: Leibel BS, Wrenshall GA, eds. *On the Nature and Treatment of Diabetes*. Excerpta Medica Foundation, Amsterdam, 1965: 679–91.

16 Gillmer M, Beard R, Brooke F, Oakley N. Carbohydrate metabolism in pregnancy. Part I. Diurnal plasma glucose profile in normal and diabetic women. *Br Med J* 1975; 3: 399–402.

17 Metzger B, Phelps R, Freinkel N, Navickas I. Effects of gestational diabetes on diurnal profiles of plasma glucose, lipids, and individual amino acids. *Diabetes Care* 1980; 3: 402–9.

18 Maresh M, Gillmer M, Beard R, Alderson C, Bloxham B, Elkeles R. The effect of diet and insulin on metabolic profiles of women with gestational diabetes mellitus. *Diabetes* 1985; 34 (Suppl. 2): 880–93.

19 Buschard K, Buck I, Molsted-Pedersen L, Hougaard P, Kuhl C. Increased incidence of true type I diabetes acquired during pregnancy. *Br Med J* 1987; 294: 275–9.

20 Persson B, Lunell N. Metabolic control in diabetic pregnancy. *Am J Obstet Gynecol* 1975; 122: 737–45.

21 Oakley N, Beard R, Turner R. Effect of sustained maternal hyperglycaemia on the fetus in normal and diabetic pregnancies. *Br Med J* 1972; 1: 466–9.

22 Salvesen D, Brudenell J, Proudler A, Crook D, Nicolaides K. Fetal pancreatic β-cell function in pregnancies complicated by maternal diabetes mellitus. Relationship to fetal acidemia and macrosomia. *Am J Obstet Gynecol* 1993; 168: 1363–9.

23 Milner R, Hales C. Effect of intravenous glucose on concentration of insulin in maternal and umbilical cord plasma. *Br Med J* 1965; 1: 284–6.

24 Milner R, Ashworth M, Barson A. Insulin release from human fetal pancreas in response to glucose, leucine and arginine. *J Endocrinol* 1972; 52: 497–505.

25 Pedersen J. *The Pregnant Diabetic and Her Newborn—Problems and Management*. Munksgaard, Copenhagen, 1977.

26 Van Assche F, Aerts L. The fetal endocrine pancreas. *Contrib Gynecol Obstet* 1979; 5: 44–57.

27 Hales C, Barker D *et al*. Fetal and infant growth and impaired glucose tolerance at age 64. *Br Med J* 1991; 303: 1019–22.

28 Ravelli A, van der Meulen R *et al*. Glucose tolerance in adults after prenatal exposure to famine. *Lancet* 1998; 351: 173–7.

29 Widness J, Susa J *et al*. Increased erythropoiesis and elevated erythropoietin in infants born to diabetic mothers and in hyperinsulinaemic rhesus fetuses. *J Clin Invest* 1981; 67: 637–42.

30 Widness J, Teramo K, Clemons G. Direct relationship of antepartum glucose control and fetal erythropoietin in human type I (insulin-dependent) diabetic pregnancy. *Diabetologia* 1990; 33: 378–83.

31 Salvesen D, Brudenell M, Nicolaides K. Fetal polycythemia and thrombocytopenia in pregnancies complicated by maternal diabetes mellitus. *Am J Obstet Gynecol* 1992; 166: 1287–93.

32 Salvesen D, Brudenell J, Snijders R, Ireland R, Nicolaides K. Fetal plasma erythropoietin in pregnancies complicated by maternal diabetes mellitus. *Am J Obstet Gynecol* 1993; 168: 88–94.

33 Damm P, Molsted-Pedersen L, Kühl C. High incidence of diabetes mellitus and impaired glucose tolerance in women with previous gestational diabetes (Abstract). *Diabetologia* 1989; 32: 479A.

34 Kucera J. Rate and type of congenital anomalies among offspring in diabetic women. *J Reprod Med*, 1971; 7: 61–70.

35 Molsted-Pedersen L, Tygstrup I, Pedersen J. Congenital malformations in newborn infants of diabetic women. Correlation with maternal diabetic vascular complications. *Lancet* 1964; i: 1124–6.

36 Pedersen J, Molsted-Pedersen L. Early growth retardation in diabetic pregnancy. *Br Med J*, 1979; 1: 18–19.

37 Leslie R, Pyke D, John P, White J. Haemoglobin A1 in diabetic pregnancy. *Lancet* 1978; ii: 958–9.

38 Miller E, Hare J *et al*. Elevated maternal haemoglobin A1C in early pregnancy and major congenital anomalies in infants of diabetic mothers. *N Engl J Med* 1981; 304: 1331–4.

39 Ylinen K, Aula P, Stenman U, Kesaniemi-Kuokkanen T, Teramo, K. Risks of minor and major fetal malformations in diabetics with high haemoglobin A1C values in early pregnancy. *Br Med J* 1984; 289: 345–6.

40 Stubbs S, Doddridge M, John P, Steel J, Wright A. Haemoglobin A1 and congenital malformation. *Diabet Med* 1987; 4: 156–9.

41 Mills J, Knopp R *et al*. Lack of relation of increased malformation rates in infants of diabetic mothers to glycemic control during organogenesis. *N Engl J Med* 1988; 318: 671–6.

42 Fuhrmann K, Reiher H, Semmler K, Fischer F, Fischer M, Glockner E. Prevention of congenital malformations in infants of insulin dependent diabetic mothers. *Diabetes Care* 1983; 6: 219–23.

43 Steel J, Johnstone F, Hepburn D, Smith A. Can prepregnancy care of diabetic women reduce the risk of abnormal babies? *Br Med J* 1990; 301: 1070–4.

44 The Diabetes Control and Complications Trial Research Group. Pregnancy outcomes in the Diabetes Control and Complications Trial. *Am J Obstet Gynecol* 1996; 174: 1343–53.

45 Deuchar E. Culture *in vitro* as a means of analysing the effect of maternal diabetes on embryonic development in rats. In: Elliott K, O'Conner M, eds. *Pregnancy Metabolism Diabetes and the Fetus. Ciba Foundation Symposium*, no. 63 (new series). Excerpta Medica, Amsterdam, 1979: 181–97.

46 Lewis N, Akazawa S, Freinkel N. Teratogenesis from B-hydroxybutyrate during organogenesis in rat embryo organ culture and enhancement by subteratogenic glucose. *Diabetes* 1983; 32 (Suppl. 1): 11A.

47 Baker L, Egler J, Klein S, Goldman A. Meticulous control of diabetes during organogenesis prevents congenital lumbosacral defects in rats. *Diabetes* 1981; 30: 955–9.

48 Eriksson U, Dahlstrom E, Hellerstrom C. Diabetes in pregnancy. Skeletal malformations in the offspring of diabetic rats after intermittent withdrawal of insulin in early gestation. *Diabetes* 1983; 32: 1141–5.

49 Buchanan T, Schemmer J, Freinkel N. Embryotoxic effects of brief maternal insulin-hypoglycemia during organogenesis in the rat. *J Clin Invest* 1986; 78: 643–9.

50 Akazawa A, Hashimoto M *et al*. Effects of hypoglycaemia on early embryogenesis in rat embryo organ culture. *Diabetologia* 1987; 30: 791–6.

51 Steel J, Johnstone F, Smith A. Prepregnancy preparation. In: Sutherland HW, Stowers JM, Pearson DWM, eds. *Carbohydrate Metabolism in Pregnancy and the Newborn IV*. Springer-Verlag, Berlin, 1989: 129–39

52 Freinkel N. The Banting Lecture 1980: Of pregnancy and progeny. *Diabetes* 1980; 29: 1023–35.

53 Eriksson U, Borg L. Diabetes and embryonic malformations: role of substrate-induced free-oxygen radical production for dysmorphogenesis in cultured rat embryos. *Diabetes* 1993; 42: 411–19.

54 Malins J. Fetal anomalies related to carbohydrate metabolism. The epidemiological approach. In: Sutherland HW, Stowers JM, eds. *Carbohydrate Metabolism in Pregnancy and the Newborn*. Springer-Verlag, Berlin 1979: 229–46.

55 Yssing M. Long term prognosis of children born to mothers diabetic when pregnant. In: Camerini-Davalos RA, Cole HS, eds. *Early Diabetes in Early Life. Proceedings of the 3rd International Symposium, Madeira*. Academic Press, New York, 1975: 575–86.

56 Churchill J, Berendes H, Nemore J. Neuropsychological deficits in children of diabetic mothers. *Am J Obstet Gynecol* 1969; 105: 257–67.

57 Stehbens J, Baker G, Kitchell M. Outcome at ages 1, 3 and 5 years of children born to diabetic women. *Am J Obstet Gynecol* 1977; 127: 408–13.

58 Naeye R, Chez R. Effects of maternal acetonuria and low pregnancy weight gain on childrens' psychomotor development. *Am J Obstet Gynecol* 1981; 139: 189–93.

59 Rizzo T, Metzger B, Burns W, Burns K. Correlations between antepartum maternal metabolism and intelligence of offspring. *N Engl J Med* 1991; 325: 911–16.

60 Miodovnik M, Lavin J, Knowles H, Holroyde J, Stys S. Spontaneous abortion among insulin-dependent diabetic women. *Am J Obstet Gynecol* 1984; 150: 372–6.

61 Miodovnik M, Mimouni F, Tsang R, Ammar E, Kaplan L, Siddiqi T. Glycemic control and spontaneous abortion in insulin-dependent diabetic women. *Obstet Gynecol* 1986; 68: 366–9.

62 Mills J, Simpson J *et al*. Incidence of spontaneous abortion among normal women and insulin-dependent diabetic women whose pregnancies were identified within 21 days of conception. *N Engl J Med* 1988; 319: 1617–23.

63 Dicker D, Feldberg D, Samuel N, Yeshaya A, Karp M, Goldman J. Spontaneous abortion in patients with insulin-dependent diabetes mellitus. The effect of preconceptional diabetic control. *Am J Obstet Gynecol* 1988; 158: 1161–4.

64 Drury M. Management of the pregnant diabetic—are the pundits right? *Diabetologia* 1986; 29: 10–12.

65 Hadden D, Traub A. Centralisation of care leads to better outcome. *Br Med J* 1998; 316: 550.

66 Maresh M, Dawson A *et al*. Pregnancy outcome with Type I diabetes in seven tertiary centres in the United Kingdom. *J Obstet Gynaecol*, 2000; 20 (Suppl. 1): S63.

67 Bradley R, Brudenell J, Nicolaides K. Chronic fetal hypoxia in diabetic pregnancy. *Br Med J* 1988; 296: 790.

68 Johnstone F, Steel J, Haddad N, Hoskins P, Greer I, Chambers S. Doppler umbilical artery flow velocity waveforms in diabetic pregnancy. *Br J Obstet Gynaecol* 1992; 99: 135–40.

69 Salvesen D, Higueras M, Mansur C, Freeman J, Brudenell J, Nicolaides K. Placental and fetal Doppler velocimetry in pregnancies complicated by maternal diabetes mellitus. *Am J Obstet Gynecol* 1993; 168: 645–52.

70 Salvesen D, Higueras M, Brudenell J, Drury P, Nicolaides K. Doppler velocimetry and fetal heart rate studies in nephropathic diabetics. *Am J Obstet Gynecol* 1992; 167: 1297–303.

71 Fox H. The placenta in diabetes mellitus. In: Sutherland HW, Stowers JM, Pearson DWM, eds. *Carbohydrate Metabolism in Pregnancy and the Newborn IV*. Springer-Verlag, Berlin, 1989: 109–17

72 Madsen H. Fetal oxygenation in diabetic pregnancy. *Dan Med Bull* 1986; 33: 64–74.

73 Shelley H, Bassett J, Miller R. Control of carbohydrate metabolism in the fetus and newborn. *Br Med Bull* 1975; 31: 37–43.

74 Susa J, Schwartz R. Effects of hyperinsulinaemia in the primate fetus. *Diabetes* 1985; 34 (Suppl. 2): 36–41.

75 Carson B, Phillips A, Simmons M. Effects of a sustained insulin infusion upon glucose uptake and oxygenation of the ovine fetus. *Pediatr Res* 1980; 14: 147–52.

76 Oppenheimer E, Esterly J. Thrombosis in the newborn: comparison between diabetic and nondiabetic mothers. *J Pediatr* 1965; 67: 549.

77 O'Sullivan J. Prospective study of gestational diabetes and its treatment. In: Stowers JM, Sutherland HW, eds. *Carbohydrate Metabolism in Pregnancy and the Newborn*. Churchill Livingstone, Edinburgh, 1975: 195–204.

78 O'Sullivan J, Charles D, Mahan C, Dandrow R. Gestational diabetes and perinatal mortality rate. *Am J Obstet Gynecol* 1973; 116: 901–4.

79 Pettitt D, Knowler W, Baird H, Bennett P. Gestational diabetes: infant and maternal complications of pregnancy in relation to third-trimester glucose tolerance in the Pima Indians. *Diabetes Care* 1980; 3: 458–64.

80 Jarrett R. Should we screen for gestational diabetes. *Br Med J* 1997; 315: 736–7.

81 Soares J, Dornhorst A, Beard R. The case for screening for gestational diabetes. *Br Med J* 1997; 315: 737–9.

82 Sermer M, Naylor D *et al.* Impact of increasing carbohydrate intolerance on maternal-fetal outcomes in 3637 women without gestational diabetes. *Am J Obstet Gynecol* 1995; 173: 146–56.

83 Keller J, Metzger B, Dooley S, Tamura R, Sabbagha R, Freinkel N. Infants of diabetic mothers with accelerated fetal growth by ultrasonography: Are they all alike? *Am J Obstet Gynecol* 1990; 163: 893–7.

84 Raychaudhuri K, Maresh M. Glycemic control throughout pregnancy and fetal growth in insulin-dependent diabetes. *Obstet Gynecol* 2000; 95: 190–4.

85 Whitelaw A. Subcutaneous fat in newborn infants of diabetic mothers: an indication of quality of diabetic control. *Lancet* 1977; i: 15–18.

86 Stubbs S, Leslie R, John P. Fetal macrosomia and maternal diabetic control in pregnancy. *Br Med J* 1981; 282: 439–40.

87 Fallucca F, Gargiulo P *et al.* Amniotic fluid insulin, C peptide concentrations, and fetal morbidity in infants of diabetic mothers. *Am J Obstet Gynecol* 1985; 153: 534–40.

88 Cardell B. Hypertrophy and hyperplasia of the pancreatic islets in new born infants. *J Pathol Bacteriol* 1953; 66: 335–8.

89 Wang H, Chard T. The role of insulin like growth factor-1 and insulin-like growth factor-binding protein-1 in the control of human fetal growth. *J Endocrinol* 1992; 132: 11–19.

90 Whittaker P, Stewart M, Taylor A, Howell R, Lind T. Insulin-like growth factor 1 and its binding protein 1 during normal and diabetic pregnancies. *Obstet Gynecol* 1990; 76: 223–9.

91 Maresh M, Beard R, Bray C, Elkeles R, Wadsworth J. Factors predisposing to and outcomes of gestational diabetes. *Obstet Gynecol* 1989; 74: 342–6.

92 O'Sullivan J, Gellis S, Dandrow R, Tenney B. The potential diabetic and her treatment in pregnancy. *Obstet Gynecol* 1966; 27: 683–9.

93 Roversi G, Gargiulo M *et al.* A new approach to the treatment of diabetic pregnant women: 479 cases (1963–75). *Am J Obstet Gynecol* 1979; 135: 567–76.

94 Buchanan T, Kjos S *et al.* Use of fetal ultrasound to select metabolic therapy for pregnancies complicated by mild gestational diabetes. *Diabetes Care* 1994; 17: 275–83.

95 Langer O, Rodriguez D, Xenakis E, McFarland M, Berkus M, Arredondo F. Intensified versus conventional management of gestational diabetes. *Am J Obstet Gynecol* 1994; 170: 1036–47.

96 Bourbon J, Farrell P. Fetal lung development in the diabetic pregnancy. *Pediatr Res* 1985; 19: 253–67.

97 Piper J, Langer O. Does maternal diabetes delay fetal pulmonary maturity? *Am J Obstet Gynecol* 1993; 168: 783–6.

98 James D, Chiswick M, Harkes A, Williams M, Tindall V. Maternal diabetes and neonatal respiratory distress. II. Prediction of fetal lung maturity. *Br J Obstet Gynaecol* 1984; 91: 325–9.

99 Kalhan S, Savin S, Adam P. Attenuated glucose production rate in newborn infants of insulin-dependent diabetic mothers. *N Engl J Med* 1977; 296: 375–6.

100 Gillmer M, Beard R, Brooke F, Oakley N. Carbohydrate metabolism in pregnancy. Part II. Relation between maternal glucose tolerance and glucose metabolism in the newborn. *Br Med J* 1975; 3: 402–4.

101 Ylinen K, Raivio K, Teramo K. Haemoglobin A1C predicts the perinatal outcome in insulin-dependent diabetic pregnancies. *Br J Obstet Gynaecol* 1981; 88: 961–7.

102 Mimouni F, Miodovnik M, Siddiqi T, Butler J, Holroyde J, Tsang R. Neonatal polycythemia in infants of insulin-dependent diabetic mothers. *Obstet Gynecol* 1986; 68: 370–2.

103 Kitzmiller J, Cloherty J *et al.* Diabetic pregnancy and perinatal morbidity. *Am J Obstet Gynecol* 1978; 131: 560–80.

104 Persson B, Gentz J, Stangenberg M. Neonatal problems. In: Sutherland HW, Stowers JM, eds. *Carbohydrate Metabolism in Pregnancy and the Newborn.* Springer-Verlag, Berlin, 1978: 376–91.

105 Persson B, Gentz J, Lunell N. Diabetes in pregnancy. In: Scarpelli EM, Cosmi EV. *Reviews in Perinatal Medicine*, Vol. 2. Raven Press, New York, 1979: 1–55.

106 Tsang R, Strub R, Brown D, Steichen J, Hartman C, Chen I-W. Hypomagnesemia in infants of diabetic mothers: Perinatal studies. *J Pediatr* 1976; 89: 115–19.

107 Leslie J, Shen S, Strauss L. Hypertrophic cardiomyopathy in a midtrimester fetus born to a diabetic mother. *J Pediatr* 1982; 100: 631–2.

108 Gutgesell H, Mullins C, Gillette P, Speer M, Rudolph A, McNamara D. Transient hypertrophic subaortic stenosis in infants of diabetic mothers. *J Pediatr* 1976; 89: 120–5.

109 Halliday H. Hypertrophic cardiomyopathy in infants of poorly-controlled diabetic mothers. *Arch Dis Child* 1981; 56: 258–63.

110 Gutgesell H, Speer M, Rosenburg H. Characterization of the cardiomyopathy in infants of diabetic mothers. *Circulation* 1980; 61: 441–50.

111 Jovanovic L, Druzin M, Peterson C. Effect of euglycaemia on the outcome of pregnancy in insulin-dependent diabetic women as compared with normal control subjects. *Am J Med* 1981; 71: 921–7.

112 Beard R, Lowy C. The British Survey of Diabetic Pregnancies. Commentary. *Br J Obstet Gynaecol* 1982; 89: 783–6.

113 O'Sullivan J, Mahan C, Charles D, Dandrow R. Screening criteria for high risk gestational diabetic patients. *Am J Obstet Gynecol* 1973; 116: 895–900.

114 Hadden D. Screening for abnormalities of carbohydrate metabolism in pregnancy 1966–77: the Belfast experience. *Diabetes Care* 1980; 3: 440–6.

115 Gillmer M, Oakley N, Beard R, Nithyanawthan R, Cawston M. Screening for diabetes during pregnancy. *Br J Obstet Gynaecol* 1980; 87: 377–82.

116 Sutherland H, Stowers J, McKenzie C. Simplifying the clinical problem of glycosuria in pregnancy. *Lancet* 1970; i: 1069–71.

117 American Diabetes Association. Gestational diabetes mellitus. *Diabetes Care* 1999; 22 (Suppl. 1): S74–S76.

118 Jardine Brown C, Dawson A *et al.* Report of the pregnancy and neonatal care group. *Diabet Med* 1996; 13: S43–S53.

119 Naylor C, Sermer M, Chen E, Farine D. Selective screening for gestational diabetes mellitus. *N Engl J Med* 1997; 337: 1591–6.

120 Perucchini D, Fischer U, Spinas G, Huch R, Huch A, Lehmann R. Using fasting plasma glucose concentrations to screen for gestational diabetes mellitus: prospective population based study. *Br Med J* 1999; 319: 812–15.

121 Mortensen H, Molsted-Pedersen L, Kuhl C, Backer P. A screening procedure for diabetes in pregnancy. *Diabete Metab* 1985; ii: 249–53.

122 Jowett N, Samanta A, Burden A. Screening for diabetes in pregnancy: Is a random blood glucose enough? *Diabet Med* 1987; 4: 160–3.

123 Reichelt A, Spichler E, Branchtein L, Nucci L, Franco L, Schmidt M, The Brazilian Study of Gestational Diabetes Working Group. Fasting plasma glucose is a useful test for the detection of gestational diabetes. *Diabetes Care* 1998; 21: 1246–9.

124 Lind T, Anderson J. Does random blood glucose sampling outdate testing for glycosuria in the detection of diabetes during pregnancy? *Br Med J* 1984; 289: 1569–71.

125 Nasrat A, Johnstone F, Hasan S. Is random plasma glucose an efficient screening test for abnormal glucose tolerance in pregnancy? *Br J Obstet Gynaecol* 1988; 95: 855–60.

126 Hennings J. Diabetes in pregnancy: lessons for the multidisciplinary team. *J Diabetes* 1998; 2: 77–84.

127 Scottish Intercollegiate Guidelines Network (SIGN). *Management of Diabetes in Pregnancy.* Royal College of Physicians, Edinburgh, 1996.

128 Jovanovic-Peterson L, Peterson C *et al.* Maternal postprandial glucose levels and infant birth weight: The Diabetes in Early Pregnancy Study. *Am J Obstet Gynecol* 1991; 164: 103–11.

129 Combs C, Gunderson E, Kitzmiller J, Gavin L, Main E. Relationship of fetal macrosomia to maternal postprandial glucose control during pregnancy. *Diabetes Care* 1992; 15: 1251–7.

130 Mazze R, Shamoon H *et al.* Reliability of blood glucose monitoring by patients with diabetes mellitus. *Am J Med* 1984; 77: 211–17.

131 Essex N, Pyke D, Watkins P, Brudenell J, Gamsu H. Diabetic pregnancy. *Br Med J* 1973; 4: 89–93.

132 Clinical Standards Advisory Group. *Standards of Clinical Care for People with Diabetes.* British Diabetic Association, London, 1994.

133 Steel J, West C. Intrauterine death during continuous subcutaneous infusion of insulin. *Br Med J* 1985; 290: 1787.

134 British Diabetic Association. Dietary recommendations for people with diabetes. An update for 1990s. *Diabet Med* 1992; 2: 189–202.

135 Fraser R, Ford F, Milner R. A controlled trial of a high dietary fibre intake in pregnancy—effects on plasma glucose and insulin levels. *Diabetologia* 1983; 25: 238–41.

136 Williamson D. Regulation of the utilisation of glucose and ketone bodies by brain in the perinatal period. In: Camerini-Davalos RA, Cole HS, eds. *Early Diabetes in Early Life.* Academic Press, New York, 1975: 200.

137 Fraser R. High fibre diets in pregnancy. In: Campbell DM, Gillmer MDG, eds. *Nutrition in Pregnancy.* Royal College of Obstetricians and Gynaecologists, London, 1983: 269–77.

138 Sutherland H, Bewsher P *et al.* The effect of moderate dosage of chlorpropamide in pregnancy on fetal outcome. *Arch Dis Child* 1974; 49: 283–91.

139 Coetzee E, Jackson W. Metformin in management of pregnant insulin-dependent diabetes. *Diabetologia* 1979; 16: 241–5.

140 Coustan D, Lewis S. Insulin therapy for gestational diabetes. *Obstet Gynecol* 1978; 51: 306–10.

141 Coustan D, Imarah J. Prophylactic insulin treatment of gestational diabetes reduces the incidence of macrosomia, operative delivery and birth trauma. *Am J Obstet Gynecol* 1984; 150: 836–42.

142 de Veciana M, Major C *et al.* Postprandial versus preprandial blood glucose monitoring in women with gestational diabetes mellitus requiring insulin therapy. *N Engl J Med* 1995; 333: 1237–41.

143 Jovanovic L, Peterson C. Insulin and glucose requirements during the first stage of labour in insulin-dependent diabetic women. *Am J Med* 1983; 75: 607–12.

144 Whichelow M, Doddridge M. Lactation in diabetic women. *Br Med J* 1983; 287: 649–50.

145 Alban Davies H, Clark J, Dalton K, Edwards O. Insulin requirements of diabetic women who breast feed. *Br Med J* 1989; 298: 1357–8.

146 O'Sullivan J. The Boston gestational diabetes studies: review and perspectives. In: Sutherland HW, Stowers JM, Pearson DWM, eds. *Carbohydrate Metabolism in Pregnancy and the Newborn.* Springer-Verlag, London, 1989: 287–94.

147 Kitzmiller J, Brown E *et al.* Diabetic nephropathy and perinatal outcome. *Am J Obstet Gynecol* 1981; 141: 741–51.

148 Paterson K, Lunan C, MacCuish A. Severe transient nephrotic syndrome in diabetic pregnancy. *Br Med J* 1985; 291: 1612.

149 Weinstock R, Kopecky R, Jones D, Sunderji S. Rapid development of nephrotic syndrome, hypertension, and hemolytic anemia early in pregnancy in patients with IDDM. *Diabetes Care* 1988; 11: 416–21.

150 Biesenbach G, Zazgornik J. Incidence of transient nephrotic syndrome during pregnancy in diabetic women with and without pre-existing microalbuminuria. *Br Med J* 1989; 299: 366–7.

151 Dibble C, Kochenour N, Worley R, Tyler F, Swartz M. Effect of pregnancy on diabetic retinopathy. *Obstet Gynecol* 1982; 59: 699–704.

152 Moloney J, Drury M. The effect of pregnancy on the natural course of diabetic retinopathy. *Am J Ophthalmol* 1982; 93: 745–56.

153 Jovanovic R, Jovanovic L. Obstetric management when normoglycaemia is maintained in diabetic pregnant women with vascular compromise. *Am J Obstet Gynecol* 1984; 149: 617–23.

154 Price J, Hadden D, Archer D, Harley J. Diabetic retinopathy in pregnancy. *Br J Obstet Gynaecol* 1984; 91: 11–17.

155 Forrester J, Towler H, Pearson D. Pregnancy and diabetic retinopathy. In: Sutherland HW, Stowers JM, Pearson DWM, eds. *Carbohydrate Metabolism in Pregnancy and the Newborn.* Springer-Verlag, London, 1989: 189–200.

156 Macleod A, Smith S, Sönksen P, Lowy C. The problem of autonomic neuropathy in diabetic pregnancy. *Diabet Med* 1990; 7: 80–2.

157 Pedersen J, Molsted-Pedersen L. Congenital malformations. the possible role of diabetes care outside pregnancy. In: Elliott K, O'Connor KM, eds. *Pregnancy, Metabolism, Diabetes and the Fetus (Ciba Symposium 63).* Excerpta Medica, Amsterdam, 1979: 265–81.

158 Pedersen J, Molsted-Pedersen L. Early fetal growth delay detected by ultrasound marks increased risk of congenital malformations in diabetic pregnancy. *Br Med J* 1981; 283: 269–71.

159 Cousins L, Key T, Schorzman L, Moore T. Ultrasonographic assessment of early fetal growth in insulin-treated diabetic pregnancies. *Am J Obstet Gynecol* 1988; 159: 1186–90.

160 Lowy C, Beard R, Goldschmidt J. Congenital malformations in babies of diabetic mothers. *Diabet Med* 1986; 3: 458–62.

161 Wald N, Cuckle H, Boreham J, Stirrat G, Turnbull A. Maternal serum alpha-fetoprotein and diabetes mellitus. *Br J Obstet Gynaecol* 1979; 86: 101–5.

162 Wald N, Cuckle H, Densem J, Stone R. Maternal serum unconjugated oestriol and human chorionic gonadotrophin levels in pregnancies with insulin-dependent diabetes: implications for screening for Down's syndrome. *Br J Obstet Gynaecol* 1992; 99: 51–3.

163 Landon M, Mintz M, Gabbe S. Sonographic evaluation of fetal abdominal growth: Predictor of the large-for-gestational-age infant in pregnancies complicated by diabetes mellitus. *Am J Obstet Gynecol* 1989; 160: 115–21.

164 Pedersen J, Molsted-Pedersen L. Sonographic estimation of fetal weight in diabetic pregnancy. *Br J Obstet Gynaecol* 1992; 99: 475–8.

165 Teramo K, Ammala P, Ylinen K, Raivio K. Pathological fetal heart rate associated with poor metabolic control in diabetic pregnancies. *Obstet Gynecol* 1983; 61: 559–65.

166 Salvesen D, Freeman J, Brudenell J, Nicolaides K. Prediction of fetal acidaemia in pregnancies complicated by maternal diabetes mellitus by biophysical profile scoring and fetal heart rate monitoring. *Br J Obstet Gynaecol* 1993; 100: 227–33.

167 Dicker D, Feldberg D, Yeshaya A, Peleg D, Karp M, Goldman J. Fetal surveillance in insulin-dependent diabetic pregnancy. Predictive value of the biophysical profile. *Am J Obstet Gynecol* 1988; 159: 800–4.

168 Johnson J, Lange I, Harman C, Torchia M, Manning F. Biophysical profile scoring in the management of the diabetic pregnancy. *Obstet Gynecol* 1988; 72: 841–6.

169 Cousins L. Pregnancy complications among diabetic women: review 1965–85. *Obstet Gynecol Surv* 1987; 42: 140–9.

170 Molsted-Pedersen L. Preterm labour and perinatal mortality in diabetic pregnancy. Obstetric considerations. In: Sutherland HW, Stowers JM, eds. *Carbohydrate Metabolism in Pregnancy and the Newborn.* Springer-Verlag, Berlin, 1979: 392–406.

171 Titus R. Diabetes and pregnancy from the obstetric point of view. *Am J Obstet Gynecol* 1937; 33: 386–92.

172 Usher R, Allen A, Maclean F. Risk of respiratory distress syndrome related to gestational age, route of delivery and maternal diabetes. *Am J Obstet Gynecol* 1971; 111: 826–9.

173 Skouby S, Molsted-Pedersen L, Petersen K. Contraception for women with diabetes: an update. In: Oats, JN. *Diabetes in Pregnancy. Bailliere's Clinical Obstetrics and Gynaecology.* WB Saunders, London, 1991: 5; 493–503.

174 Steel J, Duncan L. Contraception for the insulin-dependent diabetic woman: the view from one clinic. *Diabetes Care* 1980; 3: 557–60.

175 Skouby S, Molsted-Pedersen L, Kuhl C. Low dosage oral contraception in women with previous gestational diabetes. *Obstet Gynecol* 1982; 59: 325–8.

176 Kjos S, Peters R, Xiang A, Thomas D, Schaefer U, Buchanan T. Contraception and the risk of type 2 diabetes mellitus in Latina women with prior gestational diabetes mellitus. *J Am Med Assoc* 1998; 280: 533–8.

177 Skouby S, Molsted-Pedersen L, Kosonen A. Consequences of intrauterine contraception in diabetic women. *Fertil Steril* 1984; 42: 568–73.

178 Hod M, Merlob P, Friedman S, Schoenfeld A, Ovadia J. Gestational diabetes mellitus: a survey of perinatal complications in the 1980s. *Diabetes* 1991; 40 (Suppl. 2): 74–8.

179 O'Sullivan J. Diabetes mellitus after GDM. *Diabetes* 1991; 40 (Suppl. 2): 131–5.

180 Hagbard L, Svanborg A. Prognosis of diabetes mellitus with onset during pregnancy. *Diabetes* 1960; 9: 296–302.

181 Mestman J, Anderson G, Guadalupe V. Follow-up study of 360 subjects with abnormal carbohydrate metabolism during pregnancy. *Obstet Gynecol* 1972; 39: 421–5.

182 Konradi L, Matveeva O. Prognostic value of disorders of glucose intolerance in pregnant women. *Prob Endokrinol* 1974; 20: 10–13.

183 Hadden D. Asymptomatic diabetes in pregnancy. In: Sutherland HW, Stowers JM, eds. *Carbohydrate Metabolism in Pregnancy and the Newborn.* Springer-Verlag, Berlin, 1979: 407–24.

184 Stowers J, Sutherland H, Kerridge D. Long-range implications for the mother. *Diabetes* 1985; 34 (Suppl. 2): 106–10.

185 Metzger B, Bybee D, Freinkel N, Phelps R, Radvany R, Vaisrub N. Gestational diabetes mellitus. Correlations between the phenotypic and genotypic characteristics of the mother and abnormal glucose tolerance during the first year postpartum. *Diabetes* 1985; 34 (Suppl. 2): 111–15.

186 Grant P, Oats J, Beischer N. The long-term follow-up of women with gestational diabetes. *Aust NZ J Obstet Gynaecol* 1986; 26: 17–22.

187 Efendic S, Hansson U, Persson B, Wajngot A, Luft R. Glucose tolerance, insulin release, and insulin sensitivity in normal-weight women with previous gestational diabetes mellitus. *Diabetes* 1987; 36: 413–19.

188 Damm P, Molsted-Pedersen L. Significant decrease in congenital malformations in newborn infants of an unselected population of diabetic women. *Am J Obstet Gynecol* 1989; 161: 1163–7.

189 Ali Z, Alexis S. Occurrence of diabetes mellitus after gestational diabetes mellitus in Trinidad. *Diabetes Care* 1990; 13: 527–9.

190 Kjos S, Buchanan T, Greenspoon J, Montoro M, Bernstein G, Mestman J. Gestational diabetes mellitus: the prevalence of glucose intolerance and diabetes mellitus in the first two months post partum. *Am J Obstet Gynecol* 1990; 163: 93–8.

191 Dornhorst A, Bailey P, Anyaoku V, Elkeles R, Johnston D, Beard R. Abnormalities of glucose tolerance following gestational diabetes. *Q J Med* 1990; 284 (New Series 77): 1219–28.

192 Milner R, Richards B. An analysis of birthweight by gestational age of infants born in England and Wales 1967–71. *J Obstet Gynaecol Br Commonwealth* 1974; 81: 956–67.

193 O' Sullivan JB, Mahan CM. Criteria for the oral glucose tolerance test in pregnancy. *Diabetes* 1964; 13: 278–85.

12 Thyroid disease and pregnancy

Joanna Girling

Thyroid disease is relatively common in women of child-bearing age. Fetal and neonatal thyroid disease may occur as a consequence of maternal thyroid dysfunction, or independently, but in both cases the diagnosis and management can be challenging. This chapter will discuss the physiology of the maternal pituitary–thyroid axis in both the non-pregnant and the pregnant state, the development of the fetal pituitary–thyroid axis, the influence of the placenta on maternal and fetal thyroid function, and the management of thyroid diseases in pregnancy.

Maternal physiology

Regulation of thyroid function occurs both as part of the hypothalamus–pituitary–thyroid feedback mechanism and at an intrathyroid level. Thyroid-stimulating hormone (TSH) is a glycoprotein consisting of an α subunit shared with other anterior pituitary hormones and a unique β subunit. It is released from the anterior pituitary in 1–2-hourly pulses, and also in a circadian rhythm, which peaks just before sleep. TSH increases synthesis and release of the thyroid hormones, thyroxine (T4) and triiodothyronine (T3), by increasing iodide transport, iodide organification, release of thyroglobulin into the follicular lumen and increased endocytosis of colloid. T3 and T4 are mostly protein bound in the circulation; only the unbound portions have biological activity. The predominant binding proteins are thyroid binding globulin (TBG), albumin and transthyretin (previously named thyroid binding prealbumin). The amount of thyroid hormone bound to each of these proteins depends upon their affinities and their concentrations. TBG has the greatest affinity for T4 and T3, and therefore despite having the lowest concentration, 75% of thyroid hormones are bound to it. Overall, only 0.04% T4 and 0.5% T3 are free.

The basic unit of the thyroid gland is the thyroid follicle, a spherical structure consisting of a single layer of thyroid follicular cells and a lumen for the storage of thyroglobulin-rich colloid. Iodide is essential for thyroid hormone synthesis. The thyroid regulates the amount of iodide it takes up, actively trapping a variable proportion of the extracellular pool to maintain synthesis of thyroid hormone at a steady rate and thereby obviating potential problems of variable dietary intake of iodide. The active process of iodide uptake is not fully characterized, but is enhanced by TSH. After trapping, iodide is oxidized at the apical surface of the follicular cell by hydrogen peroxide produced by thyroid peroxidase, to iodine and then incorporated into the tyrosine residues of thyroglobulin in the lumen. This process is termed iodide *organification*, and results in hormonally inactive compounds mono-iodotyrosine and diiodotyrosine. Subsequently, thyroid peroxidase plays a key role in coupling these iodotyrosyl residues to form T4 (two diiodotyrosine molecules) and T3 (one monoiodotyrosine molecule and one diiodotyrosine molecule), the only active thyroid compounds.

Thyroglobulin is synthesized by the follicular cell, released into the lumen by exocytosis for organification and then re-enters the cell following engulfment by pseudopodia. There the thyroid hormones are liberated and enter capillary circulation via the basal surface of the follicular cells. In the presence of normal levels of iodide, each thyroglobulin molecule carries three or four molecules of T4, but only one in five molecules of thyroglobulin carry a molecule of T3. Most circulating T3 is produced by peripheral deiodination of T4; it is three times more potent than T4, and although its production is much lower than that of T4, it is available as a free and active compound in a higher proportion. The fractional rate of turnover of T4 is 10% per day (half-life 6.7 days), and of T3 is 60% per day (half-life 18 h).

There are three deiodinases. They regulate the metabolism of T4 and T3. Activation of T4 to T3 in target tissues maintains a stable T3 concentration in critical tissues during periods of reduced thyroid hormone production; inactivation of T3 and T4 is important during hyperthyroidism. Each enzyme is expressed in particular tissues and this provides further local regulation of thyroid hormone concentration (Table 12.1).

Advances in molecular biology have allowed the characterization of the thyroid hormone receptors. They are transmembrane nuclear receptors with multiple isoforms. They map to two genes, one on chromosome 17 (thyroid hormone receptor α (TRα)) and one on chromosome 3 (thyroid hormone receptor β (TRβ)), and each has two major isoforms, TRα-1, TRα-2, TRβ-1 and TRβ-2. Each isoform has a characteristic tissue distribution. TRβ-2 is the most regulated, occurring in only the pituitary and

certain areas of the central nervous system. TRα-1 has been identified in placental tissue.

Changes in thyroid physiology during pregnancy

In normal pregnancy a number of changes occur in relation to the pituitary thyroid axis as follows.

ALTERED THYROID BINDING GLOBULIN PRODUCTION

Variability in the carbohydrate content of TBG influences its rate of metabolism. In pregnancy, increased oestrogen synthesis results in greater sialylation of carbohydrate moieties on TBG, extending its half-life from 15 min to 3 days [1]. Thus, TBG begins to increase in the first 2 weeks of pregnancy and reaches a plateau by 20 weeks' gestation [2], the TBG extracellular pool increasing from 2700 to 7400 nmol. This results in increased total T4 and T3 production, with enhanced daily T4 production of 1–3% above baseline until the new steady-state plateau is reached.

IODINE DEFICIENCY

The extrathyroidal inorganic iodine pool is in dynamic equilibrium with the thyroid and the kidneys. In pregnancy, increased glomerular filtration from early in the first trimester results in increased renal loss of iodide. In iodine-replete areas, circulating iodine concentration is not reduced [3]; in iodine-depleted parts of the world it

	Type I	Type II	Type III
Action	Activates T4 to T3	Activates T4 to T3	Inactivates T4 to rT3; T3 to T2
Site	Liver, kidney thyroid pituitary	Pituitary, brain, keratinocyte, placenta (decidua + chorion)	Placenta (trophoblast), brain, epidermis
Effect of pregnancy	No change	Increases with gestation	Increases with gestation
Effect of PTU	Inhibits	Insensitive	Insensitive
Effect of hypothyroidism		Increased	Decreased
Effect of hyperthyroidism		Decreased	Increased
Effect of iodine contrast agent, iopanoic acid	Inhibits	Inhibits	

Table 12.1 Comparison of properties of deiodinase enzymes.

PTU, propylthiouracil.

is [4]. The thyroid compensates by increasing the proportion of iodide from the circulation that it takes up. In areas of relative iodide deficiency, these changes may result in enlargement of the thyroid during pregnancy and the appearance of goitre; for example, Dillon and Milliez found that 42% of pregnant women had a goitre compared with 34% of matched non-pregnant controls [4]. Transport of iodide to the fetus occurs as fetal thyroid activity commences early in the second trimester, and this too depletes the maternal iodide pool. In humans it is likely that the mechanism involves diffusion along a concentration gradient, rather than active transport as has been detected in sheep.

In areas of iodine deficiency, the iodine-concentrating mechanisms of the maternal iodine-deficient goitre override those of the placenta, so that fetuses are more likely to be afflicted by cretinism. During the first trimester the fetus is dependent upon maternal T4 and it is precisely during this time that increasing total T4 necessitates a greater maternal requirement for iodine: where iodine is in short supply, maternal hypothyroxinaemia may occur, which can adversely effect fetal brain development. Maternal hypothyroidism, fetal hypothyroidism, fetal iodine deprivation and neonatal hypothyroidism may all occur to some degree in such areas, causing as many as 10% of newborns to be hypothyroid (see later) [5].

HUMAN CHORIONIC GONADOTROPHIN PRODUCTION

Human chorionic gonadotrophin (hCG) and TSH share a common α subunit and their unique β subunits have considerable similarity. Further, their receptors are also similar. It is thought that the high levels of hCG in the first trimester may result in a hormone 'spillover' syndrome, in which hCG stimulates the TSH receptor. Observations of an association with hyperthyroidism initially in women with molar pregnancy and subsequently other pathological conditions in which there are also high levels of hCG suggested that hCG may have thyroid-stimulating activity. Subsequently an inverse association between hCG and TSH levels has been shown in women with normal pregnancy [2,6], a decrease in TSH occurring with peak hCG levels, and free T4 (fT4) having a linear relationship with hCG levels. It is estimated that an increment of hCG of 10000 U/L results in an increase of fT4 of 0.6 pmol/L and a decrease in TSH of 0.1 mU/L. Hence clinically measurable change in thyroid hormone concentration is only likely if hCG levels are around 50 000–75 000 or more. Even so this is likely to be a minor effect, not least because peak hCG levels are sustained for only a short period. This subject is considered in more detail in the section on hyperemesis gravidarum (see below).

There is some evidence that certain fractions of hCG have greater TSH-like activity than others. Partially desialated hCG has the greatest activity, and is often raised in molar pregnancy [7]. Recently a mother and daughter pair have been reported with a total of six pregnancies, all complicated by severe nausea and vomiting and three having documented hyperthyroidism which resolved after delivery on each occasion; hCG concentration was not elevated. Both women were found to be heterozygous for a mutation of the TSH receptor, which made it more responsive than usual to hCG whilst maintaining its sensitivity to TSH. This is the first report in which pregnancy induced hyperthyroidism occured because of a mutant TSH receptor rather than because of inappropriate production of hCG [8]. It raises interesting questions concerning the aetiology of recurrent hyperemesis in pregnancy, particularly in relation to the advice that should be given to the female offspring of such women.

DEIODINATION OF THYROID HORMONES (see Table 12.1)

Type I deiodinase activity does not seem to be altered during pregnancy. Type II deiodinase is located mainly in the decidua and chorion, rather than the amnion; this allows placental conversion of T4 to T3 and as in other tissues this increases as the availability of T4 decreases, presumably in order to optimize thyroid bioactivity in times of reduced availability. Type III deiodinase is found in trophoblast tissue [9] where it prevents excess transfer of maternal T4 and T3 to the fetus and may also metabolize fetal T4 and T3. Fetal serum T3 concentrations are lower than those of neonates [10] (see later). Placental type III deiodinase increases with advancing gestation [11] and this may contribute to the fall in maternal fT4 concentration often seen in later pregnancy, the decreased transfer of T4 to the fetus at this time and the increasing placental availability of iodine for transfer to the fetus.

Biochemical assessment of thyroid function in pregnancy

Free T4, free T3 (fT3) and TSH should be analysed when assessing maternal thyroid function; total T4 and total T3 should not be used in pregnancy. When deciding whether to change the dose of treatment, more weight should be placed upon fT4 and fT3 concentrations, as these reflect the actual thyroid status more accurately, rather than the stimulating hormone TSH. In cases of hypothyroidism, the latter may remain elevated despite normal fT4 and fT3 for some time after the correct dose of T4 is initiated or because of poor compliance with therapy.

Conversely, TSH may remain suppressed once fT4 and fT3 return to normal in hyperthyroidism.

Typical reference ranges for thyroid function tests during pregnancy are given in Table 12.2. The absolute values given for pregnancy should not necessarily be transferred directly to an individual unit, but rather extrapolated to make allowance for the hospital's own non-pregnant reference range.

The physiological changes of thyroid function with gestation during uncomplicated pregnancy are debated, and not universally accepted. It is possible that there is a minor fall in TSH and increase in fT4 concentrations in the first trimester of normal pregnancy, due to an effect of hCG. If this is so, the increase in fT4 may be part of the mechanism for providing the fetus with T4 in the first trimester before fetal thyroid activity is established, since transplacental transfer if it does occur, is probably gradient dependent. The absence of placental type III deiodinase activity at this gestation would also facilitate transfer of T4 to the fetus, by maximizing the concentration of T4 presented to the placenta. Hyperemesis gravidarum, molar pregnancy and trophoblastic disease may result in an exaggeration of this physiological biochemical change (see later).

There is a fall in T4 concentration with advancing gestation, the onset being in the second half of pregnancy, with most marked effect in the third trimester. In the third trimester the lower limit of normal for fT4 is below that defined for a non-pregnant woman. Some authors [12] have also found a rise in TSH concentration in the third trimester, although others have not [13]. Increasing concentrations of placental deiodinase type III contribute to the fall in maternal T4 concentrations whilst enhancing the availability of iodine for the fetus. Increasing concentrations of type II deiodinase enhance the intracellular conversion of T4 to T3, thereby raising at the cellular level the thyroid activity for a given concentration of fT4. In an evolutionary sense, this economy of maternal metabolism prior to the exertions of labour and lactation may enhance self-preservation. It does not usually indicate new-onset hypothyroidism or the need for an increased dose of T4 in established cases of hypothyroidism.

Theoretically, an increasing concentration of TBG preferentially augments the supply of T4 to target tissue with a high T4 flux across capillary walls; this would also contribute to the fall in fT4 with gestation [14].

Use of serum screening for trisomy 21 in women with thyroid dysfunction

Alpha-fetoprotein (α-FP) is a fetal plasma protein produced predominantly in the first half of pregnancy until fetal liver maturation allows production of albumin instead. TSH and T3 are important in the regulation of the transcriptional switch from α-FP to albumin during fetal development. *In vitro* studies on fetal liver have suggested that TSH can increase α-FP production up to threefold and reduce albumin production, and that T3 can inhibit production of α-FP up to 75% and increase albumin. Both T3 and TSH also change RNA expression [15]. *In vivo*, hypothyroid infants may have higher than average concentrations of α-FP, which fall during treatment with T4 and rise again if treatment is discontinued. In part, this is due to altered metabolism of α-FP, the half-life being 12 days in babies with congenital hypothyroidism and 5 days in babies with transient hyperthyrotrophinaemia [16].

Therefore, it is possible that maternal measurement of α-FP may be less accurate in women with hypothyroid fetuses, i.e. raised fetal TSH concentrations may falsely elevate both fetal and maternal serum α-FP (MSAFP), resulting in false-positive screening tests for neural tube defect or false-negative results for trisomy 21 screening. Indeed two cases of greatly elevated MSAFP (7 and 5.3 multiples of the median (MoM)) have been reported in pregnancies where postnatally a diagnosis of congenital hypothyroidism was made in the baby [17]. However, others have reported normal MSAFP in 44 out of 45 pregnancies complicated by congenital hypothyroidism in the baby, and the one abnormal result was only marginally elevated (2.9 MoM, cut-off point 2.0 MoM) [18,19]. Therefore, there is currently no need to investigate pregnancies with unexplained elevated MSAFP for fetal hypothyroidism.

It has also been suggested that maternal hypothyroidism may influence MSAFP. However, because fetal thyroid function is independent of maternal thyroid function, and indeed is only just beginning at the usual time for maternal serum screening tests, there is no reason why maternal hypothyroidism should influence fetal α-FP production or maternal α-FP concentration. Even in severe maternal hypothyroidism, there is no evidence that fetal TSH or fetal T3 concentrations are affected in iodine-replete women.

	Not pregnant	First trimester	Second trimester	Third trimester
fT4$_{pmol/L}$	11–23	11–22	11–19	7–15
fT3$_{pmol/L}$	4–9	4–8	4–7	3–5
TSH$_{mu/L}$	0–4	0–1.6	1–1.8	7–7.3

Table 12.2 Thyroid function tests in pregnancy (data from refs [12,153,154]).

Therefore MSAFP may be measured in women with hypothyroidism if clinically indicated [20].

Fetal thyroid function

Maternal thyroid disorders and their treatment, iodine intake and other circumstances can have an important effect upon the fetus, and in particular on fetal and neonatal thyroid function.

Fetal thyroid physiology

The fetal thyroid gland develops from week 5 of pregnancy, and begins to function from 10 weeks. Thyroid function in the human fetus has been studied at the time of cardiocentesis or cordocentesis performed for prenatal diagnosis. Using only fetuses that were subsequently found to be normal, Thorpe-Beeston *et al.* showed that both free and total T4 and T3, and TSH and TBG are present in fetal blood from 12 weeks' gestation and increase with advancing gestation [21]. Fetal fT4 is related to fetal TSH concentration independently of gestation. There is no association between maternal and fetal thyroid hormone levels: fetal TSH exceeds that of maternal TSH; fetal total and fT4 reach adult levels by 36 weeks' gestation; circulating T3 remains less than half the adult value, although intracellular concentrations may be higher (see below) [21]. This suggests that the peripheral conversion of T4 to T3, which accounts for most adult T3, is not active in the fetus or that placental deiodinases rapidly inactivate T3. The fetal pituitary–thyroid axis has different set points compared with the adult: either it is less sensitive to negative feedback by T4 or more dependent upon T3 whose concentration is too low to initiate negative feedback. In the fetus low levels of type I deiodinase are located in extrathyroidal tissues [22] and there are high levels of type III [23], in particular in the fetal side of the placenta [24]. The maternal side of the placenta is rich in type II deiodinase, and this increases when T4 is low and possibly with advancing gestation [9]. This, in combination with poor permeability of fetal membranes [25] to iodothyronines, makes the placenta a good barrier, minimizing transfer from the maternal circulation, especially near term [26]. These factors also contribute to the low fetal serum T3 concentration, and help to explain why circulating T3 surges in the days after delivery [10].

Human fetal brain, in particular probably neuronal precursors, contains nuclear T3 receptors and intracellular T3 from late in the first trimester, the concentration of the former increasing 10-fold between 10 and 16 weeks' gestation. Other fetal tissues including liver, heart and lung contain only T4 throughout the second trimester and not T3, supporting the concept that fetal brain T3 arises by conversion from T4 [27]. Type II and type III deiodinases have been detected in human fetal brain from 11 weeks' gestation [28] and their concentration is influenced by maternal thyroid status.

Although it has not been proved that thyroid hormone, in particular T3, is required for normal brain development, evidence from animal data makes this likely, and there is increasing *in vitro* and *in vivo* human work to support this. In the rat fetus, low serum T3 levels do not reflect the intracellular environment, which is dependent upon intracellular conversion from T4 [29]. Animal and human data show that fetal brain and pituitary, but not other tissues, have raised deiodinase II and preserved intracellular T3 levels when fetal thyroid dysfunction occurs [28]. Maternal T4 is essential for this, and helps to mitigate the neurological effects of fetal thyroid failure. Reduced placental deiodinase III probably contributes to this, by facilitating transfer of maternal T4 to the fetus in these circumstances and minimizing fetal peripheral deiodination of T4 (see later). Maternal T3 cannot provide this protection as it cannot cross the placenta nor is it taken up by the fetal brain, which relies on intracellular conversion of T3 from T4. Therefore in areas of chronic iodine deficiency where maternal T4 is often low (but T3 preserved), the fetal brain may be adversely affected (see later) [26]. These are the areas where endemic cretinism occurs due to fetal thyroid dysfunction.

Influence of maternal thyroid function on fetal thyroid function

Before 12 weeks' gestation, it is probable that small amounts of maternal T4 cross the placenta, although precisely how much reaches the fetus in the first trimester is debated. Contempre *et al.* [30] measured T4 and T3 levels in coelomic and amniotic fluids, obtained by ultrasound-guided needle aspiration. They identified T4 in the coelomic fluid from 5.8 weeks' gestation when it was 10 times more concentrated than fT4 in the maternal circulation; by 11 weeks it was 100 times more concentrated [30]. This T4 must be maternal in origin. At this gestation, maternal hypothyroxinaemia may have adverse effects on fetal brain development (see later).

Transthyretin is the fetal T4 protein carrier, and is present in the extracoelomic cavity, yolk sac and choroid plexus by 8 weeks' gestation. Its concentration increases rapidly between weeks 6 and 9 of pregnancy, and it may facilitate transfer of T4 to the embryo and in particular the developing brain [31].

It is likely that, in normal pregnancy, little if any T4 crosses the placenta in subsequent trimesters. Vulsma *et al.* [32] reported 25 neonates with total organification defect resulting in the complete absence of T4 production: at birth these babies had circulating T4 levels up to 50% normal, in an estimated maternal/fetal ratio 3:1. Some authorities have extrapolated from this pathological condition to assume the same response in normal pregnancy [33], although Vulsma himself was careful to point out that the fetal thyroid hormone status may influence placental metabolism of T4. In fact it has been suggested that in the presence of fetal hypothyroidism, placental deiodinase III is inhibited or there is extraplacental transfer of T4 to the fetus through the chorion and amnion [34], both of which would enhance transfer of T4 from mother to fetus. Perfused term human placental lobule studies indicate that transfer of maternal T4 to the fetus is very low, with fetal concentrations reaching only 0.008% of those in the maternal circulation, despite the use of supraphysiological concentrations. The addition of an inhibitor of deiodinase activity, iopanoic acid, resulted in a 2700-fold increase in T4 levels in the fetal circulation, such that fetal concentrations reached 30% of maternal levels [35]. This supports the hypothesis that placental type III deiodinase is important for regulating transfer of T4 to the fetus, and that in normal pregnancy limited maternal T4 reaches the fetus.

Only thyrotrophin-releasing hormone (TRH) and iodine are able to cross the human placenta freely [25]. The placenta is largely impermeable to TSH, T3 and T4 [36]. When 400 μg TRH is given to a pregnant woman immediately prior to delivery, cord T4 and T3 concentrations increase [37], but if given 13–36h prior to delivery, cord TSH and T3 levels are reduced suggesting rebound suppression of the fetal pituitary–thyroid axis [38]: this and other studies suggest that maternal TRH is able to influence fetal thyroid function, although its role in the physiological control of or development of the fetal hypothalamic–pituitary axis is unknown. It is likely to play only a minor role, because inactivation of maternal TRH by TRH antibody does not seem to influence fetal thyroid function [39].

In the past, TRH was administered to pregnant women to reduce the risk of respiratory distress syndrome (RDS) of the newborn in babies born prematurely. However, a prospective randomized controlled trial of 200 μg TRH and placebo found that the babies in the study arm had a higher incidence of RDS and need for ventilation, and that the mothers reported more nausea, vomiting, light-headedness and blood pressure 140/90 or more [40]. Therefore in current obstetric practice TRH is not used for this indication.

Neonatal thyroid dysfunction due to thyroid-stimulating hormone receptor mutations

Congenital hyperthyroidism is a rare disease, usually caused by the transplacental passage of TSH receptor-stimulating antibodies from women with Graves' disease (see hyperthyroidism). A small number of *de novo* germline mutations of the transmembrane [41] and extracellular [42] domains of the TSH receptor have been discovered that constitutively activate adenyl cyclase. This results in non-immune hyperthyroidism, which usually presents with restlessness, sweating, diarrhoea, frequent crying, irritability and tachycardia in the first few weeks of life or with hyperthyroidism in adolescence or adulthood. It may occur as a sporadic mutation or have autosomal dominant inheritance. Treatment of the hyperthyroidism is with the usual therapeutic options.

Conversely, loss of function mutations in the TSH receptor result in TSH resistance and either hypothyroidism or euthyroidism with elevated TSH concentration. Two of three sisters who had each inherited a different mutation on each allele of the gene for the TSH receptor from their parents (who were each heterozygous for one of the two mutations) were detected by neonatal screening. Their older sister who was 4 years old at the time had no physical or mental developmental problems, but also had a high TSH (80 mU/L) with normal fT4 [43]. This is an unusual cause of a positive Guthrie test.

Thyroid hormone resistance

Resistance to thyroid hormone (RTH) occurs in one in 50 000 live births [44], although little is known about it in relation to pregnancy. It is caused by mutation in the *TRβ* gene. The clinical manifestations are diverse, ranging from hypothyroidism to hyperthyroidism, many individuals showing features of both ends of the thyroid spectrum, and others being asymptomatic; the relationship between the genotype and phenotype is unpredictable. Biochemically, thyroid hormone concentrations are usually elevated, and TSH concentrations are normal or increased, but never suppressed. In pregnancy, symptoms should be controlled as required, usually with a β blocker, the fetus scanned serially for growth and goitre, and genetic diagnosis of the baby established neonatally [44]. The effects on the fetus of RTH are unknown, although it is suggested that when the fetus inherits RTH from the father development may be jeopardized by exposure to normal (i.e. not elevated) levels of thyroid hormone from the normal mother. However, this presumes that increased thyroid hormone concentrations if present could cross the placenta at the critical period in the first trimester. Goitre and short stature has been shown to be more common in children with RTH born to unaffected women when compared with those born to affected women [45]. One case has been reported in a pregnant woman with RTH who discontinued triiodothyrocetic acid (TRIAC) and developed a recurrence of hyperthyroid symptoms. TRIAC is a thyroid hormone analogue that inhibits secretion and biological activity of TSH with minimal effects at peripheral tissues. As TRIAC crosses the placenta, chorionic villous sampling (CVS) was performed at 17 weeks' gestation before recommencing therapy: the fetus was heterozygous for the same *TRβ* mutation as the mother, confirming a diagnosis of RTH *in utero*. TRIAC therapy was restarted, in the expectation that it would be beneficial to both the mother and fetus. The mother's thyroid status rapidly returned to normal. Interestingly, the fetus had transient hypothyroidism with very high TSH levels but low TSH bioactivity, growth restriction and goitre: fetal TSH was halved and the goitre partially alleviated by increasing the dose of TRIAC [46]. Neonatal RTH is another rare cause of a positive Guthrie test.

Iodine deficiency

Iodine deficiency results in cretinism in newborns, goitre in adults and reduced reproductive success in women. Worldwide, more than one billion people are affected by iodine deficiency, and more than 20 million have adverse neurological sequelae following fetal iodine deprivation [47].

Neurological endemic cretinism is the leading preventable cause, worldwide, of mental retardation [47], and has a major negative effect on the economy of afflicted areas. It may affect 2–10% of individuals in iodine-deficient populations; in these populations, a mild degree of mental retardation is five times more common than cretinism itself, resulting in a left shift of the IQ distribution curve by 10 points. Cretinism is characterized by deaf–mutism, intellectual deficiency, spastic motor disorder and in some cases hypothyroidism. Although the precise pathophysiology of the insult on the neurological system is poorly understood, the combination of maternal iodine deficiency and hypothyroxinaemia with, as a consequence of the former, fetal hypothyroidism, lasting throughout the pregnancy are devastating to the fetus. The developing cochlea, cerebral neocortex and basal ganglia are most sensitive to iodine deficiency, and all are growing rapidly during the second trimester. In myxoedematous cretinism, hearing, speech and motor function are spared, and the clinical picture is similar to that of untreated congenital hypothyroidism: the degree of maternal iodine deprivation is less severe, and the mother is capable of transferring either

sufficient iodine or T4 or both to the fetus at the critical stages of neurological development to ensure normal development of these functions.

In areas of endemic iodine deficiency, the usual maternal findings are goitre in association with normal T3, low or very low T4 and raised TSH; neurological cretinism is common in the offspring, suggesting that maternal T3 alone is insufficient to protect the fetal brain, and that fetoplacental deprivation of iodine and possibly of T4 may be important regarding the long-term neurological effects in the offspring (see above). This is not surprising because fetal brain utilizes T3 derived from intracellular T4 by the action of high concentrations of deiodinase II; T4 production is impaired when there is iodine deficiency. Iodine administered to women before conception or up to the end of the second trimester improves neurological status and protects the fetal brain [48,49]. As a single small oral dose of iodized oil normalizes TSH and T4 levels for 6–12 months, it is possible that this beneficial effect for the fetus may continue in pregnancies conceived some time after its administration [50]. It is likely therefore that iodination of drinking water, salt or flour, or annual administration of iodine to women of reproductive age would have a major reduction in the incidence of this devastating condition. Sadly the prospects of a theoretically simple and effective preventative programme being implicated remain remote for many iodine-deficient areas of the world.

Almost 5000 women in Senegal, West Africa, participated in a study to estimate the effects of iodine deficiency on their reproductive capacity. Thirty-two per cent of the women had a goitre, and urinary iodine measurement indicated that the population had moderate iodine deficiency. There was no delay in the age of menarche in iodine-deficient women. However, iodine deficiency was associated with increased incidence of both repeated (three or more) miscarriage and stillbirth, and this was dependent upon the degree of iodine deficiency: thus, 49% of women with severe iodine deficiency, 27% with moderate, 22% with mild and 21% with none, had one of these outcomes. Malnutrition and illiteracy significantly worsened the reproductive outcome in iodine-deficient women [4]. Pre-pregnancy iodine supplementation improves pregnancy outcome, reducing pregnancy loss form 24% to 16% in Papua New Guinea [49], and reducing stillbirth from 20 per 1000 to 12 per 1000 in Tasmania [51] and 18 per 1000 to nine per 1000 in Zaire [52].

Iodine excess

Excessive maternal iodine ingestion can result in fetal iodine-induced hypothyroidism, probably because of failure to escape the acute inhibition of thyroid hormone synthesis induced by high concentrations of intrathyroid iodine (Wolff–Chaikoff effect) [53]. Pregnant women should therefore avoid taking large quantities of iodine-containing preparations such as some cough medicines and eye drops. The iodide released from iodinated contrast dyes used in radiological procedures also crosses the placenta, and could induce fetal hypothyroidism or goitre. It is not known whether iopanoic acid and sodium iopodate themselves cross the placenta: as they inhibit type II and type III deiodinases, if they did reach the fetus they may result in decreased intracellular concentrations of T3. These agents should be avoided in pregnancy.

Radioactive iodine is totally contraindicated in women who are, or are planning to be, pregnant or are lactating (see hyperthyroidism) [54]. Transplacental passage of the radioactive iodine results in irreversible destruction of the fetal thyroid gland. As adverse radiation effects can occur even before active fetal thyroid concentration of iodine occurs, it is particularly important that radioactive iodine is not given to women even in very early pregnancy; the dose accumulated increases 8000-fold from early pregnancy to term. There is also some evidence of increased childhood malignancy in those whose mothers were given radioactive iodine in pregnancy.

Amiodarone is iodine-rich, containing 37% iodine; a single 200-mg tablet contains 75 mg iodine, the average iodine intake for 50 days in North America [55]. It inhibits deiodinases, reducing peripheral conversion of T4 to T3, and blocks the interaction of T3 with its pituitary receptor, which may result in hyperthyroidism or hypothyroidism. These effects and those in the fetus are not dose or duration dependent. It crosses the placenta, as does its major active metabolite [56]. As amiodarone and it active metabolite each have half-lives exceeding 7 weeks, fetal exposure may persist for sometime after maternal ingestion is discontinued. Only 35 cases have been reported in the literature [57]. The risk of transient neonatal hyperthyroidism is 9% and of hypothyroidism is 9–13%. It has also been associated with fetal and neonatal goitre secondary to placental transfer of excessive iodine. There are no data relating to long-term follow-up of infants exposed to amiodarone *in utero*. Amiodarone should be avoided when possible in pregnancy. However, if life-threatening arrhythmias can only be relieved by amiodarone, full neonatal assessment in relation to thyroid dysfunction must be carried out.

Transient hyperthyroidism of hyperemesis gravidarum (see also Chapter 10)

Hyperemesis gravidarum is vomiting in pregnancy of sufficient severity to require intravenous rehydration and cause weight loss; it may be associated with ketonuria, thiamine deficiency and abnormal liver or thyroid function tests. It is estimated that in 40% of cases of hyperemesis gravidarum, thyroid function will be abnormal, most commonly with elevated T4 or suppressed TSH or both [58]. The finding of abnormal thyroid function tests is an indicator of severe hyperemesis. The degree of abnormality of the thyroid function may reflect the severity of vomiting [59]. Free T4 levels may be extremely high, concentrations of 80 pmol/L being not uncommon, with TSH fully suppressed.

The thyroid dysfunction in hyperemesis is purely biochemical and not due to an intrinsic thyroid abnormality; fT4 returns to normal as the vomiting settles, although the TSH may take some time to do so. This return to normality should be confirmed, to ensure that the rare case of true hyperthyroidism is not overlooked. Although vomiting may occasionally be the sole presenting complaint in thyrotoxicosis, the clinical picture of hyperemesis is otherwise quite different from that of thyrotoxicosis. The typical patient with hyperemesis is washed out, tired, lacking in energy and deflated; there is no goitre, tremor or eye signs; if present, tachycardia is secondary to dehydration, weight loss to poor nutritional intake, and warm peripheries to the vasodilatation of pregnancy; the symptoms are clearly of recent onset and do not antedate the pregnancy. When there is clinical doubt concerning the differential diagnosis of the thyroid dysfunction, the absence of thyroid antiperoxidase and antithyroglobulin autoantibodies, and of TSH receptor antibodies supports the diagnosis of hyperemesis.

It seems unlikely that vomiting itself causes thyroid stimulation or that hyperthyroidism causes the vomiting. It is probable that both hyperemesis and the associated hyperthyroidism are caused by actions of hCG. hCG and TSH share α subunits; their β subunits are thought to have considerable homology and to share similar three-dimensional structure. In addition, there is also considerable similarity between the TSH and hCG receptors. *In vitro* work on animal and human models has demonstrated a thyrotrophic action for hCG. *In vivo* in normal pregnancy, hCG has one ten-thousandth of the action of TSH [60]. However, the term 'hCG' actually refers to a mixture of molecules, which each have differing amounts of thyrotrophic activity. These include intact hCG, nicked hCG, asialo hCG, free β-unit and free α-unit hCG and hCG lacking the carboxy terminal peptide on the β subunit (β-CTP). The β-CTP is a 31 amino acid extension, which distinguishes β-hCG from the otherwise identical β unit of luteinizing hormone (LH); LH and hCG missing β-CTP have 10-fold increase in thyrotrophic activity compared with intact hCG [61]. Nicked hCG, in which a hydrophobic loop is altered by the loss of a peptide link, may result from degradation of hCG; its thyrotrophic activity is almost double that of hCG [62]. The oligosaccharide side chains of glycoproteins such as hCG make a major contribution to their heterogeneity and changes in them, such as deglycosylation and desialylation enhance the thyrotrophic activity of hCG [63]. Women with hyperemesis have been found to have increased circulating concentrations of asialo hCG [64]. Therefore, in hyperemesis gravidarum, although the total hCG concentration as measured by routine laboratory assays may not be elevated, increased proportions of pro-thyrotrophic hCG portions can result in increased TSH-like activity, and therefore a situation of biochemical thyrotoxicosis.

Treatment of hyperemesis is centred on correcting the metabolic insults of prolonged vomiting and on preventing vomiting. There is no place for the use of antithyroid medication in hyperemesis: the thyroid abnormality is not usually long-lasting, and the fundamental problem is not one of increased intrinsic thyroid overactivity. Indeed, if antithyroid drugs are used for the treatment of hCG-induced hyperthyroidism, they are either ineffective or require extremely high doses to achieve biochemical euthyroidism [65]. There is then the worry of fetal hypothyroidism caused by drugs given to the mother crossing the placenta (see hyperthyroidism, below).

Recently an interesting cause of familial hyperemesis and hyperthyroidism has been described. A woman and her mother both had recurrent severe hyperemesis and hyperthyroidism in pregnancy. They were each found to have a mutation in the gene encoding the TSH receptor, which made it more sensitive to hCG than the wild-type receptor [8]. This raises interesting questions about hyperemesis that is recurrent, and may influence the advice given to a woman with a family history of severe hyperemesis.

Hyperthyroidism

Hyperthyroidism is not uncommon in women of reproductive age. Although conception is unusual in women with untreated acute thyrotoxicosis, once the disease is under control, fertility and libido return. The incidence is about two per 1000 pregnancies [66].

The aetiology in pregnancy reflects the most common causes in this age group. Thus, autoimmune thyrotoxicosis, Graves' disease, is the most frequent diagnosis, accounting for 95% cases. Graves' disease is characterized by a diffuse hypertrophic and hyperplastic goitre, IgG thyrotrophin receptor-stimulating antibodies, other thyroid autoantibodies such as antiperoxidase antibodies and hyperthyroidism, frequently in the presence of eye signs.

Other less common causes of hyperthyroidism include toxic nodular goitre, solitary toxic nodule, subacute thyroiditis, and well-differentiated thyroid carcinoma. Somatic mutations of the TSH receptor gene have been identified in some individuals with autonomous thyroid adenomas and in some cases of familial hyperthyroidism [67] (see above). In pregnancy, if a new diagnosis of thyrotoxicosis is suspected, hyperemesis gravidarum and molar pregnancy should be considered high in the differential diagnosis.

Pregnancy does not seem to influence the long-term course of hyperthyroidism, whatever the aetiology. However, typically, Graves' disease remits in the second and third trimesters, resulting in a reduced requirement for antithyroid medication, and in 30% cases [68] treatment may be discontinued. The first trimester and puerperium may be associated with a flare of Graves' disease [69]. These changes are thought to reflect the altered maternal immune state, and are probably exacerbated in the first trimester by reduced absorption of medication secondary to maternal vomiting and by high hCG concentrations (see above). Clinical disease activity follows the titre of thyrotrophin receptor-stimulating antibodies, which increase in the first trimester, fall in the second and third trimesters, and rise again in the puerperium, such that up to 75% of women whose disease has not completed its clinical course by the end of pregnancy, need an increased dose of treatment in the puerperium and some have a clinical relapse. There is also evidence that the balance of thyrotrophin receptor-stimulating and inhibitory antibodies changes progressively during pregnancy in favour of the latter, accounting for the fall in disease activity during pregnancy [70].

Clinical diagnosis of hyperthyroidism

The clinical assessment of thyroid disease activity is difficult in pregnancy. Failure to gain weight particularly in the presence of a good appetite and maternal tachycardia greater than 100 beats per minute which fails to slow with Valsalva manoeuvre are helpful indicators of hyperthyroidism. Eye signs and pretibial myxoedema do not reflect the activity of Graves' disease, although onycholysis, the elevation of the distal nail, a rare sign, does. Other symptoms and signs of thyrotoxicosis are not useful clinical discriminators between pregnancy and hyperthyroidism: fatigue, anxiety, emotional lability, heat intolerance, sweating, warm extremities and amenorrhoea are common in both. So in practice the diagnosis is made in a woman with history and physical findings compatible with hyperthyroidism who has elevated fT4 and/or fT3 by pregnancy criteria and where the TSH is suppressed (Table 12.2).

Outcome of pregnancies complicated by maternal hyperthyroidism

If thyrotoxicosis is well controlled before and throughout pregnancy, the outcomes for both mother and baby are generally good. However, a number of observational studies suggest that if hyperthyroidism is poorly controlled, both maternal and fetal complications such as thyroid storm, congestive cardiac failure, hypertensive disease of pregnancy, premature labour, small for gestational age infants and stillbirth seem to be increased. The outcome is worse in those pregnancies where thyroid disease is never controlled, compared with those where euthyroidism is achieved during pregnancy, but both of these groups have poorer outcome than pregnancies where thyroid disease is controlled before conception [71]. Although these studies may be flawed with confounding variables, and lack appropriate control subjects, it is unlikely that rigorous randomized controlled studies will or should be performed. Therefore, it seems prudent to ensure optimal control both before conception and throughout pregnancy.

Treatment of hyperthyroidism

Ideally, optimal disease control should be secured before contraception is discontinued. In general terms, the management of thyrotoxicosis in pregnancy is similar to that outside pregnancy, except that radioactive iodine is completely contraindicated. Medical therapy is usually the first treatment option. Partial or total thyroidectomy may be considered for failure of or allergy to medical therapy, suspicion of or definite diagnosis of thyroid cancer or compressive symptoms secondary to goitre; it is not usually used for women in whom poor compliance with medical therapy is an issue because the incidence of hypothyroidism requiring medical treatment after thyroid surgery is 50% [72] or more and it is likely that these women will again be poorly compliant with replacement T4. Surgery is usually carried out in the second trimester.

Before surgery for active thyroid disease, thyrotoxicosis must be controlled, to reduce the risk of postoperative thyroid storm (see below). This is usually achieved with antithyroid drugs, iodine and propranolol. Propranolol is effective in cases of allergy to or failure of medical therapy as it relieves symptoms of thyrotoxicosis over 4 days and makes the thyroid less vascular (see below). Iodine is given as an oral solution for 10–14 days prior to surgery, enhancing control and reducing vascularity (see below); it should not be used for longer than this as its antithyroid effect diminishes with time.

In the non-pregnant state, radioactive iodine is often used in the treatment of hyperthyroidism due to Graves' disease, toxic nodular goitre or toxic adenoma either as an adjunct to medical therapy or as first-line treatment. The decision to use radioiodine therapy is based on a number of factors including patient and doctor preference. However, pregnancy and lactation are absolute contraindications to its use [54].

MEDICAL TREATMENT OF HYPERTHYROIDISM

Propylthiouracil (PTU) and carbimazole are the mainstays of medical treatment of thyrotoxicosis in pregnancy. They block thyroid hormone synthesis and have an immunosuppressive effect, reducing the titre of TSH receptor antibodies, and thereby directly influencing the course of Graves' disease [73]. It used to be widely accepted that, because PTU is heavily protein-bound, it crosses the placenta less readily than the relatively unbound carbimazole [74], and therefore it was the drug of choice in the management of thyrotoxicosis in pregnancy. However, a number of studies have now suggested little difference between the drugs, and there is no longer any need to change pregnant women from carbimazole to PTU. Using isolated perfused human term placental lobules, Mortimer *et al.* [75] showed that PTU and methimazole (the active metabolite of carbimazole) have similar placental transfer kinetics, and indicated that contrary to general belief, PTU does cross the placenta readily. Momotani *et al.* [76] measured cord thyroid function in 77 babies whose mothers had been taking either methimazole or PTU in doses ranging from 2.5 to 20 mg and 25 to 200 mg, respectively. They found no difference in thyroid function at delivery between babies whose mothers had been taking methimazole and those who had been taking PTU, nor any apparent dose-dependent effect.

An observational study of 135 pregnancies during which antithyroid drug was taken has suggested that PTU and methimazole are equally effective in the control of maternal hyperthyroidism: one-third of women taking either drug remain hyperthyroid at delivery; in those pregnancies in which a euthyroid state is achieved, the mean time after commencing antithyroid treatment is 7–8 weeks. Euthyroidism was considered to have been achieved if indicated by clinical features and biochemical assessment, although the use of a fT4 index would no longer be considered the most appropriate test to perform [77].

The dose of antithyroid medication is titrated against maternal well-being and biochemical assessment of thyroid status. It is usual to aim for fT4 at the upper end of normal provided the patient is clinically euthyroid, thereby minimizing the dose required. Thyroid function tests should be measured 4–6-weekly in women with well-controlled Graves' disease, but more frequently if she has a new diagnosis or a relapse. Many women with well controlled Graves' disease will reduce or even discontinue (30%) treatment during the second and third trimester of pregnancy [67]. They should be monitored clinically and biochemically during the puerperium too, as they may need to return to their previous dose if the Graves' disease has not burnt out. Pregnant women should be reminded of the risk of drug-induced agranulocytosis, and to report sore throat immediately. β blockers may be used for the control of tremor and tachycardia if clinically indicated: data on propranolol for control of hypertension suggest that it is safe to use in pregnancy [78].

THYROID STORM

Thyroid storm is an uncommon life-threatening crisis, which requires immediate emergency medical treatment; aggressive therapy has reduced the mortality rate to around 10%. It is characterized by an acute exacerbation of thyrotoxicosis, usually in a patient with pre-existing hyperthyroidism. It has been reported in 20% of untreated pregnant women with thyrotoxicosis and 2% of those on medical therapy [79]. There is often a precipitating factor such as surgery, infection, anaesthesia, abrupt withdrawal of antithyroid drug therapy, or administration of radioactive iodine to a severely hyperthyroid patient. For pregnant women, labour and delivery are stress events that could precipitate a thyroid storm.

Clinical presentation is varied. Typically, the patient exhibits extreme symptoms of thyrotoxicosis with pyrexia and changes in the mental state, ranging from irritability and agitation to frank psychosis or coma. Cardiovascular symptoms are pronounced, with tachycardia and tachyarrythmias, and sometimes cardiac failure. There may be gastrointestinal symptoms such as nausea, vomiting or diarrhoea.

The diagnosis of thyroid storm is clinical rather than biochemical, as the thyroid function tests are not different from those in uncomplicated thyrotoxicosis. There may be a leucocytosis, which should be differentiated from that of normal pregnancy, elevated liver enzymes or hypercalcaemia.

Management of thyroid storm consists of both general supportive measures and specific treatment to control the thyroid dysfunction. Precipitating factors should be sought and removed if possible or treated. There should be a thorough investigation for infection, including a lumbar puncture if mental agitation cannot clearly be differentiated from meningitis or encephalitis; there should be a low threshold for administering intravenous antibiotics. Pyrexia must be controlled with rectal paracetamol, tepid sponging and a fan. Aspirin should be avoided, predominantly because it displaces thyroid hormones from TBG, increasing concentrations of free hormones. At the dose required for control of pyrexia, aspirin may also have adverse effects on the fetus, although in this context that risk is relatively insignificant. Chlorpromazine, 25–50 mg p.o. or i.v. 6- to 8-hourly acts as a useful sedative, which also has an antipyretic action. Intravenous fluid support is required, as fluid loss from sweating can be massive, but invasive monitoring may be required particularly if pulmonary oedema is present. Large volumes of glucose may be required because of the high metabolic requirements of the condition.

Specific control of the hyperthyroidism is usually achieved with PTU, which not only inhibits thyroid hormone synthesis but also reduces the conversion of T4 to T3 peripherally. A large loading dose is required, up to 1000 mg, which is given orally or via a nasogastric tube; alternatively, particularly if ileus is present, methimazole could be administered as a suppository, although it may not be readily available in the UK. This is followed by oral PTU, 150–300 mg 6-hourly. One to two hours after the first dose of PTU, iodide should be given to inhibit the release of further thyroid hormones from the thyroid gland. Iodide should not be given before PTU has been commenced, as this may result in the build-up of T4 (and T3) in the thyroid, and an exacerbation of the thyroid crisis if this excess is suddenly released. The usual regimens are Lugol's iodine, 500 mg 6-hourly by mouth or sodium iodide 500 mg as an intravenous infusion 8- to 12-hourly. Dexamethasone 2 mg 6-hourly is given for the first 24 h to block the peripheral conversion of T4 to T3; if the gestation is less than 36 weeks, the usual obstetric regimen to enhance fetal lung maturation could be used instead. Tachycardia and tachyarrhythmias are treated with propranolol provided there is no evidence of cardiac failure. It is given either intravenously, 0.5–1 mg over 1 min, repeated at 2-min intervals if required, to a maximum dose of 10 mg, or in high doses orally; 40 mg three times daily should be continued as maintenance. Monitoring with continuous electrocardiography is required, especially when intravenous propranolol is used, but also throughout the acute management of the storm. In addition, propranolol reduces peripheral conversion of T4 to T3, and renders the thyroid gland less vascular, which is helpful prior to surgery. If rapid atrial fibrillation has resulted in heart failure, oxygen, digoxin and diuretics may be required.

When thyroid storm occurs beyond fetal viability, continuous cardiotocography (CTG) should be employed. Little is written about the fetal effects of maternal thyroid storm. Maternal pyrexia is likely to result in fetal tachycardia, and severe maternal dehydration could reduce placental perfusion. Prolonged maternal hypoxia could also have adverse effects on the fetus. Nevertheless, when the maternal condition is brought under control, there is a good chance of fetal survival. However, if the CTG indicates sustained severe fetal distress in a woman near term who is not in advanced labour, very careful and clear consideration will need to be given to the correct course of action: an emergency caesarean section in the presence of a fulminating thyroid storm is likely to be a very dangerous procedure for the woman. Continuing aggressive correction of the maternal metabolic insults can usually be expected to improve the fetal condition, and may be the safest option (for the mother).

BLOCKING-REPLACEMENT REGIMEN

In the non-pregnant state the blocking-replacement regimen has been used with the intention of quickly achieving a long-lasting euthyroid state, with minimal risk of iatrogenic hypothyroidism. A relatively high dose of antithyroid medication is given to render the patient hypothyroid, and T4 is added to ensure she remains euthyroid. Eighteen months after the initiation of treatment, antithyroid treatment is stopped and T4 alone continued. The rationale behind this regimen depends upon a number of features:

1 production of TSH receptor-stimulating antibodies might be enhanced by TSH during treatment of Graves' disease—T4 might counteract this effect of TSH by suppressing TSH production;

2 the immunosuppressive effect of antithyroid medication on TSH receptor antibody titre is postulated to be dose dependent;

3 in pregnancy, the addition of T4 is thought to reduce the risk of a postpartum flare of Graves' hyperthyroidism [80].

Initial reports of its success were encouraging. In a placebo-controlled trial of 109 Japanese patients with Graves' disease, Hashizume *et al.* [81] found that the use of T4 reduced the 3-year relapse rate from 35% to 2% and resulted in lower antibody concentrations compared with the placebo group. Therefore, in some centres this method of treatment has been used widely. However, it is not recommended for use in pregnancy. First, although the woman is euthyroid, a relatively high dose of antithyroid medication is given (rendering her hypothyroid) with T4 being added to ensure she is euthyroid: as only the antithyroid medication crosses the placenta and not T4, the risk of fetal hypothyroidism is increased. In a study of 20 pregnancies treated with this regimen, the babies had higher cord TSH values than the control group of normal

pregnancies and one had a goitre; they were also 500 g lighter (after matching for gestational age at delivery) but this difference did not reach statistical significance, possibly because of the small numbers involved [82]. Secondly, there is increasing evidence that the blocking-replacement regimen is not effective: McIver *et al.* [83] found no difference in recurrence of Graves' disease or of TSH receptor antibody titres in a group of 111 Scottish patients randomized to either carbimazole alone or carbimazole plus T4.

TERATOGENESIS

Neither PTU nor carbimazole is thought to be teratogenic. There is some evidence that babies are less likely to have congenital abnormality if their mother's disease is controlled by antithyroid treatment than if the thyrotoxicosis is untreated. External examination of 643 liveborn babies whose mothers had Graves' disease revealed six congenital abnormalities, all in different systems. These babies were allocated to groups according to maternal thyroid status in the first trimester: three mothers had untreated hyperthyroidism (6%), two were hyperthyroid and treated with methimazole (including one earlobe abnormality not attributable to therapy as it would have occurred before medical treatment was started) (1.7%) and one was untreated and euthyroid (0.3%); none were euthyroid and on treatment ($p < 0.01$, hyperthyroid vs. euthyroid, both untreated and total) [84]. This study included only those pregnancies that reached term with a liveborn baby, and excluded miscarriages and stillbirth; it also excluded congenital abnormalities not detected by external examination made at the first visit after delivery, and provided no other details about the pregnancy that may be relevant to outcome. However, it seems reasonable to cautiously extrapolate that control of Graves' disease including the use of methimazole in the first trimester may protect against congenital abnormality. There is further evidence for a lack of drug-induced teratogenicity, including the more recent work from Wing *et al.* [77] on 185 women with hyperthyroidism: 3% babies (three of 99) whose mothers took PTU had congenital heart defects: in each, the mother was hyperthyroid at presentation and did not commence treatment until the second trimester; one of 36 babies whose mothers took methimazole (prior to conception) had a congenital inguinal hernia.

It has been widely believed that aplasia cutis of the scalp is associated with the first-trimester use of antithyroid drugs. However, no cases of aplasia cutis were described in either Momotani *et al.* [84] or Wing *et al.*'s [77] studies totalling 378 pregnancies where the mother took either methimazole or PTU. Likewise in a Dutch prevalence study of scalp defects in 49 000 babies conducted over 27 years, 13 cases were detected (0.03%) and none of the mothers had taken antithyroid drugs; 24 women who had taken antithyroid medication had normal babies [85]. Amongst the small number of cases described, it is possible that some are due to an autosomal dominant familial scalp defect, rather than antithyroid drugs [85]. Overall, either the association between antithyroid drugs and aplasia cutis is spurious or the risk is extremely small [86].

LACTATION

Both PTU and carbimazole cross into breast milk, the latter more than the former. Nine lactating women were given 400 mg PTU: 0.025% (range 0.007–0.077%) of the maternal dose was found in breast milk in the 4 h after maternal administration; no change in neonatal thyroid function was detected when one woman took PTU 200–300 mg daily for 5 months [87]. Low et al. [88] gave 10 mg of radiolabelled carbimazole to a lactating woman, and over 24 h found 0.47% of the maternal dose of methimazole reached breast milk; similarly, 0.077% of a radiolabelled dose of 100 mg PTU was found in breast milk. Several other small studies have shown normal neonatal thyroid function when lactating women take a low dose of either PTU or carbimazole: for example, Lamberg et al. [89] studied 11 fully lactating women taking 5–15 mg carbimazole and one taking PTU 125 mg, and demonstrated normal neonatal TSH and T4 concentrations in the first 3 weeks of life. Eight lactating women taking between 50 and 300 mg PTU had babies with mild biochemical hypothyroidism at delivery (secondary to the transplacental passage of PTU it is presumed) which resolved when they were tested 18 days to 8 months postpartum, indicating that the amount of PTU transmitted in breast milk does not suppress neonatal thyroid function [90]. Nevertheless, there is concern that high doses of antithyroid medication, particularly carbimazole, may cause neonatal thyroid suppression. If doses greater than 15 mg carbimazole or 150 mg PTU are required, consideration should be given to splitting the dose throughout the day, feeding before a dose when possible, clinically monitoring neonatal well-being and measuring neonatal thyroid function.

FETAL AND NEONATAL RISKS OF MEDICAL THERAPY

As both PTU and carbimazole cross the placenta, they may influence fetal thyroid function. It is therefore appropriate to use the minimal dose possible to control the maternal condition. It is usual to achieve this by aiming for a fT4 level at the upper limit of normal. Both drugs block the synthesis of thyroid hormones but do not prevent release of preformed hormone. They do this by blocking organification of iodine and coupling of iodotyrosyl molecules, and PTU also inhibits the conversion of T4 to T3 by deiodinase type I. These effects can occur in the fetus. However, fortunately the thionamides do not influence deiodinases II and III, which are crucial to maintaining fetal brain development. Therefore, even if the fetus becomes hypothyroid as a consequence of treatment, provided his or her iodine intake is sufficient the fetus should be able to maintain intracellular T3 levels in the brain, and therefore neurodevelopmental status should be preserved.

Babies of mothers taking PTU or methimazole had lower cord T4 levels than those whose mothers had discontinued treatment prior to delivery. They were more likely to have low T4 or high TSH in cord samples than their mothers when maternal control was achieved by antithyroid medication, but not if thyroid medication had been discontinued. This suggests that controlling the maternal disease too tightly may increase the risk of fetal hypothyroidism. Indeed, all 10 women with treatment-induced hypothyroxinaemia had suppressed cord fT4 concentrations [91]. Subsequently the same group looked at 43 women taking methimazole and 34 taking PTU, and showed no difference in the fetal risk of temporary neonatal hypothyroidism between the drugs, nor any correlation between drug dose and fetal risk. The mothers of the five (13%) babies born with transient biochemical (and asymptomatic) hypothyroidism were taking 50 or 100 mg PTU, or 2.5–10 mg methimazole. However, as only a small proportion of mothers were taking higher doses of medication, it is possible that a dose-related effect was inadvertently overlooked [76].

Overall, 10–20% babies born to mothers taking these medications have transient biochemical hypothyroidism [76], which is only rarely symptomatic; it resolves by day 4–5 [92]. The effect if any of this neonatal, and by extrapolation, fetal hypothyroxinaemia on future brain development of the children is uncertain. Initially it may mask neonatal hyperthyroidism, a potentially dangerous condition (see later). Neonatal goitre is uncommon when antithyroid drugs are used alone and without iodine therapy, occurring in two of 109 reported cases [76,82,92]. One of the mothers of these babies was taking 400 mg of PTU, the other 200 mg PTU plus 300 μg T4. The goitres were small and not obstructive, and resolved in less than 2 weeks and a few days, respectively.

A number of small retrospective studies have attempted to assess whether antithyroid drugs have any long-term adverse effects on children exposed to them in utero. The results are reassuring, demonstrating comparable physical and psychological development and no differences in thyroid size or function, when compared with a group of children whose mothers were euthyroid following thyroidectomy before pregnancy. However, only 101 children are included in four separate studies. The studies have insufficient power to detect small differences, which could therefore have been overlooked [93]. Transplacental exposure to antithyroid drugs has not been reported to cause neonatal neutropenia, fever, rash, hepatitis or other adverse effects associated with the use of these agents in adults.

Fetal and neonatal Graves' disease

In pregnancies where the woman has active Graves' disease, maternal TSH receptor-stimulating antibodies may result in fetal or neonatal thyrotoxicosis.

Fetal Graves' disease is uncommon, and although some authorities report it in up to 16% of their pregnancies that are complicated by Graves' disease, in my experience it is less frequent. Fetal risk is proportional to the titre of TSH receptor-stimulating antibodies. The fetal thyroid is unable to respond to these passively acquired maternal antibodies before 20–24 weeks' gestation [94]. After this gestation, it is important to monitor pregnancies complicated by Graves' disease, or where there is a maternal history of Graves' disease, for signs of fetal hyperthyroidism. In practice, this implies regular clinical assessment of fetal well-being by maternal detection of fetal movements, measurement of symphyseal fundal height to check fetal size and determination of fetal heart rate, a persistent tachycardia greater than 160 beats per minute being suggestive of fetal thyrotoxicosis. In addition, I do an ultrasound scan at 34 weeks' gestation to exclude fetal goitre or clinically undetected intrauterine growth restriction. If fetal hyperthyroidism is suspected, cordocentesis should be considered, and fetal TSH and fT4 measured: the normal ranges for fetal thyroid function are known [21]. This provides a more reliable estimation of fetal thyroid function than amniocentesis, and allows clear discrimination between fetal goitre associated with fetal hypothyroidism and fetal hyperthyroidism.

Fetal hyperthyroidism may cause serious complications such as premature delivery (90%), craniosynostosis and intellectual impairment, hydrops fetalis and intrauterine death; large fetal goitre may cause polyhydramnios due to oesophageal obstruction or neck extension and subsequent malposition in labour. These complications may be reduced either by delivering the baby if the pregnancy is at or approaching term, or by treating the fetus with maternally administered antithyroid agents. The dose should be titrated against fetal heart rate, fetal movement and growth

rate. Occasionally the mother may become hypothyroid and require T4 therapy that does not readily cross the placenta and therefore would not interfere with the success of the fetal therapy. Insufficient cases have been reported to be sure that this is the optimal way of treating the condition or monitoring it. Nevertheless, the risks associated with serial cordocentesis if used to monitor therapy may not be justified. It has also been reported that the fetal goitre in fetal thyrotoxicosis has an increased vascularity, which is detectable by ultrasonography and resolves as the fetal thyroid function returns to normal [95]. This may be useful for distinguishing the goitre of fetal thyrotoxicosis from that of fetal hypothyroidism, especially if cordocentesis is either unavailable or undesirable.

Neonatal hyperthyroidism is also rare, occurring in up to 1% babies [66]. It occurs most frequently in babies whose mothers have a history of Graves' disease, and although the literature reports a 2–10% risk of hyperthyroidism in these babies [96], in clinical practice it seems much less frequent. It is a consequence of the transplacental passage of TSH receptor-stimulating antibodies. These antibodies have a half-life of 21 days, considerably longer than that of PTU and carbimazole, and therefore the clinical effects of neonatal hyperthyroidism may not become apparent until the child is 7–10 days old if the mother has taken antithyroid medication during pregnancy. Thyroid function tests should be measured in cord blood, to provide a baseline, and the paediatricians informed of the delivery: local protocols will dictate surveillance and monitoring. Parents should be aware of the symptoms of neonatal hyperthyroidism and should have a low threshold for seeking medical advice. Symptoms of hyperthyroidism are non-specific, but may include jitteriness, failure to gain weight, poor feeding, poor sleeping, bossing of frontal bones, liver dysfunction and jaundice and in extreme or unrecognized cases, high output cardiac failure. Goitre may cause respiratory embarrassment or feeding difficulties. Mortality occurs in up to 25% if not recognized. Treatment is usually with antithyroid drugs, β blockers and fluid support, and is titrated against neonatal well-being and thyroid function tests; it is rarely required for more than a few months.

Recently guidelines for the measurement of TSH receptor antibodies have been published [96]. They are based on 454 women with Graves' disease, whose pregnancies were reported in nine publications from four continents; reports where there were no cases of neonatal Graves' disease were excluded. The authors concluded that TSH receptor antibodies (or if available TSH receptor-stimulating antibodies) should be measured in early (to detect fetal thyrotoxicosis) and late (to detect neonatal thyrotoxicosis) pregnancy in women with active Graves' disease or a history of Graves' disease treated by surgery or radioactive iodine (but not by medical treatment alone). If antibodies are low or absent, fetal or neonatal thyrotoxicosis is unlikely; if positive, cord and day 4–7 thyroid function tests with close clinical surveillance is recommended [96]. However, no data are given for the strength of these assertions, which can only be based on a small number of affected babies who may be derived from very select populations. In addition, in clinical practice, TSH receptor-stimulating antibody titres may not be readily available, in which case 'common sense' management such as that outlined above seems safe.

Hypothyroidism

Hypothyroidism is relatively common in women of reproductive age. It is not surprising therefore that it is the commonest pre-existing endocrine disorder in pregnant women [97]. Hypothyroidism that has been diagnosed prior to conception occurs in nine per 1000 pregnancies [98]. Amongst American women who accepted serum screening for α-FP at 15–18 weeks' gestation, 0.3% (six in the cohort of 2000 tested) had biochemical hypothyroidism with elevated TSH and low fT4 [99]. The most common aetiology is autoimmune Hashimoto's thyroiditis. However, hypothyroidism secondary to treatment of thyrotoxicosis with radioactive iodine or surgery, or thyroidectomy are also common. Increasingly, women taking T4 continuously for treatment of postpartum thyroiditis, mistakenly diagnosed as 'permanent' hypothyroidism, are also being seen in subsequent pregnancies.

Pituitary causes of hypothyroidism are rare. Pit-1 is a pituitary-specific transcription factor regulating somatotrophe, lactotrophe and thyrotrophe function. A few individuals have been identified with Pit-1 deficiency, and one pregnancy in a Pit-1-deficient woman has been reported. The baby developed growth restriction, hydrops fetalis with polyhydramnios and an uncomplicated baseline bradycardia. After delivery the baby was found to be growth hormone, prolactin, TSH and T4 deficient, and was subsequently diagnosed as having the same Pit-1 gene mutation as her mother. She was profoundly hypothyroid, and her psychomotor development was severely delayed despite early initiation of replacement T4 therapy. The unexpected severity of her condition suggested a negative influence of the maternal Pit-1-deficient environment [100].

Pregnancy outcome

Several substantial but now old studies have suggested that there is an increased risk of miscarriage, stillbirth, prematurity and congenital abnormality when women have untreated or insufficiently treated hypothyroidism in pregnancy. More than 30 years ago a prospective study of 168 hypothyroid women and 1253 controls showed an increased incidence of congenital anomaly and both mental and somatic developmental problems in the study group [101]. However, the biochemical assays available for monitoring thyroid function were less accurate than those currently employed, and treatment was therefore less precise. More recently in a study of 68 women with hypothyroidism, inadequately treated hypothyroidism was linked with an increased frequency of gestational hypertension and iatrogenic prematurity, compared with adequately treated hypothyroidism; even with attainment of euthyroidism, the incidence of hypertension was greater than in the general population [102]. Spontaneous premature delivery, intrauterine growth restriction, congenital anomaly, maternal anaemia and postpartum haemorrhage were not associated with hypothyroidism. Unfortunately the management of these women was based on TSH levels rather than fT4, and there is also the possibility of a type 2 error. Nevertheless, the study does suggest that with adequate control of hypothyroidism a good outcome can be expected [102].

Previously, miscarriage has been linked with hypothyroidism [103], and indeed there was a vogue for performing thyroid function tests in women with recurrent miscarriage. However, it now seems that mild subclinical hypothyroidism is not associated with pregnancy loss, and routine thyroid testing of healthy women who have experienced a miscarriage is not recommended [104]. Elevated antiperoxidase and antithyroglobulin antibodies are associated with miscarriage, although this may not be independent of maternal age [105].

Recently a rare complication of hypothyroidism was reported in a woman with congenital absence of the thyroid gland who had discontinued replacement therapy for several years before conception. She presented at 12 weeks' gestation with severe ovarian hyperstimulation syndrome (OHS), undetectable fT4 and fT3 levels, and TSH >350 μU/mL. Ovarian granulosa cells have TRα and TRβ receptors that are stimulated by TSH, resulting in increased oestriol production and the clinical scenario of OHS [106].

Diagnosis of hypothyroidism in pregnancy

A new diagnosis of hypothyroidism is rarely made in pregnancy because symptomatic hypothyroidism is usually associated with subfertility and/or poor libid. More commonly, the clinical dilemma is to determine whether treatment of pre-existing hypothyroidism is adequate. The diagnosis of either new hypothyroidism or of inadequate treatment of existing hypothyroidism in pregnancy based on assessment of maternal symptoms and signs is particularly difficult because of their non-specific nature and the considerable overlap with the changes that frequently occur in normal pregnancy. In particular, features such as tiredness, constipation, weight gain, anaemia, carpal tunnel syndrome and thinning of the hair are poor discriminators. Therefore there is a high dependence upon biochemical measurements, which must be interpreted according to pregnancy-specific reference ranges (see Table 12.2).

Management of hypothyroidism in pregnancy

T4 therapy is the mainstay of medical treatment of hypothyroidism in pregnancy. T4 is generally considered to be safe in pregnancy and lactation; there is no evidence of teratogenicity, nor do significant amounts pass into breast milk. The dose of T4 should be titrated against the biochemical results. Thyroid function tests should be measured at 8–12 week intervals when the thyroid dose is stable and the woman clinically and biochemically euthyroid, the first assessment being made as early in pregnancy as possible (and ideally just before conception as well) (see below). Testing is required more frequently if the dose is being adjusted, usually every 4–6 weeks, especially if undertreatment is present in the first trimester, when testing at 2-weekly intervals is required. In general, a low fT4 concentration should be the main impetus for increasing the dose of T4, rather than a raised TSH, particularly as the latter may remain elevated for some time after the correct T4 dose has been achieved. However, as raised TSH with normal fT4 can also indicate poor compliance or erratic absorption of T4, the patient should be questioned carefully.

Some authorities have recommended a blanket increase in T4 to 200 μg daily in pregnancy, although the logic for this is unclear [107]. Others have found that the majority of patients need an increase in T4 dose: Mandel *et al.* [108] studied 12 women with hypothyroidism, and found that nine needed an increased dose during pregnancy, which was reduced again after delivery. In our experience, of 36 pregnancies only 20% of women with hypothyroidism needed to increase their T4 dosage; invariably they had been undertreated prior to conception and continued on the same increased dose postnatally. The remaining 80% of women were euthyroid at booking and remained so throughout pregnancy without a change in dose [109].

FIRST-TRIMESTER/PRECONCEPTUAL CARE

Two recent papers have been influential in determining the management of hypothyroidism in early pregnancy.

There has been a long held association between severely undertreated hypothyroidism or undiagnosed hypothyroidism in the mother and a subsequent adverse effect on child development. Nearly 30 years ago, Evelyn Man demonstrated a minor reduction in intelligence quotient (IQ) in the offspring of women who had undiagnosed or undertreated hypothyroidism in pregnancy [110–112]. T4 is now known to play an important role in the developing fetal brain. Before 12 weeks' gestation, the fetal thyroid is unable to produce hormones, and the fetus is dependent upon the small amount of maternal T4 that is able to cross the placenta. Recent work, especially using rat models, suggests that the developing fetal brain is adversely affected by maternal hypothyroxinaemia during the first trimester. Neurotransmitters may have a neurotropic role in early gestation. In hypothyroid pregnant rats, fetal neurotransmitter concentrations are lower in early pregnancy than in euthyroid rats, but concentrations equalize after the onset of fetal thyroid hormone production [113].

In human pregnancy in an iodine-replete area, Pop *et al.* suggest that amongst a group of apparently normal pregnant women, those with the lowest fT4 concentrations at 12 weeks' gestation had the greatest reduction in infant neurodevelopmental scores at age 10 months, but that T4 concentrations at 32 weeks' gestation showed no such correlation. Using multiple regression analysis, alcohol intake in pregnancy, gestational depression, low educational level and the occurrence of negative life events during the pregnancy were also associated with the subsequent low neurodevelopmental scores, so it is uncertain how great the contribution of hypothyroxinaemia alone was to their findings [114].

Haddow *et al.* [115] have also suggested that maternal hypothyroidism may be associated with adverse neurodevelopment in the child. They used stored sera from early second-trimester Down's syndrome serum screening tests on 25 000 American women to select 62 with raised TSH, 14 of whom subsequently admitted taking T4 during pregnancy, but presumably at a suboptimal dose. One hundred and twenty-four controls with TSH concentrations less than 98th percentile were selected, matched for years of education. All children had satisfactory thyroid screening in the newborn period. The 7–9-year-old offspring underwent 15 tests of neuropsychological development, two of which were significantly lower in the group with raised maternal TSH than in the control group. The study group was then subdivided into those whose mothers were taking T4 during pregnancy and those whose mothers were not, and the analysis repeated; in the comparison of the untreated group and the (euthyroid) controls, eight tests were worse in the study group including a fall in IQ of 7 points. Therefore it appears that untreated but presumably relatively mild hypothyroidism may have adverse effects on the developing fetal brain and that maternal T4 treatment in part prevents this. As TSH itself does not cross the placenta, and because it often remains high for some time after T4 concentrations return to normal, it is likely that the effect demonstrated here reflects a complication of maternal hypothyroxinaemia which was overcome by treatment with T4 because the exogenous T4 crossed the placenta in the first trimester and so protected the fetal brain [115].

The cautious extrapolation for clinical practice from these studies is that T4 therapy should be optimized before conception in women with hypothyroidism; in clinical practice this also infers referral early in pregnancy to an obstetrician or a physician (or a combined clinic) with an interest in this field so that T4 dose can be monitored in the first trimester. More exciting, although daunting, is the prospect of doing thyroid function screening on all women planning to conceive: this might also have direct benefit to the mother, because Haddow *et al.* [115] found that 60% of the untreated women had a diagnosis of hypothyroidism 1 to 10 years after the index pregnancy. However, the prospects of adding this to a preconceptual package of care accessible to the majority of women are unpromising.

Neonatal outcome

Although thyroid peroxidase and antithyroglobulin auto-antibodies cross the placenta they appear to have no effect on fetal thyroid development. Therefore maternal Hashimoto's hypothyroidism is not usually associated with fetal or neonatal thyroid dysfunction [116]. However, TSH receptor blocking antibodies may rarely cause fetal or transient neonatal hypothyroidism, estimated at one in 180 000 neonates, or 2% of cases of congenital hypothyroidism [117]. Rarely, women with Hashimoto's thyroiditis have had children with neonatal or even fetal thyrotoxicosis. One woman with Hashimoto's thyroiditis had three children affected in this way, and she was shown to have both stimulating TSH receptor antibodies and three different TSH binding inhibiting antibodies, blocking both stimulating TSH receptor antibodies and TSH activity [118].

It has been suggested that either T4 therapy [119] or maternal thyroid disease [120] are risk factors for neonatal encephalopathy. However, there have been concerns that in the absence of data relating to indications for or duration of use or dose of T4, the apparent association may be either a coincidence or that T4 use was a surrogate marker for another risk factor [121]. Therefore, the same group have recently published further information relating to the 13 cases of neonatal encephalopathy and three controls in which there was maternal thyroid disease [122]. Ten of these 13 women took T4 throughout pregnancy, two took thionamides and one took no thyroid-related medication. The indications for T4 therapy included auto-immune hypothyroidism and hypothyroidism secondary to treatment of hyperthyroidism. Only five pregnancies had no other risk factors for encephalopathy. In six babies there were other associated features that may have contributed to infant outcome. Two of the three control mothers required an increased dose of T4 in pregnancy as did one of the 10 case mothers: the reasons for and timings of these changes are not given, but presumably were because the woman was found to be hypothyroid. It is our experience that women who require an increased dose of T4 during pregnancy are undertreated prior to or at conception [109], and therefore by extrapolation would have a higher risk of hypothyroxinaemia during the critical stages of the first trimester when long-term neurodevelopmental delay may occur [115]. In six of the case pregnancies thyroid function tests were not recorded, so it is unknown whether euthyroidism was achieved or not. Therefore these additional data do not strengthen the association between T4 use and encephalopathy; doctors should not be deterred from prescribing T4 for pregnant women in the appropriate dose when clinically indicated.

Although the global diagnosis of maternal thyroid disease, combining cases of both hypothyroidism and hyperthyroidism, seems to be associated with neonatal encephalopathy, the mechanisms for this are uncertain; statistically the association does not persist if hypothyroidism requiring treatment with T4 is considered separately from other forms of thyroid disease, and so the situation remains unclear. Optimal control of thyroid disease remains the gold standard, and future research should consider whether suboptimally treated or indeed untreated thyroid disease results in poorer neonatal outcome [123].

Postpartum thyroiditis

Postpartum thyroiditis (PPT) is a subacute destructive autoimmune condition occurring in the first year postpartum. It may present as either hyperthyroidism or hypothyroidism, or be a purely biochemical phenomenon. The incidence appears to vary widely. This may be due to genetic or environmental variation, or to differences in diagnostic criteria and reporting: for example in New York the incidence was reported as 1.9% [124], but in Wales it was 16.7% [125]. In the New York study, 212 women were screened 4–12 weeks postpartum; four had thyroid dysfunction, and six (2.8%) had antiperoxidase antibodies. In Wales, 901 women were screened at booking, 117 (13%) were found to have thyroid autoantibodies and 100 of these were seen 6-weekly in the first year postpartum. Normality of thyroid function was compared with a control group of 120 women without thyroid autoantibody, and through a poorly explained derivation, the prevalence of postpartum thyroid dysfunction in the unselected population was estimated to be 16.7%. In both studies, the thyroid dysfunction was clinically silent.

In clinical practice, women with PPT usually present to general practitioners, and not to obstetricians or obstetric physicians. Therefore, unless general practitioners are aware of the condition, women may be given other diagnoses, such as Hashimoto's hypothyroidism or depression (see later), or become 'heartsink' patients [126]. The most common, and increasingly frequent situation in which I see women with PPT is when they conceive their next pregnancy and attend the obstetric medicine clinic with a history compatible with PPT but on long-term treatment with T4.

Pathogenesis

PPT is believed to be an autoimmune condition, which may be precipitated by the reversal of immune suppression that occurs at delivery. The condition is more common in women with other autoimmune conditions, for example those with insulin-dependent diabetes mellitus are between two and four times more likely to develop the condition than the general population [127,128].

Thyroid antiperoxidase antibodies (previously called antimicrosomal antibodies) are associated with PPT, occurring in 8–10% of most general populations, whether measured at booking or in the puerperium, and in 90% of women with the condition [129]. Thirty-three to seventy-three per cent of women who are antibody positive develop biochemical evidence of PPT [130,131] as do 0–28% of antibody-negative women [132]. In an American population, there appeared to be an association between presence of antibody and racial group: over 1000 consecutive women were studied, the overall prevalence being 7%, the prevalence in white women being 8.8%, black women 2.5% and in both Hispanic and Arabic women around 20% [133]. The titre of these antibodies increases during the postpartum period, the peak coinciding with the peak time for thyroid dysfunction [125], and the titre of the antibodies may help to predict the risk of the thyroid dysfunction [131].

The histological appearance of thyroid biopsies has been examined in 15 Japanese women with the condition. They have focal or diffuse chronic thyroiditis with lymphocytic infiltration. In addition, varying degrees of follicular destruction and follicular hyperplasia occur; fibrosis, a typical feature of Hashimoto's thyroiditis, is absent [134]. These features support the concept that PPT is a distinct autoimmune condition.

Clinical features and treatment

The condition may be purely biochemical. Large numbers of women who are diagnosed with it in clinical trials do not have symptoms or need treatment. The prevalence of the clinical condition is likely to be much lower, although it has not been clearly defined due to deficiencies in case ascertainment.

There are classically three phases of PPT. First, at 1–3 months postpartum there may be thyrotoxicosis; secondly, at 3–8 months, hypothyroidism; and finally usually by 1 year postpartum the return of normal thyroid function. An individual woman may experience any one or two of these phases, or all three.

The thyrotoxic phase is due to destruction of thyroid follicles and release of preformed thyroid hormones; there is no change in rate of production of thyroid hormones. However, increased urinary iodine excretion occurs, possibly in proportion to the degree of destruction of the thyroid gland and therefore to the severity of the thyrotoxic phase [135]. It has been suggested that dietary iodine intake determines the degree of severity of the thyrotoxic phase and accounts for the dominance of the hyperthyroid phase in iodine-replete countries such as Japan and the hypothyroid phase in iodine-depleted areas such as Sweden. But these suggestions have not been substantiated, and they may be due to case ascertainment bias. There may be no clinical symptoms; if any are present they tend to be non-specific and difficult to distinguish from normal postnatal problems, namely lack of energy, irritability and nervousness; the thyroid is not usually enlarged, and there will be no eye signs. PPT hyperthyroidism can be distinguished from Graves' thyrotoxicosis by radioactive iodine or technetium uptake tests: uptake is low in PPT and raised in Graves' disease. However, if these tests are used, lactation should be suspended. The thyrotoxic phase tends to be transient, lasting up to 1 month. Treatment is rarely required, but if indicated should be aimed at symptom relief; for example, β blockade. Antithyroid medication is not appropriate, because production of thyroid hormone is not increased and therefore does not need to be suppressed.

The hypothyroid phase occurs after the thyrotoxic phase, whether the latter has been recognized or not. It is due to excessive destruction of thyroid follicles, such that sufficient production of hormone cannot be maintained. Its severity has been predicted by the amount of iodine excreted in the urine during the hyperthyroid phase; this in itself being a marker of the extent of thyroid damage [136]. Thyroglobulin is a storage protein found in the follicular spaces of the thyroid gland, which is released into the circulation when there is follicular damage. The severity of the hypothyroid phase has also been predicted by the thyroglobulin titre at 3 months postpartum, using a laboratory technique that permits its accurate assessment despite the presence of antithyroglobulin antibodies. The presence of raised thyroglobulin increased the predictive value of raised antithyroid peroxidase antibodies from 49% to 81% with a specificity of 98% [63]. The maximum concentrations of TSH occur at the same time as the peak titres of antiperoxidase antibody. The hypothyroid phase is more frequently symptomatic than the hyperthyroid phase, and consequently more likely to be diagnosed. Symptoms however, are again non-specific and thyroid dysfunction may not be considered in the differential diagnosis unless the practitioner is aware of this condition. The symptoms include poor memory, tiredness and vague malaise with aches and pains and cold intolerance; some series report the presence of goitre. Once hypothyroidism is diagnosed, the most important condition from which it should be distinguished is Hashimoto's thyroiditis, which may be identical in presentation. The only certain way to distinguish it from PPT is to withdraw treatment when the baby is 1 year old, and observe clinically and biochemically for relapse of hypothyroidism: if this occurs the diagnosis is Hashimoto's thyroiditis, if it does not PPT is confirmed. Rarely lymphocytic hypophysitis or Sheehan's syndrome may cause confusion, but these are both extremely uncommon conditions that usually have other presenting complaints.

If treatment of the hypothyroid phase of PPT is required, T4 is used, the dose being titrated against symptoms and biochemical measurements in the usual way. The hypothyroid phase is longer and more variable in its course than the hyperthyroid phase. There are three typical pictures: resolution over 3–6 months; resolution but later recurrence of permanent hypothyroidism; no resolution. Women in the second and third categories are more likely to have had a severe hypothyroid phase of PPT, previous thyroid disease (including previous PPT), an undetected hyperthyroid phase of PPT and in some series a positive family history of thyroid disease [136]. Clearly some of these features are in themselves risk factors for hypothyroidism, and this may indicate that women who are at increased risk of hypothyroidism are more prone to PPT. The risk of permanent hypothyroidism is 5% per year for women who are antibody positive

and had hypothyroid PPT, and 3% per year for women who are antibody positive but have not had PPT. Women with PPT have a 70% recurrence in future pregnancies [137] and should be monitored appropriately in their next pregnancy; they should have long-term follow-up for the development of permanent hypothyroidism [136] such as annual TSH and fT4 measurements outside pregnancy.

Postnatal depression has been associated with antiperoxidase antibodies (regardless of thyroid function) [138]. Postnatal depression has also been associated with overt postpartum thyroid dysfunction in some studies [132] but not in others [114]. These studies show a high incidence of postnatal depression in the control groups (thyroid autoantibody negative and or no thyroid dysfunction) of 20–28%, compared with 33–43% in the study groups. There is limited evidence that T4 may relieve the depressive symptoms for women in whom depression is a major feature of hypothyroidism in PPT.

Screening

Although it has been proposed that all pregnant women be screened for thyroid autoantibodies [137], this cannot currently be recommended [139]. Thyroid autoantibodies are linked with PPT. However, PPT does not have universally agreed diagnostic criteria, nor a reliable diagnostic test, and most importantly there is little evidence that early diagnosis confers benefit. Only a small proportion of antibody-positive women develop PPT, and the majority of those who do are asymptomatic.

Thyroid nodules and cancer in pregnancy

Half of all thyroid cancers occur in women of childbearing age [140], and many present as asymptomatic thyroid nodules. However, thyroid nodules are common, estimated to occur in 5% of women during their reproductive years, and only a small proportion are malignant. It is difficult to glean precise estimates of the risk of malignancy in a nodule, because most reports relate to the experience of individual units, which by necessity reflect their referral pattern and speciality; there are no prospective population-based surveys. Thus, 30–50% of pregnant women with thyroid nodules referred to otolaryngologists, head and neck surgeons and endocrinologists have thyroid cancer [140–142]. In an unselected obstetric population, 18 women with thyroid nodules were referred to obstetric medicine clinics, giving an approximate incidence of one in 2500 pregnancies; none was found to be malignant (M. de Swiet, personal communication).

In children the sex distribution of thyroid cancer is equal, but in adults women develop clinically apparent disease two to three times more frequently than men. Interestingly, age-matched postmenopausal women have only a 1.5-fold increased risk of thyroid carcinoma compared with men, and post-mortem studies show an equal incidence of occult thyroid microcarcinomas in men and women [141]. Therefore, it has frequently been postulated that this difference is consequent upon the female hormonal environment, although oestrogen and progestogen receptors are not found in these tumours [143]. It has also been suggested that one of the risk factors for thyroid cancer is pregnancy [144,145]. Kobayashi *et al.* [146] reported two women with rapidly growing papillary carcinoma presenting in early pregnancy, and postulated that hCG played a role by stimulating TSH receptors on the tumour. However, others have suggested that pregnancy itself is not a major risk factor for thyroid cancer [147], and that it does not alter the course of the disease or increase the risk of metastases. In a review of thyroid cancer diagnosed in New Mexico, Herzon *et al.* [142] found identical survival rates in women whose thyroid cancer was diagnosed in pregnancy compared with those in whom it was diagnosed outside pregnancy. Rosvoll and Winship [148] reported 22 women with residual thyroid carcinoma in whom pregnancy did not appear to influence the tumour and 38 who were disease free during pregnancy and did not develop local or distant recurrence. Hill *et al.* [149] found that 70 women with thyroid cancer who had subsequent pregnancies had the same risk of recurrence as 109 women of similar age who did not have subsequent pregnancies.

Following treatment of thyroid carcinoma with radioactive iodine, Schlumberger *et al.* [150] observed that the rate of miscarriage was higher in the first year than when treatment is with surgery alone (40% vs. 20%). However, iodine treatment did not influence the risk of subsequent stillbirth, congenital anomaly or low birthweight. But Ayala *et al.* [151] found congenital anomaly in three of six pregnancies conceived with 1 year of treatment with radioactive iodine, and one of 33 (plus two miscarriages) conceived more than a year after treatment. Both groups cautiously concluded that pregnancy should be delayed for 1 year after treatment with radioactive iodine, which seems a sensible policy.

Pregnant women with palpable thyroid nodules should have thyroid function tests performed to see if the nodule is hyperactive and an ultrasound scan of the thyroid: in general cystic nodules associated with thyrotoxicosis are unlikely to be malignant, and are due to either a multinodular goitre or a solitary toxic adenoma; they do not need further investigation regarding malignancy. Other nodules should undergo fine needle aspiration (FNA), regardless of the gestation. Imaging with radioisotopes is contraindicated during pregnancy. The FNA results usually fall into one of three categories: benign, cellular or malignant. Further management of malignant nodules depends upon how aggressive the tumour is and on the gestation at which the diagnosis is reached. In general, an experienced surgeon can perform thyroidectomy safely in the second trimester of pregnancy, and this may be the optimal time because the risk of premature labour is low; it also obviates the need for postnatal surgery, which may be undesirable because of the disruption to lactation and general care of the baby. Following surgery, suppressive doses of T4 are given, aiming to minimize TSH concentrations and thereby preventing its stimulatory effect on residual thyroid tissue or tumour. From a fetal perspective, this is safe during pregnancy as little T4 crosses the placenta, although care must be taken not to precipitate maternal thyrotoxicosis. If radioactive iodine is required, this is postponed until after delivery, and when possible until after lactation is completed; alternatively lactation could be discontinued if the clinical indication for radioactive iodine is felt to outweigh the benefits of extended breastfeeding. The length of time taken to clear radioactive iodine from breast milk is too long to allow resumption of lactation (e.g. 120–130 days after a 100-mCi ablation dose of radioactive iodine), which is not usually recommended [152].

If the FNA reveals cellular cytology and the nodule is non-functioning, there is a 25% risk of underlying malignancy [140]. Serial clinical and ultrasound assessment of nodule size should be undertaken, with a view to operating in pregnancy if there is an increase in size. Some suggest the use of suppressive doses of T4 whilst awaiting surgery [140]. If surgery is not performed in pregnancy, the FNA should be repeated after delivery. Functional, non-malignant nodules may have a cellular aspirate. Although thyroid function tests may be helpful, in the absence of radioactive uptake tests, it can be difficult to determine whether a nodule is active or not. If high-dose T4 is prescribed, iatrogenic thyrotoxicosis may arise.

Pregnancy in women with previous thyroid cancer

Outside pregnancy, an increase in thyroglobulin concentration is used to detect relapse. However, in pregnancy, thyroglobulin concentration is elevated, and therefore the test is not useful. Suppressive doses of T4 should continue, and be titrated against thyroid function tests, aiming to render TSH below 0.3 mU/L. As T4 does not cross the placenta in significant amounts, even in high doses such treatment is not thought to be associated with fetal problems. Theoretically it could suppress fetal TSH production, but this has not been noted clinically. There is no evidence that pregnancy increases the risk of relapse, although the data for this are sparse [142]. Neck examination should be performed in the usual way and at the usual frequency. If relapse is suspected, surgery can either be performed in the second trimester or delayed until after delivery, depending upon the gestation at diagnosis.

References

1 Brent GA. Maternal thyroid function: interpretation of thyroid function tests in pregnancy. *Clin Obstet Gynecol* 1997; 40: 3–15.

2 Glinoer D, de Nayer P *et al.* Regulation of maternal thyroid during pregnancy. *J Clin Endocrinol Metab* 1990; 71: 276–87.

3 Liberman CS, Pino SC, Fang SL, Braverman LE, Emerson CH. Circulating iodide concentrations during and after pregnancy. *J Clin Endocrinol Metab* 1998; 83: 3545–9.

4 Dillon JC, Milliez J. Reproductive failure in women living in iodine deficient areas of West Africa. *Br J Obstet Gynaecol* 2000; 107: 631–6.

5 Hetzel BS. Iodine deficiency disorders and their eradication. *Lancet* 1983; 2: 1126–9.

6 Pekonen F, Alfthan H, Stenman U-H, Ylikorkala O. Human chorionic gonadotrophin and thyroid function in early human pregnancy: circadian variation and evidence for intrinsic thyrotropic activity of HCG. *J Clin Endocrinol Metab* 1988; 66: 853–6.

7 Yoshimua M, Hershman JM. Thyrotropic action of human chorionic gonadotrophin. *Thyroid* 1999; 5: 425–37.

8 Rodien P, Bremont C *et al.* Familial gestational hyperthyroidism caused by a mutant thyrotropin receptor hypersensitive to human chorionic gonadotrophin. *N Engl J Med* 1998; 339: 1823–6.

9 Hidal JT, Kalan MM. Characteristics of thyroxine-5′-deiodination in cultured human placental cells: regulation by iodothyronines. *J Clin Invest* 1985; 76: 947–55.

10 Santini F, Chiovato L *et al.* Serum iodothyronines in the human fetus and the newborn: evidence for an important role of placenta in fetal thyroid hormone homeostasis. *J Clin Endocrinol Metab* 1999; 84: 493–8.

11 Koopdonk-Kool JM, de Vijlder JJM *et al.* Type II and type III deiodinase activity in human placenta as a function of gestational age. *J Clin Endocrinol Metab* 1996; 81: 2154–8.

12 Kotarba DD, Garner P, Perkins SL. Changes in serum free thyroxine, free tri-iodothyronine and thyroid stimulating hormone reference intervals in normal term pregnancy. *J Obstet Gynecol* 1995; 15: 5–8.

13 Rodin A, Mashiter G *et al.* Thyroid function in normal pregnancy. *J Obstet Gynaecol* 1989; 10: 89–94.

14 Ekins R. Roles of thyroxine binding proteins and maternal thyroid hormones in fetal development. *Lancet* 1985: 1129–32.

15 Yale S, Span P, Sharon T, Seer T, Ben-cheroot A. The regulatory role of triiodothyronine and thyroid stimulating hormone on the production of fetal alpha-fetoprotein. *Proc Soc Gynecol Invest* 1992; 25: 121.

16 Mengreli C, Sarafidou E, Petmezaki S, Pantelakis S. Alpha fetoprotein in congenital hypothyroidism. *Biol Neonate* 1990; 58: 326–33.

17 Ben-Neriah Z, Yale S, Zelikoviz B, Bach G. Increased maternal serum alpha fetoprotein in congenital hypothyroidism. *Lancet* 1991; 337: 437.

18 Haddow JE, Knight GJ, Palomaki GE, Johnson AM. Maternal serum alpha-fetoprotein in congenital hypothyroidism. *Lancet* 1991; 337: 922.

19 Cuckle H, Jones N, Kay J, Standing S. Maternal serum alpha-fetoprotein in congenital hypothyroidism. *Lancet* 1991; 337: 922.

20 Hallak M, O'Brien JE, Isada NB, Johnson MP, Drugan A, Evans MI. Maternal thyroid function does not alter maternal serum alpha fetoprotein interpretation. *J Mat Fet Med* 1997; 6: 115–17.

21 Thorpe-Beeston JG, Nicolaides KH, Felton CV, Butler J, McGregor AM. Maturation of the secretion of thyroid hormone and thyroid stimulating hormone. *N Engl J Med* 1991; 324: 532–6.

22 Wu SY, Polk DH, Klein AH, Fisher DA. The mechanism of low serum T3 in the fetus: hepatic T4 5′ monodeiodinase versus tissue sulfhydryl content—a clarification. *J Dev Physiol* 1986; 8: 43–7.

23 Huang T, Chopra IJ, Boado R, Solomon DH, Teco C. Thyroxine inner ring monodeiodinating activity in fetal tissues of the rat. *Pediatr Res* 1988; 23: 196–9.

24 Roti E, Fang SL, Green K, Emerson CH, Braverman LE. Human placenta is an active site of thyroxine and 3,3′,5-triiodothyronine tyrosil ring deiodination. *J Clin Endocrinol Metab* 1981; 53: 498–501.

25 Roti E, Gnudi A, Braverman LE. The placental transport, synthesis and metabolism of hormones and drugs which affect thyroid function. *Endocr Rev* 1983; 4: 131–49.

26 de Escobar GM, Obregon MJ, de Ona C, del Rey F. Transfer of thyroxine from the mother to the rat fetus near term: effects on brain 3,5,3′ triiodothyronine deficiency. *Endocrinology* 1988; 122: 1521–31.

27 Bernal J, Pekonen FD. Ontogenesis of nuclear 3,5,3′-triiodothyronine receptor in the human fetal brain. *Endocrinology* 1984; 11: 577–9.

28 Karmarkar MG, Prabarkaran D, Godbole MM. 5′ monodeiodinase activity in developing human cortex. *Am J Clin Nutr* 1993; 57: 291S–4S.

29 de Ona RC, de Escobar MC, Calbo RM, del Rey EF, Obregon MJ. Thyroid hormone and 5′ deiodinase in the rat fetus in late gestation. Effects of maternal hypothyroidism. *Endocrinology* 1991; 128: 422–32.

30 Contempre B, Jauniaux E, Calvo R, Jurkovic D, Campbell S, de Escobar GM. Detection of thyroid hormones in human embryonic cavities during the first trimester of pregnancy. *J Clin Endocrinol Metab* 1993; 77: 1719–22.

31 Ferreiro B, Bernal J, Goodyear CG, Branchard CL. Estimation of nuclear thyroid hormone receptor saturation in human fetal brain and lung during early gestation. *J Clin Endocrinol Metab* 1988; 67: 853–6.

32 Vulsma T, Gons MH, de Vijlder JJM. Maternal fetal transfer of thyroxine in congenital hypothyroidism due to total organification defect or thyroid agenesis. *N Engl J Med* 1989; 321: 13–16.

33 Utiger RD. Maternal hypothyroidism and fetal development. *N Engl J Med* 1999; 341: 601–2.

34 Burrow GN, Fisher DA, Larsen PR. Mechanisms of disease: maternal and fetal thyroid function. *N Engl J Med* 1994; 331: 1072–8.

35 Mortimer RH, Galligan JP, Addison RS, Roberts MS. Maternal to fetal thyroxine transmission in the human term placenta is

limited by inner ring deiodination. *J Clin Endocrinol Metab* 1996; 81: 2247–9.

36 Calvo R, Obregon MJ, del Rey FE, de Escobar GM. The rat placenta and the transfer of thyroid hormones from the mother to the fetus. Effects of maternal thyroid status. *Endocrinology* 1992; 131: 357–62.

37 Roti E, Gnudi A *et al.* Human cord blood concentrations of thyrotropin, thyroglobulin and iodothyronines after maternal administration of thyrotropin-releasing hormone. *J Clin Endocrinol Metab* 1981; 53: 813.

38 Ballard PL, Ballard RA *et al.* Plasma thyroid hormones and prolactin in premature infants and their mothers after prenatal treatment with thyrotropin releasing hormone. *Paediatr Res* 1992; 32: 673–8.

39 Theodoropoulos T, Braverman LE, Vagenakis AG. Thyrotropin releasing hormone is not required for thyrotropin secretion in the perinatal rat. *J Clin Invest* 1979; 63: 588.

40 ACTOBAT. Study group Australian collaborative trial of antenatal thyrotropin releasing hormone (ACTOBAT) for prevention of neonatal respiratory disease. *Lancet* 1995; 345: 877–82.

41 Kopp P, van Sande J *et al.* Brief report: congenital hyperthyroidism caused by a mutation in the thyrotropin receptor gene. *N Engl J Med* 1995; 332: 150–4.

42 Gruters A, Schoneberg T *et al.* Severe congenital hyperthyroidism caused by a germ-line neomutation in the extracellular portion of the thyrotropin receptor. *J Clin Endocrinol Metab* 1998; 83: 1431–6.

43 Sunthornthepvarakul T, Gottschalk ME, Hayashi Y, Refetoff S. Brief report: resistance to thyrotropin caused by mutations in the thyrotropin-receptor gene. *N Engl J Med* 1995; 332: 155–60.

44 Weiss RE, Refetoff S. Treatment of resistance to thyroid hormone—primum non nocere. *J Clin Endocrinol Metab* 1999; 84: 401–4.

45 Brucker-Davis F, Skarulis MC *et al.* Genetic and clinical features of 42 kindreds with resistance to thyroid hormone. The National Institutes of Health prospective study. *Ann Intern Med* 1995; 123: 573–83.

46 Rajanayagam CAO, Collingwood TN *et al.* Prenatal diagnosis of thyroid hormone resistance. *J Clin Endocrinol Metab* 1999; 84: 405–10.

47 Hetzel BS. Iodine deficiency and fetal brain damage. *N Engl J Med* 1994; 331: 1770–1.

48 Cao XY, Jiang XM *et al.* Timing of vulnerability of the brain to iodine deficiency in endemic cretinism. *N Engl J Med* 1994; 331: 1739–44.

49 Pharoah PO, Buttfield IH, Hetzel BS. Neurologic damage to the fetus resulting from severe iodine deficiency during pregnancy. *Lancet* 1971; I: 308–10.

50 Tonglet R, Bourdoux P, Minga T, Ermans AM. Efficacy of low oral doses of iodized oil in the control of iodine deficiency in Zaire. *N Engl Med* 1992; 326: 236–41.

51 Potter JD, McMichael AJ, Hetzel BS. Iodinization and thyroid status in relation to stillbirths and congenital anomalies. *Int J Epidemiol* 1979; 8: 137–43.

52 Thilly C, Delange F, Standbury JB. Epidemiologic surveys in endemic goitre and cretinism. In: Standbury JB, Hetzel B, eds *Endemic Goitre and Cretinism.* John Wiley, New York, 1980: 157–79.

53 Theodoropoulos T, Braverman LE, Vegenakis AG. Iodine induced hypothyroidism. A potential hazard during perinatal life. *Science* 1979; 205: 502.

54 Lazarus J. Guidelines for the use of radioiodine in the management of hyperthyroidism: a summary prepared by the Radioiodine Audit Subcommittee of the Royal College of Physicians on Diabetes and Endocrinology and the Research Unit of the Royal College of Physicians. *J R Coll Phys Lond* 1995: 29: 464–69.

55 Gaitan E, Cooksey RC *et al.* Thyroid function in neonates from goitrous and nongoitrous iodine-sufficient areas. *J Clin Endocrinol Metab* 1989; 69: 359–63.

56 Freedman MD, Somberg JC. Pharmacology and pharmacokinetics of amiodarone. *J Clin Pharm* 1991; 31: 1061–9.

57 Magee LA, Downar E, Sermer M, Boulton BC, Allen LC, Koren G. Pregnancy outcome after gestational exposure to amiodarone in Canada. *Am J Obstet Gynecol* 1995; 172: 1307–11.

58 Bober SA, McGill AC, Tunbridge WMG. Thyroid function in hyperemesis gravidarum. *Acta Endocrinol* 1986; 111: 404–10.

59 Goodwin TM, Hershman JM. Hyperthyroidism due to inappropriate production of human chorionic gonadotrophin. *Clin Obstet Gynecol* 1997; 40: 32–44.

60 Hershman JM. Role of human chorionic gonadotrophin as a thyroid stimulator. *J Clin Endocrinol Metab* 1992; 74: 258–9.

61 Yoshimura M, Hershman JM, Pang XP, Berg L, Pekary AE. Activation of the thyrotropin (TSH) receptor by human chorionic gonadotrophin and luteinising hormone in Chinese hamster ovary cells expressing functional human TSH receptors. *J Clin Endocrinol Metab* 1993; 77: 1009–13.

62 Yoshimura M, Pekary AE, Pang XP. Effect of peptide nicking in the human chorionic gonadotrophin β-subunit on stimulation of recombinant human thyroid-stimulating hormone receptors. *Eur J Endocrinol* 1994; 130: 92–6.

63 Parkes AB, Black EG *et al.* Serum thyroglobulin: an early indicator of autoimmune postpartum thyroiditis. *Clin Endocrinol* 1994; 41: 9–14.

64 Kimura M, Amino N, Tamaki H. Gestational thyrotoxicosis and hyperemesis gravidarum: possible role of HCG with higher stimulating activity. *Clin Endocrinol* 1993; 38: 345–50.

65 Chowdhury TA, Tanchel BM, Jaganathan RS, Dodson PM. A toxic testicle. *Lancet* 2000; 355: 2046.

66 Burrow GN. The management of thyrotoxicosis in pregnancy. *N Engl J Med* 1985; 313: 562–5.

67 Duprez L, Parma J *et al.* Germline mutations in the thyrotropin receptor gene cause nonimmune autosomal dominant hyperthyroidism. *Nat Genet* 1994; 7: 396–401.

68 Mestman JH. Hyperthyroidism in pregnancy. *Clin Obstet Gynecol* 1997; 40: 45–64.

69 Amino N, Tanizawa O *et al.* Aggravation of thyrotoxicosis in early pregnancy and after delivery in Graves' disease. *J Clin Endocrinol Metab* 1982; 55: 395–401.

70 Kung AWC, Jones BM. A change from stimulatory to blocking antibody activity in Graves' disease during pregnancy. *J Clin Endocrinol Metab* 1998; 83: 514–8.

71 Millar LK, Wing DA, Leung AS, Koonings PP, Montoro MN, Mestman JH. Low birth weight and pre eclampsia in pregnancies complicated by hyperthyroidism. *Obstet Gynecol* 1994; 84: 946–9.

72 Michie W, Pegg CAS, Brewsher PD. Prediction of hypothyroidism after partial thyroidectomy for thyrotoxicosis. *Br Med J* 1972; I: 13–17.

73 Ratanachaiyavong S, McGregor AM. Immunosuppressive effects of antithyroid drugs. *Clin Endocrinol Metab* 1985; 14: 449–66.

74 Marchant B, Brownlie BEW, Hart DM, Horton PW, Alexander WD. The placental transfer of propylthiouracil, methimazole and carbimazole. *J Clin Endocrinol Metab* 1977; 45: 1187–93.

75 Mortimer RH, Cannell GR, Addison RS, Johnson LP, Roberts MS, Bernus I. Methimazole and propylthiouracil equally cross the perfused human term placental lobule. *J Clin Endocrinol Metab* 1997; 82: 3099–102.

76 Momotani N, Noh JY, Ishikawa N, Ito K. Effects of propylthiouracil and methimazole on fetal thyroid status in mothers with Graves' hyperthyroidism. *J Clin Endocrinol Metab* 1997; 82: 3633–6.

77 Wing DA, Millar LK, Cunnings PP, Montoro MN, Mestman JH. A comparison of propylthiouracil versus methimazole in the treatment of hyperthyroidism in pregnancy. *Am J Obstet Gynecol* 1994; 170: 90–5.

78 Magee LA, Elran E, Bull SB, Logan A, Koren G. Risks and benefits of beta-receptor blockers for pregnancy hypertension: overview of randomized trials. *Eur J Obstet Gynecol Repro Biol* 2000; 88: 15–26.

79 Davis LE, Lucas MJ, Hankins GDV, Roark ML, Cunningham FG. Thyrotoxicosis complicating pregnancy. *Am J Obstet Gynecol* 1989; 160: 63–70.

80 Singer PA. Will postpartum recurrence of Graves' hyperthyroidism become a thing of the past? *J Clin Endocrinol Metab* 1992; 75: 5a–5b.

81 Hashizume K, Ichikawa K *et al.* Administration of thyroxine in treated Graves' disease. Effects on the level of antibodies to thyroid stimulating hormone receptors and on the risk of recurrence of hyperthyroidism. *N Engl J Med* 1991; 324: 947–953.

82 Ramsay I, Kaur S, Krassas G. Thyrotoxicosis in pregnancy: results of treatment by antithyroid drugs combined with T4. *Clin Endocrinol* 1983; 18: 73–85.

83 McIver B, Rae P, Beckett G, Wilkinson E, Gold A, Toft A. Lack of effect of thyroxine in patients with Graves' hyperthyroidism who are treated with an antithyroid drug. *N Engl J Med* 1996; 334: 220–4.

84 Momotani N, Ito K, Hamada N, Ban Y, Nishikawa Y, Mimura T. Maternal hyperthyroidism and congenital malformation in the offspring. *Clin Endocrinol* 1984; 20: 695–700.

85 van Dijke CP, Heyendael RJ, de Klein MJ. Methimazole, carbimazole and congenital skin defects. *Ann Intern Med* 1987; 106: 60–1.

86 Mandel SJ, Brent GA, Larsen PR. Congenital skin defects and fetus papyraceous. *J Paediatr* 1994; 91: 559–64.

87 Kampmann JP, Johansen K, Hansen JM, Helweg J. Propylthiouracil in human milk: revision of dogma. *Lancet* 1980; 1: 736–8.

88 Low LCK, Lang J, Alexander WD. Excretion of carbimazole and propylthiouracil in breast milk. *Lancet* 1979, 1011.

89 Lamberg BA, Ikonen E *et al.* Antithyroid treatment of maternal hyperthyroidism during lactation. *Clin Endocrinol* 1984; 21: 81–7.

90 Momotani N, Yamashita R, Yoshimoto M, Noh J, Ishikawa N, Ito K. Recovery from foetal hypothyroidism. evidence for the safety of breastfeeding while taking propylthiouracil. *Clin Endocrinol* 1989; 31: 591–5.

91 Momotani N, Noh J, Oyanagi H, Ishikawa N, Ito K. Antithyroid drug therapy for Graves' disease during pregnancy. Optimal regime for fetal thyroid status. *N Engl J Med* 1986; 315: 24–8.

92 Cheron RG, Kaplan MM, Larsen PR, Selenkow HA, Crigler JF. Neonatal thyroid function after propylthiouracil therapy for maternal Grave's disease. *N Engl J Med* 1981; 304: 525–8.

93 Mandel SJ, Brent GA, Larsen PR. Review of antithyroid drug use in pregnancy and report of a case of aplasia cutis. *Thyroid* 1994; 4: 129–33.

94 Heckel S, Favre R, Schleinger JL, Soskin P. Diagnosis and successful in utero treatment of a fetal goitrous hyperthyroidism caused by maternal Graves' disease. *Fet Diagn Ther* 1997; 12: 54–8.

95 Luton D, Fried D *et al.* Assessment of fetal thyroid function by colored Doppler echography. *Fetal Diagn Ther* 1997; 12: 24–7.

96 Laurberg P, Nygaard B, Glinoer D, Grussendorf M, Orgiazzi J. Guidelines for TSH receptor antibody measurement in pregnancy: results of an evidence based symposium organised by the European Thyroid Association. *Eur J Endocrinol* 1998; 139: 584–6.

97 Nelson-Piercy C, Peek MJ, de Swiet M. Obstetric physicians. are they needed? The workload of a medical complications in pregnancy clinic. *J R Coll Physicians Lond* 1996; 30: 150–4.

98 Niswander KR, Gordon M. *Women and Their Pregnancies.* W.B. Saunders, Philadelphia, 1972: 246.

99 Klein RZ, Haddow JE *et al.* Prevalence of thyroid deficiency in pregnant women. *Clin Endocrinol* 1991; 35: 41–6.

100 de Zegher F, Pernasetti F, Vanhole C, Devlieger H, van den Berghe G, Martial JA. The prenatal role of thyroid hormone evidenced by fetomaternal pit-1 deficiency. *J Clin Endocrinol Metab* 1995; 80: 3127–30.

101 Jones WS, Man EB. Thyroid function in human pregnancy. VI. Premature deliveries and reproduction failure of pregnant women with low butanol extractable iodines. *Am J Obstet Gynecol* 1969; 104: 909–14.

102 Leung AS, Millar LK, Koonings PP, Montoro M, Mestman JH. Perinatal outcome in hypothyroid pregnancies. *Obstet Gynecol* 1993; 81: 349–53.

103 Greenman GW, Gabrielson MO, Flanders JH, Wessel MA. Thyroid dysfunction in pregnancy. Fetal loss and follow up evaluation of surviving infants. *N Engl J Med* 1962; 267: 426–31.

104 Clifford K, Rai R, Watson H, Regan L. An informative protocol for the investigation of recurrent miscarriage: preliminary experience of 500 consecutive cases. *Hum Reprod* 1994; 9: 1328–32.

105 Lejeune B, Grun JP, de Nayer G, Glinoer D. Antithyroid antibodies underlying thyroid abnormalities and miscarriage or pregnancy induced hypertension. *Br J Obstet Gynaecol* 1993; 100: 669–72.

106 Nappi RG, Di Naro E, D'Aries AP, Nappi L. Natural pregnancy in hypothyroid woman complicated by spontaneous ovarian hyperstimulation syndrome. *Am J Obstet Gynecol* 1998; 178: 610–11.

107 Hall R, Richards CJ, Lazarus JH. The thyroid and pregnancy. *Br J Obstet Gynaecol* 1993; 100: 512–15.

108 Mandel SJ, Larsen PR, Seely EW, Brent GA. Increased need for thyroxine during women with primary hypothyroidism. *N Engl J Med* 1990; 323: 91–6.

109 Girling JC, de Swiet M. Thyroxine dosage during pregnancy in women with primary hypothyroidism. *Br J Obstet Gynaecol* 1992; 99: 368–70.

110 Man EB, Holden RH, Jones WS. Thyroid function in human pregnancy VII Development and retardation of 4-year-old progeny of euthyroid and hypothyroxinaemic women. *Am J Obstet Gynecol* 1971; 109: 12–19.

111 Man EB, Jones WS, Holden RH, Mellits ED. Thyroid function in human pregnancy. VIII. Retardation of progeny aged 7 years; relations to maternal age and maternal thyroid function. *Am J Obstet Gynecol* 1971; 111: 905–16.

112 Man EB, Serunian SA. Thyroid function in human pregnancy. IX. Development or retardation of 7-year-old progeny of hypothyroxinaemic women. *Am J Obstet Gynecol* 1976; 125: 949–57.

113 Evans IM, Sinha AK, Pickard MR, Edwards PR, Leonard AJ. Maternal hypothyroxinaemia disrupts neurotransmitter

metabolic enzymes in developing brain. *J Endocrinol* 1999; 161: 273–9.

114 Pop VJM, de Rooy HAM, van der Heide D, van Son MM, Komproe IH. Microsomal antibodies during gestation in relation to postpartum thyroid dysfunction and depression. *Acta Endocrinol* 1993; 129: 26–30.

115 Haddow JE, Palomaki GE *et al*. Maternal thyroid deficiency during pregnancy and subsequent neuropsychological development of the child. *N Engl J Med* 1999; 341: 549–555.

116 Fisher D. Fetal thyroid function. Diagnosis and management of fetal thyroid disorders. *Clin Obstet Gynecol* 1997; 40: 25.

117 Brown RS, Bellisario RL *et al*. Incidence of transient congenital hypothyroidism due to maternal thyrotropin receptor-blocking antibodies in over one million babies. *J Clin Endocrinol Metab* 1996, 81: 1147–51.

118 Kohn LD, Suzuki K *et al*. Characterization of monoclonal thyroid-stimulating and thyrotropin binding-inhibiting autoantibodies from a Hashimoto's patient whose children had intrauterine and neonatal thyroid disease. *J Clin Endocrinol Metab* 1997; 82: 3998–4009.

119 Adamson SJ, Alessandri LM, Badawi N, Burton PR, Pemberton PJ. Predictors of neonatal encephalopathy in full term infants. *Br Med J* 1995; 311: 598–602.

120 Badawi N, Kurinczuk JJ, Keogh JM. Antepartum risk factors for newborn encephalopathy: the Western Australia case control study. *Br Med J* 1998; 317: 1549–53.

121 Girling JC, de Swiet M. Predictors of neonatal encephalopathy in full term infants. More information needed about possible role of thyroxine. *Br Med J* 1996; 312: 580.

122 Badawi N, Kurinczuk JJ *et al*. Maternal thyroid disease: a risk factor for newborn encephalopathy in term infants. *Br J Obstet Gynaecol* 2000; 107: 798–801.

123 Girling JC, de Swiet M. Maternal thyroid disease: a risk factor for newborn encephalopathy. *Br J Obstet Gynaecol* 2001; 108: 769–70.

124 Freeman R, Rosen H, Thysem B. Incidence of thyroid dysfunction in an unselected postpartum population. *Arch Intern Med* 1986; 146: 1361–4.

125 Fung HYM, Kologlu M *et al*. Post partum thyroid dysfunction in Mid Glamorgan. *Br Med J* 1988; 296: 241–4.

126 Evans SME. The heartsink patient. *Br Med J* 2000; 320: 1513.

127 Alvarez-Marfany M, Roman SH *et al*. Long term prospective study of postpartum thyroid dysfunction in women with insulin dependent diabetes mellitus. *J Clin Endocrinol Metab* 1994; 79: 10–16.

128 Gerstein HC. Incidence of postpartum thyroid dysfunction in patients with type 1 diabetes. *Ann Intern Med* 1993; 118: 419–23.

129 Walfish JG, Meyerson J, Provias JP, Vargas MT, Papsin FR. Prevalence and characteristics of postpartum thyroid dysfunction: results of a survey from Toronto, Canada. *J Endocrinol Invest* 1992; 15: 265–72.

130 Feldt-Rasmussen U, Hoier-Madsen M, Rasmussen NG, Hegedus L, Hornnes P. Antithyroid peroxidase antibodies during pregnancy and postpartum. Relation to postpartum thyroiditis. *Autoimmunity* 1990; 6: 211–14.

131 Solomon BL, Fein HG, Smallridge RC. Usefulness of antimicrosomal antibody titres in the diagnosis and treatment of postpartum thyroiditis. *J Family Pract* 1993; 36: 177–82.

132 Pop VJM, de Rooy HAM, Vader HL. Postpartum thyroid dysfunction and depression in an unselected population. *N Engl J Med* 1991; 324: 1815–16.

133 Hayslip CC, Fein HG, O'Donnell VM, Friedisen DS, Klein TA, Smallridge RC. The value of serum antimicrosomal antibody

134 Mizukami Y, Michigishi T, Nonomura A. Postpartum thyroiditis. A clinical, histologic and immunopathologic study of 15 cases. *Am J Clin Pathol* 1993; 100: 200–5.

135 Jansson R, Safwenberg J, Dahlberg PA. Influence of the HLA DR4 antigen and iodine status on the development of autoimmune postpartum thyroiditis. *J Clin Endocrinol Metab* 1985; 60: 168–73.

136 Othman S, Phillips DIW *et al*. A long term follow up of postpartum thyroiditis. *Clin Endocrinol* 1990; 32: 559–64.

137 Lazarus JH, Ammari F, Oretti R, Parkes AB, Richards CJ, Harris B. Clinical aspects of recurrent postpartum thyroiditis. *Br J Gen Pract* 1997; 47: 305–8.

138 Harris B, Othman S *et al*. Association between postpartum thyroid dysfunction and thyroid antibodies and depression. *Br Med J* 1992; 305: 152–6.

139 Ball S. Antenatal screening of thyroid autoantibodies. *Lancet* 1996; 348: 906–7.

140 Rosen IB, Korman M, Walfish PG. Thyroid nodular disease in pregnancy: current diagnosis and management. *Clin Obstet Gynecol* 1997; 40: 81–9.

141 Doherty CM, Shindo ML, Rice DH, Montero M, Mestman JH. Management of thyroid nodules during pregnancy. *Laryngoscope* 1995; 105: 251–5.

142 Herzon FS, Morris DM, Segal MN, Raunch G, Parnell T. Coexistent thyroid cancer and pregnancy. *Arch Otolaryngol Head Neck Surg* 1994; 120: 1191–3.

143 Jacklic B, Rushin J, Ghosh B. Estrogen and progesterone receptors in thyroid lesions. *Ann Surg Oncol* 1995; 2: 429–34.

144 Preston-Martin S, Bernstein I, Pike MC, Maldonado AA, Henderson BE. Thyroid cancer amongst young women related to prior thyroid disease and pregnancy history. *Br J Cancer* 1987; 55: 191–5.

145 Galanti M, Lam M *et al*. Risk of thyroid cancer. *Can Causes Cont* 1995; 6: 37–44.

146 Kobayashi K, Tanaka Y, Ishiguro S, Mori T. Rapidly growing thyroid carcinoma during pregnancy. *J Surg Onc* 1994; 55: 61–4.

147 McTiernan AM, Weiss NS, Daling JR. Incidence of thyroid cancer in women in relation to previous exposure to radiation therapy and history of thyroid disease. *J Nat Cancer Inst* 1984; 73: 575–81.

148 Rosvoll RV, Winship T. Thyroid carcinoma and pregnancy. *Surg Gynecol Obstet* 1965; 121: 1039.

149 Hill CS, Clark RL, Wolf M. Effect of subsequent pregnancy on patients with thyroid carcinoma. *Surg Gynecol Obstet* 1966; 122: 1219.

150 Schlumberger M, de Vatharie F *et al*. Exposure to radioactive iodine-131 for scintigraphy or therapy does not preclude pregnancy in thyroid cancer patients. *J Nucl Med* 1996; 37: 606–12.

151 Ayala C, Navarro E, Rodriguez JR, Silva H, Venegas E, Astorga R. Conception after iodine 131 therapy for differentiated thyroid cancer. *Thyroid* 1998; 8: 1009–11.

152 Dydek GJ, Blue PW. Human breast milk excretion of iodine 131 following diagnostic and therapeutic administration to a lactating patient with Graves' disease. *J Nucl Med* 1988; 29: 407–10.

153 Chan BY, Swaminathan R. Serum thyrotrophin hormone concentration measured by sensitive assays in normal pregnancy. *Br J Obstet Gynaecol* 1988; 95: 1332–6.

154 Parker JH. Amerlex free tri-iodothyronine and free thyroxine levels in normal pregnancy. *Br J Obstet Gynaecol* 1985; 92: 1234–8.

13 Diseases of the pituitary and adrenal gland

Michael de Swiet

Pituitary gland

During pregnancy, diseases of the pituitary gland may manifest themselves either because of the associated endocrine disturbance or because a tumour arising from the pituitary gland causes local pressure; an effect that either specifically damages the optic nerve or generally causes a rise in intracerebral pressure. Secretion of one or more of the hormones produced by the gland may be increased (usually as a result of a tumour) or decreased. Because underactivity may also be due to the local pressure of a pituitary tumour or its treatment, the presentation of patients with these tumours can be very varied. Nevertheless, there are specific clinical syndromes associated with pituitary disease.

Pituitary tumours

Pituitary tumours comprise 10% of all cerebral tumours [1]. They may secrete any or a mixture of the hormones of the anterior pituitary: prolactin, growth hormone, adrenocorticotrophic hormone (ACTH), follicle-stimulating hormone (FSH), luteinizing hormone (LH) or thyroid-stimulating hormone (TSH). However, only tumours secreting the first three hormones are at all common clinically, and these will be considered in this chapter. In the past, pituitary tumours have been classified on the basis of their reactions with haematoxylin and eosin stains. Prolactin- and growth hormone-secreting tumours may be chromophobic or acidophilic; ACTH-secreting tumours are basophilic [2]. However, pituitary tumours are now classified on the basis of the hormones that they produce.

Hyperprolactinaemia

For general reviews see [2–8]. About 12% of non-pregnant women with secondary amenorrhoea during their reproductive life have the pituitary prolactinoma syndrome [9]; this proportion rises to 50% if galactorrhoea is also present [9,10]. Hyperprolactinaemia may be due to drugs that interfere with dopamine function (e.g. reserpine, methyldopa, phenothiazines), renal or liver disease, hypothyroidism, or disease of the pituitary gland itself. This may be a macroadenoma (>10 mm in diameter), which can extend beyond the pituitary fossa, or a microadenoma (<10 mm in diameter) [2]. Note that large nonfunctioning pituitary tumours can also interfere with dopamine release or transport and cause hyperprolactinaemia (stalk effect). Under these circumstances the prolactin levels are low relative to those in patients with a similar sized adenoma [11]. In the absence of any other cause, hyperprolactinaemia is usually considered to be due to pituitary disease, even if the lesion cannot be imaged [12].

The standard technique for the anatomical diagnosis of pituitary tumours used to be tomography of the pituitary fossa, with air encephalography in suspicious cases, to demonstrate upward or lateral expansion of the tumour. Computed tomography (CT), with or without contrast enhancement [13–15], markedly improved discrimination, but this in turn has been superseded by magnetic resonance imaging (MRI), which does not involve ionizing radiation and gives better definition. Using gadolinium for enhancement the sensitivity of detection of surgically proven microadenomata by MRI approaches 100% [16]. The question of radiation exposure is important because these patients often need several assessments over the years and there is a finite limit to the amount of radiation that can be given in the region of the pituitary fossa.

An alternative approach in those with doubtful or negative pituitary tomography was to consider the absolute level of prolactin. A normal level is up to 1000 mU/L

(30 ng/mL) [4]. A basal level in excess of 1500 mU/L (45 ng/mL) is suggestive of pituitary tumour, although patients with tumours may have lower levels than this [17]. It is also believed that patients with adenomata are less likely to show a further rise in prolactin when challenged with thyrotrophin-releasing hormone (TRH) or metoclopramide [18]; however, the value and specificity of these tests has been questioned and in general they were replaced first by the availability of CT and then by MRI.

THE EFFECT OF PREGNANCY ON PROLACTIN-SECRETING TUMOURS

The pituitary prolactinoma syndrome can be treated in over 80% of women by dopamine agonists such as bromocriptine [15], thus these patients frequently become pregnant. They may also become pregnant spontaneously [20]. The main problem in their management in pregnancy is that, under the influence of oestrogen stimulation, the pituitary adenoma (if present) may enlarge—threatening vision or even life. (Increase in prolactin concentration and episodes of visual loss in patients with a prolactin-secreting adenoma, while taking an oestrogen-containing contraceptive, have also been reported [21,22].)

Before bromocriptine therapy and prolactin estimations were available, it was possible to achieve pregnancy in about 80% of patients with amenorrhoea and galactorrhoea, using gonadotropin, and Gemzell [23] reported the outcome of pregnancy in 250 of 700 anovulatory women who became pregnant with pituitary stimulation. In the light of modern knowledge, it is likely that the 250 women who did succeed in becoming pregnant would have included a number with hyperprolactinaemia. In only four of these pregnancies (1.5%) were there symptoms of tumour expansion in pregnancy, and only one patient required neurosurgery. Thorner *et al.* [12] cited literature reports of 32 cases of visual field defects in patients with tumours around the pituitary fossa, and a number of unreported cases. Of the 32 cases, 29 had pituitary tumours, and the remainder had a craniopharyngioma or a meningioma. Some of these 32 cases have been reported to the manufacturers, who have given details of over 800 pregnancies achieved with the aid of bromocriptine [24]. There was evidence of pituitary tumour in 116 completed pregnancies, and amongst these are nine tumour-related complications (7.8%). Gemzell and Wang [2], on the basis of a questionnaire sent to interested doctors, suggest that the risk of tumour-related complications in pregnant patients with previously untreated microadenomata is 5.5%; however, in 56 pregnancies with previously untreated macroadenomata they

found an incidence of tumour-related complications in 37.5%. In a more recent review based on 246 pregnancies in the literature, Molitch [6] estimated that the overall risk of symptomatic tumour expansion in pregnancy is 1.6%; this increases to 4.5% if asymptomatic enlargement shown by CT scanning is taken into account. The data of Gemzell and Wang [2] suggest that patients who have macroadenomata are much more likely to suffer from expansion of their tumours in pregnancy than those who have microadenomata and this was confirmed by Molitch [6] who found that symptomatic tumour expansion occurred in 15% of such patients. However, Lamberts *et al.* [25] believe that it is not possible to predict which tumours will enlarge sufficiently in pregnancy to cause symptoms. This may possibly be related to the varied prolactin response that was found by White *et al.* [26] when they gave oestrogen (oestradiol benzoate) to women with prolactinomata. Nevertheless, the patients with the largest tumours studied by White *et al.* [26] did appear to increase their prolactin levels most when given oestrogen.

Other studies of prolactin-secreting tumours in pregnancy with minimal or zero tumour-related complications are those of Zarate *et al.* [27], Jewelwicz and Van de Wiele [28] and Hancock *et al.* [29]. In a specific study of visual field abnormalities, Kupersmith *et al.* [30] found that none of 57 women with microadenomata <1.0 cm developed abnormalities in pregnancy, whereas six of eight with macroadenomata >1.1 cm did.

The response of women with prolactin-secreting tumours in successive pregnancies can be quite varied [2], although Thorner *et al.* [12] found that, in women with visual field defects in one pregnancy, the defects increased in succeeding pregnancies.

If the risk of tumour-related complications in pregnancy is considered to be greater in those with macroadenomata than in those with microadenomata, the question arises whether they should be managed differently before they become pregnant.

First, all patients with hyperprolactinaemia who are treated with bromocriptine should be warned of the risks of tumour expansion if they become pregnant. As we have seen, these risks vary depending on whether or not there is a demonstrable tumour, and how large it is. In the past, a number of treatments have been used for the pituitary prolactinoma syndrome, including both external [12] and internal radiation with yttrium-90 [31] and surgery [32]. It was particularly advocated that 'definitive' treatment be performed before pregnancy, because of the risk of tumour complications in pregnancy. However, more recently, the consensus of opinion is that the dopamine agonist bromocriptine can be used to decrease prolactin secretion and the size of the tumour in all patients with the pituitary prolactinoma syndrome [33]. If tumour-related complications do develop in pregnancy, they can usually be treated with further bromocriptine (see below). Patients with macroadenomata should defer pregnancy until their tumours have been shown to shrink by CT or MRI scanning following bromocriptine therapy, and the risk of tumour-related complications in pregnancy is lower. Some authors including Molitch [6] have argued that patients with macroadenomata with suprasellar extension should be treated surgically before pregnancy, citing evidence that such patients who are treated are less likely to have tumour expansion in pregnancy than those treated by bromocriptine alone. The arguments against surgery in general are given below; furthermore Tan and Jacobs [34] have convincingly challenged the data that suggest that treatment with bromocriptine alone is associated with a higher risk of tumour expansion: it is not clear whether ovulation was induced by pituitary stimulation rather than bromocriptine in those patients whose tumours expanded, and also tumour size was not shown to have regressed before pregnancy was embarked on [35]. I therefore agree that bromocriptine should be used before pregnancy in all patients with prolactinomata regardless of size and that surgery should be reserved for the few cases where bromocriptine has failed to reduce tumour size.

Many would prefer to use cabergoline rather than bromocriptine to treat hyperprolactinaemia because cabergoline has fewer side-effects and only has to be given once or twice per week [36]. The manufacturers of cabergoline advise against its use in pregnancy even though there is no evidence of teratogenesis. There is now also sufficient experience of the safety of cabergoline in pregnancy to recommend continuing with this drug if it has been used before conception. If it is necessary to instigate treatment *de novo* in pregnancy it would seem sensible to use bromocriptine in the first instance because there is even greater experience with this drug.

Alternative forms of therapy, such as radiation, are unpleasant for the patient, and surgery is not always effective in treating the condition [20,37,38] or in preventing complications in pregnancy [25]; it may also result in permanent hypopituitarism [32,37,39]. Recurrence of hyperprolactinaemia may occur in 25–50% of patients at a mean follow-up time of 6 years after trans-sphenoidal microsurgery [40], although others have reported better results particularly following more extensive resection [41,42] with a 73% success rate at 10 years [43]. More recent surgical series have also reported more favourable outcomes in pregnancy [44,45].

Although external irradiation has enthusiastic advocates [46] it has been reported to cause sarcoma and damage to other intracerebral structures, i.e. loss of vision [47] and bone necrosis. There is also a 1–5% chance of developing a second brain tumour in patients treated with radiotherapy and followed up to 20 years. This is a ninefold increase in risk compared to the general population [48]. In addition external irradiation may also be ineffective in preventing tumour complications in pregnancy, particularly if the tumour is large [49].

Pituitary tumours may remit in up to 40% of patients following bromocriptine-induced pregnancy [50,51]. The larger the tumour, the less likely this is to occur.

THE EFFECT OF PROLACTIN-SECRETING TUMOURS ON PREGNANCY

The overall incidence of the specific complications of prolactin-secreting tumours in pregnancy has been considered above. The most common and clearly documented complication is a visual field defect, typically bitemporal hemianopia. Patients may also complain of headache, due presumably to raised intracerebral pressure. Very occasionally diabetes insipidus or pituitary apoplexy [52] occurs. All these complications are more likely after 30 weeks' gestation, but they have been reported in the first months of pregnancy [12,52]. They almost invariably regress after delivery.

The incidence of spontaneous abortion is between 13% and 32% of pregnancies that have been confirmed by elevated human chorionic gonadotrophin (hCG) levels [2,12,53]. This is rather higher than the 10% suggested by Lewellyn-Jones [54] possibly due to the inhibiting effect of prolactin on progesterone synthesis [55]. However, it must be remembered that the majority of these women will have been infertile before taking bromocriptine, pregnancy is more likely to be diagnosed early, and therefore there will be very few cases of abortion that are 'missed'. The incidence of abortion is also about 25% in pregnancies following clomiphene or pergonal treatment for other causes of ovulatory failure.

Kelly *et al.* [10] found a high incidence of operative delivery in their series of patients with pituitary tumour, but the indications for intervention were varied, and they, and others, have not found any specific complication of pregnancy. Assuming that there is not a miscarriage, there are no specific fetal complications.

MANAGEMENT OF PREGNANCY IN PATIENTS WITH HYPERPROLACTINAEMIA

All patients with previous hyperprolactinaemia should be followed carefully in pregnancy, because tumour expansion has occurred in some patients where there was no previous radiological abnormality [56]. Patients have usually conceived while taking bromocriptine or another dopamine agonist although some conceive with no treatment [20]. They should have been shown before pregnancy to have otherwise normal anterior pituitary function. Alternatively, the appropriate therapy for hypopituitarism with thyroxine and/or cortisone should have been started (see below). When the pregnancy is confirmed, bromocriptine should be discontinued [28] except in the unlikely event that a patient with a large pituitary tumour conceives without prior therapy. Here, I believe, the risk of tumour-related complication is so much higher (see above) that bromocriptine or cabergoline should be continued throughout pregnancy [57].

There is considerable experience in the use of bromocriptine in pregnancy, and no association with congenital abnormalities has been documented in up to 1973 pregnancies [6,24]. The long-term development of the children also appears to be normal [57]. At one time [31], bromocriptine was even continued for the first 12 weeks of pregnancy, because of the suggestion that prolactin depressed progesterone levels. In the series by Child *et al.* [31] there was no excess teratogenicity, confirming the safety of bromocriptine in early pregnancy. This experience has been repeated by Konopka *et al.* [58] who also used bromocriptine throughout 10 pregnancies. This experience is being echoed by the use of cabergoline in pregnancy [59]. I believe that this dopamine agonist should also be considered safe in pregnancy.

At least every month an experienced observer should plot the visual fields in patients with macroadenomata. With modern computerized equipment such testing is much less observer dependent and much less tedious than was the case previously. This objective documentation is helpful, although most patients know when their visual acuity or visual fields are deteriorating. In patients with microadenomata, history and clinical examination by direct confrontation are probably sufficient to exclude any expansion of the tumour. Particular note should be taken of any headaches (raised intracerebral pressure) or thirst (diabetes insipidus): these symptoms are an indication for further investigation if necessary, by CT or preferably MRI scanning. Some clinicians have followed serum prolactin levels in an attempt to monitor tumour

activity during pregnancy [60]. However, prolactin levels rise rather variably during pregnancy, and the within-patient, hour-to-hour variability is also much greater in pregnancy than in the non-pregnant state [61]. Reported values for prolactin in normal pregnancy are shown in Table 13.1. The considerable variability is evident in the large standard deviations. Also tumour expansion is not necessarily associated with a rise in prolactin level [62]. Therefore, there is little if any value in routine estimation of prolactin levels [6].

If there is evidence of tumour expansion during pregnancy, the patient should start or restart bromocriptine therapy [53]. Injectable bromocriptine has been used in patients unable to take oral therapy because of vomiting [63]. Additional treatment that may be indicated includes therapeutic abortion, early delivery, the use of dexamethasone [64] or hydrocortisone [25], and pituitary surgery [25]. Also, those centres that use yttrium-90 implants have successfully controlled tumour expansion in pregnancy in this way [31]. Whether any of these additional measures is necessary depends on the severity of the condition, and which treatment is used depends on the maturity of the fetus. Blindness in early pregnancy would be an indication for abortion, followed probably by surgery, although very severe visual field abnormalities [22,60] and pituitary apoplexy have been treated successfully surgically without interruption of the pregnancy. Deteriorating visual fields at 38 weeks' gestation could be managed by early delivery [65] since visual field defects regress after delivery [65]. Diabetes insipidus has responded to intranasal synthetic vasopressin, and it also usually regresses after delivery [53].

No special precautions are necessary in labour in the majority of cases. However, patients with macroadenomata or complications of tumour expansion should be delivered electively by forceps because of the rise in intracerebral pressure caused by maternal effort [52]. Labour itself proceeds normally, despite the possible interruption of the pathways from the hypothalamus to the posterior pituitary [10], and possible interference with oxytocin release. There should be no problem with breast-feeding [10,28] which should be encouraged; there is no evidence that breastfeeding causes pituitary tumours to enlarge. Presumably they are insensitive to the stimuli

		Pregnant				
	Non-pregnant	3 weeks	12 weeks	25 weeks	36 weeks	
μg/L	2–15	7 ± 3	20 ± 9	106 ± 39	147 ± 65	
mmol/L	0.08–6.0	0.28 ± 0.13	0.82 ± 0.38	4.25 ± 1.55	5.90 ± 2.62	
mm/L	60–450	210 ± 98	612 ± 285	3185 ± 1161	4426 ± 1962	

Table 13.1 Serum prolactin levels in 20 normal pregnancies [61] and in the non-pregnant state [214]. Data are ranges or means ± SD.

that, in normal women, cause a further rise in prolactin during the first few weeks of lactation. Certainly prolactin levels do not rise on suckling in these patients [60]. The risk of tumour expanding during lactation is likely to be considerably less than the already small risk of expansion during pregnancy [6].

Obviously bromocriptine or cabergoline should not be restarted after delivery if the patient wishes to breastfeed; and indeed care is necessary with the use of bromocriptine in the puerperium in all patients [66]. This is because of occasional reports of severe hypertension and dysrhythmia particularly in patients with known vascular disease [67]. Psychosis has also been noted. In about one-third of patients hyperprolactinaemia remits in the long term [68] and pregnancy may be one of the triggering factors inducing remission [68,69]. Symptoms and measurement of prolactin levels should therefore guide when and whether to restart bromocriptine or cabergoline after delivery.

CONTRACEPTION

Because of the remote risk of tumour expansion caused by the oestrogen component of oral contraception [22], barrier methods are theoretically preferable. In practice, many patients have used oral contraceptives without any problems. The low-dose combined preparations where progesterone may antagonize the effect of oestrogen are particularly suitable [21]. The risk of tumour expansion is greater with high-dose prolonged oestrogen treatment [70].

Prolactin deficiency

Isolated prolactin deficiency is very rare. It has been associated with failure of lactation in one family [71].

Acromegaly

In normal individuals, growth hormone secretion is inhibited by somatostatin, and stimulated by a peptide growth hormone releasing factor. Acromegaly is caused by excess secretion of growth hormone from the anterior pituitary, most commonly because of the presence of an adenoma, but possibly because of loss of hypothalamic control [72]. Some mixed tumours may secrete both growth hormone and prolactin [73], and prolactin may be elevated in patients with tumours that only produce growth hormone because of the mechanical effect causing loss of hypothalamic control.

Estimation of growth hormone in pregnancy is complicated by possible cross-reaction with human placental lactogen [74]. However, Yen *et al.* [74a] using a specific antiserum to human growth hormone showed that growth hormone levels were no different in pregnancy compared to the non-pregnant state. Nevertheless, the placenta also secretes a growth hormone and in the second half of pregnancy this is the dominant variety of growth hormone present. Because the placental secretion of growth hormone is non-pulsatile, growth hormone levels in the second half of pregnancy are steady and do not fluctuate as they do in the non-pregnant state [76]. The diagnosis of growth hormone excess is made by demonstration of elevating fasting levels, above $4\,\mu mol/L$ ($2\,ng/mL$) [15] which are not suppressed by a glucose load of $1\,g/kg$ bodyweight [72]. In the non-pregnant state measurement of insulin growth factor 1 levels correlates better with disease activity than does isolated growth hormone determinations [77] but the normal rise in insulin growth factor 1 in pregnancy precludes its use for diagnosis in pregnancy.

Before puberty and epiphyseal fusion, hypersecretion of growth hormone causes gigantism; after puberty it causes coarsening of the features, acromegaly. Acromegaly may also be associated with diabetes mellitus and hypertension; patients frequently complain of headache. The pituitary tumour, like the prolactinoma, can cause hypopituitarism by compression of other pituitary cells, visual field defects, and symptoms and signs of raised intracranial pressure.

The same forms of treatment are used as have been discussed in the treatment of prolactinomata: transsphenoidal microsurgery [78], internal and external irradiation [79] and bromocriptine [80]. In addition somatostatin analogues have been used [81], without complication when given in early pregnancy in one case [82]. The somatostatin analogue octreotide used to shrink macroadenomas before surgery has also been given inadvertently in pregnancy. There was no apparent harm to the fetus [83], despite placental transfer [84].

Patients with acromegaly whether treated or not rarely become pregnant [85]. For example, in the series of Gemzell and Wang [2] there were only three women with growth hormone or ACTH-secreting adenomata amongst 187 patients with pituitary adenoma. These three each had their tumours treated before pregnancy, which was subsequently uncomplicated. Not only are growth hormone-secreting tumours rarer than prolactinomata, but ovulation is also suppressed, either because of pressure effects on other pituitary cells or because of concomitant hyperprolactinaemia. Therefore acromegaly has been diagnosed for the first time in pregnancy on only a few occasions [86].

During pregnancy in treated patients, the tumour may expand or symptoms may recur [87]. These complications should be managed in the same way as tumour expansion in prolactinomata, with the resumption of bromocriptine therapy, irradiation or surgery.

To ensure that the mother is not hyperglycaemic, it is advisable to perform a blood sugar profile at 12 weeks' gestation or on presentation, and repeat it at 28 and 36 weeks' gestation. If the patient has more than one blood glucose in excess of 8 mmol/L, or two between 7.5 and 8 mmol/L, she should be managed as a diabetic (Chapter 11). The infants may be growth retarded [87] or macrosomic [85], possibly because of maternal hyperglycaemia. Growth hormone does not cross the placenta [88]. However, pregnancy is usually normal, producing an appropriately sized infant.

Fetal growth occurs normally even in the absence of growth hormone, either in the mother or in the fetus [89], possibly due to the presence of human placental lactogen, the 'growth hormone of pregnancy'. Those patients with isolated growth hormone deficiency also lactate normally. Indeed in a large series of 16 women with known growth hormone deficiency who had 25 pregnancies, no deleterious effects could be found with regard to the outcome of pregnancy [90].

Cushing's syndrome

Cushing's syndrome is the clinical condition caused by excess cortisol or cortisol-like substances. There are a number of causes. Cushing's syndrome has been included in the pituitary rather than the adrenal section of this chapter, because of the findings that in 80% of non-pregnant cases the primary pathology is in the pituitary gland (Cushing's disease) or possibly the hypothalamus [15]. A pituitary adenoma secretes excess ACTH which inappropriately stimulates the adrenal glands to produce glucocorticoids. ACTH production by the pituitary is in part controlled by corticotrophin-releasing hormone (CRH) itself produced in the hypothalamus. In pregnancy, levels of CRH are markedly elevated because of CRH production by the placenta [91]. An autonomous non-ACTH dependent benign or malignant tumour in the adrenal cortex is the other major cause of Cushing's syndrome. Primary pathology in the adrenal gland is considerably more common in Cushing's syndrome in pregnancy than in the non-pregnant state. In pregnancy, only 44% of cases are of pituitary origin, 56% are of adrenal origin and of these 21% (12% of all pregnant women with Cushing's syndrome) are due to adrenal cancer [92]. The reason why adrenal causes of Cushing's syndrome should be more common in pregnancy is not clear. However, pregnancy itself often mimics a mild form of hypercortisolism and it may be that the milder forms of Cushing's syndrome which are typically the

pituitary forms, pass undetected. Adrenal tumours and particularly adrenal carcinoma are much more florid and are more likely to be detected in pregnancy.

Neoplasms arising outside the hypothalamopituitary–adrenal axis and producing ACTH may also cause Cushing's syndrome, but this is very uncommon in pregnancy [93]. It has been recognized in one case of ovarian teratoma coincidental with pregnancy [94]. Treatment with corticosteroid drugs, obesity and alcoholism can also reproduce the clinical features of Cushing's syndrome.

Cushing's syndrome is exceedingly rare in pregnancy. Even amongst 187 patients with microadenomata of the pituitary in pregnancy, there were at most three ACTH-producing tumours [2] and about 100 cases of Cushing's syndrome in pregnancy have been reported in the world literature [2,92,95–97].

Because of the associated infertility, patients do not usually present with Cushing's syndrome *de novo* in pregnancy. More commonly the condition has been diagnosed before pregnancy and only partially treated, or a relapse has occurred during pregnancy [98].

Cushing's syndrome has been reported to appear in pregnancy, and then remit after delivery [99–101]; it is not clear to what extent pregnancy is a specific risk factor in the development of Cushing's syndrome [98].

The clinical features of Cushing's syndrome in women include bruising, myopathy, hypertension, plethora, oedema, hirsutism, red striae, menstrual irregularity, truncal obesity, headaches, acne, general obesity and impaired glucose tolerance. The presence of these does not necessarily indicate that the patient has Cushing's syndrome; the first three are the most powerful discriminators [102]. Some of these features occur in normal pregnancy.

The diagnosis of Cushing's syndrome in pregnancy, as in the non-pregnant state, depends on imaging and the results of biochemical tests, the choice of imaging depending on what biochemical abnormalities are found. All relevant biochemical parameters are changed in pregnancy [103,104]; the normal pregnant woman has total cortisol levels similar to those seen in Cushing's syndrome; this is partly due to the oestrogen-mediated increase in cortisol binding globulin [105], but there is also an increase in plasma free cortisol. Normal values for total and free plasma cortisols, free urinary cortisol and ACTH in pregnancy and the non-pregnant state are given in Table 13.2. Note the higher levels at 9.00 a.m. than those at midnight, i.e. diurnal variation persists despite the higher total levels of plasma cortisol. Table 13.2 also shows the normal range for 24-h urinary free cortisol in pregnancy. This is an estimate of the daily cortisol production rate. If, as is likely, there are not the facilities for

Table 13.2 Morning and evening plasma cortisol, urinary free cortisol and plasma adrenocorticotrophic hormone (ACTH) in pregnancy and the non-pregnant state. Values are mean ± SD or (range).

| | | First trimester | Second trimester | Labour‡ | | |
	Non-pregnant			Third trimester	Onset	Delivery
Total cortisol*	9.00 a.m.	324 ± 100		1029 ± 200	1490± 630	2120 ± 65
nmol/L	midnight	103 ± 76		470 ± 124		
Free cortisol*	9.00 a.m.	18 ± 9		38 ± 12		
nmol/L		midnight 6 ± 4		17 ± 5		
Urinary free cortisol*						
nmol/day		103 (13–256)		348 (229–680)		
ACTH ng/mL		(15–70)	30 (20–70)†	50 (20–120)†		

*[103].
†[104].
‡[215].

estimation of plasma free cortisol, urinary cortisol estimation should be performed, particularly in pregnancy, because of varying levels of cortisol binding globulin. Alternatively estimation of salivary glucocorticoid and aldosterone levels gives a good estimate of their free plasma concentrations [106], although note that aldosterone levels are markedly variable in pregnancy [107].

In light of the above information, the biochemical investigation of a woman with suspected Cushing's syndrome in pregnancy can be considered as follows.

Random estimations of cortisol are very variable and affected by stress. In addition total cortisol levels increase in pregnancy. Therefore arrange two 24-h urine estimations of free cortisol and confirm the completion of collection by also measuring 24-h urine creatinine (should be 0.13–0.22 mmol/kg bodyweight/day). The two figures for 24-h free cortisol should agree to within 10% [108] and if clearly elevated (Table 13.2) indicate hypercortisolism in pregnancy and not stress. If in doubt give dexamethasone 0.5 mg every 6 h for 48 h (2 mg suppression test) and collect urinary free cortisol for the last 24 h and plasma cortisol 6 h after the last dose. In normal patients these values will be <230 nmol/day and 300 nmol/L, respectively. Note that normal pregnant women do not suppress fully following dexamethasone 1 mg (Table 13.3 [95]).

If hypercortisolism is confirmed, distinguish ACTH dependency (pituitary tumour, ectopic ACTH) from ACTH independency (adrenal tumour) by the 8 mg high-dose dexamethasone suppression test. Give dexamethasone 2 mg every 6 h for 48 h. Collect 24-h urinary free cortisol and plasma cortisol as in the 2 mg dexamethasone suppression test. Suppression of these values to <230 nmol/day and 300 nmol/L indicates an ACTH-dependent cause. If there are facilities for measurement of ACTH, this will be elevated in ACTH-dependent causes. The ACTH will fall following high-dose dexamethasone in pituitary adenoma and may or may not fall in ectopic ACTH syndrome. Inferior petrosal sinus sampling for ACTH estimation following CRH has also been performed in pregnancy [109].

In the non-pregnant state the response of cortisol production to exogenous CRH has been used to distinguish between the various forms of Cushing's syndrome. Patients with pituitary tumour show a rise in cortisol (plasma or 24-h urinary) following CRH whereas those with adrenal tumour or ectopic ACTH production do not [110]. This test was still helpful in one case in pregnancy with pituitary tumour [111] despite the very high endogenous CRH levels due to placental production of CRH [91].

On the basis of biochemical tests, the diagnosis is likely to be a pituitary or adrenal tumour (more likely adrenal in pregnancy).

If an adrenal tumour is suspected the best imaging technique is MRI and this should be arranged. If MRI is unavailable, ultrasound may demonstrate the tumour. However, note that non-functioning adrenal tumours are common, 'incidentalomas', being found in 2–11% of abdominal CT studies or necropsies [112]. Therefore, the clinical and laboratory pictures should be consistent with the diagnosis. If not, unnecessary surgery may be undertaken.

If a pituitary cause is suspected, MRI scanning of the pituitary should be arranged. If a tumour is found, definitive treatment can be considered (see below). If a pituitary tumour is not found, further investigation can be postponed until after delivery. This is in contrast to the situation concerning adrenal tumour where because of the high maternal and fetal morbidity and mortality, treatment in pregnancy is essential.

Control	After dexamethasone			Table 13.3 Plasma cortisol—diurnal variation and response to dexamethasone 1 mg in normal late pregnancy. Values given are means with range in parentheses. (Data from [95].)
	8.00 a.m.	8.00 a.m.	5.00 p.m.	
Normal pregnant nmol/L	830 (560–1070)	520 (360–600)	450 (320–560)	
Non-pregnant nmol/L	(200–700)	(100–400)		

The treatments that have been employed have been best evaluated in non-pregnant patients and depend on the primary cause of the condition. For pituitary tumour, bilateral adrenalectomy entails lifelong corticosteroid therapy. Also because there is considerable morbidity associated with the procedure, and because of the subsequent possible development of ACTH-secreting pituitary adenomata (Nelson's syndrome) it is becoming less popular [15] and is now rarely used. Irradiation of the pituitary fossa is not always successful in curing the condition [15]. Therefore, pituitary microsurgery is the optimal treatment for those with pituitary-dependent Cushing's syndrome where an adenoma can be demonstrated [113,114], although the results vary from centre to centre [115]. It may be safely performed in pregnancy.

If pituitary surgery is not performed, either because the diagnosis is not certain, or because of reluctance to operate in pregnancy, and the patient needs to be treated, cyproheptadine, a serotonin antagonist that decreases ACTH activity is one alternative. Kasperlik-Zaluska *et al.* [116] reported two pregnancies in a patient after treatment with cyproheptadine. Griffith and Ross [117] have also reported a successful case following cyproheptadine therapy. Medical therapy is also possible with ketoconazole [118,119], which inhibits cortisol synthesis. Ketoconazole crosses the placenta and is likely to inhibit cortisol synthesis in the fetus further increasing the risk of neonatal collapse (see below) but this has not been a problem in the three cases described so far.

Cushing's syndrome due to adrenal tumour should be treated surgically in pregnancy. These patients invariably develop hypertension, which is often severe [92–94] leading to pulmonary oedema and death [120]. In addition there is the worry that 21% of the adrenal tumours are malignant [92]. Metastasis following resection of adrenal carcinoma may respond to the adrenal cytotoxic agent mitotane [121] but the pregnancy should be terminated first. Postoperatively the patient may become temporarily cortisone deficient and this will require hydrocortisone replacement therapy.

Although metyrapone therapy has been used successfully in pregnancy [122,123] to decrease cortisol synthesis, its use has also been associated with severe hypertension, possibly due to increased 11-deoxycorticosterone (DOC) levels [31]. Therefore, metyrapone should only be used

with considerable caution and where other forms of therapy are deemed unsuitable.

In addition the fetal outcome is not good in Cushing's syndrome, with fetal loss in 10 of 25 cases (400 per 1000), where pregnancy was not interrupted [95]. The reason for this high fetal loss rate is not known but, because there were four stillbirths, maternal hyperglycaemia may also be a factor. Certainly the fetus may be macrosomic, as in non-Cushing's diabetic pregnancy [95].

Another possible cause of fetal and neonatal mortality is suppression of the fetal hypothalamo pituitary–adrenal axis [124]. Kreines and Devaux [125] reported marked hypoplasia of the fetal zone of the adrenal cortex in two stillborn babies born to mothers with Cushing's syndrome. Although neonatal adrenal insufficiency appears to be a risk in these circumstances, it is exceptionally rare in the neonates of patients taking therapeutic steroids in pregnancy, occurring in only one of 260 cases studied by Bongiovanni and McPadden [126] (see Chapter 1). Because the elevated levels of cortisol binding globulin that are present in pregnancy limit placental transfer of cortisol, the mechanism of suppression of the fetal hypothalamopituitary–adrenal axis may be other than simple transference of glucocorticoids across the placenta.

If pregnancy does continue in the presence of Cushing's syndrome, treated or not, patients should be checked for hyperglycaemia, as in acromegaly (see above) and for hypertension. If there is any possibility of a pituitary tumour, the visual fields should be checked regularly. The newborn infant should be carefully watched for adrenal failure.

Lactation has been discouraged [116] because of: (i) the possibility of permanent galactorrhoea [95]; (ii) the justifiable concern that drugs such as cyproheptadine may be secreted in breast milk; and (iii) the unjustified concern that lactation will maintain the 'Cushingoid state of pregnancy'.

Hypopituitarism

The classical studies of Sheehan have shown that the pituitary gland is very vulnerable during pregnancy and the puerperium and that severe postpartum haemorrhage can cause permanent hypopituitarism by avascular necrosis [127,128]. The vulnerability of the anterior pituitary during pregnancy is presumably related to its two- to threefold increase in size at this time. Several hundred cases of Sheehan's syndrome have been reported, with 39 subsequent pregnancies in 19 well-documented cases reviewed by Grimes and Brooks [129]. Almost invariably it is the anterior pituitary that is affected by postpartum haemorrhage, possibly because its blood supply is via the superior hypophyseal artery, whereas the posterior pituitary and hypothalamus are supplied by the inferior hypophyseal artery and the circle of Willis [130]. Only two cases of diabetes insipidus following postpartum haemorrhage have been reported [130,131]. Hypopituitarism may follow pregnancy in which there has not been overt postpartum haemorrhage and in these patients in particular, the condition may only affect some functions of the pituitary gland [132]. Other rare causes of hypopituitarism in pregnancy are the pressure effect of pituitary tumours—adenoma (see above) or craniopharyngioma [75]—and eosinophilic granuloma, histiocytosis X or Hand–Schueller–Christian disease [133,134]. More recently, lymphocytic hypophysitis has been described affecting the anterior pituitary after delivery (see below). Occasionally no cause can be found [135].

Antepartum pituitary infarction has also been described in eight cases but only in insulin-dependent diabetics [136]. The patient develops a severe headache, usually in the third trimester, and her insulin requirements decrease markedly. She is then very liable to hypoglycaemic episodes. After delivery, she does not lactate, and has other features of hypopituitarism, most frequently lack of growth hormone and gonadotropins.

In those cases of Sheehan's syndrome presenting during the puerperium, there is usually a history of severe postpartum haemorrhage and hypotension, followed by lack of lactation. The patients rapidly become apathetic and are often thought to be depressed. Subsequently, there is persistent amenorrhoea, with loss of axillary and pubic hair, and the symptoms and signs of hypothyroidism and adrenocortical insufficiency. The diagnosis is rarely made during the puerperium, but any patient with a history of severe postpartum haemorrhage and impaired lactation should be followed for at least 1 year with this complication in mind. However, in one series, assessment of 17 women who had had severe blood loss from abruption did not show any cases of impaired pituitary function [137] 1 week after delivery. Therefore severe blood loss alone is a poor predictor of hypopituitarism at least as assessed in the puerperium.

The diagnosis of hypopituitarism is confirmed by demonstrating impaired secretion by the pituitary target organs (low thyroxine and plasma cortisol, etc.) with low levels of the pituitary hormones (TSH, ACTH, FSH, LH and growth hormone) that do not rise on provocative stimulation. The provocative tests that have been used include administration of LH- and TSH-releasing hormones (LHRH and TRH). The ability of the hypothalamo-pituitary axis to secret ACTH, growth hormone and prolactin is tested by insulin-induced hypoglycaemia. The dose of insulin is 0.1 unit/kg bodyweight, or 0.05 unit/kg if hypopituitarism is strongly suspected. Insulin hypoglycaemia is not without risk, because patients who are deficient in glucocorticoids, either because of adrenal or pituitary failure, can have very severe hypoglycaemic reactions. The test should not be performed unless an intravenous infusion has already been set up for subsequent emergency administration of glucose and hydrocortisone. Occasionally metyrapone, which is a metabolic inhibitor of cortisol synthesis, may be used to test ACTH secretion by the hypothalamopituitary axis.

Diabetes insipidus is diagnosed by demonstrating a high urine volume with low osmolality, which is maintained as the plasma osmolality increases with water deprivation. Water deprivation tests should also only be performed in controlled circumstances with a fixed limit placed on the maximum permissible weight loss. Pituitary-dependent diabetes insipidus is reversed by giving a synthetic analogue of vasopressin, DDAVP (deamino-D-arginine vasopressin); nephrogenic diabetes insipidus is not (see diabetes insipidus, below).

Because patients may have a wide spectrum of disease, with only one or all pituitary hormones affected, each aspect of pituitary function should be studied as far as possible. Any patient who is considered to have hypopituitarism should have an assessment of the visual fields, and MRI to exclude pituitary tumour.

Most patients with hypopituitarism become pregnant with the diagnosis already made; pregnancy without treatment is unusual. However, the condition can present in pregnancy for the first time even if, in retrospect, it is clear that the patient had some evidence of prior hypopituitarism [129]; this is particularly likely if the syndrome is incomplete [138,139].

Most indices of pituitary function have now been tested in pregnancy in patients with hypopituitarism. Grimes and Brooks [129] demonstrated levels of TSH that were not elevated despite subnormal thyroxine values. It is said that the pituitary is more sensitive to TRH in pregnancy than in the non-pregnant state [140]. Low ACTH levels [141], which did not rise above 20 pg/mL (normal range 10–70 pg/mL) during antepartum haemorrhage, have also been reported [129]—the assumption being that the hypothalamopituitary axis was unable to react to the stress of hypotension. It has been suggested that the response to metyrapone is blunted in pregnancy [142]. However, the outcome of the test was judged by a relative lack of increase in urinary steroids rather than the direct assay of ACTH. In early pregnancy, the cortisol and ACTH response to insulin hypoglycaemia (0.1 unit/kg) is similar to that in non-pregnant individuals [143].

In patients with hypopituitarism diagnosed and treated before pregnancy the outcome of pregnancy is good (Table 13.4). Where treatment is absent or inadequate the mother is at risk, and three fatalities have been reported [139,144].

Hypoglycaemia is of course a feature of hypopituitarism. Apart from glucocorticoid deficiency (hypopituitarism, Addison's disease) the differential diagnosis of hypoglycaemia in pregnancy includes hypothyroidism, insulinoma [145] and self-administration of insulin; thyroxine and insulin levels should be measured to exclude these conditions. Other causes of hypoglycaemia such as liver failure (acute fatty liver of pregnancy, see Chapter 9) are usually obvious. Overwhelming infection with falciparum malaria treated with quinine is a further cause of hypoglycaemia in pregnancy ([146], see Chapter 16).

For patients with anterior pituitary deficiency, replacement therapy with hydrocortisone up to 30 mg/day, and thyroxine up to 300 μg/day should be sufficient. It may be necessary to start this therapy, particularly hydrocortisone, before a precise diagnosis is made. It is unlikely to cause any harm, and may be life-saving [139]. In contrast to patients with Addison's disease, these patients usually secrete sufficient mineralocorticoid not to need fludrocortisone. Additional parenteral hydrocortisone 100 mg 6-hourly should be given to cover the acute stresses of labour and intercurrent illness. However, parenteral treatment may also be necessary in more chronic conditions, such as hyperemesis. Exogenous gonadotrophin may be necessary before pregnancy to stimulate ovulation, but once the patient is pregnant, replacement gonadotrophin, oestrogen and progesterone will not be necessary because of their production by the fetoplacental unit.

Abortion is the major fetal risk in untreated hypopituitarism (Table 13.4). Stillbirth has also been reported [147]. Lactation may also be impaired because of prolactin deficiency [129].

Lymphocytic hypophysitis

This condition is being recognized with increasing frequency in patients presenting after delivery or during pregnancy with hypopituitarism or a mass effect in the pituitary [148–150]. Occasionally patients present remote from pregnancy and then they may also have hyperprolactinaemia. The presence of autoantibodies to pituitary lactotrophs [151] suggests an autoimmune condition, although understandably few histological studies have been performed. Lymphocytic hypophysitis cannot be distinguished from adenoma by imaging [152], although it has been suggested that early contrast enhancement on MRI scanning may be helpful [153]. However, in general, prolactin levels are lower in lymphocytic hypophysitis, and subsequent spontaneous pregnancy is more likely, although ovulation induction may still be necessary [154]. Abnormalities of thyroid and adrenal function are more common and the patients are more likely to be symptomatic with headache and visual field disturbance [152]. The condition can regress spontaneously. In patients with severe symptoms, corticosteroid and surgical debulking therapies have been used but in the absence of visual field symptoms, replacement steroid therapy may be all that is necessary, awaiting spontaneous recovery [155]. Lymphocytic hypophysitis does not necessarily reoccur in subsequent pregnancies [155].

Diabetes insipidus

Diabetes insipidus may also be present in pregnancy when it can be a sign of tumour expansion—either pituitary adenoma (see above) or craniopharyngioma [75,156]. Lymphocytic hypophysitis (see above) is another possibility. It may also be caused by skull trauma that has occurred in pregnancy [157] and it may be idiopathic [157]. Any of the rare causes of hypopituitarism listed above such as histiocytosis X may also cause diabetes insipidus in pregnancy [158].

Hime and Richardson [159] have reviewed the subject and commented on 67 cases of diabetes insipidus in pregnancy in the world literature. Patients with pre-existing, isolated diabetes insipidus have no impairment of fertility

	Without therapy	With therapy
Pregnancies	24	15
Live births	13 (54)	13 (87)
Spontaneous abortion	10 (42)	2 (13)
Stillbirth	1 (4)	0
Maternal death	3 (12)	0

Table 13.4 Outcome of pregnancy in patients with Sheehan's syndrome. The figures in parenthesis are the proportions (%) of the total number of pregnancies in each case. (Data from [129].)

and the incidence of the disease in pregnancy is about the same as in the general population, i.e. one in 15 000 [159]. Hime and Richardson [159] found that, in 67 cases, 58% deteriorated in pregnancy, 20% improved, and 15% remained the same. There were inadequate data to assess the remaining 7%. A number of reasons have been put forward why diabetes insipidus should deteriorate in pregnancy; these include the increase in glomerular filtration rate (Chapter 7), the production of vasopressinase from the placenta, and the possibility that certain eicosanoids related to increased renal prostaglandin production may also antagonize vasopressin [160]. Similar reasons have been entertained to account for the phenomenon of transient diabetes insipidus, which may occur in pregnancy [161–163] or immediately postpartum [164]. Barron *et al.* [160] suggest that this is most likely to be due to resistance to vasopressin; however, some, although not all [165], of these patients undoubtedly do have excess vasopressinase [166] and there may well be other factors involved because impaired liver function has also been noted in several of these cases [99,161]; diabetes insipidus has also been seen in overt acute fatty liver of pregnancy [167,168] (see Chapter 9). Transient diabetes insipidus usually regresses within a few days of delivery. It has been suggested that patients with transient diabetes insipidus are particularly susceptible to epileptic seizures and that these seizures are resistant to treatment for eclampsia (magnesium and diazepam).

Diabetes insipidus presents with excessive thirst and polyuria. It is a very rare cause of oligohydramnios [169]. After exclusion of diabetes mellitus, diagnosis is made as above. However, to achieve maximum urine concentration, fluid deprivation is necessary for 22 h [170], which is very distressing for the patient. The synthetic analogue of vasopressin DDAVP is therefore frequently used for primary diagnosis [171]. DDAVP is not metabolized by vasopressinase and therefore the response to DDAVP is not usually altered in transient diabetes insipidus. Hutchon *et al.* [171] have compared the responses to DDAVP (20 µg intranasally) and 15-h fluid deprivation. Although the 15-h of fluid deprivation was a greater stimulus to urine concentration in the non-pregnant state, DDAVP was an equally effective stimulus in pregnancy, and these authors conclude that this should be the method of choice for diagnosis of diabetes insipidus in pregnancy. The maximum urine concentration achieved in normals was about 1000 mosmol/kg. Any value over 700 mosmol/kg in the 11 h after instillation of DDAVP should be considered normal [171].

A possible risk of DDAVP late in pregnancy for the diagnosis of diabetes insipidus is premature labour, even though it has minimal oxytocic action (see below). Van Der Wilt *et al.* [75] infused 1 µg in one patient at 36 weeks' gestation, and noted a marked increased in uterine contractility. The patient went into labour 3 days later. A further theoretical risk is that of thrombosis because DDAVP increases the levels of clotting factors, particularly Factor VIII and has been used for the therapy of acquired and congenital bleeding conditions. However, no excess cases of thrombosis have been reported to the manufacturers, nor has there been any difference in the thrombosis rate in meta-analysis of the controlled trials where DDAVP has been used to reduce bleeding [172]. No adverse fetal effects have been found in 29 infants whose mothers took DDAVP throughout pregnancy [173].

Treatment of diabetes insipidus in pregnancy should be with DDAVP [174,175]. The drug is given as intranasal drops 10–20 µg, two to three times daily. Its particular advantage in pregnancy is that it has 75 times less oxytocic action than preparations of arginine vasopressin [176]. However, Van Der Wilt *et al.* [75] did find that DDAVP caused some uterine contraction when given at 36 weeks' gestation (see above). DDAVP is also less likely to cause abdominal pain than vasopressin, which, in turn, can cause rhinitis and allergic pulmonary lesions [177]. Patients with some residual pituitary function, and those with nephrogenic diabetes insipidus, have been treated with chlorpropamide [178]. This drug increases the renal responsiveness to endogenous vasopressin, but it should not be used in pregnancy because of the risk of fetal hypoglycaemia (Chapter 11). Carbamazepine acts in a similar way [179], and is reasonably safe in pregnancy (Chapter 15).

Labour proceeds normally in patients with diabetes insipidus; breastfeeding is usually successful [75,134, 175].

Adrenal gland (see also Conn's syndrome, Chapter 6)

Addison's disease

Addison's disease is characterized by atrophy of the adrenal cortex and subsequent lack of glucocorticoid and mineralocorticoid activity. The clinical picture—of weight loss, vomiting, hypotension and weakness with hyperpigmentation due to excess ACTH secretion—is well known, although less florid cases are often not diagnosed. At one time, the commonest cause was tuberculosis, with autoimmune destruction of the adrenal gland accounting for a minority of cases. The situation is now reversed and patients may have other autoimmune conditions such as pernicious anaemia [180].

Interestingly the autoantigens in immune Addison's disease have been identified as key enzymes in steroid biosynthesis, 21-hydroxylase in patients with adult-type late-onset disease [181] and 17-hydroxylase in early-onset disease (type 1 polyendocrine autoimmunity syndrome) [182].

The most comprehensive historical account of the interaction between Addison's disease and pregnancy was given by Davis and Plotz [183]. Before hormone therapy was possible, there were 18 cases reported with a maternal mortality of 77%; when extracts of the adrenal cortex became available, there were 17 cases with a maternal mortality of 30%. Once deoxycorticosterone could be used, the mortality dropped to 11% in 34 cases. Now that we have experience of the use of full steroid replacement therapy, pregnancy should not be any risk in cases with previously diagnosed Addison's disease, and there should be no excess maternal mortality [184]. Patients are at risk from the nausea and vomiting of early pregnancy, from labour (when they will not be able to increase their output of steroids from the adrenal glands), and during the puerperium when the physiological diuresis may cause profound hypotension. All of these complications can be treated with extra parenteral hydrocortisone, and with intravenous saline if there is any question of hypovolaemia. Labour should be managed with intramuscular hydrocortisone 100 mg 6-hourly; because of the risk of hypovolaemia in the puerperium, this dose should be reduced only slowly in the first 6 days following delivery.

The only consistently recorded fetal complication is intrauterine growth restriction [185]. Baum and Chantler [128] reported one case of fetal hyperinsulinism, which they thought was due to fetal hypoglycaemia secondary to a temporary Addisonian state, caused by transplacental passage of maternal antibodies.

The diagnosis of Addison's disease in pregnancy is difficult, because so many of the features of Addison's disease may be associated with normal pregnancy (vomiting, syncope, weakness, hyperpigmentation). However, persistence of nausea and vomiting after 20 weeks' gestation and weight loss should be considered abnormal. The diagnosis will be made on the basis of high levels of endogenous ACTH and low plasma cortisol levels (see above) which do not rise 30 min after the patient is given intramuscular synacthen 0.25 mg. Fortunately, most patients with undiagnosed Addison's disease usually tolerate pregnancy well. The diagnosis is often made when they suffer Addisonian collapse after delivery [186] or following an obstetric catastrophe such as abruption [180] (see Chapter 4 for causes of collapse).

Patients who are being treated with corticosteroids for other reasons such as bronchial asthma (Chapter 1) or systemic lupus erythematosus (Chapter 8) should be managed during labour or in other crises in the same way as patients with Addison's disease. They do not require increased steroid medication for the same period after delivery; 24 h is usually sufficient.

Acute adrenal failure

This is a rare complication, not necessarily associated with Addison's disease, which is said to result from thrombosis or haemorrhage in the adrenal glands. It normally follows some obstetric catastrophe, such as eclampsia or postpartum haemorrhage. The patient presents with rigors, abdominal pain, circulatory collapse and vomiting. It is almost invariably fatal. The largest review is that of MacGillivray [187], which describes nine patients who died, all with haemorrhage of the adrenal glands. It may well be that acute adrenal failure is not a specific entity, but another manifestation of disseminated intravascular coagulation (Chapter 3).

Congenital adrenal hyperplasia

This term covers a group of inborn errors of metabolism affecting glucocorticoid and mineralocorticoid synthesis. Due to the absence or reduced levels of these hormones, the pituitary gland produces large quantities of ACTH, which stimulates the adrenal gland to produce excessive quantities of alternative steroid hormones; these have virilizing and hypertensive actions. For management and diagnostic purposes, the level of 17-hydroxyprogesterone is usually monitored. In 90% of cases there is a deficiency of 21-hydroxylase; other causes are 11-hydroxylase, 3β-hydroxysteroid dehydrogenase and 17-hydroxylase deficiencies [188]. Nevertheless, even within the group with 21-hydroxlase deficiency, there is a spectrum of disease depending on which of the many mutations is present [189].

This condition is inherited as an autosomal recessive. If a woman has had one child with congenital adrenal hyperplasia, she has a one in four chance that subsequent pregnancies will be affected. If the patient herself has the condition and her husband is a carrier (risk of one in 200 to one in 400) there is a one in two chance that her children will be affected [140]. Prenatal diagnosis has been helped by the finding that human leucocyte antigen (HLA) and complement genes are closely linked to those involved with congenital adrenal hyperplasia [190]. If the fetus has the same HLA and complement status as its previously affected sibling, it is likely that it will also have congenital adrenal hyperplasia. However, these test have been made redundant by advances in the molecular genetics of these conditions [191] and it is now possible to make a prenatal diagnosis with a battery of gene probes [192] on material obtained by chorionic villous sampling.

In addition, couples are understandably anxious to test the zygosity of the unaffected partner, if one partner has congenital adrenal hyperplasia. About 30% of heterozygotes have a gene deletion abnormality that can be detected easily, but unfortunately the remaining 70% have point mutations that arise *de novo* (about 400 have been detected [193]) and these mutations are mimicked by a 'pseudogene' that is present in normal individuals. So even if the laboratory detects the mutation it is not certain whether this is significant or not. Nevertheless, the absence of the gene deletion reduces the *a priori* risk of heterozygosity from one in 50 to one in 70 which some couples find helpful. Also the mutations can be grouped according to clinical severity [193]. The risk that late-onset congenital adrenal hyperplasia detected in the mother only in adult life would interact with any form of congenital adrenal hyperplasia mutation in the father to cause serious disease in their child is about 0.5% (A. Wedell, personal communication). This assumes that the parents are not related.

An alternative approach has been to study the levels of various adrenal steroids following corticotrophin stimulation. Peter *et al.* [194] claim that it is possible to detect all congenital adrenal hyperplasia heterozygotes by such specific steroid analysis, without examining the index case.

The diagnosis is usually made in infancy, either because of the presence of ambiguous genitalia in a female child, or because the child becomes acutely ill due to hyponatraemia. Children [195] and perhaps adults are also at risk from hypoglycaemia. Treatment is with glucocorticoids and sometimes mineralocorticoid replacement with sodium supplementation as indicated. This reduces pituitary secretion of ACTH and subsequent formation of alternative steroid hormones. In addition, reconstructive surgery may be necessary for the ambiguous female genitalia.

The occurrence of congenital adrenal hyperplasia in one child raises the possibility of prenatal diagnosis in subsequent pregnancies with a view to intrauterine treatment, not only to prevent masculinization of the genitalia of a female fetus but also because of worries about the female child's subsequent gender orientation (see below). The majority of this work has been performed in fetuses at risk for 21-hydroxylase deficiency. Antenatal diagnosis cannot be made by estimation of 17-hydroxyprogesterone and androgen levels in amniotic fluid or HLA typing of cultured amniotic cells until about 17 weeks. Earlier diagnosis is now available at about 10 weeks by chorionic villous sampling but even by this age masculinization of the genitalia of a female fetus may have occurred (differentiation at 9–16 weeks). David and Forest [196] have

therefore suggested treating all pregnancies subsequent to one in which the infant has been affected by congenital adrenal hyperplasia. Both hydrocortisone and dexamethasone have been given [196–198], the rationale being that in contrast to prednisone [198] (see Chapter 1) these steroids will cross the placenta and suppress excessive fetal ACTH production, thus removing the cause of fetal masculinization. The effectiveness of such therapy in suppressing fetal (and maternal) steroid production, although disputed [199], has been demonstrated by depression of maternal oestriol (and cortisol) levels [198]. Dexamethasone has been preferred to hydrocortisone because of its greater effect in suppressing ACTH production in adults with congenital adrenal hyperplasia [200]. Current recommendations [201,202] are to start dexamethasone 1.5 mg/day not later than the fifth week of gestation. Maternal compliance should be checked by showing depressed urinary cortisol and oestriol levels. Fetal material should be obtained as early in gestation as possible preferably by chorionic villous sampling at 8–10 weeks rather than amniocentesis at 16 weeks. Such material should be analysed for fetal sex and zygosity for 21α-hydroxylase deficiency. If these investigations suggest congenital adrenal hyperplasia and if the fetus is female, treatment should be continued until delivery to avoid possible neuroendocrine effects of excess androgens as well as late masculinization of female genitalia. Because congenital hyperplasia is less serious in the male, such treatment should be discontinued if the fetus is shown to be male or if it is not thought to be affected. In pregnancies where dexamethasone treatment is continued, amniocentesis should be performed at mid-gestation and if 17-hydroxyprogesterone and androgen levels are elevated, the dose of dexamethasone should be increased.

Extra steroid therapy, intravenous hydrocortisone 100 mg 6-hourly, will be necessary to cover the stress of labour. The fetus will require glucocorticoid therapy after delivery, not only as treatment for its presumed metabolic defect, but also because its adrenal glands will have been suppressed *in utero*. In the first 15 female affected pregnancies in which intrauterine suppressive therapy was reported, five of the girls had normal genitalia [202]. In six there was partial virilization and in the remaining four there was a marked virilization. The degrees of virilization did not appear to be related to the degree of suppression, which appeared complete even in some of the severe failures [202]. Suppression of the fetal pituitary–adrenal axis is therefore not the only factor controlling masculinization of the female fetus. Marked variability in phenotype has been demonstrated in sisters with apparently identical genotypes with regard to the 21-hydroxlase mutation [203].

This form of intrauterine therapy is still very much in its infancy, and further studies must be performed concerning the prenatal diagnosis of congenital adrenal hyperplasia and the dose, timing, route and monitoring of steroid therapy. The informed consent of the mother is particularly important in such cases [198].

EFFECT ON PREGNANCY

Management in pregnancy has been reviewed by Garner [204]. In two series [205,206] menarche was delayed by about 2 years compared to normal girls. Although the incidence of regular menstruation is related to the degree with which the condition is controlled by hormone replacement therapy, this rule is not invariable, because some patients do not menstruate, despite adequate biochemical control. The fertility of these patients is therefore reduced. Klingensmith *et al.* [205] found that of 14 patients who wished to become pregnant, six were unable to do so. Grant *et al.* [206] reported a lower proportion, four of 53 patients. However, the necessity for plastic surgery is not a bar to pregnancy. For example, Andersen *et al.* [124] studied one individual who was originally named as a boy and then, after hormone therapy and construction of an artificial vagina, had a successful pregnancy. In a study of 80 women with 21-hydroxylase deficiency, Mulaikal *et al.* [207] identified the following reasons for the low fertility rate of only 13 (16%) normal pregnancies.

1 Presence of the salt-losing variety (only one pregnancy in 40 patients and that terminated), which was associated with marked masculinization and the necessity for major plastic surgery. Despite this, the vaginal introitus was inadequate for intercourse in 35% of patients.

2 Poor compliance with endocrine therapy (25%).

3 Irregular or no menstruation (39%).

4 The majority (68%) were single.

5 Infrequent heterosexual intercourse.

Subsequent to Mulaikal's review there have been a few successful pregnancies in women with salt-losing congenital adrenal hyperplasia [208,209] and more encouraging results have been reported from elsewhere [210].

Nevertheless, it is quite clear that these patients can have serious physical and emotional difficulties preventing successful pregnancy. Both these factors may relate to the women's intrauterine exposure to sex hormones [211].

The outcome of pregnancy, where it has been reported, is shown in Table 13.5. Because there has only been a total of 38 pregnancies reported, it is difficult to be certain about the likely outcome of pregnancy in patients with congenital adrenal hyperplasia. There is no reason to believe that the steroid replacement therapy with prednisolone, hydrocortisone or fludrocortisone is teratogenic (see Chapter 1).

MANAGEMENT OF PREGNANCY

In patients who are not pregnant, the dose of steroid replacement therapy is usually based on clinical judgement, and assays of serum 17-hydroxyprogesterone and androstenedione; the aim being to achieve a level of 17-hydroxyprogesterone <10 nmol/L and normal androstenedione level, without the patient becoming Cushingoid; however, if this cannot be achieved and it may be difficult, 17-hydoxyprogesterone levels of 20–40 nmol/L are probably acceptable. An alternative that is currently being considered is bilateral adrenalectomy and adrenal replacement therapy.

During pregnancy, the level of 17-hydroxyprogesterone is unreliable as an estimate of adrenal suppression, but Klingensmith *et al.* [205] did not find it necessary to change the dose of steroid replacement, and this has also been the author's experience [212]. Others have found it necessary to increase steroid therapy particularly in patients with salt-losing disease [208]. There will also be concern that the high levels of maternal androgen in uncontrolled congenital adrenal hyperplasia will masculinize a female fetus; this did not occur in the one fetus with high maternal androgen levels reported by Lo *et al.* [208] perhaps because of aromatization of the androgens to oestrogen in the placenta and before transfer to the fetus.

Reference	Normal pregnancy	Abortion	Termination	Comments	Total
[205]	8	3	2	1 premature and spastic 1 multiple congenital abnormalities	15
[206]	4		1	1 eclampsia	6
[124]	1				1
[207]	13	1	2	79% LSCS rate	16
Totals	26	4	5	3	38

Table 13.5 Outcome of pregnancy in 38 patients with congenital adrenal hyperplasia. (LSCS; Lower Segment Caesarean Section)

It has been reported that fetal congenital adrenal hyperplasia due to the rare deficiency of desmolase may be associated with low maternal oestriol levels [213]. This was of importance when oestriol levels were still used for assessment of fetal well-being because it added to the other causes, anencephaly, sulphatase deficiency and maternal steroid therapy where low oestriol levels do not indicate fetal compromise. It may also be important for prenatal diagnosis not only of congenital adrenal hyperplasia but also of Down's syndrome where maternal serum oestriol is used as a marker for the 'at-risk' patient.

Some of these patients may be hypertensive, and can require antihypertensive therapy. Despite this, one of our patients developed postpartum eclampsia, but her lack of cooperation may also have contributed [212]. Another of our patients lost a pregnancy because of severe intrauterine growth restriction. My impression is that these are very high-risk patients.

Labour should be covered by increased and parenteral steroid medication. Our usual practice in these and all patients who may have depression of the hypothalamopituitary axis is to give intramuscular hydrocortisone 100 mg 6-hourly, while the patient is in labour. This will also contain sufficient mineralocorticoid activity if the patient is also taking fludrocortisone at other times.

There is controversy concerning the need for caesarean section in these patients; Klingensmith et al. [205] reported nine caesarean sections for disproportion, possibly due to the presence of an android pelvis caused by the masculinizing influence of abnormal hormone secretion. Grant et al. [206] reported only one caesarean section (for severe pre-eclampsia), but they only studied six pregnancies in four women. Mulaikal et al. [207] observed a 79% caesarean section rate in 16 pregnancies.

References

1 Russell DS, Rubenstein LJ. *Pathology of Tumours of the Nervous System*. Edward Arnold, London, 1971.
2 Gemzell C, Wang CF. Outcome of pregnancy in women with pituitary adenoma. *Fertil Steril* 1979; 31: 363–72.
3 Franks S. Modern management of pituitary prolactinomas. *Curr Obstet Gynaecol* 1991; 1: 84–92.
4 Jeffcoate SL. The pituitary prolactinoma syndrome and the mythology of hyperprolactinaemia. *Clin Reprod Fertil* 1982; 1: 209–17.
5 Klibanki A, Zervas NT. Diagnosis and management of hormone-secreting pituitary adenomas. *N Engl J Med* 1991; 324: 822–31.
6 Molitch ME. Pregnancy and the hyperprolactinaemic woman. *N Engl J Med* 1985; 312: 1364–9.
7 Hammond CB, Haney AF et al. The outcome of pregnancy in patients with treated and untreated prolactin-secreting pituitary tumors. *Am J Obstet Gynecol* 1983; 147: 148–57.
8 Molitch ME. Management of prolactinomas during pregnancy. *J Reprod Med* 1999; 44 (12 Suppl.): 1121–6.
9 Jeffcoate SL. Diagnosis of hyperprolactinaemia. *Lancet* 1978; ii: 1245–7.
10 Kelly WF, Doyle FH et al. Pregnancies in women with hyperprolactinaemia: clinical course and obstetrics complications of 41 pregnancies in 27 women. *Br J Obstet Gynaecol* 1979; 86: 698–705.
11 Soule SG, Jacobs HS. Prolactinomas: present day management. *Br J Obstet Gynaecol* 1995; 102: 178–81.
12 Thorner MO, Edwards CRW et al. Pregnancy in patients presenting with hyperprolactinaemia. *Br Med J* 1979; ii: 771–4.
13 Jung RT, White MC et al. CT abnormalities of the pituitary in hyperprolactinaemic women with normal or equivocal sellae radiologically. *Br Med J* 1982; 285: 1078–81.
14 McGregor AM, Scanion ME, Hall R, Hall K. Effects of bromocriptine on pituitary tumour size. *Br Med J* 1979; ii: 700–3.
15 Zervas NT, Martin JB. Management of hormone secreting pituitary adenomas. *N Engl J Med* 1980; 302: 210–14.
16 Levy A, Lightman SL. Diagnosis and management of pituitary tumours. *Br Med J* 1994; 308: 1087–91.
17 Jacobs HS, Franks S et al. Clinical and endocrine features of hyperprolactinaemic amenorrhoea. *Clin Endocrinol* 1976; 5: 439–54.
18 Cowden EA, Thomson JA et al. Tests of prolactin secretion in diagnosis of prolactinomas. *Lancet* 1979; i: 1156–8.
19 Editorial. PG-synthetase inhibition in obstetrics and after. *Lancet* 1980; ii: 185–6.
20 Ch'ng JL, Rosenstock J, Mashiter K, Joplin CF. Pregnancy in untreated hyperprolactinaemic women. *J Obstet Gynaecol* 1983; 3: 258–61.
21 Franks S. Regulation of prolactin secretion by oestrogens: physiological and pathological significance. *Clin Sci* 1983; 65: 457–62.
22 Mills RP, Harris AB, Heinfichs L, Burry KA. Pituitary tumor made symptomatic during hormone therapy and induced pregnancy. *Ann Ophthalomol* 1979; 11: 1672–6.
23 Gemzell C. Induction of ovulation in infertile women with pituitary adenoma. *Am J Obstet Gynecol* 1975; 121: 311–15.
24 Griffith RW, Turkalj I, Braun P. Pituitary tumours during pregnancy in mothers treated with bromocriptine. *Br J Clin Pharmacol* 1979; 7: 393–6.
25 Lamberts SWJ, Klijen JGM et al. The incidence of complication during pregnancy after treatment of hyperprolactinaemia with bromocriptine in patients with radiologically evident pituitary tumours. *Fertil Steril* 1979; 31: 614–19.
26 White MC, Anapliotu M et al. Heterogeneity of prolactin response to oestradiol benzoate in women with prolactinomas. *Lancet* 1981; i: 1394–6.
27 Zarate A, Canales ES et al. The effect of pregnancy and lactation on pituitary prolactin-secreting tumours. *Acta Endocrinol* 1979; 92: 407–12.
28 Jewelwiez R, Van de Wiele RL. Clinical course and outcome of pregnancy in twenty-five patients with pituitary microadenomas. *Am J Obstet Gynecol* 1980; 136: 339–43.
29 Hancock KW, Scott JS et al. Conservative management of pituitary prolactinomas: evidence of bromocriptine-induced regression. *Br J Obstet Gynaecol* 1980; 87: 523–9.
30 Kupersmith MJ, Rosenberg C, Kleinberg D. Visual loss in pregnant women with pituitary adenomas. *Ann Intern Med* 1994; 121 (7): 473–7.
31 Child DF, Cordon H, Mashiter K, Joplin GF. Pregnancy, prolactin and pituitary tumours. *Br Med J* 1975; ii: 87–9.

32 Hardy J, Baeuregard H, Robert F. Prolactin-secreting pituitary adenomas: transsphenoidal microsurgical treatment. In: Rolyn C, Harter M, eds. *Progress in Prolactin Physiology and Pathology.* Elsevier North-Holland Biomedical Press, Amsterdam, 1978: 361–70.

33 Editorial. Prolactinomas: bromocriptine rules OK? *Lancet* 1982; i: 430–1.

34 Tan SL, Jacobs HS. Management of prolactinomas. *Br J Obstet Gynaecol* 1986; 93: 1025–9.

35 Homburg R, West C *et al.* A double-blind study comparing a new non ergot, long acting doparnine agonist CV205–502 in women. *Clin Endocrinol* 1990; 32: 565–72.

36 Webster J. Dopamine agonist therapy in hyperprolactinemia. *J Reprod Med* 1999; 44 (12 Suppl.): 1105–10.

37 Franks S, Jacobs HS *et al.* Management of hyperprolactinaemic amenorrhoea. *Br J Obstet Gynaecol* 1977; 84: 241–53.

38 Shearman RP, Fraser K. Impact of the new diagnostic methods on the differential diagnosis and treatment of secondary amenorrhoea. *Lancet* 1977; i: 1195–7.

39 Werder KV, Fahlbusch R *et al.* Treatment of patients with prolactinomas. *Endocrinol Invest* 1978; 1: 47–58.

40 Serri O, Rasio E *et al.* Recurrence of hyperprolactinaernia after selective transsphenoidal adenomectomy in women with prolactinoma. *N Engl J Med* 1983; 309: 280–3.

41 Scanlon MF, Peters JR *et al.* Management of selected patients with hyperprolactinaerma by partial hypophysectomy. *Br Med J* 1985; 291: 1547–50.

42 Thomson JA, Teasdale GM *et al.* Treatment of presumed prolactinoma by transsphenoidal operation: early treatment and results. *Br Med J* 1985; 291: 1550–3.

43 Thomson JA, Davies DL, McLaren EH, Teasdale GM. Ten year follow up of microprolactinoma treated by transsphenoidal surgery. *Br Med J* 1994; 309: 1409–10.

44 Richards AM, Bullock MRR *et al.* Fertility and pregnancy after operation for a prolactinoma. *Br J Obstet Gynaecol* 1986; 93: 495–502.

45 Samann NA, Leavens ME *et al.* The effects of pregnancy on patients with hyperprolactinaemia. *Am J Obstet Gynecol* 1984; 148: 466–73.

46 Grossman A, Cohen BL *et al.* Treatment of prolactinomas with megavoltage radiotherapy. *Br Med J* 1984; 288: 1105–9.

47 Harries JR, Levene MB. Visual complications following irradiation for pituitary adenomas and craniopharyngiomas. *Radiology* 1976; 120: 167–71.

48 Brada M, Ford D *et al.* Risk of second brain tumour after conservation surgery and radiotherapy for pituitary adenoma. *Br Med J* 1992; 304: 1343–6.

49 Lamberts SWJ, Seldenlath JH, Kwa HG, Birkenhager JC. Transient bitemporal hemianopia during pregnancy after treatment of galactorrhoea–amenorrhoea syndrome with bromocriptine. *J Clin Endocrinol Metab* 1977; 44: 180–4.

50 Daya S, Shewchuk AB, Bryceland N. The effect of multiparity on intrasellar prolactinomas. *Am J Obstet Gynecol* 1984; 148: 512–15.

51 Mornex R, Hugues B. Remission of hyperprolactinemia after pregnancy. *N Engl J Med* 1991; 324: 60.

52 O'Donovan PA, O'Donovan PJ *et al.* Apoplexy in a prolactin secreting macroadenoma during early pregnancy with successful outcome. Case report. *Br J Obstet Gynaecol* 1986; 93: 389–91.

53 Bergh T, Nillius SJ, Wide L. Clinical course and outcome of pregnancies in amenorrhoeic women with hyperprolactinaemia and pituitary tumours. *Br Med J* 1978; i: 875–80.

54 Lewellyn-Jones D. *Fundamentals of Obstetrics and Gynaecology.* Faber and Faber, London, 1969: 157.

55 McNeilly AS. Prolactin and human reproduction. *Br J Hosp Med* 1974; 12: 57–62.

56 Kajtar T, Tomkin GH. Emergency hypophysectomy in pregnancy after induction of ovulation. *Br Med J* 1971; iv: 88–90.

57 De Wit W, Bennink HJTC, Gerards LJ. Prophylactic bromocriptine treatment during pregnancy in women with macroprolactinomas: report of 13 pregnancies. *Br J Obstet Gynaecol* 1984; 91: 1059–69.

58 Konopka P, Raymond JP, Merceron RE, Seneze J. Continuous administration of bromocriptine in the prevention of neurological complications in pregnant women with prolactinomas. *Am J Obstet Gynecol* 1983; 146: 935–8.

59 Jones J, Bashir T, Olney J, Wheatley T. Cabergoline treatment for a large macroprolactinoma throughout pregnancy. *Br J Obstet Gynaecol* 1997; 17: 375–6.

60 Dommerholt HBR, Assies J, Van Der Werf AJ. Growth of a prolactinoma during pregnancy. Case report and review. *Br J Obstet Gynaecol* 1981; 88: 62–70.

61 Whittaker PG, Wilcox T, Lind T. The effect of stress upon serum prolactin concentrations in pregnant and non-pregnant women. *J Obstet Gynaecol* 1982; 2: 149–52.

62 Divers WM, Yen SSC. Prolactin-producing microadenomas in pregnancy. *Obstet Gynaecol* 1983; 62: 426–9.

63 Landolt AM, Del Pozo E, Mayek J. Injectable bromocriptine to treat acute oestrogen-induced swelling of invasive prolactinoma. *Lancet* 1984; ii: 111.

64 Jewelwicz R, Zimmerman EA, Carmel PW. Conservative management of pituitary tumour during pregnancy following induction of ovulation with gonadotrophins. *Fertil Steril* 1977; 28: 35–40.

65 Thorner MO, Besser GM *et al.* Bromocriptine treatment of female infertility: report of 13 pregnancies. *Br Med J* 1975; iv: 694–7.

66 Morgans D. Bromocriptine and postpartum lactation suppression. *Br J Obstet Gynaecol* 1995; 102: 851–3.

67 Iffy L, O'Donnell J, Correia J, Hopp L. Severe cardiac dysrhythmia in patients using bromocriptine postpartum. *Am J Ther* 1998; 5 (2): 111–15.

68 Jeffcoate WJ, Pound N, Sturrock ND, Lambourne J. Long-term follow-up of patients with hyperprolactinaemia. *Clin Endocrinol Oxf* 1996; 45 (3): 299–303.

69 Badawy SZ, Marziale JC, Rosenbaum AE, Chang JK, Joy SE. The long-term effects of pregnancy and bromocriptine treatment on prolactinomas—the value of radiologic studies. *Early Pregnancy* 1997; 3 (4): 306–11.

70 Bevan JS, Sussman J *et al.* Development of an invasive macroprolactinoma: a possible consequence of prolonged oestrogen replacement. Case report. *Br J Obstet Gynaecol* 1989; 96: 1440–4.

71 Zargar AH, Massodi SR, Laway BA, Shah NA, Salahudin M. Familial puerperal alactogenesis: possibility of a genetically transmitted isolated prolactin deficiency. *Br J Obstet Gynaecol* 1997; 104: 629–31.

72 Lawrence AM, Goldfine ID, Kirstens L. Growth hormone dynamics in acromegaly. *J Clin Endocrinol Metabolism* 1970; 31: 239–47.

73 Nabarro JDN. Pituitary prolactinomas. *Clin Endocrinol* 1982; 17: 129–55.

74 Hytten FE, Lind T. *Diagnostic Indices in Pregnancy.* Documenta Geigy, Basle, 1973.

74a Yenn SSC, Samaan N, Pearson OH. Growth hormone levels in pregnancy. *J Clin Endocrinol Metab* 1967; 27: 1341–7.

75 Van Der Wilt B, Draver JIM, Eskes TAB. Diabetes insipidus in pregnancy as a first sign of a craniopharyngioma. *Eur J Obstet Gynecol Reprod Biol* 1980; 10: 269–74.

76 Eriksson L, Frankenne F *et al.* Growth hormone 24-h serum profiles during pregnancy—lack of pulsatility for the secretion of the placental variant. *Br J Obstet Gynaecol* 1989; 96: 949–53.

77 Barkan AL, Beitins R, Kelch RP. Plasma insulin-like growth factor-1/somatomedin-C in acromegaly: correlation with the degree of growth hormone hypersecretion. *J Clin Endocrinol* 1988; 67: 69–73.

78 Wilson CB, Dampsey LC. Transsphenoidal removal of 250 pituitary adenomas. *J Neurosurg* 1978; 48: 13–22.

79 Eastman RC, Corden P, Roth J. Conventional supervoltage irradiation is an effective treatment for acromegaly. *J Clin Endocrinol Metab* 1979; 48: 931–40.

80 Wass JAH, Mpult PJA *et al.* Reduction of pituitary tumour size in patients with prolactinomas and acromegaly treated with bromocriptine with or without radiotherapy. *Lancet* 1979; i: 66–9.

81 Lamberts SWJ. The role of somatostatin in the regulation of anterior pituitary hormone secretion and the use of its analogs in the treatment of human pituitary tumours. *Endocrinol Rev* 1988; 9: 417–36.

82 Landolt AM, Schmid J, Karlsson ERC, Boerlin V. Successful pregnancy in a previously infertile woman treated with SMS-201–995 for acromegaly. *N Engl J Med* 1989; 320: 671–2.

83 Mozas J, Ocon E, Lopez de la Torre M, Suarez AM, Miranda JA, Herruzo AJ. Successful pregnancy in a woman with acromegaly treated with somatostatin analog (octreotide) prior to surgical resection. *Int J Gynaecol Obstet* 1999; 65 (1): 71–3.

84 Caron P, Gerbeau C, Pradayrol L. Maternal-fetal transfer of octreotide. *N Engl J Med* 1995; 333: 601–2.

85 Fisch RO, Prem KA *et al.* Acromegaly in a gravida and her infant. *Obstet Gynaecol* 1974; 43: 861–5.

86 Yap AS, Clouston WM, Mortimer RH, Drake RF. Acromegaly first diagnosed in pregnancy: The role of bromocriptine therapy. *Am J Obstet Gynecol* 1990; 163: 477–8.

87 O'Herlihy C. Pregnancy in an acromegalic after bromocriptine therapy. *Irish J Med Sci* 1980; 149: 281–2.

88 King KC, Adam PAJ, Schwartz R, Teramo K. Human placental transfer of human growth hormone. *Pediatrics* 1971; 48: 534–9.

89 Rimoin DL, Holzman GB *et al.* Lactation in the absence of human growth hormone. *J Clin Endocrinol Metab* 1968; 28: 1183–8.

90 Curran AJ, Peacey SR, Shalet SM. Is maternal growth hormone essential for a normal pregnancy? *Eur J Endocrinol* 1998; 139 (1): 54–8.

91 Goland RS, Wardlaw SL *et al.* High levels of corticotropin-releasing hormone immunoactivity in maternal and fetal plasma during pregnancy. *J Clin Endocrinol Metab* 1986; 63: 1199–203.

92 Pickard J, Jochen AL, Sadur CN, Hofeldt FD. Cushing's syndrome in pregnancy. *Obstet Gynecol Surv* 1990; 45: 87–93.

93 Jones SE, Carr D, Hoffman J, Macaulay J, Tait P. Cushing's syndrome in pregnancy due to an adrenocorticotropin secreting islet cell tumour. *J Obstet Gynaecol* 1999; 19: 303.

94 Pricolo VE, Monchik JM *et al.* Management of Cushing's syndrome secondary to adrenal adenoma during pregnancy. *Surgery* 1990; 108: 1072–8.

95 Anderson KJ, Walters WAW. Cushing's syndrome and pregnancy. *Australian and New Zealand J Obstet Gynaecol* 1976; 14: 225–30.

96 Sheeler LR. Cushing's syndrome and pregnancy. *Endocrinol Metab Clin North Am* 1994; 23 (3): 619–27.

97 Wallace C, Toth EL, Lewanczuk RZ, Siminoski K. Pregnancy-induced Cushing's syndrome in multiple pregnancies. *J Endocrinol* 1996; 81: 15–21.

98 Semple CG, McEwan M *et al.* Recurrence of Cushing's disease in pregnancy. Case report. *Br J Obstet Gynaecol* 1985; 92: 295–8.

99 Aron DC, Schnall AM, Sheeler LIZ. Spontaneous resolution of Cushing's syndrome after pregnancy. *Am J Obstet Gynecol* 1990; 162: 472–4.

100 Calodney L, Eaton RP, Black W, Cohn F. Excerbation of Cushing's disease during pregnancy. Report of a case. *J Clin Endocrinol Metabolism* 1973; 36: 81–6.

101 Kreines K, Perin E, Saizer R. Pregnancy in Cushing's syndrome. *J Clin Endocrinol Metabolism* 1964; 24: 75.

102 Ross EJ, Linch DC. Cushing's syndrome—killing disease: discriminatory value of signs and symptoms during early diagnosis. *Lancet* 1983; ii: 646–9.

103 Galvao-Teles A, Burke CW. Cortisol levels in toxaemic and normal pregnancy. *Lancet* 1973; i: 737–40.

104 Rees LH, Lowry PJ. ACTH and related peptides. In: James FVT, Serio M, Guisli G, Martini L, eds. *Endocrine Function of the Human Adrenal Cortex.* Academic Press, London, 1978: 330.

105 Doe RP, Fernandez R, Seal US. Measurement of corticosteroid-binding globulin in man. *J Clin Endocrinol Metab* 1964; 24: 1029–39.

106 Few JD, Paintin DB, James VHT. The relation between aldosterone concentrations in plasma and saliva during pregnancy. *Br J Obstet Gynaecol* 1986; 93: 928–32.

107 Stevens Kj Paintin DB, Few JD. Aldosterone is secreted intermittently during pregnancy. *Br J Obstet Gynaecol* 1989; 96: 80–7.

108 Orth DN. Differential diagnosis of Cushing's syndrome. *N Engl J Med* 1991; 325: 957–9.

109 Pinette MG, Pan YQ, Oppenheim D, Pinette SG, Blackstone J. Bilateral inferior petrosal sinus corticotropin sampling with corticotropin-releasing hormone stimulation in a pregnant patient with Cushing's syndrome. *Am J Obstet Gynecol* 1994; 171: 563–4.

110 Editorial. CRH test in the 1990s. *Lancet* 1990; 336: 1416.

111 Ross RJ, Chew SL, Perry L, Erskine K, Medbak S, Afshar F. Diagnosis and selective cure of Cushing's disease during pregnancy by transsphenoidal surgery. *Eur J Endocrinol* 1995; 132: 722–6.

112 Nasir J, Walton C. Adrenal mass with virilisation: importance of endocrine investigation. *Br Med J* 1996; 313: 872–3.

113 Gold EM. The Cushing syndrome: Changing views of diagnosis and treatment. *Ann Intern Med* 1979; 90: 829–44.

114 Tyrell JB, Brooks RM *et al.* Cushing's disease: selective transsphenoidal resection of pituitary microadenomas. *N Engl J Med* 1978; 298: 753–8.

115 Burch W. A survey of results with transsphenoidal surgery in Cushing's disease. *N Engl J Med* 1983; 308: 103–4.

116 Kasperlik-Zaluska A, Migdalska B *et al.* Two pregnancies in a woman with Cushing's syndrome treated with cyproheptadine. Case report. *Br J Obstet Gynaecol* 1980; 87: 1171–3.

117 Griffith DN, Ross EJ. Pregnancy after cyproheptadine treatment for Cushing's disease. *N Engl J Med* 1981; 305: 893–4.

118 Prebtani APH, Donat D, Ezzat S. Worrisome striae in pregnancy. *Lancet* 2000; 355: 1692.

119 Berwerts J, Verheslt J, Maherl C, Abs R. Cushing's syndrome in pregnancy treated by ketocanozole: case report and review of the literature. *Gynecol Endocrinol* 1999; 13: 175–82.

120 Koerten JM, Morales WJ, Washington SR, Castaldo TW. Cushing's syndrome in pregnancy: a case report and literature review. *Am J Obstet Gynecol* 1986; 154: 626–8.

121 Luton JP, Cerdas S *et al*. Clinical features of adrenocortical carcinoma, prognosis factors, and the effect of mitotane therapy. *N Engl J Med* 1990; 322: 1195–201.

122 Gormley MJJ, Madden DR *et al*. Cushing's syndrome in pregnancy—treatment with metyrapone. *Clin Endocrinol* 1982; 16: 283–93.

123 Close CF, Mann MC, Watts JF, Taylor KG. ACTH-independent Cushing's syndrome in pregnancy with spontaneous resolution after delivery: control of the hypercortisolism with metyrapone. *Clin Endocrinol Oxf* 1993; 39: 375–9.

124 Andersen M, Andreasen E, Jest P, Larsen S. Successful pregnancy in a woman with severe congenital 21–hydroxylase deficiency of the salt losing type. *Pediatr Adolesc Gynecol* 1983; 1: 47–52.

125 Kreines K, Devaux WD. Neonatal adrenal insufficiency associated with maternal Cushing's syndrome. *Pediatrics* 1971; 47: 516–9.

126 Bongiovanni AM, McPadden AJ. Steroids during pregnancy and possible fetal consequences. *Fertil Steril* 1960; 11: 181–6.

127 Sheehan HL. Post partum necrosis of the anterior pituitary. *J Pathol Bacteriol* 1937; 45: 189–214.

128 Baum JD, Chantler C. Hyperinsulinaemic child of mother with Addison's disease. *Proc R Soc Med* 1968; 61: 1261–2.

129 Grimes HG, Brooks MH. Pregnancy in Sheehan's syndrome. Report of a case and review. *Obstet Gynecol Surv* 1980; 35: 481–8.

130 Bayliss PH, Milles JJ, London DR, Butt WR. Post partum cranial diabetes insipidus. *Br Med J* 1980; 280: 20.

131 Collins ML, O'Brien P, Cline A. Diabetes insipidus following obstetric shock. *Obstet Gynaecol* 1979; 53 (Suppl.): 16S–17.

132 Giustina C, Zuccato F, Salvi A, Candrina R. Pregnancy in Sheehan's syndrome corrected by adrenal replacement therapy. Case report. *Br J Obstet Gynaecol* 1985; 92: 1061–2.

133 Almeida OD, Menderson J, Kitay DZ. Hand–Schueller–Christian disease and pregnancy. *Am J Obstet Gynecol* 1984; 149: 906–7.

134 Ogburn PL, Cefalo RC, Nagel T, Okagaki T. Histiocytosis X. and pregnancy. *Obstet Gynaecol* 1981; 58: 513–51.

135 Gossain VV, Rhodes CE, Rovner DR. Pregnancy in hypothalamic hypopituitarism. *Obstet Gynaecol* 1980; 56: 762–6.

136 Dorfman SG, Dillaplain RP, Gambrell RD. Ante partum pituitary infarction. *Obstet Gynaecol* 1979; 53 (Suppl.): 12S–24.

137 Norman RJ, Joubbert SM, Mobbs CM. Effects of severe postpartum haemorrhage on puerperal pituitary function. *J Obstet Gynaecol* 1987; 7: 197–200.

138 Satterfield RG, Williamson HO. Isolated ACTH deficiency and pregnancy. *Obstet Gynaecol* 1976; 48: 693–6.

139 Smallridge RC, Corrigan DE, Thomason AM, Blue PW. Hypoglycemia in pregnancy. *Arch Intern Med* 1980; 140: 564–5.

140 Burrow GN. Pituitary, adrenal, and parathyroid disorders. In: Burrow G, Ferris TF, eds. *Medical Complications During Pregnancy*, 2nd edn. W.B. Saunders, Philadelphia, 1982, 215–34.

141 Bowers JH, Jubiz W. Pregnancy in a patient with hormone deficiency. *Arch Intern Med* 1974; 133: 312–14.

142 Beck P, Eaton Q, Young K, Upperman HS. Metyrapone response in pregnancy. *Am J Obstet Gynecol* 1968; 100: 327–30.

143 Kauppila A, Ylikorkalama O, Jarvinen PA, Haapalahti J. The function of the anterior pituitary-adrenal cortex axis in hyperemesis gravidarum. *Br J Obstet Gynaecol* 1976; 83: 11–16.

144 Israel SL, Conston AS. Unrecognised pituitary necrosis (Sheehan's syndrome). A cause of sudden death. *J Am Med Assoc* 1952; 148: 189–93.

145 Serrano-Rios M, Cifuentes J *et al*. Insulinoma in a pregnant woman. *Obstet Gynaecol* 1976; 47: 361–4.

146 White NJ, Warrell DA *et al*. Severe hypoglycaemia and hyperinsulinemia in falciparum malaria. *N Engl J Med* 1983; 309: 61–6.

147 Schneeberg NG, Perloff WH, Israel SL. Incidence of unsuspected Sheehan's syndrome. Hypopituitarism after postpartum haemorrhage and/or shock—clinical and laboratory study. *J Am Med Assoc* 1960; 172: 20–7.

148 Thodou E, Asa SL, Kontogeorgos G, Kovacs K, Horvath E, Ezzat S. Clinical case seminar: lymphocytic hypophysitis: clinicopathological findings. *J Clin Endocrinol Metab* 1995; 80: 2302–11.

149 Hashimoto K, Takao T, Makino S. Lymphocytic adenohypophysitis and lymphocytic infundibuloneurohypophysitis. *Endocr J* 1997; 44: 1–10.

150 Buckland RHB, Popham PA. Lymphocytic hypophysitis complicated by post-partum haemorrhage. *Int J Obstet Anaesth* 1998; 7: 263–6.

151 Bottazzo GF, Poulard A, Florin-Christensen A, Doniach D. Autoantibodies to prolactin-secreting cells of human pituitary. *Lancet* 1975; ii: 97–101.

152 Pressman EK, Zeidman SM, Reddy UM, Epstein JI, Brem H. Differentiating lymphocytic adenohypophysitis from pituitary adenoma in the peripartum patient. *J Reprod Med* 1995; 40: 251–9.

153 Powrie JK, Powell M, Ayers AB, Lowy C, Sonksen PH. Lymphocytic adenohypophysitis: magnetic resonance imaging features of two new cases and a review of the literature. *Clin Endocrinol Oxf* 1995; 42: 315–22.

154 Verdu LI, Martin-Caballero C, Garcia-Lopez G, Cueto MJ. Ovulation induction and normal pregnancy after panhypopituitarism due to lymphocytic hypophysitis. *Obstet Gynecol* 1998; 91 (5, Part 2): 850–2.

155 Gagneja H, Arafah B, Taylor HC. Histologically proven lymphocytic hypophysitis: spontaneous resolution and subsequent pregnancy. *Mayo Clin Proc* 1999; 74: 150–4.

156 Hiett AK, Barton JR. Diabetes insipidus associated with craniopharyngioma in pregnancy. *Obstet Gynaecol* 1990; 76: 982–4.

157 Phelan JP, Guay AT, Newman C. Diabetes insipidus in pregnancy. *Am J Obstet Gynecol* 1978; 130: 365–6.

158 DiMaggio LA, Lippes HA, Lee RV. Histiocytosis X and pregnancy. *Obstet Gynecol* 1995; 85: 806–9.

159 Hime MC, Richardson JA. Diabetes insipidus and pregnancy. A case report, incidence and review of literature. *Obstet Gynecol Surv* 1978; 33: 375–9.

160 Barron WM, Cohen LM *et al*. Transient vasopressin resistant diabetes insipidus of pregnancy. *N Engl J Med* 1984; 310: 442–4.

161 Goodman M, Sachs BP, Phillippe M, Moore T. Transient nephrogenic diabetes insipidus. *Am J Obstet Gynecol* 1984; 149: 910–12.

162 Harrower ADB, Galloway RK. Transient diabetes insipidus in pregnancy. *Br Med J* 1984; 289: 162.

163 Iwaski Y, Oiso Y *et al*. Aggravation of subclinical diabetes insipidus during pregnancy. *N Engl J Med* 1991; 324: 522–4.

164 Raziel A, Rosenberg T *et al*. Transient postpartum diabetes insipidus. *Am J Obstet Gynecol* 1991; 164: 616–18.

165 Williams DJ, Metcalfe KA, Skingle L, Stock AI, Beedham T, Monson JP. Pathophysiology of transient cranial diabetes insipidus during pregnancy. *Clin Endocrinol* 1993; 38: 595–600.

166 Doyle F, Mclachlan M. Radiological aspects of pituitary-hypothalamic disease. *Clin Endocrinol Metab* 1977; 6: 53–81.

167 Cammu IL, Velkeniers B *et al*. Idiopathic acute fatty liver of pregnancy associated with transient diabetes insipidus. Case report. *Br J Obstet Gynaecol* 1987; 94: 173–8.

168 Kennedy S, Hall PM, Seymour AE, Hague WM. Transient diabetes insipidus and acute fatty liver of pregnancy. *Br J Obstet Gynaecol* 1994; 101: 387–91.

169 Hanson RS, Powrie RO, Larson L. Diabetes insipidus in pregnancy: a treatable cause of oligohydramnios. *Obstet Gynecol* 1997; 89: 816–17.

170 Miles BE, de Paton A, Wardener HE. Maximum urine concentration. *Br Med J* 1954; ii: 901–4.

171 Hutchon DJR, Van Zijl JAWM, Campbell-Brown BM, McFayden IR. Desmopressin as a test of urinary concentrating ability in pregnancy. *J Obstet Gynaecol* 1982; 2: 206–9.

172 Mannucci PM, Lusher JM. Desmopressin thrombosis. *Lancet* 1989; ii: 675–6.

173 Kallen BA, Carlsson SS, Bengtsson BK. Diabetes insipidus and use of desmopressin (Minirin) during pregnancy. *Eur J Endocrinol* 1995; 132: 144–6.

174 Oravec D, Lichardus B. Management of diabetes insipidus in pregnancy. *Br Med J* 1972; iv: 114–15.

175 Sack J, Friedman E, Katznelson D, Frenkel Y. Long-term treatment of diabetes insipidus with a synthetic analog of vasopressin during pregnancy. *Israel J Med Sci* 1980; 16: 406–7.

176 Vavra IM, Machova A *et al*. Effects of synthetic analogue of vasopressin in animals and in patients with diabetes insipidus. *Lancet* 1968; i: 948–51.

177 Editorial. Diabetes insipidus—turning off the tap. *Br Med J* 1977; i: 1050.

178 Arduino F, Ferrar FPJ, Rodrigues J. Antidiuretic action of chlorpropamide in idiopathic diabetes insipidus. *J Clin Endocrinol Metab* 1966; 26: 1325–8.

179 Meinders AE, Cejka V, Robertson CL. The antidiuretic action of carbamazepine in man. *Clin Sci* 1974; 47: 289–99.

180 Seaward PGR, Guidozzi F, Sonnendecker EWW. Addisonian crisis in pregnancy. Case report. *Br J Obstet Gynaecol* 1989; 96: 1348–50.

181 Winqvist O, KarIsson FA, Kampe O. 21–hydroxylase, a major autoantigen in idiopathic Addison's disease. *Lancet* 1992; 339: 1559–62.

182 Krohn K, Uibo R *et al*. Identification by molecular cloning of an autoantigen associated with Addison's disease as steroid 17-hydroxylase. *Lancet* 1992; 339: 770–3.

183 Davis ME, Plotz E. Hormonal inter-relationship between maternal adrenal, placental and fetal adrenal functions. *Obstet Gynaecol* 1956; 2: 1.

184 Khunda S. Pregnancy and Addison's disease. *Obstet Gynaecol* 1972; 39: 431–4.

185 Osler M. Addison's disease and pregnancy. *Acta Endocrinol* 1962; 4: 67.

186 Brent F. Addison's disease in pregnancy. *Am J Surg* 1950; 79: 645.

187 MacGillivray I. Acute suprarenal insufficiency in pregnancy. *Br Med J* 1951; ii: 212.

188 Kaplan SA. Disorders of the adrenal cortex. *Pediatr Clin North Am* 1979; 26: 77.

189 Wedell A, Thilen A, Ritzen EM, Stengler B, Luthman H. Mutational spectrum of the steroid 21-hydroxylase gene in Sweden: implications for genetic diagnosis and association with disease manifestation. *J Clin Endocrinol Metab* 1995; 78: 1145–52.

190 Pollack MS, Levine LS, Pang S. Prenatal diagnosis of congenital adrenal hyperplasia (21-hydroxylase deficiency) by HLA typing. *Lancet* 1979; i: 1107–8.

191 White PC, New MI, Dupont B. Congenital adrenal hyperplasia. *N Engl J Med* 1987; 316: 1580–6.

192 Strachan T, Sinnott PJ *et al*. Prenatal diagnosis of congenital adrenal hyperplasia. *Lancet* 1987; ii: 1272–3.

193 Wedell A. An update on the molecular genetics of congenital adrenal hyperplasia: diagnostic and therapeutic aspects. *J Pediatr Endocrinol Metab* 1998; 11: 581–9.

194 Peter M, Sippell WG *et al*. Improved test to identify heterozygotes for congenital adrenal hyperplasia without index case examination. *Lancet* 1990; 335: 1269–99.

195 Hinde FRS, Johnstone DI. Hypoglycaemia during illness in children with congenital adrenal hyperplasia. *Br Med J* 1984; 289: 1603–4.

196 David M, Forest MG. Prenatal treatment of congenital adrenal hyperplasia resulting from 21-hydroxylase deficiency. *J Pediatr* 1984; 105: 799–803.

197 David M, Forest MG, Betuel M. Prenatal treatment of congenital adrenal hyperplasia (CAH): Further studies in mothers and CAH unaffected infants. *Pediatr Res* 1985; 19: 617.

198 Evans MI, Chrousos GP *et al*. Pharmacologic suppression of the fetal adrenal gland in utero. Attempted prevention of abnormal external genital masculinization in suspected congenital adrenal hyperplasia. *J Am Med Assoc* 1985; 253: 1015–20.

199 Charnvises S, de Fenci M, M *et al*. Adrenal steroids in maternal and cord blood after dexamethasone administration at mid-term. *J Clin Endocrinol Metab* 1985; 61: 1220–2.

200 Khalid BAK, Burke CW *et al*. Steroid replacement in Addison's disease and in subjects adrenalectomized for Cushing's disease: Comparison of various glucocorticoids. *J Clin Endocrinol Metab* 1982; 55: 551.

201 Editorial. Prenatal treatment of congenital adrenal hyperplasia. *Lancet* 1990; 335: 510–11.

202 Pang S, Pollack M, Marshall RN, Immken L. Prenatal treatment of congenital adrenal hyperplasia to 21-hydroxylase deficiency. *N Engl J Med* 1990; 322: 111–15.

203 Hughes IA. Congenital adrenal hyperplasia—a continuum of disorders. *Lancet* 1998; 352: 752–4.

204 Garner PR. Congenital adrenal hyperplasia in pregnancy. *Semin Perinatol* 1998; 22: 446–56.

205 Klingensmith GJ, Garcia SC *et al*. Glucocorticoid treatment of girls with congenital adrenal hyperplasia: Effects of height, sexual maturation and fertility. *J Pediatr* 1977; 90: 996–1004.

206 Grant D, Muram D, Dewhurst J. Menstrual and fertility patterns in patients with congenital adrenal hyperplasia. *J Adolesc Gynecol* 1983; 1: 97–103.

207 Mulaikal RM, Migeon CJ, Jock JA. Fertility rates in female patients with congenital adrenal hyperplasia due to 21-hydroxylase deficiency. *N Engl J Med* 1987; 316: 178–82.

208 Lo JC, Schwitzgebel VM *et al*. Normal female infants born of mothers with classic congenital adrenal hyperplasia due to 21-hydroxylase deficiency. *J Clin Endocrinol Metab* 1999; 84: 930–6.

209 Zacharin M. Fertility and its complications in a patient with salt losing congenital adrenal hyperplasia. *J Pediatr Endocrinol Metab* 1999; 12: 89–94.

210 Premawardhana LDKE, Hughes IA, Read GF, Scanlon MF. Longer term outcome in females with congenital adrenal hyperplasia (CAH): the Cardiff experience. *Clin Endocrinol* 1997; 46: 327–32.

211 Federman DD. Psychosexual adjustment in congenital adrenal hyperplasia. *N Engl J Med* 1987; 316: 209–11.

212 Porter RJ, de Swiet M. Pregnancy in a patient with congenital adrenal hyperplasia. *Pediatr Adolesc Gynecol* 1983; 1: 39–45.

213 Hardy MJ, Ragbeer MS, Goodwin JW. Low maternal blood oestriol levels resulting from congenital adrenal hyperplasia in a female baby. *J Obstet Gynaecol* 1984; 5: 84–6.

214 Sinha YA, Salby FW *et al*. A homologous radioimmunoassay for human prolactin. *J Clin Endocrinol Metab* 1973; 36: 509.

215 Haddad PF, Morris NF. Maternal plasma cortisol levels during labour. *J Obstet Gynaecol* 1986; 6: 158–61.

14 Bone disease, disease of the parathyroid glands and some other metabolic disorders

Barry N.J. Walters and Michael de Swiet

The association of disease of the skeletal system with pregnancy is by no means common in the Western world. Even so, there are notable changes in bone physiology, calcium and phosphate homeostasis in pregnancy. An understanding of these changes and their derangements is necessary for a full appreciation of such problems as do occur from time to time in pregnancy. The first part of this chapter is devoted to: (i) a consideration of normal physiology in the non-pregnant state; (ii) the changes seen in pregnancy; and (iii) the relevant clinical problems that may be seen. The second part of the chapter is concerned with various skeletal and inherited metabolic disorders of significance in pregnancy.

Bone structure and function

The tissue comprising the skeletal framework of the body is in a state of constant metabolic activity. Simultaneous processes of new bone formation and dissolution of older bone accomplish ongoing remodelling of individual bones in response to changing needs.

Further, bone acts as the major repository for calcium and phosphate in the body. Regulation of the plasma concentration of these ions is effected largely through changes in bone mediated by certain hormones.

Bone is composed of bone cells, protein matrix and mineral. The matrix comprises about half the bone volume, and bone cells only about 3%. Osteoblasts synthesize and mineralize bone. Osteocytes are osteoblasts incorporated in the bony matrix they have secreted. The osteoclast, probably of macrophage origin, appears as a multinucleate cell responsible for bone resorption.

After epiphyseal closure, the cellular activity of bone represents a dynamic balance between resorption and synthesis; remodelling begins when osteoblasts and osteoclasts appear at a focus on the bone's surface. The osteoclasts dissolve bone, leaving a bay (Howship's lacuna), into which the osteoblasts nestle and deposit new bone matrix, which later undergoes mineralization. This organic matrix (osteoid) is 90–95% collagen but also contains mucopolysaccharides and lipids. Mineralization is part of the function of the osteoblast and involves deposition of calcium and phosphorus as amorphous salts. Over days, these assume a more crystalline structure resembling dihydroxyapatite, $Ca_{10}(PO_4)_6(OH)_2$, the dominant mineral found in mature bone. The majority of the mineral phase is accommodated in spaces interspersed throughout the collagen fibrils.

Osteoblasts are rich in alkaline phosphatase. Its level rises in the blood when their activity increases as in conditions of rapid bone turnover. It is possible that alkaline phosphatase locally inactivates inhibitors of precipitation (such as inorganic pyrophosphate) resulting in the formation of crystals.

Calcium and phosphate

The total body calcium content is 25–30 mol (1000–1500 g) and 99% of this is incorporated in bone crystals. This pool is in equilibrium with the extracellular fluid calcium. Total exchange of the ions of extracellular fluid occurs several times daily. Bone deposition, and resorption, which also contribute to calcium economy, proceeds much more slowly.

The daily dietary intake of calcium averages 25 mmol (1 g). Of this, only 6 mmol is absorbed by active transport in the proximal small bowel. Under normal circumstances, 98% of calcium filtered by the kidney is reabsorbed in the proximal tubule. Calcium economy is effected by adjustments in this tubular reabsorption.

Total serum calcium includes protein-bound (45%) and free ionized fractions. A small amount is present as diffusible complexes. Binding is largely to albumin, and variations in albumin concentration will lead to misinterpretation of effective calcium concentration unless corrective calculations are performed. The biological activity of calcium relates to its free ionized concentration, and a low serum calcium may be due to a low albumin concentration, in which event serum ionized calcium should be normal.

The normal serum calcium in the non-pregnant state, after correction for albumin concentration, is 2.25–2.65 mmol/L. The normal ionized calcium is 1.1–1.4 mmol. Many clinical laboratories now measure ionized calcium directly. If this cannot be measured, it can be derived from the total serum calcium, albumin and globulin concentrations by the following equations:

% protein-bound calcium =
0.8 × albumin (g/L) + 0.2 × globulin (g/L) + 3
% ionized calcium = 100−% protein-bound calcium

It should be noted that the accuracy of the first equation in pregnancy has not been established.

Of the total body phosphorus, 85% is in the skeleton and the remainder is inside cells elsewhere. One-third of the plasma phosphorus is present as inorganic phosphate (0.8–1.4 mmol/L), whilst two-thirds is in phospholipid form. In contrast to calcium, about 88% of inorganic phosphate is free and not protein bound. Phosphate concentration is labile and alters from hour to hour. After eating, plasma phosphate falls because phosphate enters the cells with glucose under the influence of insulin. For these reasons samples for phosphate estimation should be taken early in the morning with the patient fasting.

Phosphate is abundant in normal foods. Its absorption is very efficient and dietary privation, short of actual starvation, does not lead to deficiency. Even so, non-absorbable antacids, if taken in large amounts, can interfere with phosphate absorption by binding it in the gut lumen. Under normal circumstances, the daily requirement of 40 mmol is easily satisfied by gastrointestinal absorption.

The kidney plays a major role in regulating phosphate balance. After glomerular filtration, 80–90% of phosphate is reabsorbed in the proximal convoluted tubule. A rise in plasma phosphate is countered by increased renal excretion. Parathyroid hormone (PTH) achieves this by inhibiting proximal tubular phosphate reabsorption. Bone uptake and release of phosphate also contribute to homeostasis, but the renal mechanism predominates.

Hormonal regulation of calcium, phosphate and bone

The functions of bone, kidney and the alimentary tract in calcium and phosphate homeostasis are regulated chiefly by PTH and vitamin D. Thyroid and adrenal hormones, as well as glucagon, growth hormone and sex steroids also have influence. The place of calcitonin in this system has not been fully characterized.

VITAMIN D

The healing effect of ultraviolet light on rachitic bone lesions was recognized in 1919. Soon afterwards, it was demonstrated that sunlight activates a sterol in the skin that then becomes the antirachitic agent. This process is the photochemical conversion of 7-dehydrocholesterol to cholecalciferol or vitamin D_3 (Fig. 14.1). The diet, although to a much lesser extent, also contributes to the body stores of vitamin D but about 90% of circulating vitamin D is skin derived [1]. Natural dietary sources include fish oils, eggs, butter and liver and these yield both vitamin D_3 and vitamin D_2 (ergocalciferol). Absorption from the proximal small intestine is aided by bile salts as for other fat-soluble vitamins.

Vitamin D is transported to the liver bound to a specific vitamin D binding globulin. In the liver, its first metabolic activation step yields 25-hydroxycholecalciferol (25-OHD)—the dominant circulating form of the vitamin. The serum concentration of 25-OHD is an index of vitamin D nutritional status. The same transport protein conveys 25-OHD to the kidney, the only known site of the 1α-hydroxylase enzyme in the non-pregnant state,

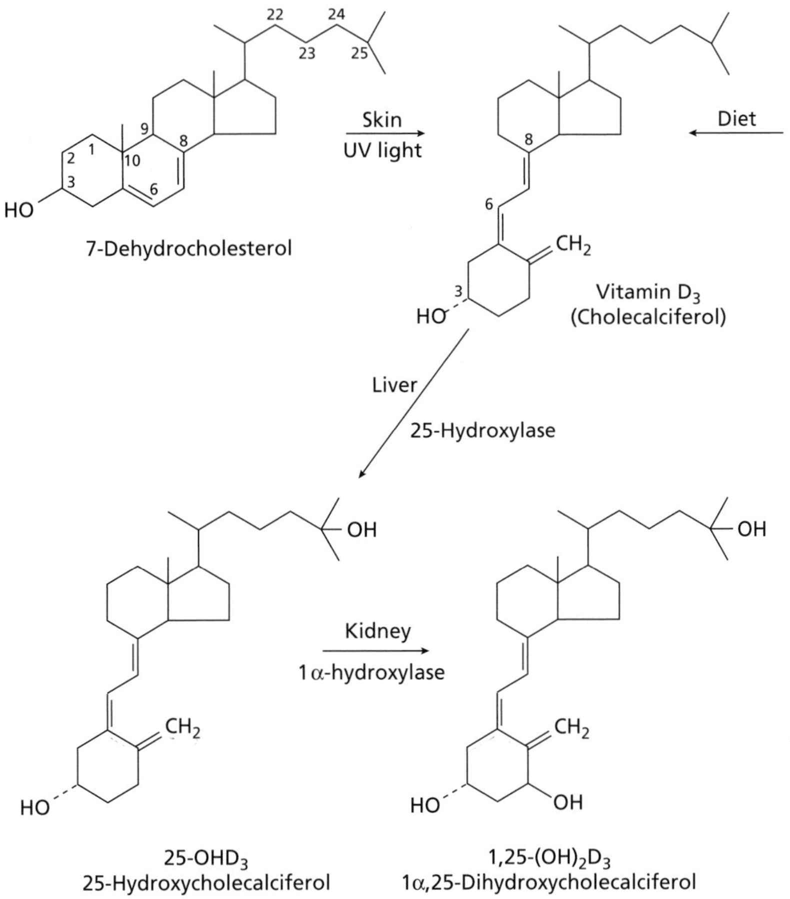

Fig 14.1 Metabolic activation of vitamin D to 1,25-OHD. In addition the kidney also synthesizes 24,25-OHD, but its function is uncertain.

although there are extrarenal sites in pregnancy, the placenta in particular [2,3]. Hydroxylation at either the C1 or C24 position takes place in cells of the proximal convoluted tubule producing 1α-25-OHD and 24,25-OHD. The latter is elaborated when vitamin D, calcium and phosphate are abundant. It is a major vitamin D metabolite, second to 25-OHD, but its biological importance is undefined. It may have a role in bone mineralization as its synthesis is favoured by hypercalcaemia, which inhibits 1,25-OHD formation. The reverse situation pertains when serum calcium is low [4]. However, 1,25-OHD clearly has a very significant role and is the most potent vitamin D metabolite. Its serum concentration (30–40 pg/mL) is 1000 times less than that of 25-OHD (20–30 ng/mL) but, in its absence, the complete syndrome of vitamin D deficiency develops. As it is synthesized in the kidney, secreted into the bloodstream, and exerts its chief effects elsewhere in the body, it can correctly be

regarded as a hormone. Several other vitamin D metabolites of weaker activity exist, but will not be considered here.

The prime function of 1,25-OHD is to sustain plasma levels of calcium and phosphate. This permits mineralization of newly forming bone. The vitamin acts on at least three target organs: gut, bone and kidney (Fig. 14.2). Its major function is in the small intestine where it induces synthesis of brush border proteins that bind calcium and phosphate, promoting their active transport from lumen to bloodstream. In the absence of vitamin D, gut absorption of these ions virtually ceases.

In the kidney, the action of vitamin D is uncertain in significance, although a direct action on the proximal convoluted tubule leads to enhanced calcium and phosphate reabsorption. However, even in the absence of vitamin D, 99% of all calcium filtered at the glomerulus can still be reabsorbed. In X-linked familial hypophosphataemia,

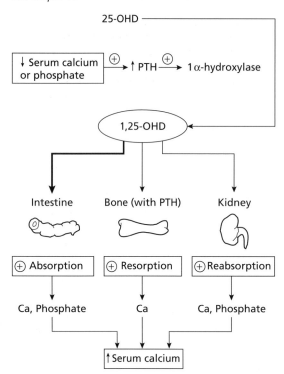

Fig 14.2 Actions of 1,25-dihydroxyvitamin D. Hypocalcaemia stimulates PTH secretion which activates renal 1α-hydroxylase, thus increasing production of 1,25-OHD. The actions of 1,25-OHD on intestine, bone and renal tubule are directed at returning serum calcium to normal range (⊕ = stimulant effect).

where the tubule does not respond to vitamin D, phosphate is lost in the urine and rickets results.

Although vitamin D clearly has effects on the skeleton, its action is complex.

The various metabolites have disparate effects and no explanation is yet available to integrate them all. 1,25-OHD is a potent direct stimulator of bone absorption [5,6], but the physiological effect of this is not established. Vitamin D is also essential for normal growth and mineralization of the skeleton. Whether it has a direct growth-promoting action or acts only indirectly by providing the optimum milieu for bone growth is not certain. Production of 1,25-OHD is enhanced at times of rapid growth, pregnancy and lactation, which are accompanied by an increased need for calcium and phosphorus.

Hypocalcaemia, by stimulating PTH secretion, activates renal 1α-hydroxylase. This increases production of 1,25-OHD synthesis (but without the mediation of PTH). This reduces phosphate excretion. The gonadal steroids, growth hormone, human placental lactogen (HPL) and prolactin as well as PTH and phosphate deficiency all have the capacity to stimulate 1α-hydroxylase [7,8].

PARATHYROID HORMONE

PTH is the second major hormone influencing calcium balance and bone. Its effects are mediated by intracellular cyclic adenosine monophosphate (cAMP) and its physiological function is to sustain, within narrow limits, extracellular fluid calcium concentration. Any fall in ionized calcium is countered by secretion of PTH. The fall in calcium is checked by the direct effects of PTH on bone and kidney, and its indirect stimulation of calcium absorption from the gut mediated by 1,25-OHD.

In bone, PTH stimulates the activity of osteoclasts and osteoblasts causing bone resorption with calcium and - phosphate mobilization. As it stimulates secretion of osteoclast collagenases and similar lytic enzymes, it acts to accomplish metabolic destruction of the bony matrix. This is reflected in increased urinary and plasma hydroxyproline. In general, remodelling activity is stimulated, but osteoclast function predominates. However, the action of PTH on bone is more complex than this and not yet fully elucidated.

In the kidney, PTH acts initially to inhibit phosphate reabsorption by the proximal tubule. Phosphate released from bone is thereby rapidly excreted with resulting hypophosphataemia and hyperphosphaturia in states of PTH excess. By a different mechanism, probably operating distally in the tubule, PTH tends to increase calcium reabsorption. Nevertheless, the flood of calcium from bone exceeds the capacity for calcium reabsorption so that hypercalciuria ensues. PTH also inhibits proximal tubular reabsorption of bicarbonate so that states of PTH excess are often accompanied by a mild metabolic acidosis.

CALCITONIN

In the absence of thyroid and parathyroid glands, the response to an intravenous calcium load is blunted and the return to normocalcaemia delayed. This observation suggested the existence of a hypocalcaemic factor, which is now known to be the hormone calcitonin. It is secreted by the parafollicular C cells of the thyroid. Its output is stimulated by a rise in ionized calcium concentration but also by the gut hormones gastrin and cholecystokinin. Hypocalcaemia has the opposite effect. The effect of calcitonin in lowering serum calcium is accompanied by a fall in serum phosphate and both probably result from a direct inhibition of bone breakdown. Also calcitonin inhibits the bone reabsorption produced by a number of substances, including PTH and vitamin D metabolites. The role of calcitonin in the complex system of calcium balance is not yet certain. In medullary carcinoma of the thyroid, where there is hypersecretion of this hormone, there are no overt bony changes and no disturbances of calcium or phosphate levels. An intriguing observation has been that of osteopetrosis in the newborn babies of women with medullary carcinoma, but this may represent genetic linkage of two disorders rather than causation [9].

Changes in calcium and phosphate homeostasis during pregnancy

The requirement for many nutrients including minerals increases during pregnancy. If exogenous sources are insufficient, the mother's system will be called upon to satisfy the demands. In particular, the maternal calcium repository found in her bone mass is available and therefore vulnerable. The fetus accumulates 30–40 g of calcium and half as much phosphorus in its own tissues [10]. Of the calcium accumulation 70% occurs in the third trimester when fetal skeletal growth is maximal with 5–6 mmol (200–250 mg) of calcium being deposited daily into the fetal skeleton. Without an anticipatory rise in calcium absorption, the necessary calcium could be drawn from the maternal skeleton, and some of it probably is. Of course, lactation prolongs the calcium demand. Human milk contains 6–9 mmol of calcium per litre [11] (two to three times the maternal serum level) and the intake of a normal 3-kg infant is 2–3 L/week, increasing with age. Furthermore, there may even be a need for increased bone deposition to provide the added structural support made necessary by the increased bodyweight of pregnancy. What then are the physiological changes which have evolved in pregnancy and how are they achieved?

In regard to dietary calcium intake, clearly this will be highly variable around the world. At least in affluent white Americans who volunteered for a study into calcium balance in pregnancy [12], dietary calcium was increased by about 20% above non-pregnant intake. However, this is at best only one of the complex of changes relating to calcium, and would certainly not operate in many other population groups. In most normal pregnant women, one or both of two additional compensatory mechanisms must come into play to preserve the maternal skeleton. The first is that urinary loss of calcium might decrease. In fact the opposite occurs and urinary calcium excretion is increased 50–300% as pregnancy proceeds [12,13].

The second possibility is that the fraction of calcium absorbed from the gut might increase. Indeed, this adjustment does occur. In a recent longitudinal study, gut absorption of calcium in early pregnancy increased by 50–60% over that observed in the same women before

conception [12]. It had doubled by the beginning of the third trimester. This finding confirms earlier careful work [13a]. Whether or not calcium absorption remains increased during lactation was a matter of some dispute. Some studies did show calcium absorption to continue to be elevated in the puerperium during lactation [14,15], but more recent investigations reveal that it quickly declines to pre-pregnant levels [12,13a,16].

Despite the dramatic antenatal increase, the two recent studies referred to above [12,16] and older studies [13a,14,17] concur that urinary calcium loss decreases in the puerperium with lactation. This seems to occur even in women who are not lactating and therefore cannot be explained by the hormonal milieu of that state [17a].

Thus, the components of calcium economy change during and after gestation. Firstly, there is an increase in urinary calcium loss and in gastrointestinal calcium absorption during pregnancy. After delivery, however, renal conservation of calcium is the rule, whilst absorption falls back to non-pregnant levels.

Inorganic phosphorus economy in pregnancy is based upon an increase in its renal tubular maximal reabsorption, likely related to diminished PTH levels, and enhanced intestinal absorption mediated by 1,25 vitamin D [17b]. This is important as inorganic phosphorus, no less than calcium, is essential for the growing fetus.

What is the mechanism of the enhanced calcium absorption during pregnancy? It probably is explained by the rise in plasma 1,25-OHD that occurs early and continues throughout gestation [17,17b,18,19,20,20a] (Fig. 14.3).

The increase is large, 250% above non-pregnant levels in the most recent of these investigations [17b]. After delivery in the lactating mother, the level falls promptly but remains slightly higher than in non-pregnant women.

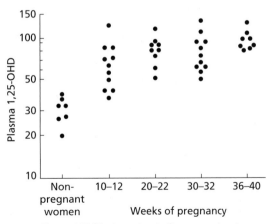

Fig 14.3 Plasma 1,25-dihydroxyvitamin D concentrations in control women and during pregnancy [20]. Units are ng/L.

The concentration of 1,25-OHD in cord blood is appreciably lower than in maternal blood [18,21,22] but, by 24 h of age, the level in the neonate has risen significantly [23]. This can be seen as an adaptive response by the baby to the new need to absorb calcium from its own intestinal lumen.

The gestational increase in 1,25-OHD activity suggests that maternal 1α-hydroxylase activity is stimulated. There are several potential stimulators of the enzyme. Oestrogens are known to do this, at least in postmenopausal osteoporotic women [28,29] and egg-laying birds [30]. The stimulatory effect in the bird is fortified by the presence of progesterone [31]. Both these hormones of course are high in pregnancy, and fall promptly after delivery. Prolactin or HPL may be involved or even growth hormone [7] which bears structural similarity to HPL. Another potent stimulator of the enzyme is lowered plasma phosphate (see below).

Furthermore, the increase in biologically active 1,25-OHD in pregnancy may come from synthesis of the hormone by the placenta itself [3].

Whether PTH rises in pregnancy [25,26], is unchanged [17,20], or decreases [16,17b,20a] has been disputed. A previous notion was of a state of mild physiological 'hyperparathyroidism' in pregnancy but this seems to have been an artefact of earlier less valid methods of measurement. The most recent studies examine the intact PTH molecule by means of a two-site immunoradiometric assay [17b,20a] and are consistent in finding that levels of the hormone are decreased in normal pregnancy but rise early in the puerperium, though some work suggests the rise occurs in the third trimester, before delivery.

Total serum calcium and phosphorus fall in pregnancy (Fig. 14.4). The fall in calcium continues from soon after conception until at least the middle of the third trimester [17] but there may be a slight rise thereafter [25]. Phosphate falls in the first trimester and then falls even further to reach low levels in the third trimester [17,133]. It is likely that the fall in serum proteins accounts for the decline in calcium and the closely parallel patterns for calcium and albumin support this. Furthermore, it has been demonstrated in longitudinal studies that the fall must be due to the protein-bound fraction as ionized calcium either rises very slightly [33] or remains quite constant [17,25], with a minimal decline near delivery [34].

Early in gestation fetal serum calcium is lower than maternal serum calcium [35,36]. At term, however, fetal levels exceed maternal by 0.25–0.5 mmol/L both for total serum calcium [22,35] and free ionic calcium [34]. This has been confirmed early in the third trimester by direct fetal blood sampling [35]. The existence of a placental active transport mechanism seems likely.

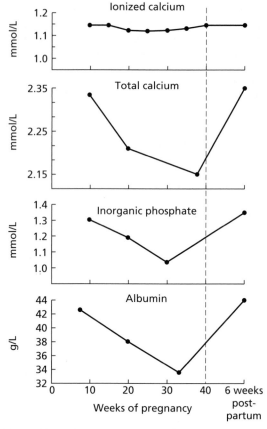

Fig 14.4 Maternal serum concentrations of ionized calcium, total calcium, inorganic phosphate and albumin during and after pregnancy. (From [25].)

Experimental data lend support to this idea [37]. Further circumstantial evidence lies in the observation that serum calcium levels fall promptly in the newborn after separation from placental supply [23,38]. Perhaps maternal 1,25-OHD stimulates a carrier protein to accomplish transplacental passage in the same way that it stimulates transmucosal importation of calcium from the gut lumen.

It is also likely that the fetus can control its calcium influx. This may be through fetal production of 1,25-OHD and there is evidence for this in an umbilical arteriovenous concentration gradient for 1,25-OHD [22,39] with higher arterial levels.

A study in sheep has suggested that it is PTH which promotes the active transport of calcium from mother to fetus and that the calcium pump cannot function in its absence, even where 1,25-OHD levels are sustained [40]. This was also postulated in a human study which showed high fetal levels of bioactive PTH [26].

The state of vitamin D nutrition is conveniently assessed by the plasma level of 25-OHD. This is no different in pregnancy from the non-pregnant range, at least in Caucasian women [20,41,42]. However, levels fluctuate seasonally [43]. A careful longitudinal study [42] (Fig. 14.5) demonstrated a fall during the third trimester when it occurred in winter (January–March). The implication was that, in normal Caucasian women, vitamin D levels are maintained in pregnancy except when the period of greatest demand (third trimester) coincides with the time of least supply (winter). Thus the major determinant is exposure to sunlight and this has been confirmed in Finland [44], North America [45] and by implication in Saudi Arabia [46,47], where local customs of dress lead to reduced exposure.

It appears that maternal vitamin D status is largely dependent on skin exposure even in sunny environments such as Saudi Arabia and Australia. In Saudi Arabia, 'extraordinarily low' 25-OHD concentrations were found in shrouded mothers and their babies in 1984 [46,47]. In Melbourne, not the sunniest part of Australia, but less gloomy than sites studied in the Northern Hemisphere, levels of 25-OHD below the reference range were demonstrated in 80% of 82 veiled or dark-skinned pregnant women raising concern about vitamin D deficiency in mother and baby [51,230]. Possible seasonal variation in 25-OHD levels was not studied. In the same city, a study identified 55 infants treated for vitamin D deficiency rickets [231]. Of these children 54 were born to mothers with 'ethnocultural risk factors' for vitamin D deficiency and 80% of the mothers assayed had low 25-OHD levels. These studies confirm, in the Southern Hemisphere, the old findings mentioned above.

The linear relationship between maternal and cord blood concentrations of 25-OHD suggests direct transfer across the placenta [42,48,49]. Conversely, 1,25-OHD is

significantly lower in the newborn baby than in maternal blood at delivery and bears no relationship to it [49]. This certainly implies that it does not cross the placenta freely.

A definite rise in calcitonin secretion can be detected during pregnancy and lactation [20,50]. Bearing in mind the considerable ability of calcitonin to inhibit bone resorption, even that caused by PTH and vitamin D, it is possible that it has a role in protecting the maternal skeleton from demineralization. The newborn baby also has high calcitonin levels [51,52].

Table 14.1 summarizes the changes in normal pregnancy discussed above. The levels may not reflect true activity as there may be changes in end-organ responsiveness to these hormones in pregnancy. If this were so, there could be changes in metabolism without quantifiable changes in serum levels of the hormones.

Bone density in pregnancy and lactation

Does either pregnancy or lactation, or the combination, have a lifelong influence on bone density and the tendency to subsequent osteoporosis?

The net effect of pregnancy and lactation on the skeleton has been studied extensively over many years. There is a good deal of variation in the findings available. This may be attributed to one or several of a host of variables. For example, there are changes in ethnic predisposition to osteoporosis. The reports of pregnancy osteoporosis are largely Caucasian in origin. The latitude in which studies are conducted is significant in that vitamin D insufficiency, as we have noted, is more prevalent as the Equator recedes in the distance and in wintry seasons. Notwithstanding this observation, the habit of some ethnic groups of covering most of the skin surface seems to override the advantage to the bones of a sunny climate. The consump-

Fig 14.5 (a) Plasma 25-OHD concentrations before, during and after pregnancy in 26 women (mean ± 1.96 SD). (b) Seasonal variation (Northern Hemisphere) of plasma 25-OHD concentration before or during pregnancy in 26 women (mean ± 1.96 SD). (From [42].)

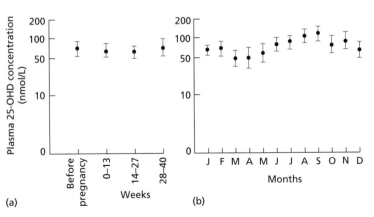

	Non-pregnant	Third trimester
Total calcium (mmol/L)	2.48 [229]	2.34 [43,229]
Ionized calcium (mmol/L)	1.18 [33]	1.22 [33]
Urinary calcium (mg/24 h)	90 [17]	300 [17]
Total phosphate (mmol/L)	1.24 [229]	1.05 [43,229]
25-OHD (μg/L)	14 [71,210]	15 [19,71]
1,25-OHD (ng/L)	50 [17,20]	120 [17,20]

Table 14.1 Mineral metabolism: changes in serum concentrations in normal pregnancy. Values are representative means from the literature. Individual studies show wide variation and are referenced in square brackets.

tion of dairy products varies between populations, as do national policies in regard to the supplementation of milk with vitamin D as is extant in the USA, for example, but not practised in Australia. Moreover, routine calcium supplementation is recommended in many antenatal populations and not in others.

Quite apart from variation in the patients studied, there has been considerable debate as to the appropriate methodology to be employed in measuring bone density, and which sites in the body should be measured. Furthermore, the technology utilized for this purpose has improved over the years. Is it surprising, then, that some studies show pregnancy and lactation lead to bone loss whilst others do not?

Bone changes during pregnancy

In normal pregnancy, radiographic methods of bone densitometry have been eschewed for obvious reasons. However, there are some studies. X-ray spectrophotometry was used in a prospective investigation [59] and showed a small but significant loss of mineral from trabecular but not cortical bone during pregnancy. Ultrasonic bone propagation velocity has been used in recent investigations, scanning the proximal phalanges of fingers [237] and the os calcis [239,238]. These concurred in describing a small but significant fall in bone mineral density (BMD) in the third trimester. The former also showed significantly lower bone density in the third trimester in women with low calcium intake.

A British study in 2000 used dual energy X-ray absorptiometry (DEXA) and studied 10 women longitudinally in considerable detail. The hip and spine were measured before pregnancy and postpartum, whilst forearm density was measured also at 14 and 28 weeks. From pre-conception to postpartum BMD decreased 3.5% at the hip and 2% at the lumbar spine. Forearm density did not change significantly [238a]. A nearby study [238b] also measured DEXA at various sites, before, during and after pregnancy. BMD increased in this study by 2.8%, whilst pelvis and lumbar spine densities fell by 3.2% and 4.6% respectively. In a prospective cohort study of 49 women in Sweden,

BMD of the forearm fell by about 1% between 12 weeks gestation and 5 months postpartum. An older American study [136] examined BMD in six women longitudinally before, 6 weeks and 6 months after pregnancy. They were compared with 25 matched (age, weight, height, activity level, calcium intake) non-pregnant women. BMD decreased about 3% in the femoral neck, radius and lumbar spine.

On balance of the available literature, it appears that there is a small loss of bone throughout pregnancy, of between 1 and 4%, in the pelvis and lumbar spine. There is less than universal agreement about the forearm, but a smaller fall seems likely.

As mentioned above, biochemical indices of bone turnover are increased in the third trimester, and more so in women with multiple gestation [240]. Two recent studies [238a,238b] concur that there is good evidence for increased bone turnover in pregnancy. The net result, however, is a definite increase in bone resorption based on biochemical markers (urinary pyridinium crosslinks and N- telopeptide). Although biochemical markers of bone formation were also increased (bone specific alkaline phosphatase, propeptides of type I collagen), the increase was only in the third trimester [238a].

Bone changes with lactation

In the short term, after childbirth, however, there are quite different findings, although they do not finally provide grounds to contradict the statement above. The period after delivery, of lactation and then weaning, has been carefully studied in a number of locations over the years. An early investigation used photon scanning of the femur in 10 lactating women and suggested mineral losses of 2.2% over 100 days [56]. Distal bone mass in the forearm, assessed by single photon densitometry in 1986, was nearly 20% lower in a long-term lactation group (three to four children averaging 11 months lactation) than in a short lactation group [57]. Furthermore, there is evidence that some adolescent mothers demonstrate greater than the usual bone demineralization after 16 weeks of lactation, perhaps because of low dietary intake of calcium and phosphorus [58].

From a cluster of more recent studies, the conclusion is that women lose 3–6% in bone mineral density during lactation, most of it in the first 3 months [17b,234,230a, 231a]. The amount of bone lost is independent of calcium intake over a wide range [60,235], but was positively related to the assessed volume of breast milk produced and the effect was more pronounced in taller women in an English study [66, 234]. The consistent finding of a major decrement in bone density in a short time would be of great concern were it not for the demonstrated fact that within 6 months of weaning, there is a comparable gain in bone density to attain previous levels [21,67,68 17b,230a,231a]. In seeking a role of the calciotrophic hormones PTH, 25-OHD and 1,25-OHD in the bone loss of lactation, no consistent correlation was found, a striking finding given that these are the hormones considered dominant in the regulation of calcium homeostasis. Thus it seems that other mechanisms must be responsible. It is possible that the hypoestrogenic milieu of lactation provides part of the reason for bone loss.

It should be noted that many biochemical indices of bone turnover have been measured in lactating women, and during the antepartum period [16,239,238,240]. These include peptides of type I collagen, osteocalcin, hydroxyproline, pyridinoline and tartrate-resistant acid phosphatase [237]. They usually demonstrate increased bone turnover or remodelling, both before delivery and with lactation. PTH-related peptide (PTH-rP) has also been found elevated in lactation together with bone loss, but its function is not certain [236].

Metabolic bone diseases

Metabolic bone diseases are those that affect the whole skeleton, though often the involvement is not uniform. We will discuss here a number of disorders which are important in pregnancy and which can be understood on the basis of aberrations in normal functions considered above. Complete descriptions of each clinical entity in the non-pregnant state can be found elsewhere. For a woman with any of the following disorders, pre-pregnancy counselling to explain the clinical significance, obstetric and genetic implications of her medical problem is highly desirable.

Rickets and osteomalacia have been classified by Harrison [61] into two types. Type I is secondary to deficiency of 1,25-OHD, either on the grounds of inadequate nutrition or malabsorption, and an important feature is secondary hyperparathyroidism. Type II rickets (and osteomalacia) is the result of hypophosphataemia, most

commonly due to impaired renal tubular phosphate reabsorption. Secondary hyperparathyroidism is not a prominent feature. The pathological disorders within each type are listed in Box 14.1. Most of them are discussed here.

Nutritional osteomalacia

Delay in or failure of bone mineralization is the hallmark of osteomalacia. If it occurs in childhood before closure of the epiphyses, it results in the characteristic disorder of rickets. The rachitic epiphysis, with widened growth plate and distorted architecture, demonstrates hyperosteoidosis, i.e. the presence of excess unmineralized osteoid. The same histopathological features are seen in adults with osteomalacia, but in different sites. The epiphyses having closed, changes can be seen throughout the skeleton wherever remodelling occurs.

There are many causes of osteomalacia, but all exert their pathological effects through abnormalities in vitamin D metabolism or through hypophosphataemia (see Table 14.1). The biochemical triad of low serum calcium and phosphate combined with high alkaline phosphatase (heat-labile or bone component to be distinguished from the heat-stable placental component in pregnancy) is generally seen with osteomalacia. Urinary hydroxyproline is almost always raised. The diagnosis of nutritional osteomalacia, however, should also include low plasma 25-

---

Box 14.1 Classification of rickets and osteomalacia [61]

Type I
- Vitamin D deficiency:
  sunlight deficiency
  dietary deficiency
- Vitamin D malabsorption
- Liver disease
- Drug-induced:
  anticonvulsants
  corticosteroids
- Renal insufficiency

Type II
- Fanconi's syndrome
- Renal tubular acidosis:
  cystinosis
  tyrosinosis
  idiopathic
- Familial primary hypophosphataemia (vitamin D-resistant rickets)
- Acquired primary hypophosphataemia

OHD and high PTH concentrations (reflecting secondary hyperparathyroidism). X-ray features will not be discussed here.

In pregnant Asians in Britain, nutritional osteomalacia seems to be common, although it is often unrecognized. The appearance of clinical osteomalacia with fractures in a pregnant woman may be a presenting feature of vitamin D deficiency [62,63] as may be the birth of a baby with rickets [64,65] or hypocalcaemia in the first week of life [66]. Enamel defects may develop in the teeth later in life [43,67], particularly after neonatal hypocalcaemic tetany.

In an investigation of maternal factors relevant to neonatal hypocalcaemia, Watney *et al.* [68] demonstrated lower serum calcium levels in Asian women than in Caucasian women at booking, 36 weeks and 6 weeks after delivery. The Asian babies had lower serum calcium levels on the sixth day of life. Elsewhere, it was shown prospectively that 25-OHD levels in Asians were lower than in Caucasians at every occasion when they were sampled throughout late pregnancy [69] (Fig. 14.6). Brooke *et al.* [70] showed that vegetarian Asians had significantly lower levels on each occasion studied and 70% of them had undetectable 25-OHD levels after pregnancy (compared with 12% of non-vegetarians). Nearly half of the babies of vegetarian women had hypocalcaemia whilst none of the other babies developed the problem. These studies supported the findings of a number of previous investigations into the vitamin D and calcium status of pregnant Asian women in the UK [48,66,71,72].

Studies from Pakistan [73] and India [74] have shown a high prevalence of subclinical and even overt osteomalacia in pregnant women. In Saudi Arabia, many women and their babies have very low levels of 25-OHD and serum calcium [46,47] indicating vitamin D deficiency. This is chiefly attributed to lack of exposure to sunlight owing to the traditional custom of women being entirely covered by their clothes.

Certainly vitamin D supplementation in pregnancy can ameliorate these changes. If pregnant Asians are given 1000 units daily, the 25-OHD level in cord blood is higher than after unsupplemented pregnancy. Even so there was no difference in bone mineral content of neonatal forearms as assessed by photon absorptiometry [75]. The conclusion was that fetal mineralization is not impaired by maternal vitamin D deficiency. Unfortunately, as neither maternal 1,25-OHD nor 25-OHD was measured, this conclusion may not be justified. In a similar study [76], 25-OHD levels were higher in both cord and maternal serum after supplementation in pregnancy but there was no attempt to assess neonatal bone density.

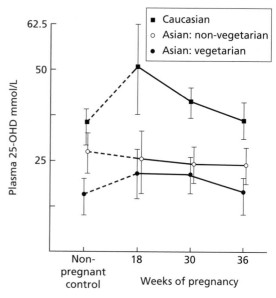

Fig 14.6 Plasma 25-OHD concentrations in non-pregnant women and during pregnancy. (From [71].)

Others also have disputed that pregnancy leads to an increased requirement for vitamin D. Dent and Gupta [71] showed that 25-OHD levels were low in a group of Asian women and remained so throughout pregnancy without further fall. They argued that this suggested there was no increased need for vitamin D in pregnancy.

Nevertheless, the association between pregnancy and osteomalacia, at least in Asians [77,78], is undeniable. It may be that pregnancy brings a vitamin D-deficient woman to medical attention for the first time by coincidence rather than causation. What is still unknown is whether women with very low vitamin D levels can furnish the normal pregnancy rise in 1,25-OHD concentration. If there is a tendency for pregnancy to unmask latent osteomalacia, it may be explicable on this basis.

It is established that low maternal 25-OHD levels are associated with neonatal morbidity [43,66,68] and impaired first year growth in some groups [79]. This underlies the recommendation that vitamin D supplements be given routinely to all Asian women in the UK from the Indian subcontinent or East Africa during pregnancy. A dose of 400 IU daily from 20 weeks or 1000 IU from 30 weeks is probably sufficient [79]. The basis for their deficiency seems to lie in dietary inadequacy (even in non-vegetarians, the diet usually contains little vitamin D) and equally, if not more so, in lack of skin exposure to sunlight. Of course indoor dwelling, northern latitudes, poor diet and the winter season all tend to aggravate the problem in many patients, and a valid argument can be made for supplementing all women in these circumstances.

The World Health Organization [80] and the US National Academy of Sciences [81] recommend 400 IU (10 μg) of vitamin D daily during pregnancy and lactation. In the absence of widespread milk supplementation with vitamin D, as practised in the USA, prescription of vitamin D by doctors is necessary. In a controlled trial [43] 400 IU of ergocalciferol was as effective at preventing neonatal problems as 1000 IU has been [48]. The preferred dose would therefore seem to be 400 IU. Moreover, it is of great interest that perhaps even a single dose of vitamin D at the beginning of the third trimester will suffice. In a French study this was the case, with maternal and cord 25-OHD levels being no lower than after daily supplementation [82].

The added loss of calcium in milk in the puerperium makes the consumption of either 0.6–1.2 L (1–2 pints) of milk per day, supplemental calcium or a high calcium diet advisable in all lactating women.

Rickets

Rickets is very rare in developed nations at the turn of the 20th century. References to its complications in childbirth, however, are easily found in earlier texts of obstetrics, when it was much feared as a cause of maternal morbidity, and fetal mortality and morbidity as a result of dystocia. These problems had their origins in childhood rickets, which results in stunting of bone growth so that the pelvis may not attain normal size and structure. This often results in reduction of the pelvic diameters. In particular the anteroposterior diameter of the brim is reduced (Fig. 14.7). Subsequent mechanical problems in vaginal delivery are well established. Whilst the bone structure cannot be improved in the short term, it remains essential that these women receive vitamin D during pregnancy as the fetus is at risk of bone disease.

Mention has been made above (see vitamin D) of neonatal rickets in mothers deficient in vitamin D. Attention must be drawn to another possible aetiology of this problem in the use of long-term magnesium sulphate for tocolysis, in this instance in the USA. The report [83] refers to five mothers treated with intravenous magnesium sulphate initiated in the second trimester and continued for weeks. The observed radiographic abnormalities of rickets in two of the infants were ascribed to fetal parathyroid gland suppression by the magnesium, and so rare and serious is this occurrence that it is impossible to escape a conclusion of causation by the drug. Further studies are necessary if this potentially dangerous therapy becomes widespread.

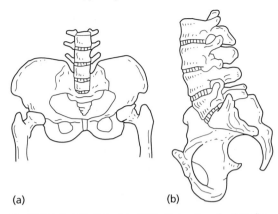

(a)   (b)

Fig 14.7 (a) Rachitic flat pelvis. (b) Sagittal section of rachitic flat pelvis with false promontory and reduced diameter of pelvic inlet.

Gastrointestinal and hepatic osteomalacia

Osteomalacia due to vitamin D and calcium deficiency may complicate any disorder of intestinal absorptive function (see Chapters 9 and 10 for an account of these conditions). Patients with inflammatory bowel disease, particularly Crohn's disease after intestinal resection, are at high risk. Seventy per cent of patients with Crohn's disease in an American series had subnormal 25-OHD levels [84]. Moreover, these patients may need very high doses of vitamin D (20 000–50 000 IU) to reverse the bone disease [69], probably because little of the administered dose is absorbed. Vitamin D may be given weekly due to its long duration of action. Patients may also have osteoporosis related to corticosteroid therapy and complex metabolic disturbances, as well as osteomalacia. Despite these potential problems, neither bony complications nor hypocalcaemia in mother or baby have been noticed in pregnancies complicated by Crohn's disease [85]. Nevertheless, it is advisable to monitor calcium and phosphate levels of women who have had bowel resection and thus may be subject to malabsorption. Vitamin D should be given in the usual recommended dose, and a larger dose, which may be monitored by serum calcium or 25-OHD levels, should be given if the mother has had prior evidence of vitamin D deficiency. Also the infant should be monitored for hypocalcaemia. One study of Asian mothers who did not have inflammatory bowel disease [68] indicated that elevated maternal heat-labile alkaline phosphatase and lowered serum phosphate are predictors of neonatal hypocalcaemia. These findings may be relevant to the pregnant patient with Crohn's disease.

Depression of serum 25-OHD, possibly temporary, has been seen in 33–60% of patients after jejuno-ileal bypass for morbid obesity, in spite of supplementation with 800 IU of vitamin D/day [86,87], and bone loss also occurs in these patients. A larger number of such women are now becoming pregnant and supplementation is warranted, with monitoring of mother and baby as detailed above.

Gluten-sensitive enteropathy (coeliac disease) also affects vitamin D absorption [88], and osteomalacia is a risk. There is a suggestion that 25-OHD may be better absorbed than vitamin D itself in this condition. Of course, the first prerequisite of care must be the obsessional adherence to a gluten-free diet. Such dietary treatment can reverse infertility, and normal pregnancies have been reported [89] (see Chapter 10).

Modern treatment of cystic fibrosis of the pancreas allows increasing numbers of women to successfully conceive and complete pregnancy (see Chapter 1). Whilst bone disease is far from the most serious problem, it can exist, and low 25-OHD levels with decreased bone mass have been detected, even after dietary vitamin D supplementation [90]. Exocrine pancreatic enzyme replacement must be continued throughout pregnancy, and vitamin D may have to be given parenterally.

As the liver is the site of synthesis of 25-OHD, liver diseases are often associated with low serum 25-OHD concentrations. However, osteomalacia is seen more frequently with cholestatic liver disorders than with hepatocellular disease. This probably reflects lack of bile salts in the intestinal lumen rendering vitamin D absorption inadequate. Even so, malabsorption is not the sole problem because, even if vitamin D is given parenterally, large doses (100 000 IU/month) are required to elevate 25-OHD levels in patients with primary biliary cirrhosis [91].

The only cholestatic disease seen with any frequency in pregnancy is obstetric cholestasis (Chapter 9). Although a temporary deficit of 25-OHD might be expected in this condition, it has not been reported.

Renal bone disease

Bone lesions are common in long-standing kidney disease. They are seen in two different clinical settings. First, osteomalacia with retardation of growth in children, resulting from conditions causing renal tubular acidosis. There may also be renal calculi and nephrocalcinosis. The bone lesions probably result from calcium and phosphate loss in the urine, but may be related to the acidosis itself, causing osteolysis with liberation of calcium. Secondly, in the presence of chronic renal failure, the pathogenesis of osteomalacia is related to deficiency of 1,25-OHD. There is phosphate retention and hypocalcaemia causing secondary hyperparathyroidism in chronic renal failure. Treatment includes administration of vitamin D and calcium, and lowering of phosphate absorption from the gut using non-absorbable antacids. The more potent forms of vitamin D (e.g. calcitriol) are needed and careful monitoring is necessary to avoid hypercalcaemia in these cases.

Pregnancy is occasionally encountered in women with chronic renal failure (see Chapter 7). Congenital rickets has been reported as a complication in their babies [92]. Certainly, vitamin D should be administered (and calcitriol is preferred), but the exact dose is not yet established and monitoring of maternal calcium is essential.

Drug-induced osteopenia

Drugs that affect bone and that may be used in pregnancy are the anticonvulsants, heparin and corticosteroids. Steroids will not be discussed here, because steroid-induced bone disease is rarely a problem in pregnancy; specifically, BMD studies have shown no impact on bone density of dexamethasone given for fetal lung maturity in doses up to 10–12-mg injections [93]. Heparin-induced osteopenia is considered in Chapter 4.

ANTICONVULSANTS

Anticonvulsant osteomalacia results from drug-induced disturbance of vitamin D metabolism, and disordered mineral ion transport in bone and intestine. Most of the currently used anticonvulsants have been implicated and the changes are dose dependent.

Many anticonvulsants stimulate activity of the hepatic microsomal oxidase enzymes, thereby converting vitamin D and 25-OHD to inactive metabolites [94]. Furthermore, phenytoin may also inhibit calcium transport from the intestinal lumen [95]. Phenytoin and phenobarbitone can inhibit bone resorption caused by PTH and 25-OHD [96]. The usual manifestations of this are slightly low serum calcium and a distinctly low serum 25-OHD levels, often with elevated alkaline phosphatase [94]. Bone loss can be detected by radiology, by photon absorption, and of course, by bone biopsy. Only in the most severe cases will the complete picture of osteomalacia (or rickets in children) develop.

Christiansen *et al.* [97] found that the bone content of epileptic gravidae was 86% of that of age-matched controls at 18 weeks. This difference persisted at 8 days and at 6 months postpartum. The bone content of the babies was no different from a control group. It is noteworthy that all epileptics and controls received vitamin D supplements throughout. Fleischman *et al.* [98] reported reduced 25-OHD levels in epileptic mothers and their babies, and hypocalcaemia in one infant. These findings were reproduced in a longitudinal study of epileptic women in pregnancy. Those on phenytoin had lower 25-OHD and 1,25-OHD values than controls, both in maternal and cord serum, but the levels in carbamazepine-treated mothers tended to be intermediate [99]. All mothers had received 400 IU of vitamin D_3 daily. None of the women or their babies had clinical evidence of hypocalcaemia or bone disease.

It is regarded as advisable, at least in the UK, to give supplements to all women on anticonvulsant drugs [100] in a dose of 400 IU daily from early in the second trimester, or 1000 IU daily in the third trimester. It is established that supplements of this dose are safe, and do not cause hypercalcaemia of infancy which may have resulted from the much higher doses used some decades ago [101].

Osteoporosis of pregnancy and the puerperium

Significant osteoporosis is rare in pregnant women, but three forms have been recognized, including that associated with heparin (see Chapter 4). The two major varieties are detailed here.

1 *Postpregnancy spinal osteoporosis* presents with severe back pain and loss of height due to vertebral compression fractures, possibly at a number of levels in late pregnancy or the puerperium. Over three decades at least 27 cases have been documented [41,127–130]. Most of these have had full investigation, including bone biopsy, with no cause for osteoporosis having been found. In all cases subsequent pregnancy was uneventful, with no further fractures, but lactation was usually proscribed. This is rational as lactation is associated with at least temporary bone loss in many women [131]. Fortunately, elevated bone formation, in excess of resorption, seems to follow weaning allowing restoration of bone mass [13]. Calcium intake of at least 1400 mg daily is necessary. Other studies of normal lactating women suggest that bone turnover is accelerated [132] but that significant bone loss usually does not occur. It may occur, however, in adolescents or in women with an as yet undefined propensity to osteoporosis. It is postulated that such women develop osteoporosis of pregnancy. The existence of this entity has been disputed by Dent and Friedman [41] whose contention was that the association with pregnancy is coincidental. They believed that women with idiopathic osteoporosis had developed fractures consequent to the weight gain of normal pregnancy and that it was unlikely that the physiological changes of normal pregnancy were of sufficient magnitude to cause significant bone loss in an otherwise healthy woman.

There are unusual elements in pregnancy osteoporosis, such as the focal nature of the disease. In some of the cases described in a 24 year series of 24 patients [132a], bone biopsy from one site was normal despite radiological and clinical evidence of recent collapse of several vertebrae with loss of centimetres in height.

2 *Transient hip osteoporosis of pregnancy*. Curtiss and Kincaid described this in 1959 [24]. The neck of the femur is also susceptible to osteoporosis in pregnancy. Many women complain of pain in the hip, but radiographic studies are seldom performed in pregnancy. Many patients have pelvic diastasis, separation of the pubic rami at the symphysis, but some of these patients may have osteoporosis [134]. For example, severe hip pain in late pregnancy was studied recently by bone mineral content estimation. In six women with severe pain undergoing six femoral bone density studies each (three on each femur), 33% of the densities were decreased. Conversely in 20 normal women studied, only 10% of the bone densities were decreased. Many other cases have been reported with symptoms limited to pregnancy and the puerperium [135,136]. The pain may be in one or both hips, worse with weight bearing and usually begins around 35 weeks' gestation. Radiology may demonstrate pronounced loss of cortical bone in the hip joint but spontaneous recovery is usual. Prudence dictates cessation of lactation, although no studies have proven this. Calcitonin has been used to reduce bone resorption.

Progression to femoral head necrosis is very uncommon, and resembles that seen after steroid ingestion. There are some cases occurring in pregnancy where no cause was apparent [137,138]. These women complain of increasingly severe pain in the hip, which may be of sudden onset.

In summary, the diagnosis of osteoporosis should be considered in any woman with persistent and severe back or hip pain in late pregnancy or the puerperium, who has appropriate radiological findings. A complete search for other causes is necessary before ascribing a diagnosis of idiopathic osteoporosis of pregnancy.

Due largely to its rarity, and the frequency of other benign aches and pains in pregnancy, the diagnosis is often overlooked and many women have undergone unnecessary suffering due to delay in recognition of the problem. It is important to consider this diagnosis in any patient with back or hip pain, as many simple measures may help, such as reassurance, bed rest, simple analgesia and aids to locomotion in severely disabled women. An article in 1996 has reviewed the subject of osteoporosis in pregnancy [132].

Finally, *osteitis pubis* is a rare but serious disorder seen in the latter half of pregnancy and characterised by fluffy opacities and sometimes necrosis at the pubic symphysis in pregnant women. Walking becomes extremely painful, with local pain triggered by each step, and there is tenderness over the symphysis. After delivery, radioisotope bone scans show increased uptake at the site and plain radiology, CT or MRI may show abnormalities. This condition is probably a local example of avascular necrosis of bone. Management is very difficult and patients often need a wheelchair until some time after delivery, the usual course being one of slow improvement over the weeks following.

Parathyroid disease

PRIMARY HYPERPARATHYROIDISM

Most patients with hypercalcaemia are asymptomatic, unless the level of calcium is extremely high. Symptoms may then comprise tiredness, thirst, polyuria, muscle and bone aches, or symptoms of complications of the hypercalcaemia, such as ureteric colic from passage of a stone, or pancreatitis. A number of these symptoms are experienced by normal pregnant women and the chance that hypercalcaemia will be diagnosed on clinical grounds is therefore very low. What is much more likely is that the disturbance will be detected by a multichannel analysis of blood sent for another purpose during evaluation of a pregnant woman. The most common cause of asymptomatic hypercalcaemia in a pregnant population is hyperparathyroidism, but it is certainly not common and is present in no more than 0.3% of this group. It should be remembered that the total serum calcium is lowered in pregnancy and a corrective factor for the low albumin concentration should be applied (see above). Thus, total calcium levels within the normal non-pregnant range may represent hypercalcaemia in a pregnant woman.

Hyperparathyroidism in pregnancy is a serious condition associated with a high rate of fetal loss and increased perinatal morbidity and mortality. Several literature reviews [102–105] have reiterated the high risks, which comprise neonatal tetany, stillbirth, neonatal death and abortion. In fact the mother's hyperparathyroidism is occasionally diagnosed only after suspicion provoked by tetany in her newborn baby [106].

Wagner *et al.* [107] found the presence of maternal bone disease (osteitis fibrosa or bone cysts) to be a worrying feature. It was in this group of women that the risk of perinatal mortality was increased. Conversely, pregnancy outcome was not correlated with renal involvement.

Neonatal hypocalcaemia is a result of parathyroid suppression by high ambient calcium levels during intrauterine life. Recovery of normal parathyroid gland function appears to take a considerable time in these infants, and hypocalcaemia may continue for many weeks [106]. Intra-

uterine death may relate to severe hypercalcaemia, as fetal calcium levels exceed maternal [23] because of active transport of calcium across the placenta.

Most women with hyperparathyroidism tolerate pregnancy well. In fact pregnancy may offer some protection against hypercalcaemia because of the low serum albumin and calcium transfer to the fetus. Even so, there are several reports of hypercalcaemic crisis in pregnancy [108–110]. What might seem more likely is postpartum crisis; but this has been reported only three times [111–113]. One case was fatal [113]. The nausea and vomiting of hypercalcaemia may be confused with hyperemesis gravidarum and a case of this, caused by hyperparathyroidism, has been reported [114]. Hyperparathyroidism may also be complicated by acute pancreatitis (see Chapter 9). There is no doubt that the definitive treatment of hyperparathyroidism is surgical. Moreover, neck exploration has proved a relatively safe procedure in pregnancy. In 16 cases reported by Shangold, operation was performed during pregnancy with only one stillbirth, at 26 weeks [110]. The remaining 27 of the 28 fetal losses described occurred in the absence of surgical treatment, as did all of the 35 cases of neonatal tetany. The reviews of Kristoffersson *et al.* [102] and Wilson *et al.* [105] have also concluded that there is a higher risk of fetal and neonatal complications when parathyroidectomy is not performed antenatally. For the fetus therefore maternal parathyroidectomy seems to be the best course of action. Ultrasound may successfully locate a parathyroid adenoma. Isotope studies are contraindicated in pregnancy and often the adenoma or hyperplasia is not located until surgery. If for any reason neck exploration cannot be performed, medical treatment with low calcium diet, high fluid intake and oral phosphate should be commenced. Montoro *et al.* [115] reported success with this therapy. Of course women with mild asymptomatic hypercalcaemia may be followed throughout pregnancy without operation and with good outcome [103].

A recent comprehensive review of this disorder, and other parathyroid problems, is available [27].

HYPOPARATHYROIDISM

In young women this usually represents a complication of thyroid surgery. Rarely, it is part of an autoimmune disorder where antibodies are directed against adrenal, thyroid, gastric and ovarian tissue as well. Treatment is intended to maintain serum calcium within normal limits with vitamin D and oral calcium supplements. In pregnancy the requirement for vitamin D has been seen to increase two- to threefold, as its behaviour in normal pregnancy might suggest [116,117]. For the fetus, the consequences of untreated maternal hypoparathyroidism are serious. There is evidence that severe hypocalcaemia is associated with mid-trimester abortion [118]. Also, intrauterine parathyroid overactivity has been reported [119–121] and neonatal rickets may occur [122]. In those cases where the maternal condition has been undiagnosed or inadequately treated, maternal hypocalcaemia leads to fetal hypocalcaemia, secondary parathyroid hyperplasia and bone demineralization [120,121].

Maternal therapy with oral vitamin D and calcium prevents deleterious effects in the fetus [123,242]. The successful use of oral 1,25-OHD has been reported [116, 124], but this must be monitored carefully as one baby showed increased density of skull and long bones consistent with excessive mineralization [117]. Frequent estimation of maternal calcium and phosphate is necessary and vitamin D is safest given as 1α-OHD or 1,25-OHD. These have the shortest half-life (6–8 h) thereby allowing titration of dose against response. As mentioned, it will usually be necessary to increase the dose to maintain normocalcaemia as pregnancy progresses. However, there is also the danger of provoking hypercalcaemia, particularly if using the potent synthetic analogue of vitamin D, dihydrotachysterol [125] or calcitriol. Moreover, continuation of these high doses into the puerperium is hazardous. When the dose is not decreased after delivery, serious maternal hypercalcaemia may ensue and has also been reported in a breastfed infant [126]. Calcium monitoring is indicated.

In pseudohypoparathyroidism there is end-organ resistance to the actions of PTH resulting in hypocalcaemia and renal resistance to the phosphaturic effect of PTH. The implications for pregnancy are the same as in hypoparathyroidism [124,126]. The therapy is identical although patients have been described in whom prior vitamin D dependency disappeared in pregnancy without treatment, suggesting placental production of 1,25-OHD.

Other inherited skeletal and metabolic disorders

Osteogenesis imperfecta

This is a generalized disorder affecting connective tissue. The most common variety (tarda) has autosomal dominant inheritance with very variable penetrance and expression. Less common is osteogenesis imperfecta congenita, which is inherited as an autosomal recessive but which is lethal with death occurring *in utero* or in the immediate neonatal period. Second-trimester diagnosis of osteogenesis imperfecta congenita by ultrasound is now an established technique in pregnancies at risk [139]. Pope *et al.* [140] have characterized a deletion within a collagen gene in four cases of lethal congenital osteogenesis imperfecta, which makes it likely that prenatal diagnosis from chorion biopsy material will soon be available [141].

In osteogenesis imperfecta tarda, the basic defect is not known but the fully developed syndrome involves blue sclerae, deafness from otosclerosis, multiple fractures, joint laxity and heart valve abnormalities. Metabolic abnormalities include impaired platelet function and hyperpyrexia during general anaesthesia [142].

The bones are porotic and fragile, and repeated fractures leave the sufferer with skeletal deformity. The pelvis is often misshapen with subsequent cephalopelvic disproportion. Ultrasound or radiography of the fetus should be performed before delivery. If the baby is affected, it is best to minimize birth trauma and this usually means delivery by caesarean section.

Because of the potential complications of general anaesthesia (hyperpyrexia, skeletal injury to the unconscious patient, respiratory embarrassment from kyphoscoliosis), a lumbar epidural is the anaesthesia of choice, although accurate needle placement may be difficult due to bony deformity [143].

Scoliosis is the most common deformity. If severe, it is accompanied by diminished lung volume, as in the case of Sengupta *et al.* [144]. Despite the fact that respiratory difficulties have not been prominent in the reported cases, pulmonary function should be monitored.

No therapy is of proven benefit in this disorder. Even so, all patients should be given calcium supplements as a propensity for hypocalcaemia in pregnancy has been demonstrated [145].

Achondroplasia

Inheritance is autosomal dominant, but many cases represent new mutations. Women with this bony disorder tend to have an early menopause. They have an increased prevalence of uterine fibroids.

During pregnancy, cardiorespiratory compromise due to restriction of lung volume is a risk as the fetus grows larger. All women with achondroplasia require caesarean section because of pelvic contraction. The choice of anaesthetic technique is not easy. Tracheal intubation for general anaesthesia may be impossible because of abnormalities of the airway [146,147]. But also spinal stenosis can make epidural block difficult. Epidural block is probably the better of two difficult options [148]. Fetal achondroplasia may be diagnosed by ultrasound, even early in the second trimester [149,150], with detection of abnormal limbs.

Other rare, inherited bone disorders

There are a number of very rare bone dysplasias. They will not be discussed here but details can be found in the articles of Hall [146] and Allanson and Hall [151].

Marfan's syndrome

This generalized disorder of connective tissue displays autosomal dominant inheritance. It has recently been shown that Marfan's syndrome is due to a defect in fibrillin synthesis. In Marfan's syndrome (but not in some other marfanoid conditions such as contractural arachnodactyly) this defect is due to mutations of a fibrillin gene on chromosome 15 [152]. Definitive diagnosis in the index case and prenatal diagnosis in fetuses of patients with Marfan's disease is now possible in many families.

The chief defects in Marfan's syndrome are in the skeletal, ocular and cardiovascular systems. The cardiovascular problems are dominant particularly in pregnancy and these are considered in Chapter 5 where the similar problems of Ehlers–Danlos syndrome are also discussed.

There is an increase in length of the tubular bones and also there are weak, yielding ligaments leading to joint laxity and kyphoscoliosis. These abnormalities usually cause no problem in pregnancy; neither is there any severe structural problem with the pelvis. Women with Marfan's syndrome have an increased risk of spontaneous abortion with low-birthweight babies [153] and also of preterm labour [154]. Spontaneous uterine inversion in association with Marfan's syndrome has been reported [155] and so has the formation of rectovaginal fistula [156].

Homocystinuria

Homocystinuria is a condition in which deficiency of cystathionine β synthase results in increased plasma levels of homocysteine and methionine and decreased plasma cysteine. It is inherited as an autosomal recessive but there is considerable heterogeneity in its expression because some patients, more severely affected, do not respond to pyridoxine whilst others do. Hyperhomocysteinaemia is a separate condition causing elevated homocysteine levels. It is considered in Chapter 4. The major clinical effects of homocystinuria are mental retardation and seizures, dislocation of the optic lens, osteoporosis and thromboembolism, the last being the most frequent cause of mortality [157]. The mechanism of thromboembolism is not known. Treatment is by methionine restriction and pyridoxine administration in those patients responsive to pyridoxine.

The condition has been reviewed in 629 patients on the basis of an international questionnaire by Mudd *et al.* [157]. These authors also discussed 108 pregnancies amongst 47 homocystinuric women [157]. The majority (88%) occurred in pyridoxine-responsive women, either because of their higher intelligence and better general health, or because of some undefined factor acting against fertility in pyridoxine-resistant patients. The overall poor results (40% pregnancy loss rate) are dominated by three patients who between them lost 22 pregnancies. These women may also represent a subset with a specific abnormality mitigating against successful pregnancy. However, patients with modestly elevated homocysteine levels who are heterozygotes for homocystinuria also have high perinatal mortality rates [158], and recurrent abortion and placental abruption have been reported in association with hyperhomocysteinaemia in general [159]. (Homocysteine levels may also be elevated because of abnormalities in folate and vitamin B_{12} metabolism.) Hyperhomocysteinaemia is a known risk factor for premature vascular disease [160]. Therefore, by analogy with patients with the antiphospholipid syndrome (see Chapter 8) who are also at risk from stillbirth and thromboembolism, the abnormality in homocystinuria may cause extensive placental infarction, although this suggestion remains speculative.

Thromboembolism is the other cause for concern. In non-pregnant patients thromboembolism is a major cause of mortality and it may also occur postoperatively [157]. There have been at least two cases of cerebrovascular disease reported in pregnancy; one a fatal case in a woman with a poor obstetric history [161] and the other occurring in a heterozygote following caesarean section [162]. Yet Brenton *et al.* [163] have reviewed seven pregnancies under their care that were all uncomplicated. The patients were able to maintain normal methionine levels taking pyridoxine with no change in their biochemical control during pregnancy.

So the decision concerning thromboprophylaxis in pregnancy is difficult. Standard 'high-risk' prophylaxis would involve giving heparin throughout pregnancy but this would increase the risk of osteoporosis (see Chapter 4) to which these patients are already exposed. The cases of thromboembolism that have occurred have both been after delivery. Perhaps the best compromise would be antenatal low-dose aspirin (75 mg/day). This has been used in the non-pregnant state [157] in homocystinuria and also may improve the fetal outcome (see above and Chapter 8). At delivery patients could be treated with low-dose subcutaneous heparin continuing for at least 1 week postpartum with a further 5 weeks of subcutaneous heparin or warfarin (see Chapter 4). Patients who have already had thromboembolism, who have a poor family history, who have ultrasound evidence of pre-existing vascular disease [164] or who are unable to maintain normal methionine levels may need to consider subcutaneous heparin treatment throughout pregnancy.

Pseudoxanthoma elasticum

Pseudoxanthoma elasticum is inherited as an autosomal recessive condition, although dominant inheritance has been reported. It is characterized by degeneration and calcification of elastic tissue causing characteristic skin, which is very lax and appears prematurely aged particularly around the neck. In addition abnormalities may be seen in the retina on fundoscopy (angioid streaks) and are present in blood vessels leading to premature cerebral, coronary and peripheral vascular disease. Hypertension was present in 22% of 200 cases [165]. Weakness of splanchnic arteries may lead to gastrointestinal bleeding. Mitral valve prolapse is common [166]. Until 1987 there had been about 28 pregnancies reported in 11 women [167,168]. Haematemesis was common and often required blood transfusion. It was clearly the major risk in pregnancy, although patients are not necessarily more susceptible to haemorrhage in pregnancy than in the non-pregnant state. Because many patients have hypertension and because they are at risk from cerebrovascular disease, any additional hypertension due to pre-eclampsia should be treated aggressively [168]. However, in 1987 a large study was reported from South Africa concerning pseudoxanthoma elasticum in 54 pregnancies [169]. The risk of haemorrhage was not confirmed although the risk of hypertension was. First-trimester miscarriage and the cosmetic problems of lax abdominal skin in multigravidae were additional features. Further review [170] also suggests that pseudoxanthoma elasticum may not be as dangerous as previously thought.

Phenylketonuria

Classical phenylketonuria (PKU) results from an inborn error of metabolism, inherited as an autosomal recessive, whereby phenylalanine is not metabolized to tyrosine because of the absence of phenylalanine hydroxylase. Its metabolic precursor, phenylpyruvic acid, is then excreted in the urine. It is usually diagnosed in the newborn by the Guthrie test, which detects the excess of phenylalanine in the blood, although rarely, the diagnosis is suspected in an adult who escaped detection at birth. The diagnosis is confirmed by quantifying the high level of phenylalanine and low level of tyrosine. There exist a wide variety of genetic aberrations resulting in hyperphenylalaninaemia, of which classical PKU is the prototype and most severe.

If a pregnant woman with PKU is left untreated, the risk to the offspring of severe intellectual handicap is 92%, microcephaly 73% and congenital heart disease 12% [175]. These outcomes are entirely avoidable by means of appropriate diet instituted from early infancy.

Since phenylalanine is present in nearly all proteins, dietary treatment consists of virtual elimination of natural proteins, and substitution of an hydrolysate of amino acid with very low phenylalanine content. Children must continue the diet and amino acid supplement throughout childhood to at least early adolescence to allow normal neurological development. Neonatal screening and early dietary intervention are so efficient that it is now very unusual to see children with severe mental handicap from PKU who were diagnosed in the newborn period [172]. When the children return to a normal diet, at between 10 and 15 years of age, blood levels of phenylalanine rise again. There is some controversy concerning the need for lifelong continuation of the diet. Many believe that general well-being, intellectual, psychological and neurological functions are improved if the diet is reinstituted in adulthood. The traditional view has been that there is no need to follow the diet after mid-teenage, when brain development is complete. As yet, there is no controlled trial evidence to confirm either of these views, and return to diet should be seen as an option, albeit an expensive one, for those who believe they feel improved by adhering to it.

Many girls with PKU previously treated in childhood are now reaching reproductive age. In addition some individuals with milder forms of previously undiagnosed hyperphenylalaninaemia are being detected in screening programmes [173]. It is now realized that PKU is quite an heterogeneous condition. More than 40 different mutations of the phenylalanine hydroxylase gene have been identified [174] resulting in a range of phenylalanine levels from only just over those found in heterozygotes to 20 times the normal level.

In regard to the implications for pregnancy, it is known that high levels of maternal phenylalanine <1.2 mmol/L ('classical PKU') transmitted across the placenta result in problems. These include a very high incidence of abortion, intrauterine growth retardation, fetal congenital abnormalities, almost exclusively congenital heart disease [175] and in particular tetralogy of Fallot [176], microcephaly and mental retardation [173,177–179]. The risk of microcephaly and mental retardation appears to be 75% in the infants of women with phenylalanine levels between 0.96 and 1.2 mmol/L [172]. The association is not complete. Some normal infants have been born to mothers with moderate to severe hyperphenylalaninaemia in pregnancy [180] but the chance of producing a normal infant in these circumstances is very low, and severity of adverse outcome is, in general, directly proportional to the mean phenylalanine level during the pregnancy. The Maternal PKU Collaborative Study reported on 576 women in 2000. In pregnancies where control (less than 0.6 mmol/L) was established preconceptionally or before 8–10 weeks, congenital heart disease and microcephaly were at normal population incidence [232].

Previously, Levy and Waisbren [177] found that the child's IQ was proportional to maternal IQ and inversely to maternal phenylalanine level. With one exception amongst 53 children they found mental retardation only where the maternal phenylalanine level was >1.1 mmol/ L [177]. However, as others have pointed out [181,182] in the data of Levy and Waisbren [177] there was a steady decline of IQ levels with increasing maternal phenylalanine >0.4 mmol/L. The 1987 report of the Maternal PKU Collaborative Study showed neurological outcome proportional to average levels down to 0.36 mmol/L. Below that, the chance of neurological sequelae or cardiac abnormality was remote [241]. The most recent report, of 253 children at age 4 years, was published in 2000. This report also noted that delayed development in the children of women with PKU is associated with lack of control before and early in pregnancy. Nearly 50% of offspring had a General Cognitive Index score 2 standard deviations below the norm when metabolic control was not achieved by 20 weeks [233]. It is clear that if dietary therapy is to be effective, it must be started before conception [183].

Fetal neurological development does not depend upon the PKU genotype of the baby. The absence of the PKU gene in a fetus did not improve its outcome, at least in a comparison of phenylketonuric and non-phenylketonuric siblings born to a woman with untreated PKU in pregnancy [171]. Both babies were exposed to high intrauterine phenylalanine levels, but low postnatal levels, in one resulting from postnatal diet therapy, in the other from the fact that PKU was absent. The neurological outcome was similarly abnormal in both, demonstrating the irreversibility of intrauterine damage.

The reintroduction of dietary therapies can certainly improve the fetal prognosis [184,185] even if started in the third trimester [186] though the latter has been disputed [187]. However, abnormal babies have occasionally been born to women taking adequate dietary therapy [188,189], including one case of congenital heart disease in a woman who started a diet at 6 weeks' gestation [190] An earlier collaborative international study of 64 pregnancies [183] suggested that the fetus will not be grossly affected if the maternal diet results in a phenylalanine concentration <600 μmol/L at the time of conception and if this diet is maintained through pregnancy.

Since there is some suggestion that low maternal tyrosine levels may also harm the fetus [193], dietary tyrosine supplementation has also been used [185,192]. The diet will also require supplementation with glucose, vitamins and minerals [185]. Since the reintroduction of a low phenylalanine diet may be difficult, and, since conception may be unexpected, girls should be encouraged to continue the diet into adult life, at least in a modified form if not as diligently as in childhood [194]. The question of lifelong adherence to the diet as an item of necessity is yet to be resolved.

Some children with PKU may be lost to follow-up and, because of the evidence that moderate elevations of phenylalanine in the blood do not cause PKU but are still harmful to the fetus [173], there is a case for a routine screening test in pregnancy [195]. Ideally, the test should be for hyperphenylalaninaemia [173]. The Guthrie test has been used [188] as have urine screening tests [184]. Since the maximum gain appears to be from treatment instituted before conception, such a screen should really be part of a pre-pregnancy or premarital screening service [188,196]. Nevertheless, the yield of such screening tests is low: one in 10 000 Guthrie tests performed in pregnancy in Glasgow [188]. Screening may be more worthwhile in populations where the risk of PKU is greater. Hyanek *et al.* [173] found nine cases of abnormal amino acid metabolism in 15 000 women screened by blood paper chromatography in Czechoslovakia. Screening for maternal PKU should be part of the investigation of any microcephalic infant or fetus.

It was estimated that there were 500 fertile women with PKU in the UK in the year 2000 [183]. There are no specific pregnancy complications in maternal PKU, apart from a slight excess of intrauterine growth retardation. However, the emotional strain put on the mother, by worrying about the fetal outcome, by having to undergo frequent blood monitoring and by having to follow a demanding and in many ways unappetizing diet, may be considerable. Analysis of maternal levels of phenylalanine should be undertaken every 1–2 weeks during pregnancy, with dietary adjustment proceeding through the different stages. For example, with vomiting in early pregnancy and reduced energy intake, the woman may catabolize her own protein stores resulting in elevated levels of phenylalanine despite apparent dietary compliance. The dietitian will need to arrive at strategies to deal with such variations during the pregnancy. Even relatively minor intercurrent illness, such as urinary infection, may be enough to promote a catabolic state.

It is important to perform a detailed scan of the fetus early in gestation to diagnose congenital heart disease and other abnormalities which may ensue [176]. Breastfeeding can be allowed, since the increased dietary load of phenylalanine in breast milk will not cause hyperphenylalaninaemia in the newborn [185], assuming PKU is not present. The chance of PKU in the newborn is 1–2%, given the population prevalence of the carrier state in the partner. In the future, transfer of normal genes for phenylalanine hydroxylase to liver cells may allow patients to maintain normal phenylalanine levels without dietary therapy [172].

Finally but most importantly, it is essential that young girls after menarche be educated time and again as to the dangers to the developing infant resulting from their conceiving with high levels of phenylalanine. PKU, as we have discussed, represents the paradigm of a condition demanding preconception counselling. Poor control in early pregnancy has an even higher risk of adverse fetal consequences than that of poorly controlled diabetes.

Thus, referral of women with PKU to a specialist clinic for preconception counselling, including dietary treatment to continue over the time of conception [191], is highly advisable. Attendance only after conception may be after damage has been sustained. The consequences of delivering a damaged infant after uncontrolled PKU in pregnancy are dire and will dominate the family's life for many years after that pregnancy. Dietary advice requires the assistance of a dietitian with experience in the management of this disorder, one of the most technically difficult to treat of all the diseases requiring dietetic assistance.

Hyperxanthinuria, hyperglycinaemia, hypertyrosinaemia, 3-MGA aciduria

In the few cases of hyperxanthinuria reported in pregnancy there has been no evidence of excess fetal abnormalities [197,198]. Nevertheless, one patient lost two out of three pregnancies, both associated with prematurity [197]. Mothers are at risk from the formation of xanthine urinary stones. Maternal uric acid levels—which are helpful in the management of hypertensive disease in pregnancy (see Chapter 6)—cannot be relied upon because of the impairment of uric acid formation, which is part of the metabolic block [197].

Hyanek et al. [173] report that one of two cases of maternal hyperglycinaemia was associated with mental retardation in the newborn. Two children from a woman with hypertyrosinaemia were normal. 3-methylglutaconic aciduria (3-MGA aciduria) is another aminoaciduria with several hypothesized inborn errors of metabolism. A group of seven children born to six mothers with 3-MGA aciduria has been described. All had microcephaly and mental retardation; no normal children were recorded born to mothers with 3-MGA aciduria. In some families, parental consanguinity may have been a factor [198a].

Glycogen storage diseases (Gaucher's disease, Forbe's disease)

The glycogen storage diseases are characterized by various abnormalities in the synthesis of glycogen. The abnormal glycogens are deposited in the monocytes and macrophages of the reticuloendothelial system so that affected patients suffer chronic ill-health due to abnormalities of the liver, spleen and bone marrow. The glycogen storage diseases are much more common in Ashkenazi Jews, and prenatal diagnosis is usually available to detect homozygotes [199].

Gaucher's disease is an autosomal recessive disorder in which there is a deficit of acid β-glucosidase. The genetic basis of the disease has now been characterized and it is possible to detect heterozygotes for counselling and homozygotes for prenatal diagnosis [200]. Enzyme therapy is available at the staggering cost of US $550 000 per year [201]; in the near future gene replacement therapy is likely to be a realistic option [201].

Goldblatt and Beighton [199] have reviewed 21 pregnancies in their personal series of more than 50 patients. They conclude that there is no evidence that pregnancy affects the course of Gaucher's disease or that fertility is affected by Gaucher's disease. Potential problems in pregnancy relate to haematological and orthopaedic complications and the worry about splenic rupture. Most patients have a mild chronic anaemia. This may become more obvious in pregnancy but apart from giving extra folate and iron, no specific therapy is necessary; transfusion is very rarely indicated [199]. Thrombocytopenia is more worrying because it has been associated with postpartum haemorrhage in seven pregnancies in two patients of the South African series [199]. Prophylactic crossmatching and early transfusion are indicated. Platelet transfusion is generally unhelpful because the platelets are rapidly destroyed by the enlarged spleen. Similar results in pregnancy have been reported in 47 pregnancies from Jerusalem [202].

Although there may be considerable skeletal deformities in Gaucher's disease, these do not usually affect the pelvis and only one patient in the South African series required delivery by caesarean section for cephalopelvic disproportion [199]. Splenomegaly, which may become more marked in pregnancy, is obviously of concern because of the possibility of rupture [203]. However, there have been no cases of splenic rupture in association with labour and Goldblatt and Beighton [199] conclude that the only indication for splenectomy should be haematological [204]; if elective splenectomy is to be performed in pregnancy, the second trimester is preferred [199].

In Forbe's disease, the abnormality is a deficiency of amylo-1,6-glucosidase. In addition to the problems above,

Confino *et al.* [205] have drawn attention to the associated problems with glucose metabolism that may be exaggerated by pregnancy. It is not clear whether such patients are particularly at risk of developing diabetes but whether they are or not, their pregnancies have the potential for being complicated by gestational diabetes as does any other pregnancy. If they do require insulin for blood glucose control, they are particularly likely to develop hypoglycaemia because their metabolic abnormalities impair glucose release from glycogen. In some forms of glycogen storage disease (e.g. von Gierke's disease) cornstarch may be preferable as a source of carbohydrate in pregnancy [206] because by contrast with glycogen, debranching enzymes can release glucose from cornstarch.

Hereditary angioneurotic oedema

Hereditary angioneurotic oedema is inherited as an autosomal dominant. The inheritance of recurrent attacks of abdominal pain and oedema of the extremities, face and larynx was first described by Osler [207]. Laryngeal oedema may be fatal. More recently it has been demonstrated that the condition is due to an abnormality of the serum inhibitor of the activated first component of complement (C1-esterase inhibitor). If C1-esterase inhibitor is either reduced in concentration (common form) or abnormal in function (variant form) the complement cascade can be activated by mild and often undetected trigger factors causing angioneurotic oedema. Attacks of abdominal pain are thought to be due to oedema of the intestines. Alteration of C1-inhibitor genes in both common [208] and variant forms have been reported but it is not clear to what extent these spectacular advances in the 'new biology' should be applied to antenatal diagnosis of a condition compatible with normal lifespan.

The first treatment used to prevent attacks was ε-aminocaproic acid (EACA), which inhibits the fibrinolytic system in general and also inhibits C1 activation [209]. However, such treatment has been limited by muscle pain, weakness and the potential for thromboembolism [209], and the latter would be of particular concern in pregnancy. EACA therapy has largely been superseded by androgens, particularly danazol, because they have been shown to reduce the frequency of attacks and increase the plasma level of C1-esterase inhibitor [210]. More recently, concentrates of C1-esterase inhibitor have been made available, and although these are very expensive and must be given intravenously, they should be used to treat acute attacks [211]. Fresh frozen plasma may be used [212] if the concentrate is unavailable. Corticosteroid therapy and adrenaline (epinephrine) are not effective. In life-threatening episodes endotracheal intubation or tracheostomy should be used.

There is no consensus concerning the interaction between pregnancy and hereditary angioneurotic oedema in the cases that have been reported [209,213–220]. It has been suggested that studies of the molecular form of high molecular weight kininogen present in pregnancy may predict the 'at-risk' patient [214] but this remains to be confirmed. If there is any tendency, pregnancy decreases the frequency of attacks [209] and that has certainly been our experience in one patient. However, in another the attacks became more frequent. Nevertheless, danazol therapy should be discontinued because of the risk of masculinization of a female fetus.

Clinicians should be aware that abdominal pain in pregnancy may or may not be due to the condition. As always, history is of vital importance. One of our patients who had a concealed accidental haemorrhage was able to indicate that the pain had a different character from that of her usual attacks of abdominal pain thus facilitating her treatment. Although trauma may initiate attacks of hereditary angioneurotic oedema and one patient has died from laryngeal oedema following vaginal delivery [219], it does not seem that vaginal delivery is associated with any greater risk of angio-oedema [220]. On this basis caesarean section should be reserved for the usual obstetric indications. Epidural anaesthesia is preferred to general anaesthesia because intubation may itself precipitate an attack of laryngeal angio-oedema [218]. Patients should be given prophylactic treatment with C1-esterase inhibitor concentrate or failing that, 2 units of fresh frozen plasma before any abdominal surgery. There is no reason why such patients should not breast feed.

Porphyria

The porphyrias are disorders of haem synthesis, which may be inherited or acquired. Porphyrins are intermediates in the haem synthetic pathway formed from δ-aminolevulinic acid and porphobilinogen and different porphyrins accumulate in the various disorders.

The chief clinical manifestations are acute attacks of neurological dysfunction (the acute porphyrias) or chronic cutaneous photosensitivity (the cutaneous porphyrias).

The acute porphyrias, acute intermittent porphyria (AIP), variegate porphyria (VP) and hereditary coproporphyria (HC), are of significance in pregnancy. Each of these may present acutely with abdominal pain, fever and leucocytosis, which may mimic other intra-abdominal conditions. Labile hypertension and tachycardia are further confusing features and some patients have symptoms

Table 14.2 Drugs that may precipitate an acute porphyric attack.

Barbiturates	Methyldopa
Carbamazepine	Metoclopramide
Chlordiazepoxide	Metronidazole
Chlormethiazole	Nitrazepam
Clonidine	Oestrogens
Danazol	Oral contraceptives
Dimenhydrinate	Pancuronium
Ergot derivatives	Phenytoin
Erythromycin	Progesterone
Ethanol	Ranitidine
Frusemide (furosemide)	Steroids
Halothane	Sulphonamides
Hydralazine	Theophylline
Lidocaine	

of nervous system involvement such as neuropathy or psychiatric disturbance. Neuropathy typically follows the abdominal symptoms by at least 3 days.

A review in 1971 [221] described 72 cases in pregnancy with a 27% mortality rate. However, a later study of 50 women with acute porphyria recorded only one death [222]. Fetal loss was 13% in this study. Just over half of the women with AIP had an attack during pregnancy and the babies from these pregnancies weighed an average of 800 g less than in pregnancies free from attack. About 25% of the attacks occurred after delivery and frequently were precipitated by intrapartum barbiturate therapy. The effects of pregnancy on HC and VP were less pronounced with only 25% and 33%, respectively, having attacks.

The activity of erythrocyte porphobilinogen deaminase activity in AIP is not affected by pregnancy [223]. However, the incidence of acute porphyric attacks is increased in pregnancy, and both oestrogens and progestogens are known to provoke attacks in non-pregnant women. Attacks can also be precipitated by alcohol excess and fasting, and many drugs may activate an acute attack. Some drugs that may be met in obstetric practice and should be avoided are listed in Table 14.2. Before the use of any drug in a patient with porphyria it is strongly advisable to seek assistance from a specialist in the field. Kantor and Rolbin [224] have discussed the drugs used in anaesthesia.

Treatment of the acute attack is firstly supportive with careful monitoring of fluid and electrolyte balance. Intravenous glucose at a rate of 20 g/h is recommended and, if no improvement within 48 h is seen, an intravenous infusion of haematin may be tried though this improves the biochemical abnormalities more than the clinical features [225,226]. β blockade is used for tachycardia and hypertension. Of course close fetal monitoring is necessary when a woman has an acute attack.

Ornithine carbamoyltransferase deficiency

This is a rather rare X-linked disorder of urea synthesis, which usually presents to paediatricians when newborn boys die from hyperammonaemic coma. But it has recently been reported that female carriers are also susceptible to cortical impairment varying from subtle abnormalities of cognitive thinking to fatal coma; and that coma is particularly likely to occur after delivery [227]. Arn *et al.* [227] described five such women who between them had six episodes of coma, four of which occurred between 3 and 8 days postpartum and two of which were fatal. In each postpartum case the fetus was not affected so perhaps the fetus had been providing ureagenic activity for its mother. The condition should be considered in any woman who becomes comatose for no obvious reason after delivery. There may be decorticate posturing and raised intracranial pressure. The diagnosis is suggested by elevated ammonia levels in the presence of normal liver function and confirmed by high levels of glutamine and low levels of citrullin and arginine. Treatment is with intravenous sodium benzoate, sodium phenylacetate and arginine hydrochloride [227]. A biochemical screening test using allopurinol is available for screening female carriers [228].

References

1 Arnaud SB, Matthusen M *et al.* Components of 25-hydroxyvitamin D in serum of young children in upper midwestern United States. *Am J Clin Nutr* 1977; 30: 1082–6.
2 Gray TK, Lester GE *et al.* Evidence for extrarenal 1-hydroxylation of 25-hydroxyvitamin D3 in pregnancy. *Science* 1979; 204: 1311–13.
3 Halhai A, Diaz L, Sanchez I *et al.* Effects of IGF-I on 1, 25 dihydroxyvitamin D(3) synthesis on human placenta in culture. *Mol Hum Reprod* 1999, 5: 771–6.
4 Goodwin D, Noff D *et al.* 24,25-Dihydroxyvitamin D is a metabolite of vitamin D essential for bone formation. *Nature* 1978; 276: 517.

5 Holtrop ME, Cox KA *et al.* 1,25-Dihydroxycholecalciferol stimulates osteoclasts in rat bones in the absence of parathyroid hormone. *Endocrinology* 1981; 108: 2293–301.

6 Raisz LC, Trummel CL *et al.* 1,25-Dihydroxycholecalciferol: a potent stimulator of bone reabsorption in tissue culture. *Science* 1972; 175: 786–9.

7 Brown DJ, Spanos E *et al.* Role of pituitary hormones in regulating renal vitamin D metabolism in man. *Br Med J* 1980; 280: 277–8.

8 Spanos E, Pike JW *et al.* Circulating 1 alpha, 25 dihydroxyvitamin D in the chicken: enhancement by injection of prolactin and during egg laying. *Life Sci* 1976; 19: 1751–6.

9 Verdy M, Beaulieu R *et al.* Plasma calcitonin activity in a patient with thyroid medullary carcinoma and her children with osteopetrosis. *J Clin Endocrinol* 1971; 32: 216–21.

10 Hytten FE, Leitch I. *The Physiology of Human Pregnancy*, 2nd edn. Blackwell Scientific Publications, Oxford, 1971: 383.

11 Feeley RM, Eitenmiller RR *et al.* Calcium, phosphorus, and magnesium contents of human milk during early lactation. *J Pediatr Gastroenterol Nutr* 1983; 2: 262–7.

12 Ritchie LD, Fung EB *et al.* A longitudinal study of calcium homeostasis during human pregnancy and lactation and after resumption of menses. *Am J Clin Nutr* 1998; 67: 693–701.

13 Sowers M, Corton G *et al.* Changes in bone density with lactation. *J Am Med Assoc* 1993; 269: 3130–5.

13a Kent GN, Price RI *et al.* The efficiency of intestinal calcium absorption is increased in late pregnancy but not in established lactation. *Calcif Tissue Int* 1991; 48: 293–5.

14 Heaney RP, Skillman TG. Calcium metabolism in normal human pregnancy. *J Clin Endocrinol Metabolism* 1971; 33: 661–70.

15 Shenolikar IS. Absorption of dietary calcium in pregnancy. *Am J Clin Nutr* 1970; 23: 63–7.

16 Cross NA, Hillman LS *et al.* Calcium homeostasis and bone metabolism during pregnancy, lactation, and postweaning: a longitudinal study. *Am J Clin Nutr* 1995; 61: 514–23.

17 Gertner JM, Coustan DR *et al.* Pregnancy as a state of physiologic absorptive hypercalciuria. *Am J Med* 1986; 81: 451–6.

17a Sowers M, Zhang D *et al.* Role of calciotrophic hormones in calcium mobilization of lactation. *Am J Clin Nutr* 1998; 67: 284–91

17b Weiss M, Eisenstein Z et al. Renal reabsorption of inorganic phosphorus in pregnancy in relation to the calciotropic hormones. *Br J Obstet Gynaecol* 1998; 105: 195–9.

18 Kumar R, Cohen WR *et al.* Elevated 1,25-dihydroxyvitamin D plasma levels in normal human pregnancy and lactation. *J Clin Invest* 1979; 63: 342–4.

19 Reddy GS, Norman AW *et al.* Regulation of vitamin D metabolism in normal human pregnancy. *J Clin Endocrinol Metabolism* 1983; 56: 363–70.

20 Whitehead M, Lane G *et al.* Interrelations of calcium regulating hormones during normal pregnancy. *Br Med J* 1981; 283: 10–12.

20a Seely EW, Brown EM et al. A prospective study of calciotropic hormones in pregnancy and postpartum: reciprocal changes in serum intact parathyroid hormone and 1,25-dihydroxyvitamin D. *Am J Obstet Gynecol* 1997; 176: 214–17

21 Lund B, Selnes A. Plasma 1,25-dihydroxyvitamin D levels in pregnancy and lactation. *Acta Endocrinol* 1979; 92: 330–5.

22 Wieland P, Fischer JA *et al.* Perinatal parathyroid hormone, vitamin D metabolites and calcitonin in man. *Am J Physiol* 1980; 239: E38590.

23 Steichen JJ, Tsang RC *et al.* Vitamin D homeostasis in the perinatal period. *N Engl J Med* 1980; 302: 315–19.

24 Curtiss PH, Kincaid WE. Transitory demineralization of the hip in pregnancy: a report of three cases. *J Bone Joint Surg* 1959; 41: 1327–30.

25 Pitkin RM, Reynolds WA *et al.* Calcium metabolism in normal pregnancy. A longitudinal study. *Am J Obstet Gynecol* 1979; 133: 781–91.

26 Allgrove J, Adami S *et al.* Cytochemical bioassay of parathyroid hormone in maternal and cord blood. *Arch Dis Child* 1985; 60: 110–15.

27 Mestman JH. Parathyroid disorders of pregnancy. *Semin Perinatol* 1998; 22: 485–96.

28 Gallagher JC, Riggs BL *et al.* Effect of estrogen therapy on calcium absorption and vitamin D metabolism in postmenopausal osteoporosis. *Clin Res* 1987; 26: 415A.

29 Nordin BEC, Heyburn PJ *et al.* Osteoporosis and osteomalacia. *Clin Endocrinol Metab* 1980; 9: 177–205.

30 Castillo L, Tanaka Y *et al.* Production of 1,25-dihydroxyvitamin D3 and formation of medullary bone in the egg-laying hen. *Endocrinology* 1979; 104: 1598–601.

31 Tanaka Y, Castillo L *et al.* Synergistic effect of progesterone, testosterone, and estradiol in the stimulation of chick renal 25-hydroxyvitamin D-1 alpha-hydroxylase. *Endocrinology* 1978; 103: 2035–9.

32 Newman RL. Serum electrolytes in pregnancy, parturition and the puerperium. *Obstet Gynecol* 1957; 10: 51–5.

33 Fogh-Anderson N, Schultz-Larsen P. Free calcium ion concentration in pregnancy. *Acta Obstet Gynecol Scand* 1981; 60: 309–12.

34 Martinez ME, Sanchez C *et al.* Ionic calcium levels during pregnancy, at delivery and in the first hours of life. *Scand J Clin Lab Invest* 1986; 46: 27–30.

35 Moniz DF, Nicolaides KM *et al.* Normal reference ranges for biochemical substances relating to renal, hepatic, and bone function in fetal and maternal plasma throughout pregnancy. *J Clin Pathol* 1985; 38: 468–72.

36 Westin B, Kaiser IH *et al.* Some constituents of umbilical venous blood of previable human fetuses. *Acta Paediatr Scand* 1959; 48: 609–13.

37 Whitsett JA, Tsang RC. Calcium uptake and binding by membrane fractions of human placenta: ATP-dependent calcium accumulation. *Pediatr Res* 1980; 14: 769–75.

38 Tsang R, Abrams L *et al.* Ionised calcium in neonates in relation to gestational age. *J Pediatr* 1979; 94: 126–9.

39 Kuoppala T, Tiumala R *et al.* Can the fetus regulate its calcium uptake? *Br J Obstet Gynaecol* 1984; 91: 1192–6.

40 Care AD, Caple IW *et al.* The effect of fetal thyro-parathyroidectomy on the transport of calcium across the ovine placenta of the fetus. *Placenta* 1986; 7: 417–24.

41 Dent CE, Friedman M. Pregnancy and idiopathic osteoporosis. *Q J Med* 1965; 34: 314–57.

42 MacLennan WJ, Hamilton JC *et al.* The effects of season and stage of pregnancy on plasma 25-hydroxyvitamin D concentrations in pregnant women. *Postgrad Med J* 1980; 56: 75–9.

43 Cockburn F, Belton NR *et al.* Maternal vitamin D intake and mineral metabolism in mothers and their newborn infants. *Br Med J* 1980; 281: 11–14.

44 Kokkonen J, Koivisto M *et al.* Seasonal variation in serum-25-OHD3 in mothers and newborn infants in Northern Finland. *Acta Paediatr Scand* 1983; 72: 93–6.

45 Hillman LS, Haddad JG. Perinatal vitamin D metabolism. III. Factors influencing late gestational human serum 25-hydroxyvitamin D. *Am J Obstet Gynecol* 1976; 125: 196–200.

46 Serenius F, Elidrissy ATH *et al.* Vitamin D nutrition in pregnant women at term and in newly born babies in Saudi Arabia. *J Clin Pathol* 1984; 37: 444–7.

47 Taha SA, Dost SM *et al.* 25-Hydroxyvitamin D and total calcium: extraordinary low plasma concentrations in Saudi mothers and their neonates. *Pediatr Res* 1984; 18: 739–41.

48 Brooke OG, Brown IRF *et al.* Vitamin D supplements in pregnant Asian women. effects on calcium status and fetal growth. *Br Med J* 1980; i: 751–4.

49 Hillman LS, Haddad JG. Human perinatal vitamin D metabolism. I. 25-hydroxyvitamin D in maternal and cord blood. *J Pediatr* 1974; 84: 742–9.

50 Stevenson JC, Hillyard CJ *et al.* A physiological role for calcitonin. Protection of the maternal skeleton. *Lancet* 1979; ii: 769–70.

51 Kovarik J, Woloszczuk W *et al.* Calcitonin in pregnancy. *Lancet* 1980; i: 199–200.

52 Samaan NA, Anderson GD *et al.* Immunoreactive calcitonin in the mother, neonate, child and adult. *Am J Obstet Gynecol* 1975; 121: 622–5.

53 Walker ARP, Richardson B *et al.* The influence of numerous pregnancies and lactations on bone dimensions in South African Bantu and Caucasian mothers. *Clin Sci* 1972; 42: 189–96.

54 Goldsmith NF, Johnston JO. Bone mineral. Effects of oral contraceptives, pregnancy and lactation. *J Bone Joint Surg Am* 1975; 57A: 657–68.

55 Nilsson BE. Parity and osteoporosis. *Surg Gynecol Obstet* 1969; 129: 27–8.

56 Atkinson PJ, West RR. Loss of skeletal calcium in lactating women. *J Obstet Gynaecol Br Commonwealth* 1970; 77: 555–60.

57 Wardlaw GM, Pike AM. The effect of lactation on peak adult shaft and ultra-distal forearm bone mass in women. *Am J Clin Nutr* 1986; 44: 283–6.

58 Chan GM, Slater P *et al.* Bone mineral status of lactating mothers of different ages. *Am J Obstet Gynaecol* 1982; 144: 438–41.

59 Lamke B, Brundin J *et al.* Changes of bone mineral content during pregnancy and lactation. *Acta Obstet Gynecol Scand* 1977; 56: 217–19.

60 Kalkwarf HJ, Specker BL *et al.* The effect of calcium supplementation on bone density during lactation and after weaning. *N Engl J Med* 1997; 337: 523–8.

61 Harrison HE. Vitamin D, the parathyroid and the kidney. *Johns Hopkins Med J* 1979; 144: 180–91.

62 Dandona F, Okonofua F *et al.* Osteomalacia presenting as pathological fractures during pregnancy in Asian women of high socioeconomic class. *Br Med J* 1985; 290: 837–18.

63 Parr JH, Ramsay I. The presentation of osteomalacia in pregnancy. Case report. *Br J Obstet Gynaecol* 1984; 91: 816–8.

64 Ford JA, Davidson DC *et al.* Neonatal rickets in Asian immigrant population. *Br Med J* 1973; iii: 211–12.

65 Moncrief MW, Fadahunsi TO. Congenital rickets due to maternal vitamin D deficiency. *Arch Dis Child* 1974; 49: 810–11.

66 Heckmatt JZ, Peacock M *et al.* Plasma 25-hydroxyvitamin D in pregnant Asian women and their babies. *Lancet* 1979; ii: 546–9.

67 Purvis RJ, Barrie WJM *et al.* Enamel hypoplasia of the teeth associated with neonatal tetany; a manifestation of maternal vitamin D deficiency. *Lancet* 1973; ii: 811–14.

68 Watney PJ, Chance GW *et al.* Maternal factors in neonatal hypocalcaemia: a study in three ethnic groups. *Br Med J* 1971; ii: 432–6.

69 Driscoll RH, Meredith S *et al.* Bone histology and vitamin D status in Crohn's disease: assessment of vitamin D therapy. *Gastroenterology* 1977; 72: 1051.

70 Brooke OG, Brown IRF *et al.* Observations of the vitamin D state of pregnant Asian women in London. *Br J Obstet Gynaecol* 1981; 88: 18–26.

71 Dent CE, Gupta MM. Plasma 25-hydroxyvitamin D levels during pregnancy in Caucasians and in vegetarian and non-vegetarian Asians. *Lancet* 1975; ii: 1057–60.

72 Polanska N, Dale RA *et al.* Plasma calcium levels in pregnant Asian women. *Ann Clin Biochem* 1976; 13: 339–44.

73 Rab SM, Baseer A. Occult osteomalacia amongst healthy and pregnant women in Pakistan. *Lancet* 1976; ii: 1211–3.

74 Risvi SNA, Vaishnava H. Occult osteomalacia in pregnant women in India. *Lancet* 1977; i: 1102.

75 Congdon P, Horsman A *et al.* Mineral content of the forearms of babies born to Asian and white mothers. *Br Med J* 1983; 286: 1233–5.

76 Delvin EE, Salle BL *et al.* Vitamin D supplementation during pregnancy. Effect on neonatal calcium homeostasis. *J Pediatr* 1986; 109: 328–34.

77 Maxwell JP. Further studies in adult rickets (osteomalacia) and foetal rickets. *Proc R Soc Med* 1934; 28: 265–300.

78 Wilson DC. The incidence of osteomalacia and late rickets in Northern India. *Lancet* 1931; ii: 10–12.

79 Brooke OG, Butters F *et al.* Intrauterine vitamin D nutrition and postnatal growth in Asian infants. *Br Med J* 1981; 283: 1025.

80 WHO. *Nutrition in Pregnancy and Lactation. Report of a WHO Expert Committee.* World Health Organization Technical Report Series, 1965; 302: 37.

81 Food and Nutrition Board. *Recommended Dietary Allowances,* 9th edn. National Research Council, National Academy of Sciences, Washington DC, 1979.

82 Mallet E, Gugi B *et al.* Vitamin D supplementation in pregnancy. A controlled trial of two methods. *Obstet Gynecol* 1986; 68: 300–4.

83 Lamm CI, Norton KI *et al.* Congenital rickets associated with magnesium sulfate infusion for tocolysis. *J Pediatr* 1988; 113: 1078–82.

84 Genant HK, Mall JC *et al.* Skeletal demineralisation and growth retardation in inflammatory bowel disease. *Invest Radiol* 1976; 11: 541–9.

85 Mogadam M, Dobbins WO, Korelitz BI, Ahmed SW. Pregnancy in inflammatory bowel disease. Effect of sulphasalazine and corticosteroids on fetal outcome. *Gastroenterology* 1981; 80: 72–6.

86 Schoen MS, Lindenbaum J *et al.* Significance of serum level of 25-hydroxycholecalciferol in gastro-intestinal disease. *Am J Dig Dis* 1978; 23: 137–42.

87 Teitelbaum SL, Halverson JD *et al.* Abnormalities of circulating 25-OH vitamin D after jejunoileal bypass for obesity and evidence of an adaptive response. *Ann Intern Med* 1977; 86: 289–93.

88 Arnaud SB, Newcomer AD *et al.* Serum 25-OHD and the pathogenesis of osteomalacia in patients with non-tropical sprue. *Gastroenterology* 1977; 72: 1025.

89 Morris IDS, Adjukiewicz AB *et al.* Coeliac infertility: an indication for dietary gluten restriction. *Lancet* 1970; i: 213–14.

90 Hahn TJ, Squires AE *et al.* Reduced serum 25-hydroxyvitamin D concentration and disordered mineral metabolism in patients with cystic fibrosis. *J Pediatr* 1979; 94: 38–42.

91 Skinner RK, Sherlock S *et al.* 25-hydroxylation of vitamin D in primary biliary cirrhosis. *Lancet* 1977; i: 720–1.

92 Savdie E, Caterson RJ *et al.* Successful pregnancies in women treated by haemodialysis. *Med J Aust* 1982; 2: 9.

93 Ogueh O, Khastgir G *et al.* Postpartum bone mineral density following antenatal dexamethasone therapy. *Br J Obstet Gynaecol* 1999; 106: 1093–5.

94 Hahn TJ, Hendin BA *et al.* Effect of chronic anticonvulsant therapy on serum 25-hydroxycalciferol levels in adults. *N Engl J Med* 1972; 287: 900–3.

95 Hahn TJ, Halstead LR. Anticonvulsant drug-induced osteomalacia: alterations in mineral metabolism and response to vitamin D3 administration. *Calcif Tissue Int* 1979; 27: 13–18.

96 Jenkins NW, Harris M *et al.* The effect of phenytoin on parathyroid extract and 25-hydroxycholecalciferol-induced bone reabsorption. *Calcif Tissue Res* 1974; 16: 163–7.

97 Christiansen C, Brandt NJ *et al.* Bone mineral content during pregnancy in epileptics on anticonvulsant drugs and in their newborns. *Acta Obstet Gynecol Scand* 1981; 60: 501–3.

98 Fleischman AR, Rosen JF *et al.* 25-hydroxyvitamin D. Serum levels and oral administration of calciferol in neonates. *Arch Intern Med* 1978; 138: 869–73.

99 Markestad T, Ulstein M *et al.* Anticonvulsant drug therapy in human pregnancy. Effects on serum concentrations of vitamin D metabolites in maternal and cord blood. *Am J Obstet Gynecol* 1984; 150: 254–8.

100 Brooke OG. Vitamin D supplements in pregnancy. *J Maternal Child Health* 1981; 1: 18–20.

101 Lightwood R. Idiopathic hypercalcaemia with failure to thrive: nephrocalcinosis. *Proc R Soc Med* 1952; 45: 401.

102 Kristoffersson A, Dahigren S *et al.* Primary hyperparathyroidism in pregnancy. *Surgery* 1985; 97: 326–30.

103 Lowe DK, Orwoll ES *et al.* Hyperparathyroidism in pregnancy. *Am J Surg* 1983; 145: 611–14.

104 Shangold MM, Dor N *et al.* Hyperparathyroidism and pregnancy: a review. *Obstet Gynecol Surv* 1982; 37: 217–28.

105 Wilson DT, Martin T *et al.* Hyperparathyroidism in pregnancy. Case report and review of the literature. *Can Med Assoc J* 1983; 129: 986–9.

106 Better O, Levi J *et al.* Prolonged neonatal parathyroid. suppression: a sequel to asymptomatic maternal hyperparathyroidism. *Arch Surg* 1973; 106: 722–4.

107 Wagner G, Transbol I *et al.* Hyperparathyroidism and pregnancy. *Acta Endocrinol* 1964; 47: 549–64.

108 Clark D, Seeds JW *et al.* Hyperparathyroid crisis and pregnancy. *Am J Obstet Gynecol* 1981; 140: 840–2.

109 Thomason JL, Sampson MB *et al.* Pregnancy complicated by concurrent primary hyperparathyroidism and pancreatitis. *Obstet Gynecol* 1981; 57: 345–65.

110 Whalley P. Hyperparathyroidism and pregnancy. *Am J Obstet Gynecol* 1963; 86: 517–21.

111 Mattias GSH, Helliwell TR *et al.* Postpartum hyperparathyroid crisis. Case report. *Br J Obstet Gynaecol* 1987; 94: 807–10.

112 Salam R, Taylor S. Hyperparathyroidism in pregnancy. *Br J Surg* 1979; 66: 648–50.

113 Schenker J, Kallner B. Fatal postpartum hyperparathyroid crisis. *Obstet Gynecol* 1965; 25: 705–9.

114 Gould CS, O'Malley BP *et al.* Endocrine hyperemesis—the need for a high index of clinical suspicion. *J Obstet Gynaecol* 1984; 4: 191–2.

115 Montoro MN, Collea JV *et al.* Management of hyperparathyroidism in pregnancy with oral phosphate therapy. *Obstet Gynecol* 1980; 65: 431–4.

116 Sadeghi-Nejad A, Wolfsdorf JI *et al.* Hypoparathyroidism and pregnancy: treatment with calcitriol. *J Am Med Assoc* 1980; 243: 254–5.

117 Salle BL, Berthezene F *et al.* Hypoparathyroidism during pregnancy: treatment with calcitriol. *J Clin Endocrinol Metab* 1981; 52: 810–12.

118 Eastell R, Edmonds CJ *et al.* Prolonged hypoparathyroidism presenting eventually as second trimester abortion. *Br Med J* 1985; 291: 955–6.

119 Goldberg E, Winter ST *et al.* Transient neonatal hyperparathyroidism associated with maternal hypoparathyroidism. *Israel J Med Sci* 1976; 12: 199–201.

120 Landing BH, Kamoshita S. Congenital hyperparathyroidism: secondary to maternal hypoparathyroidism. *J Pediatr* 1970; 77: 842–7.

121 Sann L, David L *et al.* Congenital hyperparathyroidism and vitamin D deficiency secondary to maternal hypoparathyroidism. *Acta Paediatr Scand* 1976; 65: 381–5.

122 Gradus D, Le Roith D *et al.* Congenital hyperparathyroidism and rickets secondary to maternal hypoparathyroidism and vitamin D deficiency. *Israel J Med Sci* 1981; 17: 705–9.

123 Graham WP, Gordon GS *et al.* Effect of pregnancy and of the menstrual cycle on hypoparathyroidism. *J Clin Endocrinol Metab* 1964; 24: 512–16.

124 O'Donnell D, Costa J *et al.* Management of pseudohypoparathyroidism in pregnancy. Case report. *Br J Obstet Gynaecol* 1985; 92: 639–41.

125 Jensen LP, Ras G *et al.* Hypercalcaemia in pregnancy. A case report. *S Afr Med J* 1980; 57: 712–13.

126 Glass EJ, Barr DG. Transient neonatal hyperparathyroidism secondary to maternal pseudo-hypoparathyroidism. *Arch Dis Child* 1981; 56: 566–8.

127 Gutteridge DH, Doyle FH *et al.* Two types of osteoporosis in younger women natural history and relationship to pregnancy and lactation. *Calcif Tissue Intl* 1986; 39 (Suppl. 2): A133.

128 Lose C, Lindholm P. Transient painful osteoporosis of the hip in pregnancy. *Int J Gynaecol Obstet* 1986; 24: 13–16.

129 Nordin BEC, Roper A. Post-pregnancy osteoporosis, a syndrome? *Lancet* 1955; i: 431–4.

130 Smith R, Stevenson JC *et al.* Osteoporosis in pregnancy. *Lancet* 1985; i: 1178–80.

131 Kent GN, Price RI *et al.* Human lactation. forearm trabecular bone loss, increased bone turnover, and renal conservation of calcium and inorganic phosphate with recovery of bone mass following weaning. *J Bone Miner Res* 1990; 5: 361–9.

132 Khovidhunkit W, Epstein S. Osteoporosis in pregnancy. *Osteoporosis Int* 1996; 6: 345–54.

132a Smith R, Athanasou NA, Ostlere SJ, Vipond SE. Preganacy-associated osteoposis. *QJM* 1995; 88: 865–78.

133 Cushard WG, Creditor S *et al.* Calcium, magnesium, phosphorus and parathyroid hormone interrelationships in pregnancy and newborn infants. *J Clin Endocrinol Metab* 1972; 34: 767–71.

134 Longstreth PL, Malinak LR *et al.* Transient osteoporosis of the hip in pregnancy. *Obstet Gynecol* 1973; 41: 563–9.

135 Brodell JD, Burns JE *et al.* Transient osteoporosis of the hip of pregnancy. *J Bone Joint Surg Am* 1989; 71A: 1252–7.

136 Drinkwater BL, Chesnut CH. Bone density changes during pregnancy and lactation in active women: a longitudinal study. *Bone Miner* 1991; 14: 153–60.

137 Kay NRM, Park WM *et al.* The relationship between pregnancy and femoral head necrosis. *Br J Radiol* 1972; 45: 828–31.

138 Zolla-Pazner S, Pazner SS *et al*. Osteonecrosis of the femoral head during pregnancy. *J Am Med Assoc* 1980; 244: 689–90.

139 Merz E, Goldhofer W. Sonographic diagnosis of lethal osteogenesis imperfecta in the second trimester. Case report and review. *J Clin Ultrasound* 1986; 14: 380–3.

140 Pope FM, Cheam KSE *et al*. Lethal osteogenesis imperfecta and a 300 base pair deletion for an (I)-like collagen. *Br Med J* 1984; 288: 431–4.

141 Ries L, Frydman M *et al*. Prental diagnois of a novel col1A1 mutation in osteogensis imperfecta type I carried through full term pregnancy. *Prenat Diagn* 2000; 20: 876–80.

142 Roberts JM, Solomons CC. Management of pregnancy in osteogenesis imperfecta: new perspectives. *Obstet Gynecol* 1975; 45: 168–70.

143 Price J, Reynolds F. Management of pregnancy complicated by severe osteogenesis imperfecta. *J Obstet Gynaecol* 1987; 7: 178–80.

144 Sengupta BS, Sivapragasam S *et al*. Osteogenesis imperfecta: its physiopathology in pregnancy. *J R Coll Surg Edin* 1977; 22: 358–64.

145 Freda VJ, Vosburgh GJ *et al*. Osteogenesis imperfecta congenita. *Obstet Gynecol* 1961; 18: 535–47.

146 Hall JG. Disorders of connective tissue and skeletal dysplasia. In: Simpson JL, Shulman JD, eds. *Genetic Disorders in Pregnancy*. Academic Press, New York, 1981: 57–87.

147 Mather JS. Impossible direct laryngoscopy in achondroplasia. A case report. Anaesthesia. 1966; 21: 244–8.

148 Beilin Y, Leibowitz AB *et al*. Controversies of labor epidural analgesia. *Anesth Analg* 1999; 89: 969–78.

149 Graham D, Tracey J *et al*. Early second trimester sonographic diagnosis of achondrogenesis. *J Clin Ultrasound* 1983; 11: 336–8.

150 Kurtz AB, Filly RA *et al*. *In utero* analysis of heterozygous achondroplasia: variable time of onset as detected by femur length measurements. *J Ultrasound Med* 1986; 5: 137–40.

151 Allanson JC, Hall JG. Obstetric and gynecologic problems in women with chondrodystrophies. *Obstet Gynecol* 1986; 67: 74–8.

152 Tsipouras P, Del Mastro R *et al*. Genetic linkage of the Marfan syndrome, ectopia lentis and congenital contractural arachnodactyly to the fibrillin genes on chromosomes 15 and 5. *N Engl J Med* 1992; 326: 905–9.

153 Pyeritz RE. Maternal and fetal complications of pregnancy in the Marfan syndrome. *Am J Med* 1981; 71: 784–90.

154 Liang ST. Marfan syndrome, recurrent preterm labour and grandmultiparity. *Aust NZ J Obstet Gynaecol* 1985; 25: 288–9.

155 Quinn RJ, Mukerjee B. Spontaneous uterine inversion in association with Marfan's syndrome. *Aust NZ J Obstet Gynaecol* 1982; 22: 163–4.

156 Lind J, Hoynck-van-Papendrecht HP. Obstetrical complications in a patient with the Marfan syndrome. *Eur J Obstet Gynecol Reprod Biol* 1984; 18: 161–8.

157 Mudd SH, Skovby F *et al*. The natural history of homocystinemia due to cystathionine β-synthetase deficiency. *Am J Hum Genet* 1985; 37: 1–31.

158 Burke G, Robinson K *et al*. Intrauterine growth retardation, perinatal death, and maternal homocysteine levels. *N Engl J Med* 1992; 326: 69–77.

159 Steegers-Theunissen RPM, Boers GHJ *et al*. Hyperhomocysteinaemia and recurrent spontaneous abortion or abruptio placentae. *Lancet* 1992; i: 1122–3.

160 Clarke R, Daly L *et al*. Hyperhomocystinemia: An independent risk factor for vascular disease. *N Engl J Med* 1991; 324: 1149–55.

161 Constantine G, Green A. Untreated homocystinuria: a maternal death in a woman with four pregnancies. *Br J Obstet Gynaecol* 1987; 94: 803–6.

162 Minkhorst AG, van Dongen PW *et al*. Cerebral infarction after caesarean section due to heterozygosity for homocystinuria; a case report. *Eur J Obstet Gynecol Reprod Biol* 1991; 40: 241–3.

163 Brenton DP, Cusworth DC *et al*. Pregnancy and homocystinuria. *Ann Clin Biochem* 1977; 14: 161–2.

164 Rubba P, Faccenda F *et al*. Ultrasonographic detection of arterial disease in treated homocystinuria. *N Engl J Med* 1989; 321: 1759–60.

165 Eddy DD, Farber EM. Pseudoxanthoma elasticum. Internal manifestations. A report of cases and a statistical review of the literature. *Arch Dermatol* 1962; 86: 729.

166 Lebwohl MG, Distefano D *et al*. Pseudoxanthoma elasticum and mitral valve prolapse. *N Engl J Med* 1982; 307: 228–31.

167 Berde C, Wilks DC *et al*. Pregnancy in women with pseudoxanthoma elasticum. *Obstet Gynecol Surg* 1983; 38: 332–44.

168 Lao TT, Walters BNJ *et al*. Pseudoxanthoma elasticum and pregnancy. A report of two cases. *Br J Obstet Gynaecol* 1984; 91: 1049–50.

169 Viljoen DL, Beatty S *et al*. The obstetric and gynaecological implications of pseudoxanthoma elasticum. *Br J Obstet Gynaecol* 1987; 94: 884–8.

170 Yoles A, Phelps R *et al*. Pseudoxanthoma elasticum and pregnancy. *Cutis* 1996; 58: 161–4.

171 Levy HL, Lobbregt D *et al*. Comparison of phenylketonuric and nonphenylketonuric sibs from untreated pregnancies in a mother with phenylketonuria. *Am J Genet* 1992; 44: 439–42.

172 Medical Research Council Working Party on Phenylketonuria. Phenylketonuria due to phenylalanine hydroxylase deficiency: an unfolding story. *Br Med J* 1993; 306: 115–19.

173 Hyanek J, Homolka J *et al*. Results of screening for phenylalanine and other amino add disturbances among pregnant women. *J Inher Metab Dis* 1979; 2: 59–63.

174 Konecki DS, Lichter-Konecki V. The phenylketonuria locus. current knowledge about defects and mutations of the phenylalanine hydroxylase gene in various populations. *Hum Genet* 1991; 87: 377–88.

175 Lenke RR, Levy HL. Maternal phenylketonuria and hyperphenylalaninemia. An international survey of the outcome of untreated and treated pregnancies. *N Engl J Med* 1980; 303: 1202–8.

176 Copel JA, Pilu G *et al*. Congenital heart disease and extracardiac anomalies: Associations and indications for fetal echocardiography. *Am J Obstet Gynecol* 1986; 154: 1121–32.

177 Levy MI, Waisbren SE. Effects of untreated maternal phenylketonuria and hyperphenylalaninemia on the fetus. *N Engl J Med* 1983; 309: 1269–74.

178 Mabry CC, Denniston JC *et al*. Mental retardation in children of phenylketonuric mothers. *N Engl J Med* 1966; 275: 1331–6.

179 Yu JS, O'Halloran MT. Children of mothers with phenylketonuria. *Lancet* 1970; i: 210–12.

180 Woolf LI, Ounsted C *et al*. Atypical phenylketonuria in sisters with normal offspring. *Lancet* 1961; ii: 464–5.

181 Buist NRM, Tuerck J *et al*. Effects of untreated maternal phenylketonuria and hyperphenylalaninemia on the fetus. *N Engl J Med* 1984; 311: 52–3.

182 Kirkman HW, Hicks RE. More on untreated maternal hyper-phenylalaninemia. *N Engl J Med* 1984; 311: 1125.

183 Drogani E, Smith I *et al*. Timing of strict diet in relation to fetal damage in maternal phenylketonuria. *Lancet* 1987; ii: 927–30.

184 Arthur LJG, Hulme SRD. Intelligent, small-for-dates baby born to oligophrenic phenylketonuric mother after low phenylalanine diet during pregnancy. *Pediatrics* 1970; 46: 235–9.

185 Davidson DC, Isherwood DM *et al*. Outcome of pregnancy in a phenylketonuric mother after low phenylalanine diet introduced from the ninth week of pregnancy. *Eur J Pediatr* 1981; 137: 45–8.

186 Zaleski A, Casey RE *et al*. Maternal phenylketonuria: dietary treatment during pregnancy. *Can Med Assoc J* 1979; 12: 1591–4.

187 Platt LD, Koch R *et al*. Maternal phenylketonuria collaborative study, obstetric aspects and outcome: the first 6 years. *Am J Obstet Gynecol* 1992; 166: 1150–60.

188 Scott TM, Morton Fyfe W *et al*. Maternal phenylketonuria: abnormal baby despite low phenylalanine diet during pregnancy. *Arch Dis Child* 1980; 55: 634–9.

189 Smith J, Macartney FJ *et al*. Fetal damage despite low-phenylalanine diet after conception in a phenylketonuric woman. *Lancet* 1979; i: 17–18.

190 Bouvierre-Lapierre M, Saint-Dizier C *et al*. Deux enfants nés de mère phenylcetonurique. Echec d'un regime pauvre en phenylalanine institue pendant la deuxieme grossesse. *Pediatrie* 1974; 29: 51–72.

191 Smith I, Glossop J *et al*. Fetal damage due to maternal phenylketonuria. Effects of dietary treatment and maternal phenylalanine concentrations around the time of conception (an interim report from the UK Phenylketonuria Register). *J Inher Metab Dis* 1990; 13: 651–7.

192 Thompson GN, Francis DE *et al*. Pregnancy in phenylketonuria: dietary treatment aimed at normalising maternal plasma phenylalanine concentration. *Arch Dis Child* 1991; 66: 1346–9.

193 Bessman SP, Williamson ML *et al*. Diet, genetics and mental retardation interaction between phenylketonuric heterozygous mother and fetus to produce non-specific diminution of IQ: evidence in support of the justification hypothesis. *Proc Natl Acad Sci USA* 1978; 75: 1562–6.

194 Murphy D, Troy EM. Maternal phenylketonuria. *Irish J Med Sci* 1979; 48: 310–13.

195 Tolmie JL, Harvie A *et al*. The teratogenic effects of undiagnosed maternal hyperphenylalaninaemia: a case for prevention? *Br J Obstet Gynaecol* 1992; 99: 347–8.

196 Luke B, Keith LG. The challenge of maternal phenylketonuria screening and treatment. *J Reprod Med* 1990; 35: 667–73.

197 Curiel P, Bandinelli R. Pregnancy in a woman with xanthinuria. Study of amniotic fluid uric acid. *Am J Obstet Gynecol* 1979; 134: 721–2.

198 McKeran RO. Xanthinuria and pregnancy. *Lancet* 1977; ii: 86–7.

198a de Konig TJ, Duran M *et al*. Maternal 3-methylgutaconic aciduria associated with abnormalities in offspring. *Lancet* 1996; 384: 887–8.

199 Goldblatt J, Beighton P. Obstetric aspects of Gaucher's disease. *Br J Obstet Gynaecol* 1985; 92: 145–9.

200 Mistry PK, Smith SJ *et al*. Genetic diagnosis of Gaucher's disease. *Lancet* 1992; 339: 889–92.

201 Beutler E. Gaucher's disease. *N Engl J Med* 1991; 325: 1354–60.

202 Zlotogora J, Sagi M *et al*. Gaucher disease type 1 and pregnancy. *Am J Med Genet* 1989; 32: 475–7.

203 Young KR, Payne MJ. Obstetric aspects of Gaucher's disease. *Br J Obstet Gynaecol* 1985; 92: 993.

204 Rose JS, Grabowski GA *et al*. Accelerated skeletal deterioration after splenectomy in Gaucher type I disease. *Am J Roentgenol* 1982; 139: 1202–4.

205 Confino E, Pauzner D *et al*. Pregnancy associated with amylo-1,6-glucosidase deficiency (Forbe's disease) Case report. *Br J Obstet Gynaecol* 1984; 91: 494–7.

206 Johnson MP, Compton A *et al*. Metabolic control of von Gierke disease (glycogen storage disease type Ia) in pregnancy: maintenance of euglycamia with cornstarch. *Obstet Gynecol* 1990; 75: 507–10.

207 Osler W. Hereditary angio-neurotic edema. *Am J Med Sci* 1888; 95: 362.

208 Stoppa-Lyonnet D, Tosi M *et al*. Inhibitor genes in type 1 hereditary angioedema. *N Engl J Med* 1987; 317: 1–6.

209 Frank MM, Sergent JS *et al*. Epsilon aminocaproic acid therapy of hereditary angioedema. *N Engl J Med* 1972; 286: 803.

210 Gelland JA, Sherins RJ *et al*. Treatment of hereditary angioedema with danazol. Reversal of clinical and biochemical abnormalities. *N Engl J Med* 1976; 95: 1444.

211 Gadek JE, Mosea SW *et al*. Replacement therapy of hereditary angioedema. Successful treatment of acute episodes of angioedema with partly purified CI-INH. *N Engl J Med* 1980; 302: 542.

212 Frank MM, Gelfand JA *et al*. Hereditary angioedema. The clinical syndrome and its management. *Ann Intern Med* 1976; 4: 580.

213 Chappatte O, de Swiet M. Hereditary, angioneurotic oedema and pregnancy. Case reports and review of the literature. *Br J Obstet Gynaecol* 1988; 95: 938–42.

214 Chhibber G, Cohen A *et al*. Immunoblotting of plasma in a pregnant patient with hereditary angioedema. *J Lab Clin Med* 1990; 115: 112–21.

215 Ferlazzo B, Barrile A *et al*. Clinical contribution to the problem of correlations between hereditary angioneurotic edema and pregnancy. *Minerva Ginecol* 1990; 42: 351–6.

216 Hardy F, Ngwingtin L *et al*. Hereditary angioneurotic edema and pregnancy. *J Gynecol Obstet Biol Reprod* 1990; 19: 65–8.

217 Hopkinson RB, Sutcliffe AJ. Hereditary angioneurotic oedema. *Anaesthesia* 1979; 34: 183–6.

218 Peters M, Ryley D *et al*. Hereditary angioedema and immunoglobulin A deficiency in pregnancy. *Obstet Gynecol* 1988; 72: 454–5.

219 Postnikoff IM, Pritzker KPH. Hereditary angioneurotic edema. An unusual cause of maternal mortality. *J Forensic Sci* 1979; 24: 473–8.

220 Stiller RJ, Kaplan BM *et al*. Hereditary angioedema and pregnancy. *Obstet Gynecol* 1984; 64: 133–5.

221 Hunter DJ. Acute intermittent porphyria and pregnancy. *J Obstet Gynaecol Br Commonwealth* 1971; 78: 746–50.

221a Kritz-Silverstein D, Barrett-Connor E, Hollenbach KA. Pregnancy and lactation as determinants of bone mineral density in post menopausal women. *Am J Epidemiol* 1992; 136: 1052–9.

222 Brodie MJ, Moore MR *et al*. Pregnancy and the acute porphyrias. *Br J Obstet Gynaecol* 1977; 84: 726–31.

223 Sassa S, Kappas A. Lack of effect of pregnancy or hematin therapy on erythrocyte porphobilinogen deaminase activity in acute intermittent porphyria. *N Engl J Med* 1989; 321: 192–3.

224 Kantor G, Rolbin SH. Acute intermittent porphyria and caesarean delivery. *Can J Anaesthesia* 1992; 39: 282–5.

225 Gorchein A, Webber R. Delta-aminolaevulinic acid in plasma, cerebrospinal fluid, saliva and erythrocytes: studies in normal, uraemic and porphyric subjects. *Clin Sci* 1987; 72: 103–12.

226 Herrick AL, McColl KEL *et al.* Controlled trial of haem arginate in acute hepatic porphyria. *Lancet* 1989; i: 1295–7.

227 Arn PH, Hauser ER *et al.* Hyperammonemia in women with a mutation at the ornithine carbamoyltransferase locus. *N Engl J Med* 1990; 322: 1652–5.

228 Hauser ER, Finkelstein JE *et al.* Allopurinol-induced orotidinuria. A test for mutations at the ornithine carbamyltransferase locus in women. *N Engl J Med* 1990; 322: 1641–5.

229 Turton CWG, Stanley P *et al.* Altered vitamin D metabolism in pregnancy. *Lancet* 1977; i: 279–5.

230 Grover SR, Morley R. Vitamin D deficiency in veiled or dark-skinned pregnant women. *Med J Australia* 2001; 175: 251–2.

230a Kalkwarf HJ, Specker BL. Bone mineral loss during lactation and recovery after weaning. *Obstet Gynecol* 1995; 86: 26–32

231 Nozza JM, Rodda CP. Vitamin D deficiency in mothers of infants with rickets. *Med J Australia* 2001; 175: 253–5.

231a Polatti F, Capuzzo E, Viazzo F, Colleoni R, Klersy C. Bone mineral changes during and after lactation. *Obstet Gynecol* 1999; 94: 52–6.

232 Platt LD, Koch R *et al.* The international study of pregnancy outcome in women with maternal phenylketonuria: report of a 12 year study. *Am J Obstet Gynecol* 2000; 182: 326–33.

233 Waisbren SE, Hanley WB *et al.* Outcome at age 4 years in offspring of women with maternal phenylketonuria: the Maternal PKU Collaborative Study. *J Am Med Assoc* 2000; 283: 756–62.

234 Laskey MA, Prentice A *et al.* Bone changes after 3 mo of lactation: influence of calcium intake, breast-milk output, and vitamin D-receptor genotype. *Am J Clin Nutr* 1998; 67: 685–92.

235 Prentice A, Jarjou LM *et al.* Calcium requirements of lactating Gambian mothers: Effects of a calcium supplement on breast-milk calcium concentration, maternal bone mineral content, and urinary calcium excretion. *Am J Clin Nutr* 1995; 62: 58–67.

236 Sowers MF, Hollis BW *et al.* Elevated parathyroid hormone-related peptide associated with lactation and bone density loss. *J Am Med Assoc* 1996; 276: 549–54.

237 Aguado F, Revilla M *et al.* Ultrasonographic bone velocity in pregnancy: a longitudinal study. *Am J Obstet Gynecol* 1998; 178: 1016–21

238 Gambacciani M, Spinetti A, Gallo R, Cappagli B, Teti GC, Facchini V. Ultrasonographic bone characteristics during normal pregnancy. Longitudinal and cross-sectional evaluation. *Am J Obstet Gynecol* 1995; 173: 890–3.

238a Black AJ, Topping J *et al.* A detailed assessment of alterations in bone turnover, calcium homeostasis, and bone density in normal pregnancy. *J Bone Mineral Res.* 2000; 15(3):557–63.

238b Naylor KE, Iqbal P *et al.* The effect of pregnancy on bone density and bone turnover. *J Bone Mineral Res.* 2000; 15(1):129–37.

239 Yamaga A, Taga M, Minaguchi H, Sato K. Changes in bone mass as determined by ultrasound and biochemical markers of bone turnover during pregnancy and puerperium: a longitudinal study. *J Clin Endocrinol Metab* 1996; 81: 752–6

240 Okah FA, Tsang RC, Sierra R, Brady KK, Specker BL. Bone turnover and mineral metabolism in the last trimester of pregnancy: effect of multiple gestation. *Obstet Gynecol* 1996; 88: 168–73.

241 Rouse B, Azen C *et al.* Maternal Phenylketonuria Collaborative Study (MPKUCS) offspring: facial anomalies, malformations, and early neurological sequelae. *Am J Med Genet* 1997; 69: 89–95.

242 Callies F, Arlt W, Scholz HJ *et al.* Management of hypoparathyroidism during pregnancy—report of 12 cases. *Eur J Endocrinol* 1998; 139: 284–9.

15 Neurological disorders

James O. Donaldson

Active obstetricians each year encounter women with some major or minor neurological condition, and during a lifetime of active practice will participate in the care of women with many of the disorders discussed in this chapter. However, most obstetricians do not have an extensive experience with any one neurological disorder and must rely upon the collective experience in order to answer questions concerning diagnostic procedures, management and prognosis. In some instances all concerned are thrust into a complex medical, ethical and legal situation, such as the fate of the fetus after a woman has lost function of her cerebrum and brain stem due to a disastrous car accident [1,2]. Although obstetricians have an important role in preventing and detecting neurological conditions in the fetus, this chapter focuses upon the more common maternal neurological disorders.

Diagnostic tests

Before considering specific neurological conditions it is important to mention neurodiagnostic procedures during pregnancy. The best, most important and cheapest procedure is a probing history and a detailed examination by a skilled neurologist. The neurologist's task is to localize the lesion, which *per se* often limits the list of diagnostic possibilities. Thereafter, additional studies may be needed to define the diagnosis. Only after an accurate diagnosis has been secured can physicians properly advise a pregnant woman and her family concerning the management and prognosis of her condition.

Electromyography (EMG) and electroencephalography (EEG) are without risk. Pregnancy alters neither the composition of cerebrospinal fluid (CSF) nor the indications for examination of CSF [3].

However, far too often the author has been presented with cases in which treating physicians have shied away from neuroradiological procedures just because the patient was pregnant, only to have found themselves in a quandary when something unexpected later endangered the patient. Pregnancy is not an absolute contraindication for any neuroradiological study, although it is prudent to limit fetal X-ray exposure, especially during the first trimester. An increased risk of malformation can be detected with fetal exposure to more than 0.015 Gy (1.5 rad). The absolute risk of malformation is increased 1% with exposure to more than 0.1 Gy (10 rad). Compare this to background fetal radiation exposure of 0.75 mGy (75 mrad). Abdominal lead shielding reduces fetal radiation from plain radiographs and computed tomography (CT) of the head and neck to right-angle scatter, approximately 0.01 mGy (1 mrad). Transfemoral cerebral angiography adds exposure during fluoroscopy, which can be limited if the procedure is performed by an experienced angiographer with 'good hands'. Plain films of the thoracic and lumbar spine expose the fetus to 5 mGy (500 mrad) and 10 mGy (1000 mrad), respectively. Lumbar myelography involves at least 0.015 Gy (1.5 rad) plus fluoroscopy time plus (often) lumbar CT, another 7 mGy (700 mrad).

Magnetic resonance imaging (MRI) has no radiation exposure and apparently little, if any, risk to the fetus. Thus, in most instances MRI is preferred during pregnancy for imaging of the head and of the thoracic and lumbar spine.

Epilepsy

Epilepsy occurs in one in 200 women of childbearing age and is the most common major neurological disorder to be encountered by obstetricians. A unit delivering 3000 mothers a year will have about 15 pregnant women with epilepsy on their books at any one time. Although much has been learned about the complex interactions amongst the different types of epilepsy, anticonvulsant metabolism, birth defects, genetics and socio-economic and environmental factors, much of this immense literature is contradictory, and controversies abound. The following is my assimilation of that literature and my current approach to this clinical situation.

Oral contraception

Although oestrogens can lower seizure threshold and aggravate the condition of some women with intractable epilepsy, oral contraceptives can be used by almost all epileptic women. Some women with epilepsy become unexpectedly pregnant while taking conventional doses of oral contraceptives because most first-choice anticonvulsants, with the probable exception of valproic acid, induce hepatic hydroxylating enzymes and thereby accelerate oestrogen catabolism [4]. Thus, breakthrough bleeding and pregnancy are more likely to occur if a low oestrogen-containing contraceptive is used.

Effect of pregnancy

The effect of pregnancy upon epilepsy can be estimated according to the degree of control achieved beforehand. The longer a woman has been seizure free, the less likely she will convulse during pregnancy. Almost all women with an average seizure frequency of >1 per month will worsen during pregnancy, whereas only 25% who did not convulse in the 9 months preceding pregnancy will convulse during pregnancy [5]. Sleep deprivation in the last month of pregnancy may induce seizures, even in well-controlled epilepsy [6]. An epileptic woman has a 1% chance of convulsing during labour with hyperventilation as a probable factor. Aggravation of epilepsy by lactation is extremely rare.

Pregnancy-induced change in anticonvulsant metabolism is the most important manageable factor affecting the course of epilepsy during pregnancy [7,8]. In the era before blood levels of anticonvulsants could be easily monitored, approximately 50% of patients deteriorated during pregnancy [9]. If daily dosages are adjusted so as to maintain blood levels within a range found to be therapeutic before pregnancy, only approximately 10% will experience more seizures during pregnancy.

The course of pregnancy is unaffected by epilepsy for most women. Other maternal diseases, parity, socio-economic status and the quality of prenatal care are more important factors. The rate of spontaneous abortion is not increased [10]. Although the risk of almost any complication can be found to be increased in one survey or another, maternal epilepsy is not consistently associated with any obstetric complication of pregnancy with the possible exception of third-trimester bleeding, which may be secondary to anticonvulsant-induced folate deficiency [11] and/or alteration in the metabolism of vitamin K-dependent blood clotting agents. Maternal epilepsy is rarely an indication for caesarean section unless either a seizure occurs during the second stage of labour or the patient cannot cooperate with vaginal delivery.

Epilepsy and the fetus

The fetus is remarkably tolerant of isolated maternal grand mal convulsions although it can be assumed that the hypoxia and lactic acidosis that accompany a seizure cannot be good for it. Fetal bradycardia occurs during and for 20 min after a maternal convulsion. In rare instances fetal death and intraventricular haemorrhages have been attributed to a maternal convulsion. However, the effect of maternal convulsions may be remote, and only detected in intellectual performance years later as Gaily et al. [12] suggest. Status epilepticus is a certain threat to both mother and fetus with a doubling of risk of maternal death and a 50% chance of fetal wastage.

Neonatal coagulopathy

A neonatal bleeding disorder due to a deficiency of vitamin K-dependent clotting factors has been reported with maternal use of phenytoin, phenobarbital and primidone. Maternal coagulation studies are usually normal.

Birth defects

Birth defects are not unusual in the general population, and occur in 3–5% of all babies depending upon methodology and the population studied. The risk of some malformation increases, perhaps doubles, for the offspring of women with treated epilepsy. The largest controlled series, a Norwegian study with 3879 infants in each group, found the absolute risk increased from 3.5% to 4.4% if the mother was epileptic [13]. The risk of birth defects increases with the number of anticonvulsants used. However, a fundamental problem is difficulty distinguishing the risk of congenital malformation due to the severity of the maternal trait of epilepsy from the risk due to treatment.

OROFACIAL CLEFTS

Orofacial clefting is the most common major malformation that has been attributed to anticonvulsants, particularly phenytoin. The relative risk is approximately 5. However, a genetic link between epilepsy and orofacial clefts is suspected because epileptics have twice the expected incidence of orofacial clefts. Furthermore epilepsy is more common than expected in the extended families of children with orofacial clefts [14]. Thus, an important part of counselling sessions is taking a detailed family history concerning congenital malformations especially orofacial clefts, neural tube defects and congenital heart disease.

NEURAL TUBE DEFECTS

Surveillance studies have found a 1–2% risk of neural tube defects amongst infants exposed *in utero* to valproic acid [15]. The relative risk is approximately 10. A smaller but increased risk has been reported due to carbamazepine [16]. Fortunately prenatal diagnosis of serious neural tube defects can be made in the second trimester. High-resolution ultrasonography at 18–19 weeks plus serum α-fetoprotein determination will be diagnostic in most instances [17]. Quantification of α-fetoprotein in amniotic fluid is preferred by some centres but the procedure carries a 1% risk of miscarriage.

DYSMORPHIC FEATURES AND DIGITAL HYPOPLASIA

Craniofacial dysmorphic features plus hypoplasia of fingertips and fingernails have been attributed to all major anticonvulsants [18]. Distal digital hypoplasia and hypertelorism are most strongly associated with phenytoin exposure. It should be emphasized that most babies with these 'minor malformations' regarded as typical of the fetal anticonvulsant syndrome grow out of these features, with the possible exception of hypertelorism.

NEURODEVELOPMENTAL DELAY

There has been concern for several years that maternal anticonvulsant therapy might affect brain development of the fetus. However it has been very difficult to separate the possible relative contributions of maternal epilepsy itself, the drugs used to treat it and postnatal influences. However a recent retrospective survey of women attending a regional epilepsy clinic in the UK does suggest that maternal valproate therapy may carry a specific risk for additional educational needs (AEN) when the children go to school. The odds ratio for AEN in all children exposed to antiepileptic drugs and compared to those born to mothers not taking antiepileptic drugs was 1.5, not significantly raised. But the odds ratio for AEN in children exposed to valproate monotherapy compared to no treatment was significantly elevated (3.4, 95% CI 1.6–7.1). By contrast there was no significant effect of carbamazepine therapy (odds ratio 0.3, 95% CI 0.01–1.1) [18a]. Although these are preliminary findings and need to be confirmed in a prospective study, they are suggestive and should be included in patient counselling. However, note the comments below about the effectiveness of valproate therapy in some patients.

Pathogenesis

The increased risk of congenital malformations in the offspring of epileptic mothers is probably multifactorial. The role of genetics in the 'fetal anticonvulsant syndrome' is well illustrated by the remarkable case of heteropaternal dizygotic twins simultaneously exposed to phenytoin throughout gestation [19]. One baby had the syndrome; the other did not. Other aspects sometimes ascribed to the fetal anticonvulsant syndrome may have a genetic basis if families are studied. For instance epicanthus in exposed infants was strongly associated with epicanthus in the mothers [18]. Similar studies of head circumference and stature of the infants of epileptic mothers show genetics to be the major factor [20].

One mechanism could be an inherited deficiency of epoxide hydrolase which in the case of phenytoin could increase arene oxides [21]. Polytherapy can shift metabolism to potentially teratogenic pathways [22]. For instance, the combination of valproic acid plus carbamazepine plus phenobarbitone appears to be associated with an exceptionally high rate of major congenital malformations. Thus, monotherapy could lessen the risk of birth defects.

A second proposed teratogenic mechanism is folate deficiency [23]. Folate malabsorption is most commonly associated with phenytoin and phenobarbitone therapy but also occurs with carbamazepine and valproic acid.

Therapy with multiple drugs causes the lowest levels of folate. Folic acid supplementation before conception appears to decrease birth defects in children of epileptic and non-epileptic mothers. Folate deficiency could be one way in which socio-economic status affects the malformation rate. The optimal daily dose of folate has not been determined but 5 mg is reasonable.

Counselling and management

The best management of epilepsy during pregnancy begins with counselling of the prospective parents before conception [17]. First, confirm the diagnosis. Not infrequently patients with syncope, panic attacks, hyperventilation and sometimes more complex pseudoseizures have been mislabelled as epileptics and treated inappropriately with anticonvulsant drugs. In other instances the previous investigation of true seizures may not have been thorough enough to exclude a condition, such as an arteriovenous malformation (AVM), which could significantly alter management of both epilepsy and pregnancy. The author recommends measuring erythrocyte folate levels at pre-pregnancy counselling sessions and starting vitamins, which typically contain folate before pregnancy occurs. Often women stop oral contraceptives and start prenatal vitamins with folate.

The primary objective is to keep the prospective mother seizure free with the fewest drugs at the lowest dosage that is effective. Monotherapy is recommended if at all possible. The time to change medication is before conception. None of the most commonly used anticonvulsants is preferred just because pregnancy is contemplated. Trimethadione and paramethadione are strongly teratogenic and best avoided by teenagers and women of childbearing age. A statistically significant comparison of the outcomes of pregnancies of epileptic mothers taking different anticonvulsant drugs in monotherapy has never been done.

The author's first choice for an anticonvulsant drug is dictated by the type of seizure disorder and the patient's potential for compliance. The latest generation of anticonvulsants appear to have a low risk of birth defects, at least from animal studies and limited experience in humans. Indeed lamotrigene has become an acceptable alternative to valproic acid for the treatment of juvenile myoclonic epilepsy. However, if valproic acid in monotherapy successfully controls a seizure disorder whereas polytherapy in several regimes was unsuccessful, the author recommends continuing treatment with valproic acid provided the woman understands the risks. Avoiding high peak blood levels of valproic acid may lessen the risk of neural tube defects and can be accomplished by changing the customary twice daily doses to smaller doses three or four times daily.

Anticonvulsant blood levels should be checked if a convulsion occurs. The author prefers to monitor blood levels approximately each month during pregnancy so that daily dosages can be adjusted in an attempt to keep the level in that patient's predetermined therapeutic range. Free protein-unbound anticonvulsant blood levels are preferred during pregnancy because protein binding decreases during pregnancy. Thus, lower blood levels due to increased metabolism during pregnancy are partially offset by decreased binding and higher free drug levels. For instance, although total blood phenytoin may drop 56%, free phenytoin declines only 31%. This effect is not as great for carbamazepine, with a 42% decrease in total blood level accompanied by a 28% decrease in the protein unbound amount [24].

Vitamin K should be given during the last month of pregnancy as prophylaxis for the neonatal bleeding disorder reported with maternal use of phenytoin, phenobarbitone and primidone. The lowest effective dose is undetermined, but it is known that 20 mg/day orally will prevent this disorder [25].

If anticonvulsant dosages were increased during pregnancy, remember to decrease the dosage postpartum. Blood levels of phenytoin increase quickly after childbirth. The rebound in carbamazepine and phenobarbitone levels is slower. The pre-pregnancy dosage is usually re-established at 6–8 weeks postpartum.

All anticonvulsants are present in breast milk, but only in some instances with phenobarbitone and the benzodiazepines does the combination of the amount ingested plus slow neonatal metabolism produce sedation. Usually babies cannot ingest enough milk to cause any effect. Beginning at about 1 week after birth, infants of women taking phenobarbitone or primidone can experience withdrawal symptoms if they are not breastfed. These symptoms are hyperexcitability, tremor, high-pitched cry, feeding problems and continual hunger [20]. Withdrawal symptoms may also occur with other anticonvulsant drugs.

Cerebrovascular disease

Cerebrovascular disease is a major cause of maternal mortality and morbidity. Unusual types of cerebrovascular disease are relatively common during pregnancy. For instance, the most common cause of hypertensive encephalopathy is eclampsia. At least 30% of eclamptic deaths are attributed to cerebral pathology. During delivery acute blood loss may infarct the pituitary gland (Sheehan's syndrome), the optic chiasm and cerebral watersheds. Air and amniotic fluid embolisms are dramatic and often fatal. Cerebral venous thrombosis is a rare condition that principally occurs in the puerperium. Rupture of a cerebral aneurysm is a more common disaster. Ischaemic stroke is less likely to cause death but can cause significant impairment.

Ischaemic stroke

The incidences of transient ischaemic attacks (TIAs) and strokes during pregnancy are debated, and they may not be increased as once suggested. An increased risk in the early puerperium is generally accepted.

The risk of a cerebral ischaemic event increases with age in both pregnant and non-pregnant women. Few pregnancy-associated strokes are due to premature atheromatous disease, and these events usually occur in women in their 30s with long-standing diabetes mellitus and hypertension who are also at risk for other complications of pregnancy. It is said that no underlying cause can be found in one-quarter, but that proportion may be reduced by more extensive investigation. The majority of strokes are caused by one of an ever-increasing list of relatively unusual causes of cerebral ischaemia including mitral valve prolapse, peripartum cardiomyopathy, subacute bacterial endocarditis, sickle cell disease, syphilis, vasculitis (including Takayasu's arteritis), thrombotic thrombocytopenic purpura, moya moya disease, fibromuscular dysplasia, carotid artery dissection and choriocarcinoma. Although antiphospholipid antibodies (the 'lupus anticoagulant' and anticardiolipin antibodies) are a leading cause of stroke in non-pregnant young women, this and some other hypercoagulable states are associated with fetal wastage due to placental ischaemia and thus are a less frequent cause of stroke during pregnancy than would be expected (see Chapter 4 and 8).

Almost all strokes associated with pregnancy occur in the carotid distribution. In young adults strokes are rarely in the vertebrobasilar system, with the exception of strokes associated with the use of oral contraceptives. A pregnancy-associated stroke in the posterior circulation is usually due to dissection of a vertebral artery [29]. Approximately 30% of pregnancy-associated strokes are concentrated during the first week postpartum with equal shares for each in the second and third trimesters. Strokes during pregnancy have a greater than expected incidence of occlusions of a middle cerebral artery, and are sometimes bilateral [29]. This suggests an embolus of cardiac origin. Strokes after delivery have a greater than expected incidence of carotid occlusion. The author suspects that many of these postpartum strokes are caused by paradoxical emboli from peripheral veins and the pelvic venous

beds. Transoesophageal echocardiography is superior to trans-sternal echocardiography in both instances and should be used in the investigation of pregnancy-associated cerebral ischaemic events. The physician must be circumspect and should not avoid angiography because the patient is pregnant. Rarities are often found serendipitously during angiography.

Paradoxical embolism is an overlooked diagnosis that should be suspected whenever right atrial pressure is increased, such as following pulmonary embolism [30]. If right atrial pressure exceeds left atrial pressure, an anatomically patent but usually physiologically closed foramen ovale can open, clots can cross to the left side of the heart and thence to the brain, kidneys and peripheral arteries. Sometimes pieces of clot trapped in the foramen ovale can intermittently be the source of emboli. A saddle embolus at the carotid bifurcation may be surgically removed sometimes with immediate recovery, if the condition is diagnosed and the embolectomy performed within 4 h. Thrombolytic agents are relatively contraindicated during pregnancy and the early puerperium (see Chapter 4).

Treatment and prognosis depend upon the diagnosis. If anticoagulation is necessary in multiple unexplained TIAs heparin, or preferably low molecular weight heparin is the obvious choice (see Chapters 4 and 5).

A woman who, whilst taking an oral contraceptive or whilst pregnant, had a cerebral ischaemic event that remained unexplained after a thorough evaluation does not appear to be at greater risk of having another ischaemic event during a subsequent pregnancy. This observation is most important when counselling women who have previous stroke and are considering pregnancy or further pregnancy.

Cerebral venous thrombosis

Aseptic cerebral venous thrombosis is strongly associated with the use of oral contraceptives and with the puerperium. Most cases of late postpartum eclampsia in the antiquarian literature were probably cerebral venous thromboses [31]. This is a rare condition in Western Europe and North America with an incidence of perhaps one per 10 000 deliveries. In these areas the condition typically presents in the second and third weeks postpartum within a range of 4 days to 4 weeks. In India puerperal cerebral venous thrombosis is a public health problem with an incidence of 40–50 per 10 000 deliveries [32]. In most cases, women delivered at home present within days of childbirth. The reason appears to be dehydration because midwives restrict water intake for the first day. Some puerperal cases have been associated with hypercoagulable states including antiphospholipid antibodies (see Chapter 8), protein C deficiency, Factor V Leiden and prothrombin gene mutation [33] (see Chapter 4), homocystinuria (see Chapter 4) and paroxysmal nocturnal haemoglobinuria (see Chapter 2). Cerebral venous thrombosis may coexist with thrombophlebitis in the legs and pelvis.

The clinical presentation depends upon which veins are occluded and how fast the clot propagates. Sometimes there is a stuttering course for a week before the disease declares itself. Usually a severe persistent headache or a seizure demand explanation. There are two typical presentations depending upon where the clot starts. In the instance of a cortical vein thrombosis, increasingly severe headache precedes focal or generalized convulsions that are followed by aphasia, weakness and other focal neurological signs, in some instances with stupor. The propagation of clot through the cortical veins can provoke more seizures and neurological deficits. The faster the progression, the poorer the prognosis because collateral circulation is obstructed and the risks of venous infarction and intracerebral bleeding increase. Increased intracranial pressure may be caused by either the mass effect of intracerebral bleeding or the obstruction of CSF absorption by clot in the superior sagittal sinus.

The second presentation is a thrombosis in the superior sagittal sinus or the right lateral sinus. Headache is due to intracranial hypertension. Sometimes clot spreads into the parasagittal motor cortex causing primarily leg weakness and focal convulsions and into the occipital cortex causing hemianopia or on occasion cortical blindness if both occipital lobes are affected.

The diagnosis is confirmed by neuroimaging studies. CT is the best method to detect acute intracerebral bleeding. MRI is better able to show established venous clots in cortical veins and sinuses. Because intracerebral haemorrhage is always part of the differential diagnosis CT scans are often performed first followed by MRI. If there is any doubt, the gold standard is angiography, preferably digital subtraction angiography, which can simultaneously study both hemispheres and requires little contrast material.

The treatment of cerebral venous thrombosis is controversial and evolving. Anticoagulation is being used more aggressively even in patients with some haemorrhage and cerebral oedema. The historical mortality rate is 20–30% if not treated. With the exception of one dissenting study, treatment with heparin decreased the mortality rate to <10% without appreciably increasing the risk of intracerebral haemorrhage. The use of thrombolytic agents carries an indisputable risk of bleeding and should be considered to be experimental, especially in the early puerperium.

Survivors usually do well because the supply of oxygenated blood continues to reach brain tissue. Cerebral venous thrombosis has recurred in subsequent pregnancies but this is extremely rare. Prophylactic anticoagulation during pregnancy is not indicated because this condition is a postpartum phenomenon.

Subarachnoid haemorrhage

Spontaneous subarachnoid haemorrhage complicates only one or two in 10 000 pregnancies but causes as much as 10% of maternal mortality [36,37]. The principal cause of subarachnoid haemorrhage in women under 25 years is an AVM; most are primigravidae [38,39]. AVMs are more common in Asians than Caucasians. Older women are more likely to have a ruptured berry aneurysm. Cocaine abuse has precipitated rupture of aneurysms and AVMs (see Chapter 19) [40]. Although rupture of a berry aneurysm or an AVM together cause the majority of cases, at all ages approximately one-third of cases are due to other causes including bleeding disorders, vasculitis, subacute endocarditis, sickle haemoglobinopathy and metastatic choriocarcinoma. No cause will be established in approximately 5%. Unless a woman with a subarachnoid haemorrhage is in active labour, she should be evaluated as if she were not pregnant. Four-vessel angiography will be needed in the case of an aneurysm.

The initial haemorrhage of an AVM usually occurs during the second trimester or during childbirth. Oestrogen dilates other arteriovenous shunts, as is clinically apparent in pregnant women and alcoholics with spider naevi and palmar erythema. Blood oestrogen levels reach a plateau during the second trimester. Haemorrhage during childbirth is probably related to haemodynamic abnormalities produced by the Valsalva manoeuvre, which accompanies strong labour pains. Venous angiomata, which are now detected frequently by MRI, are not associated with haemorrhage although sometimes a venous angioma is in the vicinity of a cavernous AVM (cavernoma). The morbidity due to the rupture of an AVM is proportional to its size and related to location. If possible the AVM should be excised during the second trimester. Then the woman can be delivered vaginally without special precautions. Although some studies conclude that vaginal delivery is possible for a woman with an inoperable AVM, the author continues to recommend an elective caesarean section near to term for women with a large AVM.

The initial haemorrhage from berry aneurysms, and aneurysms at other sites throughout the body, increases with each trimester of pregnancy. The peak period is from

32 to 36 weeks. Rarely does an initial haemorrhage occur intrapartum, although rebleeding does occur during labour. The risk of death increases as the patient's stupor increases, and is approximately 20% even if the patient survives the first bleed with little more than a headache and a stiff neck. If possible the offending aneurysm should be clipped or otherwise surgically cured during pregnancy. Hypothermia and controlled hypotension can be used safely during pregnancy [33]. In a few instances a caesarean section has been immediately followed by neurosurgery [42]. If multiple aneurysms exist, as occurs in 10 per cent, the offending aneurysm can be handled during pregnancy and the remainder can be treated several months postpartum, with the possible exception of large aneurysms, with diameters >810 mm. If curative surgery is not performed, most women are delivered by elective caesarean section. If a multiparous woman with a proven pelvis can avoid bearing down by panting and regional analgesia, vaginal delivery is an option.

Eclamptic hypertensive encephalopathy
(see also Chapter 6)

Eclamptic seizures are often preceded by headache, brisk reflexes and the perception of flashing lights. The convulsions are generalized sometimes with superimposed clinical features of multiple foci activated in succession. For example, clonic movements in a leg due to a focus in one hemisphere and aversive eye movements to a focus in the other hemisphere can irregularly punctuate successive seizures or a prolonged eclamptic convulsion.

Eclamptic seizures are probably caused by patches of small haemorrhages and microinfarctions in the cerebral cortex [31]. Similar lesions in the visual cortex cause visual hallucinations and, if multiple lesions accumulate, cortical blindness. Sometimes multiple petechial haemorrhages are compacted into 'haematomata' in the subcortex, pons, caudate nucleus and other deep central grey matter. Streak haemorrhages occur in the corona radiata. The classic microscopic lesion is a ring haemorrhage about a thrombosed capillary or precapillary. In addition large haematomata, which may be correlated with disseminated intravascular coagulation (DIC), often cause sudden coma and need not occur during a convulsion. The mortality associated with eclampsia is greater than that of severe pre-eclampsia, in part because other organs are more seriously involved. Cerebral pathology causes 30–60% of eclamptic and pre-eclamptic deaths.

The onset of brain lesions sometimes precedes the first eclamptic convulsion. The traditional diagnostic criteria for eclampsia excludes both visual hallucinations and cortical blindness even though these are manifestations

of lesions in the occipital cortex which are identical to the lesions which elsewhere are associated with convulsions. The traditional definition also excludes pre-eclamptic women who suddenly become comatose due to a large intracerebral haematoma without convulsing. Furthermore, CT, MRI [43] and positron-emission tomography (PET) scanning have demonstrated changes in the brain in pre-eclamptic women who have not convulsed.

NEURODIAGNOSTIC STUDIES

Neurodiagnostic studies and the input of a neurologist are usually not needed unless the patient has atypical features such as focal deficits, impaired consciousness following a fit, or convulsions occurring more than 24 h after childbirth [44,45]. In those instances an imaging study is indicated. CT has the advantage of faster scanning, and detects major acute haemorrhages better than MRI [46]. MRI is better than CT in detecting oedema in the cortical mantle and elsewhere in the brain, and gadolinium enhancement denotes breaks in the blood–brain barrier. Both techniques can be normal, show diffuse cerebral oedema with slit-like ventricles, or show regions with decreased density denoting increased brain water [44,47]. Sometimes, arcuate bands of oedema course through the internal and external capsules. Cerebral oedema can be apparent on CT immediately after the eclamptic crisis and often disappears in a few days. This timing is compatible with vasogenic cerebral oedema and is unlike the delay of several days in the CT appearance of cytotoxic cerebral oedema following a common ischaemic stroke. Single-photon emission computed tomography (SPECT) shows increased perfusion adjacent to abnormal regions on CT and MRI [48].

Special note should be made concerning late postpartum eclampsia, i.e. eclamptic convulsions starting more than 24 to 30 h after delivery. The differential diagnosis of postpartum convulsions is complex and includes thrombotic thrombocytopenic purpura (see Chapter 3) and cerebral venous thrombosis (see above). Arteriography can suggest the diagnosis of late postpartum eclampsia by demonstrating smooth vasospasm in large- and medium-calibre cerebral arteries, which resembles spasm following rupture of a berry aneurysm [49]. In Europe this entity is called postpartum angiopathy [51].

Other tests usually have a lower priority but can be important in certain instances. CSF pressure is normal or increased [34]. The concentration of protein in CSF is typically 0.5–1.5 g/L. A few red cells or pink-tinged fluid is not unusual. A grossly bloody CSF is a poor prognostic sign. The EEG reflects the status of the patient ranging from mild slowing of the background activity to prominent δ activity in stuporous patients. Slowing is often more prominent in the posterior regions [52]. Transcranial Doppler studies have shown a marked increase in the velocity of flow in the middle cerebral arteries of women who developed postpartum eclampsia or who have severe pre-eclampsia. This is compatible with vascular spasm.

PATHOGENESIS

In 1928 Oppenheimer and Fishberg [53] understood that the classic form of the eclamptic attack consisted of epileptiform seizures in every way analogous to those occurring in acute glomerulonephritis, and included both as causes of hypertensive encephalopathy in usually normotensive young patients [53]. In physiological terms, blood pressure has exceeded the zone of blood pressures within which cerebral blood flow remains constant. The upper limit of this cerebral autoregulation is directly dependent upon an individual's customary blood pressure and inversely dependant upon arterial Pco_2. The variability in these functions is probably the reason why obstetricians have difficulty in determining strict blood pressure criteria for various degrees of pre-eclampsia.

Although generations of American obstetricians have been wedded to magnesium sulphate as an anticonvulsant for toxaemic women [55], its use until now has been empirical and without scientific support [56]. However, a recent large international multicentre study confirms the superiority of magnesium compared to diazepam or phenytoin in preventing further convulsions in eclamptic women [57]. Nevertheless, it must be stressed that no anticonvulsant drug will be 100% effective for eclamptic convulsions unless hypertension is adequately controlled.

The ideal antihypertensive drug for eclamptic hypertensive encephalopathy would lower systemic vascular resistance without affecting cerebral vessels, thereby allowing *pari passu* a decrease in cerebral vasoconstriction by the autoregulatory mechanism. Blood pressure should be lowered rapidly to within the range of autoregulation but in a controlled manner in order to prevent overshooting that range.

The targeted zone of blood pressure can be estimated from knowledge of an individual patient's customary blood pressure. If this is unknown, mean arterial blood pressure should be lowered by 20–25%. Each agent has its advantages and disadvantages. Usually obstetricians use the agent with which they are most familiar.

Mild vasogenic cerebral oedema accompanying eclamptic hypertensive encephalopathy usually abates soon after blood pressure is controlled. In more severe cases with stupor, active management is needed [58]. Hyperventilation appears to be an obvious first measure because it both decreases intracranial pressure and increases the upper limit of autoregulation. Corticosteroid therapy could be effective as it is for vasogenic cerebral oedema surrounding tumours metastatic to brain. If no contraindication exists, dexamethasone therapy is reasonable. Nimodipine, a relatively specific cerebral vasodilator, has also been used in these circumstances [59]. In some cases, often in eclamptic women with intracerebral haemorrhages, intracranial pressure may need to be monitored and more aggressive treatment may be needed including CSF drainage, hypothermia and barbiturate coma. Surgical evacuation is rarely indicated.

Mannitol can be predicted to be ineffective and sometimes dangerous. The effectiveness of mannitol as an osmotic agent depends upon the integrity of the blood–brain barrier formed by the tight junctions between capillary endothelial cells. Vasogenic cerebral oedema occurs because those junctions are leaky. Leakage of mannitol with its sphere of hydration into brain could worsen patients with widespread vasogenic cerebral oedema.

Tumours

Pregnancy and brain tumours profoundly affect one another. Tumours of virtually every type have been reported to coexist with pregnancy [60]. Yet the coincidence is only 38% of expected, perhaps because the developing tumour affects libido or fertility. Nevertheless, brain tumours cause approximately 5% of maternal deaths if the first 6-month postpartum period is counted. During pregnancy, tumours grow faster and are more vascular in part in response to stimulation of oestrogen and progesterone receptors that have been found in meningiomata, neurofibromata and some gliomata. After childbirth this effect can regress, at least temporarily. Symptoms of some benign tumours (e.g. acoustic neuromata and meningiomata) have regressed enough after one pregnancy to escape attention until a recurrence during a subsequent pregnancy.

Exact diagnosis is crucial. Abscess and metastatic cancer should be kept in mind even though they are unlikely. Choriocarcinoma is a special consideration during and for a few years after pregnancy. Fixed guidelines for the management of these cases do not exist because every instance is different. Nevertheless, trends emerge. Benign tumours tend to be operated upon after delivery because tumours are smaller and the operative field less bloody. Patients suspected of having a supratentorial astrocytoma presenting during pregnancy usually proceed to diagnostic biopsy and sometimes excision of the tumour. Interruption of an early pregnancy is often recommended for women with malignant gliomata, especially those with uncontrollable convulsions. Childbirth in the face of intracranial hypertension due to a mass lesion is usually accomplished by caesarean section, although a few multiparous women have been delivered vaginally.

Choriocarcinoma

Choriocarcinoma is relatively rare in Western Europe and North America when compared to Nigeria, the Philippine Islands and elsewhere in the tropics. Patients with choriocarcinoma usually present after miscarriage or a molar pregnancy with uterine enlargement and vaginal bleeding. Approximately 15% occur during or after a normal pregnancy. In some there will be no evidence of tumour in the uterus.

A few patients present with neurological symptoms [61]. Most but not all of these cases also have pulmonary spread. Cerebral metastases present in three manners:
1 a solitary mass lesion with or without Jacksonian seizures;
2 single or multiple strokes due to occlusion of arteries of any size including the carotid artery; and
3 haemorrhage into any intracranial compartment.

For instance, the cause of a fatal acute subdural haematoma 9 months following a normal pregnancy was one small nidus of choriocarcinoma. Tumour can also invade the sacral plexus and spine. Serum levels of β-human chorionic gonadotrophin (β-hCG) may be higher than expected for late pregnancy, and are particularly helpful in diagnosing and following postpartum cases. A serum to CSF β-hCG ratio <60 : 1 is highly suggestive of a brain metastasis.

Whole-brain irradiation and aggressive chemotherapy can be very successful in what was once a fatal situation.

Pituitary adenoma (see also Chapter 13)

Pregnancy induces enlargement of both a normal pituitary gland and pituitary tumours; however, only growth of a tumour causes symptoms. Headache typically precedes the constriction of visual fields by 1 month. Large tumours can cause diabetes insipidus and compromise the release of other pituitary hormones. Rarely pituitary apoplexy occurs.

Until the era of CT and MRI allowed the easy detection of microadenomata, many infertile women with small prolactin-secreting adenomata were not diagnosed until after ovulation was induced and pregnancy accomplished. Now women with prolactinomata can be managed according to the size of the tumour [27]. Patients with suprasellar tumours are candidates for surgery before pregnancy if the tumour does not shrink sufficiently with initial bromocriptine or cabergoline treatment. Thirty-five per cent of women with macroadenomata >10 mm in diameter will become symptomatic during pregnancy;

whereas fewer than 5% of women with microadenomata will develop symptoms. Thus, bromocriptine therapy is usually discontinued for women with microadenomata once they have become pregnant.

Lymphocytic hypophysitis (see also Chapter 13)

Lymphocytic hypophysitis is a rare autoimmune disorder, which typically presents postpartum as an intrasellar mass or as hypopituitarism without a history of intrapartum haemorrhage and shock [62].

Benign intracranial hypertension (pseudotumour cerebri)

Pregnancy-associated pseudotumour cerebri (benign intracranial hypertension) usually begins in the third to fifth month of pregnancy and lasts a few months before spontaneously remitting [35]. A few cases persist until the puerperium. Women with pre-existing pseudotumour cerebri typically worsen with the onset of pregnancy. Obesity is characteristic of both pregnant and nonpregnant patients, and rapid excess weight gain is common amongst the pregnant cohort. Headache, often retro-orbital, is the universal presenting complaint. Unless the examining physician is thorough enough to inspect the optic fundi and discover papilloedema, the diagnosis will be missed because these patients can be neurologically normal, although some will have diplopia due to abducens palsy. CT or MRI easily rule out hydrocephalus and intracranial space-occupying lesions. CSF pressure is increased. Commonly the CSF level of protein is <0.2 g/L.

Management is aimed at preserving vision. The author weighs the patient, examines the optic fundi and determines visual acuity and visual fields each week. Failing colour vision and visual obscurations are to be reported immediately.

Treatment starts with limitation of weight gain to ordinary increments. Repeated CSF drainage affords some temporary relief. Corticosteroid therapy should be started if visual acuity diminishes or visual fields become restricted when the inferior nasal quadrants may be the first area affected. A reasonable regimen would be prednisone 10 mg three times daily in pregnancy. Lumboperitoneal shunting or fenestration of the optic nerve sheath should be considered for recalcitrant cases.

Hydrocephalus

An increasing number of women with indwelling shunts for the treatment of hydrocephalus are becoming pregnant [63,64]. Presumably their offspring are at an increased risk of developing hydrocephalus. Thus, ultrasonography and assays for α-fetoprotein are recommended as for the detection of neural tube defects.

Both ventriculoperitoneal and ventriculoatrial shunts have malfunctioned during pregnancy and have required replacement, which has been accomplished without special problems. Some patients have received intrapartum prophylactic antibiotics, but whether this is necessary is not clear at present. In the case of shunts to the peritoneal space, caesarean section is recommended only for very definite obstetric indications.

Multiple sclerosis

Disseminated sclerosis is a demyelinating disease of the central nervous system that is characterized by exacerbations and spontaneous remissions. The disease has a propensity to occur in women during their fertile years. Pregnancy alters the natural history of multiple sclerosis [41]. Both initial episodes and exacerbations are less likely to occur with each successive trimester of pregnancy. However, the relapse rate in the first 3–6 months after delivery is much greater than expected. Retrospective studies, which may underestimate this effect, generally estimate the risk of a postpartum exacerbation at 40%. Thus, the relapse rate for a pregnancy year including the first 3 months of the puerperium is at least equal to if not greater than the risk in a non-pregnancy year. Breastfeeding is an indeterminant factor. Neither the number of pregnancies nor the timing of those pregnancies *vis-à-vis* the onset of multiple sclerosis appears to affect eventual disability [65].

Multiple sclerosis rarely affects fertility but it profoundly alters family patterns. After the diagnosis of multiple sclerosis has been determined, more women remain unmarried, have more elective abortions, and elect to have either fewer children or no additional children. The divorce rate increases with the degree of disability. Young women with mild disease and no children usually decide to proceed with a pregnancy, whereas older women with children and either significant disability or a progressive course do not.

Treatment with either interferon β or glitamer acetate has improved the prognosis of multiple sclerosis. Pregnant and lactating women are advised not to use these drugs. Many women elect not to breastfeed their babies in favour of restarting interferon β soon after delivery.

Uncomplicated multiple sclerosis has little effect on the management of pregnancy. Patients with difficulty walking often experience more problems during the second half of pregnancy when their centre of balance is changed by the increasing abdominal weight. Furthermore, an enlarging uterus can complicate the function of a neurogenic bladder and increase the risk of cystitis. Spasticity often fluctuates during pregnancy. Extensor or flexor spasms can be triggered by labour pains. There is no significant change in the incidence of spontaneous abortion, premature delivery, difficult delivery, pre-eclampsia or stillbirth. Nor is the risk of birth defects altered. Experience with epidural analgesia is limited but favourable. Spinal anaesthesia is usually avoided in patients with multiple sclerosis.

Headache

Headache is a common neurological symptom during pregnancy [50]. Headache appearing for the first time should be viewed with suspicion for it can be symptomatic of one of a long list of serious conditions including pre-eclampsia, subarachnoid haemorrhage, tumours, pseudotumour cerebri and cerebral venous thrombosis in addition to more mundane afflictions of sinuses, ears and teeth. Once again a careful history and a neurological examination including inspection of the eye grounds is the important first step in sorting through the list of possibilities.

Muscle contraction headache

The most common headache during pregnancy is muscle contraction headache. This includes bruxism in which increased resting muscle tension exists in the muscles of mastication. Although postural changes predispose some women to generalized muscle contraction headache, the majority are symptomatic of situational stress and depression. The treatment of an occasional acute muscle contraction headache consists of paracetamol, muscle massage and ice packs. Sometimes codeine preparations are needed. Paracetamol is preferred to aspirin for frequent use for chronic headache during pregnancy [66]. Frequent recurrent muscle contraction headache may warrant psychological assessment and prophylaxis with a tricyclic antidepressant such as amitriptyline or imipramine. Both drugs have been used extensively during pregnancy in psychiatric patients at dosages higher than the 50 or 75 mg that is often effective for these headaches (see Chapter 21).

Classic migraine

Classic migraine is affected by hormonal change, typically oestrogen withdrawal around the time of menstruation [67]. Fortunately 80% of women with classic migraine

improve during pregnancy but equally migraine presenting for the first time is a common cause of headache in
pregnancy. The first trimester is the usual time for classic
migraine to worsen or to present. Not infrequently this is
an unusual variety such as hemiplegic migraine, middle
cerebral artery migraine or basilar migraine [68,69]. The
differential diagnosis can be complicated. During pregnancy, an occasional classic migraine is usually treated
with analgesics and, if necessary, an antiemetic. If classic
migraine occurs more than twice monthly, prophylactic
therapy can be considered. Aspirin 75 mg daily is the
obvious first choice. Propranolol, 40–160 mg daily in
divided doses, is also effective and reasonably safe during
pregnancy [70] (see Chapter 6). Calcium-channel blockers
and tricyclic antidepressant agents are third choices.
Ergot alkaloids are not used during pregnancy and lactation. Sumitriptan and related drugs are not recommended
during pregnancy or while breastfeeding. Nevertheless, a
prospective study of 96 women who were exposed to
sumitriptan during the first trimester found neither an
adverse effect on pregnancy nor an increase in birth
defects.

Neuropathy

Bell's palsy

Acute unilateral facial paralysis is 10-fold more common
than expected during the third trimester and the first 2
weeks postpartum [71]. This plus the association of Bell's
palsy in non-pregnant women with the pre-luteal stage of
the menstrual cycle suggests a hormonal mechanism.
Cases occurring just before term have an excellent prognosis. A short course of corticosteroid therapy (e.g. prednisone 40 mg/day in divided doses lapsing to zero over 2
weeks) is reasonable for women with complete facial
weakness. Bilateral Bell's palsy suggests the Guillain–
Barré syndrome, or sarcoid or Lyme disease.

Carpal tunnel syndrome

Nocturnal acroparaesthesia is experienced by one-third of
pregnant women [72,73]. Bilateral symptoms are reported
by the majority. However, only a few pregnant women
develop true entrapment of the median nerve at the wrist,
the carpal tunnel syndrome. Progression to weakness of
the abductor pollicus brevis is uncommon during pregnancy, but such weakness is an indication for surgical
division of the transcarpal ligaments. Most pregnant
women with carpal tunnel syndrome can expect their
symptoms to regress after delivery. Nocturnal splinting
of the wrist in mid-position is usually effective, although

some find that an injection of corticosteroid is needed to
carry the patient over to the puerperium.

Meralgia paraesthetica

Unilateral or bilateral meralgia paraesthetica develops in
the last 10 weeks of pregnancy due to entrapment of the
lateral femoral cutaneous nerve at the inguinal ligament by
an enlarging abdomen. For most it is a nuisance that remits
within 3 months after childbirth if excess weight is lost [26].

Intrapartum lumbosacral plexopathy

Intrapartum entrapment of peripheral nerves within the
pelvis can be caused by the fetal head and the application
of forceps [74]. The typical patient is a short, overweight
primipara with dystocia due to cephalopelvic disproportion.

The most common syndrome is footdrop due to compression of the lumbosacral trunk (L4, L5) against the
pelvic brim. Sometimes elements from the S1 root are
involved if the point of compression is lower. Although
a few bilateral cases have been reported, this syndrome is
characteristically unilateral and contralateral to the presentation of the occiput. Footdrop may also be caused by
compression of the common peroneal nerve between leg
holders and the fibular head.

Femoral (anterior crural) and obturator neuropathies
are bilateral in about 25%, with no preference as to right
or left side for the unilateral cases. Arrest of labour in a
transverse lie is frequent.

The prognosis depends upon the severity of the nerve
injury. Complete recovery within 2 months is expected in
neuropraxis in which only the myelin sheath has been
distorted. If axons have been crushed, improvement is
slower and sometimes incomplete. Furthermore, women
with axonal lesions are probably at greater risk if nerves
are again damaged during a subsequent delivery. Thus,
women with EMG evidence of denervation are future
candidates for a caesarean section, whereas women with
neuropraxis are more likely to have a trial of labour,
especially with a smaller fetus.

Guillain–Barré syndrome

The concurrence of acute inflammatory polyneuropathy
and pregnancy is coincidental. The incidence may be
increased in the puerperium [62]. The course of pregnancy and the fetus are unaffected. Plasmapheresis early
in the course of the illness in severely affected patients
improves the prognosis by decreasing the duration of
assisted ventilation and complications due to immobility.

Plasmapheresis has been performed in all three trimesters of pregnancy [75]. Amongst non-pregnant patients intravenous immune globulin is at least as effective as plasmapheresis. There is sufficient experience with the use of immunoglobulin in pregnancy compounded by immune thrombocytopenia (see Chapter 3) to allow its use in Guillain–Barré syndrome also. Immunoglobulin has also been used during pregnancy in the treatment of chronic inflammatory demyelinating polyneuropathy [60].

Muscle disease

Polymyositis

Polymyositis is a subacute inflammatory disease of multiple aetiologies that typically worsens during pregnancy [76]. Aggressive treatment with corticosteroids is warranted. Fetal wastage is approximately 50%. However, infants thrive once removed from the hostile milieu.

Myasthenia gravis

Myasthenia gravis is an autoimmune disease affecting nicotinic acetylcholine receptors of motor endplates of striated muscle. Its severity fluctuates. During pregnancy the chances of worsening, improving or remaining unchanged are approximately equal [54]. The effect of one pregnancy does not predict the effect of the next. In distinction, postpartum exacerbations are common. Previous thymectomy decreases the risk of pregnancy-associated exacerbations [77]. Myasthenic crises have been shortened by plasmapheresis in all three trimesters [75].

Myasthenia gravis does not increase the risk of uterine inertia or uterine involution and usually does not prolong labour and delivery. This is because smooth muscle and myometrium are not affected. Magnesium sulphate is contraindicated because it can precipitate a myasthenic crisis [78]. Obstetric analgesia and anaesthesia are more complicated. Narcotics should be administered judiciously because they reduce respiratory drive. If an inhalation anaesthetic is needed, ether is usually avoided. Regional anaesthesia is preferred. If the patient is being treated with anticholinesterase agents, large amounts of procaine and related compounds, as used with paracervical and pudendal blocks, should be avoided because their hydrolysis by plasma cholinesterase has been blocked. Lidocaine is recommended because it is metabolized by a different pathway.

NEONATAL MYASTHENIA GRAVIS

At least 12% of the offspring of women with generalized myasthenia gravis will develop self-limited neonatal my-

asthenia gravis [28]. The condition lasts approximately 3 weeks and is occasionally life threatening because of respiratory paralysis in the neonate. It is important to be aware that symptoms may not present until 4 days after delivery therefore all at-risk babies of mothers with myasthenia need to be kept under close observation for the first week of life. Mothers with mild weakness can have severely affected babies, and vice versa. A high maternal titre of antibody to acetylcholine receptor is the best predictor. Antibody titres in maternal blood and cord blood are approximately equal. Unlike other IgG-mediated disorders, there are no manifestations of fetal myasthenia such as polyhydramnios or arthrogryposis. Indeed, women report vigorous intrauterine movement. The explanation appears to be a fetoprotein that inhibits the antigen-antibody reaction and protects the infant until its concentration drops.

Myotonic muscular dystrophy

Myotonic muscular dystrophy is the most common inherited disorder of muscle in women of childbearing age. It is an autosomal dominant disease. A woman can be so mildly affected that her diagnosis may only be established during the evaluation of her floppy baby.

Myotonic dystrophy does affect pregnancy [79]. Polyhydramnios is due to defective fetal swallowing. Smooth muscle and myometrium are also dystrophic. This causes prolonged labours, uterine inertia and delays uterine involution with postpartum haemorrhage. Oxytocin does stimulate contractions. Obstetric anaesthesia is complicated [80]. It is important to be aware that hypoventilation and chronic respiratory acidosis may exist. Regional anaesthesia in preferred. Depolarizing muscle relaxants can precipitate severe spasms and hyperthermia. Curariform agents are preferred.

Paraplegia

Paraplegia does not prevent a young woman from becoming pregnant, although orgasm cannot be achieved if both spinothalamic tracts are affected. The manifestations of a spinal cord transection vary with the level of the lesion, and so does its influence upon pregnancy and childbirth [81]. All patients have sacral anaesthesia. Women with lesions of the cauda equina have relaxed perineal muscles. Women with lesions above uterine sensory afferents (T11, T12, L1) have painless labour. Some can time their contractions by a periodic increase in spasticity. Autonomic hyperreflexia occurs if the level is above the splanchnic autonomic outflow (T5/6). In that case the paroxysmal release of catecholamines causes periodic tachycardias, hypertension, flushing and throbbing headache, symptoms that have been mistaken for pre-eclampsia. Both autonomic and somatic hyperreflexia can be treated by interrupting reflex arcs with regional anaesthesia including epidural and spinal anaesthesia.

Paraplegic women are prone to have premature labour, especially those with lesions above T11. Frequent vaginal examinations are warranted during the third trimester in order to detect early cervical dilatation and effacement. Hospitalization is warranted at least 4 weeks before term or if any changes are detected. Sometimes multiparae are admitted after the 30th week even without any cervical changes.

The principal complications are urinary tract infections and compromise of the function of neurogenic bowels and bladder.

Women with profound immobility are at particular risk of deep vein thrombosis and should be given low molecular weight heparin prophylaxis throughout pregnancy (see Chapter 4). Anaemia lowers resistance to pressure sores and is an indication for transfusion at haemoglobin levels that would not ordinarily justify transfusions. Nonabsorbable suture material should be used to repair the skin in perineal tears or incisions because buried catgut can cause sterile abscesses.

Chorea gravidarum

Chorea gravidarum is now exceptionally rare even in developing countries and it has become much milder. The obstetrician/gynaecologist is more likely to see chorea subsequent to prescribing the oral contraceptive [82]. Even in pregnancy chorea is not necessarily of rheumatic origin, but may be the first manifestation of Huntingdon's chorea, or be a complication of antiphospholipid syndrome [42].

Successful management of the pregnancy and labour complicated by rheumatic chorea depends largely on any associated cardiac lesion. Adequate rest, quiet and reassurance will help the chorea but sedation by a benzodiazepine may be required. Termination of pregnancy is now unlikely to be necessary.

References

1 Bernstein IM, Watson M *et al.* Maternal brain death and prolonged fetal survival. *Obstet Gynecol* 1989; 74: 434–7.
2 Loewy EH. The pregnant brain dead and the fetus. Must we always try to wrest life from death? *Am J Obstet Gynecol* 1987; 157: 1097–101.
3 Davis LE. Normal laboratory values of CSF during pregnancy. *Arch Neurol* 1979; 36: 443.
4 Mattson RH, Cramer JA *et al.* Use of oral contraceptives by women with epilepsy. *J Am Med Assoc* 1986; 256: 238–40.
5 Knight AH, Rhind EG. Epilepsy and pregnancy. A study of 153 pregnancies in 59 patients. *Epilepsia* 1975; 16: 99–110.
6 Schmidt D, Canger R *et al.* Change of seizure frequency in pregnant epileptic women. *J Neurol Neurosurg Psychiatr* 1983; 46: 751–5.
7 Hopkins A. Epilepsy and anticonvulsant drugs. *Br Med J* 1987; 294: 497–501.
8 Leppik IE, Rask CA. Pharmacokinetics of antiepileptic drugs during pregnancy. *Semin Neurol* 1989; 8: 240–6.
9 Donaldson JO. *Neurology of Pregnancy*, 2nd edn. WB Saunders, London, 1989.
10 Annegers JF, Baumgartner KB *et al.* Epilepsy, anticonvulsant drugs, and the risk of spontaneous abortion. *Epilepsia* 1988; 29: 451–8.
11 Hiilesmaa VK, Bardy A, Terano R. Obstetric outcome in women with epilepsy. *Am J Obstet Gynecol* 1985; 152: 499–504.
12 Gaily EK, Kantola-Sorsa E, Granstrom M-L. Specific cognitive dysfunction in children with epileptic mothers. *Dev Med Child Neurol* 1990; 32: 403–14.
13 Bjerkedal T. Outcome of pregnancy in women with epilepsy, Norway, 1967–78: congenital malformations. In: Janz D, Dam M, Richens A *et al.*, eds. *Epilepsy, Pregnancy and the Child.* Raven Press, New York, 1982: 289–95.
14 Friis ML, Holm NV *et al.* Facial clefts in sibs and children of epileptic patients. *Neurology* 1986; 36: 346–50.
15 Oakeshott P, Hunt GM. Valproate and spina bifida. *Br Med J* 1989; 298: 1300–1.
16 Rosa FW. Spina bifida in infants of women treated with carbamazepine during pregnancy. *N Engl J Med* 1991; 324: 674–7.
17 Delgado-Escueta AV, Janz D. Consensus guidelines: preconception counseling, management, and care of the pregnant woman with epilepsy. *Neurology* 1992; 42 (Suppl. 5): 149–60.
18 Gaily E, Granstrom M-L *et al.* Minor abnormalities in offspring of epileptic mothers. *J Pediatr* 1988; 112: 520–9.
18a Adab N, Jacoby A *et al.* Additional educational need in children born to mothers with epilepsy. *J Neurol Neurosurg Psych* 2001; 70: 15–21.
19 Phelan MC, Pellock MM, Nance EW. Discordant expression of fetal hydantoin syndrome in heteropaternal twins. *N Engl J Med* 1982; 397: 397–9.
20 Gaily E, Granstrom M-L. A transient retardation of early postnatal growth in drug-exposed children of epileptic mothers. *Epilepsy Res* 1989; 4: 147–55.
21 Buehler BA, Delimont D *et al.* Prenatal prediction of risk of fetal hydantoin syndrome. *N Engl J Med*, 1990; 322: 1567–72.
22 Lindhout D. Pharmacokinetics and drug interactions: role in antiepileptic-drug-induced teratogenesis. *Neurology*, 1992; 42 (Suppl. 5): 443–7.
23 Dansky LV, Rosenblatt DS, Andermann E. Mechanisms of teratogenesis: folic acid and antiepileptic therapy. *Neurology* 1992; 42 (Suppl. 5): 32–42.
24 Yerby MS, Friel PN *et al.* Pharmacokinetics of anticonvulsants in pregnancy: alterations in plasma protein binding. *Epilepsy Res* 1990; 5: 223–8.
25 Deblay MF, Vert P *et al.* Transplacental vitamin K prevents haemorrhagic disease of infant of epileptic mother. *Lancet* 1982; i: 126–8.
26 Massey EW. Mononeuropathies in pregnancy. *Semin Neurol* 1988; 8: 193–6.

27 Molitch ME. Pregnancy and the hyperprolactinemic woman. *N Engl J Med* 1985; 312: 1364–70.

28 Morel E, Eymard B *et al*. Neonatal myasthenia gravis: a new clinical and immunological appraisal of 30 cases. *Neurology* 1988; 38: 138–42.

29 Cross JN, Castro PO, Jennett WB. Cerebral strokes associated with pregnancy and the puerperium. *Br Med J* 1968; iii: 214–17.

30 Webster MWI, Chancellor AM *et al*. Patent foramen ovale in young stroke patients. *Lancet* 1988; ii: 11–12.

31 Sheehan HL, Lynch JB. *Pathology of Toxaemia of Pregnancy*. Churchill Livingstone, Edinburgh, 1973.

32 Srinivasan K. Puerperal cerebral venous and arterial thrombosis. *Semin Neurol* 1988; 8: 222–5.

33 Minielly R, Yuzde AA, Drake CG. Subarachnoid hemorrhage secondary to ruptured cerebral aneurysm in pregnancy. *Obstet Gynecol* 1979; 53: 64–70.

34 Fish SA, Morrison JC *et al*. Cerebral spinal fluid studies in eclampsia. *Am J Obstet Gynecol* 1972; 112: 502–12.

35 Digre KB, Varner MW, Corbett JJ. Pseudotumor cerebri and pregnancy. *Neurology* 1984; 34: 721–9.

36 Dias MS, Selchar LN. Intracranial hemorrhage from aneurysms and arteriovenous malformations during pregnancy and the puerperium. *Neurosurgery* 1990; 27: 855–66.

37 Wiebers DO. Subarachnoid hemorrhage in pregnancy. *Semin Neurol* 1988; 8: 226–9.

38 Hurton JC, Chambers WA *et al*. Pregnancy and the risk of hemorrhage from cerebral arteriovenous malformations. *Neurosurgery* 1990; 27: 867–72.

39 Sadasivan B, Malik GM *et al*. Vascular malformations and pregnancy. *Surg Neurol* 1990; 33: 305–13.

40 Mercado A, Johnson G *et al*. Cocaine, pregnancy, and postpartum intracerebral hemorrhage. *Obstet Gynecol* 1989; 73: 467–78.

41 Korn-Lubetski I, Kahana E *et al*. Activity of multiple sclerosis during pregnancy and puerperium. *Ann Neurol* 1984; 16: 229–31.

42 Whitburn RH, Laishley RS, Jewkes DA. Anaesthesia for simultaneous caesarean section and clipping of intracerebral aneurysm. *Br J Anaesthesiol* 1990; 64: 642–5.

43 Lau SPC, Chan FL *et al*. Cortical blindness in toxaemia of pregnancy: findings on computed tomography. *Br J Radiol* 1987; 60: 347–9.

44 Royburt M, Seidman DS *et al*. Neurologic involvement in hypertensive disease of pregnancy. *Obstet Gynecol Surg* 1991; 46: 656–64.

45 Sibai BM, Spinnato JA *et al*. Eclampsia IV. Neurological findings and future outcome. *Am J Obstet Gynecol* 1985; 152: 184–92.

46 Dahmus MA, Barton JR, Sibai BM. Cerebral imaging in eclampsia: magnetic resonance imaging versus computed tomography. *Obstet Gynecol* 1992; 67: 935–41.

47 Richards A, Graham D, Bullock R. Clinicopathological study of neurological complications due to hypertensive disorders of pregnancy. *J Neurol Neurosurg Psychiatr* 1988; 51: 416–21.

48 Schwartz RB, Jones KM *et al*. Hypertensive encephalopathy: findings on CT, MR imaging, and SPECT imaging in 14 cases. *Am J Roentgenol* 1992; 159: 379–83.

49 Lewis LK, Hinshaw DB *et al*. CT and angiographic correlation of severe neurological disease in toxemia of pregnancy. *Neuroradiology* 1988; 30: 59–64.

50 Reik L. Headaches in pregnancy. *Semin Neurol* 1988; 8: 187–92.

51 Bogousslavsky J, Despland PA *et al*. Postpartum cerebral angiopathy: reversible vasoconstriction assessed by transcranial Doppler ultrasounds. *Eur Neurol* 1989; 29: 102–5.

52 Aguglia U, Tinuper P *et al*. Electroencephalographic and anatomo-clinical evidences of posterior cerebral damage in hypertensive encephalopathy. *Clin Electroencephalogr* 1984; 15: 53–60.

53 Oppenheimer BS, Fishberg AM. Hypertensive encephalopathy. *Arch Intern Med* 1928; 41: 264–78.

54 Fennell DF, Ringel SP. Myasthenia gravis and pregnancy. *Obstet Gynecol Surv* 1987; 41: 414–21.

55 Sibai BM, Ramanathan J. The case for magnesium sulfate in preeclampsia-eclampsia. *Int J Obstet Anesth* 1992; 1: 167–75.

56 Donaldson JO. The case against magnesium sulfate for eelamptic convulsions. International. *J Obstet Anesth* 1992; 1: 159–66.

57 Collaborative Eclampsia Trial. Which anticonvulsant for women with eclampsia? Evidence from the Collaborative Eclampsia Trial. *Lancet*, 1995; 345: 1455–63.

58 Richards AM, Moodley J *et al*. Active management of the unconscious eclamptic patient. *Br J Obstet Gynaecol* 1986; 93: 554–62.

59 Horn EH, Filshie M, Kerslake RW, Jaspan T, Worthington BS, Rubin PC. Widespread cerebral ischaemia treated with nimodipine in a patient with eclampsia. *Br Med J* 1990; 301: 794.

60 Roelvink NCA, Kamphorst W *et al*. Pregnancy-related primary brain and spinal tumors. *Arch Neurol* 1987; 44: 209–15.

61 Kanazawa K, Takeuchi S. Clinical analysis of intracranial metastases in gestational choriocarcinoma. a series of 15 cases. *Aust NZ J Obstet Gynaecol* 1985; 25: 16–22.

62 Cosman F, Post KD *et al*. Lymphocytic hypophysitis: report of three new cases and review of the literature. *Medicine* 1989; 68: 240–56.

63 Cusimano MD, Meffe FM *et al*. Ventriculoperitoneal shunt malfunction during pregnancy. *Neurosurgery* 1990; 27: 969–71.

64 Hassan A, El Mouman AW. Pregnancy and ventriculoperitoneal shunt. Report of a case and literature review. *Acta Obstet Gynaecol Scand* 1988; 67: 669–70.

65 Weinshenker BG, Hader W *et al*. The influence of pregnancy on disability from multiple sclerosis: a population-based study in Middlesex County, Ontario. *Neurology* 1989; 29: 1438–40.

66 Rudolph AM. Effects of aspirin and acetaminophen in pregnancy and the newborn. *Arch Intern Med* 1981; 141: 358–63.

67 Silberstein SD, Merriam GR. Estrogens, progestins, and headache. *Neurology*, 1991; 41: 786–93.

68 Jacobson S-L, Redman CWG. Basilar migraine with loss of consciousness in pregnancy: case report. *Br J Obstet Gynaecol* 1989; 96: 495.

69 Wright DS, Patel MK. Focal migraine and pregnancy. *Br Med J* 1986; 293: 1557–8.

70 Rubin PC. Beta-blockers in pregnancy. *N Engl J Med* 1981; 305: 1323–6.

71 Hilsinger RL, Adour KK, Doty HE. Idiopathic facial paralysis, pregnancy, and the menstrual cycle. *Ann Otol Rhinol Laryngol* 1975; 84: 433–42.

72 Ekman-Ordeberg G, Salgeback S, Ordebert G. Carpal tunnel syndrome in pregnancy. *Acta Obstet Gynaecol Scand* 1987; 66: 233–5.

73 McLeannan HG, Oats JN, Walstab JE. Survey of hand symptoms in pregnancy. *Med J Aust* 1987; 147: 542–4.

74 Feasby TE, Burton SR, Hahn AF. Obstetrical lumbosacral plexus injury. *Muscle Nerve* 1992; 15: 937–40.

75 Watson WJ, Katz VL, Bowes WA. Plasmapheresis during pregnancy. *Obstet Gynecol* 1990; 76: 451–7.

76 Rosenzweig BA, Rotmensch S *et al*. Primary idiopathic polymyositis and dermatomyositis complicating pregnancy: diagnosis and management. *Obstet Gynecol Surv* 1989; 44: 162–70.

77 Eymard B, Morel E *et al*. Myasthenie et grossesse: one étude clinique et immunologique de 42 cas (21 myasthenies neonatales). *Rev Neurol (Paris)* 1989; 45: 696–70.

78 Bashuk RG, Krendel DA. Myasthenia gravis presenting as weakness after magnesium administration. *Muscle Nerve* 1990; 13: 708–12.

79 Jaffe R, Mock M *et al*. Myotonic dystrophy and pregnancy: a review. *Obstet Gynecol Surv* 1986; 41: 272–8.

80 Camann WR, Johnson MD. Anesthetic management of a parturient with myotonia dystrophica: a case report. *Reg Anesth* 1990; 15: 41–3.

81 Hughes SJ, Short DJ *et al*. Management of the pregnant woman with spinal cord injuries. *Br J Obstet Gynaecol* 1991; 98: 513–18.

82 Pulsinelli WA, Hamill RW. Chorea complicating oral contraceptive therapy. *Am J Med* 1978; 65: 557–9.

16 Fever and non-viral infectious diseases

Geoffrey L. Ridgway[1]

Irrespective of race or climate, the body temperature normally lies within the range 37.0–37.5°C, with diurnal variation such that evening temperatures are from 0.5–1.0°C higher than the morning level. Oral and axillary temperatures are approximately 0.5°C and 1.0°C lower than the core temperature. Persistent elevation of core temperature above these levels defines fever or pyrexia. Fever is a non-specific indicator of disease, whether infective or non-infective in origin, and as such is analogous with other non-specific indicators such as the erythrocyte sedimentation rate or serum C-reactive protein level. Central control of thermal regulation resides in the hypothalamus. Products of tissue injury, however caused, termed endogenous pyrogens, appear to mediate disturbance of thermoregulation. In infective causes of fever, bacterial products such as endotoxin are the cause of cell injury resulting in the release of endogenous pyrogens from granulocytes, monocytes and fixed macrophages. The resulting fever may be characterized by rises followed by precipitous falls with sweating and peripheral dilatation of blood vessels. Increased muscle activity may lead to rigors, resulting in peripheral vasoconstriction and the cold clammy skin that is the hallmark of severe septicaemia, particularly with Gram-negative organisms. The majority of acute-onset fevers are likely to be microbial in origin. Many are self-limiting, often viral, and frequently an aetiological diagnosis is not achieved. A useful account of the pathophysiology of septicaemia is given by Gilstrap and Faro [1]. For prolonged fever, both infective and non-infective causes must be considered. Table 16.1 lists the most important non-infectious causes of prolonged pyrexia. The term fever (pyrexia) of unknown origin (F(P)UO)

is used strictly to describe the condition of fever in excess of 38°C for at least 3 weeks and following 1 week of relevant investigations. However, common usage applies a broader definition of simply 'undiagnosed fever'. Infective conditions associated with prolonged fever in Western cultures are listed in Table 16.2. See also individual chapters for accounts of infection in the respiratory and gastrointestinal systems etc.

The pregnant woman may be exposed to any of the common causes of infection. Women in labour and during the puerperium are particularly susceptible to serious infection of the genitourinary tract. In addition, breast and wound infections may occur. Puerperal sepsis (child bed fever) rightly remains the most fearful complication of childbirth, still with a significant mortality and morbidity. Table 16.3 summarizes the non-viral causes of fever complicating pregnancy and the puerperium.

The investigation of fever in pregnancy requires attention not only to the specific infections of pregnancy, but also to the common causes in the community. Therefore, the need for careful history taking cannot be overemphasized. Questions must include symptoms, chronology, recent travel, eating habits, pets and contacts with others with fever. Careful examination of the whole patient is neccessary, with particular attention to the genitourinary tract, skin rashes, palpable masses and heart murmurs. Investigation should be relevant and thorough, and include vaginal swabs, urine (with microscopy), and blood cultures. Serum for antibody tests, preferably paired specimens at least 10 days apart, even if the second specimen is after recovery, should be obtained to confirm an aetiological diagnosis. Relevant history must be included on the request form to ensure that full investigations are carried out. This is particularly important for both high vaginal swabs, which in the absence of relevant history

---

[1]The section on Malaria (pp. 510–511) was written by Dr Stephen Wright and Professor Michael de Swiet.

Neoplasia
Metastatic carcinoma
Melanoma
Lymphomata
Leukaemias
Retroperitoneal sarcoma
Tumours of lung, liver, kidney, pancreas, heart

Connective tissue disease
Rheumatic fever
Systemic lupus erythematosus
Rheumatoid arthritis

Miscellaneous
Drug fever
Embolic disease
Sarcoidosis
Haemolytic disease

Table 16.1 Non-infective diseases associated with prolonged fever.

Tuberculosis
Systemic fungal infection
Gallbladder infection
Abdominal abscesses
Appendicitis
Pelvic inflammatory disease
Upper urinary tract infection (pyelitis)
Retroperitoneal infection
Septicaemia
Infective endocarditis
Leptospirosis and relapsing fever
Viral infections
Parasitic infections

Table 16.2 Infective conditions associated with prolonged fever in Europe and the USA.

Non-specific	Specific
Puerperal or postabortal Endometritis Pelvic abscess Chorioamnionitis Thrombophlebitis Intraperitoneal abscess Amniotic fluid embolus	Disseminated gonococcal infection Syphilis Listeriosis Tuberculosis Tetanus Severe infection consequent on HIV
Septicaemia/bacteraemia Mastitis and breast abscess Wound infection Infective endocarditis	

Table 16.3 Non-viral infective causes of fever in pregnancy and the puerperium.

may only be screened for *Trichomonas vaginalis* and yeasts, and for urine, which may otherwise not receive microscopy.

Before considering the causes of fever and infection further, it is necessary to delineate the normal vaginal flora of women in the reproductive phase.

Normal vaginal flora

The vaginal flora during the reproductive phase is a moist complex ecosystem of aerobic and anaerobic Gram-positive and Gram-negative bacteria coexisting in close symbiosis. Under the influence of oestrogen, the vaginal epithelium contains glycogen, which favours colonization by large

Gram-positive rods (Döderlein's bacilli, *Lactobacillus* spp.), and other acid-tolerant bacteria, which metabolize glycogen to form lactic acid [2]. The resulting pH of less than 4.5 suppresses the growth of potential pathogens, assisted by the production of hydrogen peroxide by lactobacilli. Other bacteria commonly present in large numbers (approximately 10^7/mL vaginal fluid) include anaerobic and non-β-haemolytic streptococci, diphtheroids (*Corynebacterium* spp.) and coagulase-negative staphylococci (including the novobiocin-resistant *Staphylococcus saprophyticus*, a common cause of urinary tract infection) [1,3]. Common commensal organisms that are potentially pathogenic include *Candida* spp., β-haemolytic streptococci (Lancefield Group B, *Streptococcus agalactiae* is found in 5–30% of normal vaginas [1], and rarely Group A *Str. pyogenes*), *Staphylococcus aureus* and *Actinomyces* spp. Mycoplasmas are also frequent commensals, with *Ureaplasma urealyticum* present in over 50% of sexually active women, and *Mycoplasma hominis* in some 15% [4,5]. Other organisms, for example coliforms, anaerobic Gram-negative rods and *Gardnerella vaginalis* are often present in low numbers.

Vaginal discharge in pregnancy

Abnormal vaginal discharge is a common problem in both the non-pregnant and pregnant woman. Its particular importance in pregnancy reflects the effect on both outcome, and on the puerperium. The infective causes of abnormal discharge include viral (herpes simplex), protozoal (*Trichomonas vaginalis*), fungal (*Candida* spp.) and bacterial infections. Bacterial causes are cervical infection by *Neisseria gonorrhoeae* and/or *Chlamydia trachomatis*, and the altered state of microbial flora that characterizes bacterial vaginosis.

Bacterial vaginosis

Bacterial vaginosis (BV) presents as a greyish watery discharge with an offensive odour in the absence of localized inflammation. Diagnosis is made by the application of Amsel's criteria (Table 16.4) [6]. The routine request for *G. vaginalis* culture has no place in the diagnosis of BV. In the past BV has been dismissed as a trivial complaint. This

is not so. BV is a risk factor for premature rupture of membranes with or without labour, preterm labour with intact membranes, chorioamnionitis, postpartum endometritis and late miscarriage [7–9]. Fetal and neonatal infection has also been reported [10].

The underlying cause of BV is not understood. The consequence is a fall in the absolute number of hydrogen peroxide-producing lactobacilli leading to a rise in pH, and an increase in the absolute number of *G. vaginalis*, anaerobic Gram-negative rods (*Bacteroides* spp., *Prevotella* spp. and *Porphyromonas* spp.), *Mobiluncus* spp. and *Mycoplasma hominis*. The metabolic activity of *Mobiluncus* spp. leads to a release of trimethylamine, producing the foul fishy odour. Exfoliation of vaginal epithelial cells with their adherent *G. vaginalis* results in the characteristic 'clue cells' seen on microscopy of the vaginal discharge [2,3]. An association between pregnancy, BV and human immunodeficiency virus (HIV) infection has recently been reported [11]. A longitudinal study of BV in pregnancy suggests that women do not commonly develop BV after 16 weeks of pregnancy. Spontaneous remission is also likely in women acquiring BV early in pregnancy [12]. The authors suggest that in the light of these findings, treatment of symptomatic women should be initiated no later than the beginning of the second trimester.

Treatment is problematic, and there is actually no evidence that it affects outcome. The best available antibiotic is metronidazole, given as either a single oral dose or a 5-day course [3]. The single dose has the advantage of better compliance, but response is lower than with the 5-day course (95% compared with 84%). Metronidazole should not be prescribed in the first trimester because of potential chromosomal effects, although extensive reporting has not yielded any convincing evidence of fetal damage to date. Patients must be warned concerning interaction with alcohol, producing nausea and vomiting. Alternate therapy is with topical 2% clindamycin cream, but this drug is also not licensed for use in pregnancy. A novel approach is to use biotherapeutic agents. The treatment of women with BV in the first trimester with intravaginal commercial yoghurt may be helpful. However, it should be noted that the lactobacilli in yoghurt (*Lactobacillus acidophilus*) are not the predominating species found in the human vagina.

Table 16.4 Amsel's criteria for diagnosis of bacterial vaginosis.

Three out of four of the following criteria should be present:
- A white/grey homogenous discharge with offensive odour, and no local inflammation
- A vaginal discharge pH of >4.5
- A positive amine test (drop of 10% potassium hydroxide added to drop of discharge on a slide produces fishy odour)
- Microscopy demonstrates 'clue cells'

Trichomonas vaginalis

Trichomonas vaginalis also causes a raised vaginal fluid pH. The organism may cause considerable discomfort and a foul greenish frothy discharge. Diagnosis is readily made on microscopical examination of the discharge. The raised pH may predispose to an increase in the absolute numbers of abnormal anaerobic bacteria, and the risk of premature rupture of membranes, and low-birthweight infants [13]. The only effective therapy is metronidazole, and treatment should therefore be deferred until after the first trimester [14].

Candidiasis

Candida spp. is a common vaginal commensal. It is estimated that some 75% of all women will have at least one episode of *Candida* vaginitis [15]. The vaginal pH is more acid in pregnancy, leading to an increased risk of symptomatic infection [16]. Asymptomatic carriage in pregnancy occurs in 30–40%, compared with 10–20% of non-pregnant women. *Candida* vaginitis in pregnancy is not associated with adverse outcome. The vaginal discharge is usually white and odourless. The vaginal pH is normal or *reduced* in contrast to trichomoniasis or BV. Several species of *Candida* are involved, but *C. albicans* predominates (>90%). Treatment is no more difficult than in the non-pregnant woman, but the choice of agent is restricted. Topical nystatin and topical imidazoles (e.g. clotrimazole, econazole, miconazole) are safe and effective. The orally active drugs flucytosine and the triazole fluconazole should not be used. Amphotericin B is reserved for the rare systemic fungal infection.

Gonorrhoea

The overall prevalence of genital tract infection with *Neisseria gonorrhoeae* in pregnancy is generally reported as between 2% and 7%. In common with uncomplicated gonococcal infection in the non-pregnant woman, asymptomatic cervical infection is the commonest form, responsible for up to 80% of infections. Infection in pregnancy is associated with premature rupture of membranes and preterm delivery. There may also be an increased risk of pelvic inflammatory disease (PID) and disseminated gonococcal infection (DGI). PID is less likely after the first trimester, owing to physical obstruction of the cervical os by the products of infection. DGI classically presents with oligoarthritis involving the hands, feet and elbows. Fever and skin rash make up the classic triad.

The most important consequence to the neonate is gonococcal ophthalmia neonatorum. Disseminated infection with arthritis and meningitis occurs, but is rare. The classical prophylaxis of 1% silver nitrate solution (Credé's drops) is no longer justified in the UK, because prevalence is low, and the drops may cause a chemical conjunctivitis. Management nowadays concerns identification and antibiotic treatment of the infected mother, and antibiotic treatment of the baby if it is found to be infected.

Women presenting with vaginal discharge, or risk factors such as previous history of sexually transmitted disease (STD), recent partner change or relevant lifestyle, should be screened by culture of a cervical swab specimen (*not* a vaginal swab). The gonococcus does not travel well, and a suitable transport medium should be used (e.g. Stuart's), even for a short transfer. Alternatively, the specimen should be direct plated on to an antibiotic-screened enriched medium (e.g. Thayer Martin), and transported in a candle extinction jar or commercial system to ensure enhanced levels of carbon dioxide in the culture atmosphere.

The recommended treatment for uncomplicated gonorrhoea in pregnancy is one of the following: 3 g amoxicillin plus 1 g probenecid orally (if penicillin resistance in the region where infection is thought to have been acquired is <5%), or ceftriaxone 250 mg i.m., or cefotaxime 500 mg i.m., or spectinomycin 2 g i.m. [17] Fluoroquinolones and tetracyclines should be avoided in pregnancy. None of the above regimens is adequate to treat concurrent chlamydial infection, which is likely in up to 50% of women with gonococcal infection (see below).

Chlamydial infection

Chlamydia trachomatis is the commonest bacterial cause of sexually transmitted infection. A recent study of asymptomatic cervical carriage in English women aged 18–35 years yielded a prevalence of 2.6% [18]. Higher prevalence rates have been reported in certain specific groups, for example 8–12% in women presenting for termination of pregnancy [19,20]. The reported prevalence in antenatal patients ranges from 2 to 30% [21]. *Chlamydia trachomatis* is also the commonest cause of secondary infertility, consequent upon an attack of overt or covert PID. The risk of ectopic pregnancy is increased by 7–10 times following chlamydial PID. As is the case with gonorrhoea, over 70% of infected women will be asymptomatic, and 35–45% of women with gonorrhoea will have a concurrent chlamydial infection [22]. Risk factors for infection in pregnancy include young age, recent partner change, multiple partners and being unmarried. The routine screening of all pregnant women during the first trimester is recommended.

The effect of chlamydial infection on the pregnancy *per se* is not well understood. Apart from causing a vaginal discharge consequent on mucopurulent cervicitis, the main concern is with ascending genital tract infection, leading to amnionitis and perinatal endometritis. Acute non-gonococcal salpingitis is unusual in pregnancy. *Chlamydia trachomatis* may infect the urethra, and should be considered in women with dysuria and frequency who have negative bacterial cultures on conventional media.

The role of chlamydial infection in fetal wastage is not proven. *Chlamydia trachomatis* has been associated with premature rupture of membranes, prematurity and perinatal death in some studies [23,24], but not in others [25]. A recent serological study by Gencay *et al.* [26] found an association between raised maternal antichlamydial IgM and increased incidence of chorioamnionitis, prematurity and perinatal mortality.

True congenital infection of the fetus has not been described. Infection has occurred following caesarean section, but is unusual, and usually follows ruptured membranes. However, acquisition of the organism during vaginal birth is common. Up to 70% of babies born to infected mothers will become colonized. In 30–40% this will manifest as conjunctivitis, and in 10–20% as a characteristic pneumonitis. Infection of the vagina, rectum and pharynx may also occur, but may be delayed for up to 7 months, and persist for over 2 years [27].

Chlamydial ophthalmia neonatorum is much commoner than gonococcal, and is clinically indistinguishable. Up to 50% of babies with gonococcal conjunctivitis will have concurrent chlamydial infection. The incubation period of chlamydial ophthalmia is 6–21 days, in contrast to the 48 h incubation period of gonococcal infection. Symptoms and signs may vary from a 'sticky eye' to florid mucopurulent conjunctivitis with pronounced periorbital oedema.

Chlamydial pneumonitis presents between 3 weeks and 3 months of birth, and is characterized by dyspnoea and staccato cough. Chest radiograph reveals diffuse alveolar infiltration. Peripheral blood examination will demonstrate eosinophilia, and raised specific antichlamydial IgM antibodies. In one study 30% of affected children subsequently developed asthma [28].

The diagnosis of chlamydial infection has been revolutionized by the introduction of nucleic amplification (NAA) technology, for example polymerase chain reaction (PCR) and ligase chain reaction (LCR) [29]. These tests are highly sensitive and specific, but are relatively expensive when compared with the older and less sensitive enzyme immunoassays. Chlamydial NAA tests can be carried out as a non-invasive test on urine samples from women. Pregnancy can cause inhibition of NAA tests on urine, leading to false-negative results [30]. It is important that the test manufacturer's instructions concerning obtaining and transporting specimens are followed closely, and that the testing protocol has been agreed with the diagnostic laboratory.

Because tetracyclines and quinolones are contraindicated in pregnancy, oral erythromycin is the current treatment of choice [31]. However, nausea and vomiting can be a problem, and the preferred dose is 500 mg twice daily for 14 days, rather than the more conventional 500 mg four times daily for 7 days. Compliance requires careful supervision. Amoxicillin provides alternative therapy in pregnancy, 500 mg three times daily for 7 days. There are concerns about the latter regimen causing suppression rather than eradication of chlamydial infection but a meta-analysis supported its use [32]. A test of cure should be performed 3 weeks after completion of treatment. Although not yet licensed for use in pregnancy, the azalide macrolide azithromycin appears to be safe, and can be prescribed as a single 1-g oral dose. A study involving 146 pregnant women with proven chlamydial infection gave a 95% cure rate and no adverse sequelae on the fetus [33].

Chlamydial infection in neonates is best treated with erythromycin 50 mg/kg divided into four oral doses daily for at least 10–14 days. Topical antibiotic therapy alone is inadequate for treatment, and unnecessary with systemic therapy. Local toilet should be applied.

Mycoplasmas

Although *M. hominis* isolated from a case of bartholinitis was the first human mycoplasma isolate, the role of the genital mycoplasmas in disease is ill-defined. As noted above, both *M. hominis* and *U. urealyticum* are normal constituents of the genital tract flora. They are associated with acute chorioamnionitis, but whether their role is causal remains unclear. Both organisms have been isolated in pure culture from the blood of 10–15% of women with postpartum or postabortal pyrexia.

There is an apparent association with low birthweight, but this finding is clouded by the association of BV *per se* with this condition. *Ureaplasma urealyticum* is implicated as a cause of chronic respiratory problems in preterm infants, and along with *M. hominis*, is an occasional cause of neonatal meningitis [34].

Mycoplaasma hominis can be isolated from blood using conventional blood culture medium, and blood agar incubated microaerophilically with 10% CO_2. *Ureaplasma urealyticum* is best isolated using a specific mycoplasma medium. There is no justification for routine screening for mycoplasmas during pregnancy.

Mycoplasma are classically sensitive to tetracyclines, but these drugs should not be used during pregnancy or lactation. *Ureaplasma urealyticum* is sensitive to erythromycin and other macrolides, but is resistant to clindamycin (a lincosamine), whereas *M. hominis* is resistant to erythromycin and sensitive to clindamycin. This important difference should be borne in mind when a postpartum pyrexia fails to respond to either erythromycin or clindamycin.

Syphilis

Pregnancy appears to have a modifying effect on syphilis, although the effect on the fetus may be disastrous. Between 70% and 100% of pregnant women with early syphilis will transmit infection to the fetus, and in up to one-third of cases this will result in stillbirth. Maternal symptoms are often mild or non-existent, and the longer the woman has had untreated syphilis before the first pregnancy, the less likely *in utero* death will occur, and the more likely a congenitally syphilitic live child will be born. The longer the duration of untreated illness, and the more pregnancies, the less likely that a subsequent fetus will be infected. The mother becomes immune to infection by the baby, even if the latter has mouth lesions (Colles' Law).

The primary lesion is the ulcer or chancre at the site of inoculation, which may be extragenital. The lesion heals in 6–8 weeks, and is followed by the secondary phase of systemic spread. The most important sign is a rash (characteristically involving the palms and soles in addition to elsewhere) with constitutional upset. Other signs include patchy alopecia, cervical lymphadenopathy, and flat warty lesions termed condylomata lata. However, symptoms and signs may be transient or absent. The disease then enters the latent phase, divided into early (the first year), and late, when the disease is relatively quiescent. Subsequently, after several years, the cardiological and neurological manifestations of tertiary syphilis may develop in up to one-third of untreated patients.

Screening for syphilis remains mandatory during pregnancy, because of the importance of identifying infected women early in pregnancy before fetal wastage or damage has occurred, and the availability of effective therapy. Screening is generally carried out either using a non-specific reagin test such as the rapid plasma reagin test (RPR) or venereal disease research laboratory test (VDRL), or a treponemal specific test such as the *Treponema pallidum* haemagglutination test (TPHA), or *T. pallidum* particle agglutination test (TPPA). A positive test with any of these requires confirmation by another unrelated test (reagin or specific), and an adsorbed fluorescent treponemal antigen test (FTA-Abs). The latter test should also be carried out if early syphilis is suspected, for example presence of a genital ulcer, because it may become positive early in the disease before the other tests (Table 16.5). A potential disadvantage of the reagin tests is the biological false positive (BFP), where other unrelated conditions such as acute viral infection or collagen vascular diseases, and even pregnancy itself may give a positive reaction. BFPs need to be distinguished from the positive results given by other treponemal diseases such as yaws and pinta, which cannot be differentiated from syphilis by any currently available laboratory test. Screening tests generally remain positive for life, even in patients adequately treated in the past for syphilis or other treponemal infection. If active syphilis cannot be excluded, then the woman must receive contemporaneously an adequate course of therapy.

Treatment regimens differ substantially between the UK and USA. Authorities in the USA favour a single injection with a depot penicillin such as benzathine penicillin 2.4 mega units [35], in contrast with the UK preference for a course of procaine penicillin at 600 000 units i.m. for 10 days in early syphilis. Depot preparations of penicillin are becoming increasingly difficult to obtain in the UK. Currently available is bicillin, a combination preparation containing procaine penicillin G and sodium penicillin G (equivalent

	Reagin tests (e.g. VDRL, RPR)	Specific tests (e.g. TPHA, TPPA)	FTA-Abs
Early primary syphilis	Negative	Negative	Positive
Late primary syphilis	Positive	Positive	Positive
Secondary syphilis	Strong positive	Strong positive	Positive
Latent syphilis	Positive	Positive	Positive
Treated syphilis	Positive	Positive	Positive
Yaws, pinta (treated or untreated)	Positive	Positive	Positive
Biological false positive	Positive	Negative	Negative

Table 16.5 Serological tests for syphilis.

VDRL, venereal disease research laboratory; RPR, rapid plasma reagin; TPHA, *Treponema pallidum* haemagglutination test; TPPA, *Treponema pallidum* particle agglutination test; FTA-Abs, absorbed treponemal antigen test.

to 600 000 units procaine penicillin G). For penicillin-allergic patients, desensitization should be considered, as there are no trials confirming the efficacy of alternate therapies. Erythromycin 500 mg p.o. four times daily for 14 days has been used, but careful follow-up of the mother and neonate is essential. As in the non-pregnant state, patients should be warned of the possibility of a Jarisch–Herxheimer reaction manifesting as an acute febrile response with rigors within 24 h of starting treatment. Fetal distress and premature labour have been reported [36].

Acute chorioamnionitis

This condition is poorly defined. Histological examination demonstrates infiltration of organisms and polymorphonuclear leucocytes between the layers of chorion and amnion. Clinically, the term is used to describe pyrexia of uncertain cause in late pregnancy, particularly accompanied by lower abdominal pain. Other than maternal pyrexia, there is little by way of confirmatory tests, other than sampling of amniotic fluid, which may reveal an increased white cell count. Other tests such as peripheral blood count and C-reactive protein may add nonspecific weight to the diagnosis. There seems little doubt that maternal and fetal morbidity are increased by this condition, and hence early administration of relevant antibiotics, and progression of labour are important.

Bacteria from the vagina will be implicated, including group B streptococci (GBS), coliforms, anaerobes and *M. hominis*. Depending on the clinical condition, antibiotics with relevant activity include co-amoxyclav (amoxicillin plus clavulanic acid) as a single agent, or a second-generation cephalosporin such as cefuroxime, or ceftriaxone plus metronidazole. In severe circumstances, parenteral therapy with penicillin, clindamycin and gentamicin is required. For further information and discussion on this condition see Gilstrap and Faro [1].

Postpartum pyrexia and puerperal (postabortal) sepsis

Any sustained pyrexia in the 14 days after childbirth is a puerperal (postpartum) pyrexia (UK definition), and an indication for a full infection screen in addition to any other measures indicated at the time of examination. Irrespective of the subsequent bacterial cause of puerperal sepsis, the empirical parenteral antibiotic therapy must cover not only the classical group A streptococcus (GAS) but also other relevant organisms including coliforms and anaerobic bacteria.

Postpartum pyrexia is not uncommon, and rarely proceeds to puerperal sepsis. However, it is mandatory that it

is always regarded seriously, and fully investigated and treated because of the potentially disastrous consequences. To this end an infection screen should be dispatched to the laboratory, and the intensity of monitoring the patient should be increased, with the early (but not necessarily initial) administration of appropriate antibiotics by an appropriate route.

Classical puerperal fever (i.e. generalized systemic infection with *Streptococcus pyogenes* (GAS) is unusual these days, but does still occur. The source of the organism can be either endogenous from a carrier site in the patient, or exogenous from procedures or attendants. The genital carriage of GAS is uncommon in women, but the perianal skin may be colonized following infection at other sites such as the throat and nose. GAS is today still the commonest bacterial cause of a sore throat. Outbreaks and isolated cases of puerperal sepsis associated with GAS still occur from time to time; hence the importance of maintaining basic standards of hygiene in the delivery room.

Symptoms of GAS endometrial infection are severe. The patient is critically ill, with all the hallmarks of uncontrolled septicaemia, including abdominal pain, prostration, pyrexia and hypotension. The lochia may or may not be offensive, nor will it necessarily be obvious. Indeed, if a pyometra (the uterus being full of inspissated pus) has developed, the clinician may be lulled into a false sense of security by the absence of significant discharge. This condition is an obstetrical emergency, and rapid intervention with full resuscitation measures, appropriate antibiotics and serious consideration of emergency hysterectomy are necessary to avoid the high mortality of this condition [37].

Puerperal or postabortal sepsis associated with *Clostridium perfringens (welchi)* infection is now very rare. The patient will be extremely toxic, and radiography may reveal the cardinal sign of myometrial gas formation. Resuscitation, antibiotic therapy and surgical intervention will be required promptly.

The more common form of puerperal or postabortal infection seen today is essentially acute endometritis (infection of the uterus). This is usually an ascending infection from the patient's genital tract, and is characteristically a mixed infection of coliforms and anaerobic organisms. Other organisms, including *Staph. aureus* may be associated, particularly if infection follows instrumentation. It is unusual, but by no means unknown for this form of infection to spread outside the genital tract.

Antimicrobial chemotherapy must be started early. In the absence of symptoms of septicaemia, a β-lactamase-stable penicillin with activity against anaerobic organisms as well is indicated, for example co-amoxyclav (amoxicillin plus clavulanic acid). Alternatively, the same spectrum of activity can be achieved using a second-generation cephalosporin such as cefuroxime, cefotaxime or ceftriaxone with metronidazole to give anaerobic cover. In the presence of signs of severe sepsis, penicillin, clindamycin and an aminoglycoside such as gentamicin should be prescribed in full dosage.

In addition, the other causes of postpartum pyrexia need to be considered, including urinary infection (common), bacteraemia from other genital tract organisms without underlying endometritis (e.g. genital mycoplasmas—see above, GBS infection—see below), infection of any wounds (e.g. episiotomy, caesarean section scar), mastitis and postoperative chest infection. There are a number of non-infectious causes of pyrexia in the puerperium such as thromboembolism, which should not be overlooked.

Group B streptococcus

Group B, β-haemolytic streptococcus (GBS) (*Streptococcus agalactiae*) is a common vaginal commensal. The prevalence varies in different reports but is generally quoted as within the range 4.5–36%. Carriage may occur in one or more of vagina, rectum and perineal skin. Furthermore, it is well established that carriage is intermittent. Thus, it is impossible to exclude carriage of the organism on a single examination.

The main reason for concern about GBS carriage is that neonatal infection can be severe. Between 28% and 72% of babies born to colonized mothers acquire GBS, yet the incidence of neonatal septicaemia is only 0.3–3.7 cases per 1000 live births [38].

Carriage of GBS in the vagina *per se* is not usually associated with symptoms, and the presence of the organism is not necessarily a requirement to treat with specific antibiotic therapy. Indeed, one of the problems is failure of penicillin therapy to eradicate reliably the organism from carrier sites. The reasons for this are probably multiple, including recolonization from other carrier sites, for example rectum, transmission from colonized sexual partners, and inability of antibiotic to act against mucosal colonization.

Two forms of neonatal GBS infection are recognized. The early-onset form occurs within 48 h of delivery, and is characterized by rapid onset of bacteraemic shock, and respiratory distress with or without meningitis. Lethargy and poor feeding are also present. In addition to maternal colonization, predisposing factors include maternal complications in labour such as premature or prolonged rupture of membranes, prematurity, maternal pyrexia and a previous baby with GBS disease. The mortality is high.

Late-onset disease is less likely to be bacteraemic, and more likely to be meningitic. The onset is more insidious, and the prognosis generally better providing diagnosis and treatment are prompt. Late-onset disease is not associated with maternal carriage, nor with prematurity. Nosocomial infection is most likely.

Controversy surrounds the best course for identification and management of women at risk of transmitting GBS infection to their baby. The discussion has not been helped by litigation in what cannot be an exact science. There is little point in routine antenatal screening of women for carriage, because a negative result does not exclude colonization, and a positive result including swabbing of the vagina in late pregnancy is poorly predictive of the likelihood of neonatal infection. Furthermore, attempts at eradication of the organism during pregnancy are unlikely to be successful owing to recolonization. At the other extreme, giving all babies a single dose of a penicillin during labour will expose a large number of infants to an unnecessary antibiotic, with the risk (albeit small) of anaphylaxis or sensitization.

A compromise strategy seems most logical, based for example on perceived risk. Women presenting with any of the following should receive intrapartum antibiotic prophylaxis: premature labour, prolonged rupture of membranes in labour, maternal pyrexia in labour and a previous history of GBS neonatal infection, or GBS urogenital infection in this pregnancy. In addition, women with prolonged rupture of membranes not in labour should receive a course of relevant antibiotic until their GBS carriage status is established. In all cases, a lower vaginal swab must be sent for culture.

Advocates of a screening approach to identification of potential GBS infection recommend vaginal swab tests at 35–37 weeks' gestation. Women found to harbour the organism are offered intrapartum penicillin [39].

Patients not allergic to penicillin should receive either amoxicillin or benzyl-penicillin intravenously. Clindamycin or erythromycin are suitable alternatives.

GBS infection in adults is well recognized. In the postpartum woman, endometritis is the most likely manifestation, and is commoner in women delivered by caesarean section. In most cases, onset of fever and abdominal (uterine) pain occurs within 48 h of delivery. Treatment is with a penicillin, to which the organism is at present always susceptible. Later complications such as pelvic abscess and septic shock, are rare.

Urinary tract infection (see also Chapter 7)

Urinary tract infection will occur in 3–8% of pregnant women, a rate similar to that found in non-pregnant women of the same age. Management of both covert and symptomatic urinary tract infection is important, in order to prevent possible preterm birth, intrauterine growth restriction and stillbirth. Acute pyelonephritis, leading to fetal loss in 16–30% was previously found, but the condition is now unusual owing to early diagnosis and treatment.

Listeriosis

Listeria monocytogenes is a small Gram-positive rod, morphologically resembling a diphtheroid. The organism is ubiquitous in nature, with a wide range of temperature tolerance. It is frequently found in soil, and survives and multiplies at 4°C. Contaminated food will not be protected in a domestic refrigerator, and the organism will survive inadequate pasteurization.

There are about 16 serotypes of *L. monocytogenes*, but only a few are associated with human infection, usually types 4b, 1/2a and 1/2b [40].

Infection in pregnancy is characterized by a biphasic febrile illness in the third trimester. The first stage is usually only considered retrospectively, consisting of non-specific symptoms such as headache, malaise, backache and abdominal or loin pain, pharyngitis and conjunctivitis—essentially 'flu'-like symptoms. The patient may or may not receive antibiotics that by chance are active against *L. monocytogenes*, and recovers. The second attack occurs within 10–15 days of premature delivery, and may reflect reinfection from the contaminated placenta. In about one-third of cases maternal pyrexia in labour will have occurred. Maternal disease can be severe, leading to respiratory distress. However, meningitis (a feature of adult disease) is unusual in pregnancy.

Listeriosis affects approximately one in 30 000 live and stillbirths in the UK. The neonatal mortality in one series was 22.6% [41], but is higher in babies born at gestational age less than 37 weeks. Babies infected during pregnancy are ill at birth or within hours, whereas babies infected at birth will develop late-onset disease 5–7 days later. Predominant features include respiratory distress, bradycardia or apnoea, cyanosis, hepatosplenomegaly and jaundice. In one-third of babies a papular rash is found. The cardinal feature of infection is miliary necrosis of the tissues, best seen as white nodules on the cut surface of the placenta, or abscesses on the maternal surface [42].

Listeria monocytogenes is sensitive to a number of antibiotics *in vitro*. Optimal therapy is with ampicillin or amoxicillin plus gentamicin depending on severity. Treatment should be prolonged for 1 week after fever falls.

Emphasis is on prevention, and all pregnant women should be counselled on the importance of food hygiene and the potential risks of unpasteurized foods such as soft cheeses and paté.

Toxoplasmosis

Toxoplasma infection is a common benign infection in immunocompetent persons. The illness may be asymptomatic, or present as a febrile illness with lymphadenopathy. Untreated, the condition is self-limiting as the parasitaemia subsides and the organisms become dormant in the tissues, commonly brain, heart and skeletal muscle. They may remain viable for the life of the host, and become reactivated should immunosuppression occur, such as following infection with HIV. The importance of this ubiquitous infection lies in the potential for primary infection in pregnancy to lead to congenital infection of the fetus.

Toxoplasma gondii is an obligate intracellular coccidian protozoan parasite. The definitive host is the domestic cat. Tissue cysts from infected animals, or infectious oocysts ingested from soil release viable organisms in the gut of the cat. These trophozoites undergo both asexual (schizogony) and sexual reproduction. The latter results in the release of non-infectious oocysts into the environment. These mature into infectious oocysts by sporulation over 3–4 days. There is no extraintestinal cycle in the cat. However, consumption of oocysts containing viable sporocysts or of tissue cysts by animals or humans leads to an abortive life cycle of tissue invasion in the abnormal host. Humans are usually infected by consumption of infected undercooked meat, particularly lamb and pork.

The consequence to the fetus depends on the time of maternal primary infection in relation to gestation. The earlier the infection, the lower the chance of fetal infection, but the more likely severe involvement (Table 16.6) [43]. Maternal infection is frequently unnoticed, or presents as a self-limiting non-specific illness.

Establishment of infection in the placenta may lead to congenital infection. Severe early infection may lead to abortion or stillbirth. The classic triad of intracranial calcification, hydrocephalus and choroidoretinitis is the most extreme form, but is not common. The majority (>90%) of babies are asymptomatic at birth. Manifestations of the disease are numerous, including encephalitis, epilepsy, mental and growth retardation, jaundice, hepatosplenomegaly, thrombocytopaenia and skin rashes.

Estimates of maternal infection are unreliable, and observed rates are much lower than expected rates. About 14 cases were reported to the British Paediatric Surveillance Unit between 1989 and 1990, compared with an expected 30–40 severely affected [44].

Time of maternal infection	Fetal infection rate (%)	Severe disease at birth (%)	Ocular sequelae (%)
Preconception	Unknown	Unknown	–
First trimester	25	75	45–65
Second trimester	50	55	45–65
Third trimester	65	<5	45–65

Table 16.6 Transmission of toxoplasmosis in pregnancy. (From [43].)

Testing for toxoplasmosis is far from straightforward. Preconception testing will establish those who have previously been infected, and will not therefore have an infected child, or those susceptible who can be counselled concerning contact with cats, uncooked food and general hygiene. The problem surrounds the interpretation of tests performed during pregnancy. The most widely used test is the serum *Toxoplasma* latex agglutination test (Eiken test). Unfortunately this test is prone to false-negative results in active disease because antibody may take several weeks to appear. Rheumatoid factor or non-specific IgM may result in false-positive results. Therefore, in pregnancy, serum should always be sent to a reference laboratory for determination of specific antitoxoplasma IgM, and the definitive *Toxoplasma* dye test. IgM can be determined using the immunosorbent agglutination assay (ISAGA). IgM-positive serum indicates recent infection, but the problem is to determine how recent, in order to guide the clinician and patient regarding the probability of severe congenital infection. Avidity tests have gone some way to assisting, in that low avidity seems to indicate recent acute infection (<3 months), whereas high-avidity IgG indicates chronic infection. The only certain way of positively identifying acute infection is the demonstration of seroconversion.

If acute infection of the mother is likely, then ultrasound and cordocentesis should be considered, and serology carried out on cord blood to determine whether congenital infection is established. Although not without risk, the result is important because it may influence the choice of anti-infective drugs and whether to continue with pregnancy.

Mothers thought to be suffering from acute *Toxoplasma* infection who either do not seek termination, or in whom termination is not indicated, require antimicrobial therapy for the duration of the pregnancy. The drug of choice is the macrolide spiramycin, which can safely be given throughout pregnancy. Firm evidence of congenital infection should lead to therapy with short courses of sulfadiazine and pyrimethamine alternating with spiramycin until delivery. It should be noted that although studies indicate a reduction in congenital infection with these regimens, there are no double-blind placebo-controlled trials reported.

Controversy continues over whether antenatal screening should be routine. However, the imprecision of the currently available tests would suggest that the extra uncertainty and anxiety would not justify any possible benefit.

Malaria[2]

Plasmodium infection should be considered in any patient with fever and/or jaundice who has recently travelled through Africa, South-East Asia, India or South America. Pregnant women have an increased incidence of infection, and parasitaemia may be great [45] probably due to impaired host defences [46]. In addition, chondroitin sulphate A, present in the placenta, binds *Plasmodium falciparum* infected red blood cells [47]. Haemolytic anaemia which can cause jaundice may be severe in pregnancy, and hepatorenal syndrome is often the cause of death. Malaria may infect the placenta leading to maternal anaemia, spontaneous abortion, still birth and low birthweight. Malaria parasites may cross the placenta, particularly in non-immune mothers [48] leading to congenital malaria. Immune primigravidae are prone to relapse in the second trimester [49]. The placentae of patients treated for malaria in pregnancy should always be examined histologically for the presence of parasites. If these are present, the neonate is at risk and should be given a course of antimalarial therapy.

Prophylaxis and treatment depend on the local area, the dominant Plasmodium type and pattern of drug resistance. In theory, chloroquine would be the treatment of choice for severe infestation with *Plasmodium falciparum* in chloroquine-sensitive areas [50], even though this drug has been suspected of causing neonatal deafness if used in the first trimester [49], it is not a major teratogen [51]. Quinine is less safe in pregnancy, although in a collaborative perinatal study of 106 women exposed to quinine in early pregnancy there was no increase in frequency of congenital malformation [52].

Quinine does not increase the risk of preterm labour [53] but in pregnancy in particular, patients are at risk from

[2]The section on Malaria was written by Dr Stephen Wright and Professor Michael de Swiet.

quinine-induced hyperinsulinaemia [53] which has caused fatal hypoglycaemia [54]. If 50% dextrose is not effective, somatostatin analogues such as SMS 201–995 that inhibit insulin release are the treatment of choice for quinine-induced hypoglycaemia and they may be the only effective therapy [55]. Despite these concerns about quinine, falciparum malaria is so dangerous and the prevalence of chloroquine resistance is so high that all pregnant patients with falciparum malaria should be treated with quinine and Fansidar (pyrimethamine with sulfadoxine) whatever the source of infection—possible pregnancy-related risks are trivial by comparison with the risks of the disease.

In chloroquine-resistant areas, the combination of pyrimethamine and dapsone (Maloprim) has been used for prophylaxis in pregnancy and is probably safe providing extra folate (10 mg/day) is given [56] (pyrimethamine and proguanil are folate antagonists). Fansidar (sulphadoxine-pyrimethamine) has also been used alone for malaria prophylaxis in a high-risk area (Kenya) [57]. Pyrimethamine is excreted in breast milk, but appears harmless to the breastfed infant. The sulphone drug, dapsone, and various sulphonamides, are often used in combination with trimethoprim, pyrimethamine or primaquine, but haemolysis may occur in neonates and adults with glucose-6-phosphate dehydrogenase deficiency.

The British National Formulary at the time of writing advises that halofantrine and doxycycline (causes dental discoloration) should not be used in pregnancy, and that mefloquine and Fansidar (despite comments above) are best avoided until further information is available [58].

Patterns of resistance to antimalarials change so rapidly that expert advice should always be sought regarding treatment and prophylaxis. It is likely that proguanil and chloroquine are the safest drugs in pregnancy.

Malaria prophylaxis with chloroquine or proguanil should be continued throughout pregnancy and visitors to high-risk (holoendemic) areas should continue with their prophylaxis for at least the last trimester and preferably until after delivery [59]. The crucial importance of compliance must be stressed and advice must be given on the avoidance of mosquito bites. Importation of malaria is increasing in the UK. Health advice for travellers outside the European Community is available in pamphlet form from the Department of Health and is also accessible on Prestel.

References

1 Gilstrap LC, Faro S. *Infections in Pregnancy*. Wiley-Liss, New York.

2 Macsween KF, Ridgway GL. The laboratory investigation of vaginal discharge. *J Clin Pathol* 1998; 51: 564–7.

3 Sobel JD. Vaginitis. *N Engl J Med* 1997; 337: 1896–902.

4 Taylor-Robinson D, McCormack WM. The genital mycoplasmas I. *N Engl J Med* 1980; 302: 1003–10.

5 Taylor-Robinson D, McCormack WM. The genital mycoplasmas II. *N Engl J Med* 1980; 302: 1063–7.

6 Amsel R, Totten PA et al. Non-specific vaginitis. Diagnostic criteria and microbiologic and epidemiologic associations. *Am J Med* 1983; 74: 14–22.

7 Gravett MG, Hummel D et al. Preterm labour associated with subclinical amniotic fluid infection and with bacterial vaginosis. *Obstet Gynecol* 1986; 67: 229–37.

8 Hay PE, Lamont RF et al. Abnormal bacterial colonisation of the genital tract and subsequent pre-term delivery and late miscarriage. *Br Med J* 1994; 308: 295–8.

9 Hillier SL, Nugent RP et al. Association between bacterial vaginosis and preterm delivery of a low birth weight infant. *N Engl J Med* 1995; 333: 1737–42.

10 Furman LM. Neonatal *gardnerella* infection. *Paediatr Infect Dis J* 1988; 7: 890.

11 Royce RA, Thorp J, Granados JL, Savitz DA. Bacterial vaginosis associated with HIV infection in pregnant women from North Carolina. *J AIDS Hum Retrotirol* 1999; 20: 382–6.

12 Hay PE, Morgan DJ et al. A longitudinal study of bacterial vaginosis in pregnancy. *Br J Obstet Gynecol* 1994; 101: 1048–53.

13 Cotch MF, Pastorek JG et al. *Trichomonas vaginalis* associated with low birth-weight and preterm delivery. *Sex Transm Dis* 1997; 24: 353–60.

14 Saurina GR, McCormack WM. Trichomoniasis in pregnancy. *Sex Transm Dis* 1997; 24: 361–2.

15 Sobel JD. *Candida* vulvo-vaginitis. *Clin Obstet Gynecol* 1993; 36: 153–66.

16 Mårdh P-A. The vaginal ecosystem. *Am J Obstet Gynecol* 1991; 165: 1163–8.

17 Clinical Effectiveness Group. National guidelines for the management of gonorrhoea in adults. *Sex Transm Infect* 1999; 75: S13–15.

18 Grun L, Tassano-Smith J et al. Comparison of two methods of screening for genital chlamydial infection in women attending in general practice: cross sectional survey. *Br Med J* 1997; 315: 226–30.

19 Fish ANJ, Fairweather DV, Oriel J, Ridgway GL. *Chlamydia trachomatis* infection in a gynaecology clinic population: identification of high risk groups and the value of contact tracing. *Eur J Obstet Gynecol Reprod Biol* 1989; 31: 67–74.

20 Ridgway GL, Mumtaz G, Stephens RA, Oriel JD. Therapeutic abortion and chlamydial infection. *Br Med J* 1983; 286: 1478–9.

21 Hammerschlag MR. *Chlamydia trachomatis* infection and pregnancy. In: Reeves P, ed. *Chlamydial Infections*. Berlin: Springer-Verlag, 1987: 56–71.

22 Schachter J, Ridgway GL, Collier L. Chlamydial diseases. In: Collier L, Balows A, Sussman M, eds (edition), Hausler WJ, Sussman M, eds (volume). *Topley and Wilson's Microbiology and Microbial Infections*, Vol. 3. Arnold, London, 1998: 977–94.

23 Gravett M, Nelson H et al. Independent association of bacterial vaginosis and *Chlamydia trachomatis* infection with adverse pregnancy outcome. *J Am Med Assoc* 1987; 256: 1899–903.

24 Martin D, Koutsky L et al. Prematurity and perinatal mortality in pregnancy associated with maternal *Chlamydia trachomatis* infection. *J Am Med Assoc* 1982; 247: 1585–8.

25 Sweet RL, Lander D et al. *Chlamydia trachomatis* infection and pregnancy outcome. *Am J Obstet Gynecol* 1987; 156: 824–33.

26 Gencay M, Koskiniemi M *et al. Chlamydia trachomatis* seropositivity during pregnancy is associated with perinatal complications. *Clin Infect Dis* 1995; 21: 424–6.

27 Bell TA, Stamm WE *et al.* Delayed appearance *Chlamydia trachomatis* infections acquired at birth. *Paediatr Infect Dis* 1987; 6: 928–31.

28 Weiss SG, Newcombe RW, Beem MO. Pulmonary assessment of children after chlamydial infection of infancy. *J Paediatr Infect* 1986; 108: 59–64.

29 Davies PO, Ridgway GL. The role of polymerase chain reaction and ligase chain reaction for the detection of *Chlamydia trachomatis. Int J STD Aids* 1997; 8: 731–8.

30 Mahony J, Chong S *et al.* Urine specimens from pregnant and non-pregnant women inhibitory to amplification of *Chlamydia trachomatis* nucleic acid by PCR, ligase chain reaction, and transcription mediated amplification: identification of urinary substances associated with inhibition and removal of inhibitory substances. *J Clin Microbiol* 1998; 36: 3122–6.

31 Clinical Effectiveness Group. National guidelines for the management of *Chlamydia trachomatis* genital tract infection. *Sex Transm Infect* 1999; 75: S4–8.

32 Turrentine MA, Newton ER. Amoxicillin or erythromycin for the treatment of antenatal chlamydial infection: a meta-analysis. *Obstet Gynecol* 1995; 86: 1021–5.

33 Miller JM. Efficacy and tolerance of single dose azithromycin for the treatment of chlamydial cervicitis during pregnancy. *Infect Dis Obstet Gynecol* 1995; 3: 189–92.

34 Taylor-Robinson D, Bradbury J. Mycoplasma diseases. In: Balows A, Collier L, Hausler WJ, Sussman M, eds. *Topley and Wilson's Microbiology and Microbial Infections*, 3. London: Arnold, 1998: 1013–37.

35 Centers For Disease Control and Prevention. 1998 guidelines for treatment of sexually transmitted diseases. *MMWR* 1998: 47 (RR1).

36 Clinical Effectiveness Group. National guidelines for the management of early syphilis. *Sex Transm Infect* 1999; 75: S29–33.

37 Gergis H, Barik S, Lim K, Porter W. Life-threatening puerperal infection with Group A streptococcus. *J R Soc Med* 1999; 92: 412–13.

38 Ridgway GL. Bacterial infections. In: Chamberlain G, ed. *Modern Antenatal Care of the Foetus*. Oxford: Blackwell Scientific Publications, 1990: 221–3.

39 Schuchat A. Epidemiology of Group B streptococcal disease in the United States: shifting paradigms. *Clin Microbiol Rev* 1998; 11: 497–513.

40 Lorber B. Listeriosis. *Clin Infect Dis* 1997; 24: 1–11.

41 Relier JP. Listeriosis. *J Antimicrob Chemother* 1979; 5 (Suppl. A): 51–7.

42 Ridgway GL. Bacterial infections. In: Chamberlain G, ed. *Modern Antenatal Care of the Foetus*. Oxford: Blackwell, 1990: 217–18.

43 Holliman RE. Congenital toxoplasmosis. prevention, screening and treatment. *J Hosp Infect* 1995; 30 (Suppl.): 179–90.

44 Hall SM. Congenital toxoplasmosis. *Br Med J* 1992; 305: 291–7.

45 Bray RS, Anderson MJ. Falciparum malaria and pregnancy. *Trans Roy Soc Trop Med Hyg* 1979;73:427–31.

46 Gilles HM, Lawson JB *et al.* Malaria, anaemia and pregnancy. *Ann Trop Med Parasit 1969; 63:245–63*

47 Fried M, Duffy PE. Adherence of *Plasmodium falciparum* to chondroitin sulfate A in the human placenta. *Science* 1996; 272: 1502–4.

48 Jelliffe EEP. Placental malaria and foetal growth failure. In: Aysen RN (ed). *Nutrition and Infection*. CIBA Foundation Study Group, No 31, Churchill, London, 1967.

49 Trusell RR, Beeley L. Infestations. In: *Clinics in Obstetrics and Gynaecology: Prescribing in Pregnancy*, Volume 8. WB Saunders, London, 1981: 333–340.

50 Lancet editorial. Malaria in pregnancy. *Lancet* 1983; ii: 84–5.

51 Wolfe MS, Cordero JF. Safety of chloroquine in chemosuppression of malaria during pregnancy. *Br Med J* 1985; 290: 1466–7.

52 Heinonen OP, Slone D *et al. Birth Defects and Drugs in Pregnancy*. Publishing Sciences Group Inc, Littleton, Massachusetts: 1977.

53 Looareesuwan S, Philips RE *et al.* Quinine and severe falciparum malaria in late pregnancy. *Lancet* 1985; ii: 4–7.

54 White NJ, Warrell DA *et al.* Severe hypoglycaemia and hyperinsulinaemia in falciparum malaria. *N Engl J Med* 1983; 309: 61–6.

55 Philips RE, Warrell DA *et al.* Effectiveness of SMS 201–995, a synthetic long acting somatostatin analogue, in treatment of quinine induced hyperinsulinaemia. *Lancet* 1986; i: 713–6.

56 Bruce-Chwatt LJ. Malaria and pregnancy. *Br Med J* 1983; 296: 1457–8.

57 Shulman CE, Dorman EK *et al.* Intermittent sulphadoxine-pyrimethamine to prevent severe anaemia secondary to malaria in pregnancy: a randomised placebo-controlled trial. *Lancet* 1999; 353: 632–63.

58 BNF 39: British National Formulary. The British Medical Association and the Royal Pharmaceutical Society of Great Britain. London, 2000: 299.

59 Bruce-Chwatt LJ. *Essential Malariology*. Heinemann Medical, London 1980.

Further reading

Infections and pregnancy. MacLeon A, Regan L & Corrington D. 2001; RCOG Press, London.

17 Viral infections in pregnancy
Jangu E. Banatvala

The prevalence, severity and outcome of virus infections in pregnancy is dependent on such variables as the patient's nutritional state, often poor in many developing countries, compounded by the lack of facilities for the appropriate management of persons who may have some of the more severe forms of such exotic infections as Japanese encephalitis, virally induced haemorrhagic fevers and infection by hepatitis E virus. It is possible that abnormal pulmonary ventilation (see Chapter 1) in the late stages of pregnancy may contribute to the development of severe pulmonary complications in such infections as influenza A and varicella.

Immunological factors may also play a part. Thus, it is known that some cell-mediated immune responses may be suppressed during pregnancy, reverting to normal postpartum. This may provide an explanation, for example, as to why genital warts may increase considerably in size during pregnancy but regress markedly in the puerperium. There is as yet no consensus as to the exact mechanisms involved in maternal immunosuppression. Increased concentration of placental hormones, fetal products that may be immunosuppressive or the production of cytokines and other uncharacterized serum factors that suppress lymphocyte-activated responses to mitogens may be possible factors [1]. Severe and sometimes fatal maternal infections are more likely to occur during the last trimester; such infections often result in premature delivery and fetal death.

Virus infections that may be unduly severe in pregnancy

Table 17.1 lists viral infections that may be severe or fatal in pregnancy, together with preventive measures.

With regard to smallpox, although not listed since it was eradicated worldwide in 1979, such complications as unduly severe disease (including haemorrhagic smallpox frequently resulting in death) occurred four to five times more frequently among pregnant women. Nevertheless, the potential for use of smallpox by bioterrorists should be considered. Vaccination against smallpox was effective in preventing infection, however, if carried out during pregnancy, vaccinia virus could be transmitted transplacentally to the fetus resulting in fetal vaccinia or delivery of an infant with evidence of active lesions or scarring.

The classification and characteristics of other viruses of significance in pregnancy are listed in Table 17.2.

Influenza (Fig. 17.1)

The major epidemics of influenza A occurring in 1918 (H1N1) and in 1957 (H2N2) were associated with an increased mortality in pregnancy among patients with chronic cardiac disease, particularly valvular heart disease. An analysis of 200 deaths occurring in New York City following the 1957 epidemic showed that 25% of 93 deaths among those aged 50 or less were among pregnant women [2]. Deaths occurred more infrequently during the last trimester.

Virus infection	Comments	Prevention
Influenza A (B)	Increased mortality in 1918 and 1957 associated with chronic heart disease	Influenza vaccine (disrupted or subunit)
Varicella	Mortality associated with pneumonia among adults. Possibly more severe in pregnancy	Varicella-zoster immune globulin preferably within 10 days (preferably sooner) of contact. (Treat established infections if severe with aciclovir systemically)
Poliomyelitis	Spinal paralysis increases with gestational age	Polio vaccine for travellers to remaining endemic areas if not already immunized
Measles	Increased mortality and complications in pregnancy	In the absence of previous vaccination or history of measles give normal human immunoglobulin to contacts
Hepatitis E	10–17% mortality with fetal death in last trimester. Endemic in many developing countries	Trials in progress with recombinant derived vaccines
Lassa fever	70–90% mortality with fetal death in last trimester. Endemic in West Africa	? Prophylactic ribivarin to pregnant household contacts. (Treat patient with ribivarin systemically)
Japanese B encephalitis	Up to 30–40% mortality; higher in pregnancy with fetal death. Widely distributed in South-East Asia and the Far East	Vaccine available on named patient basis for travellers to endemic areas

Table 17.1 Virus infections that may be severe or fatal in pregnancy. (*Basic Science in Obstetrics and Gynaecology. A Textbook for MRCOG Part I*, 3rd edn. de Swiet M, Chamberlain G, Bennett P (eds). Churchill Livingstone, Edinburgh, 2002: 126–127; with permission.)

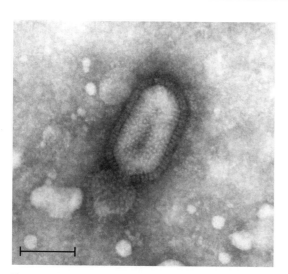

Fig 17.1 Electron micrograph of influenza virus (negative staining with 3% sodium phosphotungstate, pH 6.0). Bar = 100 nm. (By kind permission of Dr Ian L Chrystie, Department of Infection (Virology), Guy's, King's and St Thomas' School of Medicine, King's College London, London.)

Influenza A and B may be prevented by immunization; there is no contraindication because currently licensed vaccines, which provide 70–80% protection against infection, are either inactivated and purified or are 'split virus vaccines' consisting of surface antigens (haemagglutinin and neuraminidase) prepared from disrupted influenza particles [3].

Although such drugs as amantadine and rimantadine may be used to prevent or treat influenza A (but not B) and ribavarin may be effective in reducing the symptoms of both influenza A and B, these drugs are not licensed for use in pregnancy. More recently, zanamivir (which works by inhibiting influenza viruses neuraminidase) has been shown to be effective in reducing the duration of influenza symptoms [4]. Although the drug has been shown to be safe and well tolerated among adults, there is no information relating to its effects on the developing human fetus.

Herpes virus infections (Fig. 17.2)

Although eight human herpes viruses have been identified, only varicella zoster virus (VZV) and herpes simplex

Table 17.2 Classification and characteristics of viruses of significance in pregnancy. (*Basic Science in Obstetrics and Gynaecology. A Textbook for MRCOG Part I*, 3rd edn. de Swiet M, Chamberlain G & Bennett P (eds). Churchill Livingstone, Edinburgh, 2002: 126–127; with permission.)

Virus	Maternal, intrauterine or perinatal infection	Classification	Genome	Properties of virus symmetry	Size (nm)	Envelope
Herpes simplex virus type 1 and 2,	Perinatal	Herpesvirus*	ds DNA	Cubic	120–300	Yes
Varicella zoster virus	Maternal, intrauterine, perinatial	Herpesvirus*	ds DNA	Cubic	180–200	Yes
Cytomegalovirus	Intrauterine, perinatial	Herpesvirus†	ds DNA	Cubic	150–200	Yes
Hepatitis B virus	Perinatal	Hepadnavirus	ds DNA	Cubic	40–42	Yes
Hepatitis C virus	Perinatal	Hepacivirus	(+) ss RNA	Cubic	not known	Yes
Hepatitis E virus	Maternal	Calicivirus	(+) ss RNA	Cubic	27–34	No
Human immunodeficiency virus type I and II	Intrauterine, perinatal	Retrovirus	(+) ss RNA	Cubic	110	Yes
Rubella virus	Intrauterine	Rubivirus	(+) ss RNA	Cubic	58	Yes
Human parvovirus B19	Intrauterine	Parvovirus	(+) or (−) ss DNA	Cubic	18–26	No
Human papillomavirus	Perinatal	Papovavirus	ds DNA	Cubic	55	No
Enteroviruses	Intrauterine, perinatal	Picornavirus	(+) ss RNA	Cubic	24–30	No
Influenza virus A and B	Maternal	Orthomyxovirus	(−) ss RN	Helical	120	Yes
Japanese encephalitis virus	Maternal	Flavivirus	(+) ss RNA	Cubic	40–60	Yes
Lassa virus	Maternal	Arenavirus	ambisense ss RNA	Cubic	90–110	Yes
HTLV1	Perinatal	Retrovirus	(+) ss RNA	Cubic	110	Yes
HTLV 2	?	Retrovirus	(+) ss RNA	Cubic	110	Yes

*Herpes simplex viruses and varicella zoster viruses are subclassified as α herpes viruses. These herpes viruses have a variable host range, grow rapidly in cell culture, efficiently destroying infected cells, and establish latency *in vivo* primarily in sensory ganglia.
†Cytomegalovirus is subclassified as a β herpes virus. These herpes viruses usually have a restricted host range, grow slowly in cell culture, infected cells often show cytomegalic inclusions both *in vivo* and *in vitro*. They establish latency in a variety of tissues including secretory glands, the kidney and lymphoreticular cells.

virus (HSV) have been shown to be unduly severe in pregnancy. The epidemiology of varicella (chickenpox) exhibits a changing pattern in the UK [5]. There is now not only a higher incidence in preschool children (perhaps because of the increased use of day-care centres and playgroups) but also an increased incidence among adults. Thus, in 1975, approximately 10% of adults were susceptible but, by 1990, the percentage had doubled. This may in part reflect the fact that there is now a significant proportion of adults who were born in and spent some of their childhood days in such developing parts of the world as Africa, India and South-East Asia where up to 30% of adults may be susceptible to varicella. Indeed, in South-East Asia and the Caribbean, 25–60% of adults are susceptible; in Singapore, the peak incidence shifted from those aged 5–14 in 1982 to 15–24 by 1990. For reasons that are not understood, there appears to be little transmission among younger children in many developing parts of the world.

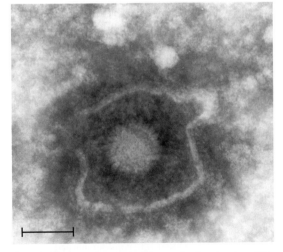

Fig 17.2 Electron micrograph of herpes simplex virus (negative staining with 3% sodium phosphotungstate, pH 6.0). Bar = 100 nm. (By kind permission of Dr Ian L Chrystie, Department of Infection (Virology), Guy's, King's and St Thomas' School of Medicine, King's College London, London.)

Varicella among adults may be considerably more severe than among children, and there is therefore some doubt as to whether infection in pregnancy is more severe than among non-pregnant adults. Those who are immunosuppressed as a result of disease or treatment may experience particularly severe infection, and varicella pneumonitis occurs more commonly and severely among smokers.

Varicella zoster immunoglobulin (VZIG) should be administered to pregnant women who give no history of having had varicella or who have been shown by serological tests to be susceptible. A latex agglutination test can give a result within minutes although the sensitivity of different reagent batches varies. Enzyme immunoassays are more reliable, and results are generally available within a day or so. VZIG is used not only to reduce the severity of infection in pregnancy but theoretically also to reduce viral load, thereby reducing the risk of malformation in pregnancy. VZIG should be given within 10 days of exposure. This may attentuate, but not necessarily preventing infection. VZIG is not effective once varicella has developed but, because infection may be severe and life-threatening among some adults, consideration should be given to treating patients, including those who are pregnant, with systemically administered aciclovir [6]. For medicolegal reasons, patients should be told that this drug is not licensed for use during pregnancy but that an adverse outcome is not expected since over 200 women have now been treated in the first trimester and their infants showed no excess of fetal malformations. It is important to remind mothers not to attend antenatal clinics until their lesions have crusted.

In contrast with varicella, infection by HSV type 1 (HSV-1) is acquired in childhood in most developing countries. However, in industrialized countries, only about 30–40% of adults (particularly those in the higher socio-economic groups) are immune. Studies conducted in London have shown that acquisition of antibodies to HSV type 2 (HSV-2) correlates with the age of sexual activity as well as ethnicity. Among women of childbearing age, the presence of antibodies to HSV-2 is uncommon among Asians from the Indian Sub-Continent but the proportion among Afro-Caribbeans and Africans is about 50% [7]. Most infections in pregnancy are the result of reactivation of latent HSV-1 or HSV-2. Primary infections, if clinically overt, may be particularly severe and usually involve the oropharynx or the genital tract. Primary genital lesions may be associated with considerable oedema, and urinary retention may occur. However, there have been a small number of reports of particularly severe infection in pregnancy associated with liver disease accompanied by thrombocytopenia, leucopenia, coagulation defects and encephalitis. Although severe infections in pergnancy are rare, they are associated with a high mortality and fetal death is common (reviewed in [8]). Severe infections should be treated with aciclovir.

Hepatitis viruses

Infection by hepatitis A, B or C is not associated with a significantly increased mortality rate in pregnancy, although the severity of hepatitis A increases with age. However, hepatitis C may result in deterioration in liver histopathology during pregnancy, although it is not known whether this improves post partum [9]. In contrast, hepatitis E, which like hepatitis A is transmitted by the oro-faecal route may be severe in pregnancy and mortality rates from 10 to 17% have been described in developing countries. Mortality rates increase in successive trimesters. Outbreaks of water-borne infection are common in developing countries. Infection is rare in industrialized countries and, if reported, is the result of infection being acquired abroad [10].

Poliomyelitis

As a result of the World Health Organization's WHO immunization campaigns, poliomyelitis has not only been eliminated from the Western Hemisphere but also from many developing parts of the world. However, polio is still endemic in parts of Central Africa and, to a lesser extent, in parts of the Indian Sub-Continent. Where polio is still endemic, severe disease may occur among unvaccinated adults. During pregnancy, the severity of paralytic disease increases with gestational age [11].

There is no evidence to suggest that the administration of attenuated polio vaccine results in fetal infection or damage and, although it is recommended that live vaccines should not be administered during pregnancy, it would be prudent to vaccinate pregnant women who have not had a full course of vaccine (or who are uncertain about this) should they be visiting polio-endemic parts of the world.

Blood-borne viral infections

The prevalence and risks to the mother and fetus of blood-borne infections caused by the various hepatitis viruses are considered in Chapter 9.

Japanese encephalitis

Infection is mosquito borne and caused by a flavivirus. Infection is widely distributed in South-East Asia and the

Far East, and occurs more commonly in rural areas, particularly where paddy fields and pig farming coexist. Generally, infection occurs during the monsoon. Although most infections are asymptomatic, about one in 200 may be associated with an encephalitis carrying a mortality rate of 30–40%; a high proportion of survivors have permanent neurological sequelae.

Pregnancy is associated with particularly high maternal and fetal mortality rates. Japanese encephalitis (JE) virus has been shown to cross the placenta [12]. Although immunization with a formalin-inactivated whole-cell vaccine is recommended for those who will be residing in JE-endemic countries for longer than a month, the vaccine may occasionally induce severe allergic as well as local reactions at the injection site. Immunization could therefore upset an unstable pregnancy, although such risks must be evaluated against the risks of acquiring infection, particularly in rural areas during or after the rainy season. Three doses of vaccine are required and since some reactions may occur as late as 10 days after any one of the three injections, vaccinees are advised to avoid long-haul flights until at least 10 days have elapsed [13]. Emphasis should be placed on preventing infection by ensuring that appropriate clothing is worn and use is made of insect repellents.

Viral haemorrhagic fevers (Fig. 17.3)

These include infections caused by arenaviruses (e.g. Lassa fever, Bolivian haemorrhagic fever and Argentinean haemorrhagic fever), filoviruses (Marburg and Ebola) and yellow fever (flavivirus). Dengue may be associated with a haemorrhagic diathesis in severe cases, mostly in children but occasionally in adults including pregnant women who may deliver infants prematurely. Very occasionally their newborn infants may have, or develop, manifestations of haemorrhagic disease [14].

Pregnant women are at increased risk of dying from haemorrhagic fevers, particularly if acquired during the last trimester. In those who survive, fetal death is likely to occur [15–17].

There is more information relating to Lassa fever in pregnancy than for other viruses causing acute haemorrhagic fevers. In general, infection occurs in rural areas in West Africa where humans are exposed to the secretions and excretions of *Mastomys natalensis*, a rodent that is the natural reservoir. A study carried out in Sierra Leone showed that, during a Lassa fever epidemic, it was responsible for 25% of maternal deaths and that, among patients who suffered spontaneous abortion or in whom the uterus was evacuated, there was a fourfold increase in the maternal fatality rate [18]. Ribavarin provides

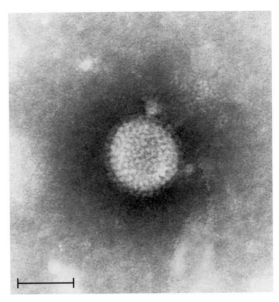

Fig 17.3 Electron micrograph of Lassa virus (negative staining with 3% sodium phosphotungstate, pH 6.0). Bar = 100 nm. (By kind permission of Dr David S Ellis, London School of Hygiene and Tropical Medicine, London.)

effective treatment but must be given early in the course of infection; health-care workers sustaining percutaneous injury to blood or other body fluids should be given oral ribavarin prophylactically.

Viral vaccines in pregnancy

Inactivated, subunit or recombinantly derived vaccines are unlikely to be teratogenic, although those that may be reactogenic could, because of fever or because of the induction of other factors, result in miscarriage.

Administration of attenuated vaccines should whenever possible be avoided in pregnancy. There is no evidence, however, to suggest that such live vaccines as polio, yellow fever or rubella are teratogenic or cause fetal death. As stated above, risks of acquiring such severe infections as polio or yellow fever in those who have to travel to endemic areas should be weighed against the hypothetical risks of administration of live vaccines during pregnancy. Indeed, if attenuated polio vaccine posed any risk, it could not be used as a vaccine because infants and children who are given this vaccine excrete the virus and may transmit it to susceptible contacts, thereby immunizing them. It must be borne in mind that attenuated yellow fever virus is neurotropic in animals. Furthermore, transplacental transmission (but without fetal damage) has been recorded and these factors justify the caution that must be exercised in administering this vaccine in pregnancy [19,20].

Although the administration of live attenuated rubella vaccine to pregnant women is contraindicated, no abnormalities compatible with congenitally acquired rubella have been detected in more than 500 infants delivered of such women. However, in about 3%, there is virological evidence of congenital infection, namely the presence of a virus-specific IgM and/or the persistence of rubella IgG beyond the time that maternal antibodies should have disappeared. Pregnant women, inadvertantly vaccinated should be counselled and should they wish to continue with their pregnancy, reassured. Thus, therapeutic abortion is not indicated.

The diagnosis of intrauterine and perinatal infections: the virological approach

It is essential to ensure close collaboration between clinical and laboratory personnel to ensure that appropriate specimens, including follow-up ones, are collected by those who have the necessary skills in obtaining them. Most laboratories retain serum samples obtained at antenatal booking clinics for at least a year and often longer. Such specimens may be useful for comparison of serological responses with blood obtained from the mother at delivery or shortly thereafter.

Prenatal diagnoses may be made by the detection of virus-specific IgM in fetal blood, culturing the virus or, perhaps more appropriately today, by detecting its nucleic acid by gene amplification techniques in fetal blood or chorionic villus samples. Because virus-specific IgM does not cross the placenta, its presence is indicative of an intrauterine infection. However, such investigations are limited by the fact that responses are unlikely to be detected until the fetus is of about 22 weeks gestational age and, even after then, a negative response cannot exclude an intrauterine infection.

Although gene amplification techniques such as polymerase chain reaction (PCR) are of great sensitivity, this in itself is a limiting factor, because contamination from maternal blood may occur, thereby producing a false-positive result. Molecular techniques including dot blot hybridization and PCR on fetal blood obtained by cordocentesis or by amniocentesis are of value in establishing a diagnosis of prenatal infection by human parvovirus B19, if there is evidence of falling haemoglobin levels and hydramnios, because consideration can then be given to intrauterine blood transfusion. PCR may be used to detect cytomegalovirus (CMV) in amniotic fluid in order to establish a diagnosis of an intrauterine infection, although maternal CMV infections (whether the result of a primary infection or

reactivation) are usually subclinical; consequently those caring for such patients will not be alerted to the occurrence of such an infection. However, intrauterine infection does not provide evidence of fetal damage (see below). Because maternal rubella almost invariably results in fetal infection during the first trimester, little will be gained by attempting to establish a prenatal diagnosis. Attempts to detect rubella virus in chorionic villus biopsies following maternal infection after the first trimester have not been shown to be sufficiently reliable for diagnostic purposes [21]. The detection of rubella virus RNA in amniotic fluid and fetal blood seems more promising: sensitivities of 87.5% and positive predictive values of 100% were obtained when these specimens were tested by the reverse transcription PCR of Bosma *et al.* [22] (G. Enders & D. Betzel, personal communication).

Unfortunately, many clinicians still request a TORCH (toxoplasmosis, rubella, CMV, herpes) screening test for the serological diagnosis of infants who may have intrauterine or perinatal infections. A Public Health Laboratory Service (PHLS) Working Party has recommended that the use of the acronym TORCH should be discouraged [23,24]. This is because the acronym TORCH relates only to toxoplasma, rubella, CMV and HSV. As can be seen from Table 17.3, the list of viruses that may induce intrauterine and perinatal infections is more extensive [25]. Furthermore, apart from rubella, specific IgM tests may be negative in cord or early samples collected in the first few days of life. Consequently, additional blood may need to be tested during the next 2–4 weeks.

In addition to serological tests, it is of importance to collect excretions or secretions to identify viruses neonatally. Thus, such techniques as cell culture or PCR may be used to identify neonatal HSV, enteroviruses, CMV and human parvovirus B19. Since infants infected with CMV, particularly those manifesting clinical features, excrete very high concentrations of virus, herpes virus particles may be detected by electron microscopy within a few minutes of processing the sample. Identification of viruses neonatally is of importance not only diagnostically but also for infection control because such viruses as HSV and enteroviruses may spread readily to other infants as well as staff working in nurseries for the newborn. Such infections need to be identified rapidly; tests to detect virus-specific IgM may become positive in due course but, by that time, infection may have spread to susceptible contacts.

Mother-to-baby transmission of human immunodeficiency virus (HIV) may occur *in utero* or, more frequently, perinatally; a combination of serological and molecular biological techniques (PCR) is required to establish a diagnosis of HIV in infancy (see Chapter 18).

Table 17.3 Viruses that may infect or damage the fetus/neonate. (*Basic Science in Obstetrics and Gynaecology. A textbook for MRCOG Part I*, 3rd edn. de Swiet M, Chamberlain G & Bennett P (eds). Churchill Livingstone, Edinburgh, 2002: 126–127; adapted with permission.)

Virus infection	Birth defects	Persistent infection	Fetal death
Rubella	Yes	Yes	Yes
Cytomegalovirus	Yes	Yes	Yes
Varicella	Yes	Occasional	Yes
Herpes simplex 1 and 2	Rare	No	Neonate
Human parvovirus B19	No	Yes	Yes
HIV 1 and 2	No	Yes	Yes
Hepatitis B	No	Yes	No
Hepatitis C	No	Yes	Unknown
Hepatitis E	No	Insufficient data	Yes
Poliomyelitis	No	No	Yes
Coxsackie B virus	No	No	Yes
Japanese B encephalitis	Unknown	Unknown	Yes
Lassa fever	No	No	Yes
HTLV1	No	Yes	No
HTVL2	No	?	No

Virus infections that may damage the fetus if acquired in early pregnancy

Rubella (Fig. 17.4)

Most industrialized countries have adopted a rubella vaccination programme, and rubella is now a rare infection. Nevertheless, the proportion of women of childbearing age who are susceptible to rubella in the UK is <2–3%. Outbreaks of rubella may still occur if the proportion of susceptible women of childbearing age increases as a result of poor uptake of rubella vaccination. For example, in parts of California, infection was introduced by migrating workers from Mexico, and in the UK a sizeable epidemic which occurred in 1996, was largely confined to young adult males who had never been offered rubella vaccine. The augmentation of the UK rubella vaccination programme in 1988 in which MMR was offered to preschool children of both sexes had not, of course, reduced the susceptibility rate of adult males by 1996. Rubella epidemics have also occurred in parts of Eastern Europe, including the Ukraine, as a result of less attention and fewer resources being focused on preventive medicine than had hitherto been the case.

In developing countries, the proportion of susceptible women (15–20%) is little different from that in industrialized countries in the pre-vaccination era, and a recent report showed that susceptibility rates of more than 25% were reported from 12 of 45 countries. Furthermore, studies conducted after rubella outbreaks in developing countries have shown that the incidence of congenital rubella syndrome (CRS) per 1000 live births was often higher than in the UK during the early years of rubella vaccination programmes [26,27]. It has been suggested that about 230 000–240 000 cases of CRS occur annually in developing countries, although, during epidemics, this number may increase 10-fold [26]. The burden induced by CRS in developing countries, which imposes a considerable strain on scarce resources, is insufficiently recognized.

WHO is now developing a programme aiming to eliminate rubella in many developing countries. High quality surveillance of both post-natally and congenitally acquired rubella will be part of this programme. Since measles elimination programmes are in progress in many developing countries, this should provide an ideal opportunity to implement rubella vaccination because measles vaccination uptake rates now approach about 80% or more and many regions have adopted measles elimination goals. In countries with sustained measles coverage of at least 80% a single dose of combined measles and rubella vaccine could be given to all children, preferably aged 1 to 2 years [28].

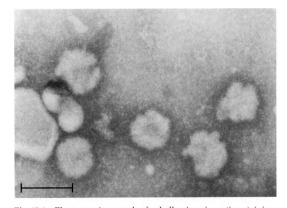

Fig 17.4 Electron micrograph of rubella virus (negative staining with 3% sodium phosphotungstate, pH 6.0). Bar = 100 nm. (By kind permission of Dr Ian L Chrystie, Department of Infection (Virology), Guy's, King's and St Thomas' School of Medicine, King's College London, London.)

The fetus is at risk during maternal viraemia, which occurs prior to the onset of the clinical features of maternal infection. Confirmation of the diagnosis is of importance because rubella frequently presents atypically, and rubella-like rashes may be caused by such infections as human parvovirus B19, enteroviruses and by arbovirus infections such as dengue, Ross River and Chikunguya. In developing countries, clinicians may sometimes find it difficult to distinguish rubella from dengue and measles.

During the first trimester, fetal infection is almost inevitable and, although there is a high risk of spontaneous abortion and stillbirth, congenital abnormalities may be present in 80–90% of infants who survive. Such infants have evidence of a generalized and persistent infection, and multisystem defects are likely to be present, particularly if infection is acquired during the first 8 weeks of pregnancy, i.e. during the critical phase of organogenesis [29]. Congenitally infected infants may excrete virus for 6–12 months. Despite having persistent neutralizing antibody responses, they may also exhibit defects in cell-mediated immune responses [30,31].

Congenitally acquired anomalies may be divided into transient (low birthweight, hepatosplenomegaly, cloudy corneas, thrombocytopenic purpura), developmental (sensorineural deafness, mental retardation, endocrine disorders particularly insulin-dependent diabetes mellitus), and those that persist for life unless corrected. These include ocular anomalies (including cataract, glaucoma and retinopathy) and cardiac defects, which include myocarditis, ventricular septal defects and pulmonary stenosis (reviewed in [29]). If rubella occurs after the first trimester, congenitally acquired anomalies are much less common and less severe, occurring in about 15% of infants whose mothers acquire rubella between 13 and 16 weeks. After this period, defects are very rare. When acquired after the first trimester, rubella is not associated with a persistent and generalized infection and there is no virus excretion at birth.

The fetus is not infected if rubella is acquired prior to conception [32]. Maternal reinfection following naturally acquired and vaccine-induced immunity has been reported but such infections are only rarely associated with maternal viraemia. This may perhaps be associated with a rubella-specific defect in the maternal immune mechanism. Although this risk has not been quantified, pregnant women known to be immune who have been exposed should be reassured that the risk to the fetus is probably no more than 5%.

Assessment of women who have been exposed to or who have developed rubella-like illnesses in pregnancy requires close collaboration between obstetric staff and the laboratory. In order to interpret serological investigations among women who have been exposed to rubella-like illnesses in pregnancy, it is important to have precise details relating to the dates and nature of exposure (e.g. family or casual contact), history of vaccination and results of screening tests for rubella in previous pregnancies. Those with rubella-like illnesses should be tested for rises in antibody titre and/or rubella-specific IgM. Such tests should be carried out within a few days of onset of illness in order to confirm or refute the diagnosis, thereby reducing the period of anxiety on the part of the patient to a minimum.

A diagnosis of congenitally acquired rubella can readily be established by detecting a rubella-specific IgM response during the first 3 months and/or the presence of virus during the first 6 months of life, occasionally longer. Recently non-invasive techniques have been used for serological tests. Thus, specific IgG and IgM antibodies may be detected reliably in saliva and this technique is likely to be of value for establishing a diagnosis among children in developing countries [28]. After the first 3 months of life, evidence of congenitally acquired rubella may be obtained by finding rubella antibodies of low avidity [31]. In addition, rubella RNA has been identified by PCR in lens aspirates from cataracts removed surgically from Indian children [21]. This technique is promising because it may be useful in older children. Rubella virus had previously been isolated from cataracts of children up to 3 years of age [33].

Cytomegalovirus (Fig. 17.5)

CMV belongs to the β subfamily of herpes viruses and, in common with all other herpes viruses establishes a state of latency following a primary infection. For CMV the site of latency is in the B and possibly T lymphocytes; reactivation occurs commonly not only in severely immunocompromised patients but also in pregnancy.

In industrialized countries, about 50–60% of women of childbearing age have developed antibodies to CMV but in developing countries infection occurs commonly in infancy and childhood so that, by early adult life, almost all persons have been infected. Maternally acquired CMV infection increases in successive pregnancies, indicating that children's excretions/secretions may infect their mothers [34]. In general, women working in day-care centres also have a high prevalence of seroconversion, although those nursing children in hospitals do not appear to be at increased risk; this probably reflects the high standards of hygiene and infection control.

In immunocompetent persons, CMV infection (whether primary or the result of reactivation) is usually subclinical. Thus, in contrast with rubella, there is little to

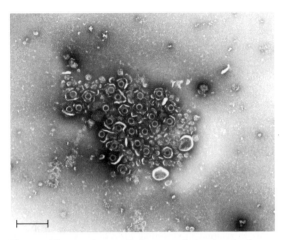

Fig 17.5 Electron micrograph of cytomegalovirus in urine from a congenitally infected infant (negative staining with 3% sodium phosphotungstate, pH 6.0). Note the high concentration of virus particles. Bar = 500 nm. (By kind permission of Dr Ian L Chrystie, Department of Infection (Virology), Guy's, King's and St Thomas' School of Medicine, King's College London, London.)

pinpoint infection, e.g. the development of an illness with rash, albeit often atypical, or contact with a person with a rubella-like infection.

CMV may be transmitted to the fetus during maternal viraemia and infants may also be infected during delivery via cervical secretions or postdelivery via breastfeeding. Although the fetus may be infected *in utero* as a result of both primary infection and reactivation or even reinfection with another CMV strain, CMV-induced sequelae are less common in infants delivered of mothers who are antibody positive before pregnancy. Reinfection demonstrates that maternal antibody is only partially protective and that when it does occur, may result from infection from a close household contact, particularly a child, although it must be appreciated that maternal viraemia may persist for periods up to three years or more. Follow-up studies on infants whose mothers were reinfected by CMV have

shown that about 8% have evidence of intrauterine transmission and symptomatic congenital disease [35]. The risks of reinfection have yet to be defined accurately.

In contrast to rubella, in which severe damage is restricted to about the first 16 weeks of pregnancy, CMV-induced anomalies occur over a much wider gestational age.

Following a primary maternal infection CMV is transmitted transplacentally in about 30–40% of cases but only about 5–7% of congenitally infected infants will be symptomatic at birth. However, when followed up, a further 10–15% are likely to have hearing defects or some degree of psychomotor retardation. It is not known what determines whether transplacental transmission of virus and fetal damage will occur, although it has been suggested that this may be due to a specific CMV-induced defect in maternal cell-mediated immunity [36] or a reflection of a high viral load. Indeed, recent studies employing quantitative PCR assays (Table 17.4) have shown that a high CMV DNA load in amniotic fluid is a good indicator of symptomatic congenital infection [39]. Infants who are symptomatic at birth classically present with intrauterine growth restriction, jaundice, hepatosplenomegaly, a petechial or thrombocytopenic rash, chorioretinitis and encephalitis. Microcephaly may be present at birth or develop during the early months of life. Areas of periventricular calcification may be seen radiologically. Table 17.4 compares the public health burden induced by congenitally acquired CMV in the USA and the UK. The total number of damaged infants, most of whom will have central nervous system (CNS) anomalies, indicates that congenitally acquired CMV is the second commonest known cause of motor retardation after Down's syndrome [40]. Perhaps the commonest abnormality in congenitally acquired CMV is the presence of sensorineural deafness; indeed, it has been estimated that it is a more frequent cause of deafness than bacterial meningitis (even prior to introduction of *Haemophilus influenzae* vaccine), congenitally acquired rubella and genetic causes put together [40].

Table 17.4 Annual public health impact of congenital cytomegalovirus. (From [37,38].)

	USA	UK
Number of live births	4 000 000	700 000
Proportion congenitally infected	1%	0.3%
Number congenitally infected	40 000	2100
Number with cytomegalic inclusion disease (5–7%)	2800	147
Number fatal (12%)	336	18
Number with sequelae (90%)	2218	132
Number asymptomatic (93%)	37 200	1953
Number with sequelae (15%)	5580	293
Total number damaged	8134	443

If acquired intrapartum or via breastfeeding, rather than damaging the infant, acquisition of CMV may be beneficial because it is a method by which infants can be immunized naturally.

The diagnosis of congenitally acquired CMV infection may be established by demonstrating the presence of CMV-specific IgM as well as by detecting virus in the urine or nasopharyngeal secretions. Virus is identified by culture, detection of early antigens by immunofluorescence, or PCR. A rapid diagnosis may also be established by electron microscopy of urine, which may show numerous herpes particles because infants excrete particularly high concentrations of virus (Fig. 17.5). Detection of virus should be carried out in the first 2–3 weeks of life because, after this period, detection of virus may be the result of infection acquired intrapartum or via breastfeeding. In contrast to congenitally acquired rubella, where virus excretion may persist for 6–9 months (occasionally longer), infants infected congenitally by CMV may excrete virus for periods up to 5–7 years.

Screening pregnant women serologically for CMV is not recommended because frequent visits to collect sequential samples would be necessary. It would be difficult to predict whether virus was transmitted transplacentally and if so whether this would result in damage. Detection of virus-specific IgM in a single serum sample obtained at booking clinics would be of limited value because specific IgM responses may persist for some months. Thus, its presence may be indicative of a primary infection at some time prior to conception. Furthermore, large numbers of routine CMV-specific IgM tests may provide a hazard because false-positive results may be reported. However, in the event of a pregnant woman having clinically overt CMV infection (e.g. an infectious mononucleosis-like illness), a prenatal diagnosis may be established by detecting virus in amniotic fluid.

Perhaps the best hope for preventing CMV infection in pregnancy lies in the development of a vaccine. The epitopes involved in inducing neutralizing antibodies and cytotoxic T-cell responses have been identified (glycoprotein B (gB)) [41] and there is consequently hope for developing recombinant-derived vaccines which could be expressed in such vectors as Canary Pox.

Although such drugs as ganciclovir, foscarnet and cidoforvir are licensed for life-threatening infections in immunocompromised patients, their toxicity (particularly if used long term) contraindicates their use in CMV-infected infants. It must also be borne in mind that their tissues contain particularly high concentrations of virus which would make it difficult or impossible for most drugs to induce a significant prolonged reduction in virus replication.

Varicella

VZV belongs to the α subfamily of herpes viruses, its site of latency being in the sensory nerve ganglia.

Advice is sought more frequently from clinical virologists in relation to maternal varicella and infections by human parvovirus B19 than for any other infections. However, there is only a 1% risk of embryopathy following maternal varicella, this being confined overall to the first 20 weeks of pregnancy with a slightly higher risk (2%) between weeks 13 and 20 [42]. In addition a small proportion of infants whose mothers acquired varicella during pregnancy may develop zoster in early childhood, this occurring more frequently when maternal infection was acquired 25–36 weeks into pregnancy (1.7%) than between 13 and 24 weeks (0.8%) [42]. It is believed that the cicatricial skin scarring is the result of reactivation of VZV in the developing fetus. Table 17.5 shows some of the clinical features associated with varicella embryopathy.

Maternal zoster (shingles) is not associated with risk to the fetus because there is little or no viraemia, and infection is associated with a rapid varicella/zoster IgG booster response.

In contrast to rubella and CMV, a varicella-specific IgM response can only be detected in about 25% of infants with embryopathy, the detection rate increasing with gestational age. Furthermore, persistent IgG responses occur even less frequently (8%), and specific IgG and IgM responses are often discordant. Pregnant women who have been exposed to varicella may be protected by the administration of VZIG (see above). However, before VZIG is given, patients should be asked if they have a history of varicella; a reliable history is predictive of immunity in about 85–90% of cases. About 60% of women who give no history of varicella will be

---

- Intrauterine growth restriction
- Dermatological—skin loss or scarring
- Skeletal—including hypoplasia of bone and muscle, often with rudimentary digits
- CNS—including cortical and cerebella atrophy, microcephaly
- Ophthalmic—including microphthalmia, chorioretinitis, optic atrophy and cataracts
- Gastrointestinal and genitourinary malformations

Table 17.5 Varicella embryopathy.

shown to be immune. Thus, women who give no history of varicella (or those who express doubt) should be assessed serologically (see above).

Women who develop varicella may be treated with orally administered aciclovir (see above and Chapter 1), although, if patients have respiratory symptoms or other complications, consideration should be given to intravenous administration.

Although varicella-specific IgM may occasionally be detected in fetal blood, and VZV DNA has been found in amniotic fluid and chorionic villus samples, such findings may not be indicative of fetal damage. Such investigations are difficult to assess because varicella embryopathy is only rarely encountered. However, high-resolution ultrasonography may be of value in detecting some of the more obvious malformations listed in Table 17.5; repeat ultrasound examinations may be necessary.

A live attenuated varicella vaccine has been licensed in the USA for routine administration in childhood. In the UK, this vaccine is only available for the immunocompromised on a named patient basis. It is encouraging that studies conducted in Japan have shown that the antibody response is of up to 20 years' duration [43] and does not increase the risk of subsequent zoster (shingles). This vaccine is unlikely to be licensed for administration to women of childbearing age who may become pregnant but widespread use of the vaccine among children would reduce the risks of virus transmission to adults who may be pregnant. Better vaccines are now being prepared using viral glycoproteins that may be expressed in similar vectors to those being tried for CMV vaccines.

Human parvovirus B19 (Fig. 17.6)

Parvoviruses infect a number of different species, particularly humans, cats, dogs, pigs, rodents and birds. Parvoviruses have an affinity for rapidly dividing cells and, in the human fetus, this applies particularly to erythroid progenitor cells. The receptor for human parvovirus B19 (the P antigen) has now been identified (see Table 17.6.)

Table 17.6 Expression of human parvovirus B19 receptor (P antigen). (Adapted from [44].)

- Mature erythrocytes
- Erythroid progenitor cells
- Fetal cardiac myocytes
- Placenta
- Endothelial cells
- Megakaryocytes

Infection occurs worldwide; in temperate climates, outbreaks usually occur in the spring and summer. In industrialized countries about 50% of women are immune, with an annual seroconversion rate of about 1.5%. Children are usually infected between the ages of 4 and 10 years, although, in developing countries, this occurs earlier. Maternal B19 infections often result from exposure to children, usually within the household or, if working in a school, to pupils [45]. Clinically, erythema infectiosum (fifth disease) and rubella-like rash sometimes associated with arthritis are common presenting features. Occasionally, outbreaks of rubella and parvovirus B19 occur concurrently but, because the management of each in pregnancy differs, it is essential to establish a virological diagnosis. B19 infection may precipitate aplastic crises in patients with sickle cell disease and induce persistent infections in the immunosuppressed. However, subclinical infection is common, occurring in about 30–40% of cases (reviewed in [46]). Figure 17.7 demonstrates the virological, haematological and clinical features of infection in a susceptible volunteer challenged with B19. Viraemia occurs within a few days of exposure, this being associated with pharyngeal virus excretion. At this time, infection may be transmitted to other susceptible persons. Reduction in the number of reticulocytes and a fall in haemoglobin occur at this stage and may persist for 2–3 weeks. Rash and arthralgia, should they be present, occur relatively late in the infection cycle, being associated with the development of virus-specific immune responses.

Fetal infection may occur during maternal viraemia. Table 17.7 summarizes the risks of an adverse outcome

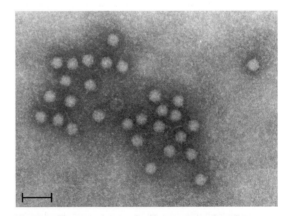

Fig. 17.6 Electron micrograph of human parvovirus virus (negative staining with 3% sodium phosphotungstate, pH 6.0). Bar = 50 nm. (By kind permission of Dr Ian L Chrystie, Department of Infection (Virology), Guy's, King's and St Thomas' School of Medicine, King's College London, London.)

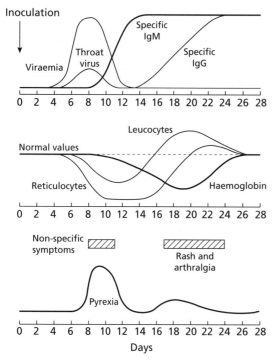

Fig 17.7 Virological, haematological and clinical events during B19 virus infection of volunteers. (From [71].)

following a maternal B19 infection in pregnancy during epidemic and non-epidemic periods. Spontaneous abortion or intrauterine deaths usually occur in the second or third trimesters. Hydrops fetalis results from severe fetal anaemia or myocarditis. A recent report suggests that up to 15% of intrauterine fetal deaths, but without hydrops fetalis, may be associated with B19 infection [47]. However, not only was the number of cases reported small but it must be appreciated that the placental and fetal tissues contain maternal blood. Consequently the presence of B19 by a sensitive PCR may reflect residual maternal viraemia which may persist for many months following clinical recovery from B19 infection. Table 17.8 provides guidelines relating to the management of B19 infections in

pregnancy in which serological studies, ultrasonography and haematological investigations play an important part. There is some evidence to suggest that echocardiography is of prognostic significance because fetal deaths are associated with enlarged biventricular outer dimensions in diastole [48]. Intrauterine transfusions for infants with hydrops fetalis may reduce fetal deaths by 50% [49].

Fortunately, B19 does not induce developmental defects, and follow-up studies conducted on infants infected *in utero* for periods up to 10 years have shown normal development.

A virological diagnosis of intrauterine infection can be established by detecting B19 DNA by dot blot hybridization or PCR on fetal blood or amniotic fluid and, at birth, evidence of infection can sometimes be confirmed by detecting the presence of B19-specific IgM or IgA, although such investigations are relatively insensitive. Persistence of B19-specific IgG in blood or saliva beyond a time at which maternal antibodies would have disappeared is more reliable.

Although parvovirus vaccines are used in veterinary practice, B19 is difficult to grow to high titres in cell culture. However, recent studies have shown that the capsid protein, VP1, induces protective antibodies, and studies are in progress to determine whether recombinant-derived vaccine expressed in a bacculovirus vector can be used as a vaccine; such a preparation induces neutralizing antibodies experimentally in rabbits.

Infections acquired in later pregnancy and intrapartum

Varicella

Twenty-five to thirty per cent of infections among infants whose mothers acquire varicella (but not zoster) near term may have severe disease with haemorrhagic manifestations. There was a high fatality rate prior to the availability of VZIG or treatment with aciclovir. VZIG should be given to infants whose mothers develop varicella (but not herpes zoster) in the period 8 days before to 28 days after delivery, as well as to infants who lack

Risk of acquiring B19	1 in 400
Excess fetal loss	9% (confined to the first 20 weeks of pregnancy)
Risk of spontaneous abortion or IUD	50–60 per year (300–350 during epidemics)
Risk of hydrops fetalis	~15 (45–60 during epidemics)
No. congenitally infected	20% (persistent salivary IgG)
Outcome in survivors at birth and at 7–10 years	No abnormalities consistent with B19 infection

Table 17.7 PHLS study 1985–88 and 1992–95 on outcome of human parvovirus B19 among 427 pregnant women. (Adapted from [70].)

Table 17.8 Management of human parvovirus B19 in pregnancy.

Following contact: screen booking blood for B19 IgG	
If positive:	reassure
f negative:	look for seroconversion/rising IgG (3–4 weeks after contact)
	look for specific IgM (lasts 8–12 weeks)
If maternal infection is diagnosed:	serial ultrasound 1–2 weekly for 12–14 weeks elevation of maternal serum α-fetoprotein
If fetal hydrops develops:	cordocentesis for parvovirus B19, Hb, karyotype, WBC and platelets consider fetal blood transfusion*

*Requirement for fetal blood transfusion is dependent on degree of anaemia rather than the presence or degree of hydramnios.

maternal antibody exposed to varicella or herpes zoster in the first month of life. VZIG is more likely to attenuate rather than prevent infection. Aciclovir, which should be administered parenterally, can be used if, despite the administration of VZIG, severe manifestations of neonatal varicella appear to be developing. Premature infants born before 28 weeks of gestation, or with a birth weight <1000 g may not have acquired maternal antibodies despite their mothers being immune. VZIG should be given to such infants [50].

Herpes simplex virus types 1 and 2

Genital herpes is one of the most common infections presenting in genitourinary medicine clinics in many industrialized countries. However, the true extent of infection is difficult to quantify because many patients have asymptomatic and undiagnosed infections. Genital lesions may be caused by either HSV-1 or HSV-2 and, although clinically indistinguishable, infection by HSV-1 is less likely to result in recurrent infections [51]. Despite the high and increasing incidence of genital HSV infection, neonatal herpes (which carries high morbidity and mortality rates) is rare. In the UK it is estimated that the infection rate is about 1.65 per 100 000 live births annually [52]. In the USA the incidence may be higher, particularly in some of the southern states.

Newborn infants may acquire infection as a result of contact with genital lesions during delivery or via an ascending infection if membranes rupture early. Infection may also be introduced from mother to baby via fetal scalp monitoring and blood sampling, or postpartum via non-genital maternal lesions. Nosocomial infection may be the result of infection being transmitted via infected health-care personnel.

Infection is readily transmitted during vaginal delivery via primary maternal lesions because they contain high concentrations of virus, which may persist for 2–3 weeks. The overall transmission rate in these circumstances (five studies) was 19 cases out of 46 (41%) (reviewed in [53]). It was previously recommended that, if pregnant women or their partners had a history of recurrent herpes, attempts should be made to culture virus before delivery. This practice has now largely been discontinued because the presence of virus antepartum does not appear to predict risk of transmission to the neonate. Conversely, some infants have been shown to be infected despite negative maternal cultures [50].

Some authorities recommend the use of prophylactic aciclovir during the last trimester for women with a history of frequent episodes of genital herpes in order to reduce the risk of virus shedding near delivery, although, as is the case for maternal varicella, the drug is not licensed for use in pregnancy.

Caesarean section should be carried out if active genital lesions are present, providing membranes are intact or have been ruptured for less than 6 h. This markedly reduces but may not always prevent neonatal infection by HSV. If there is thought to be a risk of an ascending infection, infants should be given prophylactic intravenous aciclovir. Although it is established practice to deliver infants by caesarean section in a mother with a history of recurrent genital lesions who has an active lesion during labour, obstetricians in the Netherlands no longer carry out caesarean section for such cases having shown that there was no significant difference in the incidence of neonatal herpes among infants delivered vaginally or by caesarean section [54].

Asymptomatic shedding of HSV-2 is much commoner than had hitherto been thought among women who have antibodies to the virus. Thus, studies conducted in the USA showed that, of women who had been taught how to collect their own specimens on a daily basis and examine their genitalia for herpetic lesions, 78% excreted HSV-2 and 62% reported typical lesions [55]. Although these findings may not be applicable elsewhere, it is perhaps surprising that neonatal infection is uncommon, although this may be a reflection of the relatively lower concentration and duration of virus excreted by women experiencing recurrent infection.

The onset of neonatal HSV usually occurs 5–17 days (occasionally longer) after delivery by which time infants will usually no longer be in hospital. Infants with localized herpes encephalitis as their initial manifestation of infection, although typically presenting in the second or third week of life, may present as late as 4–6 weeks of age. Consequently, infants should be followed up carefully if intrapartum exposed to HSV or after delivery. Although infants may present with vesicular lesions of the skin and mucous membranes, in 70% of cases without treatment HSV will disseminate to cause a generalized and frequently fatal infection. Some infants may present with evidence of a generalized infection whereas others may present with CNS manifestations alone. An adverse outcome is associated with prematurity, infection by HSV-2 rather than HSV-1, seizures and the presence of coma at presentation. Despite treatment, some infants still die during the first year of life or are left with some residual sequelae. In general, treated infants infected with HSV-1 experience fewer long-term sequelae than those with HSV-2 infections [8]. Infants who are treated with aciclovir within 48 h of onset of clinical features have a much more favourable outcome than those in whom treatment is delayed, usually because there is a lack of awareness of the possible diagnosis [56].

Newly described human herpes viruses (types 6, 7 and 8)

There is as yet little information as to the role of these viruses in inducing congenitally acquired infections although evidence of infection by human herpes virus type 6 (HHV-6) has been detected in 1.6% of 300 babies delivered of healthy mothers. HHV-6 DNA was detected in cord blood indicating that infection had occurred *in utero*. Steps were taken to exclude maternal contamination of cord blood [57].

Recent studies conducted in French Guiana, which has a high prevalence (15%) of seropositivity for HHV-8 among persons aged between 15 and 40 years (both sexes), showed that HHV-8 transmission occurred mainly within families, including mother to child but not during pregnancy, delivery or via breastfeeding [58]. Further information is awaited to determine the significance, if any, of the role of HHV-7 and HHV-8 in congenital infections.

Enteroviruses (Fig. 17.8)

Enteroviruses are ubiquitous and, although infection occurs commonly in childhood, particularly in developing countries, all age groups may be infected. Sixty-six serotypes have now been identified among which are included polioviruses 1–3, coxsackie A viruses 1–23, coxsackie B 1–6, echoviruses 1–34, and a number of additional enteroviruses which are now designated numerically rather than listed with the other groups of enteroviruses.

Enteroviruses may be transmitted *in utero*, often the result of an asymptomatic maternal infection, or during delivery via blood, faeces or saliva. Infection may also be transmitted from other infected infants in nurseries for the newborn.

Mothers may present with Bornholm's disease, aseptic meningitis, myocarditis or non-specific febrile illnesses associated with abdominal pain or respiratory symptoms. Poliomyelitis, although increasingly rare even in many developing countries, may result in miscarriage or, if acquired near term, stillbirth or delivery of a child with paralytic disease. The most frequently reported enterovirus infections in pregnancy are coxsackie B 2–5 and various echovirus infections (particularly echovirus 11). Infants may be delivered with, or develop shortly after birth, clinical features of enterovirus infections, usually within 3–7 days of delivery. The early features of infection may be mild or non-specific but transient respiratory distress or listlessness

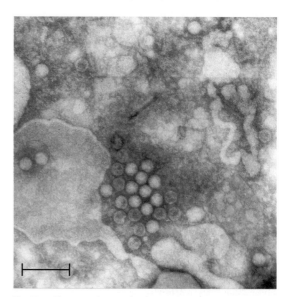

Fig 17.8 Electron micrograph of enterovirus (negative staining with 3% sodium phosphotungstate, pH 6.0). Bar = 100 nm. (By kind permission of Dr Ian L Chrystie, Department of Infection (Virology), Guy's, King's and St Thomas' School of Medicine, King's College London, London.)

may follow, with or without a febrile response. However, this may be followed by a fulminating and generalized infection in which CNS involvement and myocarditis are prominent features. Circulatory collapse, bleeding and hepatic necrosis may occur.

Scandinavian studies [59,60] suggest that infants delivered of mothers who have evidence of an enterovirus-specific IgM response at delivery, indicative of a current or recent enterovirus infection, may develop insulin-dependent diabetes mellitus in early childhood.

Mothers and infants with clinical features suggestive of enterovirus infection should be investigated by attempting to detect virus in culture or by PCR. Nasopharyngeal aspirates, stools, blood and cerebrospinal fluid (CSF) should be tested. Mothers and babies are likely to develop enterovirus-specific IgM responses within 3–4 days of the onset of symptoms.

Human normal immunoglobulin contains antibodies to many of the commoner enteroviruses. Consequently, it has been used and shown to be effective prophylactically in preventing infection among infants in nurseries for the newborn in which infants have been exposed to infection.

A rapid diagnosis is of importance, not only in preventing nosocomial spread, but also for instituting prompt therapy; treatment of potentially life-threatening infections may be achieved with an antiviral agent, pleconaril, which has recently been shown to be promising [61].

Human papillomaviruses (Fig. 17.9)

About 100 genotypes have been identified, human papillomavirus (HPV) 6 and 11 being associated with genital warts (condylomata acuminata). The incidence of genital warts has increased markedly in recent years, particularly among those with multiple sexual partners. HPV-6 and -11 may be transmitted intrapartum, and infected infants may subsequently develop recurrent juvenile papillomatosis, which, despite the frequency of infection with these genotypes, is rare.

HPV-16 and -18 are the genotypes implicated in the pathogenesis of cervical malignant disease. Recent studies have shown that infection may not only be transmitted from mother to baby but also persist in the buccal mucosa for periods extending to 2 years [62]. Studies among 3–11-year-old London school children have shown that about 40% have HPV-16 in their buccal mucosa, although it cannot be determined whether this results from infection acquired intrapartum or horizontally in later childhood. Because HPV vaccines are under development, it is of importance to know whether such children are immunologically competent or tolerant.

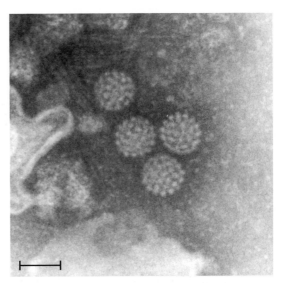

Fig 17.9 Electron micrograph of human papillomavirus (negative staining with 3% sodium phosphotungstate, pH 6.0). Bar = 50 nm. (By kind permission of Dr Ian L Chrystie, Department of Infection (Virology), Guy's, King's and St Thomas' School of Medicine, King's College London, London.)

Hepatitis B virus (Fig. 17.10) (see also Chapter 9)

Hepatitis B virus (HBV) is a 42-nm spherical double-shelled particle surrounded by a lipoprotein envelope. Hepatitis e antigen (HBeAg) is a soluble antigen associated with a high rate of viral replication, viraemia and high infectivity, and is present in those with acute infection as well as carriers who are likely to transmit infection. In contrast, those developing antibodies to the HBe antigen (HBeAb) or who have no HBV 'e' markers are less likely to transmit infection.

It has been estimated that there are some 300–350 million HBV carriers worldwide. High carrier rates with a prevalence ranging from 10% to 20% occur in many developing countries, particularly in Sub-Saharan Africa, the Far East and many Pacific Islands. In such parts of the world, the carrier state is the result of perinatal transmission or infection acquired in infancy or early childhood.

In the UK, HBV carrier rates among pregnant women vary from about 0.1% to 0.5%, although, in some inner city areas, a 1% carrier rate has been reported [63]. This reflects the high proportion of women who originate from parts of the world which have a high endemicity hepatitis of B.

About 90–95% of infants delivered of mothers who have markers of high infectivity (HBeAg or HBV DNA)

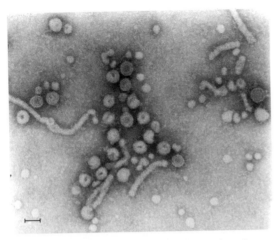

Fig 17.10 Electron micrograph of hepatitis B virus (negative staining with 3% sodium phosphotungstate, pH 6.0). Bar = 50 nm. (By kind permission of Dr Ian L Chrystie, Department of Infection (Virology), Guy's, King's and St Thomas' School of Medicine, King's College London, London.)

will not only be infected but also develop prolonged HBV carriage. The carrier state appears in only about 5% of infants whose mothers are anti-HBe positive. Infants acquiring HBV infection during delivery are usually asymptomatic, although rarely an acute or even a fulminating hepatitis may occur in infants whose mothers are anti-HBe positive. This is usually the result of the mothers having a particular precore mutant, which results in the virus retaining its infectivity but not being able to synthesize HBeAg.

Infants are usually infected via contact with maternal blood during delivery, although, in about 5% of cases, HBV infection is transmitted transplacentally. It has been suggested that maternal antibody to the core antigen (anti-HBc) may suppress viral replication in the fetus, immune responses to HBV associated antigens being delayed until after delivery when maternal antibodies decline.

In order to prevent the long-term carrier state associated with the risks of developing chronic liver disease, the WHO has taken active steps to promote universal vaccination against HBV in infancy or adolescence. About 110 countries now have such programmes, although in Europe, only the UK, the Netherlands and Scandinavian countries do not as yet recommend universal immunization. However, the UK Department of Health strongly recommends that all mothers should be tested for hepatitis B surface antigen (HBsAg) whilst attending antenatal clinics and infants of those who are HBsAg and HBeAg positive or who, although HBsAg positive have no 'e'

markers, should be given a full course of hepatitis B vaccination commencing within 24 h of birth but including simultaneous administration of hepatitis B immunoglobulin (HBIG) at that time [64]. Infants delivered of mothers who are both HBsAg and anti-HBe positive should be protected by a full course of vaccination but without HBIG. An accelerated course may be useful in protecting infants because rapid acquisition of immunity can be useful in preventing perinatal infection among families who may be poor clinic attenders. Thus, vaccine can be given at birth, and at 1 and 2 months of age with a booster dose at 12 months.

Recent attention has been focused on HBsAg surface mutants because not only may they not be recognized by conventional diagnostic tests for HBsAg which employ monoclonal antibodies, but also there is a potential risk of currently available vaccines failing to protect against these mutants. Infants who have been given a full course of hepatitis B vaccine have been infected via their mothers' surface mutants and have acquired infection by HBV despite developing vaccine-induced immune responses. Although surface mutants have been described in all continents, fortunately, as yet, they appear to be relatively rare. Surveillance is required in order to determine whether they are of increasing frequency because modification to existing vaccines may be necessary.

Hepatitis C virus (see also Chapter 9)

Although detailed information about the genomic configuration of hepatitis C virus (HCV) is available, its fine structure has not as yet been visualized. Six genotypes are recognized, types 1, 2 and 3 being the predominant ones in Europe, including the UK, and the USA. There are also a number of subtypes of each genotype.

It is estimated that there are about 170 million chronic HCV carriers throughout the world, of whom about 4 million are in the USA and 5 million in Western Europe. Acute HCV infection is asymptomatic in about 75–80% of cases, although infection is likely to develop into a chronic carrier state in about 80% of cases. Chronic liver disease, including cirrhosis and primary hepatocellular carcinoma, develops in approximately 60–70% of HCV-infected patients, although the interval between acquiring infection and developing serious liver disease exhibits considerable variation and may extend to 20 years or more.

In Britain the prevalence of antibodies to HCV among pregnant women ranges from about 0.14 to 0.21% in cities apart from London; in London it is of the order of 0.5% [65,66]. About 75% of such persons will be shown to be viraemic when tested by PCR. The incubation period is about 6–8 weeks, but antibodies may not appear for a further 4–6 weeks.

Vertical transmission of HCV is uncommon, and transmission rates from mother to child are of the order of 6%. Mothers who have antibodies to HCV, but who have no viral RNA by PCR, rarely transmit. However, transmission rates of 36% have been reported among mothers who are coinfected with HIV [67]. Mothers who acquire acute HCV infection in the last trimester have a high risk of transmitting infection. Pregnancy is not contraindicated in HCV-infected women and, currently, routine screening for HCV is not recommended during pregnancy. Recent studies conducted on a large number (441) of mothers who were HCV positive, showed that elective caesarean section significantly reduced transmission of HCV from mother to baby, which suggests that viral transmission usually occurs around the time of delivery [68]. Breast-feeding is not contraindicated for mothers who are known to be HCV positive.

Infants delivered of mothers known to be HCV positive should be tested for HCV by PCR at or shortly after birth and, if negative, the tests should be repeated at 3–6 months. Because maternal antibodies persist for up to a year, infants who are PCR and antibody negative may be considered not to have been infected. However, infants whose blood has been found to be positive for HCV by PCR on two occasions should be considered to have been infected, although it is possible that some may clear infection after a variable interval. Recent evidence suggests that children who have been infected by HCV following blood transfusion appear to clear infection more readily than adults [69].

As yet there is no vaccine against HCV, and results of treatment in infancy and childhood with interferon or combination therapy with ribavirin have yet to completed and evaluated.

Human T-cell lymphotrophic Viruses (HTLV)

These viruses are a subfamily of retroviruses consisting of HTLV-I and HTLV-II. The viruses share about 70% sequence homology but in contrast to HIV-1 (see Chapter 18), the genomes of HTLV viruses are highly conserved.

HTLV-I is widely distributed globally; there are about 20 million carriers worldwide. Particularly high prevalence rates are found in Japan, where up to 15% of the population are sero-positive in the South West parts of the country. Other endemic areas are found in parts of sub-Saharan Africa (particularly Central, West and South Africa), the Caribbean, Melanesia, the South Eastern States of the USA, and Brazil [71]. Studies in London have shown that the prevalence of infection by HTLV-I among pregnant women whose parents were born in non-endemic regions, was of the order of 0.06 to 0.12 per 100 000. However, the sero-prevalence among infants whose mothers were born in the Caribbean or West and Central Africa, was markedly increased, being 3.2 per 1000 and 6.8 per 1000 respectively [72].

HTLV-I is associated with adult T-cell leukaemia/lymphoma and tropical spastic paraparesis; there are much less conclusive reports suggesting that polymyositis, inflammatory arthropathy, Sicca syndrome and uveitis may also be associated. Although HTLV-II was originally isolated from a few patients with a typical hairy-cell leukaemia, there is, as yet, insufficient evidence linking HTLV-II with this or any other disease.

Although HTLV-I may be transmitted from mother to baby during delivery, the virus is closely cell associated and is usually transmitted by breastfeeding. High maternal HTLV-I pro-viral loads and elevated maternal antibody titres, are associated with mother-to-child transmission and girls are more frequently infected than boys [73]. Maternal antibodies protect breastfeeding infants until their concentration begins to decline. Thus, infants who are breast fed over a short period are not more frequently infected than babies who are formula fed, but if breast-feeding is continued for 6 months or more, higher rates of transmission are reported. Data relating to transmission of HTLV-II from mother to baby are limited and somewhat conflicting, although studies in Brazil suggest that mother-to-infant transmission may be as high as 30–50% [74].

There is considerable debate about recommending universal screening for HTLV-I in Britain. However, since transmission rates are of the order of only 5% within 3 months of breastfeeding, about one-third of mothers do not breastfeed at all, and because there is only about a 1% life time risk of developing malignant disease and even less of developing tropical spastic paraparesis, both of which may take as long as 20 to 40 years to develop, there is a less compelling case for screening than for HIV (see Chapter 18). Indeed, 80% of mother-to-child HTLV-I transmission, which is responsible for most cases of adult T-cell leukaemia, can be prevented by avoiding breastfeeding [75]. The prevalence of HTLV-II has increased markedly among intravenous drug users in many European countries, but since disease associations have yet to be established, little consideration has been given for screening antenatal patients for this virus.

The diagnosis of infection by HTLV-I or II, is usually made serologically. Gel particle agglutination provides a rapid although relatively insensitive test. Enzyme immunoassays employing recombinant derived antigens, are more specific and can distinguish between HTLV-I and II, although results should be confirmed by Western blotting.

References

1 Daunter B. Immunology of pregnancy: towards a unifying hypothesis. *Eur J Obstet Gynecol Reprod Biol* 1992; 43: 81–95.

2 Greenberg M, Jacobiner H, Pakter J, Weisl BAG. Maternal mortality in the epidemic of Asian Influenza, New York City, 1957. *Am J Obstet Gynecol* 1958; 76: 897–902.

3 Department of Health, Welsh Office, Scottish Home Office and Health Departments, DHSS (Northern Ireland). *Immunisation Against Infectious Diseases*. HMSO, London, 1996: 113–20.

4 Monto AS, Fleming DM *et al.* Efficacy and safety of the neuraminidase inhibitor zanamivir in the treatment of influenza A and B virus infections. *J Infect Dis* 1999; 180: 254–61.

5 Miller E, Vurdien J, Farrington P. Shift in age in chickenpox. *Lancet* 1993; 341: 308–9.

6 Andrews EB, Yankasbas BC, Cordero JF, Schoeffler K, Hampp S. and the Aciclovir in Pregnancy Registry Advisory Committee. Aciclovir in Pregnancy Registry: six years' experience. *Obstet Gynecol* 1992; 79: 7–13.

7 Ades AE, Peckham CS, Dale GE, Best JM, Jeansson S. Prevalence of antibodies to herpes simplex virus types 1 and 2 in pregnant women, and estimated rates of infection. *J Epidemiol Commun Health* 1989; 43: 53–60.

8 Whitley RJ. Perinatal herpes simplex virus infections. *Rev Virol* 1991; 1: 101–10.

9 Fontaine H, Nalpas B, Carnot F, Brechot C, Pol S. Effect of pregnancy on chronic hepatitis C: a case control study. *Lancet* 2000; 356: 1328–9.

10 Seibert D, Locarnini S, Cunningham A. Viral hepatitis in pregnancy. In: Jeffries DJ, Hudson CN, eds. *Viral Infections in Obstetrics and Gynaecology*. London: Edward Arnold, 1999: 165–217.

11 Siegel M, Greenberg M. Incidence of poliomyelitis in pregnancy. Its relation to maternal age, parity and gestational period. *N Engl J Med* 1955; 253: 841–7.

12 Chaturvedi UC, Mathur A, Chandra A, Das SK, Tandon HO, Singh UK. Transplacental infection with Japanese encephalitis virus. *J Infect Dis* 1980; 141: 712–15.

13 UK Department of Health. *Immunisation against Infectious Diseases*. HMSO, 1996.

14 Carles G, Talarmin A, Peneau C, Bertsch M. Dengue fever and pregnancy: A study of 38 cases in French Guiana. *J Gynecol Obstet* 2000; 8: 758–62.

15 Briggiler AM, Levis S, Enria D, Ambrosio AM, Maiztegui JI. Argentine hemorrhagic fever in pregnant women. *Medicine (Buenos Aires)* 1990; 50: 443.

16 Johnson KM, Halstead SB, Cohen SN. Hemorrhagic fevers of South-east Asia and South America: a comparative appraisal. *Prog Med Virol* 1967; 9: 105–58.

17 Douglas RG, Wiebenga NH, Couch RB. Bolivan hemorrhagic fever probably transmitted by personal contact. *Am J Epidemiol* 1965; 82: 85–91.

18 Price ME, Fisher-Hoch SP, Craven RB, McCormick JB. A prospective study of maternal and fetal outcome in acute Lassa fever infection during pregnancy. *Br Med J* 1988; 297: 584–7.

19 Tsai TF, Paul R, Lynberg MC, Letson GW. Congenital yellow fever virus infection after immunization in pregnancy. *J Infect Dis* 1993; 168: 1520–3.

20 Tsai TF, Paul R, Lynberg MC, Letson GW. Congenital yellow fever virus infection after immunization in pregnancy. *J Infect Dis* 1994; 170: 251.

21 Bosma TJ, Corbett KM, Eckstein MB, O'Shea S, Vijayalakshmi P, Banatvala JE. Use of PCR for prenatal and postnatal diagnosis of congenital rubella. *J Clin Microbiol* 1995; 33: 2881–7.

22 Bosma TJ, Corbett KM, O'Shea S, Banatvala JE, Best JM. Use of the polymerase chain reaction for the detection of rubella virus RNA in clinical samples. *J Clin Microbiol* 1995; 33: 1075–9.

23 Sutherland S, ed. *TORCH Screening Reassessed; the Report of a PHLS Working Party on Diagnostic Tests for Congenital Infections*, 2nd edn. Public Health Laboratory Service, London, 1993.

24 Best JM, Sutherland S. Diagnosis and prevention of congenital and perinatal infections, TORCH screening should be discouraged. *Br Med J* 1990; 301: 888–9.

25 Best JM, Banatvala JE. Congenital virus infections: more viruses are now known to infect the fetus. *Br Med J* 1990; 300: 1151–2.

26 Cutts FT, Robertson SE, Diaz-Ortega J-L, Samuel R. Control of rubella and congenital rubella syndrome (CRS) in developing countries, Part 1: burden of disease from CRS. *Bull WHO* 1997; 75: 55–68.

27 Robertson SE, Cutts FT, Samuel R, Diaz-Ortega J-L. Control of rubella and congenital rubella syndrome (CRS) in developing countries, part 2: vaccination against rubella. *Bull WHO* 1997; 75: 69–80.

28 World Health Organisation. *Report of a meeting on preventing congenital rubella syndrome; immunization strategies, surveillance needs*. Departments of Vaccines & Biologicals, Geneva, 2000.

29 Best JM, Banatvala JE. Rubella. In: Zuckerman AJ, Banatvala JE, Pattison JR, eds. *Principles and Practice of Clinical Virology*, 4th edn. John Wiley and Sons, Chichester, 2000: 387–418.

30 O'Shea S, Best J, Banatvala JE. A lymphocyte transformation assay for the diagnosis of congenital rubella. *J Virol Meth* 1992; 37: 139–48.

31 Thomas HIJ, Morgan-Capner P, Enders G, O'Shea S, Caldicott DM, Best JM. Persistence of specific IgM and low avidity specific IgG following primary rubella. *J Virol Meth* 1992; 39: 149–55.

32 Miller E, Cradock-Watson JE, Pollock TM. Consequences of confirmed maternal rubella at successive stages of pregnancy. *Lancet* 1982; ii: 781–4.

33 Menser MA, Harley JD, Hertzberg R, Dorman DC, Murphy AM. Persistence of virus in lens for three years after prenatal rubella. *Lancet* 1967; ii: 387–8.

34 Stagno S, Pass RF *et al.* Primary cytomegalovirus infection in pregnancy. Incidence, transmission to fetus, and clinical outcome. *J Am Med Assoc* 1986; 2566: 1904–8.

35 Boppana SB, Rivera LB, Fowler KB, Mach M, Britt WJ. Intrauterine transmission of cytomegalovirus to infants of women with preconceptional immunity. *N Engl J Med* 2001; 344:1366–71.

36 Pass RF, Stagno S, Britt WJ, Alford CA. Specific cell mediated immunity and the natural history of congenital infection with cytomegalovirus. *J Infect Dis* 1983; 148: 953–61.

37 Griffiths PD. Cytomegalovirus. In: Zuckerman AJ, Banatvala JE, Pattison JR, eds. *Principles and Practice of Clinical Virology*, 3rd edn. John Wiley and Sons, Chichester, 1995: 69–108.

38 Stagno S. Cytomegalovirus. In: Remington JS, Klein JO, eds. *Infectious Diseases of the Fetus and Newborn Infant*. WB Saunders, Philadelphia, PA: 1990: 240–81.

39 Lazzarotto T, Varani S, Guerra B, Nicolosi A, Lanari M, Landini MP. Prenatal indicators of congenital cytomegalovirus infection. *J Pediatr* 2000; 137(1): 90–5.

40 Griffiths PD. Cytomegalovirus. In: Zuckerman AJ, Banatvala JE, Pattison JR, eds. *Principles and Practice of Clinical Virology*, 4th edn. John Wiley and Sons, Chichester, 2000: 79–116.

41 Adler SA, Plotkin SA *et al.* A canarypox vector expressing cytomegalovirus (CMV) glycoprotein B primes for antibody responses to a live attenuated CMV vaccine (Towne). *J Infect Dis* 1999; 180: 843–6.

42 Enders G, Miller E, Cradock-Watson J, Bolley I, Ridehalgh M. Consequences of varicella and herpes zoster in pregnancy: prospective study of 1739 cases. *Lancet* 1994; 343: 1548–51.

43 World Health Organization. Varicella vaccines: WHO position paper. *Weekly Epidemiol Record* 1998; 73: 241–8.

44 Brown KE, Young NS. Human parvovirus B19 infections in infants and children. *Adv Pediatr Infect Dis* 1998; 13: 101–26.

45 Harger JH, Adler ST, Koch WC, Harger GF. Prospective evaluation of 618 pregnant women exposed to parvovirus B19: Risks and symptoms. *Obstet Gynecol* 1998; 91 (3): 413–20.

46 Pattison JR. Human parvovirus B19. In: Zuckerman AJ, Banatvala JE, Pattison JR, eds. *Principles and Practice of Clinical Virology*, 4th edn, pp. John Wiley and Sons, Chichester, 2000: 645–58.

47 Tolfvenstam T, Papodogiannakis N, Norbeck O, Petersson K, Broliden K. Frequency of human parvovirus B19 infection in intrauterine fetal death. *Lancet* 2001; 257: 1494–97.

48 Carlson DE, Platt LD, Mecearis AL, Horenstein J. Prognostic indicators of the resolution of nonimmune hydrops fetalis and survival of the fetus. *Am J Obstet Gynaecol* 1990; 163: 1785–7.

49 Fairley CK, Smoleniec JS, Caul OE, Miller E. Observational study of effect of intrauterine tranfusions on outcome of fetal hydrops after parvovirus B19 infection. *Lancet* 1995; 346: 1335–7.

50 Arvin A, Hensleigh PA *et al.* Failure of antepartum maternal cultures to predict the infants risk of exposure to herpes simplex virus at delivery. *N Engl J Med* 1986; 315: 796–800.

51 Benedetti J, Corey L, Ashley R. Recurrence rates in genital herpes after symptomatic first-episode infection. *Ann Intern Med* 1994; 121: 847–54.

52 Tookey PA, Peckham CS. Neonatal herpes simplex virus infection: the British Isles. *Paediatric Perinatal Epidemiol* 1996; 10: 432–42.

53 Smith JR, Cowan FM, Munday P. The management of herpes simplex virus infections in pregnancy. *Br J Obstet Gynaecol* 1998; 105: 255–60.

54 van Everdingen JJE, Peeters MF, ten Have P. Neonatal herpes policy in the Netherlands: five years after a consensus conference. *J Perinat Med* 1993; 21: 371–5.

55 Wald A, Zeh J *et al.* Reactivation of genital herpes simplex virus type 2 infection in asymptomatic seropositive persons. *N Engl J Med* 2000; 342: 844–50.

56 Arvin AM, Whitley RJ. Herpes simplex virus infections. In: Remmington JS, Kline JO, eds. *Infections of the Fetus and Neonate*, 5th edn. WB Saunders Co, Philadelphia, 2000: 425–46.

57 Adams O, Krempe C, Kogler G, Wernet P, Scheid A. Congenital infections with human herpesvirus 6. *J Infect Dis* 1999; 179: 1046–7.

58 Plancoulaine S, Abel L *et al.* Human herpesvirus 8 transmission from mother to child and between siblings in an endemic population. *Lancet* 2000; 356: 1062–5.

59 Hyoty H, Hiltunen M *et al.* A prospective study of the role of coxsackie B and other enterovirus infections in the pathogenesis of IDDM. Childhood Diabetes in Finland (DiMe) Study Group. *Diabetes* 1995; 44: 652–7.

60 Dahlquist G, Frisk G, Ivarsson SA, Svanberg L, Forsgren M, Diderholm H. Indications that maternal coxsackie B virus infection during pregnancy is a risk factor for childhood-onset IDDM. *Diabetologia* 1995; 38: 1371–3.

61 Rotbart HA, Webster AD. Treatment of potentially life-threatening enterovirus infections with pleconaril. *CID* 2001; 32; 228–35.

62 Rice PS, Cason J, Best JM, Banatvala JE. High risk genital papillomavirus infections are spread vertically. *Rev Med Virol* 1999; 9: 15–21.

63 Chrystie IL, Sumner D, Palmer SJ, Kenney A, Banatvala JE. Screening of pregnant women for evidence of current hepatitis B infection: selective or universal? *Health Trends* 1992; 24 (1): 13–15.

64 Department of Health, Welsh Office, Scottish Home Office and Health Departments, DHSS (Northern Ireland). *Immunisation Against Infectious Diseases*. HMSO, London, 1996: 95–108.

65 Ades A,E, Parker S, Walker J, Cubitt WD, James R. HCV prevalence in pregnant women in the United Kingdom. *Epidemiol Infect* 2000; 125: 399–405.

66 Unlinked Anonymous Surveys Steering Group. *Prevalence of HIV in the UK in 1998. Report of the Unlinked Anonymous Seroprevalence Monitoring Programme in England and Wales*. Department of Health, Public Health Laboratory Service, Scottish Centre for Infection and Environment Health, Institute of Child Health, London, 1999.

67 Zanetti AR, Tanzi E *et al.* Mother to infant transmission of hepatitis C virus. Lombardy Study Group on Vertical HCV Transmission. *Lancet* 1995; 345: 289–91.

68 Gibb DM, Goodall RL *et al.* Mother-to-child transmission of hepatitis C virus: evidence for preventable peripartum transmission. *Lancet* 2000; 356: 904–7.

69 Vogt M, Lang T *et al.* Prevalence and clinical outcome of hepatitis C infection in children who underwent cardiac surgery before the implementation of blood-donor screening. *N Engl J Med* 1999; 341: 866–70.

70 Miller E, Fairley CK, Cohen BJ, Seng C. Immediate and long term outcome of human parvovirus B19 infection in pregnancy. *Br J Obstet Gynaecol* 1998; 105: 174–6.

71 Taylor GP. Human T-cell lymphotrophic viruses. In *Principles and Practice of Clinical Virology*, ed. Zucherman AJ, Banatvala JE & Pattison JR. John Wiley & Sons, Chichester, 696–710.

72 Ades AE, Parker S, Walker J, Edginton M, Taylor GP, Weber JN. Human T cell leukaemia/lymphoma virus infection in pregnant women in the United Kingdom: population study. *BMJ* 2000; 320: 1497–1501.

73 Ureta-Vidal A, Angelin-Duclos C *et al.* Mother to child transmission of human T-cell leukaemia/lymphoma virus type I: implication of high antiviral antibody titer and high proviral load in carrier mothers. *Int J Cancer* 1999; 82: 832–6.

74 Ishak R, Harrington WJ Jr *et al.* (1995) Identification of human T cell lymphotropic virus type IIa infection in the Kayapo, an indigenous population of Brazil. *AIDS Res Hum Retroviruses*, II, 813–21.

75 Hino S, Sugiyama H *et al.* (1987) Breaking the cycle of HTLV-I transmission via carrier mothers' milk (Letter). *Lancet* ii 158–9.

18 HIV infection

Frank D. Johnstone, Laurent Mandelbrot and Marie-Louise Newell

Human immunodeficiency virus (HIV) has dominated public and scientific attention in the late 20th century. In many countries, deaths from HIV disease are significantly reducing life expectancy for women and children, and the HIV epidemic remains a global calamity. At the same time the enormous research drive has made this the most evidence-based subject in obstetrics, with success relating to prevention of vertical transmission. However, the speed of development of new drugs has outpaced the testing of safety in pregnancy, hindering decision making. With new information accumulating rapidly, much pregnancy management is about effective communication, up-to-date knowledge and expertise in managing HIV. This chapter reviews aspects of HIV infection that are relevant to pregnancy, and suggests how these relate to pregnancy management, based on available evidence at the time of writing (November 1999, updated November 2001). See also Chapter 9 concerning acquired immune deficiency syndrome (AIDS), HIV and the liver; and Chapter 17 about the human T-cell lymphotrophic virus (HTLV) and pregnancy.

Information about this fast moving subject is increasingly web based. There are excellent websites, often updated regularly, and allowing easy access to guidelines, published work, and abstracts and reviews from recent conferences. For example there is a wealth of information from the US Public Health Service on http://www.hivatis.org/, from the excellent BHIVA site on http://aidsmap.com, for epidemiology at UNAIDS (see below) and from Medscape on http://hiv.medscape.com

Epidemiology

It has been suggested that the source of virus was one subspecies of chimpanzee, *Pantroglodytes troglodytes* (Gao *et al.* 1999). This host species has probably harboured the virus for hundreds of thousands of years, although infection does not result in disease in these animals. Phylogenetic analysis suggests that the interspecies jump to humans occurred on at least three occasions, as recently as 50–60 years ago (Zhu *et al.* 1998). How this occurred is the subject of debate. Whatever the source, the unique feature of HIV has been the initial long transmission chain, and the rapidity of subsequent spread (Hooper 1999).

From this original epicentre, the relentless march of HIV/AIDS as a predominantly sexually transmitted disease (STD) has shown few signs of abating. Estimates relating to December 2000 suggest that more than 1% of all sexually active adults are now infected and that 6000 more women become infected each day. (These figures and several others in this section have been taken from the excellent website from UNAIDS, http://hivinsite.ucsf.edu/social/un/2098.3cee.html)

The greatest impact has been in sub-Saharan Africa, where 10 million women of childbearing age are currently infected. Indeed, of people living with HIV around the world, it is estimated that eight in every 10 adult women, and nine of every 10 children infected are in sub-Saharan Africa. Rates of infection throughout Southern Africa have risen rapidly in recent years, with prevalence in many antenatal clinics greater than 25%. Mortality throughout the continent has risen dramatically and tragically. It is claimed that AIDS has cut life expectancy in sub-Saharan Africa by a quarter (Logie 1999).

With overall numbers of infected people in some parts of the world stabilizing (Europe, North America, Latin America) it is the explosive exponential increase in parts of the Asia-Pacific Region that is defining the scale of the pandemic for this century. With 60% of the world's population, this part of the world currently has a number of sharply focused epidemics, against an overall background of very low HIV prevalence. Foci of intense HIV spread in the region include large metropolitan areas in western and southern India; the India/Nepal border area; the 'Golden Triangle' (encompassing northern Thailand, eastern Myanmar, Manipur in India, and Yunnan in China); and the Mekong delta area of Cambodia and Vietnam.

HIV infection remains a leading cause of mortality in young women in large urban areas of America and Europe, particularly since mortality from other causes at these ages is generally low. In the USA, the overall prevalence in childbearing women was estimated to be 0.15% in 1994. However, the infection is more common in some urban districts, such as along the Atlantic coast and in the South, and among poor and vulnerable women. Rates of infection are much higher in black and Hispanic women. In Europe the highest prevalence in childbearing women is found in countries of the south-west, initially related particularly to injection drug use with heterosexual transmission more common in recent years. The highest prevalences were seen in Spain, Italy, Portugal, the south of France and Switzerland (Cazein *et al.* 1998). Recently, increases have been especially pronounced in Eastern Europe, where Russia is the country with the fastest growing HIV epidemic. Immigrants and refugees from Africa make up a significant proportion of infected women in major cities such as Paris and London. In Paris, the prevalence has been stable (0.49% in 1995) from 1991 to 1997 and is consistently higher in women who terminate their pregnancy than in those who deliver (0.98% vs. 0.28%, respectively). The UK is one of many European countries with low overall prevalence, at around one in 6500 births excluding London, but with significant prevalence in Inner London, of one in 200 births.

At the millennium 36 million adults and children were living with HIV or AIDS. On current trends, by 2020 HIV will be the second leading cause of death in adults in their prime years in the developing world (currently third). This will result in serious demographic distortions. Eight million children have already been orphaned by AIDS mortality, and this number is expected to increase rapidly in the near future. This has strained the ability of extended families and communities to provide for their children's needs. Orphanhood will therefore impact on children in many serious and socially disruptive ways.

Despite the medical advances, treatment is not available for most infected individuals, and this remains a fatal disease. Ninety per cent of those with HIV live in sub-Saharan Africa and the developing countries of Asia, the very countries that can least afford to deal with the prob-

lem. HIV also exacerbates existing disease patterns. This is a particular problem for the 30–70% of young adults in developing countries who are infected with *Mycobacterium tuberculosis*. The synergy between these organisms on the one hand increases tuberculosis (TB) disease (between 5 and 10% of dually infected adults will develop TB each year) and on the other hand enhances replication of HIV disease, probably leading to more rapid progression of HIV in those who develop TB.

Human immunodeficiency virus infection

Virology

Within 2 years of the recognition of AIDS as a disease, the aetiological agent human immunodeficiency virus type 1 (HIV-1) had been discovered. Since then its scrap of genetic information (less than 10 000 nucleotides) has been exposed to the full power of contemporary molecular biology. Knowledge of HIV greatly supersedes that of any other virus. A separate, but related virus (HIV-2) was reported in 1986. This virus (believed to have crossed species much earlier from the West African monkey, the sooty mangabey) causes a slower, less virulent clinical disease and is less likely to be vertically transmitted. However, the two viruses both result in progressive immunodeficiency.

HIV-1 (subsequently referred to here as HIV) contains two copies of a single-stranded RNA genome, and it is only with conversion of the genetic material into DNA that the viral genes can be transcribed and translated into proteins in the usual way. This is accomplished by a viral DNA polymerase with a ribonuclease (together called reverse transcriptase) and it is this reversal of the normal flow of genetic information that classifies HIV as a retrovirus. Once in the form of double-stranded DNA, the viral genetic information is spliced into the DNA of the host cell. It then serves as a template for viral gene transcription leading to production of new virus. Infection of that cell and its progeny will then be permanent.

Several steps are necessary before HIV can enter and infect a cell. The virion is surrounded by a lipid membrane from which protrudes the envelope extracellular glycoprotein. This mediates binding of virus to the surface of the target cell through an interaction with the target cell receptor CD4 ('cluster designation 4'). However, a further interaction with a chemokine receptor to form a trimolecular complex appears to trigger the final conformational changes in the envelope protein. This leads to fusion between viral and cellular membranes, hence allowing infection to proceed.

Two principal chemokine coreceptors for HIV have been described, CCR5 and CXCR4. CCR5 is used preferentially by macrophage-tropic strains of virus. These strains are responsible for transmission and are the prevalent viral type isolated from asymptomatic individuals. CXCR4 is the coreceptor required by T-cell tropic strains, the emergence of which, late in disease history, correlates with accelerated disease progression (Mummidi *et al.* 1998; Zhu *et al.* 1998; Horuk 1999). CCR5 polymorphism explains some of the variations in susceptibility to infection, and in rate of progression to illness. The importance of these coreceptors for viral cell entry also offers a further possible target for treatment.

In untreated disease there is an enormous viral production, about a billion virions each day (Ho *et al.* 1995). There is also a high rate of emergence of mutant forms. This rapid turnover and generation of viral diversity makes for problems with resistance to antiviral drugs. Much recent understanding of the virology has come from studies following treatment with highly active antiretroviral therapy, HAART (see below).

Pathogenesis

After infection the body mounts a very aggressive cell-mediated and humoral immune response. HIV manages, to a greater or lesser extent, to evade this, and viral replication stabilizes around a steady state. Different individuals display different 'set points' of persisting viraemia, the level of which determines the speed of disease progression (Feinberg 1996). HIV targets CD4 receptor bearing cells, in particular the T-helper subset of lymphocytes. These cells interact with antigen-presenting cells, which display antigen on their own cell membrane, together with class 2 major histocompatibility complex glycoproteins. Helper T cells then initiate an immune response against other cells bearing the antigen, and thus occupy a pivotal position in overall cell-mediated immune response. Although the CD4$^+$ lymphocyte is the main target, a proportion of peripheral monocytes (that mature to become macrophages), follicular dendritic cells and Langerhans' cells express CD4 and can be infected by HIV, as can microglial cells.

Defects in HIV infection are not restricted to the depletion of CD4$^+$ lymphocytes. Activation of lymphocytes is a consistent feature, even in early HIV infection, and qualitative abnormalities have been demonstrated in B cells and monocytes. However, the pathognomonic feature is the progressive attrition in CD4$^+$ lymphocyte number, with an average yearly decrease in CD4$^+$ lymphocytes of around 60×10^6/L. When numbers are critically reduced in end-stage disease, the individual is open to opportunistic infections and malignancies (that would normally be controlled by the immune system). The type of opportunistic infection varies in different parts of the world depending on locally prevalent conditions. AIDS used to be defined in terms of these infections or neoplasms. The Centers for Disease Control and Prevention has since expanded the AIDS case definition to include all HIV-infected patients with CD4$^+$ counts of less than 200×10^6/L regardless of clinical status, although the European AIDS case definition is still based on clinical symptoms and signs only.

The mechanisms underlying the progressive decline in CD4$^+$ lymphocyte number are not completely understood. It was previously argued that CD4$^+$ cell number was maintained initially because of massive replacement of the destroyed cells. This occurred only because of a huge production rate by the haemopoietic system, and this process eventually became exhausted. The metaphor of a sink with the tap and drain equally wide open was used (Ho *et al.* 1995). The current picture of T-cell turnover in HIV infection suggests that both CD4$^+$ and CD8$^+$ cells are dying prematurely, but at a much slower rate than previously thought. The fundamental problem seems to be that T-cell production is inadequate, either because of failure of generation of lymphocyte precursors from the bone marrow, or thymic dysfunction, or a combination of the two (Wolthers *et al.* 1998; Hellerstein *et al.* 1999; Pantaleo 1999; Rowland-Jones 1999). The current metaphor is that the sink empties because the tap is damaged, and when the drain is slightly more open, the system is unable to maintain homeostasis (Wolthers *et al.* 1998).

Natural history and plasma viraemia

Untreated, most infected people show a progressive decline in immunocompetence, and are ultimately diagnosed with AIDS, a combination of symptoms and signs. About 5% remain well for prolonged periods and in the short to medium term do not display the same characteristic reduction in CD4$^+$ cell number. Cohort studies have indicated that approximately 50% of individuals with HIV infection will progress to AIDS after 10 years.

In recent years, follow-up and treatment have been transformed by the availability of quantitative measurements of plasma viraemia using HIV RNA measurements. This gives a direct measure of viral replication, and is an important prognostic marker for progression of disease. CD4$^+$ cell counts also remain an important measure of disease progression, highly correlated with the risk of opportunistic infections. In studies performed before the introduction of effective antiretroviral drugs, the combination of CD4 count and plasma HIV RNA was shown to be predictive of progression to AIDS and death over a 10-year period. Plasma HIV RNA measurements, and particularly CD4 counts (Hogg *et al.* 2001) are also the key markers used to monitor the effectiveness of treatment.

A word of caution is required here. Mismatches between the probes used in commercial assays and RNA target sequences can result in falsely low estimates of viral load. This happens with some assays developed primarily using the B subtype, where the ability to quantify non-B subtypes is limited. In the UK for example, 78% of infections in women attending antenatal clinics are non-B (Parry *et al.* 2001, discussed in BHIVA guidelines 2001).

Antiretroviral therapy

Zidovudine (ZDV) was the first drug to be licensed for the treatment of HIV infection. Early short-term studies using monotherapy in patients with symptomatic disease showed that survival was enhanced (Moore & Chaisson 1999). However, a large European study (the Concorde trial) failed to demonstrate a prolongation in the time to progression to AIDS or survival for asymptomatic patients followed for longer than a year. It became clear that benefits were very time limited. The development of additional drugs allowed combination therapy, and the clinical availability of estimates of viral load opened up the possibility of effective monitoring of treatment.

HAART is based on such use of combinations of several drugs. These typically include two reverse transcriptase inhibitors plus a protease inhibitor, but there is now an increasing array of combinations, including the above classes, and also non-nucleoside reverse transcriptase inhibitors. HAART first entered clinical trials in 1995 and impressive results were evident by early 1996. HAART substantially and quickly reduces viral load, and also acts to release the constraints on $CD4^+$ cell production. Even outside the research setting, HAART reduces plasma viraemia to undetectable levels in most patients, prolongs life and reduces morbidity. Indeed the effectiveness of HAART is dramatically demonstrated by the fact that AIDS hospices are closing. Such a huge decrease in mortality and morbidity in such a short time has few precedents in medicine (Hirschel & Opravil 1999).

But the news is not all good. Initial hopes that non-detectable viraemia might equate with complete eradication of virus from the body have not been fulfilled (Ledergerber *et al.* 1999; Pomerantz 1999b). Rebound viraemia occurs rapidly and vigorously on stopping treatment. Recent measurements of half-life decay with current HAART regimens translate to eradication of virus in ap-

proximately 60 years. Attention has focused on explanatory paradigms, including viral reservoirs, long-lived cells, reduced inhibition of proximal activation and transmission and ongoing HIV replication in multiple local bursts (Grossman *et al.* 1998; Pomerantz 1999a; Siliciano 1999).

In addition there are problems with toxicity. A syndrome of lipodystrophy (peripheral fat wasting and/or central fat accumulation) hyperlipidaemia and insulin resistance develops with HAART, even after short-term use. This was initially attributed to protease inhibitor therapy (Carr *et al.* 1998) but could be mitochondrial toxicity due to reverse transcriptase inhibitors (Brinkman *et al.* 1999). This complication has also been associated with myocardial damage. Treatment with nucleoside analogue reverse transcriptase inhibitors is certainly known to be associated with a range of pathologies due to mitochondrial toxicity (Brinkman *et al.* 1998). Some of these conditions are reversible on stopping treatment but others, including lactic acidosis, liver steatosis and pancreatitis, have been fatal.

Partly related to toxicity and side-effects, but also due to the complexity of the regimens, there are serious problems in strict adherence to treatment schedules (Chesney *et al.* 1999). Adhering to a life-long therapy is always problematic for patients who are asymptomatic. Furthermore, these regimens may involve taking 20 or more pills a day, with timing related to meals and fat content. These are probably the most complex regimens ever prescribed for continuous treatment of a large patient population. Lack of adherence quickly results in viral breakthrough and also in the rapid emergence of drug-resistant strains.

Viral resistance is increasing, and reduced antiviral drug susceptibility is beginning to emerge even in patients with primary HIV infection (Pomerantz 1999b). Drug-resistant quasi-species emerge mostly following suboptimal therapy, and this could cast a shadow over the future efficacy of these treatments. Follow-up of patients receiving first-line HAART with good adherence suggests that effective suppression of virus replication reduces the risk of resistant strains emerging. Multiple drug treatment also raises difficulties for management in pregnancy (see below).

Interaction of human immunodeficiency virus and pregnancy

Interpreting the associations between HIV and pregnancy is complicated. Possible confounding variables include adverse lifestyle factors and other STDs. Women who are ill and immunocompromised are likely to have different outcomes from women who are well. The experience in Africa may be different from that in the developed world.

Two systematic reviews conclude that HIV adversely affects pregnancy outcome and that pregnancy increases the rate of progression of HIV disease. However, the associations are not strong and the authors acknowledge that these could be due to bias (Brocklehurst & French 1998; French & Brocklehurst 1998). These reviews are important, but of somewhat limited clinical value because they do not disentangle the key variables of place and degree of illness.

Effect of pregnancy on disease progression

Concerns that pregnancy would cause HIV to progress more rapidly were based partly on the concept of pregnancy as an immunodeficient state. While pregnancy does cause basic changes in the immune system, the case that infectious diseases are more aggressive during pregnancy is perhaps more selective and less emphatic than once thought (Landers *et al.* 1997). CD4$^+$ lymphocyte count does fall by 100×10^6/L in normal early pregnancy, but only 2% of CD4$^+$ lymphocytes are found in the peripheral blood system and this may represent redistribution rather than loss (Johnstone *et al.* 1994).

In Africa, many women enter pregnancy in a vulnerable nutritional state, have an increased load of other infectious diseases (particularly malaria and TB), and will most commonly present with weight loss if they have advancing disease. It is plausible that the additional demands of pregnancy under these circumstances could increase the subsequent rate of progression of maternal disease. However there is no strong evidence to substantiate this.

In the developed world, in women who are immunocompetent, pregnancy does not seem to have any long-term effect on the rate of decline of CD4$^+$ count or progression to AIDS (Brettle *et al.* 1995; Hocke *et al.* 1995; Saada *et al.* 2000). Also, the natural history of HIV in women is similar to that in men, suggesting that pregnancy does not substantially influence progression of disease (Phillips *et al.* 1994; Chaisson *et al.* 1995).

Effect of human immunodeficiency virus on pregnancy

FERTILITY

A number of direct and indirect estimates from studies in Uganda show a consistent pattern of reduced fertility (Gray *et al.* 1998; Gregson *et al.* 1999). Two plausible reasons for this are: (i) that HIV infections are more likely

in women with existing low fertility (due to other STDs such as gonorrhoea and *Chlamydia*); and/or (ii) that HIV has a direct influence on fecundity, particularly through increased early pregnancy loss. Lower fertility has an impact on demographic data, such as orphanhood and early childhood mortality, and the implications are explored by Gregson *et al.* (1999). There is also a comparison of pregnancy rates in HIV-infected women living in France, before and after HIV diagnosis (Fourquet *et al.* 2001). Among European women the incidence of deliveries and terminations decreased after diagnosis, but in African women it increased among those with fewer than two children. This highlights the importance of allowing for cultural background when assessing fertility patterns.

SPONTANEOUS ABORTION

A number of studies based on history of spontaneous abortion have suggested an increase in women infected with HIV (Desgrees *et al.* 1998; Temmerman *et al.* 1992; D'Ubaldo *et al.* 1998). In the largest prospective study to date (Temmerman *et al.* 1992) HIV antibody status was assessed in 195 women admitted with abortion to a hospital in Kenya. Although there are methodological problems, particularly associated with selection of a control group, attempts were made to account for other variables, and HIV was still statistically more common in the abortion group.

At present it is uncertain whether HIV is a direct cause of spontaneous abortion. Most published information suggests a trend in that direction, but the studies are either retrospective or there is doubt about whether the findings could be explained by a correlated variable, such as positive syphilis serology or other infectious disease; also there is a difficulty in distinguishing spontaneous and induced abortions in settings where voluntary terminations are illegal. Nevertheless, the consistency of the reports, and the plausible mechanism (alteration in decidual immune cells which could affect implantation and subsequent trophoblast proliferation) may indicate that this is a real effect.

LATER PREGNANCY COMPLICATIONS

Adequately controlled studies from the developed world have shown no significant increase in pregnancy complications, except for infectious complications of the mother (Bucceri *et al.* 1997). However, these studies were based on small numbers, and lack statistical power to address the issue of relatively infrequent pregnancy complications. In the large European Collaborative Study, HIV-infected women with evidence of severe immune deficiency were more likely to deliver early than those who were less severely immunosuppressed (European Collaborative Study 1998; O'Shea *et al*. 1998). In addition, multivariate analysis adjusted for risk factors showed an increased risk of prematurity for infants exposed to combination therapy, whether or not this included a protease inhibitor (European Collaborative Study 2000).

Studies from Africa provide information for both infected and uninfected women, suggesting that HIV seropositivity is associated with preterm delivery and an increase in perinatal mortality (Temmermann *et al*. 1990; Desgrees *et al*. 1998). A large case–controlled study from Nairobi focused on adverse pregnancy outcome; 373 women who delivered a preterm baby, 324 who delivered a baby small for gestational age, 120 who had an intra-uterine death, and 69 with an intrapartum death were compared for HIV status with 711 controls (Temmermann *et al*. 1990). HIV was more common in the case groups but so were other, potentially confounding, features such as primiparity, lack of antenatal clinic attendance and maternal syphilis infection. However, linear logistic regression retained HIV status as a statistically significant associated outcome with modestly increased odds ratios of 2.1 (preterm birth), 2.3 (small for gestational age), 2.7 (intrauterine death) and 2.9 (intrapartum death).

Regardless of whether preterm delivery is due directly to HIV disease, or is related to associated confounding variables, it is clinically important. Preterm delivery is an important obstetric risk factor for HIV transmission and it has been argued that prevention of preterm delivery may account for some of the effect of ZDV (European Collaborative Study 1998). The background links between local infection, preterm delivery and perinatal HIV transmission have been reviewed (Goldenberg *et al*. 1998).

A contrast between data from the developed world and Africa is also seen with regard to birthweight. All studies from Africa are consistent in showing a decrease in birthweight in pregnancies from HIV-infected mothers (reviewed in Johnstone 1993; Desgrees *et al*. 1998). On the other hand, most of the small controlled studies from Europe and the USA do not suggest that maternal HIV infection has any impact on birthweight, when taking into account other factors such as smoking, street drug use and poor socio-economic conditions (Bucceri *et al*. 1997). However, multivariate analysis in one study did retain HIV as having a statistically significant but modest effect on fetal growth (Johnstone *et al*. 1996), and in some large European cohort studies the mean birthweight of HIV-infected infants was lower than for those not infected (Blanche *et al*. 1997), although this is not necessarily a causal relation (European Collaborative Study 1998). There is some evidence that decrease in size is related to the stage of maternal disease. Any effect on birthweight does not seem to be mediated through anticardiolipin antibodies. These antibodies are common in HIV-infected women (about a quarter have raised levels above the normal range), but these infection-stimulated antibodies do not produce adverse pregnancy or thrombotic events (Johnstone *et al*. 1992).

Mother-to-child transmission

Rates of transmission and determinants

Before specific treatment, the estimated rate of vertical transmission of HIV-1 ranged from 15% to 20% in Europe, 15% to 30% in the USA and 25% to 35% in Africa. However, most of this infection is now theoretically preventable.

Transmission of HIV-2 is less frequent than for HIV-1, on the order of 1–4% in the absence of prophylaxis (O'Donovan *et al*. 2000).

In recent years the maternal plasma HIV-1 RNA level has been identified as the best single predictor of the risk of perinatal transmission of HIV-1 (European Collaborative Study 1996; Sperling *et al*. 1996; Mayaux *et al*. 1997a; Garcia *et al*. 1999; Mofenson *et al*. 1999; Shaffer *et al*. 1999). However there is great overlap in the HIV-1 RNA levels between transmitting and non-transmitting mothers, and clearly, many other factors are relevant (European Collaborative Study 1999). Although several studies have shown no transmission where maternal plasma viral levels have been undetectable (Garcia *et al*. 1999; Mofenson *et al*. 1999; Shaffer *et al*. 1999) this has been reported to occur (Sperling *et al*. 1996; Mayaux *et al*. 1997b; Ioannidis *et al*. 2001). Just as transmission can (rarely) occur at low plasma levels of maternal viral RNA, there is no upper threshold of maternal viraemia that is always associated with transmission. Clinical factors shown in some studies to be associated with transmission are often those associated with high viral load (seroconversion during pregnancy, advanced HIV disease, low CD4 count). The prognostic significance of CD4 count and plasma HIV RNA are only known in the absence of prophylaxis and in the presence of ZDV monotherapy (Mofenson *et al*. 1999). In women receiving more potent combination therapies, transmission rates are lower and therefore the relationships between low CD4 count and/or high viral load and transmission risk are less clear (Dorenbaum *et al*. 2001).

Importantly, the degree of exposure to maternal virus will depend on more than simply maternal plasma viraemia. Increased exposure to virus seems to underlie the observations of increased transmission following invasive procedures during pregnancy (Mandelbrot *et al.* 1996a), and vaginal delivery as opposed to elective caesarean section (European Mode of Delivery Collaboration 1999; International Perinatal HIV Group 1999). Similarly, increased transmission has been associated with presence of ruptured membranes for more than 4 h (Landesman *et al.* 1996; Garcia *et al.* 1999). Recently, results from a large meta-analysis showed this effect to be gradual, with each 1-h increase in time since the membranes ruptured increasing by 2% the risk of vertical transmission (International Perinatal HIV Group 2001). As well as the issue of degree of contamination with maternal fluids, the disassociation between the concentrations of virus in maternal plasma and vaginal fluids may be relevant (Chuachoowong *et al.* 2000). Importantly, genital tract HIV-1 shedding was found in 33% (27/83) of women with less than 500 copies/ml plasma RNA (Kovacs *et al.* 2001). Maternal smoking also seems to increase risk of transmission (Turner *et al.* 1997).

The timing of transmission is now well known (Newell 1998). The baby can be infected before, during or after birth. Studies using polymerase chain reaction (PCR) to detect the virus in the infant from birth onwards, and a backtracking mathematical model, have all concurred in estimating that around two-thirds of cases probably occur around delivery (Simonon *et al.* 1994; Dunn *et al.* 1995; Rouzioux *et al.* 1995; Kalish *et al.* 1997). These studies were performed in non-breastfeeding populations. Although *in utero* transmission accounted for about one-third of cases of transmission, studies in second-trimester fetuses indicate that transmission in early pregnancy is rare in uneventful pregnancies (Mandelbrot *et al.* 1996a). Most *in utero* transmission probably occurs in the last weeks or days of pregnancy. In women receiving antiretroviral therapies, there are recent data (Dorenbaum *et al.* 2001) indicating that more than half of the residual cases of transmission occurred *in utero*.

The actual mechanisms of vertical transmission are more difficult to establish. Fetuses swallow, and macaque neonates can easily be infected with the related simian immunodeficiency virus given orally (Baba *et al.* 1995). HIV is often detected in gastric aspirates of neonates (Ait-Khaled *et al.* 1998; Mandelbrot *et al.* 1999). This is therefore a possible site of entry. In one report from Kenya a significant relationship was found between presence of virus in the aspirate and actual HIV transmission (Gaillard *et al.* 2000) though this was not found in other studies (Ait-Khaled *et al.* 1998; Mandelbrot *et al.* 1999). Ocular or pulmonary surfaces are other possible sites of entry. Where twins are discordant for infection, the first twin is more likely than the second twin to be infected (Duliege *et al.* 1995), suggesting that it is the degree of exposure to

infected maternal blood and other fluids during delivery that is a main determinant of transmission. Transmission may also occur via the placenta. Although infection of trophoblast has been obtained *in vitro*, there are no data showing infection *in vivo*. Transfer of free virus or infected cells may occur by transcytosis, or through microtransfusions, which occur at the end of pregnancy and mostly during labour and delivery.

Chorioamnionitis may be a major underlying obstetric risk factor for transmission of HIV (Goldenberg *et al.* 1998). This would explain the increased risk associated with preterm birth and prolonged rupture of the membranes. A plausible hypothesis is that bacterial invasion of the uterus initiates massive cytokine response, in turn attracting a large number of leucocytes into the amniotic fluid and thereby enhancing viral replication and transmission, as has been suggested in monkeys. Under this hypothesis, the use of antibiotics may have a role in the prevention of vertical transmission.

These factors have been well reviewed (Newell 1998; Gibb & Tess 1999, Mofenson & Fowler 1999).

Strategies for prevention of mother-to-child transmission

There is now a wide array of strategies for prevention. These include:

- reducing maternal plasma viral load by antiretrovirals;
- reducing exposure of the fetus during delivery by caesarean section (or by reducing viral load in the genital tract);
- pre- and postexposure prophylaxis by antiretrovirals crossing the placenta administered during pregnancy and delivery, and antiretrovirals in the neonate;
- avoiding postnatal transmission via breast milk.

In recent years, the rate of mother-to-infant HIV-1 transmission has been reduced to 1–2% in cohort studies from industrialized countries. A large proportion of the cases of infection are attributable to lack of appropriate prenatal care, refusal of prevention measures by the mother, or obstetrical complications such as very preterm delivery.

ZIDOVUDINE

ACTG 076 (AIDS Clinical Trials Group Protocol 076) was a randomized, placebo-controlled, double-blind trial carried out in 43 centres in the USA and France (Connor *et al.* 1994; Sperling *et al.* 1996). Treatment with ZDV 500 mg daily or placebo was started at a median of 26 weeks. Women also received ZDV or placebo intravenously during labour and their infants received ZDV syrup.

There was a 68% reduction in the frequency of transmission, from 25.5% in the placebo group to 8.3% in the ZDV group.

There has been ample confirmation that this intervention is effective, with reduced vertical transmission throughout the developed world. In addition there is considerable evidence that even abbreviated regimens are effective in a general population, and outside a trial setting (Wade *et al.* 1998; Bulterys *et al.* 1999). If an HIV-infected woman did not receive ZDV during pregnancy, it appears from these studies that ZDV given only intrapartum and neonatally still has a substantial effect on the risk. Neonatal treatment on its own appears effective, provided it is given within 24 h (Bulterys *et al.* 1999; Wade *et al.* 1998).

Abbreviated regimens have now been well tested, and this makes use of the drug more feasible in developing countries. In Bangkok, Thailand, a double-blind, placebo-controlled, randomized controlled trial (RCT) examined a much simpler regimen. ZDV was given to the mother only from 36 weeks' gestation, twice daily, and was given orally every 3 h in labour. None of the women breastfed. Mother-to-child transmission was reduced by 51%, from 18.9% in the placebo arm to 9.4% in the ZDV arm (Shaffer *et al.* 1999). In another trial in Thailand (Lallemant *et al.* 2000), shortened regimens were compared with the full ACTG 076-derived regimen. The 'short-short' regimen (as used in the Bangkok trial) was less effective than the full 'long-long' ACTG regimen, but both the 'short-long' regimen starting at 28 weeks and the 'long-short' regimen with only 1 week of postnatal prophylaxis, were as effective as the full ACTG regimen.

Two other similarly designed trials in West Africa examined the effect of short course oral ZDV in breast-feeding populations. Both showed that ZDV was well accepted, well tolerated and still effective (Dabis *et al.* 1999, Wiktor *et al.* 1999). The reductions in infection rate found were somewhat less than seen in the Bangkok trial, which in turn showed less effect than ACTG 076, but because of the different populations, and different entry criteria, quantitative comparison of effect is not valid. It should be noted that ultra-short ZDV treatment, orally during delivery and for 1 week in the neonate, was associated with a transmission rate of 25% in Uganda, suggesting that the efficacy of this regimen is at best very poor. This trial (Guay *et al.* 1999) did not have a placebo group, and is considered in more detail below. In summary, short regimens of ZDV are of importance for developing counties, but they may be less effective than the 076 regimen, which remains the standard of care in industrialized settings.

How does ZDV work? In the Bangkok study, reduction in viral load explained 80% of the effect (Shaffer *et al.* 1999) and this may perhaps be the most important mechanism. In ACTG 076, the effect was not due simply to reduction in viral load because by the time of delivery, this reduction was only 0.3 log and was calculated to account for only 17% of the effect (Sperling *et al.* 1996). Perhaps after more prolonged therapy there may have been selection of species less fit to infect. In addition there may have been an effect from pre-exposure prophylaxis, similar to the postexposure prophylaxis used in health-care workers (Cardo *et al.* 1997). An effect through reduction in incidence of preterm delivery has been suggested (European Collaborative Study 1998).

NEVIRAPINE

Nevirapine is a non-nucleoside reverse transcriptase inhibitor (RTI), with several theoretical advantages for short-term prophylaxis around delivery. It has a potent antiviral effect, rapid oral absorption, good bioavailability, a long half-life, good placental passage, is active immediately against intracellular and extracellular virus and, as a non-nucleoside RTI, it does not inhibit the actions of γ DNA polymerase on mitochondrial DNA replication.

Now there is evidence of effectiveness. A randomized study from Kampala, Uganda, compared nevirapine and ZDV given around delivery (Guay *et al.* 1999). Because of the different half-lives, the regimens were different and the study was therefore open. Nevirapine was given as a single oral dose of 200 mg at the onset of labour, and as a single oral dose to the baby within 72 h of birth. ZDV 600 mg orally was given to the mother at the onset of labour, every 3 h until delivery, and twice daily to the baby for 7 days. The risk of infection by age 14–16 weeks was 25.1% in the ZDV group, and 13.1% in the nevirapine group, a reduction in risk of nearly 50%. Compared to some other study populations, these pregnancies were at high risk for transmission. Nearly all the babies were breastfed, and the mothers had a median plasma viral load that was five times higher than those women in ACTG 076 (Guay *et al.* 1999). Another trial, in South Africa (SAINT), compared nevirapine with ZVD and lamivudine, for use intrapartum and neonatally only, in a breastfeeding population. The efficacy of the two regimens was equivalent (McIntyre 2000). The major advantage of the two-dose nevirapine regimen is its remarkable cost effectiveness (Marseille *et al.* 1999). It is therefore an important breakthrough in resource-poor settings, above all in Africa.

The role of nevirapine as adjunct therapy in the developed world was investigated in a randomized clinical trial (PACTG 316) in the USA and Europe (Dorenbaum *et al.* 2001). Nevirapine or placebo was added (one dose at delivery and one dose in the neonate) to whatever antiretrovirals the mother was already receiving as prevention or therapy. There was no difference in transmission rate (1.4–1.5%) between the two groups. This trial was stopped prematurely because the overall rate of vertical transmission was much lower than anticipated. The recalculated sample size to test for effect was impractical.

OTHER ANTIRETROVIRAL DRUGS

In recent years, combination antiretroviral therapies have been widely used in HIV-infected pregnant women, but there have been no randomized clinical trials testing their efficacy against ZDV monotherapy or comparing different combination regimens. Because antiretroviral combinations markedly reduce maternal viral load, an effect on transmission was to be expected. There is now evidence from observational studies that various antiretroviral combinations are associated with transmission rates on the order of 1–2%. This was the case, for instance, in the above-mentioned PACTG 316 trial of nevirapine, in which the mother-to-infant HIV transmission rate was 1.4%. To date, the combination which has been most studied is ZDV–lamivudine. In a French prospective open-label intervention performed in 1997–98 (Mandelbrot *et al.* 2001a), lamivudine was added to standard ZDV prophylaxis, to mothers from 32 weeks until delivery, and to neonates for 6 weeks. In the group of 445 HIV-1-infected women treated with ZDV–lamivudine, mother-to-infant HIV-1 transmission was 1.6%. In comparison, the transmission rate was 6.8% in a historical control group of 899 women receiving ZDV monotherapy in 1994–97 as standard care. The above-mentioned PACTG 316 nevirapine trial offers the most detailed data available on transmission under combination therapy. Interestingly, there was no significant difference in transmission according to the type of maternal therapy, ZDV, lamivudine–ZDV, other combinations without protease inhibitors, or combinations with protease inhibitors. Among 512 women receiving combination therapies with protease inhibitors (HAART), 1.4% transmitted HIV to their children. The European Collaborative Study (2001a) also gives rates of vertical transmission by interventions.

SAFETY OF PERINATAL ANTIRETROVIRAL EXPOSURE

Short- and medium-term follow-up data are now available for large numbers of children exposed to ZDV perinatally. Although haematological side-effects, i.e. anaemia and/or granulocytopenia, are frequent, and sometimes severe (Connor *et al.* 1994), short-term outcome is reassuring. Nevertheless, concerns remain about long-term effects. One study giving ZDV in very high doses to pregnant mice and monkeys showed genotoxic and tumour-inducing effects (Olivero *et al.* 1997) although other animal studies have been largely reassuring (Centers for Disease Control and Prevention 1998). In addition, follow-up has shown no difference in any parameters between infants who were exposed to the ZDV regimen compared with placebo (Culnane *et al.* 1999). There were no malignancies in 734 infants with *in utero* ZDV exposure up to 6 years of age (Hanson *et al.* 1997). As discussed below, there could be a link between mitochondrial dysfunction and the perinatal administration of prophylactic nucleoside analogues (Blanche *et al.* 1999). This is potentially very serious, and intuitively plausible, but a causal link has not been established (Morris & Carr 1999). On current information, the balance of risk remains strongly in favour of use of ZDV to prevent vertical transmission.

There is still little clinical information concerning the tolerance of antiretrovirals other than ZDV, except to a certain extent 3TC. In a large prospective, open-label clinical study of ZDV + 3TC (Mandelbrot *et al.* 2001a), there was a high incidence of haematological toxicity in neonates, but few life-threatening complications at 18 months of follow-up. However, the incidence of cases for which mitochondrial dysfunction could be suspected appeared higher than in an historical control group receiving standard ZDV prophylaxis. A number of phase 1–2 trials with drugs including stavudine, nelfinavir, ritonavir, abacavir and indinavir are ongoing to investigate safety, toxicity and pharmocokinetics. All of the nucleoside analogues and non-nucleoside inhibitors cross the placenta, and 3TC has been shown to accumulate in the amniotic fluid (Mandelbrot *et al.* 2001b). In contrast, placental transfer has been demonstrated for some but not all of the protease inhibitors. In preclinical studies, none of these drugs has been proved to cause harm to the fetus, but nor are there adequate data to demonstrate safety (Centers for Disease Control and Prevention 1998). According to the US Food and Drug Administration classification ddC, d4T, 3TC, indinavir, nevirapine and delaverdine are in category C (animal studies have either not been done or have shown abnormalities); and ddI, saquinavir, ritonavir and nelfinavir are in category B (animal studies fail to show a risk to the fetus) (Tovo *et al.* 1999b). The only drug showing teratogenic potential in one animal species is efavirenz.

In the first published report on pregnancies with combination therapy, a study from Switzerland of 16 pregnancies with protease inhibitors (Lorenzi *et al.* 1998), a cluster of rather unusual adverse effects was observed, including extrahepatic biliary atresia and two cases of intracerebral haemorrhage. In another small study (McGowan *et al.* 1999), out of 13 pregnancies with protease inhibitors, there was one stillbirth at term, one baby with microcephaly and two preterm deliveries. More recently, in the large PACTG 316 trial (Dorenbaum *et al.*, unpublished data, Durban) cohort, there was no difference in the incidence of birth defects or other severe adverse events between neonates exposed *in utero* to combination therapies, with or without protease inhibitors, versus ZDV monotherapy.

The incidence of preterm delivery was found to be significantly higher in the presence of therapy with protease inhibitors, than in the presence of antiretroviral therapy without protease inhibitors or no therapy in a large prospective European study (European Collaborative Study 2000). In contrast, a review of databases from cohort studies in the USA failed to confirm an increase in preterm delivery among women receiving antiretroviral combination therapies when compared to HIV-infected women without therapy.

In addition to potential toxicity to the fetus, antiretroviral drugs may occasionally have side-effects in the mother which may impact on the pregnancy, such as glucose intolerance or diabetes, pancreatitis, hepatitis, anaemia and even lactic acidosis (Luzzati *et al.* 1999). Recently, the US Food and Drugs Administration and the European Medicines Authority advised doctors that they had received reports of three cases of lactic acidosis resulting in maternal death. There were reports of another four non-fatal cases in pregnancy. In addition, hepatotoxicity has been reported after initiation of combination therapy in pregnancy, and a further maternal death has occurred from fulminant hepatic failure (Hill *et al.* 2001). These complications seem rare, but are extremely worrying.

POSSIBLE RISKS OF MITOCHONDRIAL TOXICITY

One theoretical risk is damage to fetal mitochondria caused by nucleoside reverse transcriptase inhibitors (NRTI). All NRTIs are dideoxy analogues (ddNRTI). Five types of DNA polymerase are active in the human cell, catalysing the formation of new DNA strands from the DNA template. Whereas DNA polymerase α, δ and ϵ are insensitive to inhibition by ddNRTI (and it is DNA polymerases α and δ that are responsible for DNA duplication in the nucleus) DNA polymerases β and γ are sensitive to inhibition by ddNRTI. These enzymes are involved in DNA repair mechanisms in the nucleus, but also γ DNA polymerase appears to be the only regulating enzyme in mitochondrial DNA replication. Therefore inhibition of this by ddNRTIs could down-regulate mitochondrial production. Mitochondria are responsible for oxidative phosphorylation, generating adenosine triphosphate (ATP), the primary source of energy for most tissues. It is not surprising that toxicity causes a wide range of system failures, and this is the common pathway for adverse effects of ddNRTIs in adults (Brinkman *et al.* 1998).

Mitochondrial DNA is particularly vulnerable to acquired mutations, because it has neither an effective repair mechanism nor protective histones, and is exposed to oxygen radicals generated by the respiratory chain. Because each cell contains a large number of copies of the mitochondrial DNA genome, a large number of DNA defects have to accumulate before mitochondrial ATP production declines below the minimum energy levels necessary. Nevertheless, in monkeys treated with doses similar to those used for pregnant women, mitochondrial damage was seen on electron microscopy in skeletal and cardiac muscle (Gerschenson *et al.* 1998).

In view of this theoretical background, the report by Blanche *et al.* (1999) is particularly concerning. These authors described eight children in France with documented mitochondrial dysfunction, four exposed to combined ZDV and lamivudine and four to ZDV alone. Five of the children, two of whom died, presented with neurological symptoms. The repeated occurrence of such a rare disorder in a series of about 1700 exposed infants seems highly suggestive of a link with NRTIs. In fact, the first three cases were observed in a cohort of 445 infants exposed to ZDV + 3TC in a prospective clinical study (Mandelbrot *et al.* 2001a). The five additional cases were identified through a retrospective study, and may therefore underestimate the actual prevalence.

In contrast to these findings, investigators in the US reviewed databases concerning over 15 000 infants perinatally exposed to antiretrovirals. This report, quoted by Morris and Carr (1999), and so far unpublished, showed no excess of deaths that could have been due to mitochondrial toxicity. Morris and Carr make the point that even if the relationship was causal, NRTIs would be associated with only a 0.1% mortality and 0.4% morbidity. There have however, been a few case reports of suspected mitochondrial toxicity including lactic acidosis in perinatally exposed infants (Scalfaro *et al.* 1998).

These data suggest that the incidence of deaths due to mitochondrial toxicity is likely to be small from a public health standpoint. However, one should note that the large database reviews were retrospective, concerned mostly infants exposed to ZDV monotherapy and not combinations, and looked for excess mortality not morbidity. It is possible that mitochondrial dysfunction may range from mild biological abnormalities, to reversible clinical anomalies, and more rarely irreversible damage.

In addition to determining the incidence of mitochondrial toxicity, several theoretical issues need to be investigated. In children who suffer minor and reversible adverse events, there is concern that neurological sequelae may appear later. The mechanisms whereby mitochondrial dysfunction may occur remain to be investigated, as the consequences may differ according to whether γ-polymerase activity is inhibited, mutations in the mitochodrial or nuclear DNA occur, or another unknown mechanism is involved. The hypothesis that genetic factors may predispose some individuals to these toxicities should also be investigated.

From a clinical perspective, many questions remain unanswered. Is the potential for mitochondrial toxicity greater when two or more nucleoside analogues are used rather than one? Is it greater when there is a longer period of exposure (*in utero* and after birth)?

In addition to these issues, there are more insidious long-term theoretical risks that would be difficult to recognize. One theory is that some aspects of ageing and age-related degenerative diseases (ischaemic heart disease, Parkinson's disease and Alzheimer's disease) are due to accumulation of mitochondrial DNA defects. The suggested paradigm is that each individual is born with an initial oxidative phosphorylation capacity that declines with age. Individuals born with a low oxidative phosphorylation capacity due to deleterious mutations would cross expression thresholds earlier, and hence develop 'old age' disease symptoms while still young (Wallace 1992). Whether the very actively dividing cells of the fetus could develop a long-term acquired reduction in oxidative phosphorylation capacity appears to be unknown. Perhaps this is unlikely, based on experiments showing rapid replacement of mitochondrial DNA in depleted cell lines (King & Attardi 1989).

A second risk is that reduction of oxidative phosphorylation during fetal life could reduce cell division, which could be another mechanism for degenerative disease, or could affect brain development. There is some reassurance in the lack of any effect of ZDV on birthweight or subsequent weight of the children (Connor *et al.* 1994; Culnane *et al.* 1999).

The fetuses of women taking HAART throughout pregnancy, involving two or more ddNRTIs are at highest risk of these theoretical complications. Further information from animal studies and exposed children is urgently required. Mitochondrial toxicity is only one possible risk among many, and it may be many years—and many exposed fetuses—before these risks are resolved.

DRUG RESISTANCE ISSUES

The presence of drug-resistant virus may be due to primary infection with resistant quasi-species, or more often emerge during the course of antiretroviral therapy. Emergence of resistant virus is due mostly to insufficient suppression of viral replication. This is less likely to occur with HAART, unless compliance is poor or the regimen is underdosed, than with monotherapies or double nucleoside analogue therapies. The presence of drug-resistant virus is of concern for the mother, as it may reduce the efficacy of antiretroviral therapy in the long run, even though it is likely to be replaced by wild type when the selection pressure is removed. Furthermore, it may lead to transmission of resistant virus to the infant. Thus, the choice of antiretroviral therapy in pregnancy must take into account the risk of emerging drug resistance.

Monotherapy with ZDV will allow viral resistance to develop in patients with high viral replication treated for several months. This situation should not occur in pregnant women, because only those with low viral loads are eligible for prophylaxis with ZDV monotherapy, and because exposure is limited to only a few weeks. In fact, data from the ACTG 076 trial was quite reassuring. Although there was often long exposure to ZDV monotherapy, only one of 39 women whose viruses were wild type at codon 70 at entry, developed a codon K70R mutation during the study. None of the 42 women developed a codon K215Y/f mutation (Eastman *et al.* 1998). Furthermore, follow-up of the women enrolled in the ACTG 076 trial showed no increase in HIV progression among those in the ZDV group, compared with those in the placebo group. The overall maternal risks of a short course of ZDV monotherapy do not seem substantial.

Of greater concern is the high risk of emerging drug resistance, in case of inadequate viral suppression, when using drugs for which a single point mutation can confer resistance, i.e. lamivudine or nevirapine. In the French AZT–3TC study, one-third of the mothers had the V184V mutation, which confers resistance to 3TC, at the 6 weeks postpartum visit (Mandelbrot *et al.* 2001a). In the Ugandan single-dose nevirapine trial, 19% of the mothers developed the K103N mutation (Jackson *et al.* 2000). In the international ACTG 316 trial, among women with viral loads above 400 copies/ml at delivery, the incidence of NNRTI resistance acquisition at the 6 weeks postpartum visit was 8% (Cunningham *et al.* 2001).

CAESAREAN SECTION

Elective caesarean section substantially reduces the chance of the baby being infected. In the first randomized mode of delivery trial in obstetrics ever to have resulted in a definite conclusion, three babies were infected in the 170 pregnancies allocated to caesarean section (1.8%) and 21 babies were infected in the 200 mothers randomized to vaginal delivery (10.5%) (European Mode of Delivery Collaboration 1999). This definitive study was supported by a meta-analysis of 15 prospective cohort studies, which included 8533 mother child pairs. The adjusted odds ratio of infant infection with elective caesarean section was 0.45 (0.33–0.56) (International Perinatal HIV Group 1999).

Importantly, several studies show that the protective effect of elective caesarean section is strongest in women who receive ZDV, i.e. an additive or possibly interactive effect (Kind *et al.* 1998; Mandelbrot *et al.* 1998; European Mode of Delivery Collaboration 1999; International HIV Perinatal Group 1999). It has also been shown that the relative effect is similar for women with a viral load below the median than for those with a load above the median (European Collaborative Study 1996). Caesareans are protective only when performed before labour or before rupture of the membranes. On general principles, attempts should be made to minimize contact of the baby with maternal fluids and one method of 'bloodless caesarean section' has been described (Towers *et al.* 1998). The above studies show that the combination of prophylactic ZDV and elective caesarean section reduced the risk of transmission to less than 2%.

Caesarean delivery carries a well-known risk of postoperative complications for the mother. There is concern that complication rates may be higher in HIV-infected women than in low-risk populations (Semprini *et al.* 1995; Bulterys *et al.* 1996; Grubert *et al.* 1999; Maiques-Montesinos *et al.* 1999). While these complications are usually minor, they may lead to serious morbidity and mortality. In HIV-infected women, the rate of postpartum morbidity is of the order of 3–5 times higher than that following vaginal delivery (Watts *et al.* 2000; Read *et al.* 2001), an increase of the same magnitude as in general obstetric practice. Much of the morbidity is due to the underlying obstetric or medical conditions leading to the indication of caesarean section, rather than the operation itself, and it is lower with elective, rather than emergency caesarean section (Marcollet *et al.* 2002).

INFANT FEEDING

In populations where alternatives to breastfeeding are not safe, not affordable or not feasible, postnatal transmission through breastfeeding is a substantial route of acquisition of infection for infants of HIV-infected mothers. This remains true even when peripartum transmission can be reduced with antiretroviral prophylaxis.

Transmission of HIV through breast milk can occur in situations where the mother acquired the infection shortly after delivery, but also in established maternal infection. In an analysis of observational studies from South Africa, Brazil and Europe, the rate of transmission was twice as high in breastfed, than in formula-fed infants (Dunn *et al.* 1992). This was confirmed in a randomized clinical trial in Nairobi, which enrolled more than 400 women (Nduati *et al.* 2000). The transmission rate was nearly twice as high in the breastfed, compared to the formula-fed group (36% versus 20%, respectively). Postnatal acquisition of infection in infants born to HIV-infected mothers, who were shown to be HIV negative at 2–3 months of age, can account for a considerable proportion of paediatric infection. It is estimated that the rates of late postnatal transmission through breastfeeding after 3 months of age is more than 3% per year (Leroy *et al.* 1998).

Transmission through breastfeeding may be related to the amount of exposure, the time of exposure, the infectivity of milk or specific susceptibility of the infant. Postnatal transmission has also been linked with maternal viral load in the breast milk, mastitis and severe deficiency in vitamin A (Semba *et al.* 1999).

Variations in breastfeeding practices may also play a role in the transmission risk. Workers from Durban suggested that the risk of vertical transmission may be particularly high for young infants who receive other foods as well as breast milk, i.e. mixed feeding (Coutsoudis *et al.* 1999a). In this *post hoc* subgroup analysis, no increase in risk of HIV transmission was observed in the first 3 months of age amongst infants who were exclusively breastfed compared to infants who were exclusively formula-fed, with the highest rates observed among mixed feeders. (Mixed feeding was defined as breastfeeding with also water, juices or other types of milk.) If there is a protective effect of exclusive breastfeeding, it is possible to think of explanations. For example, there may be reduced exposure to dietary antigens and enteric pathogens, thus lessening the risk of an inflammatory process facilitating HIV transmission across the gut mucosa. Or there could be changes in specific components of breast milk, maternal hormonal or immunological factors or alterations in the integrity of epithelial tight junctions in the mammary gland. However, it is unknown whether the putative effect of exclusive breastfeeding reported in this study continued after 3 months. There is a need for other studies to confirm this finding and to extend research into this area. When infants born to HIV-infected mothers can be ensured uninterrupted access to nutritionally adequate breast-milk substitutes that are safely prepared and fed to them, they are at less risk of illness and death if they are not breastfed. However, when these conditions are not met, in particular when infectious diseases and malnutrition are common causes of infant mortality, artificial feeding substantially increases children's risk of illness and death. Of concern was the high mortality rate at 2 years of age in the above-mentioned Nairobi trial, in both the breastfed (24%) and the formula-fed (20%) group. In view of the higher number of infected children in the breastfed than in the formula-fed group, the finding that one in five children in the latter group died before reaching 2 years of age is especially disturbing. These high mortality rates need to be taken into account when considering policies relating to infant feeding in sub-Saharan Africa.

Early cessation of breastfeeding rather than prolonged breastfeeding has been suggested to reduce the risk of acquisition of infection (Kuhn & Stein 1997; Leroy et al. 1998) and the study described above suggested that with truly exclusive breastfeeding for a limited period, the risk of transmission may be similar to that in a formula-fed group (Coutsoudis et al. 1999a). However, few data are available to confirm whether it is possible to breastfeed in such a way as to minimize the risk while maximizing the benefits. More work needs to be done to confirm the finding of an increased risk of mixed feeding, and to investigate the acceptability and feasibility for mothers to change their breastfeeding habits to fully exclusive breastfeeding, which is currently rare. By providing support and counselling the prevalence of breast problems can also be reduced.

Detailed UK guidelines on HIV and infant feeding are available. These were produced in September 2001 for the Department of Health (www.doh.gov.uk/eaga).

VITAMIN THERAPY

In 1994, Semba et al. reported a strong relationship between maternal serum vitamin A levels in the HIV-infected mother, and the risk of mother-to-child transmission of HIV. These authors suggested that maternal vitamin A deficiency contributed to the risk of transmission (Semba et al. 1994). In a smaller study in the USA, no relationship was found between maternal serum vitamin A level and transmission (Burger et al. 1997). This was supported in a larger study of 449 pregnancies, where those HIV-infected women with low serum vitamin A levels were not more likely to transmit HIV. But they were at significantly higher risk of delivering preterm (Burns et al. 1999).

A large ambitious study in Tanzania had 1075 HIV-infected pregnant women as participants, and used a 2×2 factorial design to examine the effect of supplementation with multivitamins, or vitamin A, or both, on pregnancy outcome (Fawzi et al. 1998). Multivitamin supplementation, but not vitamin A, decreased the risk of fetal death, severe preterm birth, and small for gestational age at birth. The decreases were substantial, approximately 40% for each. A further randomized trial in South Africa assessed the effect of vitamin A supplementation alone (Coutsoudis et al. 1999b). Vitamin A supplementation was not found to be effective in reducing overall mother-to-child transmission, but it was associated with a lower rate of preterm delivery. Among these preterm deliveries, those assigned to the vitamin A group were less likely to be infected. In an earlier randomized trial, vitamin A supplementation for children of HIV-infected women appeared to be beneficial in reducing morbidity, particularly diarrhoea (Coutsoudis et al. 1995).

Despite a number of studies, the situation is not clear. This may be because the prevalence of vitamin A deficiency differs widely in the different populations. Vitamin A is teratogenic, and supplements in pregnancy have been associated with birth defects. Therefore it seems that at present, the evidence does not support vitamin A supplementation with the aim of preventing vertical transmission. There is no evidence supporting use of vitamins in this population in the industrialized world. Multivitamins may have an important role in reducing pregnancy complications in some parts of the developing world.

OTHER INTERVENTIONS

There are several other interventions that are intuitively plausible, but that have little support as yet from observational or randomized studies.

A vaginal wash with an antiseptic, antiviral agent during labour has many theoretical advantages. Chlorhexidine is already used in many centres for vaginal examination, and is believed to be safe. This could be built in to general obstetric practice in areas of Africa without the need for individual HIV testing, and without any special change in structure of care. It is very cheap, and would be affordable in all countries. In a study in Malawi, vaginal lavage was shown to result in significantly reduced maternal and neonatal morbidity and mortality (Taha et al. 1997). Unfortunately, in this trial, there was no overall difference in transmission of HIV (Biggar et al. 1996), although there was a significant reduction in the group with membranes ruptured for longer than 4 h before delivery. Similarly, a clinical trial in Mombasa, Kenya, showed no decrease in transmission with a chlorhexidine wash (Gaillard et al. 2001).

Benzalkonium chloride has been shown to inactivate HIV *in vitro*. However, in the French Perinatal HIV

Study, although washing with benzalkonium chloride was widely performed, it was not associated with a decreased risk of transmission (Mandelbrot *et al.* 1998). Other trials are currently exploring this intervention further. Another approach is the use of vaginal suppositories in the last weeks of pregnancy, in order to reduce viral load in the genital tract before the onset of labour. A study in West Africa (Msellati *et al.* 1999) showed a good acceptability and tolerance of this regimen, but no efficacy studies have yet been planned.

Management issues in pregnancy

Testing for human immunodeficiency virus as part of antenatal care

As treatment improves, the benefits of knowing HIV status become more emphatic. From the woman's point of view, knowledge of HIV infection will allow the following:

1 Evaluation of her clinical status to see whether she requires antiretroviral therapy or prophylaxis against opportunistic infections. Early therapy will decrease disease progression and improve life expectancy.

2 Protection of uninfected sexual partner(s).

3 An informed decision about pregnancy.

4 An informed decision about use of ZDV, other antivirals and caesarean section, to minimize the risk of perinatal transmission.

5 A decision not to breastfeed.

6 Early testing of the baby, and if the baby is infected despite the above measures, appropriate *Pneumocystis carinii pneumonia* (PCP) and antiviral prophylaxis.

Although in some ways pregnancy is not the ideal time to offer testing, many of the benefits relate to pregnancy, and at present this is the only practical opportunity for population testing.

HIV undoubtedly fulfils the criteria for an appropriate screening test. Such testing has been shown to be cost effective in a range of scenarios (Newell *et al.* 1998; Ratcliffe *et al.* 1998; Wilkinson *et al.* 1998; Ades *et al.* 1999b; Postma *et al.* 1999; Söderlund *et al.* 1999). Whether, and how, testing should be introduced in a particular population is now largely dependent on issues of cost and HIV prevalence. The first assessment is to confirm that the health structure for adequate care and treatment is in place before testing is started. Inadequate resources may mean this is not currently the case for many countries in sub-Saharan Africa. The broader issues of maternal mortality have been thoughtfully discussed by Graham and Newell (1999). The next issue is that the prevalence of unknown HIV infection in pregnant women has to be sufficient to justify the cost of screening, in comparison to competing health needs. It is clear that overall prevalence is not an adequate basis for screening strategy (Ades *et al.* 1999b). Local cost can be reduced by centralizing viral testing, and by using one package for all antenatal tests in one blood sample.

The optimal method of testing may also vary with local circumstances. In some situations (very low prevalence outside a clearly defined risk group) selective testing may be appropriate (Ades *et al.* 1999a). However, there are several general advantages to a universal screening programme. In most areas with significant prevalence, infection is no longer confined to clearly identified groups with 'risk factors'. In Europe and the USA the most rapidly increasing group of infections is via heterosexual contact, and many women are unaware that their partners are at risk of HIV infection. In addition it may be less stigmatizing to offer testing to everyone and conversely easier for the health-care provider, who no longer has to do detailed 'risk' assessments. Even so, in some circumstances take-up may be highly influenced by the health-care worker offering the test (Boyd *et al.* 1999).

In France, it has been an obligation since January 1993 to offer voluntary HIV testing to all pregnant women at the first prenatal visit. In the USA the Public Health Service currently recommends a universal approach to counselling and testing with consent for all pregnant women. This has recently been advised in the UK, with its much lower prevalence. In countries where a universal offer of testing has been established for many years, such as France and Sweden, the rate of refusal is well below 1%. There has been gradual acceptance that testing can most appropriately be 'normalized' as one of the routine antenatal tests, but with adequate written and verbal information, and the opportunity for each woman to refuse taking the test. This approach is not associated with increased anxiety or decreased information transfer (Simpson *et al.* 1998, 1999). The uptake of HIV testing in the UK is now much improved, without any obvious adverse effects on the other aspects of the maternity service.

Preconception counselling

The proportion of women who are aware of their serostatus before becoming pregnant differs between settings, but is currently on the order of 60% in most industrialized countries. Many of these women were tested for HIV in a previous pregnancy. Most HIV-infected women are under care, unless there is a breakdown in the relationship between the woman and the health-care system. Planning for pregnancy is of particular importance, to help women to avoid unwanted pregnancies and prepare themselves to confront the risks and the decisions ahead. Information should also be provided on the issues of safe conception, such as partner notification and testing and 'self-insemination' if he is HIV-negative. Treatment issues, relating to efficacy and safety should be carefully discussed. The majority of women who know that they are HIV infected receive antiretroviral therapy before the pregnancy. In some cases, for instance when aggressive antiretroviral regimens are ineffective, or there is profound immune deficiency or other active diseases, the women may be advised to defer the pregnancy. More frequently, drug therapy may be changed before conception, either to improve adherence to therapy and/or virological efficacy, reduce side-effects or in order to avoid drugs which are potentially teratogenic. The option of programmed treatment interruption during the first trimester should be discussed on a case-by-case basis. There is no consensus on this point, because there are no data showing that avoiding first-trimester exposure to any antiretroviral can reduce the risk of adverse effects. On the other hand, there are now data showing that the risks for the mother of interrupting treatment are highly dependent on the treatment history, the initial CD4 lymphocyte count and the viral load prior to therapy. Finally, the need for and choice of therapies other than antiretrovirals should be re-evaluated, as well as the need for vitamin or folic acid supplementation.

Clinical care during pregnancy

BOOKING VISIT

This may be the first contact of the infected woman with the obstetric service. The situation differs according to whether she has just discovered her HIV status or has already been under care for some time. It is important to demonstrate the obstetric team approach of empathy, support, calm, reassurance and a shared partnership of care. This is, of course, true for all pregnant women, but is especially important for a woman with HIV infection. She may have particular concerns about confidentiality, and, for various reasons, may be suspicious and apprehensive about possible discrimination and lack of knowledge or understanding. This first visit can set the scene for later care.

Because this visit may have been undertaken with some trepidation, it is often best not to make this an overwhelming experience by subjecting her to information overload. Obviously, women attend equipped with very differing degrees of knowledge, but unfortunately this may include misinformation, and this can take some

time to talk through. In some cases, if possible, it is best to discuss management over two sessions, to encourage the partner or a supportive friend to attend, to encourage her to bring notes of questions, and to give her written information and appropriate helpline telephone numbers.

At this first visit, it is important to ensure that the woman is aware of the risk of vertical transmission, and to ensure that she is definite that she wants to continue the pregnancy. If she is considering termination of pregnancy, which should be an available option, then discussion will focus on her assessment around this.

Assessment of HIV disease includes clinical staging from available history. In general, if she is asymptomatic, detailed physical examination is not necessary. But simple clinical examination of the heart, chest and mouth may disclose soft clinical indicators of disease such as oral Candida, hairy cell leukoplakia or seborrhoeic dermatitis.

Blood tests should include lymphocyte subsets, quantitative RNA PCR measurement of viral load, liver function tests, syphilis serology, Toxoplasma serology and hepatitis B and C antibody status.

Discussion at this first visit should include discussion as to who 'needs to know', i.e. disclosure to her partner, and which health-care workers should be kept informed, how information should be recorded in her hospital notes and her liaison card, and how communication should be maintained. Having made these decisions together, it can still be difficult to ensure, in the obstetric system of routines, that her wishes are actually fulfilled. This is the sort of issue that can result in loss of confidence, and strictness in this area is of great importance.

This is an opportunity to define the team responsible for the care of her pregnancy. This should be as small a number as possible, but should ensure that she has access to all necessary expertise. The team will usually include her family doctor, midwife, obstetrician, the community- or hospital-based paediatrician who will follow up the baby, and the physician caring for her HIV disease. Communication between these professionals is essential for an effective interdisciplinary approach.

Current drugs should be considered, and where indicated and wished, arrangements made for ultrasound to examine for structural abnormality at 18–20 weeks.

Other screening tests are important. Cervical cytology is required if she has not had screened for cervical intraepithelial neoplasia (CIN) in the last 6 months. Cervical and vaginal swabs to screen for STDs, group B Streptococcus and bacterial vaginosis are also necessary. This is because women with immunological compromise may be more at risk of preterm delivery and, in addition, babies delivered preterm are more likely to acquire HIV. There have also been recent reports of a stimulatory effect of bacterial vaginosis on HIV replication (Al-Harthi *et al.* 1999; Olinger *et al.* 1999). Also the chance of preterm delivery might be reduced by treating bacterial vaginosis.

Another problem which needs to be addressed in the first trimester is the issue of invasive prenatal diagnosis. In addition to the known risks of amniocentesis, the procedure carries a potential risk of viral transmission. Because clinicians have been cautious in performing such procedures in HIV-infected women, there are few data to estimate the risk or the risk factors. There is some evidence that this may be a real risk. A trend towards increased transmission was reported in a small number of patients in the era before ZDV prevention (Mandelbrot *et al.* 1996b), but no data on invasive procedures and HIV transmission have been published regarding women treated with antiretrovirals. This uncertain risk needs to be balanced against the need for prenatal diagnosis or treatment. In practice, the most common situation is routine voluntary screening for Down's syndrome. A practical approach is to inform women of the potential risk and to offer on a voluntary basis the most effective (or least ineffective) combined risk analysis upon which to make a decision. This may at present include maternal age, nuchal translucency at 11–13 weeks and biochemical markers. When the fetus is found to be at high risk for Down's syndrome and the decision is made to perform an amniocentesis, the procedure should be done under antiretroviral treatment, adapted according to maternal immune status and viral load, i.e. ZDV or combination therapy, to reduce viral load to below the detection limit. Technical precautions to avoid maternal–fetal microtransfusions include use of a thin needle and avoiding the placenta. More invasive procedures, such as chorionic villus or fetal blood sampling, should be avoided (BHIVA 2001).

LATER PREGNANCY

Pregnancy is a relatively short time in relation to the natural history of HIV disease. In practice, it is very unlikely that a woman will have any opportunistic infection if her booking CD4 count is $> 300 \times 10^6$/L, or if it remains $> 200 \times 10^6$/L throughout pregnancy. Therefore, repeat CD4 count should be performed each trimester, and more often if the maternal viral load is high. HIV RNA measurements should also be performed each trimester, with additional testing when therapy is started for maternal indications.

The difficult subject of appropriate antiretroviral therapy has been discussed above, and is authoritatively discussed in the BHIVA (2001) guidelines. Although opinions vary considerably about management of the asymptomatic woman, there is consensus that the woman with advanced disease should be treated with effective therapy, i.e. combination antiretroviral drugs.

Current guidelines distinguish three situations, according to maternal disease markers. In the first situation, there is no need for therapy for the woman's health. In the second situation, the woman is already under therapy before starting her pregnancy. In the third situation, therapy has not yet been started, but is required from the woman's standpoint.

PROPHYLAXIS IN WOMEN NOT REQUIRING THERAPY

If the woman is not already taking treatment, the best time to start ZDV is uncertain. Recruitment for ACTG 076 was between 14 and 34 weeks and the median start date was 26 weeks. The shorter the fetal exposure, the less risk of any possible long-term complications, and the less chance of selecting out ZDV-resistant species. On the other hand, preterm labour may occur and is associated with an increased rate of infection. As most infection is believed to occur in late pregnancy and around delivery, the consensus in Europe is to start ZDV in the early third trimester. In women at high risk of preterm delivery, we advise starting ZDV earlier. Care needs to be taken with the dose of ZDV in women taking opiates (where higher blood concentrations of ZDV are attained) and in women with liver disease. Treatment should be started at 100 mg twice daily in these women and built up gradually as the drug is tolerated. Early symptoms may dissuade women from continuing. In women weighing more than 85 kg, ZDV prophylaxis has been found to be less effective (Shapiro *et al.* 1999), therefore ZDV should be given at higher doses, which may be adapted by measuring residual levels of the drug and its glucuronide metabolite in plasma.

Monitoring after starting ZDV is important and one possible regimen is suggested in Table 18.1.

The main argument against combination treatment is the uncertain risk of a serious developmental problem in the non-infected children. Not only would this be a disaster for those children harmed, but it could result in reduced public acceptance of all regimens, including ZDV monotherapy.

The issues to be considered are resistance and safety. Emergence of genotypic resistance (see above) is least likely if viral replication is suppressed, most likely if 3TC or nevirapine are used in a suboptimal regimen, and is infrequent with ZDV monotherapy, when it is used as prophylaxis for a short period in women with relatively low viral loads. The safety profile of ZDV is well known, whereas use of combination therapy presumably

Monitoring in women on ZDV alone

Full blood count every 2 weeks twice, then every month

Liver function tests each month

Creatinine each month

Repeat viral load and CD4 count in the third trimester

Consider discontinuing therapy if:

    Haemoglobin is <8 g/100 mL

    Granulocytes $<750 \times 10^9$/L

    Liver enzymes are >5 times normal

    There are serious cardiac, respiratory, neurological or gastrointestinal problems

Additional monitoring in women receiving a protease inhibitor

Either fasting and postprandial glucose OR glucose tolerance testing each trimester

Additional monitoring in women receiving two or more nucleoside reverse transcriptase inhibitors

Pancreatic lipase each trimester

If a new biochemical abnormality (elevated liver or pancreatic enzymes) or second or third trimester

    symptoms of vomiting, abdominal pain and/or shortness of breath

Test for lactic acidosis, including anion gap, blood gases and fasting lactate

    measurements

exposes both the mother and the fetus to a higher risk of known or unknown adverse effect, in the short or long term.

This is a very uncertain area, and management for each woman will have to be carefully assessed. Until more data on safety are available it seems sensible to try to limit exposure of the fetus to antiviral drugs. Current US opinion puts greater emphasis on the benefits of using HAART in pregnancy and avoidance of caesarean section (Star *et al.* 1999; Stringer *et al.* 1999), whereas a European consensus is to advise caesarean section liberally and to use combination therapy only in pregnancies where there is a need for the mother to be treated.

WOMEN ALREADY TREATED BEFORE THE PREGNANCY

The general consensus is to continue therapy throughout pregnancy. Treatment should not be reduced from HAART to suboptimal double therapy for instance, because this is likely to lead to drug resistance. There are only a few indications for changing drugs, such as switching from the potentially teratogenic efavirenz to another drug, replacing stavudine by ZDV (unless there is likely to be ZDV-resistant virus), or changing because of intolerance. As mentioned above, there is controversy over the option of suspending all therapy for the first trimester (or more) of pregnancy, because of concern over the potential toxicities for the fetus. When therapy is suspended, the HIV RNA level returns to baseline. Thus, the risks of such an approach depend on the original baseline values of viral load and CD4 counts. As the indications for initiat-

ing therapy vary widely, this should be discussed with the HIV specialist and the woman on a case-by-case basis.

WOMEN NOT TREATED BUT REQUIRING THERAPY

The general rule is that therapy should not be withheld because of concern about fetal toxicity in women who clearly require to be treated. As there is no information available about the best combination in pregnancy, the choice can only be made according to the same criteria as in non-pregnant individuals. First-line therapy should be a combination that is likely to optimize adherence and that is virologically effective (usually triple). In antiretroviral-naïve women, it should include ZDV. Starting antiretroviral therapy is almost never an emergency. The objectives, side-effects and risks for the woman and child, as well as how the drugs need to be taken, must be carefully discussed with the woman. If the woman actively participates in the decision to start therapy, it is our experience that adherence to antiretroviral therapy tends to be better in pregnancy than in other periods of life. Usually, the treatment can be started in the second or third trimester. Starting earlier may unnecessarily expose the embryo and fetus, whereas starting late may increase the risk of *in utero* transmission for which women with low CD4 counts are at greater risk.

FOLLOW-UP OF COMBINATION THERAPIES IN PREGNANCY

Because the risks of adverse effects are higher than in patients receiving ZDV monotherapy, clinical and biological follow-up must be increased. In addition to the clinical, haematological and liver function follow-up described above, pancreatic lipase measurements are required. When nevirapine is used, it is started at half-dose and particular attention must be given to acute liver failure, as well as itching or eruptions because of the risk of severe and life-threatening skin reactions, including Stevens–Johnson syndrome and toxic epidermal necrolysis. When protease inhibitors are used, testing for glucose intolerance or diabetes is required. In women taking combination therapy who present with nausea, vomiting, abdominal pain or confusion, a complete biochemical work-up is necessary in addition to testing for the usual obstetric complications. Because of the risk of lactic acidosis, this work-up should include blood gas and lactic acid, as well as blood cell counts, lipase and transaminase measurements. Clinicians should be aware that a mild elevation of serum transaminase levels may precede the onset of lactic acidosis by several days or weeks. Particular attention is required in case of treatment including stavudine and didanosine.

Symptoms must also be taken seriously as they may reveal AIDS-defining illnesses. This is particularly so in women with CD4 count $< 200 \times 10^6$/L; it may thus be helpful to give a list of symptoms that could mean opportunistic infection. Weight should also be measured, and failure to gain weight, or weight loss, may be ominous.

If CD4 count is confirmed $< 200 \times 10^6$/L, then PCP prophylaxis is usually advised, in addition to combination antiviral therapy. Even though there is a small fall in CD4$^+$ count just because of pregnancy, it is reasonable to take the same threshold value for prophylaxis in pregnancy. Cotrimoxazole is best and, in spite of the theoretical risk of folate inhibition with trimethoprim, appears to be safe in later pregnancy. There has been a report suggesting a high rate of fetal anomalies with use in the first trimester together with HAART. Given just before delivery, there are possible risks of neonatal haemolysis, methaemoglobinaemia and perhaps bilirubinaemia. Standard dosage is 960 mg once daily but lower doses are effective and better near term (e.g. 480 mg once daily). Aerosolized pentamidine (300 mg given monthly) is probably safe because little is absorbed systemically but is not so effective and may be difficult to use in late pregnancy. Dapsone (50–100 mg) has not been used much in pregnancy for HIV disease but there is extensive experience in pregnancy with leprosy. With the availability of HAART, advanced disease is uncommon.

Thrombocytopenia (platelet count $< 100\,000 \times 10^9$/L) occurred in 3.2% of pregnancies in a large study in France (Mandelbrot *et al.* 1994). This usually responded to routine treatments with ZDV or gammaglobulin and only one neonate had a platelet count $< 100\,000 \times 10^9$/L.

In addition to the issue of invasive procedures discussed above, other procedures that have been suggested to increase exposure should be avoided; these include external cephalic version, membrane sweeping and amnioscopy. Cervicovaginal infections and STDs should be diagnosed and treated, and emphasis placed on the prevention of preterm labour and premature rupture of membranes.

DELIVERY

Intravenous ZDV should be used regardless of whether the mother received ZDV or any combination therapy during the pregnancy. It should be given even if ZDV-resistant virus is present. The only situation in which ZDV should not be used is a history of serious intolerance to the drug.

Women receiving combination therapies should continue taking their usual scheduled doses, even on the day of delivery. The only exceptions are stavudine, which should not be given during the ZDV infusion because of drug interaction, and SMX–TMP because of the risk of jaundice in the neonate.

The choice of when to opt for elective caesarean section is controversial. There are as yet no data to estimate the potential additional benefit of elective caesarean delivery in women receiving HAART with good virological efficacy. In many European centres, elective caesarean delivery is recommended for all HIV-1-infected women, whereas in the USA it is recommended when the maternal viral load is above 1000 copies/ml, and in France whenever viral load is above the detection limit. In addition, most obstetricians would recommend a caesarean section in any HIV-1-infected woman when the likelihood of dystocic labour is high.

When caesarean section is planned, it should be scheduled at 38 weeks in order to reduce the likelihood of spontaneous labour or membrane rupture occurring. There is some evidence that women with HIV tend to deliver earlier, particularly if using HAART, and if there are signs that labour may be imminent, the date for caesarean section should be brought forward. Caesarean section should expose the baby to as little maternal blood as possible. This can be helped by securing obvious bleeding points and by allowing the membranes to present intact along the uterine incision before rapid delivery. The stapling device (Autosuture) can make relatively bloodless caesarean section more feasible. In a term baby, the cord should be clamped quickly to avoid possible maternal–fetal transfusion during detachment of the placenta. If vaginal delivery is undertaken, this should be as conservative as possible, leaving membranes intact, avoiding scalp sampling or scalp electrodes. Forceps delivery may be preferable to vacuum extraction. The baby should be washed carefully at delivery with warm water or saline so that any maternal blood is removed. Some units prefer using antiseptic solutions, such as dilute chlorhexidine or benzalkonium chloride. Particular care should be taken to remove maternal blood with an alcohol swab before giving intramuscular vitamin K. None of these suggestions about delivery is based on secure evidence (BHIVA 2001).

One common clinical problem is the occurrence of labour or membrane rupture prior to the date planned for elective caesarean section. There is concern that it may be too late to perform the intervention, as studies have shown no benefit with non-elective caesarean delivery. When the woman presents in active labour, we suggest that vaginal delivery be considered if it is expected that she will deliver quickly. If she presents at the earliest stages of labour or immediately after membrane rupture, or if labour is likely to be prolonged, prompt caesarean section may still be protective.

In the event of preterm premature rupture of the membranes, antibiotics should be given prophylactically in all cases. The difficult choices between expectant management, labour induction or caesarean section depend on the mother's viral load, the obstetric condition, and most of all the gestational age. At early gestational ages, when management is expectant, glucocorticoids can be administered, and the mother's antiretroviral regimen should be re-evaluated in view of the increased risk of transmission.

Another important clinical problem concerns women who have had no antiretroviral therapy during the pregnancy. The principal reason is late diagnosis of HIV infection, which usually results from underlying problems in prenatal care, due to the system or to the woman's personal or social situation. In some settings, rapid HIV testing during labour is considered for high-risk women who had no access to testing during their pregnancy. Several effective methods are available, including intravenous ZDV followed by 6 weeks of oral ZDV in the infant, and single-dose nevirapine in the mother and the baby. There is consensus to offer both ZDV and nevirapine in such emergency situations. When the woman is not in active labour, caesarean section should also be offered.

POSTPARTUM CARE

Because of the potential risk of infectious morbidity in the postpartum period, prophylactic antibiotics should be used whenever there are obstetric risk factors or low CD4 counts. Particular care needs to be taken in case of caesarean delivery. In addition to antibiotic (as well as anticoagulant) prophylaxis, drainage should be used sparingly and connected to a closed suction system, and the bladder catheter should be removed as soon as possible.

Antiretroviral therapy must be re-evaluated from the point of view of long-term management. For women who did not require therapy for their own health and therefore received ZDV prophylaxis during the pregnancy, ZDV can be stopped, and careful follow-up must be organized. Women receiving HAART should continue their therapy under the surveillance of their HIV specialist or a trained general practitioner.

Following birth, the mother is faced with many issues concerning her child's future. In particular, there is the stress surrounding HIV testing of the baby and waiting for the results. The mother often needs to be reminded how and why ZDV prophylaxis and formula feeding are useful for her infant, and how and why follow-up is to be performed. She needs support and reassurance. Some women may experience a variety of personal and social problems, such as housing, drug dependence or lack of communication with the child's father, which may or may not have been anticipated by the team. Although many of these problems cannot be solved by care providers, they must be addressed in a helpful way before the child's physical and mental health becomes jeopardized.

Follow-up of children born to human immunodeficiency virus-infected mothers

In recent years, it has been possible to diagnose 90% of infected children by 1–2 months of age. Although the gold standard remains serostatus beyond the age of 18 months, diagnosis can be performed reliably on the basis of two consistent positive or negative virus tests, one of which is performed at 3 months or more. DNA PCR is the most widely used, and has largely replaced virus culture. HIV RNA tests, such as reverse transcription (RT) PCR or branched DNA (bDNA) are increasingly used, as they are more widely available outside research laboratories.

About 15% of infected and untreated children have a severe form of disease and become ill or die in the first year of life (European Collaborative Study 2001b). The remainder have a more prolonged duration of relatively asymptomatic disease, more akin to the adult model. Around 5% become ill or die each year, so that by 6 years around a quarter of babies have died but two-thirds of the children still alive only have minor symptoms (Blanche *et al.* 1997).

Because of concern over the possible side-effects of drugs used during the pregnancy and in the neonate, the child should be seen at regular visits through at least

18 months, even if found to be HIV negative by virological tests. Surveillance should include clinical, haematological and biochemical tests including liver and pancreatic enzymes. Serum lactate determinations are currently recommended in France, but are not routinely performed in most countries. Exposure to antiretroviral drugs should be reported to the appropriate registries, parents should be offered enrolment of their child in a prospective cohort, and any abnormal signs and symptoms should be reported to the national drug agency. All of these reports must be strictly anonymous. For clinicians, being involved in an interdisciplinary network with specialists can be particularly helpful.

Because PCP is most frequent in the first 6 months of life, and because a first episode can be fatal, PCP prophylaxis used to be recommended for all children of HIV-infected mothers, to start when prophylactic ZDV is stopped, and to stop as soon as it is known that the child is not infected. Nowadays, when the mother has taken up all the interventions, the risk of neonatal HIV infection is so low that in most European countries routine PCP prophylaxis would no longer be prescribed. However if the child is infected, PCP prophylaxis is recommended until 1 year of age, thereafter being led by the CD4 count. The likelihood of rapid progression is higher in children with high viral load set-points. Because perinatal HIV infection is a primary infection, as reflected by very high viral loads occurring in the perinatal period, many paediatricians recommend antiviral therapy in all infected children under the age of 12 months. Combination therapy markedly reduces mortality for infected children and adolescents, just as it has for adults (Gortmaker et al. 2001).

Infection risk to health-care workers

All staff should be aware of current guidelines for health workers suffering needle-stick exposure to HIV-infected blood (Centers for Disease Control and Prevention 1996; UK Health Department 1997). It is most important to avoid this through training in universal precautions (Shanson et al. 1992) but, if it does occur, then postexposure prophylaxis may be advisable. However, it is believed this has to be started within 1–2 h, and all workers should have considered the evidence and made up their minds as to what they would do before any accident. It is also important that these drugs are easily accessible.

Conclusion

The issues surrounding HIV infection and pregnancy have undergone profound changes over the last few years. Anti-retroviral therapies have improved the survival of HIV-infected persons, and decreased the rate of mother-to-child transmission. However, these drugs can have toxicities such as mitochondrial diseases in the mother and infant. The incidence and long-term consequences for children are still unknown. The choice of therapy should be based on an estimate of benefit/risk on a case-by-case basis. If the patient requires an effective antiretroviral combination, it should not be withheld because of the pregnancy. Interdisciplinary care must include clear information in a climate of dialogue with the mother.

The greatest challenge today is access to prevention and therapy in the developing world. Although simple and relatively low-cost methods have proved to be effective and acceptable in research settings, they are still not available in the most affected regions of the world. There is an urgent need for action by health professionals, governments, agencies and non-governmental organizations both internationally and at a local level.

References

Ades, A.E., Gupta, R. et al. (1999a) Selective versus universal antenatal HIV testing: epidemiological and implementational factors in policy choice. AIDS **13**, 271–278.

Ades, A.E., Sculpher, M.J., Gibb, D.M., Cupta, R. & Ratcliffe, J. (1999b) Cost effectiveness analysis of antenatal HIV screening in the United Kingdom. British Medical Journal **319**, 1230–1234.

Ait-Khaled, M., Lyall, H.E.G. et al. (1998) Intrapartum mucosal exposure to human immunodeficiency virus type 1 (HIV-1) of infants born to HIV-1-infected mothers correlates with maternal plasma virus burden. Journal of Infection and Disease **177**, 1097–1100.

Al-Harthi, L., Roebuck, K.A., Olinger, G.C., Landay, A., Sha, B.E., Hashemi, F.B. & Spear, G.T. (1999) Bacterial vaginosis-associated microflora isolated from the female genital tract activates HIV-1 expression. Journal of Acquired Immune Deficiency Syndromes **21**, 194–202.

Baba, T.W., Jeong, Y.S., Penninck, D., Bronson, R., Greene, M.F. & Ruprecht, R.M. (1995) Pathogenicity of live attenuated SIV after mucosal infection of neonatal macaques. Science **267**, 1820–1825.

BHIVA guidelines (2001) www.aidsmap.com

Biggar, R.J., Miotti, P.G. et al. (1996) Perinatal intervention trial in Africa: effect of a birth canal cleansing intervention to prevent HIV transmission. Lancet **347**, 1647–1650.

Blanche, S., Newell, M.-L. et al. (1997) Morbidity and mortality in European children vertically infected by HIV-1: The French Pediatric HIV Infection Study Group and European Collaborative Study. Acquired Immune Deficiency Syndrome and Human Retrovirology **14**, 442–450.

Blanche, S., Tardieu, M. et al. (1999) Persistent mitochondrial dysfunction and perinatal exposure to antiretroviral nucleoside analogues. Lancet **354**, 1084–1089.

Boyd, F.M., Simpson, W.M., Johnstone, F.D., Goldberg, D.J. & Hart, G.J. (1999) Uptake and acceptability of antenatal HIV testing: midwives make a difference. British Journal of Midwifery **7**, 151–156.

Brettle, R.P., Raab, G.M. *et al.* (1995) HIV infection in women: immunological markers and the influence of pregnancy. *AIDS* 9, 1177–1184.

Brinkman, K., Hofstede, H.J.M., Burger, D.M., Smeitink, J.A.M. & Koopmans, D.M. (1998) Adverse effects of reverse transcriptase inhibitors: mitochondrial toxicity as common pathway. *AIDS* 12, 1735–1744.

Brinkman, K., Sneitink, J.A., Romijn, J.A. & Reiss, P. (1999) Mitochondrial toxicity induced by nucleoside—analogue reverse-transcriptase inhibitors is a key factor in the pathogenesis of antiretrivirol-therapy-related lipodystrophy. *Lancet* 354, 1112–1115.

Brocklehurst, P. & French, R. (1998) The association between maternal HIV infection and perinatal outcome. A systematic review of the literature and meta-analysis. *British Journal of Obstetrics and Gynaecology* 105, 836–848.

Bucceri, A., Luchini, L. *et al.* (1997) Pregnancy outcome among HIV positive and negative intravenous drug users. *European Journal of Obstetrics, Gynecology and Reproductive Biology* 72, 169–174.

Bulterys, M., Chao, A., Dushimimana, A. & Saah, A. (1996) Fatal complications after caesarean section in HIV-infected women. *AIDS* 10, 923–924.

Bulterys, M., Orloff, S. *et al.* (1999) Impact of zidovudine post-perinatal exposure prophylaxis on vertical HIV-1 transmission: a prospective cohort study in 4 US cities. *The 2nd Conference on Global Strategies for the Prevention of HIV Transmission from Mothers to Infants.* Montreal, Canada, Abstract 015.

Burger, H., Kovacs, A. & Weiser, B. (1997) Maternal serum vitamin A levels are not associated with mother-to-child transmissions of HIV-1 in the United States. *Journal of Acquired Immune Deficiency Syndrome and Human Retrovirology* 14, 321–326.

Burns, D.N., Fitzgerald, G. *et al.* (1999) Vitamin A deficiency and other nutritional indices during pregnancy in human immunodeficiency virus infection: prevalence, clinical correlates and outcome. Women and Infants Transmission Study Group. *Clinical Infection and Disease* 29, 328–334.

Cardo, D.M., Culver, D.H. *et al.* (1997) A case-control study of HIV seroconversion in health care workers after percutaneous exposure. *New England Journal of Medicine* 337, 1485–1490.

Carr, A., Samaras, K. *et al.* (1998) A syndrome of peripheral lipodystrophy, hyperlipidaemia and insulin resistance in patients receiving HIV protease inhibitors. *AIDS* 12, F51–F58.

Cazein, F., Hamers, F. & Brunet, J.B. (1998) HIV prevalence in pregnant women in Europe: differences in assessment methods and prevalence levels across countries. *Journal of Acquired Immune Deficiency Syndrome and Human Retrovirology* 19, 296–305.

Centers for Disease Control and Prevention (1996) Update: Provisional Public Health Service recommendations for chemoprophylaxis after occupational exposure to HIV. *Morbidity and Mortality Weekly Report* 45, 468–472.

Centers for Disease Control and Prevention (1998) Public Health Service Task Force recommendations for the use of antiretroviral drugs in pregnant women for maternal health and for reducing perinatal HIV-1 transmission in the United States. *Morbidity and Mortality Weekly Report* 47, 1–30.

Chaisson, R.E., Keruly, J.G. & Moore, R.D. (1995) Race, sex, drug use and progression of human immunodeficiency virus disease. *New England Journal of Medicine* 333, 751–756.

Chesney, M.A., Ickovics, J., Hecht, F.M., Sikipa, G. & Rabkin, J. (1999) Adherence: a necessity for successful HIV combination therapy. *AIDS* 13 (Suppl. A), S271–S278.

Chuachoowong, R., Shaffer, N. *et al.* (2000) Short-course antenatal zidovudine reduces both cervicovaginal human immunodeficiency virus type 1 RNA Levels and risk of perinatal transmission. *Journal of Infectious Diseases* 181, 99–106.

Connor, E.M., Sperling, R.S. *et al.* (1994) Reduction of maternal-infant transmission of human immunodeficiency virus type-1 with zidovudine treatment. *New England Journal of Medicine* 331, 1173–1180.

Coutsoudis, A., Bobat, R.A., Coovadia, H.M., Kuhn, L., Tsai, W.Y. & Stein, Z.A. (1995) The effects of vitamin A supplementation on the morbidity of children born to HIV-infected women. *American Journal of Public Health* 85, 1076–1081.

Coutsoudis, A., Pillay, K., Spooner, E., Kuhn, L. & Coovadia, H.M. (1999a) for the South African Vitamin A Study Group. Influence of infant-feeding patterns on early mother-to-child transmission of HIV-1 in Durban, South Africa: a prospective cohort study. *Lancet* 354, 1046–1047.

Coutsoudis, A., Pillay, K., Spooner, E., Kuhn, L. & Coovadia, H.M. (1999b) Randomised trial testing the effect of vitamin A supplementation on pregnancy outcomes and early mother-to-child HIV-1 transmission in Durban, South Africa. South Africa Vitamin A Study Group. *AIDS* 13, 1517–1524.

Culnane, M., Fowler, M. & Lee, S.S. (1999) Lack of long-term effects of in-utero exposure to zidovudine among uninfected children born to HIV-infected women. *Journal of the American Medical Association* 281, 151–157.

Cunningham, C.K., Britto, P. *et al.* (2001) Genotypic resistance analysis in women participating in PACTG 316 with HIV-1 RNA > 400 copies/ ml. *Program and abstracts of the 8th Conference on Retroviruses and Opportunistic Infections*, 4–8 February 2001, Chicago, Illinois. Abstract 712. Available at: http://www.retroconference.org/2001/abstracts/abstracts/712.htm

D'Ubaldo, C., Pezzotti, P., Rezza, G., Branca, M. & Ippolito, G. (1998) Association between HIV-1 infection and miscarriage: a retrospective study. DIANAIDS Collaborative Study Group. Diagnosi Iniziale Anomalie Neoplastiche AIDS. *AIDS* 12, 1087–1093.

Dabis, F., Msellati, P. *et al.* (1999) Six-month efficacy, tolerance, and acceptability of a short regimen of oral zidovudine to reduce vertical transmission of HIV in breastfed children in Cote d'Ivoire and Burkina Faso: a double-blind placebo-controlled multicentre trial. *Lancet* 353, 786–789.

Desgrees du, L., Msellati, P. *et al.* (1998) HIV-1 infection and reproductive history: a retrospective study among pregnant women: Abidjan, Cote d'Ivoire 1995–96. *International Journal of STD and AIDS* 9, 452–456.

Dorenbaum, A., for the PACTG 316 Study Team (2001) Report of results of PACTG 316: an international phase III trial of the standard antiretroviral (ARV) prophylaxis plus nevirapine (NVP) for prevention of perinatal HIV transmission. *Program and Abstracts of the 8th Conference on Retroviruses and Opportunistic Infections*, 4–8 February 2001, Chicago, Illinois. Abstract LB7. Available at: http://www.retroconference.org/2001/abstracts/abstracts/abstracts/lb7.htm

Duliege, A.-M., Amos, C.I., Felton, S., Biggar, R.J. & Goedert, J.J. (1995) The international registry of HIV-exposed twins. Birth order, delivery route and concordance in the transmission of human immunodeficiency virus type 1 from mothers to twins. *Journal of Paediatrics* 126, 625–632.

Dunn, D.T., Brandt, C.D. & Krivine, A. (1995) The sensitivity of HIV-1 DNA polymerase chain reaction in the neonatal period and the relative contributions of intra-uterine and intra partum transmission. *AIDS* 9, F7–F11.

Dunn, D.T., Newell, M.L., Aden, A.E. & Peckham, C.S. (1992) Risk of human immunodeficiency virus type 1 transmission through breastfeeding. *Lancet* 340, 585–588.

Eastman, P.S., Shapiro, D.E., Coombs, R.W., Frenkel, L.M. & McSherry, G.D. (1998) Maternal viral genotypic zidovudine resistance and infrequent failure of zidovudine therapy to prevent perinatal transmission of human immunodeficiency virus type 1 in pediatric AIDS Clinical Trials Group Protocol 076. *Journal of Infection and Disease* 177, 557–564.

European Collaborative Study (1996) Vertical transmission of HIV-1: maternal immune status and obstetric factors. *AIDS* 10, 1675–1681.

European Collaborative Study (1999) Maternal viral load and vertical transmission of HIV-1: an important factor but not the only one. *AIDS* 13, 1377–1385.

European Collaborative Study (2001a) HIV-infected pregnant women and vertical transmission in Europe since 1986. *AIDS* 15, 761–70.

European Collaborative Study (2001b) Fluctuations in symptoms in HIV-infected children: the first 10 years of life. *Pediatrics* 108, 116–22.

European Collaborative Study (Bailey, A.J., Newell, M.-L. & Peckham, C.S.) (1998) Is zidovudine therapy in pregnant HIV-infected women associated with gestational age and birthweight? *AIDS* 13, 119–124.

European Collaborative Study and Swiss Mother and Child HIV Cohort Study (2000) Combination antiretroviral therapy and duration of pregnancy. *AIDS* 14, 2913–2920.

European Mode of Delivery Collaboration (1999) Elective caesarean section versus vaginal delivery in prevention of vertical HIV-1 transmission: a randomised clinical trial. *Lancet* 353, 1035–1039.

Fawzi, W.W., Msamanga, G.I. et al. (1998) Randomised trial of effects of vitamin supplements on pregnancy outcome and T cell counts in HIV-1 infected women in Tanzania. *Lancet* 351, 1477–1482.

Feinberg, M.B. (1996) Changing the natural history of HIV disease. *Lancet* 348, 239–246.

Fourquet, F., Le Chenadec, J., Mayaux, M.J. & Meyer, L. (2001) Reproductive behaviour of HIV-infected women living in France, according to geographical origin. *AIDS* 15, 2193–2196.

French, R. & Brocklehurst, P. (1998) The effect of pregnancy on survival in women infected with HIV: systematic review of the literature and meta-analysis. *British Journal of Obstetrics and Gynaecology* 105, 827–835.

Gaillard, P., Myanyumba, F., Verhofstede C. et al (2001) Vaginal lavage with chlorhexidine during labour to reduce mother-to-child HIV transmission: clinical trial in Mombasa, Kenya. *AIDS* 15, 389–96.

Gaillard P., Verhofstede C., Myanyumba F. et al (2000) Exposure to HIV-1 during delivery and mother-to-child transmission. *AIDS* 14, 2341–8.

Gao, F., Bailes, E. et al. (1999) Origins of HIV-1 in the chimpanzee *Pan troglodytes*. *Nature* 397, 436–441.

Garcia, P.M., Kalish, L.A. et al. (1999) Maternal levels of plasma human immunodeficiency virus type 1 RNA and the risk of perinatal transmission. *New England Journal of Medicine* 341, 394–402.

Gerschenson, M., Erhart, S.W., Paik, C.Y. et al (2000) Fetal mitochondrial heart and skeletal muscle damage in Erythrocebus patas monkeys exposed *in utero* to 3′-azido-3′-deoxythymidine. *AIDS Res Hum Retroviruses*.16, 635–44.

Gibb, D.M. & Tess, B.H. (1999) Interventions to reduce mother-to-child transmission of HIV infection: new developments and current controversies. *AIDS* 13 (Suppl. A), S93–S102.

Goldenberg, R.L., Vermund, S.H., Goepfert, A.R. & Andrews, W.W. (1998) Choriodecidual inflammation: a potentially preventable cause of perinatal HIV-1 transmission? *Lancet* 352, 1927–1930.

Gortmaker, S.L., Hughes, M. et al. (2001) Effect of combination therapy including protease inhibitors on mortality among children and adolescents infected with HIV-1. *New England Journal of Medicine* 345, 1522–1528.

Graham, W.J. & Newell, M.-L. (1999) Seizing the opportunity: collaborative initiatives to reduce HIV and maternal mortality. *Lancet* 353, 836–839.

Gray, R., Wawer, M. et al. (1998) Population-based study of fertility in women with HIV-1 infection in Uganda. *Lancet* 351, 98–103.

Gregson, S., Zaba, B. & Garnett, G.P. (1999) Low fertility in women with HIV and the impact of the epidemic on orphanhood and early childhood mortality in sub-Saharan Africa. *AIDS* 13 (Suppl. A), S249–S257.

Grossman, Z., Feinberg, M., Kuznetsov, V., Dimitrov, D. & Paul, W. (1998) HIV infection: how effective is drug combination treatment? *Immunology Today* 19, 528–532.

Grubert, T.A., Reindell, D., Kastner, R., Lutz-Friedrich, R., Behohradsky, B.H. & Dathe, O. (1999) Complications after caesarean section in HIV-1 infected women not taking antiretroviral treatment. *Lancet* 354, 1612–1613.

Guay, L.A., Musoke, P. et al. (1999) Intrapartum and neonatal single-dose nevirapine compared with zidovudine for prevention of mother-to-child transmission of HIV-1 in Kampala, Uganda: HIV NET 012 randomised trial. *Lancet* 354, 795–802.

Hanson, I.C., Antonelli, T.A., Sperling R.S. et al. (1999) Lack of tumours in infants with perinatal HIV exposure and fetal/neonatal exposure to Zidovudine. *J Acquir Immune Defic Syndr Hum Retrovirol* 20 463–7

Hellerstein, M., Hanley, M.B. et al. (1999) Directly measured kinetics of circulating T lymphocytes in normal and HIV-1 infected humans. *Nature Medicine* 5, 83–89.

Hill, J.B., Sheffield, J.S., Zeeman, G.G. & Wendel, G.D. (2001) Hepatotoxicity with antiretroviral treatment of pregnant women. *Obstetrics and Gynecology* 98, 909–911.

Hirschel, B. & Opravil, M. (1999) The year in press: antiretroviral treatment. *AIDS* 13 (Suppl. A), S177–S187.

Ho, D.D., Neumann, A.V., Perelson, A.S., Chen, W., Leonar, J.M. & Markovita, M. (1995) Rapid turnover of plasma virions and CD4 lymphocytes in HIV-1 infection. *Nature* 373, 123–126.

Hocke, C., Morlat, P., Chene, G., Groupe d'Epidemologie Clinique des SIDA en Aquitaine (1995) Prospective cohort study of the effect of pregnancy on the progression of human immunodeficiency virus infection. *Obstetrics and Gynecology* 86, 886–891.

Hogg, R.S., Yip, B. et al. (2001) Rates of disease progression by baseline CD4 cell count and viral load after initiating triple-drug therapy. *Journal of the American Medical Association* 286, 2568–2577.

Hooper, E. (1999) *The River: a Journey to the Source of HIV and AIDS*. Little, Brown, Boston, MA.

Horuk, R. (1999) Chemokine receptors and HIV-1: the fusion of two major research fields. *Immunology Today* **20**, 89–93.

International Perinatal HIV Group (1999) The mode of delivery and the risk of vertical transmission of HIV-1: a meta-analysis from fifteen prospective cohort studies. *New England Journal of Medicine* **340**, 977–987.

International Perinatal HIV Group (2001) Duration of ruptured membranes and vertical transmission of human immunodeficiency virus type 1: a meta-analysis from fifteen prospective cohort studies *AIDS* **15**, 357–368.

Ioannidis, J.P., Abrams, E.J. *et al.* (2001) Perinatal transmission of human immunodeficiency virus type 1 by pregnant women with virus loads <1000 copies/ml. *Journal of Infectious Diseases* **183**, 539–545.

Jackson, J.B., Becker-Pergola, G. *et al.* (2000) Identification of the K103N resistance mutation in Ugandan women receiving nevirapine to prevent HIV-1 vertical transmission. *AIDS* **14**, F111–F115.

Johnstone, F.D. (1993) Pregnancy outcome and pregnancy management in HIV-infected women. In: Johnstone, F.D. & Johnson, M.A., eds. *HIV Infection in Women*. Churchill Livingstone: Edinburgh, 187–198.

Johnstone, F.D., Kilpatrick, D.C. & Burns, S. (1992) Anticardiolipin antibodies and pregnancy outcome in women with human immunodeficiency virus infection. *Obstetrics and Gynecology* **80**, 92–96.

Johnstone, F.D., Raab, G.M. & Hamilton, B.A. (1996) The effect of human immunodeficiency virus infection on birth characteristics. *Obstetrics and Gynecology* **88**, 321–326.

Johnstone, F.D., Thong, K.J. & Bird, A.G. (1994) Lymphocyte subpopulations in early human pregnancy. *Obstetrics and Gynecology* **83**, 941–946.

Kalish, L.A., Pitt, J. *et al.* (1997) Defining the time of fetal or perinatal acquisition of human immunodeficiency virus type 1 infection on the basis of age at first positive culture. *Journal of Infectious Diseases* **175**, 712–715.

Kind, C., Rudin, C. *et al.* (1998) Prevention of vertical HIV transmission: additive protective effect of elective caesarean section and zidovudine prophylaxis. *AIDS* **12**, 205–210.

King, M.P. & Attardi, G. (1989) Human cells lacking mtDNA: Repopulation with exogenous mitochondria by complementation. *Science* **246**, 500–503.

Kovacs, A., Wasserman, S.S. *et al.* (2001) Determinants of HIV-1 shedding in the genital tract of women. *Lancet* **358**, 1593–1601.

Kuhn, L. & Stein, Z. (1997) Infant survival, HIV infection and feeding alternatives in less developed countries. *American Journal of Public Health* **87**, 926–931.

Lallemant, M., Jourdain, G. *et al.* (2000) A trial of shortened zidovudine regimens to prevent mother-to-child transmission of human immunodeficiency virus type 1. *New England Journal of Medicine* **343**, 982–991.

Landers, D.V., Tejada de, B.M. & Coyne, B.A. (1997) Immunology of HIV and pregnancy: the effects of each on the other. *Obstetrics and Gynecologic Clinics of North America* **24**, 821–831.

Landesman, S.H., Kalish, L.A., Burns, D.N., Minkoff, H., Fox, H.E. & Zorilla, C. (1996) Obstetrical factors and the transmission of human immunodeficiency virus type 1 from mother to child. *New England Journal of Medicine* **334**, 1617–1623.

Ledergerber, B., Egger, M. *et al.* (1999) Clinical progression and virological failure on highly active antiretroviral therapy in HIV-1 patients: a prospective cohort study. *Lancet* **353**, 863–868.

Leroy, V., Newell, M.-L. *et al.* (1998) International multicentre pooled analysis of late postnatal mother-to-child transmission of HIV-1 infection. *Lancet* **352**, 597–600.

Logie, D. (1999) AIDS cuts life expectancy in sub-Saharan Africa by a quarter. *British Medical Journal* **319**, 806.

Lorenzi, P., Masserey Spicher, V. *et al.* (1998) The Swiss Collaborative HIV and Pregnancy Study and the Swiss Neonatal HIV Study. Antiretroviral therapies in pregnancy: maternal, fetal and neonatal effects. *AIDS* **12**, F214–F247.

Luzzati, R., Del Bravo, P., Di Perri, G., Luzzani, A. & Concia, E. (1999) Riboflavine and severe lactic acidosis. *Lancet* **353**, 901–902.

Maiques-Montesinos, V., Cervera-Sanchez, J., Bellver-Pradas, J., Abad-Carrascosa, A. & Serra-Serra, V. (1999) Post-cesarean section morbidity in HIV-positive women. *Acta Obstetrica Gynecologica Scandinavica* **78**, 789–792.

Mandelbrot, L., Brossard, Y. *et al.* (1996a) Testing for in utero human immunodeficiency virus infection with fetal blood sampling. *American Journal of Obstetrics and Gynecology* **175**, 489–493a.

Mandelbrot, L, Burgard, M. *et al.* (1999) Frequent detection of HIV-1 in the gastric aspirates of neonates born to HIV-infected mothers. *AIDS* **13**, 2143–2149.

Mandelbrot, L., Landreau-Mascaro, A. *et al.* (2001a) Lamivudine-zidovudine combination for prevention of maternal-infant transmission of HIV-1. *Journal of the American Medical Association* **285**, 2083–2093.

Mandelbrot, L., Le Chenadec, J. *et al.* (1998) Perinatal HIV-1 transmission: interaction between zidovudine prophylaxis and mode of delivery in the French Perinatal Cohort. *Journal of the American Medical Association* **280**, 55–60.

Mandelbrot, L., Mayaux, M.J. *et al.* (1996b) French Pediatric HIV Infection Study Group. Obstetric factors and mother-to-child transmission of human immunodeficiency virus type 1: the French perinatal cohorts. *American Journal of Obstetrics and Gynecology* **175**, 661–667.

Mandelbrot, L., Peytavin, G., Firtion, G. & Farinotti, R. (2001b) Maternal-fetal transfer and amniotic fluid accumulation of lamivudine in human immunodeficiency virus–infected pregnant women. *American Journal of Obstetrics and Gynecology* **184**, 153–158.

Mandelbrot, L., Schlienger, I. *et al.* (1994) Thrombocytopaenia in pregnant women infected with human immunodeficiency virus: maternal and neonatal outcome. *American Journal of Obstetrics and Gynecology* **171**, 252–257.

Marcollet, A., Goffinet, F., Firtion, G., Pannier, E., Le Bret, T., Brival, M.L. & Mandelbrot, L. (2002) Differences in postpartum morbidity in HIV-infected women following elective cesarean section, emergent cesarean or vaginal delivery. *American Journal of Obstetrics and Gynecology* **186**, 784–9.

Marseille, E., Kahn, J.G., Guay, L., Mosoke, P., Fowler, M.G. & Jackson, J.B. (1999) Cost effectiveness of single-dose nevirapine regimen for mothers and babies to decrease vertical HIV-1 transmission in sub-Sahara African. *Lancet* **354**, 803–809.

Mayaux, M.J., Dussaix, E. *et al.* (1997a) Maternal viral load during pregnancy and mother-to-child transmission of human immunodeficiency virus type 1: the French perinatal cohort studies. *Journal of Infection and Disease* **175**, 143–148a.

Mayaux, M.J., Teglas, J.P. *et al.* (1997b) Acceptability and impact of zidovudine prevention on mother-to-child HIV-1 transmission in France. *Journal of Pediatrics* **131**, 857–862.

McGowan, J.P., Crane, M., Wiznia, A.A. & Blum, S. (1999) Combination antiretroviral therapy in human immunodeficiency virus-infected pregnant women. *Obstetrics and Gynecology* **94**, 641–646.

McIntyre, J. (the SAINT Study Team) (2000) Evaluation of safety of two simple regimens for prevention of mother to child transmission (MTCT) of HIV infection: nevirapine (NVP) vs. lamivudine (3TC) + zidovudine (ZDV) used in a randomized clinical trial (the SAINT Study). *XIII International AIDS Conference*, Durban, South Africa, July 2000 (abstract TuOrB356).

Mofenson, L.M. & Fowler, M.G. (1999) Interruption of materno-fetal transmission. *AIDS* **13** (Suppl. A), S205–S214.

Mofenson, L.M., Lambert, J.S. *et al.* (1999) Risk factors for perinatal transmission of human immunodeficiency virus type 1 in women treated with zidovudine. *New England Journal of Medicine* **341**, 381–393.

Moore, R.E. & Chaisson, R.E. (1999) Natural history of HIV infection in the era of combination antiretroviral therapy. *AIDS* **13**, 1933–1942.

Morris, A.A.M. & Carr, A. (1999) HIV nucleoside analogues: new adverse effects on mitochondria? *Lancet* **354**, 1046–1047.

Msellati, P., Meda, N. *et al.* (1999) Safety and acceptability of vaginal disinfection with benzalkonium chloride in HIV-infected pregnant women in West Africa: ANRS 049b phase II randomized, double blinded placebo-controlled trial. *Sexually Transmitted Infection* **75**, 420–425.

Mummidi, S., Ahuja, S.A. *et al.* (1998) Geneology of the CCR5 locus and chemokine system gene variants associated with altered rates of HIV-1 disease progression. *Nature Medicine* **4**, 786–794.

Nduati, R., John, G. *et al.* (2000) Effect of breastfeeding and formula feeding on transmission of HIV-1: a randomized clinical trial. *Journal of the American Medical Association* **283**, 1167–1174.

Newell, M.L. (1998) Mechanisms and timing of mother-to-child transmission of HIV-1. *AIDS* **12**, 831–837.

Newell, M.L., Dabis, F., Tolley, K. & Whynes, D. (1998) Cost effectiveness and cost benefit in the prevention of mother-to-child transmission of HIV in developing countries. *AIDS* **12**, 1571–1580.

O'Donovan, D., Ariyoshi, K. *et al.* (2000) Maternal plasma viral RNA levels determine marked differences in mother-to-child transmission rates of HIV-1 and HIV-2 in the Gambia. *AIDS* **14**, 441–448.

O'Shea, S., Newell, M.L. *et al.* (1998) Maternal viral load, CD4 count and vertical transmission of HIV-1. *Journal of Medical Virology* **54**, 113–117.

Olinger, G.G., Hashemi, F.B., Sha, B.E. & Spear, G.T. (1999) Association of indicators of bacterial vaginosis with a female genital tract factor that induces expression of HIV-1. *AIDS* **13**, 1905–1912.

Olivero, O.A., Anderson, L.M. *et al.* (1997) Transplacental effects of 3-azido-2,3-dideoxythymidine (AZT) tumorigenicity in mice and genotoxicity in mice and monkeys. *Journal of the National Cancer Institute* **89**, 1602–1608.

Pantaleo, G. (1999) Unravelling the strands of HIV's web. *Nature Medicine* **5**, 27–28.

Parry, J., Murphy, G. *et al.* (2001) National surveillance of HIV-1 subtypes for England and Wales: Design, methods and initial findings. *Journal of AIDS* **26**, 381–388.

Phillips, A.N., Antunes, F. & Stergious, G. (1994) A sex comparison of rates of new AIDS-defining disease and death in 2554 AIDS cases. *AIDS* **8**, 831–835.

Pomerantz, R.J. (1999a) Primary HIV-1 resistance: a new phase in the epidemic? *Journal of the American Medical Association* **282**, 1177–1179.

Pomerantz, R.J. (1999b) Residual HIV-1 disease in the era of highly active antiretrovirol therapy. *New England Journal of Medicine* **340**, 1672–1674.

Postma, M.J., Beck, E.J. *et al.* (1999) Universal HIV screening of pregnant women in England: cost effectiveness analysis. *British Medical Journal* **318**, 1656–1660.

Ratcliffe, J., Ades, A.E., Gibb, D., Sculpher, M.J. & Briggs, A.H. (1998) Prevention of mother-to-child transmission of HIV-1 infection: alternative strategies and their cost-effectiveness. *AIDS* **12**, 1381–1388.

Read, J., Tuomala, R. *et al.* (2001) Mode of delivery and postpartum morbidity among HIV-infected women: the Women and Infants Transmission Study. *Journal of AIDS* **26**, 236–245.

Rouzioux, C., Costalagliola, D., Burgard, M., Blanche, S., Mayaux, M.J., Griselli, C. & Valleron, A.J. (1995) Estimated timing of mother-to-child human immunodeficiency virus type 1 (HIV-1) transmission by use of a marker model. The HIV infection in French Collaboration Group. *American Journal of Epidemiology* **142**, 1330–1337.

Rowland-Jones, S. (1999) HIV infection: where have all the T cells gone? *Lancet* **354**, 5–7.

Saada, M., Le Chenadec, J., Berrebi, A., Bongain, A., Delfraissy, J.F., Mayaux, M.J. & Meyer, L. (2000) Pregnancy and progression to AIDS: results of the French prospective cohorts. SEROGEST and SEROCO Study Groups. *AIDS* **14**, 2355–2360.

Scalfaro, P., Chesaux, J.J. *et al.* (1998) Severe transient neonatal lactic acidosis during prophylactic zidovudine treatment. *Intensive Care Medicine* **24**, 247–250.

Semba, R.D., Kumwenda, N. *et al.* (1999) Human immunodeficiency virus load in breast milk, mastitis, and mother-to-child transmission of human immunodeficiency virus type 1. *Journal of Infectious Disease* **180**, 93–98.

Semba, R.D., Miotti, P.G. *et al.* (1994) Maternal vitamin A deficiency and mother-to-child transmission of HIV-1. *Lancet* **343**, 1593–1597.

Semprini, A.E., Castagna, C. *et al.* (1995) The incidence of complications after caesarean section in 156 HIV-positive women. *AIDS* **9**, 913–917.

Shaffer, N., Chuachoowong, R. *et al.* (1999) Short course zidovudine for perinatal HIV-1 transmission in Bangkok, Thailand: a randomised controlled trial. *Lancet* **353**, 773–780.

Shanson, D.C., Taylor, E.W. *et al.* (1992) Risks to surgeons and patients from HIV and hepatitis: Guidelines on precautions and management of exposure to blood or body fluids. *British Medical Journal* **305**, 1337–1343.

Shapiro, D.E., Sperling, R.S., Mandelbrot, L., Britto, P. & Cunningham, B.E., for the Pediatric AIDS Clinical Trials Group Protocol 076 Study Group (1999) Risk factors for perinatal human immunodeficiency virus transmission in patients receiving zidovudine prophylaxis. *Obstetrics and Gynecology* **94**, 897–908.

Siliciano, R.F. (1999) Latency and reservoirs for HIV-1. *AIDS* **13** (Suppl. A), S49–S58.

Simonon, A., Lepage, P. & Karita, E. (1994) An assessment of the timing of mother-to-child transmission of human immunodeficiency virus type 1 by means of polymerase chain reaction. *AIDS* **7**, 952–957.

Simpson, W., Johnstone, F.D., Goldberg, D., Hart, G., Boyd, F. & Prescott, R. (1998) Uptake and acceptability of antenatal HIV testing: Randomised controlled trial of different methods of offering the test. *British Medical Journal* **316**, 262–267.

Simpson, W.M., Johnstone, F.D., Goldberg, D.J., Gormley, S.M. & Hart, G.J. (1999) Antenatal HIV testing. Assessment of a routine voluntary approach. *British Medical Journal* **318**, 1660–1661.

Söderlund, N., Zwi, K., Kinghorn, A. & Gray, G. (1999) Prevention of vertical transmission of HIV: analysis of cost effectiveness of options available in South Africa. *British Medical Journal* **318**, 1650–1656.

Sperling, R., Shapiro, D.E. *et al.* (1996) Maternal viral load, zidovudine treatment, and the risk of transmission of human immunodeficiency virus type 1 from mother to infant. *New England Journal of Medicine* **335**, 1621–1629.

Star, J., Powrie, R., Cu-Uvin, S. & Carpenter, C.C.J. (1999) Should women with human immunodeficiency virus be delivered by caesarean? *Obstetrics and Gynecology* **94**, 799–801.

Stringer, J.S.A., Rouse, D.J. & Goldenberg, R.J. (1999) Prophylactic caesarean delivery for the protection of perinatal human immunodeficiency virus transmission; the case for restraint. *Journal of the American Medical Association* **281**, 1946–1949.

Taha, T.E., Biggar, R.J. *et al.* (1997) Effect of cleansing the birthcanal with antiseptic solution on maternal and newborn morbidity and mortality in Malawi: clinical trial. *British Medical Journal* **315**, 216–220.

Temmermann, M., Lopita, M.I., Sanghvi, H.C.G., Sinei, S.K.F., Plummer, F.A. & Piot, P. (1992) Association of maternal HIV-1 infection with spontaneous abortion. *International Journal of STD and AIDS* **3**, 418–422.

Temmermann, M., Plummer, F.A. *et al.* (1990) Infection with HIV as a risk factor for adverse obstetrical outcome. *AIDS* **4**, 1087–1093.

Tovo, P.-A., Newell, M.-L., Mandelbrot, L., Semprini, E. & Giaquinto, C. (1999a) Recommendations for the management of HIV-infected women and their infants—a European consensus. *Prenatal and Neonatal Medicine* **4**, 3–17.

Tovo, P.-A., Newell, M.-L., Mandelbrot, L., Semprini, E. & Giaquinto, C. (1999b) *Recommendations for the management of HIV infected women and their infants—a European consensus.* Publication of the European Commission.

Towers, C.V., Deveikis, A., Asrat, T., Major, C. & Nageotte, M.P. (1998) A 'bloodless caesarean section' and perinatal transmission of the human immunodeficiency virus. *American Journal of Obstetrics and Gynecology* **179**, 708–714.

Turner, B.J., Hauck, W.W., Fanning, T.R. & Markson, L.E. (1997) Cigarette smoking and maternal-child HIV transmission. *Journal of AIDS* **14**, 327–337.

UK Health Department (1997) *Guidelines on Post-Exposure Prophylaxis for Health Care Workers Occupationally Exposed to HIV.* Department of Health, London.

Wade, N.A., Birkhead, G.S. *et al.* (1998) Abbreviated regimens of zidovudine prophylaxis and perinatal transmission of the human immunodeficiency virus. *New England Journal of Medicine* **339**, 1409–1414.

Wallace, D.C. (1992) Mitochondrial genetics: a paradigm for aging and degenerative diseases? *Science* **256**, 628–632.

Watts, D.H., Lambert, J.S. *et al.* (2000) Complications according to mode of delivery among human immunodeficiency virus-infected women with CD4 lymphocyte counts of 500/fL. *American Journal of Obstetrics and Gynecology* **183**, 100–107.

Wiktor, S.Z., Ekpini, E. *et al.* (1999) Short course oral zidovudine for prevention of mother-to-child transmission of HIV-1 in Abidjan, Cote d'Ivoire: a randomised trial. *Lancet* **353**, 781–785.

Wilkinson, A.D., Floyd, K. & Gilks, C.F. (1998) Antiretroviral drugs as a public health intervention for pregnant HIV infected women in rural South Africa: an issue of cost-effectiveness and capacity. *AIDS* **12**, 1675–1682.

Wolthers, K.C., Schuitemaker, H. & Miedema, F. (1998) Rapid CD4+ T cell turnover in HIV-1 infection a paradigm revisited. *Immunology Today* **19**, 44–48.

Zhu, T., Korber, B.T., Nahmias, A.J., Hooper, E., Sharp, P.M. & Ho, D.D. (1998) An African HIV-1 sequence from 1959 and implications for the origin of the epidemic. *Nature* **391**, 594–597.

19 Substance abuse

Michael de Swiet

The increase in the number of young people who abuse or are addicted to drugs has brought a corresponding increase in the number of women who abuse drugs during pregnancy. This is more of a problem in the USA from where most of the large series concerning substance abuse in pregnancy have been published and reviewed by Finnegan [1–3]. However, substance abusers are frequently seen in hospitals in the UK, particularly those catering for patients from the centres of large towns. A recent study of anonymous urine testing in 1000 pregnant women attending an inner city UK maternity hospital found that 11% had evidence of substance abuse; by far the most common substance was cannabis (8.5%); other substances found were opiates (1.4%) and methadone (0.3%) together with cocaine (1.1%), cyclizine (0.4%) and dextropropoxyphene (0.3%) [4]. By contrast a nationwide survey of all maternity units in the UK performed at about the same time, asking about pregnant female drug abusers found a mean rate of 0.8% with wide regional variation between 0.1% and 5% [5].

Human immunodeficiency virus (HIV) infection, which is discussed in Chapter 18, has become the major problem in those who abuse drugs intravenously and in those who use prostitution to finance their drug habits, even if these do not involve needle sharing. For example in New York cocaine abuse increases the risk of the patient having HIV infection fivefold (and syphilis eightfold) [6]. The increasing acceptance of HIV testing for all pregnant women makes discussion of testing with the drug abuser less pejorative. Hepatitis B and C are also obvious problems that should be discussed and tested for with the patient's consent.

Intravenous drug abuse obviously increases the risk of other forms of sepsis. An echocardiographic study from New York [7] showed abnormal valve structure in 21 of 23 intravenous drug abusers with heart murmurs even though they had no other signs or symptoms of heart disease. There should therefore be a much more liberal attitude towards echocardiography in intravenous drug abusers with heart murmurs in pregnancy than in other pregnant patients (see Chapter 5). Mycotic aneurysms [8], epidural abscess [9] and a marked increase in the risk of pneumonia [10] have also been reported. The overall mortality from all those abusing drugs intravenously is estimated to be 1% annually.

In addition sharing of needles and syringes increases the risk of rhesus isoimmunization [11] presumably because rhesus-negative women receive an innoculum of blood from syringes contaminated by other rhesus-positive users.

Drug abuse is not a problem that will go away either in society or in the individual; even though individuals may become abstinent, the need of the body for the drug remains and relapse is always a threat.

Most of the following comments concern opiate, cocaine and alcohol abuse, but as drug users usually abuse several different sorts of drugs, it is difficult to be certain that the effects ascribed to the above drugs are not due to other drugs taken in addition. In recent years the literature has been dominated by the wave of cocaine abuse that has swept over the USA, which has specific pregnancy problems (see below). Also, illicit drugs are so expensive that the drug abuser is forced to adopt a very poor standard of living, often indulging in prostitution (with its associated risk of sexually transmitted disease) to pay for her drugs. An alternative viewpoint is that many women who are socially deprived lead such miserable lives that it is not surprising that they turn to drugs to relieve their misery; and the more easily available the drugs are the less severe is the precipitating social deprivation. In addition there is a very high incidence of previous sexual abuse in those who abuse drugs and other substances [12]. These nutritional and social factors must also affect the outcome of pregnancy in drug abusers. The above comments are inevitably biased because the substance abusers that come to the attention of health-care workers are those with chaotic lifestyles and other social difficulties. Yet anonymous urine testing indicates that substance abuse is widely distributed across all social classes [12] and those who are more advantaged may not suffer so much either in pregnancy or in the non-pregnant state.

The management of pregnancy in those who abuse drugs is difficult and demands teamwork; important members of the team are community worker, drug worker, general practitioner, social worker, health visitor, midwife and obstetrician. As it would not be practical for all these members to see the women simultaneously, it is especially important for there to be a good communication network; something that is often given low priority as is the whole of health care for a group that is seen to be difficult, manipulating and excessively demanding. Health-care workers need to develop a special combination of firmness and sympathy. For example, women must realize that illicit drug taking or dealing on hospital premises is absolutely forbidden and that if necessary visitors suspected of supplying drugs will be forbidden or ejected. On the positive side, women who are substance abusers may well seek and respond to health-care advice more readily in pregnancy because of their wish for a healthy baby. Certainly women are more likely to enter detoxification, residence and methadone programmes in pregnancy than in the non-pregnant state [13].

Opiates

Effect of opiate abuse on pregnancy and its outcome

Finnegan [2] quotes a number of obstetric complications of opiate abuse including abortion, abruption, breech pre-sentation, previous caesarean section, etc., but she has not controlled for the social deprivation that we have already mentioned. From this point of view, a better series is that of Ostrea and Chavez [14] who studied 830 opiate-dependent mothers delivered in one hospital in Michigan, and compared them with 400 controls matched for social class and race (86% black). The relative risks of meco-nium-stained amniotic fluid, anaemia, premature rupture of membranes, haemorrhage, multiple pregnancy and in-trauterine growth restriction are shown in Table 19.1. It can be seen that the risk of these complications for the drug abuser ranges between 1.5 and 5.5 times the risk in the control group. In addition, once born the infant has greater risk of jaundice, aspiration pneumonia (particularly meconium aspiration), transient tachypnoea and congenital abnormalities. The question of neonatal withdrawal is considered below. In contrast to earlier studies [15] the incidence of hyaline membrane disease in the preterm drug-abusing group was the same as in the preterm deliveries from the control group.

The congenital abnormalities found were varied; an excess risk has not been found in other studies [2]. At present, this should be considered a chance finding, but something to watch carefully.

It has been suggested that the frequent occurrence of meconium staining of the liquor, and hence of meconium aspiration is part of the fetal response to maternal drug withdrawal. Liu *et al.* [16] cite reports from mothers that increased fetal movements occur before subjective symptoms of withdrawal in the mother. Cardiotocographic findings, and falling maternal oestriol levels, also suggest fetal stress at the time of maternal withdrawal [16]. Experimental data in sheep [17] suggest that a fetal withdrawal syndrome can occur even within a few hours of

	Abuser (n = 830)	Controls (n = 400)	Relative risk (abuser/control)
Meconium staining	21.2	13.8	1.5
Anaemia†	13.4	8.2	1.6
Premature rupture of membranes	12.2	7.8	1.6
Haemorrhage (abruption and placenta praevia)	3.0	1.2	2.5
Multiple pregnancy	3.4	1.2	2.8
Premature delivery (<38 weeks)	18.5	9.8	1.9
Small for gestational age‡	16.5	3.0	5.5
Apgar <6 at 1 min	19.9	10.0	2.0
Perinatal mortality	2.7	1.0	2.7

Table 19.1 Antenatal problems (%) and condition of infants at birth (%) in opiate abusers compared to controls.* (From [14].)

*All differences were statistically significant $p < 0.05$.

†Haemoglobin <10 g/dL.

‡Less than 10th percentile for weight in the Lubchenco curve.

maternal opiate administration and indicate that the fetus may be continually undergoing withdrawal because of fluctuating maternal opiate levels. In addition, fetal asphyxia may be precipitated by the increased oxygen consumption caused by excessive movement in an already compromised fetus [18].

The excess rate of multiple pregnancy has also been noted by Rementeria *et al.* [19] who found an overall multiple pregnancy rate of one in 32 pregnancies—about three times their usual rate. Dizygotic twins largely accounted for the excess. Perhaps opiates stimulate the ovary to release an extra follicle, either directly or via the hypothalamus and gonadotrophin release.

Neonatal withdrawal syndrome and other effects on children

This will occur in 60–90% of infants born to drug-dependent women [20–22], at between 4 h and 2 weeks of age. The timing is related to the rate of metabolism of the drugs. This is most clearly expressed with regard to opiate dependency. Heroin and morphia are metabolized rapidly, and infants will develop signs between 4 and 24 h after delivery. Methadone is metabolized much more slowly, and signs do not occur until 1 day or even 1 week [23] or 2 weeks [2] after delivery.

The neonatal withdrawal syndrome is characterized by signs of central nervous hyperirritability (increased reflexes and tremor) with gastrointestinal dysfunction (continual finger sucking, with regurgitation of feeds and diarrhoea) and respiratory distress [2]. Paediatricians are undecided as to whether treatment should be with dilute opium solutions such as paregoric [1] or barbiturates [1]. Chlorpromazine [23] and diazepam have also been used, but the latter causes a marked impairment in sucking [1]. Nevertheless, neonatal abstinence syndrome is rarely a major problem and mothers should be reassured accordingly.

Neonatal abstinence syndrome has also been reported with other non-narcotic drugs of abuse, such as barbiturates, pentazocine, ethyl alcohol and amphetamines [2]; and indeed with drugs that are not usually abused such as other anticonvulsants (see Chapter 15).

Infants born to opiate-dependent mothers have an increased risk of dying unexpectedly from sudden infant death syndrome (SIDS). This risk varies from 1.6% [24] to 21.4% [25] compared to the overall population risk of 0.3% [26]. The overall incidence of SIDS is declining; so in a more recent study in Los Angeles, Ward *et al.* [27] found a SIDS rate of 0.9% in infants of substance abusing mothers, 0.1% in infants of controls, still a substantially increased risk. Almost identical data were reported by Durand *et al.*

[28] from Oakland also in California, where the SIDS rate was 0.9% in infants of substance abusing mothers, 0.13% in infants of controls. In a very large study of 1760 cases of SIDS the relative risk was about 3 for the infant of an opiate abuser after correction for other high-risk variables [29]. Although there must be social factors accounting, in part, for this increased incidence, it is of great theoretical importance, because of the possible interference by opiates with the normal development of cardiorespiratory control in the newborn infant, either directly or through maternal hypoventilation [30]. The fetuses of women on a methadone maintenance programme show decreased response to maternal carbon dioxide administration as judged by fetal breathing movements and when compared to controls. This response is decreased still further by acute methadone administration [31].

It is encouraging that Sardemann *et al.* [32] who studied 19 infants for 2 years after delivery from drug-abusing mothers in Denmark, did not find any evidence of behavioural disturbance, impaired intelligence or growth restriction. However, most of the children had spent long periods in institutional care.

In another study, opiate abusers were more likely to have been exposed to opiates during their birth than their non-abusing siblings [33]. The opiates were being given for therapeutic pain relief. So it is possible that opiate exposure *in utero* imprints the individual towards opiate abuse in later life.

Management of pregnancy in the opiate-dependent woman

The majority of problems that can occur in drug-dependent women during pregnancy are not specific to drug dependency and could, and do, occur in other women of low social class and poor health and nutrition. Specific problems for the attending doctor relate to the choice of which opiate should be used, and interactions between opiates and other drugs during pregnancy. One further practical problem is that drug abusers usually have very few patent, superficial veins. Indeed they may be the only people that can successfully perform venepuncture on themselves.

In 1973, Zelson *et al.* [22] described a study from New York which purported to show that heroin-exposed infants have a much better neonatal outcome than methadone-exposed infants, with less severe withdrawal symptoms and no cases of hyaline membrane disease despite their prematurity. For these reasons, they suggested that mothers should not be taken off a 'street' supply of heroin by changing them to a methadone maintenance programme. This bold suggestion made quite an impact at the time, but it was challenged, largely because the groups of methadone- and heroin-treated abusers were not necessarily comparable [34].

The general view now is that patients and their offspring are much better managed in a methadone maintenance programme, than trying to obtain heroin or other more rapidly acting opiates illegally. Such a programme will put the abuser in contact with medical and social services, and this alone can improve her standard of living sufficiently to benefit her and her infant's health [35]. She will have a stable legal supply of the drug and will therefore no longer need to prostitute herself. Methadone syrup as prescribed for opiate abusers is very difficult to inject intravenously and does not give the same 'high' as heroin so the risks of injection are avoided. However, a more recent study [36] indicates that although a methadone programme increases the number of prenatal visits in pregnancy, and reduces maternal anaemia, it does not necessarily affect the reduced birthweight or other adverse fetal outcomes in women who abuse opiates.

The reason for using methadone is that with a half-life of 18–97 h, it is metabolized much more slowly than heroin, and withdrawal symptoms do not occur until 72–96 h after the last dose. The half-life of heroin is 4–10 h, and withdrawal symptoms may occur within 24 h after the last dose. Patients may be maintained on an oral methadone regimen, and they and their fetuses are much less likely to have withdrawal symptoms than when they are taking heroin. In addition, most countries have narcotics regulations that forbid the supply of heroin to abusers, but will legalize specific individuals to give methadone in cases of drug abuse. Unfortunately, patients may not like to change from heroin to methadone, because the latter does not produce the same feelings of pleasure. Nevertheless, for the reasons outlined above, all opiate abusers should be transferred to a methadone maintenance programme during pregnancy [37]. The only exceptions are those that present in late pregnancy or during labour.

'Street' heroin is diluted to a varying extent with fillers such as lactose, making it difficult to know exactly how much heroin the abuser has in fact been taking. Therefore, transfer to an adequate methadone regimen takes time, because of the need to find the right dose and the longer duration of methadone action. There is therefore a risk of precipitating a withdrawal state during transfer, and, as indicated above, this may be particularly dangerous for the fetus. Indeed Liu *et al.* [16] have observed fetal distress in labour not due to recognized causes, which was relieved by administration of pethidine. For these reasons, it is best not to transfer to methadone the abuser who

presents late in pregnancy as an outpatient. Such patients should ideally be admitted and transferred to methadone with judicious use of short-acting narcotics, to render them symptom free, and to prevent fetal distress and preterm labour [38]. Also health-care attendants should be aware that the volume of distribution of drugs increases in pregnancy, particularly in late pregnancy so that for the same dose women will get less biological effect. Indeed methadone maintenance programmes should in pregnancy err towards generosity to ensure that patients do not attempt to get street drugs for top-up purposes [39]. Conversely the dose of drugs is likely to need reduction after delivery.

If women will not accept a methadone programme and wish to continue injecting they should at least be offered a needle exchange programme or failing that given instruction in domestic sterilization of their equipment with bleach or detergent.

Although many would prefer detoxification in the form of complete abstinence, to the regimens described above, relapse rates after detoxification are very high, of the order of 50% at 6 months so this really is not very practical in the pregnancy setting.

Fetal monitoring is difficult because the cardiotochograph often shows a non-reactive trace [40], particularly soon after ingestion of methadone or other opiates. This may lead to unnecessary intervention. Equally these are at-risk pregnancies and other characteristics such as lack of baseline variability, growth restriction and abnormal fetal Doppler studies should not be ignored.

Analgesia during labour is best given by an epidural anaesthetic. If this is not possible, opiates such as pethidine can be given, but they will be less effective in an opiate abuser. Because this effect is rather variable, it is better to give a standard dose, such as pethidine 100 mg intramuscularly more frequently, rather than a large (and possibly too large) dose at standard time intervals. Methadone is not a good analgesic. Pentazocine should not be used because it is a narcotic antagonist, and can precipitate a withdrawal reaction in an opiate abuser [38].

Overdose of opiate should be treated with the specific antagonist naloxone, which is given in an initial dose of 200 µg, followed by 100 µg every 2 min according to response. The dose given to the neonate is 5–10 µg/kg. Nalorphine should not be used because it causes respiratory depression, even though it is an opiate antagonist. All opiate antagonists may cause very severe withdrawal symptoms in the mother or her child. If necessary, these can be treated with further doses of opiate.

Narcotics interact dangerously with other drugs such as barbiturates, hypnotics, sedatives, general anaesthetics and tranquillizers causing central nervous system depression. These drugs should be given with great care, if at all, to drug abusers. In addition, muscle relaxants, such as D-tubocurarine can interact with opiates to cause severe respiratory depression.

Methadone is secreted in breast milk. The average concentration found by Blinick et al. [41] in a group of women taking an average of 52 mg/day was 0.27 μg/mL. This would be equivalent to a daily dose of 0.12 mg in an infant taking 450 mL of milk per day, or 0.04 mg/kg in a 3-kg infant. This is about one-twentieth of the maternal dose of 0.75 mg/kg for a 70-kg mother, and is clearly very little. Since there have been no reports of adverse effects of breastfeeding by drug-dependent mothers, it would seem sensible to encourage breastfeeding in these patients, particularly considering it may be difficult for them to bond to their children. However, in a British series of heroin abusers [21], only four of 23 babies were breastfed successfully and only six were living in families that had a stable relationship. Note also the danger of transmission of HIV infection by breastfeeding (see Chapter 18).

Alcohol

The fetal effects of other drugs of dependence are even harder to define than those of opiates, because their abusers do not form such a clear-cut group. However, it is indisputable that alcohol, if taken in sufficient quantities, will produce a specific fetal alcohol syndrome, first described by Jones and Smith [42]. The newborn child is growth restricted with characteristic facies, narrow palpebral fissures, epicanthal folds, short nose and long philtrum. In addition, the children are often mentally retarded, and may have other major congenital abnormalities such as club foot [43] or chromosome abnormalities [44]. The craniofacial abnormalities may regress as the child grows up but the mental abnormalities do not. Persistent retardation has been documented at age 10 [45] and major social problems have been shown in adolescence [46].

By contrast one advantage of alcohol abuse is that it appears to reduce the risk of respiratory distress syndrome presumably by increasing lung maturation [47].

Although alcohol abuse in pregnancy has been considered to be very uncommon in the UK, Beattie et al. [48] have reported 40 cases from the west of Scotland, an area with a notoriously high incidence of alcoholism. Unfortunately measurement of mean corpuscular volume (MCV) and γ-glutamyl transpeptidase (GTT) cannot be used very effectively [49] to screen for alcohol intake after the first trimester because both values decline to the normal range in heavy drinkers during the second trimester [50]. For example elevated GTT and elevated MCV predicts only 61% and 41% of adverse fetal effects, respectively [51].

Furthermore, the evidence from the Charing Cross Study [52] is that even modest alcohol consumption (1–2 glasses of wine per day) at the time of conception is associated with increased risk of low birthweight. Therefore screening in the antenatal clinic is not the answer. There must be greater awareness of the risk in the general population and in health-care professionals [53]. Although the overall incidence of alcohol consumption in pregnancy may be declining (from 32% in 1985 to 20% in 1988 in the USA [54]), this is not the case for smokers, the unmarried and younger less well-educated women [54].

It is not clear what the minimum daily alcohol intake is that affects the fetus, or the maximum daily intake that is safe. Most affected fetuses with full fetal alcohol syndrome have been born to mothers taking large quantities of alcohol: on average, 174 mL/day—the equivalent of at least 17 drinks [55]. However, growth restriction has been reported in patients taking much smaller quantities of alcohol, no more than 100–400 mL/week [56], although corrections are not always made for important confounding variables such as smoking, social class [53] and paternal alcohol intake [57]. An intake of 100–140 mL/week is between one and two glasses of wine per day. No short-term detectable effects have been shown at levels of alcohol consumption <100 mL per week [58,59].

Variation in the risk of developing fetal alcohol syndrome may relate to the metabolism of acetaldehyde, the first oxidation product of ethanol. Veghely [60] found that the blood level of acetaldehyde in mothers giving birth to a child with fetal alcohol syndrome was >40 μmol/L after a drink of alcohol whereas some heavy drinkers who had normal children had acetaldehyde levels <40 μmol/L. The validity of Veghely's measurements has been challenged [61]. The mechanism of intrauterine growth restriction is unknown. Deficiencies of zinc and copper, which may cause growth restriction in other circumstances, have been excluded [43].

It is very unlikely that the fetal alcohol syndrome is due to intercurrent consumption of other drugs, because the syndrome is specific to alcoholics, and those taking this quantity of alcohol do not, as a group, consistently abuse any other one drug. Acute intoxication of the infant at birth as would occur following unsuccessful treatment of preterm labour with alcohol infusion, has been associated with impairment of intellectual development when assessed at 4–7 years [62]. It is postulated that the intoxicated infant does not bond satisfactorily with the mother who may also be intoxicated at birth [62]. The fetal heart trace also shows loss of beat-to-beat variation at maternal blood alcohol levels of 130–290 mg/100 mL [63]. Such abnormalities should not be thought to indicate acute fetal distress or the necessity for immediate delivery [63].

Alcohol is secreted in breast milk where it achieves approximately the same concentration as in the maternal blood [64]. The dose of alcohol received by the baby will be small [64] but babies consume less milk if their mothers have been drinking [65] and there may be a minor impairment in motor but not mental development when the children are followed up at age 1 year [66]. Maternal alcohol intake also affects the flavour of milk [65]. So for all these reasons, mothers should not drink excessively when breastfeeding.

Cocaine

Possible effects of cocaine in pregnancy are of considerable importance in view of the increasing popularity of this drug both in the USA and Europe. It is estimated that 5 million Americans use cocaine regularly and that each day 5000 use it for the first time [67]. Young women are particularly likely to use the drug because it is believed to enhance sexuality. True physical dependence probably does not occur but regular abusers get very panicky if they have to quit. Screening for cocaine and other substances of abuse either by routine testing of pregnant women's urine [68,69] or by testing meconium from her neonate [70] shows that the patient history seriously underestimates the size of the problem [68–72]. The overall prevalence of cocaine abuse was about 10% in New York [68] and Pennsylvania [70], up to 25% in Washington DC [73] and up to 30% in Detroit [74], although <1% in rural Missouri where alcohol was more of a problem [69].

Cocaine blocks the presynaptic uptake of noradrenaline (norepinephrine) producing excess transmitter and marked activation of the sympathetic nervous system. In the non-pregnant this has lead to myocardial infarction, dysrhythmia, rupture of the aorta and cerebrovascular accidents [67]. In pregnancy mechanisms of adverse effect have been well reviewed by Volpe [75]. There is a small (odds ratio 1.4) risk of miscarriage of borderline statistical significance [76]. Congenital malformations reported have been sirenomelia [73], abnormalities of the genitourinary system [77,78] and limb–body abnormalities [79] possibly due to vasospasm in the fetal and uteroplacental circulations at a critical time in embryogenesis [80].

Chasnoff *et al*. [81] compared the offspring of a group of women who only abused marijuana in pregnancy with those who were also exposed to cocaine. Additional cocaine abuse was associated with an increased risk of intrauterine growth restriction; the marijuana-exposed group having reduced head size at birth alone. Several psychomotor indices remained impaired in the children at follow-up aged 2 years old [81]. This may well relate to the increased risk of cerebral infarction in the neonate of a cocaine-abusing mother shown by computed tomography (CT) scanning [82] and again thought to be due to cocaine-induced vasospasm [83].

The risks of preterm delivery, intrauterine growth restriction and accidental haemorrhage are approximately doubled in those who 'ever' abuse cocaine in pregnancy [84]. After adjusting for confounding variables such as alcohol abuse and smoking, the odds ratios for low birth-weight and growth restriction were about 1.6 in a large study of 483 women abusing cocaine in pregnancy [85]. Premature rupture of membranes and meconium staining of amniotic fluid are also more common [86]. However, it is possible that maternal cocaine abuse like maternal alcohol abuse (see above) may protect the preterm neonate from developing respiratory distress syndrome [87].

Cocaine abuse does not shorten labour as is commonly believed [88] and indeed it has been associated with acute fetal distress in labour [89].

In Portland, Oregon, neonatal cost for the infant of a cocaine-abusing mother averaged US$13 222 compared to US$1297 for the infant of a non-abusing mother [90]. These costs were largely due to the increased risk of prematurity. In another analysis [91] it was shown that between 1984 and 1988 there were an extra 4500 preterm infants born in New York compared to what would have been expected from analysis of data between 1968 and 1988. The increase in prematurity was almost certainly due to cocaine abuse; the cost of caring for these extra preterm infants was put at more than US$22 million at 1986 prices.

The most striking association between cocaine abuse and pregnancy is with accidental haemorrhage presumably related to hypertension induced by excess noradrenaline as described above. Several cases of abruption have been reported [92,93] all with large retroplacental clot and no evidence of coagulopathy, although additional thrombocytopenia has been recorded in one case [94].

Although obstetricians should be aware that hypertension in a cocaine user may be due to the drug rather than any other pathology, it is more important for them to try to stop their patients using the drug in the first place.

Benzodiazepines, lysergic acid diethylamide, cannabis, phencyclidine, amphetamines, toluene

Benzodiazepines such as temazepam are widely available as street drugs and many have become habituated from previous regular medical prescription. The latter should not be so much of a problem in women who are currently pregnant because regular benzodiazepine prescription has been discouraged for some time. In some studies use in early pregnancy has been associated with a low increased risk of birth defects, typically facial clefts and dysmorphic features; other studies have denied this association [95]. Management strategy concentrates on transferring the patient to a long-acting benzodiazepine such as diazepam and then reducing the daily intake very slowly.

Lysergic acid diethylamide (LSD) may be teratogenic. There are several isolated reports of phocomelia [96] and other typical amniotic band lesions [97,98], which have been discussed by Blanc *et al.* [99].

The use of cannabis six or more times per week during pregnancy is associated with a reduction in gestation by about 1 week after allowing for confounding variables [100]. It also causes growth restriction [101,102]. There is no direct evidence of teratogenicity in humans [103]. It remains controversial whether these agents cause chromosomal damage in humans [96]. Cannabis is secreted into breast milk [103]. Within these constraints, cannabis use in pregnancy is unlikely to be much of a problem.

Phencyclidine (PCP or 'angel dust') is a hallucinogen that is widely used by the American adolescent population. It is also used in pregnancy [104] and there have been reports of a dysmorphic fetus [105] and of neonatal withdrawal symptoms [106]. There are not sufficient data to state whether there are specific risks of phencyclidine abuse.

Amphetamine abuse has been studied in a group of 52 women [107]. The babies were growth restricted but no other abnormalities were significantly more frequent when compared to controls. Acute intravenous overdose has been implicated as a cause of intrauterine death [108].

Toluene, inhaled in patients who sniff glue, can cause renal tubular acidosis. Fetuses born from women who are acidotic at the time of delivery are compromised and usually growth restricted [109,110]. In addition the mother is at risk from hypokalaemia, cardiac dysrhythmias and rhabdomyolysis, which are exacerbated by β-sympathomimetic drugs given for preterm labour to which the patients are also susceptible.

References

1 Finnegan LP. Management of pregnant drug-dependent women. *Ann NY Acad Sci* 1978; 311: 135–46.
2 Finnegan LP. Pathophysiological and behavioural effects of the transplacental transfer of narcotic drugs to the foetuses and neonates of narcotic-dependent mothers. *Bull Narcotics* 1979; 31: 1–59.
3 Finnegan LP, ed. *Drug Dependence in Pregnancy. Clinical Management of Mother and Child.* Castle House Publications, 1980.
4 Farkas AG, Colbert DL, Erskine KJ. Anonymous testing for drug abuse in an antenatal population. *Br J Obstet Gynaecol* 1995; 102: 563–5.

5 Morrison C, Siney C. Maternity services for drug misusers in England and Wales: a national survey. *Health Trends* 1995; 27: 15–7.
6 Minkoff HL, McCalla S *et al.* The relationship of cocaine use to syphilis and human immunodeficiency virus infections among inner city parturient women. *Am J Obstet Gynecol* 1990; 163: 521–6.
7 Henderson CE, Terribile S, Keefe D, Merkatz IR. Cardiac screening for pregnant intravenous drug abusers. *Am J Perinatol* 1989; 6: 397–9.
8 Boike GM, Gove N *et al.* Mycotic aneurysms in pregnancy. *Am J Obstet Gynecol* 1987; 157: 340–1.
9 Van Winter JT, Nielsen SN, Ogburn PL Jr. Epidural abscess associated with intravenous drug abuse in a pregnant patient. *Mayo Clin Proc* 1991; 66: 1036–9.
10 Berkowitz K, LaSala A. Risk factors associated with the increasing prevalence of pneumonia during pregnancy. *Am J Obstet Gynecol* 1990; 163: 981–5.
11 Bowman J, Harman C *et al.* Intravenous drug abuse causes Rh immunization. *Vox Sang* 1991; 61: 96–8.
12 Hans SL. Demographic and psychosocial characteristics of substance-abusing pregnant women. *Clin Perinatol* 1999; 26 (1): 55–74.
13 Daley M, Argeriou M, McCarty D. Substance abuse treatment for pregnant women: a window of opportunity? *Addict Behav* 1998; 23 (2): 239–49.
14 Ostrea EM, Chavez CJ. Perinatal problems (excluding neonatal withdrawal) in maternal drug addiction. A study of 830 cases. *J Pediatr* 1979; 94: 292–4.
15 Glass L, Rajegowda BK, Evans HE. Absence of respiratory distress syndrome in premature infants of heroin addicted mothers. *Lancet* 1971; ii: 685–6.
16 Liu DTY, Tylden E, Tukel SH. Fetal response to drug withdrawal. *Lancet* 1976; ii: 588.
17 Umans JC, Szeto HH. Precipitated opiate abstinence *in utero*. *Am J Obstet Gynecol* 1983; 151: 441–4.
18 Zuspan FP, Gumpel JA *et al.* Fetal stress from methadone withdrawal. *Am J Obstet Gynecol* 1975; 122: 43–6.
19 Rementeria JL, Janakammal S, Hollander M. Multiple births in drug-addicted women. *Am J Obstet Gynecol* 1975; 122: 958–60.
20 Hill RM, Desmond MM. Management of the narcotic withdrawal syndrome in the neonate. *Pediatr Clin North Am* 1963; 10: 67–86.
21 Klenka HM. Babies born in a district general hospital to mothers taking heroin. *Br Med J* 1986; 298: 745–6.
22 Zelson C, Lee SJ, Casalino M. Neonatal narcotic addiction. Comparative effects of maternal intake of heroin and methadone. *N Engl J Med* 1973; 289: 1216–20.
23 Challis RE, Scopes JW. Late withdrawal symptoms in babies born to methadone addicts. *Lancet* 1977; ii: 1230.
24 Harper G, Concepeion GS, Blenman S. Observations on the sudden death of infants born to addicted mother. *Proceedings of the Fifth National Conference on Methadone Treatment.* National Association for the Prevention of Addiction to Narcotics, New York, 1983: 1122.
25 Peirson PS, Howard P, Kleber HD. Sudden deaths in infants born to methadone-maintained addicts. *J Am Med Assoc* 1972; 220: 1733.
26 Southall DP, Richards JM *et al.* Prospective population based studies into heart rate and breathing patterns in newborn infants: prediction of infants at risk of SIDS. *International Conference into SIDS*, Baltimore, 1982.

27 Ward SL, Bautista D *et al.* Sudden infant death syndrome in infants of substance abusing mothers. *J Pediatr* 1990; 117: 876–81.

28 Durand DJ, Espinoza AM, Nickerson BG. Association between prenatal cocaine exposure and sudden death infant syndrome. *J Pediatr* 1990; 117: 909–11.

29 Kandall SR, Gaines J, Habel L, Davidson G, Jessop D. Relationship of maternal substance abuse to subsequent sudden infant death syndrome in offspring. *J Pediatr* 1993; 123: 120–6.

30 Metcalfe J, Dunham MJ, Olsen CD, Krall MA. Respiratory and haemodynamic effects of methadone in pregnant women. *Respir Physiol* 1980; 42: 383–93.

31 Richardson BS, O'Grady JP, Olsen GD. Fetal breathing movements and the response to carbon dioxide in patients on methadone maintenance. *Am J Obstet Gynecol* 1984; 150: 400–5.

32 Sardemann H, Madsen KS, Friis-Hansen B. Followup of children of drug-addicted mothers. *Arch Dis Child* 1976; 51: 131–4.

33 Jacobson B, Nyberg K *et al.* Opiate addiction in adult offspring through possible imprinting after obstetric treatment. *Br Med J* 1990; 301: 1067–70.

34 O'Brien CP. Narcotic abuse during pregnancy. *N Engl J Med* 1974; 291: 311.

35 Rosner MA, Keith L, Chasnoff I. North Western University Drug Dependence Program: The impact of intensive perinatal care on labour and delivery outcomes. *Am J Obstet Gynecol* 1982; 144: 23–7.

36 Edelin KC, Curganious L, Golar K, Oellerich D. Methadone maintenance in pregnancy: consequences to care and outcome. *Obstet Gynecol* 1988; 71: 399–404.

37 Ward J, Hall W, Mattick RP. Role of maintenance treatment in opioid dependence. *Lancet* 1999; 353: 221–6.

38 Fultz JM, Senay EC. Guidelines for the management of hospitalized narcotic addicts. *Ann Intern Med* 1975; 82: 815.

39 Laken MP, McComish JF, Ager J. Predictors of prenatal substance use and birth weight during outpatient treatment. *J Subst Abuse Treat* 1997; 14 (4): 359–66.

40 Anyaegbunam A, Tran T, Jadali D, Randolph G, Mikhail MS. Assessment of fetal well-being in methadone-maintained pregnancies: abnormal nonstress tests. *Gynecol Obstet Invest* 1997; 43: 25–8.

41 Blinick G, Inturissi CE, Jerez E, Wallach RC. Methadone assays in pregnant women and their progeny. *Am J Obstet Gynecol* 1975; 121: 617–21.

42 Jones KL, Smith DW. Recognition of the fetal alcohol syndrome in early infancy. *Lancet* 1973; ii: 999–1001.

43 Halesmaki E, Raivo K, Ylikorkala O. A possible association between maternal drinking and fetal clubfoot. *N Engl J Med* 1985; 312: 790.

44 Gardner LI, Mitter N *et al.* Isochromosome 9q in an infant exposed to ethanol prenatally. *N Engl J Med* 1985; 312: 1521.

45 Spohr HL, Willms J, Steinhausen HC. Prenatal alcohol exposure and long term developmental consequences. *Lancet* 1993; 341: 907–10.

46 Streissguth AP, Aase JM *et al.* Fetal alcohol syndrome in adolescents and adults. *J Am Med Assoc* 1991; 265: 1961–7.

47 Ioffe S, Chernick V. Maternal alcohol ingestion and the incidence of respiratory distress syndrome. *Am J Obstet Gynecol* 1987; 156: 1231–5.

48 Beattie J, Day R, Cockburn F, Garg RA. Alcohol and the fetus in the West of Scotland. *Br Med J* 1983; 287: 17–20.

49 Halmesmaki E, Roine R, Salaspuro M. Gamma-glutamyl transferase, aspartate and alanine aminotransferases and their ratio, mean cell volume and urinary dolichol in pregnant alcohol abusers. *Br J Obstet Gynaecol* 1992; 99: 287–91.

50 Barrison IG, Wright TJ *et al.* Screening for alcohol abuse in pregnancy. *Br Med J* 1982; 285: 1318.

51 Ylikorkala O, Stenman UH, Halmesmaki E. γ-Glutamyl transferase and mean cell volume reveal maternal alcohol abuse and fetal alcohol effects. *Am J Obstet Gynecol* 1987; 157: 344–8.

52 Wright JT, Waterson EJ *et al.* Alcohol consumption, pregnancy and low birth weight. *Lancet* 1983; i: 663–5.

53 Wright JT, Toplis PJ. Alcohol in pregnancy. *Br J Obstet Gynaecol* 1986; 93: 201–2.

54 Serdula M, Williamson DF *et al.* Trends of alcohol consumption by pregnant women. *J Am Med Assoc* 1991; 265: 876–9.

55 Ouellette EM, Rosett HL, Rosman P, Weiner L. Adverse effects on offspring of maternal alcohol abuse during pregnancy. *N Engl J Med* 1977; 297: 528–30.

56 Davis PJM, Partridge JW, Storrs CN. Alcohol consumption in pregnancy. How much is safe? *Arch Dis Child* 1982; 57: 940–3.

57 Little RE, Sing CF. Association of father's drinking and infant's birth weight. *N Engl J Med* 1986; 314: 1644–5.

58 Forrest FV, Forey C *et al.* Reported social alcohol consumption during pregnancy and infants' development at 18 months. *Br Med J* 1991; 303: 22–6.

59 Sulaiman ND, Du V, Florey C, Taylor DJ, Ogston SA. Alcohol consumption in Dundee primigravidas and its effects on outcome of pregnancy. *Br Med J* 1988; 296: 1500–3.

60 Veghely PV. Fetal abnormality and maternal ethanol metabolism. *Lancet* 1983; ii: 53–4.

61 Ryle PR, Thomson AD. Acetaldehyde and fetal alcohol syndrome. *Lancet* 1983; ii: 219–20.

62 Sisenwein FE, Tejani NA, Boxer HS, DiGiuseppe R. Effects of methanol infusion during pregnancy on the growth and development of children at four to seven years of age. *Am J Obstet Gynecol* 1983; 147: 52–6.

63 Halmesmaki E, Ylikorkala O. The effect of maternal ethanol intoxication on fetal cardiotocography: a report of four cases. *Br J Obstet Gynaecol* 1986; 93: 203–5.

64 Lawton ME. Alcohol in breast milk. *Aust NZ J Obstet Gynaecol* 1985; 25: 71–3.

65 Mennella JA, Beauchamp CK. The transfer of alcohol to human milk. *N Engl J Med* 1991; 325: 981–5.

66 Little RE, Anderson KW *et al.* Maternal alcohol use during breast-feeding and infant mental and motor development at one year. *N Engl J Med* 1989; 321: 425–30.

67 Cregler LL, Mark H. Medical complications of cocaine abuse: special report. *N Engl J Med* 1986; 23: 1495–500.

68 Matera C, Warren WB *et al.* Prevalence of use of cocaine and other substances in an obstetric population. *Am J Obstet Gynecol* 1990; 163: 797–801.

69 Sloan LB, Gay JW, Snyder SW, Bales WR. Substance abuse during pregnancy in rural population. *Obstet Gynecol* 1992; 79: 245–8.

70 Schutzman DL, Frankenfield Chernicoff M, Clatterbaugh HE, Singer J. Incidence of intrauterine cocaine exposure in a suburban setting. *Pediatrics* 1991; 88: 825–7.

71 Colmorgen GH, Johnson C, Zazzarino MA, Durinzi K. Routine urine drug screening at the first prenatal visit. *Am J Obstet Gynecol* 1992; 166: 588–90.

72 McCalla S, Minkoff HL *et al.* Predictors of cocaine use in pregnancy. *Obstet Gynecol* 1992; 79 (641): 4.

73 Sarpong S, Headings V. Sirenomelia accompanying exposure of the embryo to cocaine. *South Med J* 1992; 85: 545–7.

74 Ostrea EM, Brady M, Cause S, Raymundo AL, Stevens M. Drug screening of newborns by meconium analysis: a large-scale, prospective, epidemiological study. *Pediatrics* 1992; 89: 107–13.

75 Volpe JJ. Effect of cocaine use on the fetus. *N Engl J Med* 1992; 327: 399–407.

76 Ness RB, Grisso JA *et al.* Cocaine and tobacco use and the risk of spontaneous abortion. *N Engl J Med* 1999; 340: 333–9.

77 Greenfield SP, Rutighano E, Steinhardt C, Elder JS. Genitourinary tract malformations and maternal cocaine abuse. *Urology* 1991; 37: 455–9.

78 Lutiger B, Graham K, Einarson TR, Koren G. Relationship between gestational cocaine use and pregnancy outcome: a meta-analysis. *Teratology* 1991; 44: 405–14.

79 Van Den Anker JN, Cohen Overbeek TE, Wladimiroff JW, Sauer PJJ. Prenatal diagnosis of limb-reduction defects due to maternal cocaine use. *Lancet* 1991; 338: 1332.

80 Viscarello RR, Ferguson DD, Nores J, Hobbins JC. Limb-body wall complex associated with cocaine abuse: further evidence of cocaine's teratogenicity. *Obstet Gynecol* 1992; 80: 523–6.

81 Chasnoff IJ, Griffith DR, Freier C, Murray J. Cocaine/polydrug use in pregnancy: two-year follow-up. *Pediatrics* 1992; 89: 284–9.

82 Heier LA, Carpanzano CR *et al.* Maternal cocaine abuse: the spectrum of radiologic abnormalities in the neonatal CNS. *Am J Neuroradiol* 1991; 12: 951–6.

83 Dixon SD, Bejar R. Echoencephalographic findings in neonates associated with maternal cocaine and methamphetamine use: incidence and clinical correlates. *J Pediatr* 1989; 155: 770–8.

84 Handler A, Kirstin N, Davis F, Ferre C. Cocaine use during pregnancy: perinatal outcomes. *Am J Epidemiol* 1991; 133: 818–25.

85 Sprauve ME, Lindsay MK, Herbert S, Graves W. Adverse perinatal outcome in parturients who use crack cocaine. *Obstet Gynecol* 1997; 89: 674–8.

86 Mastrogiannis DS, Decavalas GO, Verma U, Tejani N. Perinatal outcome after recent cocaine usage. *Obstet Gynecol* 1990; 76: 8–11.

87 Zuckerman B, Maynard EC, Cabral H. A preliminary report of perinatal cocaine exposure and respiratory distress syndrome in premature infants. *Am J Dis Child* 1991; 145: 696–8.

88 Dombrowski MP, Wolfe HM, Welch RA, Evans MI. Cocaine abuse is associated with abruptio placentae and decreased birthweight, but not shorter labour. *Obstet Gynecol* 1991; 77: 139–41.

89 Sztulman L, Ducey JJ, Tancer NIL. Intrapartum intranasal cocaine use and acute fetal distress. *J Reprod Med* 1990; 35: 917–8.

90 Calhoun BC, Watson PT. The cost of maternal cocaine abuse: 1. Perinatal cost. *Obstet Gynecol* 1991; 78: 731–4.

91 Joyce T. The dramatic increase in the rate of low birthweight in New York city: an aggregate timeseries analysis. *Am J Publ Health* 1990; 80: 682–4.

92 Acker D, Sachs BP, Tracey KJ, Wise WE. Abruptio placentae associated with cocaine use. *Am J Obstet Gynecol* 1983; 146: 220–1.

93 Chasnoff LJ, Burns WJ Schnoll SH, Burns KA. Cocaine use in pregnancy. *N Engl J Med* 1985; 313: 666–7.

94 Abramowicz JS, Sherer M, Woods JR Jr. Acute transient thrombocytopenia associated with cocaine abuse in pregnancy. *Obstet Gynecol* 1991; 78: 499–501.

95 Dolovitch LR, Addis A, Vaillancourt JMR, Power B, Einarson TR. Benzodiazepine use in pregnancy and major malformations or oral cleft: meta-analysis of cohort and case-control studies. *Br Med J* 1998; 317: 839–43.

96 Hecht F, Beals RK *et al.* Lysergic-acid-diethylamide and cannabis as possible teratogens in man. *Lancet* 1968; ii: 1087.

97 Assemany SR, Neu RL, Gardner LL. Deformities in a child whose mother took LSD. *Lancet* 1970; i: 1290.

98 Carakushansky G, Neu KL, Gardner LL. Lysergide and cannabis as possible teratogens in man. *Lancet* 1969; i: 150–1.

99 Blanc WA, Mattison DR, Kane R, Chauhan P. LSD, intrauterine amputations and amniotic-band syndrome. *Lancet* 1971; ii: 158–9.

100 Fried PA, Watkinson B, Willan A. Marijuana use during pregnancy and decreased length of gestation. *Am J Obstet Gynecol* 1984; 150: 23–7.

101 Frank DA, Bauchner H, Parker S. Neonatal body proportionality and body composition after *in utero* exposure to cocaine and marijuana. *J Pediatr* 1990; 117: 622–6.

102 Zuckerman B, Frank DA *et al.* Effects of maternal marijuana and cocaine use on fetal growth. *N Engl J Med* 1989; 320: 762–8.

103 Ashton CH. Cannabis: dangers and possible uses. *Br Med J* 1987; 294: 141–2.

104 Golden NL, Kulmert BR *et al.* Phencyclidine use during pregnancy. *Am J Obstet Gynecol* 1984; 148: 254–9.

105 Golden NL, Sokol RJ, Rubin K. Angel dust: possible effects on the fetus. *Pediatrics* 1980; 65: 16.

106 Strauss AA, Modanlou HD, Basu SK. Neonatal manifestations of maternal phencyclidine (PCP) abuse. *Pediatrics* 1981; 68: 550.

107 Little BB, Snell LM, Cilstrap LC. Methamphetamine abuse during pregnancy: outcome and fetal effects. *Obstet Gynecol* 1988; 72: 541–4.

108 Dearlove JC, Betteridge TJ, Henry JA. Stillbirth due to intravenous amphetamine. *Br Med J* 1992; 304: 548.

109 Goodwin TM. Toluene abuse and renal tubular acidosis in pregnancy. *Obstet Gynecol* 1988; 71: 715–18.

110 Wilkins Hang L, Gabow PA. Toluene abuse during pregnancy: obstetric complications and perinatal outcome. *Obstet Gynecol* 1991; 77: 504–9.

20 Skin diseases in pregnancy

Samantha Vaughan Jones and Martin M. Black

Pregnancy is a period of profound temporary hormonal change, which may affect the skin in numerous ways. Many are so common that they are not considered abnormal and are classified as 'physiological skin changes'. Other dermatoses occur less frequently and are specifically associated with the gravid state. Finally, pregnancy may modify pre-existing dermatological conditions. For other reviews see [1–3].

Physiological skin changes in pregnancy

There are a number of common skin changes in pregnancy that are thought to be related to hormonal changes.

Pigmentation

Hyperpigmentation is very common during pregnancy and occurs in up to 90% of women [4]. It is one of the most commonly recognized signs of pregnancy and may be generalized or restricted to areas of normal hyperpigmentation such as nipples, areolae, perineum, vulva and perianal region. The linea alba, a tendinous median line on the anterior abdominal wall, frequently hyperpigments to become the linear nigra and may extend from the symphysis pubis to xiphisternum. Pigmentation increases in the first trimester particularly in dark-haired, dark-complexioned women and fades postpartum, although it seldom returns to the pre-pregnancy level. Freckles and melanocytic naevi tend to darken and may increase in number. Recent scars may also hyperpigment.

Melasma

Irregular, sharply demarcated patches of facial pigmentation known as melasma develop in approximately 70% of women during the second half of pregnancy [4,5]. Melasma also occurs in up to 30% of women taking oral contraceptives [6] and in essentially healthy women between early adulthood and the menopause [7]. The most common pattern is centrofacial, involving the forehead, cheeks, upper lip, nose and chin. The malar pattern is limited to cheeks and nose, and the mandibular type involves the ramus of the mandible [8]. Histologically, there are two patterns of pigmentation: the epidermal type, which occurs in 72% of cases, in which the melanin is deposited mainly in the basal melanocytes, and the dermal type, which affects 13% of patients, where the melanin is mainly in the superficial and deep dermis [8]. Examination under Wood's light shows enhancement of colour contrast if melanin is primarily in the epidermis, and not if the melanin is located only in the dermis. Nearly 90% of women with chloasma due to oral contraception have a past history of melasma of pregnancy [6].

PATHOGENESIS

Oestrogen and progesterone are known to be strong melanogenic stimulants [9] and these hormones may well be responsible for the hyperpigmentation of pregnancy. Serum and urinary melanocyte-stimulating hormone (MSH) levels have been reported as elevated during pregnancy with a rapid decrease postpartum [10]. Other work has, however, demonstrated no difference in β-MSH levels in the third trimester and after parturition [11]. Levels of β-MSH were higher than the mean level obtained from non-pregnant controls but were within the normal range and therefore thought unlikely to be responsible for the pigmentary changes.

The patterns of pigmentation may relate to differences in end-organ sensitivity or distribution of melanocytes. Sun exposure may also be relevant in the development of melasma.

TREATMENT

Treatment is unsatisfactory and consists of minimizing exposure to sunlight and subsequent avoidance of oral contraceptives. Sunscreens should be used and cosmetic camouflage with non-allergic products is helpful. Depigmenting agents may be effective and Kligman and Willis [12] report success in 14 out of 16 patients using twice-daily application of 5% hydroquinone, 0.1% tretinoin and 0.1% dexamethasone in ethanol and propylene glycol for 5–7 weeks. Sanchez *et al.* [8] recommends the use of 2% hydroquinone and 0.05% tretinoin on the epidermal type of persistent melasma and believes that the dermal types respond poorly if at all to this therapy. Depigmenting agents should always be used with caution as dermatitis, further hyperpigmentation or even hypopigmentation may ensue. Melasma usually fades within 1 year of delivery [13], although in one study 30% of cases persisted after 10 years [10].

Pruritus gravidarum

This term refers to intense pruritus that occurs as a manifestation of pregnancy, without any associated rash or clinical jaundice and usually in early pregnancy. Pruritus from all causes occurs in 17% of pregnant women [4] and may be due to scabies, pediculosis, urticaria, atopic eczema, drug eruptions, candidiasis, trichomonal vaginitis or neurodermatitis. Once these underlying conditions have been excluded, a small group of patients remains whose pruritus is due to alteration in hepatic function. Such women may have mild obstetric cholestasis (OC) [14] (see Chapter 9 where OC is described in detail).

TREATMENT

Mild forms of pruritus gravidarum may be treated with bland topical antipruritic creams such as calamine. Antihistamines may be a useful adjunct. However, in some patients the pruritus may be so severe that preterm delivery is necessary.

Pruritus gravidarum and OC usually settle rapidly postpartum but may recur with subsequent pregnancies and the oral contraceptive. The maternal and fetal prognosis is normal except in those patients with frank OC (see Chapter 9).

Vascular changes

OEDEMA

Clinically apparent oedema of the face and hands occurs in approximately 50% of pregnant women, whilst oedema of the legs not associated with pre-eclampsia develops in about 80% [4]. It is usually non-pitting in nature and worse in the morning. It is probably due to several factors: increased fluid retention (approximately 2.5 L during pregnancy), increased vascular permeability, increased blood flow [15] and decreased colloid osmotic pressure of plasma.

SPIDER NAEVI

Vascular spiders develop between the second and fifth months of pregnancy and are present in about 57% of white women and 10% of black women by the third trimester [16]. This difference is probably due to difficulty in visualizing them on dark skin. In comparison, spider naevi are said to occur in 15% of normal non-pregnant white women. They occur in the areas drained by the superior vena cava on the upper trunk and face, increase in size and number throughout pregnancy and fade postpartum. The majority (75%) have disappeared by the seventh week after delivery [16]; the remainder persist and recurrence may occur at the same sites in subsequent pregnancies. Clinically they are indistinguishable from the spider naevi of chronic liver disease and consist of a central pulsating arteriole with radiating telangiectases. Treatment for persistent lesion is with cold point cautery or pulsed dye laser.

PALMAR ERYTHEMA

Palmar erythema develops during pregnancy in 70% of white women and 35% of black women [16]. Its onset is in the first trimester and it fades within 1 week of delivery. There are two clinical patterns: (i) diffuse mottling of the whole palm; and (ii) erythema confined to the thenar and hypothenar eminences. The former is the more common. It frequently occurs in patients who also have spider naevi and both are thought to be due to high oestrogen levels. The increases in blood volume and blood flow are other possible factors.

VARICES

Varices may affect as many as 40% of pregnant women and may involve the saphenous system or small superficial vessels in the legs, as well as the haemorrhoidal and vulvar networks. They are due to several factors: increased venous pressure in femoral and pelvic vessels due to compression from the gravid uterus, increase in the blood volume, increased collagen fragility and a hereditary tendency to varicose veins. Varices tend to regress postpartum, although not always completely.

Treatment is elevation of the legs and elastic support stockings. Thrombosis may occur in leg varices or in haemorrhoids. Thromboembolism in pregnancy is considered in Chapter 4.

HAEMANGIOMATA

Haemangiomata develop on the head and neck in 5% of pregnant women, appearing at the end of the first trimester and enlarging until term [13]. The 'pregnancy tumour' or telangiectatic epulis, is a similar lesion sited on oral mucosa or gingiva. It usually develops at between 2 and 5 months gestation, affects 2% of pregnant women and arises from interdental papillae on the buccal or lingual surfaces of the gingiva. It is usually associated with extensive gingivitis and may bleed or ulcerate. All these lesions may be initiated by trauma and resemble pyogenic granulomata both clinically and histologically. Pre-existing haemangiomata may increase in size. High oestrogen levels are probably an aetiological factor. Surgical removal is the treatment for lesions, which persist postpartum.

PURPURA

This may occur on the legs during the second half of pregnancy due to increased capillary permeability and fragility [13]. Vasculitis and thrombocytopenia must be excluded.

Connective tissue and collagen

STRIAE (GRAVIDARUM AND DISTENSAE)

Striae gravidarum develop during the second half of pregnancy in most women. They occur on the abdomen, breasts and thighs. Initially they are pink or violaceous linear wrinkles, which develop perpendicular to skin tension lines. They become white and atrophic with time, although never disappear completely. They are identical to the striae associated with puberty, obesity, Cushing's disease and steroid therapy.

The aetiology of striae is multifactorial: stretching is a localizing factor and striae do tend to occur more with overweight mothers or those carrying heavier babies or with multiple pregnancy [17]. There is also a familial tendency [18]. Rupture of collagen and elastic fibres [19], and increased adrenocortical activity have been considered important [17]. It has also been suggested that oestrogen and relaxin increase the collagen and sulphate-free mucopolysaccharides and that subsequent stretching leads to easier separation of collagen [18].

Histologically, striae consist of areas of broken and curled elastic fibres in the upper dermis with parallel bands of collagen and elastic fibres in the centre [20]. Fibrillin microfibrils in the elastic fibre network appear to be reduced and reorganized in skin affected by striae [21]. There is no specific treatment for striae and it is controversial as to whether emollient massage is effective in their prevention [17]. Topical tretinoin cream 0.025% does not appear to have any beneficial effect [22].

SKIN TAGS OR MOLLUSCUM FIBROSUM GRAVIDARUM

Soft, fleshy, pendunculated, skin-coloured or slightly pigmented papillomata may develop on the face, neck, upper anterior chest, axillae and under the breasts during the second half of pregnancy. They are about 1–5 mm in diameter and clinically and histologically identical to skin tags [23]. They are probably due to hormonal factors and regress postpartum. Persisting lesions may be removed by electrodesiccation.

Glandular activity

SWEAT AND APOCRINE GLANDS

Eccrine sweating is increased during pregnancy [24] and may be associated with milia (due to occlusion of the sweat ducts) and intertrigo. Palmar eccrine sweating is, however, diminished [25]. Apocrine activity is also reduced with subsequent improvement of conditions such as Fox–Fordyce disease and hidradenitis suppurativa [3], which may, however, rebound postpartum.

SEBACEOUS GLANDS

Sebaceous activity increases during the third trimester, and acne occasionally develops during pregnancy. Sebaceous glands associated with lactiferous ducts on the areolae, hypertrophy as early as 6 weeks' gestation and appear as Montgomery's tubercles. They are one of the signs of early pregnancy.

Hair changes

TELOGEN EFFLUVIUM

The proportion of hairs in anagen (the growing phase) increases during pregnancy [26]. Postpartum, the conversion from anagen hairs to telogen (resting) hairs is accelerated and postpartum hair loss or 'telogen effluvium' follows after 4–20 weeks [3]. Normally about 15% of scalp hairs are in the telogen phase and in pregnancy this falls to 5%, rising within a few months of delivery to 25%. The hair loss is generally diffuse, although may be more marked in the frontoparietal hairline in women with a tendency to male-pattern baldness. Baldness seldom, if ever, occurs, and spontaneous recovery usually takes place within 6 months of delivery [27], although it may take as long as 15 months [3]. Recovery is usually complete unless the telogen effluvium is severe, repeated in several pregnancies or associated with male-pattern alopecia. With successive pregnancies hair loss tends to be less marked.

The diagnosis is made by finding large numbers of club hairs. Histologically, the follicles in telogen are normal. Increased adrenocorticosteroids and ovarian androgens probably account for the increase in anagen hairs, and oestrogens prolong the anagen phase [5]. Telogen effluvium is probably caused by several factors including changes in endocrine balance, the stress of delivery, difficult labour and blood loss. No specific treatment is required apart from reassurance.

Some women develop male-pattern hair loss in late pregnancy while in others the loss is diffuse. This is due to inhibition of anagen in some follicles and not due to increased loss. The regrowth with the male-pattern hair loss in unlikely to be complete.

There is no significant change in the anagen/telogen ratio of body hair [28].

HIRSUTISM

Hypertrichosis, most marked on face, arms and legs, is quite common in pregnancy but marked hirsutism is rare. It resolves postpartum but recurrence in subsequent pregnancies frequently occurs.

Hirsutism may be accompanied by acne, deepening of the voice and clitoral enlargement and is probably due to increased adrenocorticosteroid and ovarian androgen secretion. Other causes of hirsutism, namely androgen-secreting ovarian tumours and polycystic ovaries, should be excluded. Treatment is with reassurance and cosmetic removal (depilatory creams, electrolysis or ruby laser).

Nails

Nail changes, consisting of transverse grooving, brittleness, distal onycholysis and subungual keratosis, may occur from the sixth week. The pathogenesis of these changes is not known. There is no effective treatment.

Breasts and nipples

Sore nipples with cracks and fissures commonly develop in the first few days of breastfeeding. The soreness may limit sucking, and stasis, mastitis or breast abscess may follow. Nipple eczema may also develop and involve the breast. Secondary infection must be excluded. Fissures and eczema are avoided by gentle washing to remove saliva and milk and by use of emollients. The breasts should be left exposed if possible and secondary infection treated with antibiotics. Severely affected patients are often atopic.

Dermatoses specific to pregnancy

A number of dermatoses are specific to pregnancy, to the puerperium or occur as a result of trophoblastic tumours. They have recently been reclassified into the following groups:
1 pemphigoid gestationis (herpes gestationis);
2 polymorphic eruption of pregnancy;
3 prurigo of pregnancy; and
4 pruritic folliculitis of pregnancy.

Pemphigoid (herpes) gestationis

Pemphigoid (herpes) gestationis (PG) is an intensely pruritic bullous eruption that occurs in one in 60 000 pregnancies [29] or in association with the trophoblastic tumours, chorioncarcinoma [30] and hydatidiform mole [31]. The eruption initially consists of pruritic erythematous urticated papules and plaques, target lesions and annular wheals. Vesicles develop after a delay varying between a few days and a month and enlarge to become tense bullae (Fig. 20.1). In 90% of patients the lesions begin in the periumbilical region and spread to involve thighs, breast, palms and soles (Fig. 20.1). The face and oral mucosa are only rarely involved. It may begin during the first or any subsequent pregnancy arising between 9 weeks' gestation and 1 week postpartum [32]. In subsequent pregnancies recurrence usually occurs with an earlier onset and more severe disease. When PG develops during the mid-trimester, there is usually a period of relative remission in the last few weeks of pregnancy followed by an abrupt postpartum flare [15]. The bullous lesions tend to resolve

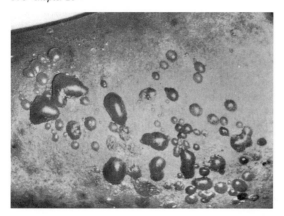

Fig 20.1 Pemphigoid gestationis. Large tense bullae on the thigh.

within a month of delivery, but the urticated plaques may persist for over a year [32].

The aetiology of PG is unknown, but recent work highlights the immunopathological findings in this disease. Paternal histocompatibility antigens (human leucocyte antigens (HLAs)) were considered important following a study in which 50% of the consorts were HLA-DR2 compared to 25% of the controls [33]. However, this was not confirmed in another study in which the frequency of paternal HLAs was normal [34]. A paternal factor is likely, as in some patients with pregnancies by several consorts the onset of PG has coincided with a change in partner, and in one case a patient had PG in her first and second pregnancies and then had an unaffected pregnancy by a new consort [34].

Maternal HLA studies have revealed a significantly increased frequency of DR3 with DR4 [33]. DR3 and DR4 are associated with other diseases with an immune pathogenesis such as Graves' disease, rheumatoid arthritis and insulin-dependent diabetes mellitus, which suggests that their presence confers an increase in immune susceptibility in the patients with PG. A recent study has confirmed the association between PG and other autoimmune diseases, particularly Graves' disease [35]. The antigenic trigger is probably paternally derived as PG occurs not only in pregnancy but also in association with hydatidiform mole and chorioncarcinoma, and in these trophoblastic tumours, the chromosomes are all paternally derived. There is also evidence that DR compatibility between mother and fetus favours a spared pregnancy [36]. Once initiated, PG is undoubtedly hormonally modulated.

Exacerbations may occur with ovulation or premenstrually, suggesting that oestrogen is responsible. It tends to be in a phase of relative remission in late pregnancy and flares postpartum when the most significant hormonal change is a fall in progesterone. Progesterone has been shown to have immunosuppressive effects similar to glucocorticoids and may exert an inhibiting effect on PG [37]. Exacerbations may also be induced by taking the contraceptive pill [37]. Holmes *et al.* [36] prescribed oral contraceptives to eight patients and four experienced exacerbations; three were given combined oestrogen and progesterone, but the patient who flared most severely was given oestrogen alone. Two patients were given progesterone alone and their PG was unaffected. There is experimental evidence that at certain concentrations oestrogen may have immunoenhancing properties [39] and this may account for its effect in PG. Holmes *et al.* [36] also demonstrated that breastfeeding was associated with a shorter and less severe postpartum illness suggesting that prolactin may have an immunosuppressant effect on the disease.

FETAL PROGNOSIS

It has been stated that PG is associated with an increased fetal and maternal risk [40], although other workers have disagreed and found that fetal prognosis was normal [41]. In a study of 50 infants from affected pregnancies, there was a significant increase in babies of low birthweight and small-for-dates babies which did not correlate with the severity or duration of PG [40,42]. There were no stillbirths or maternal deaths and none of the four neonatal deaths were ascribed to PG. One infant developed a bullous eruption resembling PG, which resolved within a week. A more recent study [35] has once again indicated a tendency for premature delivery to be associated with PG. As small-for-dates infants have a raised morbidity, it is essential that patients with PG are delivered in maternity units with access to special care facilities.

PATHOLOGY

Histologically, the early urticated lesions of PG show epidermal and papillary dermal oedema with occasional foci of eosinophilic spongiosis [43]. The bullae are subepidermal and contain numerous eosinophils. Ultrastructurally, the split occurs within the lamina lucida [43,44].

Direct immunofluorescence demonstrates C3 at the basement membrane zone in all patients with active PG [37]. Indirect immunofluorescence usually shows a C3 binding factor [44]. This PG factor is an IgG of the IgG1 or IgG3 subclass [45] and although it is only positive in 25% of cases by conventional techniques, it can be demonstrated more reliably by immunoelectron microscopy [46].

DIFFERENTIAL DIAGNOSIS

The main differential diagnoses are from the much more common polymorphic eruption of pregnancy (PEP), and from bullous pemphigoid.

PEP usually affects primigravidae, and the eruption starts in prominent striae. Urticarial plaques, wheals and vesicles may occur in both disorders but only become frankly bullous in PG [37]. Histologically there are no features of early lesions to distinguish between the two, but on direct immunofluorescence, PEP is consistently negative [32,37] (Table 20.1).

PG and bullous pemphigoid share several features. Both are characterized by pruritic, urticarial and bullous eruptions. Histological and immunofluorescent findings are also closely similar. However, the lesions of PG occur predominantly on the lower abdomen and thighs, whilst the distribution in bullous pemphigoid is more variable. The clinical activity of PG is affected by oestrogen and progesterone, but there is no evidence that these have any effect on bullous pemphigoid. Finally, the frequency of HLAs in bullous pemphigoid is normal. Nevertheless, considerable similarities between PG and bullous pemphigoid led to the suggestion that 'pemphigoid' gestationis is a more appropriate term than 'herpes' gestationis [32,37]. Two cases reported evolved from PG into bullous pemphigoid again demonstrating the close links between these two dermatoses [47].

TREATMENT

Mild cases of PG respond to treatment with antihistamines and topical fluorinated corticosteroids. Systemic steroids are indicated in more severe disease with bullae. Most cases respond to 40 mg daily of prednisolone and this can usually be reduced fairly rapidly to a daily maintenance dose of 10 mg. It should be increased again in anticipation of the postpartum flare, which occurs so frequently. Plasmapheresis should be considered for severe cases [48]. Dapsone is best avoided as it can cause haemolytic disease of the newborn [49], although it has been given safely to treat leprosy during pregnancy [50]. A single case has recently been reported of complete remission of severe PG during treatment with ritodrine commenced for premature labour [51]. However, for the present, systemic steroids remain the mainstay of treatment. Recently the use of new luteinizing hormone releasing hormone (LHRH) analogue, goserelin, led to a complete temporary remission in a long-standing case of PG [52].

MATERNAL PROGNOSIS

Once a patient has had an affected pregnancy, PG will usually recur in subsequent pregnancies [15] with an earlier onset and more severe disease. Thus, many would caution against further pregnancy. However, occasional 'skipped' pregnancies can occur and some mothers are prepared to risk another pregnancy. HLA-DR3 typing may be a useful prognostic indicator as the absence of DR3 is associated with milder disease.

Polymorphic eruption of pregnancy

This pruritic urticarial eruption develops in and around abdominal striae in approximately one in 240 pregnancies. It has previously been classified as pruritic urticarial papules and plaques of pregnancies [53,54], toxaemic rash of pregnancy [55] or late-onset prurigo of pregnancy [56,57]. It has been suggested that these are all synonyms for the same eruption and PEP has been proposed [58]. Three clinical subtypes of PEP have recently been

Table 20.1 Comparison of pemphigoid gestationis and polymorphic eruption of pregnancy. (From [32].)

	Pemphigoid gestationis	Polymorphic eruption of pregnancy
Incidence per 100 000 pregnancies	2	420
Postpartum exacerbations	75%	15%
+ve direct immunofluorescence	100%	0%
HLA-DR3	84%	46%
Associated autoimmune phenomena	+	−
Morphology		
Urticarial lesions	+	+
Vesicles	+	+
Bullae	+	−
Prominent striae	3%	81%
Umbilical lesions	87%	12%

described [59]: type I, mainly urticarial papules and plaques; type II, non-urticarial erythema; type III, papules or vesicles and combinations of the two forms. Seventy-six per cent of affected women are primigravidae, and recurrence with subsequent pregnancies is rare [58]. PEP is significantly associated with increased abdominal skin distension and multiple pregnancies [60,61]. If a second episode does occur, it is much less severe than the first, which is in direct contrast to PG. Severe cases of PEP can closely mimic the early stages of PG and thus direct immunofluorescence can be a useful diagnostic test [62].

A recent prospective study of 44 cases of PEP showed low cortisol levels compared to controls, suggesting a hormonal influence [63]. Furthermore, a male/female ratio of 2:1 was found in the offspring of affected women [63]. This may be relevant in the light of a preliminary study of male DNA detection in the skin of women with PEP [64]. The results of this study indicate that fetal cells can migrate to maternal skin during pregnancy (a phenomenon known as microchimerism). Such migration of fetal DNA may be an important factor in the pathogenesis of PEP and was not seen in the skin of pregnant women without skin disease [64].

Polymorphic eruption generally begins in the last 5 weeks of pregnancy and rarely persists for more than a few weeks. It usually begins in prominent abdominal striae and may remain confined to the abdomen with relative sparing of the umbilicus (Fig. 20.2). Sometimes it becomes widespread involving buttocks, shoulders and limbs. The lesions consist of urticarial papules, plaques and polycyclic wheals (Fig. 20.3). Vesicles occur in approximately 45% and target lesions in 19%, but the vesicles rarely enlarge beyond 2 mm [58] and thus bullous lesions as in PG are hardly ever seen.

Histology of the urticarial papules shows epidermal and upper dermal oedema with a perivascular infiltrate

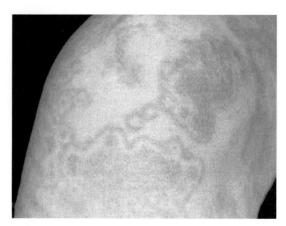

Fig 20.3 Polymorphic eruption of pregnancy. Polycyclic wheals on the knee.

of lymphocytes, histiocytes and eosinophils. With the vesicular lesions, vesicular spongiosis occurs. Immunofluorescence is consistently negative [58].

Treatment is with antihistamines and mild topical steroids. Systemic corticosteroids have been effective in extensive disease [65]. In very severe cases elective delivery may be the only way to relieve pruritus [66].

Prurigo of pregnancy

This pruritic papular eruption affects one in 300 pregnancies [57] and begins earlier in pregnancy than PEP. It is also referred to as prurigo gestationis of Besnier and 'early-onset prurigo of pregnancy'. The onset is usually between 25 and 30 weeks' gestation and although the pruritus settles at delivery, the papules tend to persist for several months. The lesions consist of groups of excoriated papules on the extensor surface of limbs and abdomen, although they may become widespread.

Histology of the lesions demonstrates parakeratosis, acanthosis and perivascular lymphocytic infiltrate. Immunofluorescence is negative.

The cause is unknown, but many patients appear to be atopic. It has been suggested that prurigo of pregnancy may be the result of pruritus gravidarum developing in atopic individuals [32].

The rash may recur in subsequent pregnancies and there is no increased risk to mother or fetus. Treatment is symptomatic with antihistamines and topical corticosteroids.

Pruritic folliculitis of pregnancy

This is a pruritic folliculitis that begins between the fourth month of gestation and term and usually resolves by 2

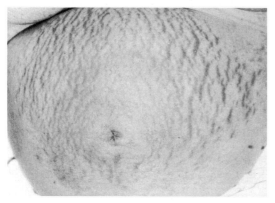

Fig 20.2 Polymorphic eruption of pregnancy. Urticarial lesions in prominent abdominal striae.

weeks postpartum [67]. The eruption is acneiform with widespread follicular erythematous papules.

As the clinical appearance resembles the monomorphic type of acne seen in some patients taking systemic corticosteroids, it is possible that pruritic folliculitis may be a form of hormonally induced acne rather than a specific dermatosis of pregnancy. Histopathology demonstrates acute folliculitis with focal spongiosis and exocytosis of polymorphonuclear and mononuclear cells. In the dermis, there is oedema and a perivascular infiltrate. Direct immunofluorescence is negative. The maternal and fetal prognosis is normal. Treatment is with topical 10% benzoyl peroxide and 1% hydrocortisone. Serum androgens do not appear to be elevated in this condition [68,69]. However, a recent prospective study of 14 cases showed a male/female ratio of 2:1 in the offspring of affected women and a significant reduction in birthweight compared to controls [68].

Papular dermatitis of pregnancy

This was described as a distinct entity by Spangler *et al.* [71] as a widespread papular dermatitis associated with a significant fetal mortality of 30% [70]. The authors found characteristic biochemical changes with elevated urinary chorionic gonadotrophin levels in the last trimester and reduced plasma cortisol and urinary oestriol. Spangler *et al.* [70] felt that the clinical feature that distinguished those with papular dermatitis of pregnancy from those with prurigo of pregnancy was that the lesions were widespread rather than grouped on the extensor surfaces of limbs. Holmes and Black [58], however, suggested that these cases of Spangler *et al.* do not justify a separate classification and may simply represent more florid examples of prurigo of pregnancy or PEP [58]. It is important to point out that similar biochemical studies have not been performed in other specific dermatoses of pregnancy. Spangler *et al.* [70,71] claimed that administration of systemic steroids or diethylstilboestrol dramatically improved the fetal mortality to approximately 12%. However, in the following year in a letter to the editor, this statement was withdrawn [72].

The fetal mortality of 30% that was reported [70] has not been confirmed subsequently. Vaughan Jones *et al.* [63] in their prospective study of 200 women with pregnancy dermatoses showed an overall fetal mortality of less than 5%. Furthermore, no cases of papular dermatitis were identified in this study. Thus, papular dermatitis is no longer considered to be a separate pregnancy dermatosis, but probably forms part of the spectrum of PEP or prurigo of pregnancy.

Autoimmune progesterone dermatitis of pregnancy

A single case of autoimmune progesterone dermatitis of pregnancy was described by Bierman [73]. It consisted of a non-pruritic acneiform eruption with papules, pustules and comedones on the fingers, arms, legs and buttocks. The eruption recurred in a subsequent pregnancy and both pregnancies terminated in spontaneous abortion. The striking histopathological features were of intense accumulation of eosinophils in hair follicles, epidermis, dermis and subcutis. Intradermal testing with aqueous progesterone produced a delayed hypersensitivity reaction, and administration of an oral contraceptive containing norethindrone and mestranol resulted in a severe flare of the eruption. No premenstrual flares occurred. The dermatitis, which resolved rapidly on treatment with conjugated oestrogens, probably represents hypersensitivity to endogenous progesterone. No similar cases have since been reported.

The more common autoimmune progesterone dermatitis not associated with pregnancy is clinically distinct and consists of a polymorphic rash with urticaria, papulopustular vesicular or erythema multiforme-like lesions that recur on the trunk and extremities in the premenstrual period [74]. It is associated with previous use of progesterone-containing oral medication, which appears to sensitize the body to endogenous progesterone [74]. There is usually a positive intradermal skin test to progesterone and treatments include conjugated oestrogens or oophorectomy [75]. Tamoxifen 30 mg has also caused complete remission but with consequent amenorrhoea [76]. The anabolic androgen danazol (200 mg twice daily given just before the onset of a period) has also proved effective in two cases [77].

The effect of pregnancy on other dermatoses

The effect of pregnancy on other skin disorders is generally unpredictable, although individual patients may react consistently.

Eczema

Atopic eczema is frequently exacerbated during pregnancy. In addition, if pruritus gravidarum develops, there may be further exacerbation with development of prurigo. A recent prospective study of 200 women with pregnancy dermatoses showed eczema to be the commonest skin complaint during pregnancy [63]. In some cases it presented *de novo* during pregnancy. Hand and nipple eczema are both common in the puerperium and often require treatment with emollients and moderately potent topical corticosteroids.

Acne vulgaris

The effect of pregnancy on acne vulgaris is variable. Some patients improve whilst others develop acne for the first time. In these patients acne is often limited to the chin and may be associated with hirsutism. Tetracyclines and retinoids frequently prescribed for acne are contraindicated during pregnancy and their withdrawal may result in a flare.

Psoriasis and impetigo herpetiformis

Psoriasis may remain unchanged, clear or worsen and may also only manifest itself during pregnancy. Impetigo herpetiformis is a rare form of pustular psoriasis, which can develop at any stage of gestation. The eruption consists of urticated erythema, which begins in the flexures especially in the inguinal region. Superficial sterile pustules form at the margins of the lesions and the eruption may become widespread with involvement of mucosal surfaces. Fever, malaise, neutrophilia, hypocalcaemia and tetany are associated.

The histopathology is similar to that of pustular psoriasis with intraepidermal and subcorneal spongiform pustules of Kogoi and a perivascular infiltrate [78].

The disease usually remits at delivery but recurs with each subsequent pregnancy and with oral contraceptive therapy [79]. The main obstetric problem is placental insufficiency, which can lead to stillbirth, neonatal death and fetal abnormalities [80]. Management requires intensive medical care with fluid and electrolyte replacement and correction of hypocalcaemia. Antibiotics are indicated for secondary infection, and systemic corticosteroids may be helpful. Low-dose methotrexate can be substituted postpartum to prevent rebound pustulation, but is contraindicated during pregnancy and lactation. Gonadotrophins are also reported to be helpful [81]. Fetal well-being should be carefully monitored and elective caesarean section may be necessary to improve fetal morbidity [82].

Condylomata acuminata

Condylomata acuminata tend to grow rapidly during pregnancy even to the extent of interfering with delivery. Treatment with podophyllin is contraindicated but electrocoagulation and curettage may be effective.

Candidiasis

Candidiasis is 10–20 times more common in pregnancy when lowered vaginal pH and increased sweating create a favourable environment. It may be associated with pruritus vulvae and intertrigo. Infants born to affected mothers are increasingly prone to infection with *Candida*. Treatment is with topical nystatin or miconazole.

Leprosy

In general, patients with leprosy (Hansen's disease) do well in pregnancy. However, the subgroups of active lepromatous and dimorphous types have an increased incidence of obstetric complications and of Hansen's disease reactions. There is also an increased incidence of twins in lepromatous patients [50]. Although the sulphone drugs may be safely used as treatment during pregnancy [50], they have caused haemolytic disease of the newborn (HDN) [49], and dapsone has also caused HDN when transmitted through breast milk [83]. Patients with glucose-6-phosphate dehydrogenase deficiency are especially susceptible.

Pregnancy and collagen disease
(see also Chapter 8)

Systemic lupus erythematosus (SLE) is no longer a contraindication to pregnancy, although it may precipitate a flare in up to 38% of patients [4]. Women in complete clinical remission, irrespective of past manifestations of SLE, have the best chance of uncomplicated pregnancy and the highest incidence of fetal survival [84,85]. Exacerbation is more likely if the disease has been active in the preceding 6 years and may occur at any stage between early pregnancy and 8 weeks postpartum. Oral contraceptives may also induce exacerbations.

There is a higher fetal morbidity and mortality (see Chapter 8), and transient skin lesions clinically and histologically resembling those of SLE have been reported in the fetus [86].

Pregnancy has no consistent effect on discoid lupus erythematosus. The fetus is not affected.

Dermatomyositis has been reported unchanged in 60%, improved in 20% and worsened in 20%. Two patients first developed dermatomyositis during pregnancy. The fetal mortality is 46%. Progesterone may aggravate dermatomyositis [87].

Systemic sclerosis and polyarteritis nodosa are commented on in Chapter 8.

Pregnancy and inflammatory skin disease

Urticaria may develop in late pregnancy, and dermographism is also common. The specific dermatoses of pregnancy such as PG and prurigo of pregnancy may have an urticarial component. Treatment is with antihistamines.

Erythema multiforme

Erythema multiforme may also develop in successive pregnancies and can be differentiated histologically and on immunofluorescence from mild PG [15]. Drugs and viral infections, especially herpes simplex, are possible precipitating causes.

Erythema nodosum and sarcoidosis are discussed in Chapter 1.

Pregnancy and benign and malignant skin tumours

Pregnancy usually has an adverse effect on neurofibromatosis (von Recklinghausen's disease). Women with neurofibromatosis have a higher than expected rate of first trimester spontaneous abortions, stillbirths and intrauterine growth restriction so that close monitoring of pregnancy is essential [88,89]. Lesions may appear for the first time or increase in size and number. Many patients have associated hypertension (see Chapter 6). Other complications include neuropathies associated with tumour growth and occasional sudden haemorrhage into neurofibromata. Major blood vessels can rupture and hypertension can occur [90].

MELANOMA

Malignant melanoma accounts for nearly 50% of metastases to the placenta and approximately 90% involving the fetus, which is nevertheless exceedingly rare (see below). Stage 1 disease survival rates are unaffected by pregnancy but stage 2 survival rates are decreased [91]. Prognosis is also worse for those patients who have had previous pregnancies associated with growth or activation of a lesion subsequently diagnosed as melanoma. Pregnancy and oral contraception is best avoided in these and patients with stage 2 melanoma [91]. Treatment is as for melanoma in the non-pregnant state and termination of pregnancy appears to offer no appreciable maternal benefit [92]. Transplacental transmission of melanoma to the fetus is extremely rare, and maternal melanoma usually has no adverse effects on the fetus [92]. Women who have had malignant melanomata excised should be advised to delay future pregnancy by at least 2 years after diagnosis, as 83% of patients with metastatic disease present within 2 years after they present with a primary melanoma [93].

Drug therapy during pregnancy

Ideally no drug should be prescribed for the first 3 months of pregnancy but potential guidelines for dermatological drug prescribing in pregnancy or the lactating period are now available [94]. Drugs of dermatological relevance that have already been considered and should not be given include methotrexate (psoriasis), tetracycline (see above, acne), podophyllin (see above, condylomata) and the vitamin A derivatives isotretinoin and etretinate (see above, acne). Although cyclosporin has been contraindicated in pregnancy, recent experience from transplant patients indicates that there is no conclusive evidence of any teratogenic effect [95]. A recent paper reported the first British case of the successful use of cyclosporin to control pustular psoriasis in pregnancy from 25 weeks' gestation [96].

There is still no evidence to suggest that psoralen and UVA (PUVA) is teratogenic when used to treat psoriasis. However, because PUVA is mutagenic, it is considered advisable to avoid PUVA as first-line treatment during pregnancy [97] even though a recent study found no adverse effects in pregnancies conceived during PUVA treatment [98].

Those drugs that should be given with caution include azathioprine, chloroquine, metronidazole and trimethoprim.

Thalidomide, now being advocated for the treatment of erythema nodosum, should never be used in pregnancy because of the well-known risk of limb reduction defects. Hydroxyurea and griseofulvin should not be used because of potential toxicity. Most of the commonly used antihistamines appear to be safe during pregnancy after the first trimester. The use of corticosteroids is discussed in Chapter 1.

Some antiviral agents such as idoxuridine are also contraindicated. Topical corticosteroids should be used sparingly in view of the risk of percutaneous absorption. Dithranol and tar appear to be safe.

In general all treatments should nevertheless be kept to a minimum, especially in the first trimester.

References

1 Catanzarite V, Quirk SG. Papular dermatoses of pregnancy. *Clin Obstet Gynecol* 1990; 33: 754–8.
2 Hayashi RH. Bullous dermatoses and prurigo of pregnancy. *Clin Obstet Gynecol* 1990; 33: 746–53.

3 Winton GB. Skin diseases aggravated by pregnancy. *J Am Acad Dermatol* 1989; 20: 1–13.

4 Fitzpatrick TB, Eisen AZ, Wolff K. *Dermatology in General Medicine*. McGraw-Hill, New York, 1987: 2082.

5 Wade TR, Wade SL, Jones HE. Skin changes and diseases associated with pregnancy. *Obstet Gynecol* 1978; 52: 233–42.

6 Resnick S. Melasma induced by oral contraceptive drugs. *J Am Med Assoc* 1967; 199: 601–5.

7 Newcomer VD, Linberg MC, Sternberg TH. A melanosis of the face 'cholasma'. *Arch Dermatol* 1961; 83: 284–97.

8 Sanchez NP, Pathak MA *et al*. Melasma; a clinical, light microscopic, ultrastructural and immunofluorescence study. *J Am Acad Dermatol* 1981; 4: 698–710.

9 Snell R. The pigmentary changes occurring in breast skin during pregnancy and following oestrogen treatment. *J Invest Dermatol* 1964; 43: 181–6.

10 Schizume K, Lerner AB. Determination of melanocyte stimulating hormone in urine and blood. *J Clin Endocrinol Metab* 1954; 14: 1491.

11 Thody AJ, Plummer NA *et al*. Plasma SS-melanocyte stimulating hormone levels in pregnancy. *J Obstet Gynaecol Br Commonwealth* 1974; 81: 875–7.

12 Kligman AM, Willis I. A new formula for depigmenting human skin. *Arch Dermatol* 1975; 111: 540–7.

13 Hellreich PD. The skin changes of pregnancy. *Cutis* 1974; 13: 82–6.

14 Aldercreutz H, Tenhunen R. Some aspects of the interaction between natural and synthetic female sex hormones and the liver. *Am J Med* 1970; 49: 630–8.

15 Iffy L, Kaminetzky HA. Skin diseases in pregnancy. In: Iffy L, Kaminerzky Ha, eds. *Principles Practice of Obstetrics and Perinatology*. John Wiley. Chichester. 1981: 1361–79.

16 Bean WB, Cogswell R *et al*. Vascular changes in the skin in pregnancy. *Surg Gynaecol Obstet* 1949; 88: 739–52.

17 Davey CMH. Factors associated with the occurrence of striae gravidarum. *J Obstet Gynaecol Br Commonwealth* 1972; 79: 113.

18 Liu DTY. Striae gravidarum. *Lancet* 1974; i: 625.

19 Shuster S. The cause of striae distense. *Acta Dermatovenereol Suppl (Stockh)* 1979; 59: 161–9.

20 Pinkus H, Keech MK, Mehregan AH. Histopathology of striae distensae with special reference to striae and wound healing in the Marfan syndrome. *J Invest Dermatol* 1966; 46: 293–9.

21 Watson REB, Parry EJ *et al*. Fibrillin microfibrils are reduced in skin exhibiting striae distensae. *Br J Dermatol* 1998; 138: 931–7.

22 Pribanich S, Simpson FG, Held B, Yarbrough CL, White SN. Low-dose tretinoin does not improve striae distensae: a double blind, placebo-controlled study. *Cutis* 1994; 54: 121–4.

23 Cummings K, Derbes VJ. Dermatoses associated with pregnancy. *Cutis* 1967; 3: 120–6.

24 Demis DB, Dobson RL, McGuire J. *Clinical Dermatology*. Harper & Row, New York, 1972.

25 MacKinnon PCB, McKinnon IL. Palmar sweating in pregnancy. *J Obstet Gynaecol Br Empire* 1955; 62: 298–9.

26 Lyndfield YL. Effect of pregnancy on the human hair cycle. *J Invest Dermatol* 1960; 35: 323–7.

27 Schiff BL, Pawtucket RI, Kern AB. Study of postpartum alopecia. *Arch Dermatol* 1963; 87: 609–11.

28 Trotter M. The activity of hair follicles with reference to pregnancy. *Surg Gynaecol Obstet* 1935; 60: 1092–5.

29 Kolodny RC. Herpes gestationis. A new assessment of incidence, diagnosis and foetal prognosis. *Am J Obstet Gynecol* 1969; 104: 39–45.

30 Tillman WG. Herpes gestationis with hydatidiform mole and chorion epithelioma. *Br Med J* 1950; i: 1471.

31 Dupont C. Herpes gestationis with hydatidiform mole. *Trans St Johns Dermatol Soc* 1974; 60: 103.

32 Holmes RC, Black MM. The specific dermatoses of pregnancy. *J Am Acad Dermatol* 1983; 8: 405–12.

33 Shornick JK, Stastny P, Gilliam JN. High frequency of histocompatibility antigens HLA-DR3 and DR4 in herpes gestationis. *J Clin Invest* 1981; 68: 553–5.

34 Holmes RC, Black MM, James DCO. Paternal responsibility for herpes gestationis. In: MacDonald DM, eds. *Immunodermatology*. Butterworths, London, 1984: 251–3.

35 Jenkins RE, Hern S, Black MM. Clinical features and management of 87 patients with pemphigoid gestationis. *Clin Exp Dermatol* 1999; 24: 255–9.

36 Holmes RC, Black MM *et al*. Clues to the aetiology and pathogenesis of herpes gestationis. *Br J Dermatol* 1983; 109: 131–9.

37 Holmes RC, Black MM *et al*. A comparative study of toxic erythema of pregnancy and herpes gestationis. *Br J Dermatol* 1982; 106: 499–510.

38 Lynch FN, Albrecht RJ. Hormonal factors in herpes gestationis. *Arch Dermatol* 1966; 3: 465–6.

39 Kenny JF, Pangburn PC, Trail G. Effect of oestradiol on immune competence: in vivo and in vitro studies. *Infect Comm* 1976; 13: 448.

40 Lawley TJ, Stingl G, Katz ST. Foetal and maternal risk factors in herpes gestationis. *Arch Dermatol* 1978; 114: 552–5.

41 Shornick JK, Bangert JL *et al*. Herpes gestationis. Clinical and histologic features of twenty eight cases. *J Am Acad Dermatol* 1983; 8: 214.

42 Shornick JK, Black MM. Fetal risk in herpes gestationis. *J Am Acad Dermatol* 1992; 26: 63–8.

43 Borrego L, Peterson EA *et al*. Polymorphic eruption of pregnancy and herpes gestationis: comparison of granulated cell proteins in tissue and serum. *Clin Exp Dermatol* 1999; 24: 213–25.

44 Provost TT, Tomasi TB. Evidence of complement activiation via the alternative pathway in skin diseases I. Herpes gestationis, systemic lupus erythematosus and bullous pemphigoid. *J Clin Invest* 1973; 52: 1779–87.

45 Kelly SE, Cerio R, Bhogal BS, Black MM. The distribution of IgG subclasses in pemphigoid gestationis: PG factor is an IgG1 autoantibody. *J Invest Dermatol* 1989; 92: 695–8.

46 Jureka W, Holmes RC *et al*. An immunoelectron microscopy study of the relationship between herpes gestationis and polymorphic eruption of pregnancy. *Br J Dermatol* 1983; 108: 147–51.

47 Jenkins RE, Vaughan Jones SA, Black MM. Conversion of pemphigoid gestationis to bullous pemphigoid—two refractory cases highlighting this association. *Br J Dermatol* 1996; 135: 595–8.

48 Van Der Wiel A, Hart H *et al*. Plasma exchange in herpes gestationis. *Br Med J* 1980; 281: 1041.

49 Hocking DR. Neonatal haemolytic disease due to dapsone. *Med J Aust* 1968; 1: 1130.

50 Lockwood DNJ, Sinha HH. Pregnancy and leprosy. A comprehensive literature review. *Int J Lepr* 1999; 167: 6–12.

51 MacDonald KJS, Raffle EJ. Ritodrine therapy associated with remission of pemphigoid gestationis. *Br J Dermatol* 1984; 111: 630.

52 Garvey MP, Handfield-Jones SE, Black MM. Pemphigoid gestationis response to chemical oophorectomy with goserelin. *Clin Exp Dermatol* 1992; 17: 443–5.

53 Andersen B, Felding C. Pruritic urticarial papules and plaques of pregnancy. *J Obstet Gynaecol* 1992; 12: 1–3.

54 Lawley TJ, Hertz KC *et al*. Pruritic urticarial papules and plaques of pregnancy. *J Am Med Assoc* 1979; 241: 1696–9.

55 Boume G. Toxaemic rash of pregnancy. *J R Soc Med* 1962; 55: 462–4.

56 Cooper AJ, Fryer JA. Prurigo of late pregnancy. *Austral J Dermatol* 1980; 21: 79–84.

57 Nurse DS. Prurigo of pregnancy. *Austral J Dermatol* 1968; 9: 258–67.

58 Holmes RC, Black MM. The specific dermatoses of pregnancy. A reappraisal with special emphasis on a proposed simplified classification. *Clin Exp Dermatol* 1982; 7: 65–73.

59 Aronson IK, Bond S *et al*. Pruritic urticarial papules and plaques of pregnancy: Clinical and immunopathologic observations in 57 patients. *J Am Acad Dermatol* 1998; 39: 933–9.

60 Bunker CB, Erskine K *et al*. Severe polymorphic eruption of pregnancy occurring in twin pregnancies. *Clin Exp Dermatol* 1990; 15: 228–31.

61 Cohen LM, Capeless EL *et al*. Pruritic urticarial papules and plaques of pregnancy and its relationship to metemal-fetal weight gain and twin pregnancy. *Arch Dermatol* 1989; 125: 1534–6.

62 Vaughan Jones SA, Dunnill MGS, Black MM. Pruritic urticarial papules and plaques of pregnancy (polymorphic eruption of pregnancy): two unusual cases. *Br J Dermatol* 1996; 135: 102–5.

63 Vaughan Jones SA, Hern S *et al*. A prospective study of 200 women with dermatoses of pregnancy correlating the clinical findings with hormonal and immunopathological profiles. *Br J Dermatol* 1999; 141: 71–81.

64 Aractingi S, Berkane N *et al*. Fetal DNA in skin of polymorphic eruptions of pregnancy. *Lancet* 1998; 352: 1898–901.

65 Yancey KB, Hall RB, Lawley T. Pruritic urticarial papules and plaques of pregnancy. *J Am Acad Dermatol* 1984; 10: 473–80.

66 Beltrani VP, Beltrani VS. Pruritic urticarial papules and plaques of pregnancy: a severe case requiring early delivery from relief of symptoms. *J Am Acad Dermatol* 1992; 26: 266–7.

67 Zoberman E, Farmer ER. Pruritic folliculitis of pregnancy. *Arch Dermatol* 1981; 117: 20–2.

68 Vaughan Jones SA, Hern S, Black MM. Pruritic folliculitis and serum androgen levels. *Clin Exp Dermatol* 1999; 24: 392–5.

69 Wilkinson S. M, Buckler H, Wilkinson N *et al*. Androgen levels in pruritic folliculitis of pregnancy. *Clin Exp Dermatol* 1995; 20: 234–6.

70 Spangler AS, Reddy W *et al*. Papular dermatitis of pregnancy. *J Am Med Assoc* 1962; 181: 577–81.

71 Spangler AS, Emerson K. Estrogen levels and estrogen therapy in papular dermatitis of pregnancy. *Am J Obstet Gynaecol* 1971; 110: 534–7.

72 Spangler AS, Emerson K. Diethylstilbestrol in the management of papular dermatitis of pregnancy. A reply to the editor. *Am J Obstet Gynaecol* 1972; 113: 571.

73 Bierman SM. Autoimmune dermatitis of pregnancy. *Arch Dermatol* 1973; 107: 896–901.

74 Hart RH. Autoimmune progesterone dermatitis. *Arch Dermatol* 1977; 113: 427–30.

75 Rodenas JM, Herranz MT, Tercedor J. Autoimmune progesterone dermatitis: treatment with oophorectomy. *Br J Dermatol* 1998; 139: 508–11.

76 Stephens CJM, Wojnarowska FT, Wilkinson JD. Autoimmune progesterone dermatitis responding to tamoxifen. *Br J Dermatol* 1989; 121: 135–7.

77 Shahar E, Bergman R, Pollack S. Autoimmune progesterone dermatitis: effective prophylactic treatment with Danazol. *Int J Dermatol* 1997; 36: 708–11.

78 Lever WF. *Histopathology of the Skin*. JB Lippincott, Philadelphia, PA, 1985: 145.

79 Oumeish OY, Farraj SE, Bataineh AS. Some aspects of impetigo herpetiformis. *Arch Dermatol* 1982; 118: 103–5.

80 Lotem M, Katzenelson V *et al*. Impetigo herpetiformis. a variant of pustular psoriasis or a separate entity? *J Am Acad Dermatol* 1989; 20: 338–41.

81 Rasmussen KA, Ehrenskjold MI. Impetigo herpetiformis. A case in a pregnant women treated with antex. *Acta Obstet Gynaecol Scand* 1965; 44: 563.

82 Beveridge GW, Harkness RA, Livingstone JRB. Impetigo herpetiformis in two successive pregnancies. *Br J Dermatol* 1966; 78: 106–12.

83 Sanders SW, Zone JJ *et al*. Haemolytic anaemia transmitted through breast milk. *Ann Intern Med* 1982; 96: 485–6.

84 Hayslett JP, Reece EA. Systemic lupus erthematosus in pregnancy. *Clin Perinatol* 1985; 12: 539–50.

85 Lundbert I, Hedfors E. Pregnancy outcome in patients with high titre anti-RNP antibodies. A retrospective study of 40 pregnancies. *J Rheumatol* 1991; 18: 359–62.

86 Vonderheid EC, Koblenzer PJ *et al*. Neonatal lupus erythematosus. *Arch Dermatol* 1976; 112: 698–705.

87 Tsai A, Lindheimer MD *et al*. Dermatomyositis complicating pregnancy. *Obstet Gynecol* 1973; 41: 570–3.

88 Segal D, Holcberg G *et al*. Neurofibromatosis in pregnancy. *Eur J Obstet Gynaecol Reprod Biol* 1999; 84 (1): 59–61.

89 Weissman A, Jakobi P *et al*. Neurofibromatosis and pregnancy. An update. *J Reprod Med* 1993; 38 (11): 890–6.

90 Braude PB, Bolan JC. Neurofibromatosis and spontaneous hemothorax in pregnancy: two case reports. *Obstet Gynecol* 1984; 63 (Suppl.): 35–8.

91 Shiu MA, Schottenfeld D *et al*. Adverse effect of pregnancy on melanoma. A reappraisal. *Cancer* 1976; 37: 181–7.

92 Colburn DS, Nathanson L, Belilos E. Pregnancy and malignant melanoma. *Semin Oncol* 1989; 16: 377–87.

93 Mackie RM, Bufalino R *et al*. Lack of effect of pregnancy on outcome of melanoma. *Lancet* 1991; i: 653–5.

94 Stockton DL, Paller AS. Drug administration to the pregnant or lactating woman: a reference guide for dermatologists. *J Am Acad Dermatol* 1990; 23: 87–103.

95 Wright S, Glover M, Baker H. Psoriasis, cyclosporin and pregnancy. *Arch Dermatol* 1991; 127: 426.

96 Finch TM, Tan CY. Pustular psoriasis exacerbated by pregnancy and controlled by cyclosporin A. *Br J Dermatol* 2000; 142: 582–4.

97 Stern RS, Lange R. Outcomes of pregnancies among women and partners of men with a history of exposure to methoxsalen photochemotherapy (PUVA) for the treatment of psoriasis. *Arch Dermatol* 1991; 127: 347–400.

98 Gunnarskog JG, Kallen AJB *et al*. Psoralen photochemotherapy (PUVA) and pregnancy. *Arch Dermatol* 1993; 129: 320–3.

21 Psychiatry in pregnancy

Peter F. Liddle and Margaret R. Oates

Psychiatric disorders in pregnancy and the puerperium reflect a complex interplay between the physiological, psychological and social aspects of conceiving, carrying, delivering and nurturing a baby, and the pre-existing psychological adjustment of the woman. To a large extent, the signs and symptoms of psychiatric disorders in pregnancy and the puerperium resemble the signs and symptoms of psychiatric disorders occurring at other times, but precipitating factors are shaped by circumstances unique to childbearing. Furthermore, the need on the one hand to achieve relatively rapid resolution of symptoms threatening the well-being of the mother and her child, whilst on the other hand avoiding unnecessary pharmacological treatment in pregnancy, presents unique challenges in the planning of treatment.

The most common disorders presenting during pregnancy are depression, anxiety and various specific phobias. In addition pre-existing psychiatric disorders require careful management planning during pregnancy. In the puerperium, the majority of women experience the transient mood disturbance known as the blues. A smaller proportion develops a depressive illness (postnatal depression), which is more sustained and can be associated with substantial adverse effects on the woman, her baby and her partner. The most severe disorder of the puerperium is postpartum psychosis, which is rare but has a potentially devastating effect on the woman and her family. Before considering each of these clinical conditions in detail, we should briefly consider some general issues regarding management of psychiatric disorder in relation to pregnancy and the early postpartum period.

Pharmacological treatment

During pregnancy, planning pharmacological treatment entails balancing of benefits against risks. For the long-established exemplars of all the major classes of psycho-trophic medication, the available evidence indicates that overt developmental abnormalities following exposure *in utero* are very unlikely, except possibly in the case of lithium, carbamazepine and perhaps other anticonvulsant mood stabilizers (see Chapter 15). However, there is also a theoretical possibility that exposure to psychotrophic medication might produce subtle alterations in the development of the central nervous system, influencing behaviour later in life. Furthermore, many psychotrophic drugs can produce toxic effects such as excitation or depression of the central nervous system, extrapyramidal motor signs and anticholinergic effects that might be harmful in the neonate. There is no reason to believe that the foetus and neonate is less likely to develop side-effects than an adult.

The risks of marked fetal malformation are greatest in the first trimester, but the neural architecture of the brain takes shape throughout intrauterine development, so potential influences on central nervous system development might not be confined to the first trimester. Thus, whilst it is most important to minimize drug exposure in the first trimester, caution is required throughout pregnancy, and in the final weeks risks of adverse influence on labour and the physiology of the newborn infant must be taken into account. When psychological treatment alone might be successful, as is the case in mild depression and simple anxiety states, it is clearly preferable to avoid pharmacological treatment. However, it is important not to underestimate the consequences for both mother and child, including the dangers of disrupted antenatal care, self-neglect or self-harm, likely to result if mental disorder in pregnancy is not treated adequately. Therefore, for severe depression, disabling anxiety and for active psychotic disorders, pharmacological treatment is justified. The question of prophylaxis in cases of prior psychotic illness demands a careful evaluation of the likelihood of relapse.

Most psychotrophic medications, including antipsychotic medication as well as antidepressants and anxiolytics, are excreted in breast milk, although in many instances a breastfeeding infant is likely to receive a very small dose. In cases of serious mental disorder in the postpartum period, such as psychosis or severe depression, pharmacological treatment is almost always essential because the dangers of inadequately treating such disorders include risk of maternal suicide and neglect or harm of the infant. For treatments with a substantial potential for toxicity, such as lithium and high doses of antipsychotic medication, the balance of risk indicates that the mother should not breastfeed. For tricyclic antidepressant medication, and low doses of antipsychotic medication there is little evidence of substantial risk to the breastfeeding infant, and the balance between the risks and benefits of breastfeeding are not clear-cut. Therefore, if the mother wishes to breastfeed while taking such medication, she should be told that the available evidence suggests low risk. However if the infant is not feeding well, failing to gain adequate weight, drowsy or otherwise giving cause for concern, medical advice should be sought and breastfeeding suspended. Some clinicians have argued that it is valuable to perform measurements of levels of the psychotrophic medication in the infant serum, but this is not a routine practice in the UK.

Psychological treatment

Usually, the major goal of treatment of mental disorder in pregnancy and the puerperium is rapid control of symptoms. For such purposes, short-term, goal-orientated psychotherapies are especially useful. The strategies and techniques required are similar to those required in other settings, but in addition, there are several features specific to pregnancy and the puerperium that demand recognition.

The worries encountered in pregnancy and the puerperium frequently reveal distorted beliefs about pregnancy and motherhood, which are fostered by cultural myths. For a woman who experiences in the second trimester a disconcerting sense that control of her life has been taken from her and who is unsure how she will cope with motherhood, the expectation of her family and friends that she should by this stage be serene and content reinforces her sense of inadequacy. It is less easy for her to confide in friends and there is danger of a vicious cycle driven by negative self-evaluation. For the primiparous mother of a 2-month-old infant who only encounters other young mothers in public settings where they manage to maintain a competent facade, her own awareness of her fragile competence at home reinforces the growing realization that she is failing to achieve the image of motherhood that had been inculcated in her since childhood. Again there is a risk of a vicious cycle in which low self-esteem creates a depressed mood that further diminishes self-esteem. In such situations, there is need for education, and for simple psychological strategies to help restore a balanced perspective. For most women suffering from mild mixed anxiety and depression or from psychological conflicts resulting from the gap between expectations and reality, psychological treatments are more rational and acceptable than pharmacological ones. Examples of evidence-based interventions include brief interpersonal psychotherapy, cognitive therapy and non-directive counselling.

It should not be forgotten that sympathetic skilled 'active listening' from midwives and health visitors or the creative use of antenatal classes may be the most appropriate help.

Social issues in management

For the economically deprived, pregnancy and parenthood present severe challenges and major stresses that can either precipitate or maintain mental illness. The clinician often needs to adopt the role of advocate exerting influence to obtain social services for the patient.

Even amongst those who are relatively well-off, for many young couples the struggle for economic security places pressure on both partners to work. Hence, when pregnancy and motherhood makes this impossible, practical economic difficulties (often compounded by the covert pressures arising from society's conflicting attitudes towards combining work and motherhood) place substantial pressures on the woman and on her relationship with her partner.

Social support and particularly a confiding relationship with a female friend and practical assistance and companionship, improves women's resilience to adversity at this time. Conversely, lack of social support in the face of personal vulnerability and adversity increases a woman's risk of becoming depressed.

Simple interventions based on social support theory, for example provided by voluntary agencies such as Homestart and Newpin, can improve women's resilience and well-being.

Psychiatric disorder in pregnancy

The antenatal period is not a time of increased risk of psychiatric disorder for the majority of women. Indeed, it is probable that for many, the happiness and hope associated with pregnancy helps enhance self-esteem and together with the rising oestradiol levels affords some protection against mental illness. However, the absence of a statistical increase in mental disorder in pregnancy conceals a more complex picture. For women in adverse social circumstances, and for those who suffered difficulty in conceiving, or who have faced persisting threat of miscarriage, pregnancy can be fraught with worry. Physical violence directed against women by their partners is also quite common in pregnancy. Even in benign circumstances, the potentially destabilizing influence of rapidly increasing hormone levels and the tiring physiological demands of pregnancy can lead to changeable mood and irritability. Thus, attention to emotional health is an important aspect of antenatal care.

Depression during pregnancy

The evidence suggests that depression is most common in the first trimester of pregnancy. Approximately 10% of women suffer depression during that time [1]. This is similar to the expected prevalence of depression in non-pregnant women, and there is no reason to propose that the pathophysiology of depression arising in pregnancy differs from that of depression at other times. However, the nature of the stresses that precipitate the episodes of depression tend to reflect the specific psychosocial stressors associated with pregnancy. The incidence of depression falls in the second and third trimester.

As in other types of depression, the cardinal clinical feature is low mood, often accompanied by anxiety. The low mood is usually associated with low self-esteem, pessimism, loss of interest and loss of capacity for enjoyment. There is usually impairment of concentration, and disturbance of sleep and appetite. Suicide is substantially less common in pregnancy than at other times but the clinician must always perform an assessment of potential suicide risk. There is a substantial overlap between the features of depression and anxiety. It is not uncommon for depression to be associated with agoraphobia. Untreated, antenatal depression may improve as the pregnancy progresses. However in some cases it may persist or be the precursor of postnatal depression.

TREATMENT

In mild cases, the most appropriate treatments are psychological, for example non-directive counselling, brief interpersonal psychotherapy or cognitive therapy. In more severe cases, such as those characterized by marked early morning wakening and/or suicidal ideas, treatment with a tricyclic antidepressant such as amitriptyline, imipramine or lofepramine is warranted. Although more recently developed antidepressants, such as the selective serotonin reuptake inhibitors (SSRIs), offer the potential advantages of fewer anticholinergic side-effects and less risk of death from overdose, less information is available about potential risk to the fetus. However, preliminary data from quite large studies are encouraging [2,3].

Tricyclic antidepressants have been in use for almost 40 years and the evidence suggests that the risk to the fetus is low. In 1972, McBride reported congenital limb deformity in the child of a mother who had taken imipramine during pregnancy [4], but a systematic large-scale survey failed to confirm an association between tricyclic antidepressants and limb deformity [5]. In 1997 a study of 80 women who had taken tricyclic antidepressants in pregnancy showed no developmental problems in their children at ages 16–86 months [3]. In view of the substantial anticholinergic effects of amitriptyline and imipramine, the neonate is at risk of neuromuscular irritability and of disturbance of visceral function if the mother has a substantial serum level at the time of delivery. Therefore, in the final weeks of pregnancy it is desirable to reduce the dose and then withdraw the drug entirely prior to delivery if possible.

Anxiety during pregnancy

Pregnancy is associated with risk, and a degree of concern about possible dangers is natural and appropriate. Normal concerns are usually best dealt with by straightforward explanation of the issues, avoiding unwarranted reassurance, as this is liable to undermine the trust that is essential for a reasonably confident approach to the pregnancy.

In cases where the worry is clearly disproportionate to the circumstances, and is accompanied by other characteristic symptoms of anxiety such that ability to function becomes impaired, the condition has crossed the boundary of normal reaction and should be regarded as an illness. The symptoms of an anxiety disorder include a subjective sense of anxiety; and somatic symptoms such as tachycardia, dyspnoea, tremor and gastrointestinal disturbance, sleep disturbance and impaired concentration. In pregnancy, gastrointestinal symptoms, especially nausea and vomiting, are a frequently encountered feature of anxiety, presumably because the normal physiological events of pregnancy predispose to such gastrointestinal disturbances.

During the first trimester anxiety disorders are at least as common as in non-pregnant women, although the incidence falls in the second and third trimester. Women with a previous history of such disorders are at risk of a recurrence of their condition during pregnancy particularly if they have stopped their medication abruptly.

Sometimes the anxiety occurs in discrete episodes of panic in which there is sudden onset of somatic symptoms of anxiety, often accompanied by fears of perceived catastrophe, such as a fear of heart attack, fainting in embarrassing circumstances or going mad. Such episodes of panic can appear to arise 'out of the blue' without obvious precipitants, but in other cases they are clearly related to specific precipitating circumstances, such as travelling in public transport or being in a public place such as a supermarket. In instances where there is a specific precipitant, the patient tends to avoid the precipitating situation, thereby reinforcing a phobic fear of that situation. Specific phobias are discussed below, but it is important to note that phobic fears, especially agoraphobia, are commonly encountered in association with more generalized anxiety.

Anxiety states are also frequently accompanied by low mood and other features of depression. It is probable that there is an intrinsic overlap between the pathophysiology of anxiety and depression, such that at least in milder cases, there is often little point in attempting to distinguish between the two conditions.

The treatment of anxiety states in pregnancy might entail either psychological treatments alone, or a combination of pharmacological and psychological treatment. In relatively mild cases, psychological treatment is usually to be preferred. The principal psychological techniques are derived from behaviour therapy and cognitive therapy. Two cardinal behavioural strategies are learning to relax in anxiety-provoking situations, and planning activities that deflect the person away from preoccupation with worrying thoughts. However, it should be noted that avoidance of a feared situation is in itself likely to enhance the fear by reinforcing the belief that avoidance is the only way of alleviating the symptoms ('safety behaviours'). Cognitive techniques entail learning to recognize the distorted thinking processes that underlie disproportionate fear, and then weighing up the evidence with the object of putting the situation in a reasonable perspective. Psychological management of anxiety is as successful as pharmacological management in mild to moderate cases. In severe anxiety disorders, such as cases where there is a persistent generalized anxiety that is disabling, or there are frequent panic attacks, it may be necessary to consider pharmacological treatment. Whilst benzodiazepines (such as diazepam) can offer short-term relief they are best avoided except in emergencies. They can result in tolerance and dependency and prevent psychological change. Early studies suggested a possible relationship between cleft lip and palate and exposure to diazepam *in utero*, though a large case–controlled study found no evidence for such an association [6]. A comparison of a large sample of malformed newborns with control infants revealed an association between use of benzodiazepines (mainly diazepam) in the first trimester and various defects including inguinal hernia, cardiac defects and pyloric stenosis [7]. A thorough study of eight infants with dysmorphic features, growth retardation and central nervous system defects who had been exposed to substantial doses of benzodiazepines (e.g diazepam 30 mg/day) during pregnancy failed to identify any plausible cause for the abnormalities other than benzodiazepine exposure [8]. On balance, the evidence suggests that diazepam poses some teratogenic risk. Because of risk of depression of respiration and of muscular hypotonia in the neonate, it is necessary to minimize use of benzodiazepines in the final weeks of the pregnancy. Tricyclic antidepressants and SSRIs are also effective anxiolytics, and are effective in reducing panic attacks.

CASE ILLUSTRATION

A woman was referred for psychiatric assessment because she had been phoning her midwife on a daily basis fearing that her blood pressure was rising. Each time she was reassured that all was well only to become anxious again the following day and seek to have her blood pressure checked again.

She had suffered from severe pre-eclampsia in her last pregnancy, necessitating the delivery of her baby at 30 weeks' gestation. Following this she was seriously ill with epileptic fits, was detained in an intensive care unit for 4 days and had persistent hypertension for some weeks. It took her 5 years to summon the courage to embark on a further pregnancy. She was anxious from the point of conception. However, following an ultrasound scan which showed equivocal results she developed palpitations and felt light headed with blurred vision. She instantly misattributed these physical symptoms of anxiety as the harbinger of pre-eclampsia. She then hyperventilated and had a panic attack thinking that she was about to die. A hospital admission and the ensuing investigations served only to reinforce her fears.

Following the assessment and diagnosis of an acute anxiety state with panic attacks, her community psychiatric nurse and psychiatrist, using cognitive techniques, were able to help her reattribute her signs and symptoms to those of panic attacks. Using behavioural techniques they helped her reduce her levels of anxiety and deal with the acute bouts of panic. In her later pregnancy she was able to engage in regular obstetric midwifery review appropriate to the management of her condition.

Obsessional disorders and phobias

Obsessional phenomena are distressing recurrent thoughts, images or fears, which the patient recognizes are unreasonable, but which intrude insistently into every-day mental activity. Phobias are unreasonable fears of specific situations or objects. Obsessions and phobias can arise in a context of more wide-ranging anxiety. They can also occur as symptoms of a primary depressive disorder. In other instances, a specific obsession or phobia occurs in relative isolation, with other symptoms such as depressed mood or generalized anxiety either absent or forming only a very minor component of the clinical picture. These conditions are as common in pregnancy as at other times. Women with a previous history may suffer from a recurrence during pregnancy.

The major component of treatment for phobias is cognitive behavioural therapy. Simple phobias, in which the subject has a specific focused fear of a particular situation, usually respond well to a behavioural approach directed at achieving exposure of the patient to the feared situation, thereby demonstrating to the patient that her irrational fears do not come to fruition. Behavioural techniques such as progressive muscular relaxation, and cognitive techniques that encourage the patient to evaluate the evidence about the fears in a balanced manner, are used to facilitate the goal of exposure.

Obsessional ruminations respond less well to traditional behavioural techniques. Although cognitive therapy is often effective, it may be necessary to combine cognitive therapy with pharmacological therapy. Antidepressant drugs can be effective in reducing the intensity and frequency of obsessional traits. Clomipramine (a tricyclic antidepressant) and more recently, SSRIs, particularly paroxetine have been demonstrated to be especially effective for treating obsessive–compulsive disorders [9].

CASE ILLUSTRATION

A professionally successful older woman was referred for a psychiatric assessment by her midwife who had noticed that she was reluctant to allow her 3-year-old child to touch objects in the consulting room and that the woman's hands were red and raw from the excessive use of bleach and detergents. When the midwife had sympathetically enquired into the reasons for this, the woman had become acutely distressed and embarrassed and revealed her fear of contamination.

During her psychiatric assessment it became clear that this woman had long-standing obsessional personality traits of perfectionism, high personal standards, a tendency to self-criticism and ruminative worry. However,

prior to the current pregnancy, these had not interfered with her functioning and she had led a full and successful life.

She had become pregnant unexpectedly and had initially been ambivalent and considered termination. During the first trimester she had a threatened miscarriage and began to worry that she might have brought this upon herself by her earlier ambivalence. She knew that this was silly but found herself unable to stop thinking about it. Some short time later, she read a newspaper article about the dangers of eating soft cheese and uncooked eggs in pregnancy. She then found herself prey to repeated intrusive, senseless but insistent ruminative thoughts that she might have inadvertently eaten such a substance without knowing it and might have damaged her baby. Her condition then deteriorated to the point at 22 weeks where she was having to scrutinize all food products entering her house for possible contamination by *Salmonella* and was using large quantities of cleaning agents in the house. She felt unable to allow her older child contact with anything that could possibly be contaminating. She was distressed and guilty about these restrictions but unable to stop herself from doing them.

After assessment, she was seen regularly by a community psychiatric nurse and a psychiatrist. Together they engaged her in using a cognitive approach explaining the nature of her condition and the chain of cognitions that had led to her problem. Using the behavioural technique of response prevention, they helped her to stop the compulsive behaviours which were serving to maintain her anxiety. She was also given clomipramine, a tricyclic antidepressant, which is known to be particularly effective in helping limit obsessional–compulsive phenomena. Using this combination of cognitive behavioural psychotherapy and clomipramine she was much improved by 28 weeks of pregnancy when the dose of clomipramine was gradually tapered off so that she was free from medication at the point of delivery. In view of the substantial risk of a relapse of her condition following delivery, her clomipramine was restarted immediately following delivery. She breastfed her baby and the clomipramine was compatible with this. She did well following delivery. Her clomipramine was gradually withdrawn between 6 months and 1 year postpartum. She was advised about the possibility of a recurrence of her condition should she embark upon a further pregnancy.

Pre-existing psychiatric disorders

In circumstances where a woman receiving long-term treatment for psychiatric disorder is considering having a baby, it is important that she and her partner are encouraged to seek advice before conception. They need to consider the effects of pregnancy and childbirth on her mental health and whether it is robust enough to weather the vicissitudes of parenthood. In addition they need to know about the effects of psychotropic medication on the developing child and risk to the woman of stopping this medication. The aim of preconception counselling should be informed choice.

Chronic depressive illness

Depression is prevalent in the general population, and in a substantial proportion of cases it runs a very chronic course. In many instances, pre-existing chronic depression has shown at best an equivocal response to prior treatment with antidepressant medication. Hence, if the patient is taking antidepressant medication prior to, or at the time of, conception, it is usually preferable to institute a trial withdrawal of this medication, replacing pharmacotherapy with supportive psychotherapy. The goal is to contain symptoms throughout the pregnancy and help the patients find pragmatic solutions to the specific psychosocial problems they encounter. If trial withdrawal of antidepressant medication leads to a substantial exacerbation of the depression, antidepressant medication should be reinstated, though if possible, recommencement should be delayed until after the end of the first trimester.

Manic–depressive illness

The lifetime risk of suffering manic–depressive illness is approximately 1–2%. It is a condition characterized by episodes of acute illness interspersed with periods of relatively normal psychological function. Prophylactic medication such as lithium carbonate helps maintain stability of mood. Carbamazepine and sodium valproate are of similar efficacy as prophylactic agents. Antipsychotics, which include phenothiazines such as chlorpromazine and trifluoperazine, and butyrophenones such as haloperidol, are also used as prophylaxis, but the main role of these drugs is in the treatment of acute episodes.

The major issues facing a woman with manic–depressive illness who wishes to have a baby are: (i) the risk that the child will inherit manic–depressive illness; (ii) the risk of psychotic relapse if prophylactic medication is discontinued during pregnancy; (iii) the high risk of a psychotic relapse in the postpartum period; and (iv) the risk of damage to the fetus if either lithium or carbamazepine is taken in the first trimester of pregnancy.

The risk that the child will suffer manic–depressive illness lies in the range 10–15%, and the risk that the mother will suffer a psychotic episode in the early post-partum period is as high as 50% if no precautions are taken. If the woman and her partner decide that they nevertheless wish to have a child, it is important to plan the management of the illness throughout pregnancy and in the postpartum period with great care, to minimize the risk of the woman suffering a psychotic relapse.

PROPHYLACTIC TREATMENT DURING PREGNANCY

Maternal treatment with lithium carbonate is associated with maldevelopment of the heart and great vessels, especially with Ebstein's anomaly, which is a maldevelopment of the tricuspid valve [10]. The severity of this abnormality ranges from incompatibility with live birth to relatively minor impairment of cardiac function. Data based on an international register of lithium-exposed pregnancies suggested that the risk of significant congenital abnormality when the mother takes lithium in the first trimester is about 10%, including 8% with cardiovascular malformation of whom half suffered Ebstein's anomaly [11]. However, a more recent multicentre prospective study [12] of 138 pregnancies in which lithium was taken in the first trimester found the prevalence of major congenital abnormality was only 2.8%, with one case of Ebstein's anomaly. In the control group, the prevalence of major abnormality was 2.4%, with no cases of Ebstein's anomaly. Thus, the risk associated with lithium exposure is probably lower than had hitherto been accepted.

Until the late 1980s, the available information suggested that carbamazepine was a potentially useful alternative to lithium for prophylaxis against manic–depressive illness in pregnancy, but more recent evidence raises the possibility of risk of harm to the developing fetus. A prospective study of 35 children of women taking carbamazepine (for epilepsy in all but one case) who expressed concern about the risk during the pregnancy, found minor craniofacial defects in 11%, fingernail hypoplasia in 26% and a degree of developmental delay in 20% [13]. The study employed several criteria for developmental delay, of which the least stringent was a score of only 1 SD below the population average. Furthermore, in the absence of a control group suffering from epilepsy, observed abnormalities cannot necessarily be attributed to treatment with carbamazepine, especially as epilepsy can be associated with fetal abnormality unrelated to medication [14]. Thus, the question of the risk associated with carbamazepine remains controversial. Nonetheless current evidence would suggest its use as a mood stabilizer should be avoided in pregnancy.

There are no clearly established teratogenic effects attributable to the principal long-established antipsychotic medications, but some studies have raised the possibility of such effects. A retrospective study of 315 infants whose mothers had been exposed to phenothiazines, mainly aliphatic phenothiazines similar to chlorpromazine, found congenital malformation in 3.5% compared with a frequency of 1.6% in a control group of 12764 women [15]. The initial reports from a large epidemiological study of the children of women treated with phenothiazines for hyperemesis, 80% of whom received prochlorperazine (a phenothiazine with a piperazine side chain that is used mainly as an antiemetic), indicated no significant excess of congenital abnormalities. However, a careful reanalysis taking account of the stage of pregnancy at which exposure to medication occurred, revealed a trend for an increase in abnormalities when the mother had taken the phenothiazine between the sixth and 10th week of gestation [16]. On the basis of these data, it is possible to conclude with 90% confidence that any excess of abnormalities associated with exposure to such medication lies in the range between 0.1% and 5%. Furthermore, there is a report of two cases of severe limb deformity in the children of women treated with prochlorperazine for hyperemesis [17].

Several other studies, including one of 472 women treated for nausea and vomiting in early pregnancy with trifluoperazine, which also belongs to the piperazine class of phenothiazines, found no excess of congenital abnormality [18]. Overall, with regard to phenothiazines, there is slight evidence that aliphatic phenothiazines and also the piperazine phenothiazine, prochlorperazine, might be associated with a small increase in the risk of congenital abnormalities, while there is even less evidence of such risk with trifluoperazine. With regard to the butyrophenones, a study of pregnancies in which there was exposure to haloperidol revealed no increase in congenital abnormalities [19], but the mean dose was only 1.2 mg/day, which is between one-fifth and one-tenth of the dose required for full antipsychotic effect.

Antipsychotics present a risk of acute toxicity in the infant, especially of extrapyramidal signs and anticholinergic effects. A 7-year follow-up study of children exposed to antipsychotic medication *in utero* found that 21.2% of the 80 children exposed for >2 months exhibited abnormal motor activity at 36–60 h after birth, compared with 11.8% of the 76 exposed for <2 months and 9.6% of 115 control children who were not exposed to medication [20].

Whilst the role of prophylactic medication is a major factor in reducing the risk of psychotic episodes, the potential role of psychosocial factors should not be underestimated. Stressful life events, and also sustained tension, play a substantial role in precipitating psychotic episodes. Hence, advice about planning life in a way that minimizes the risk of stressful events, and the use of cognitive and/or behavioural anxiety management techniques to reduce the impact of unavoidable stresses, can reduce the risk of psychotic relapse.

For the majority of women with a history of manic–depressive illness, the most appropriate management in the first trimester is a combination of psychological coping strategies with the intermittent use of antipsychotic medication such as trifluoperazine, at the first sign of the non-specific symptoms, such as agitation and sleep disturbance, that can herald the onset of a psychotic episode. However, close vigilance and a preparedness to utilize medication when required is essential, because florid psychotic relapse is likely to result in potentially irresponsible and/or dangerous behaviour and the need for large doses of medication. Furthermore, as a manic episode develops, insight is often lost, leading to great difficulty in maintaining collaboration with treatment, and to the possibility that compulsory hospital treatment will become necessary.

In the final few weeks of pregnancy, all medication should be minimized. Lithium, or the patient's usual mood stabilizer, should be recommenced on the first day postpartum [21]. Because of shifts in body fluid distribution in the immediate postpartum period, the serum level should be monitored very closely. It is not advisable to breastfeed while taking lithium but acceptable to do so on carbamazepine or sodium valproate. The management of psychotic illness in the postpartum period is discussed in the section on postpartum disorders.

TREATMENT OF ACUTE EPISODES DURING PREGNANCY

In the event of an acute manic relapse, antipsychotic medication such as trifluoperazine, haloperidol or chlorpromazine should be used as required to control symptoms. The evidence regarding congenital malformations considered above slightly favours use of high-potency phenothiazines such as trifluoperazine in preference to lower-potency phenothiazines such as chlorpromazine, but in circumstances where a marked sedative effect is required chlorpromazine might be preferable. In cases of depressive relapse, tricyclic antidepressants are likely to be beneficial. In severe cases of psychotic depression electroconvulsive therapy (ECT) may be considered, as the evidence indicates that it is both a safe and effective treatment in pregnancy [22]. However the theoretical risk of fetal hypoxia and premature labour means that it is rarely acceptable to the woman or family.

If such a relapse occurs in the last trimester of pregnancy consideration should be given to admission to a mother and baby unit. This will allow for her physical needs to be met and close liaison with the obstetrician to take place.

CASE ILLUSTRATION

A young woman, in her first pregnancy, had a 5-year history of manic–depressive illness. She had had frequent relapses of her condition necessitating hospital admission and had accidentally become pregnant whilst taking lithium carbonate. Unknown to her psychiatrist she had stopped this medication on discovering her pregnancy. At 28 weeks' gestation, she had become acutely disturbed with marked motor overactivity, pressure of speech, flight of ideas and grandiose delusions. She was admitted compulsorily to a psychiatric unit with a diagnosis of mania. It was felt after discussion with the obstetrician that the risks to the unborn child of the disturbed maternal mental state outweighed the potential hazards of using antipsychotic medication. The woman was therefore treated with haloperidol, which was reduced to the minimum possible dose as soon as compatible with improving her mental state and behaviour. She was transferred to an inpatient mother and baby unit where she was more easily managed. Close liaison with the obstetrician was maintained and she was induced at term. Lithium carbonate was reinstituted on day 1 following delivery together with a therapeutic dose of haloperidol. She was transferred from the maternity unit back to the mother and baby unit during the first day postpartum where she made a rapid and excellent recovery. She was not separated from her baby and was discharged into the community with a well-established relationship with her infant. Specialized community care following delivery enabled her to work cooperatively with the psychiatric services to ensure her continuing mental health. She was made aware of the risk of relapse.

Schizophrenia

The lifetime risk of suffering schizophrenia is approximately 1% and the majority of cases begin in young adult life. It is no longer associated with reduced fertility perhaps because of the increasing trend to community care and the newer medication regimes. The issues facing a woman suffering from schizophrenia who wishes to become pregnant are: (i) the risk that the child will inherit schizophrenia; (ii) the pressures that caring for a child will put on a schizophrenic mother; (iii) her ability to meet the needs of the child; (iv) the balance between benefits and harm from antipsychotic medication during the pregnancy; and (v) the risk of psychotic relapse in pregnancy and the postpartum period.

LONG-TERM RISKS

The risk that the child of a schizophrenic mother will suffer from schizophrenia is approximately 12%. With regard to the long-term well-being of the mother and child, estimation of the difficulties is made complex by the variability of the illness. In a small minority, the time course resembles that of manic–depressive psychosis, with periods of virtually normal psychological function between psychotic episodes. In the majority, there is a degree of residual disability between episodes of acute disturbance that ranges from mildly impaired ability to deal with stressful situations, to a markedly reduced ability to organize life in a coherent manner. Thus, each case must be assessed taking account of the clinical features of that case and the individual's wishes and social circumstances. Nevertheless, for the majority of cases it is likely that the demands of parenthood would present serious problems for a woman with schizophrenia and for her child.

STABILIZATION OF THE MENTAL STATE IN PREGNANCY

The role of antipsychotic medication in reducing the risk of schizophrenic relapse is well established. Many recent studies in non-pregnant women (reviewed in [23]) have tested strategies for minimizing the usage of long-term medication, such as reduction in dosage or targeted treatment administered only at times when prodromal symptoms emerge. However, in all of these studies, the strategy intended to reduce exposure to medication resulted in a significantly increased rate of relapse. Nevertheless, most of these studies found that relapse was rare in the first few months after reducing or stopping the medication, raising the possibility that such strategies might be useful in pregnancy.

As mentioned in the discussion of manic–depressive illness, there is equivocal evidence that antipsychotic medication in pregnancy is associated with congenital abnormality in the fetus, and in addition some risk of acute toxicity in the neonate. On balance, the evidence suggests that in cases where the illness is severe, with persisting symptoms that tend to be exacerbated by reduction in medication, it is probably best to continue antipsychotic medication throughout the pregnancy, with a cautious reduction in dose in the final few weeks. In the event of psychotic relapse during pregnancy, doses of an oral antipsychotic medication such as trifluoperazine, chlorpromazine or haloperidol adequate to control symptoms, should be given. Immediately after delivery, normal-dose antipsychotic medication should be resumed in all cases. Antipsychotic medication is excreted in the breast milk. If the dose is substantial or there is any evidence of extrapyramidal side-effects in the infant, it is preferable to advise against breastfeeding.

Psychosocial management also has a major part to play throughout the pregnancy and in the postpartum period. Sustained support, usually by a community psychiatric nurse, is essential to help resolve practical problems and to facilitate collaboration with the proposed medication strategy.

In this account of the treatment of pre-existing psychotic illness in pregnancy, schizophrenia has been considered separately from manic–depressive illness. However, whilst typical cases of schizophrenia and of manic–depressive psychosis are quite distinct, these two illnesses lie at the ends of a spectrum of disorders exhibiting mixed clinical features. Those cases lying near the midpoint of this spectrum are described as schizoaffective. The management programme for each case must be tailored for the individual. To the extent that the clinical picture is dominated by relatively poor psychological function even during stable phases of the illness, the management programme will place emphasis on the use of maintenance antipsychotic medication and close supervision by a community psychiatric nurse. On the other hand, if the dominant clinical feature is episodic disturbance, the most appropriate management programme is likely to include a combination of cognitive strategies to cope with stress: or low doses of antipsychotics at times of non-specific symptoms, and the use of prophylactic lithium carbonate, at least in the postpartum period.

RISK OF RELAPSE FOLLOWING DELIVERY

A woman with a prior diagnosis of schizophrenia faces a risk of relapse in the postpartum period of 10–15%. Re-instituting the usual medication following delivery is therefore very important.

CASE ILLUSTRATION

An older woman, with a teenage child, became unexpectedly pregnant by a fellow patient whilst being treated for chronic schizophrenia. She had been maintained in the community with depot antipsychotic medication but refused to take this medication following the confirmation of her pregnancy. Her mental state gradually deteriorated as did her relationship with the psychiatric team. She defaulted from her antenatal care. Shortly before delivery she became acutely disturbed after it was discovered she had a placenta previa. She was admitted compulsorily directly to a mother and baby unit. She remained resistant

to all forms of psychiatric treatment but could be managed conservatively within the mother and baby unit. As delivery was imminent it was felt on balance that the risks of instituting antipsychotic medication and the ensuing struggle outweighed the benefit to the mother and unborn child. She eventually agreed to a caesarean section. Treatment was then instituted immediately after the delivery of the baby. She and her infant were transferred back to the mother and baby unit. She recovered from the acute relapse within 10 days. She remained on the mother and baby unit for a sufficient period of time to demonstrate that she was a competent and affectionate mother and was then managed in the community by a specialist community team together with assistance from social services.

Disorders in the postpartum period

The blues and highs

The postpartum period is a time of psychological vulnerability. Approximately 60% of women suffer from transient disturbance of mood known as the blues during the first postpartum week [24]. The blues typically occur on the fifth postpartum day, and last for 24–36 h. Although tearfulness is the most common sign, the mood is characteristically labile. In some instances, there is a period of unnaturally elevated mood, perhaps accompanied by irritability, which is known as the highs. This period of elevated mood typically follows delivery and resolves during the first week. There is some suggestion that the blues and the highs are associated with increased risk of depression at 6 weeks postpartum [25,26].

Puerperal psychosis

Puerperal psychosis, which occurs in approximately one in 500 births [27], usually begins with an abrupt onset in the first 2 weeks after delivery. In the majority of cases the first few days of the illness are hallmarked by an acute undifferentiated psychosis with prominent confusion, perplexity and disturbance. Thereafter the clinical features resemble those of manic–depressive psychosis. There is a marked disturbance of mood, which is usually labile, fluctuating between abnormal elation, irritability and depression. This mood disturbance is accompanied by delusions and hallucinations. The content of the delusions varies greatly between cases. Grandiose or religious themes are quite common, but delusions of guilt and abnormality in the infant can also occur, especially in cases in which the mood is predominantly depressed. Hallucinations are usually auditory, but in some cases are visual. Attention is seriously impaired and in some cases there is disorientation. Sleep is usually seriously disturbed, the patient often paces about in an agitated manner, and behaviour may be disinhibited. The risk of suicide or infanticide although very low should always be considered.

AETIOLOGY

Because the majority of cases exhibit manic–depressive features and, furthermore, individuals with a past history of manic–depressive episodes are at very high risk of developing a psychotic episode in the puerperal period, it is reasonable to assume that the majority of cases reflect the interaction of a manic–depressive predisposition with the physiological and psychological events of childbirth. This proposal is supported by the finding of Wieck *et al.* of an oestrogen-related dopamine-receptor sensitivity in those who become psychotic [28]. More recently, variations in the serotonin transporter gene have been associated with a subset of women with bipolar disorder that also developed puerperal psychosis [29].

In a small minority of cases that might be described as overtly organic psychoses, the aetiology involves disturbance of brain physiology secondary to systemic metabolic disorder, infection, cardiovascular or respiratory disease, drug toxicity or drug withdrawal. Hence, the assessment of postpartum psychosis must include a history of the use of both therapeutic drugs and drugs of abuse, and an assessment of cardiovascular, respiratory, hepatic and renal function. The clinical features of psychosis with an overtly organic cause can be similar to those of idiopathic postpartum psychosis, but disorientation and/or visual hallucinations are more common and should alert the clinician to the need for an especially thorough general medical examination.

TREATMENT

Close supervision and support are essential because the woman's ability to care for herself and her baby are severely impaired. In virtually all cases, hospital admission is indicated because of behavioural disturbance and the risks of suicide or infanticide. If possible, admission should be to a mother and baby unit with the facilities and expertise to meet the needs of mother and baby whilst minimizing the need for separation of the mother from her baby. If the mother is unwilling to accept hospital admission, the need for compulsory admission under the Mental Health Act should be assessed.

The florid psychotic symptoms should be treated with antipsychotic medication such as chlorpromazine or haloperidol. ECT is likely to provide the most certain and safe resolution of symptoms, and should be considered if florid disturbance persists or presents severe management problems.

The evidence suggests that for women who have suffered from previous postpartum psychosis, or who have had repeated episodes of psychosis at any time, prophylactic treatment with lithium from the first postpartum day reduces the risk [21], although larger studies of the value of this treatment are required. However the high risk of recurrence following future childbirth underlines the importance of counselling and proactive management during the next pregnancy.

CASE ILLUSTRATION

A professional married lady was admitted compulsorily to a mother and baby unit together with her infant on the seventh postpartum day. She had been noted by her community midwife to be unduly anxious and agitated on the fifth postpartum day. She had not slept at all the night of the sixth day and in the hours preceding her admission had been found in the streets in her nightclothes clutching her infant, bewildered, frightened and perplexed. She had been admitted previously on the seventh day following the birth of her first child 4 years ago. On that occasion she had been separated from her infant and had decided not to tell her obstetrician because of her fear that this separation might happen again. If her previous history had been ascertained then the high risk of recurrence (50%) would have been recognized and perhaps preventative measures could have been taken.

For the first few days following admission, her mental state and behaviour was changeable and varied. At times she was elated, overactive and grandiose, at other times tearful, frightened and distressed, and intermittently confused and disinhibited. By the second postpartum week her mental state was more clearly that of mania. She was restless and overactive, over-talkative and unduly cheerful with markedly impaired concentration and very distractible. She found it difficult to manage her baby without considerable assistance from the nursing staff although she was affectionate and concerned. Initially she was determined to breastfeed and was given haloperidol. However, this soon proved too difficult for her to continue with and after she decided to stop breastfeeding, lithium carbonate was instituted. She rapidly improved and by the fourth postpartum week was symptom free. As soon as she was confidently competent with her baby she was discharged to the community where she was supported by a specialist community nursing team. Her lithium was continued for the postpartum year before being gradually reduced and withdrawn. She now understands that she faces a 50% risk of recurrence of her condition should she embark upon a further pregnancy and has been advised to be referred early in her next pregnancy so that a proactive management plan may be instituted.

Postnatal depression

Whilst the occurrence and special importance of depression in the postpartum period is undeniable, the question of whether or not postnatal depression should be regarded as distinct from other forms of depression still remains a subject of controversy. The best available evidence regarding prevalence, from a study of 232 postpartum women by Cox *et al.* [30], indicates that there is no significant increase in prevalence of depression during the first 6 months postpartum, in comparison with the prevalence in an equivalent time interval in a group of women from the same geographical area matched for age, marital status and number of children. In the postnatal group, the point prevalence at 6 months postpartum was 9.1% and the period prevalence in the 6 months since delivery was 13.8%. In the control group, the point prevalence at assessment 6 months after an index date was 8.2% and the period prevalence in the intervening 6 months was 13.4%.

However, there was evidence for a clustering of dates of onset of depression in the weeks shortly after delivery. In the group with postnatal depression, half had onset in the 5 weeks following delivery, one-tenth had onset during pregnancy and one-tenth had had the onset prior to becoming pregnant. In the control group, one-sixth of the cases with depression had onset in the 5 weeks after the index date, approximately one-tenth had onset in the 40 weeks prior to the index date and a little over one-quarter had onset more than 40 weeks prior to the index date. Thus, the postpartum group were less likely than the controls to have had long-standing depression, but did show evidence of an excess number having onset in the first 5 weeks postpartum.

Although there is some evidence of a temporal relationship between childbirth and onset of depression, it remains unknown whether or not postpartum depression has a specific pathophysiology or merely reflects the interaction between the stresses of childbirth and predisposition to depression acting through a mechanism similar to that mediating the relationship between other types of stressors and depression.

Depressive illness in the postpartum period, as at other times, represents a spectrum of severity and subtype.

CLINICAL FEATURES

The principal clinical features of postpartum depression, as in depression arising in other circumstances, are de-pressed or anxious mood, irritability, loss of ability to enjoy activities, self-depreciation, guilty or pessimistic preoccupations, and somatic disturbances such as poor appetite and disturbed sleep. It can be difficult to distinguish the pathological sleep disorder of depression from the disturbance due to the demands of the infant, but inability to sleep even when the baby is settled, and waking earlier than is necessary, are indicative of depression.

Features that are relatively specific to postpartum depression include preoccupation with inadequacy as a mother, undue anxiety about the infant, and, in severe cases, hopelessness about the future of the infant. These negative cognitions can in extreme cases lead to suicide or even infanticide. Whilst such serious sequelae are rare in non-psychotic depression, it is nevertheless essential for the clinician to be alert to the possibility, because failure to detect the risk can have such terrible consequences.

PROGNOSIS

The illness usually persists for many months, and often for more than a year [31], especially if untreated. Premenstrual mood disturbance can become a dominant feature that lingers on, long after the postnatal depression has resolved in some cases [32]. There is evidence for adverse effects on the baby and on the relationship with the partner. Murray *et al.* [33] have reviewed the evidence of effects on the child and conclude that there can be delayed development that is detectable at age 4 years. Many studies have shown a relationship between postnatal depression and poor marital relationships [34], although the direction of causation is unclear.

AETIOLOGY

Whilst a full account of the aetiology is unlikely until the pathophysiology of the condition has been more clearly delineated, it is possible to identify many of the contributing factors in a way that provides a foundation for a rational approach to early detection of the illness and to the formulation of a management programme. It is helpful to classify these various factors as predisposing factors, precipitating factors and maintaining factors.

Predisposing factors

A previous history of depression, either following previous childbirth or at other times, predisposes to postnatal depression [35]. This indicates that the pathophysiology of postnatal depression has at least some overlap with that of other depressive illnesses. In individual cases it is sometimes clear that social disadvantage and pre-existing marital disharmony have played a predisposing role, although it is difficult to obtain reliable statistical support for the role of any specific psychosocial stressor. It is likely that any one of a wide variety of different forms of pre-existing chronic psychosocial stress might play a role in predisposing to depression.

Precipitating factors

Precipitating factors include both the events associated with the delivery itself, especially with caesarean section [26,35], and the subsequent stresses of caring for a young infant. It is probable that the psychological response to the event of delivery can precipitate depression just as various types of major life events can precipitate depression in other circumstances. In the months following childbirth the mother experiences not only the physically exhausting demands of caring for a young baby, but in addition is vulnerable to insidious negative self-evaluation. One source of negative self-evaluation that can play a role in precipitating depression is the discrepancy between the expectations of motherhood and the reality of coping with an infant, especially if the baby's sleeping pattern or feeding proves difficult, and/or there is inadequate support from partner or family.

The role of the physiological processes of childbirth in precipitating depression is less clear. Although the puerperium is a time of rapid hormonal change, there is no clear, consistent evidence of abnormal levels of either oestrogen or progesterone in those who become depressed. Harris et al. [36] found that low levels of progesterone (measured in saliva) were associated with depression in women who were breastfeeding, whilst there was a positive correlation between progesterone level and depression in those who were bottle feeding. Rapidly falling cholesterol in the puerperium has also been implicated [37]. Mild thyroiditis occurs after about 5% of births [38], often associated with hyperthyroidism followed by hypothyroidism, which is usually transient (see Chapter 12). As both hyper- and hypothyroidism can be associated with depression, it is possible that thyroid disturbance contributes to postnatal depression in some cases.

Maintaining factors

The vicious cycle established between the mood and lack of energy, and negative evaluation of one's role as a mother can be a potent factor in the maintenance of depression. The problem can be compounded if the partner becomes demoralized or feels rejected, leading to escalating tension within the relationship.

TREATMENT

The optimum balance between social, psychological and pharmacological management depends on individual circumstances, but in most cases of moderate or greater severity, all three approaches are usually required. In one study of non-psychotic depression both fluoxetine and cognitive–behavioural counselling were equally effective as initial therapy [39].

The first issue to be addressed in formulating a management programme is ensuring there is an adequate network of support for the mother and her child, from family, friends, voluntary services or statutory services. Providing information about the nature of postnatal depression to both the woman and to her partner can itself help reduce the demoralizing sense of inadequacy. Cognitive therapy is the form of individual psychotherapy that lends itself most readily to the needs of women with postnatal depression. It can break the vicious cycle between mood and negative evaluation of self that tends to maintain the depression.

There have been no adequate trials to determine which type of pharmacological therapy is best. In depression in general, treatment with tricyclic antidepressants is associated with substantial improvement in about 70% of cases, and clinical experience suggests a similar level of efficacy in postnatal depression. Lofepramine has a lower incidence of anticholinergic side-effects than the longer-established tricyclics such as imipramine and amitryptiline, and is somewhat safer in overdose [40]. The more recently developed SSRIs, such as paroxetine and sertraline, are even safer in overdose; they produce gastrointestinal side-effects such as nausea but no anticholinergic effects.

The more recently a drug has been introduced, the greater the uncertainty about its safety in breastfeeding mothers, although the risk to the breastfeeding infant is probably low for both the tricyclics and the newer SSRIs. For tricyclic antidepressants the data suggest that the infant dose per unit of bodyweight is less than one-hundredth of the maternal dose per unit of bodyweight [41] and the available data indicate similarly low infant doses for the serotonin reuptake inhibitors, fluoxetine and fluvoxamine [42].

Hormonal treatments

On the basis of an uncontrolled trial, Dalton [43] proposed that treatment with progesterone, starting with injections for the first 5 days and then continuing with suppositories until the re-establishment of regular menstruation, is effective in preventing postpartum depression but there is no evidence from controlled trials to support this and its use either as a propylactic or treatment cannot be recommended.

There is a somewhat stronger theoretical basis and evidence to suggest that oestrogen has a therapeutic effect. The available evidence indicates that oestrogen can be used to treat depression that is not related to childbirth [44]. Furthermore, a small double-blind placebo-controlled study in women with postnatal depression found that oestrogen patches produce a significant benefit [45]. One issue that must be addressed is the risk of thrombosis granted the known increased risk in association with oestrogens in general and when used for suppression of lactation in particular. The risks of thrombosis with oestrogen patch therapy for postnatal depression have not yet been clearly established, but are probably substantially lower than with oral contraception (OC) or with oestrogen for lactation suppression. The synthetic oestrogens used in OC are several times more potent than the natural oestrogens in the oestrogen patch in inducing the liver enzymes that produce clotting factors [46].

At this stage it is difficult to draw definitive conclusions about the optimum pharmacological treatment for postnatal depression. The tricyclic antidepressants are the most firmly established, mainly on the grounds of their efficacy for treating depression in other circumstances, but recent evidence suggests that treatment with oestrogen [47] in the form of patches might also be effective. It is not clear whether or not there is a specific subgroup of cases in which hormonal factors play a more substantial role, and for which hormonal treatment might therefore offer the most rational approach.

CASE ILLUSTRATION

A woman with a 3-month-old baby, her first child, was referred by her general practitioner for a psychiatric assessment. The doctor had first suspected that this woman might be suffering from postnatal depression when she complained of feeling tired and tearful at her 6-week postnatal examination. The woman's health visitor had noticed that she was struggling to cope with the baby and voicing fears that she was an inadequate and incompetent mother. The woman was initially very reluctant to agree to a psychiatric assessment, as she feared that her baby might be removed from her. She was breastfeeding and was worried that if the psychiatrist prescribed an antidepressant that she would have to stop.

When the woman was first seen by the psychiatrist she was embarrassed and guilty and felt that she was a failure as a mother and the child might be better cared for by somebody else. She did not believe that she was de-

pressed but that she was not suited to motherhood. On questioning she revealed that she was not sleeping, waking persistently in the early hours despite the fact that her baby was still asleep. She felt particularly low in the mornings, unable to concentrate or organize her thoughts and activities, and overwhelmed by the difficulties in planning her day. She found that her mood improved somewhat as the day progressed and by the time her husband returned from work she was just able to present herself as being reasonably well and organized. Although worried about the baby, she could not relax and enjoy him and was preoccupied by concerns that this might affect his proper development. Whenever he cried or had difficulty in feeding she felt that he knew that she was not a proper mother. The psychiatrist was able to convince her, after explanation, that the way she felt was because she was depressed and not because she was a bad mother. He was able to convince her that she could safely take antidepressants and continue to breastfeed. She was started on imipramine 50 mg *nocte* which was incrementally increased over the next 2 weeks to 150 mg *nocte* and was visited regularly by a specialist community psychiatric nurse. The nurse was able to help the woman understand her own symptoms, develop coping strategies whilst she recovered and to instil hope for the future. The woman rapidly recovered and was symptom free within 8 weeks. Her medication was continued for a further 6 months before it was gradually reduced and withdrawn. She was advised about the possibility of recurrence of her condition following a further pregnancy and agreed to recontact the service when she next became pregnant.

References

1 Kumar R, Robson KM. A prospective study of emotional disorders in childbearing women. *Br J Psychiatry* 1984; 144: 35–47.
2 Chambers CD, Johnson KA, Dick LM, Felix RJ, Jones KL. Birth outcomes in pregnant women taking fluoxetine. *N Engl J Med* 1996; 335: 1010–15.
3 Nulman I, Rovet J *et al.* Neurodevelopment of children exposed *in utero* to antidepressant drugs. *N Engl J Med* 1997; 336: 258–62.
4 McBride WG. Limb deformities associated with iminodibenzyl hydrochloride. *Med J Aust* 1972; 1: 49.
5 Australian Drug Evaluation Committee. Tricyclic antidepressants and limb reduction deformities. *Med J Aust* 1973; 1: 768–9.
6 Rosenberg L, Mitchell AA, Parsells JL, Pashayan H, Louik C, Shapiro S. Lack of relation of oral clefts to diazepam use during pregnancy. *N Engl J Med* 1983; 309: 1282–5.
7 Bracken MB, Holford TR. Exposure to prescribed drugs in pregnancy and association with congenital malformations. *Obstet Gynecol* 1981; 58: 336–44.
8 Laegreid L, Olegard R, Walstrom J, Conradi N. Teratogenic effects of benzodiazepine use during pregnancy. *J Paediatr* 1989; 114: 126–31.

9 Insel TR, Mueller EA, Gilin JC, Siever L, Murphy DL. Tricyclic response in obsessive compulsive disorder. *Prog Neuropsychopharmacol Biol Psychiatry* 1984; 9: 25–31.

10 Nora JJ, Nora HA, Toews WH. Lithium, Ebstein's anomaly and other congenital heart defects. *Lancet* 1974; ii: 594–5.

11 McElhatten P. *Review of the Use of Lithium in Human Pregnancy.* Guy's Hospital Teratology Information Service, London, 1990.

12 Jacobson SJ, Jones K *et al.* Prospective multicentre study of pregnancy outcome after lithium exposure during the first trimester. *Lancet* 1992; 339: 530–3.

13 Jones KL, Lacro RV, Johnson KA, Adams J. Pattern of malformations in the children of woman treated with carbamazepine during pregnancy. *N Engl J Med* 1989; 320: 1661–6.

14 Scialli AR, Lione A. The teratogenic effects of carbamazepine. *N Engl J Med* 1989; 321: 1480.

15 Rumeau-Rouquette J, Goujard J, Huel G. Possible teratogenic effect of phenothiazines in human beings. *Teratology* 1977; 15: 57–64.

16 Edlund MJ, Craig TJ. Antipsychotic drug use and birth defects: an epidemiologic re-assessment. *Comp Psychiatry* 1984; 25: 32–7.

17 Rafla N. Limb deformities associated with prochlorperazine. *Am J Obstet Gynecol* 1987; 156: 1557.

18 Moriarty AJ, Nance NR. Trifluoperazine and pregnancy. *Can Med Assoc J* 1963; 88: 375–6.

19 Van Waes A, Van de Velde EJ. Safety evaluation of haloperidol in the treatment of hyperemesis gravidarum. *J Clin Pharmacol* 1969; 9: 224–6.

20 Platt JE, Friedhoff AJ, Broman SH, Bond R, Laska E, Lin SP. Effects of prenatal neuroleptic drug exposure on motor performance in children. *Hum Psychopharmacol* 1989; 4: 205–13.

21 Stewart DE, Klompenhouwer JL, Kendell RE, van Hulst AM. Prophylactic lithium in puerperal psychosis. The experience of three centres. *Br J Psychiatry* 1991; 158: 393–7.

22 Nurnberg HG. An overview of somatic treatment of psychosis during pregnancy and post-partum. *Gen Hosp Psychiatry* 1989; 11: 328–38.

23 Hirsch S. Pharmacological and psychosocial longterm treatment of schizophrenia. In: Brunello N, Mendelewicz J, Racagni J, eds. *New Generation of Antipsychotic Drugs: Novel Mechanisms of Action.* Karger, Basel, 1993: 77–8.

24 Pitt B. Maternity blues. *Br J Psychiatry* 1973; 122: 431–5.

25 Glover V, Liddle P, Taylor A, Adams D, Sandler M. Mild hypomania (the highs) can be a feature of the first postpartum week: association with later depression. *Br J Psychiatry* 1994; 164: 517–21.

26 Hannah P, Adams D, Lee A, Glover V, Sandler M. Links between early post-partum mood and post-natal depression. *Br J Psychiatry* 1992; 160: 777–80.

27 Kendell RE, Chalmers JC, Platz C. Epidemiology of puerperal psychosis. *Br J Psychiatry* 1987; 150: 662–73.

28 Wieck A, Kumar R, Hirst AD, Marks MN, Campbell IC, Checkley SA. Increased sensitivity of dopamine receptors and recurrence of affective psychosis after childbirth. *Br Med J* 1990; 303: 613–16.

29 Coyle N, Jones I, Robertson E, Lendon C. Variation in the serotonin transporter gene influences susceptibility to bipolar affective puerperal psychosis. *Lancet* 2000; 356: 1490–1.

30 Cox JL, Murray D, Chapman G. A controlled study of the onset, duration and prevalence of post-natal depression. *Br J Psychiatry* 1993; 163: 27–31.

31 Pitt B. Atypical depression following childbirth. *Br J Psychiatry* 1968; 114: 1325–35.

32 Warner P, Bancroft J, Dixson A, Hampson M. The relationship between premenstrual depressive mood and depressive illness. *J Affect Disord* 1991; 23: 9–23.

33 Murray L, Cooper PJ, Stein A. Post natal depression and infant development. *Br Med J* 1991; 302: 978–9.

34 O'Hara MW, Zekowski EM. Post-partum depression: a comprehensive review. In: Kumar R, Brockington F, eds. *Motherhood and Mental Illness, 2. Causes and Consequences.* Wright, London, 1988.

35 O'Neill T, Murphy P, Greene VT. Postnatal depression: aetiological factors. *Irish Med J* 1990; 83: 17–18.

36 Harris B, Johns S *et al.* The hormonal environment of post-natal depression. *Br J Psychiatry* 1989; 154: 660–7.

37 Ploeckinger B, Dantedorfer K, Ulm M, Baischer W, Derfler K, Musalek M, Dadak C. Rapid decrease of serum cholesterol concentration and postpartum depression. *Br Med J* 1996; 313: 664–9.

38 Gerstein HC. How common is postpartum thyroiditis? *Arch Intern Med* 1990; 150: 1397–400.

39 Appleby L, Warner R, Whitton A, Faragher B. A controlled study of fluoxetine and cognitive-behavioural counselling in the treatment of postnatal depression. *Br Med J* 1997; 314: 932–6.

40 Lancaster SG, Gonzales JP. Lofepramine: a review of its pharmacodynamic and pharmacokinetic properties, and therapeutic efficacy in depressive illness. *Drugs* 1989; 37: 123–40.

41 Buist A, Norman TR, Dennerstein L. Breast-feeding and the use of psychotrophic medication: a review. *J Affect Disord* 1990; 19: 197–206.

42 Wright S, Dawling S, Ashford JJ. Excretion of fluvoxamine in breast milk. *Br J Clin Pharmacol* 1991; 31: 209.

43 Dalton K. Progesterone prophylaxis used successfully in postnatal depression. *Practitioner* 1985; 229: 507–8.

44 Klaiber EL, Broverman DM, Vogal W, Kobabayashi Y. Estrogen replacement therapy for severe persistent depression in women. *Arch Gen Psychiatry* 1979; 36: 550–4.

45 Henderson AF, Gregoire AJP, Kumar R, Studd JWW. The treatment of severe post-natal depression with oestradiol skin patches. *Lancet* 1991; ii: 816.

46 Campbell S. Potency and hepatocellular effects of oestrogens after oral, percutaneous and subcutaneous administration. In: VanKeep PA, Utian WH, Vermeulan A, eds. *The Controversial Climacteric.* MTP Press, Lancaster, 1982: 103.

47 Lawrie TA, Herxheimer A, Dalton K. Oestrogens and progestogens for preventing and treating postnatal depression (Cochrane Review). In: *The Cochrane Library,* Issue 2. Update Software, Oxford, 2000.

Index